Physiotherapy for Respiratory and Cardiac Problems

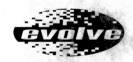

Evolve Learning Resources for Students and Lecturers:
The complete collection of over 300 images from this book in JPEG and PDF format.
Suitable for downloading and importing into applications such as Powerpoint and Word.

See the instructions and PIN code panel on the inside cover for access to the web site and your image bank.

Think o ____ k...**evolve**

D1346716

To our families, friends and to our teachers

Publisher: Heidi Harrison
Commissioning Editor: Rita Demetriou-Swanwick
Associate Editor: Siobhan Campbell
Development Editor: Veronika Watkins
Project Manager: Emma Riley
Design Direction: George Ajayi
Illustration Manager: Merlyn Harvey
Illustrator: Oxford Designers & Illustrators

Physiotherapy for Respiratory and Cardiac Problems

Adults and Paediatrics

FOURTH EDITION

Edited by

Jennifer A Pryor PhD MBA MSc FNZSP MCSP
*Senior Research Fellow in Physiotherapy, Royal Brompton & Harefield NHS Trust, London, UK;
Honorary Lecturer, University College London, UK*

S Ammani Prasad GradDipPhys MCSP
*Cystic Fibrosis Coordinator / Senior Research Physiotherapist, Respiratory Unit, Great Ormond
Street Hospital for Children NHS Trust, London, UK*

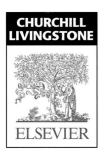

CHURCHILL
LIVINGSTONE

ELSEVIER

EDINBURGH   LONDON   NEW YORK   OXFORD   PHILADELPHIA   ST LOUIS   SYDNEY   TORONTO   2008

CHURCHILL
LIVINGSTONE
ELSEVIER

An imprint of Elsevier Limited
© Longman Group (UK) Limited 1993
© 1998, 2001, 2002, 2008, Elsevier Limited. All rights reserved.

The right of Jennifer A Pryor & S Ammani Prasad to be identified as editors of this work has been asserted by them in accordance with the Copyright, Designs and Patents Act 1988.

First edition 1993
Second edition 1998
Third edition 2002
Fourth edition 2008
    Reprinted 2009 (three times), 2010, 2011

ISBN: 9780080449852

British Library Cataloguing in Publication Data
A catalogue record for this book is available from the British Library

Library of Congress Cataloging in Publication Data
A catalog record for this book is available from the Library of Congress

Notice
Neither the Publisher nor the Editors assume any responsibility for any loss or injury and/or damage to persons or property arising out of or related to any use of the material contained in this book. It is the responsibility of the treating practitioner, relying on independent expertise and knowledge of the patient, to determine the best treatment and method of application for the patient.

The Publisher

The publisher's policy is to use **paper manufactured from sustainable forests**

Printed in China

Contents

Contributors

Paul Aurora MRCP PhD
Consultant in Respiratory Medicine and Paediatric Lung Transplantation, Great Ormond Street Hospital for Children NHS Trust, London, UK

Ian Balfour-Lynn BSc MD MBBS FRCP FRCS(Ed) FRCPCH DHMSA
Consultant in Paediatric Respiratory Medicine, Royal Brompton & Harefield NHS Trust, London, UK

Anne Ballinger MD FRCP
Senior Lecturer, Digestive Diseases Research Centre, St Bartholomew's and Royal London School of Medicine and Dentistry, London, UK

Jenny Bell BA MPhil PhD
Clinical Exercise Physiologist, England, UK

Delva Bethune MHSc DipPT DipOT RPT
Formerly Associate Professor, Queen's University, School of Rehabilitation Therapy, Faculty of Health Sciences, Division of Physical Therapy; Downtown Physiotherapy Clinic and Health Centre, Kingston, Ontario, Canada

Mandy Bryon BA MSc PhD
Consultant Clinical Psychologist, Department of Psychological Medicine, Great Ormond Street Hospital for Children NHS Trust, London, UK

Nola Cecins BAppSc(Phty) MSc
Senior Physiotherapist, Physiotherapy Department, Sir Charles Gairdner Hospital; School of Physiotherapy, Curtin University of Technology, Perth, Western Australia

Michelle Chatwin BSc MCSP PhD
Clinical Specialist Physiotherapist, Non-invasive Ventilation and Neuromuscular Disease, Royal Brompton & Harefield NHS Trust, London, UK

Connor D Collins BSc MB MRCPI FRCR
Consultant Radiologist, St Vincent's Hospital, Dublin, Ireland

Susan J Copley MD MRCP FRCR
Consultant Radiologist, The Hammersmith Hospitals NHS Trust, Hammersmith Hospital, London, UK

Elizabeth Dean PhD PT
Professor, Department of Physical Therapy, University of British Columbia, Vancouver, British Columbia, Canada

Linda Denehy PhD BAppSc(Phty) GradDipPhysio(Cardiothoracic)
Senior Lecturer, School of Physiotherapy, Faculty of Medicine, Dentistry and Health Sciences, The University of Melbourne, Victoria, Australia

Mary E Dodd DSc(Hon) FCSP
Consultant Physiotherapist, Manchester Adult Cystic Fibrosis Centre, University Hospital of South Manchester NHS Foundation Trust, Manchester, UK

Elizabeth R Ellis PhD GradDipPhty MHL
Honorary Senior Lecturer, Discipline of Physiotherapy, Faculty of Health Sciences, The University of Sydney, Sydney, NSW, Australia

Stephanie Enright MCSP MSc MPhil PhD
Senior Lecturer, School of Health Care Studies, Wales College of Medicine, Biology, Life and Health Sciences, Cardiff University, Wales, UK

Rachel Garrod PhD MSc PG Cert Ed HE Grad Dip Phys MCSP
Reader, School of Physiotherapy, St George's Hospital Medical School, London, UK

Christopher D. George FRCS FRCR
Consultant Radiologist, Department of Radiology, Epsom and St Helier University Hospitals NHS Trust, Carshalton, Surrey, UK

David M Hansell FRCP FRCR MD
Professor of Thoracic Imaging, Royal Brompton & Harefield NHS Trust, London, UK

Kathryn Harris GradDipPhys MCSP
Respiratory Clinical Specialist Physiotherapist, The Duke of Cornwall Spinal Treatment Centre, Salisbury District Hospital NHS Trust, Salisbury, Wiltshire, UK

Kate J Hayes BPhysio MPhysio(Cardio)
Senior Clinician Physiotherapist, Cardiothoracic Unit, The Alfred, Melbourne, Victoria, Australia

Ian Hudson MD FRCP
Consultant Cardiologist, Leicester General Hospital, Gwendolen Road, Leicester, UK

Diana M Innocenti FCSP
Formerly Head of Physiotherapy, Guy's Hospital, London, UK

Tomás Iolster MD
Head, Paediatric Intensive Care, Hospital Universitaris Austral, Buenos Aires, Argentina

Sue Jenkins GradDipPhys PhD
Associate Professor in Cardiopulmonary Science, School of Physiotherapy, Curtin University of Technology; Physiotherapy Department, Sir Charles Gairdner Hospital, Perth, Western Australia

Alice YM Jones PhD FACP MPhil MSc Cert PT
Professor, Department of Rehabilitation Sciences, The Hong Kong Polytechnic University, Hong Kong

Fiona Lough MPhil MCSP
Superintendent Cardiac Rehabilitation Physiotherapist, The Hatter Cardiovascular Health & Rehabilitation Institute, University College London Hospitals NHS Foundation Trust, UK

Eleanor Main BSc BA MSc PhD
Senior Lecturer in Physiotherapy, Institute of Child Health, University College London, London, UK

Sally Middleton MSc(Med) BAppSc(Phty)
Clinical Research Assistant, David Reed Laboratory, University of Sydney, Sydney, Australia

Peter G. Middleton MBBS (Hons) BSc (MED) PhD FRACP
Senior Staff Specialist & Head, Cystic Fibrosis Unit, Department of Respiratory Medicine, Westmead Hospital, Westmead, Australia

Prue E Munro BPhysio GradDipHlthMgt
Senior Clinician Physiotherapist, Heart Lung Transplant Unit, The Alfred, Melbourne, Victoria, Australia

Indra Narang MBBCh MD FRCPCH
Director Sleep Medicine, Staff Pulmonologist, The Hospital for Sick Children, Toronto, Canada

George Ntoumenopoulos PhD GradDipClinEpi BAppSc(Phty) BSc
Clinical Specialist Respiratory Physiotherapist, Physiotherapy Department, Guy's and St Thomas' NHS Foundation Trust, London, UK

Leyla P Osman PhD MCSP
Clinical Lead Physiotherapist – Respiratory, Physiotherapy Department, Guy's and St Thomas' NHS Foundation Trust, London, UK

Jennifer Paratz PhD FACP MPhty GradCertEd(Medical Sciences)
Chair and Research Fellow, Burns, Trauma and Critical Care Research Centre, School of Medicine, University of Queensland, Brisbane, Australia

Stephen Patchett MD FRCPI
Consultant Physician/Gastroenterologist, Beaumont Hospital, Dublin, Ireland

Christiane Perme PT CCS
Board Certified Cardiovascular and Pulmonary Clinical Specialist and Senior Physical Therapist, The Methodist Hospital, Houston, Texas, USA

Amanda J Piper PhD BAppSc(Phty) MEd
Senior Physiotherapist and Research Fellow, Department of Respiratory Medicine, Centre for Respiratory Failure and Sleep Disorders, Royal Prince Alfred Hospital, Camperdown, NSW, Australia; Clinical Senior Lecturer, The University of Sydney, Sydney, NSW, Australia

Fabio Pitta PT MSc PhD
*Laboratório de Pesquisa em Fisioterapia Pulmonar,
Departamento de Fisioterapia, Universidade Estadual de
Londrina, Paraná, Brazil*

Helen M Potter BAppSc(Phty) GradDipManipTherapy
MSc FACP
*Manipulative Physiotherapist, In Touch Physiotherapy,
Perth, Australia*

S Ammani Prasad GradDipPhys MCSP
*Cystic Fibrosis Coordinator/Senior Research
Physiotherapist, Respiratory Unit, Great Ormond Street
Hospital for Children NHS Trust, London, UK*

Vanessa Probst PT MSc PhD
*Laboratório de Pesquisa em Fisioterapia Pulmonar,
Departamento de Fisioterapia, Universidade Estadual de
Londrina, Paraná, Brazil*

Jennifer A Pryor PhD MBA MSc FNZSP MCSP
*Senior Research Fellow in Physiotherapy, Royal Brompton
& Harefield NHS Trust, London, UK; Honorary Lecturer,
University College London, UK*

Sally Singh PhD BA MCSP
*Professor, Faculty of Health & Life Sciences, Coventry
University, Coventry, UK; Head of Cardiac and Pulmonary
Rehabilitation, Department of Respiratory Medicine,
University Hospitals of Leicester NHS Trust, Leicester, UK*

Elizabeth Steed PhD CPsychol
*Health Psychologist, Royal Brompton & Harefield NHS
Trust, London, UK*

Linda Tagg Grad Dip Phys MCSP
*Chartered Physiotherapist, Back to Work, Basingstoke,
UK*

Robert C Tasker MA MB MD FRCP
*Consultant Paediatric Intensivist, Department of
Paediatrics, Addenbrookes Hospital, Cambridge, UK*

Ann Taylor PhD MSc BA MCSP DipTP
*Head of Department of Physiotherapy, School of Health
Sciences, University of Limerick, Limerick, Ireland*

Fiona Troup BAppSc(Phty) MCSP
*Clinical Director, Sports and Spinal Clinics, Harley Street,
London, UK*

Beatrice Tucker BAppSc(Phty) PGradDipPhty MSc
*Senior Lecturer, Office of Teaching and Learning, Curtin
University of Technology, Perth, Western Australia*

Trudy Ward MSc GradDipPhys
*Formerly Therapy Manager, The Duke of Cornwall Spinal
Treatment Centre, Salisbury District Hospital NHS Trust,
Salisbury, Wiltshire, UK*

A Kevin Webb FRCP
*Professor of Respiratory Medicine & Clinical Director,
Manchester Adult Cystic Fibrosis Centre, University
Hospital of South Manchester NHS Foundation Trust,
Manchester, UK*

Barbara A Webber FCSP DSc(Hon)
*Formerly Head of Physiotherapy, Royal Brompton Hospital,
London, UK*

Preface to fourth edition

It has given us great pleasure to once again work with colleagues who are internationally recognized as experts in their field. In the fourth edition we are delighted to have been able to widen the international scope of the book with contributions from experts in Argentina, Australia, Brazil, Canada, Hong Kong, Ireland, the United Kingdom and the United States of America.

We are grateful to the authors of previous editions and to our readers for the opportunity to undertake a fourth edition. The success of this title has been dependent on the quality of the contributors, the readers and the confidence of the Publisher.

We owe a considerable amount to all our contributors; clinicians who have full clinical loads with little time to spare and to our academic colleagues, for whom writing a chapter no longer carries the same academic kudos as the writing of a peer reviewed paper. Despite these constraints, they have found time to contribute to this text and it has been a privilege to work with them.

In today's electronic world it is easy to think that 'everything' can be accessed on-line, but we feel very strongly that there is still a place for a book that encapsulates international cardiorespiratory physiotherapy expertise. We hope that the 4th edition brings together the research evidence that underpins our current clinical practice for both an undergraduate and postgraduate audience.

J.A.P.
S.A.P.
London 2007

Preface to third edition

This third edition has a much greater emphasis on paediatrics. We have a number of new authors, for both the adult and paediatric sections, who are internationally recognized in their field. We are most grateful to all the authors who have contributed so much of their time both in writing and in updating their sections. It is owing to the multiauthor, multidisciplinary and international characteristics of this book that such a wealth of knowledge can be contained within one text.

A textbook is neither a meta-analysis nor a systematic review of each and every topic covered. Papers on particular topics will be published both during and after publication of this book. When pursuing a subject in detail it is important that the reader also searches the literature but it is hoped that this text will provide a basis for further review and research.

We wish to acknowledge the tremendous help from the many people who have advised and supported us during this project, including Guy Thorpe Beeston, Barbara Webber, Margaret Hodson, Robert Dinwiddie, Mary Dodd, Colin Wallis, Peter Pryor and the Medical Illustration Departments at the Institute of Child Health and the Royal Marsden Hospital NHS Trust, particularly Nicholas Geddes, Milena Potucek and Paul Hyett. Our thanks also to our colleagues in the Cystic Fibrosis Departments of the Royal Brompton & Harefield NHS Trust and Great Ormond Street Hospital for Children NHS Trust.

J.A.P.
S.A.P.
London 2002

Preface to second edition

During the last five years the term 'evidence-based medicine' has had an increasing profile in medicine and 'purchasers' of physiotherapy services are asking for outcomes and evidence that physiotherapy is of benefit in specific patients with specific problems.

We cannot answer all these questions but the database of clinical trials is growing. In assessing the evidence it is important to remember the definition of Sackett et al (1996): 'Evidence-based medicine involves integrating individual clinical expertise and the best external evidence available from systematic research'.

In this book we have referenced statements where possible, but there are still many areas of practice which are anecdotal. We must not lose the skills and tech-

niques in these areas if there are indications of patient benefit.

The second edition includes separate and new chapters on surgery and intensive care, and new chapters on non-invasive ventilation and pulmonary rehabilitation. Other chapters have been expanded with sections written by physiotherapy specialists in the field – manual therapy and acupuncture. All the chapters have been updated and new references included.

No text can meet every reader's need but we hope that the material here will lead the reader on to other sources and contacts and, by open exchange of information and ideas, we should be able to take the profession forward to benefit our patients.

J.A.P.
B.A.W.
London 1997

Preface to first edition

This book is intended for physiotherapy students, new graduates and postgraduate physiotherapists with an interest in patients with respiratory and cardiac problems.

Assessment of the patient should reveal the patient's problems. If some or all of these problems can be influenced by physical means, physiotherapy is indicated. Physiotherapy is also indicated when potential problems have been identified and preventative measures should be taken. The role of the physiotherapist as an educator in both the prevention and treatment of problems is another important aspect.

Diagnoses will continue to provide useful medical categories, but treatment can become prescriptive and inappropriate or ineffective if given in response to a diagnosis alone. The pathology behind the problem provides the key as to whether it is a physiotherapy problem or a medical problem.

It is by accurate assessment of the patient that short- and long-term patient goals can be identified and agreed, and an effective treatment plan outlined. Continuous reassessment of the patient and the treatment outcomes will identify the need for continuation or modification of treatment.

This book begins with assessment of the patient and the interpretation of medical investigations. This is followed by a section on mechanical support and cardio-pulmonary resuscitation.

An important part of our role is communication, counselling and health education. The skills available to the cardiorespiratory physiotherapist are many and varied. Practical skills have been outlined and referenced where possible. All skills are not yet supported by rigorous clinical studies, but it is important that we continue to use them if outcome measures support their place in clinical practice. In the future measurement tools could validate their use. Research should be an integral part of the practice of physiotherapy.

Patients' problems and their management are outlined in the context of differing pathologies. One pathological process may present as several patient problems. Pneumothorax, for example, appears under the problems of both pain and breathlessness. The characteristic problems of some patient groups and diagnostic categories are then discussed detailing the pathology, medical management, physiotherapy and evaluation of treatment.

This book should be read in conjunction with specialized texts on anatomy, physiology and pathology. Further reading is indicated within each chapter. Throughout the text, for simplicity, the patient is referred to as he/him and the physiotherapist as she/her, but it is not intended to imply that all patients are male or that all physiotherapists are female.

It is hoped that the problem-orientated approach to physiotherapy practice will facilitate the learning process for the physiotherapist and improve the quality of the care we provide.

B.A.W.
J.A.P.
London 1993

Acknowledgements

We would like to thank those who have supported us behind the scenes, in particular Guy Thorpe-Beeston, Margaret Hodson, Colin Wallis, Ranjan Suri, Peter Pryor and Barbara Webber. Our thanks also go to Denise Sheehan, Charlotte Dawson and our immediate colleagues at Royal Brompton Hospital and Great Ormond Street Hospital for Children for their constant support.

Chapter 1

Assessment and investigation of patients' problems

Sally Middleton, Peter G Middleton

INTRODUCTION

The aim of assessment is to define the patient's problems accurately. It is based on both a subjective and an objective assessment of the patient. Without an accurate assessment, it is impossible to develop an appropriate plan of treatment. Equally, a sound theoretical knowledge is required to develop an appropriate treatment plan for those problems that may be improved by physiotherapy. Once treatment has started, it is important to assess its effectiveness regularly in relation to both the problems and goals.

The system of patient management used in this book is based on the problem-oriented medical system (POMS) first described by Weed in 1968. This system has three components:

- problem-oriented medical records (POMR)
- audit
- educational programme.

The POMR is now widely used as the method of recording the assessment, management and progress of a patient. It is divided into five sections, as shown in Figure 1.1 and summarized below.

- *Database*. Here personal details, medical history, relevant social history, results of investigations and tests, together with the physiotherapist's assessment of the patient are recorded.

- *Problem list*. This is a concise list of the patient's problems, compiled after the assessment is complete. Problems are not always written in order of priority. The list includes problems both amenable to physiotherapy and problems that must be taken into consideration during treatment. The resolution of problems and the appearance of new ones are noted appropriately.

1

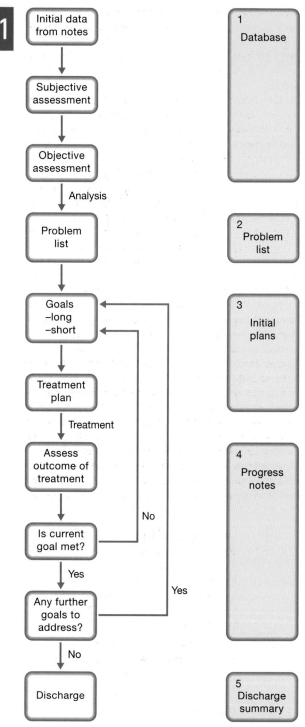

Figure 1.1 The process of problem–oriented medical records.

- *Initial plan and goals.* A treatment plan is formulated to address the physiotherapy-related problems, with consideration given to the patient's other problems. Long- and short-term goals are then formulated. Long-term goals are what the patient and the physiotherapist want to achieve finally, and should relate to the problems. Short-term goals are the stages by which the long-term goals should be achieved.

- *Progress notes.* These are written to document the patient's progress, especially highlighting any changes. The notes are written in the 'subjective, objective, analysis, plan' (SOAP) format for each problem, and provide an up-to-date summary of the patient's progress.

- *Discharge summary.* This is written when the patient is discharged from treatment or transferred to another institution. It includes presenting problems, treatment given, outcomes of treatment, together with any home programme or follow-up instructions.

DATABASE

The database contains a concise summary of the relevant information about the patient taken from the medical notes, together with the subjective and objective assessment made by the physiotherapist. The format may differ from hospital to hospital, but will contain the same information.

The first part contains the patient's personal details including name, date of birth, address, hospital number, and referring doctor. It may also contain the diagnosis and reason for referral. The second part summarizes the history from the medical notes and the physiotherapy assessment. This is often divided into several sections.

- *History of presenting condition (HPC)* summarizes the patient's current problems, including relevant information from the medical notes.

- *Previous medical history (PMH)* summarizes the entire list of medical and surgical problems that the patient has had in the past. It may be written in disease-specific groupings or as a chronological account.

- *Drug history (DH)* is a list of the patient's current medications (including dosage) taken from the medication charts. Drug allergies should also be noted.

- *Family history (FH)* includes a list of any major diseases suffered by members of the immediate family.

- *Social history (SH)* provides a picture of the patient's social situation. It is important to specifically question the patient about the level of support available at home, and to gain an idea of the patient's expected contribution to household duties. The layout of the patient's home should also be ascertained with particular emphasis on stairs. Occupation and hobbies, both past and present, give further information about the patient's lifestyle. Finally, history of smoking and alcohol use should be noted.

- *Patient examination* includes all information collected in the physiotherapist's subjective and objective assessment of the patient.

- *Test results* contain any significant findings as they become available. These may include arterial blood gases, spirometry, blood tests, sputum analysis, chest radiographs, computed tomography (CT) and any other relevant tests (e.g. hepatitis B positive).

Subjective assessment

Subjective assessment is based on an interview with the patient. It should generally start with open-ended questions *What is the main problem? What troubles you most?* allowing the patient to discuss the problems that are most important to them at that time. Indeed, by asking such questions, previously unmentioned problems may surface. As the interview progresses, questioning may become more focused on those important features that need clarification. There are five main symptoms of respiratory disease:

- breathlessness (dyspnoea)
- cough
- sputum and haemoptysis
- wheeze
- chest pain.

With each of these symptoms, enquiries should be made concerning:

- *duration* – both the absolute time since first recognition of the symptom (months, years) and the duration of the present symptoms (days, weeks)

- *severity* – in absolute terms and relative to the recent and distant past

- *pattern* – seasonal or daily variations

- *associated factors* – including precipitants, relieving factors, and associated symptoms, if any.

Breathlessness

Breathlessness is the subjective awareness of an increased work of breathing. It is the predominant symptom of both cardiac and respiratory disease. It also occurs in anaemia where the oxygen-carrying capacity of the blood is reduced, in neuromuscular disorders where the respiratory muscles are affected, and in metabolic dis-

orders where there is a change in the acid–base equilibrium (Chapter 3) or metabolic rate (e.g. hyperthyroid disorders). Breathlessness is also found in hyperventilation syndrome or dysfunctional breathing where psychological factors (e.g. anxiety) may be contributory factors.

The pathophysiological mechanisms causing breathlessness are still the subject of intensive investigation. Many factors are involved, including respiratory muscle length–tension relationships, respiratory muscle fatigue, stimulation of pulmonary stretch receptors, and alterations in central respiratory drive.

The duration and severity of breathlessness is most easily assessed through enquiries about the level of functioning in the recent and distant past. For example, a patient may say that 3 years ago he could walk up five flights of stairs without stopping, but now cannot manage even one flight. Some patients may deny breathlessness as they have (unconsciously) decreased their activity levels so that they do not get breathless. They may acknowledge breathlessness only when it interferes with important activities, e.g. bathing. The physiotherapist should always relate breathlessness to the level of function that the patient can achieve.

Comparison of the severity of breathlessness between patients is difficult because of differences in perception and expectations. To overcome these difficulties, numerous gradings have been proposed. The New York Heart Association classification of breathlessness, shown in Box 1.1, was developed for patients with cardiac disease, but is also applicable to respiratory patients. The Borg Rating of Perceived Exertion Scale (Borg 1982) is another scale that is frequently used for both respiratory and cardiac patients. No scale is universal and it is important that all staff within one institution use the same scale.

Box 1.1 The New York Heart Association classification of breathlessness

Class I	No symptoms with ordinary activity, breathlessness only occurring with severe exertion, e.g. running up hills, fast bicycling, cross-country skiing
Class II	Symptoms with ordinary activity, e.g. walking up stairs, making beds, carrying large amounts of shopping
Class III	Symptoms with mild exertion, e.g. bathing, showering, dressing
Class IV	Symptoms at rest

(Criteria Committee of the New York Heart Association 1994)

1

Breathlessness is usually worse during exercise and better with rest. An exception is hyperventilation syndrome where breathlessness may improve with exercise. Two patterns of breathlessness have been given specific names:

- *Orthopnoea* is breathlessness when lying flat
- *Paroxysmal nocturnal dyspnoea (PND)* is breathlessness that wakes the patient at night.

In the cardiac patient, lying flat increases venous return from the legs so that blood pools in the lungs, causing breathlessness. A similar pattern may be described in patients with severe asthma, but here the breathlessness is caused by nocturnal bronchoconstriction.

Further insight into a patient's breathlessness may be gained by enquiring about precipitating and relieving factors. Breathlessness associated with exposure to allergens and relieved by bronchodilators is typically found in asthma.

Cough

Coughing is a protective reflex that rids the airways of secretions or foreign bodies. Any stimulation of receptors located in the pharynx, larynx, trachea or bronchi may induce cough. Cough is a difficult symptom to clarify as most people cough normally every day, yet a repetitive persistent cough is both troublesome and distressing. Smokers may discount their early morning cough as being 'normal' when in fact it signifies chronic bronchitis.

Important features concerning cough are its effectiveness, and whether it is productive or dry. The severity of cough may range from an occasional disturbance to continual trouble. A loud, barking cough, which is often termed 'bovine', may signify laryngeal or tracheal disease. Recurrent coughing after eating or drinking is an important symptom of aspiration. A chronic productive cough every day is a fundamental feature of chronic bronchitis and bronchiectasis. Interstitial lung disease is characterized by a persistent, dry cough. Nocturnal cough is an important symptom of asthma in children and young adults, but in older patients it is more commonly due to cardiac failure. Drugs, especially beta-blockers and some other antihypertensive agents, can cause a chronic cough. Chronic cough may cause fractured ribs (cough fractures) and hernias. Stress incontinence is a common complication of chronic cough, especially in women. As this subject is often embarrassing to the patient, specific questioning may be required (see below).

Postoperatively, the strength and effectiveness of cough is important for the physiotherapist to assess.

Sputum

In a normal adult, up to 100 ml of tracheobronchial secretions are produced daily and cleared subconsciously by swallowing. Sputum is the excess tracheobronchial secretions that are cleared from the airways by coughing or huffing. It may contain mucus, cellular debris, microorganisms, blood and foreign particles. Questioning should determine the colour, consistency and quantity of sputum produced each day. This may clarify the diagnosis and the severity of disease (Table 1.1).

Table 1.1 Sputum analysis

	Description	Causes
Saliva	Clear watery fluid	
Mucoid	Opalescent or white	Chronic bronchitis without infection, asthma
Mucopurulent	Slightly discoloured, but not frank pus	Bronchiectasis, cystic fibrosis, pneumonia
Purulent	Thick, viscous: Yellow Dark green/brown Rusty Redcurrant jelly	 *Haemophilus* *Pseudomonas* *Pneumococcus, Mycoplasma* *Klebsiella*
Frothy	Pink or white	Pulmonary oedema
Haemoptysis	Ranging from blood specks to frank blood, old blood (dark brown)	Infection (tuberculosis, bronchiectasis), infarction, carcinoma, vasculitis, trauma, also coagulation disorders, cardiac disease
Black	Black specks in mucoid secretions	Smoke inhalation (fires, tobacco, heroin), coal dust

A number of grading systems for mucoid, mucopurulent, purulent sputum have been proposed. For example, Miller (1963) suggested:

M1   mucoid with no suspicion of pus
M2   predominantly mucoid, suspicion of pus
P1   1/3 purulent, 2/3 mucoid
P2   2/3 purulent, 1/3 mucoid
P3   >2/3 purulent.

However, in clinical practice sputum is often classified as mucoid, mucopurulent or purulent, together with an estimation of the volume (1 teaspoon, 1 egg cup, half a cup, 1 cup). Odour emanating from sputum signifies infection. In general, particularly offensive odours suggest infection with anaerobic organisms (e.g. aspiration pneumonia, lung abscess).

In patients with allergic bronchopulmonary aspergillosis (ABPA), asthma and occasionally bronchiectasis, sputum 'casts' may be expectorated. Classically these take the shape of the bronchial tree.

Haemoptysis is the presence of blood in the sputum. It may range from slight streaking of the sputum to frank blood. Frank haemoptysis can be life threatening, requiring bronchial artery embolization or surgery. Isolated haemoptysis may be the first sign of bronchogenic carcinoma, even when the chest radiograph is normal. Patients with chronic infective lung disease often suffer from recurrent haemoptyses.

Wheeze

Wheeze is a whistling or musical sound produced by turbulent airflow through narrowed airways. These sounds are generally noted by patients when audible at the mouth. Stridor, the sound of an upper airway obstruction, is often mistakenly called 'wheeze' by patients. Heart failure may also cause wheezing in those patients with significant mucosal oedema. Wheezing is discussed in more detail later in this chapter.

Chest pain

Chest pain in respiratory patients usually originates from musculoskeletal, pleural or tracheal inflammation, as the lung parenchyma and small airways contain no pain fibres.

Pleuritic chest pain is caused by inflammation of the parietal pleura, and is usually described as a severe, sharp, stabbing pain that is worse on inspiration. It is not reproduced by palpation.

Tracheitis generally causes a constant burning pain in the centre of the chest, aggravated by breathing.

Musculoskeletal (chest wall) pain may originate from the muscles, bones, joints or nerves of the thoracic cage. It is usually well localized and exacerbated by chest and/or arm movement. Palpation will usually reproduce the pain.

Angina pectoris is a major symptom of cardiac disease. Myocardial ischaemia characteristically causes a dull central retrosternal gripping or band-like sensation, which may radiate to either arm, neck or jaw.

Pericarditis may cause pain similar to angina or pleurisy.

A differential diagnosis of chest pain is given in Table 1.2.

Incontinence

Incontinence is a problem that is often aggravated by chronic cough (Orr et al 2001, Scottish Intercollegiate Guidelines Network 2004, Thakar & Stanton 2000). Coughing and huffing increase intra-abdominal pressure, which may precipitate urine leakage. Fear of this may influence compliance with physiotherapy. Thus, identification and treatment of incontinence is important. Questions may need to be specific to elicit this symptom: '*When you cough, do you find that you leak some urine? 'Does this interfere with your physiotherapy?'*

Other symptoms

Of the other symptoms a patient may report, a number have particular importance:

Fever (pyrexia) is one of the common features of infection, but low-grade fevers can also occur with malignancy and connective tissue disorders. Equally, infection may occur without fever, especially in immunosuppressed (e.g. chemotherapy) patients or those on corticosteroids. High fevers occurring at night, with associated sweating (night sweats), may be the first indicator of pulmonary tuberculosis.

Headache is an uncommon feature of respiratory disease. Morning headaches in patients with severe respiratory failure may signify nocturnal carbon dioxide retention. Early morning arterial blood gases or nocturnal transcutaneous carbon dioxide monitoring are required for confirmation.

Peripheral oedema in the respiratory patient suggests right heart failure, which may be due to cor pulmonale (right ventricular failure secondary to hypoxic pulmonary vasoconstriction). Peripheral oedema may also occur in patients taking high-dose corticosteroids, as a result of salt and water retention.

Functional ability

It is important to assess the patient as a whole, enquiring about their daily activities. If the patient is employed, what does the job *actually* entail? For example, a surveyor may sit behind a desk all day, or may be climbing 25-storey buildings. The home situation should also be documented, in particular the number of stairs to the

1

Table 1.2 Syndromes of chest pain		
Condition	Description	Causes
Pulmonary		
Pleurisy	Sharp, stabbing, rapid onset, limits inspiration, well localized, often 'catches' at a certain lung volume, not tender on palpation	Pleural infection or inflammation of the pleura, trauma (haemothorax), malignancy
Pulmonary embolus	Usually has pleuritic pain, with or without severe central pain	Pulmonary infarction
Pneumothorax	Severe central chest discomfort, with or without pleuritic component, severity depends on extent of mediastinal shift	Trauma, spontaneous, lung diseases (e.g. cystic fibrosis, AIDS)
Tumours	May mimic any form of chest pain, depending on site and structures involved	Primary or secondary carcinoma, mesothelioma
Musculoskeletal		
Rib fracture	Localized point tenderness, often sudden onset, increases with inspiration	Trauma, tumour, cough fractures (e.g. in chronic lung diseases, osteoporosis)
Muscular	Superficial, increases on inspiration and some body movements, with or without palpable muscle spasm	Trauma, unaccustomed exercise (excessive coughing during exacerbations of lung disease), accessory muscles may be affected
Costochondritis (Tietze's syndrome)	Localized to one or more costochondral joints, with or without generalized, non-specific chest pain	Viral infection
Neuralgia	Pain or paraesthesia in a dermatomal distribution	Thoracic spine dysfunction, tumour, trauma, herpes zoster (shingles)
Cardiac		
Ischaemic heart disease (angina or infarct)	Dull, central, retrosternal discomfort like a weight or band with or without radiation to the jaw and/or either arm, may be associated with palpitations, nausea or vomiting	Myocardial ischaemia, onset at rest is more suggestive of infarction
Pericarditis	Often retrosternal, exacerbated by respiration, may mimic cardiac ischaemia or pleurisy, often relieved by sitting	Infection, inflammation, trauma, tumour
Mediastinum		
Dissecting aortic aneurysm	Sudden onset, severe, poorly localized central chest pain	Trauma, atherosclerosis, Marfan's syndrome
Oesophageal	Retrosternal burning discomfort, but can mimic all other pains, worse lying flat or bending forward	Oesophageal reflux, trauma, tumour
Mediastinal shift	Severe, poorly localized central discomfort	Pneumothorax, rapid drainage of a large pleural effusion

front door and within the house. With whom does the patient live? What roles does the patient perform in the home (shopping, housework, cooking)? Finally, questions concerning activities and recreation often reveal areas where significant improvements in quality of life can be made.

Quality of life

Assessment of quality of life (QOL) is becoming increasingly important to assess the impact of disability on the patient and as a measure of response to treatment. QOL scales measure the effect of an illness and its management upon a patient as perceived by the patient. Often there is little correlation between physiological measures (e.g. lung function) and QOL. A number of both generic, for example SF-36 (Ware & Sherbourne 1992) and disease-specific QOL scales are available which allow data to be gathered principally by self-report questionnaires or interview. QOL scales available for assessment of patients with respiratory or cardiovascular disease are reviewed elsewhere (Juniper et al 1999, Kinney et al 1996, Mahler 2000, Pashkow et al 1995). The choice of a QOL measure requires an evaluation of QOL scales with respect to their reliability, validity, responsiveness and appropriateness (Aaronson 1989).

Disease awareness

During the interview it is important to ascertain the patient's knowledge of his disease and treatment. The level of compliance with treatment, often difficult to assess initially, may become evident as rapport develops. These issues will influence the goals of treatment.

Objective assessment

Objective assessment is based on examination of the patient, together with the use of tests such as spirometry, arterial blood gases and chest radiographs. Although a full examination of the patient should be available from the medical notes, it is worthwhile to make a thorough examination at all times, as the patient's condition may have changed since the last examination, and the physiotherapist may need greater detail of certain aspects than is available from the notes. A good examination will provide an objective baseline for future measurement of the patient's progress. By developing a standard method of examination, the findings are quickly assimilated and the physiotherapist remains confident that nothing has been omitted. This chapter refers mainly to assessment of the adult patient, although much of the information is also relevant to the paediatric population. Specific details for the assessment of infants and children and normal values can be found in the relevant paediatric sections (Chapters 9 & 10).

General observation

Examination starts by observing the patient from the end of the bed. Is the patient short of breath, sitting on the edge of the bed, distressed? Is he obviously cyanosed? Is he on supplemental oxygen? If so, how much? What is the speech pattern – long fluent paragraphs without discernible pauses for breath, quick sentences, just a few words, or are they too breathless to speak? When he moves around or undresses, does he become distressed? With a little practice, these observations should become second nature and can be noted while introducing yourself to the patient.

In the intensive care patient there are a number of further features to be observed. The level of ventilatory support must be ascertained. This includes both the mode of ventilation (e.g. supplemental oxygen, continuous positive airway pressure, intermittent positive pressure ventilation) and the route of ventilation (mask, endotracheal tube, tracheostomy). The level of cardiovascular support should also be noted, including drugs to control blood pressure and cardiac output, pacemakers and other mechanical devices. The patient's level of consciousness should also be noted. Any patient with a decreased level of consciousness is at risk of aspiration and retention of pulmonary secretions. In those patients who are not pharmacologically sedated, the level of consciousness is often measured using the Glasgow Coma Scale (Box 1.2). This gives the patient a score (from 3 to 15) based on his best motor, verbal and eye responses.

Box 1.2 The Glasgow Coma Scale		
Eye opening	Spontaneous	4
	To speech	3
	To pain	2
	None	1
Best verbal response	Oriented	5
	Confused speech	4
	Inappropriate words	3
	Incomprehensible sounds	2
	None	1
Best motor response	Obeys commands	6
	Localizes to pain	5
	Withdraws (generalized)	4
	Flexion	3
	Extension	2
	No response	1
Maximum total score is 15; minimum total score is 3 (Teasdale and Jennett 1974)		

The patient's chart should then be examined for recordings of temperature, pulse, blood pressure and respiratory rate. These measurements are usually performed by the nursing staff immediately on admission of the patient and regularly thereafter.

Body temperature. Body temperature can be measured in a number of ways. Oral temperatures are the most convenient method in adults, but should not be performed for at least 15 minutes after smoking or consuming hot or cold food or drink. Aural, axillary and rectal temperature may also be measured.

Body temperature is maintained within the range 36.5–37.5°C. It is lowest in the early morning and highest in the afternoon.

Fever (pyrexia) is the elevation of the body temperature above 37.5°C, and is associated with an increased metabolic rate. For every 1°C rise in body temperature, there is an approximately 10% increase in oxygen consumption and carbon dioxide production (Manthous et al 1995). This places extra demand on the cardiorespiratory system, which causes a compensatory increase in heart rate and respiratory rate.

Heart rate. Heart rate is most accurately measured by auscultation at the cardiac apex. The pulse rate is measured by palpating a peripheral artery (radial, femoral or carotid). In most situations, the heart rate and pulse rate are identical; a difference between the two is called the 'pulse deficit'. This indicates that some heartbeats have not caused sufficient blood flow to reach the periphery and is commonly found in atrial fibrillation and some other arrhythmias. The normal adult heart rate is 60–100 beats per minute.

Tachycardia is defined as a heart rate greater than 100 beats/min at rest in adults. It is found with anxiety, exercise, fever, anaemia and hypoxia. It is also common in patients with cardiac disorders. Medications such as bronchodilators and some cardiac drugs may also increase heart rate.

Bradycardia is defined as a heart rate less than 60 beats/min. It may be a normal finding in athletes and may also be caused by some cardiac drugs (especially beta-blockers).

Blood pressure (BP). With every contraction of the heart (systole) the arterial pressure increases, with the peak called the 'systolic' pressure. During the relaxation phase of the heart (diastole), the arterial pressure drops, with the minimum called the 'diastolic' pressure. Blood pressure is usually measured non-invasively by placing a sphygmomanometer cuff around the upper arm, and listening over the brachial artery with a stethoscope. The cuff width should be approximately one-half to two-thirds of the length of the upper arm, otherwise readings may be inaccurate. Cuff inflation to above systolic pressure collapses the artery, blocking flow. With release of the air, the cuff pressure gradually falls to a point just below systolic. At this point, the peak pressure within the artery is greater than the pressure outside the artery, so flow recommences. This turbulent flow is audible through the stethoscope. As the cuff is further deflated the noise continues. When the cuff pressure drops to just below diastolic, the pressure within the artery is greater than that of the cuff throughout the cardiac cycle, so turbulence abates and the noise ceases. The gauge to measure BP was previously a column of mercury, but with the increasing awareness of the risks of mercury, many devices now use pressure gauges or totally digital systems. Blood pressure is recorded as systolic/ diastolic pressure. Normal adult blood pressure is between 95/60 and 140/90 mmHg.

Hypertension is defined as a blood pressure greater than 145/95 mmHg, usually due to changes in vascular tone and/or aortic valve disease.

Hypotension is defined as a blood pressure less than 90/60 mmHg. It is often a normal finding during sleep. Daytime hypotension may be due to heart failure, blood loss or decreased vascular tone.

Postural hypotension is a drop in blood pressure of more than 5 mmHg between lying and sitting or standing, and may be due to decreased circulating blood volume, or loss of vascular tone.

Pulsus paradoxus is the exaggeration of the drop in blood pressure that occurs with inspiration. Normally, during inspiration the negative intrathoracic pressure reduces venous return and drops cardiac output slightly. Exaggeration of this normal response where blood pressure drops by more than 10 mmHg is seen in situations where the intrathoracic pressure swings are greater, as occurs in severe airway obstruction.

Respiratory rate. Respiratory rate should be measured with the patient seated comfortably. The normal adult respiratory rate is approximately 12–16 breaths/min.

Tachypnoea is defined as a respiratory rate greater than 20 breaths/min, and can be seen in any form of lung disease. It may also occur with metabolic acidosis and anxiety.

Bradypnoea is defined as a respiratory rate of less than 10 breaths/min. It is an uncommon finding, and is usually due to central nervous system depression by narcotics or trauma.

Body weight. Weight is often recorded on the observation chart. Respiratory function can be compromised by both obesity and severe malnourishment. As ideal body weight has a large normal range, the body mass index (BMI) is a more valid measurement and is often expressed as a standard deviation score. This is calculated by dividing the weight in kilograms by the square of the height in metres (kg/m^2); the normal range is 20–25 kg/m^2. Patients with values below 20 are underweight, those with values of 25–30 are overweight, and those with values over 30 are classified as obese.

Malnourished patients often exhibit depression of their immune system with increased risk of infection. They also have weaker respiratory muscles, which are more likely to fatigue. Obesity causes an increase in residual volume (RV) and a decrease in functional residual capacity (FRC) (Rubinstein et al 1990). Thus tidal breathing occurs close to closing volumes. This is particularly important postoperatively, where the obese are more prone to subsegmental lung collapse.

An accurate daily weight gives a good estimate of fluid volume changes, as any change in weight of more than 250 g/day is usually due to fluid accumulation or loss. Daily weights are commonly used in intensive care, renal and cardiac patients to assess fluid balance.

Other measures. In the intensive care patient there is a plethora of monitoring that can be performed. As well as the parameters listed above, measures of central venous pressure (CVP), pulmonary artery pressure (PAP) and intracranial pressure (ICP) will need to be reviewed as part of the physiotherapy assessment. Many intensive care units now record this information on bedside computer terminals. Further details of intensive care monitoring can be found in Chapters 8 & 9.

Apparatus. The presence of lines and tubes should be noted. Venous lines provide constant direct access to the bloodstream, and vary widely in site, complexity and function. The simplest cannula in a small peripheral vein, usually in the forearm, is called a 'drip'. It is used for the administration of intravenous (IV) fluids and most IV drugs. At the other end of the spectrum are the multilumen lines placed in the subclavian, internal jugular or femoral veins, ending in the venae cavae close to the heart. These central lines allow simultaneous administration of multiple drugs and can be used for central venous pressure monitoring. Central lines can be potentially dangerous, as disconnection of the line can quickly suck air into the central veins, causing an air embolus, which may be fatal.

Some patients, especially those in intensive care, may have an arterial line for continuous recording of blood pressure and for repeated sampling of arterial blood. These lines are usually inserted in the radial or brachial artery. If accidentally disconnected, rapid blood loss will occur.

After cardiac surgery, most patients have cardiac pacing wires that exit through the skin overlying the heart. In most cases these wires are not required and are removed routinely before discharge. In the event of clinically significant cardiac arrhythmias, these wires are connected to a pacing box that electrically stimulates the heart. In medical patients, pacemaker wires are introduced through one of the central veins and rest in the apex of the right ventricle. Care must be taken with all pacing wires as dislodgement may be life threatening.

Postoperatively, drains may be placed at any operation site (e.g. abdomen) to prevent the collection of fluid or blood. These are generally connected to sterile bags. Nasogastric tubes are placed for two reasons: soft, fine-bore tubes are used to facilitate feeding, while firm, wider-bore tubes allow aspiration of gastric contents.

Intercostal drains are placed between two ribs into the pleural space to remove air, fluid or pus which has accumulated. They are also used routinely after cardio-thoracic surgery. In general, the tube is attached to a bottle partially filled with sterile water, called an 'underwater seal drain' (Chapter 11). The bottle should be positioned at least 0.5 metres below the patient's chest (usually on the floor). Bubbling indicates that air is entering the tube from the pleural space at that time. Frequent observations must be made of the fluid level within the tube, which should oscillate or 'swing' with every breath. If the fluid does not swing, the tube is not patent and requires medical attention. In certain situations the bottle may be connected to continuous suction, which will dampen the fluid 'swing'. Those patients who are producing large volumes of fluid or pus may be connected to a double bottle system, where the first bottle acts as a reservoir to collect the fluid and the second provides the underwater seal. Fully enclosed disposable plastic systems are now available. Any patient with a chest drain should have a pair of large forceps available at all times to clamp the tube if any connection becomes loosened.

The hands. Significant findings can be identified by observing and examining the hands. A fine tremor will often be seen in association with high-dose bronchodilators. Warm and sweaty hands with an irregular flapping tremor may be due to acute carbon dioxide retention. Weakness and wasting of the small muscles in the hands may be an early sign of an upper lobe tumour involving the brachial plexus (Pancoast's tumour). Examination of the fingers may show nicotine staining from smoking.

Clubbing is the term used to describe the changes in the fingers and toes as shown in Figure 1.2. The first sign of clubbing is the loss of the angle between the nail bed and the nail itself. Later, the finger pad becomes enlarged. The nail bed may also become 'spongy', but this is a difficult sign to elicit. A summary of the diseases associated with clubbing is given in Box 1.3. The exact

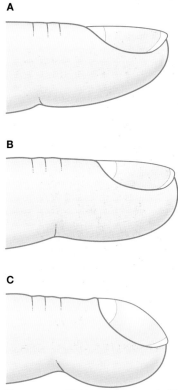

A

B

C

Figure 1.2 Clubbing: (**A**) normal; (**B**) early clubbing; (**C**) advanced clubbing.

Box 1.3   Causes of clubbing

Lung disease	Infective (bronchiectasis, lung abscess, empyema) Fibrotic Malignant (bronchogenic cancer, mesothelioma)
Cardiac disease	Congenital cyanotic heart disease Bacterial endocarditis
Other	Familial Cirrhosis Gastrointestinal disease (Crohn's disease, ulcerative colitis, coeliac disease)

---

cause of clubbing is unknown. It is interesting to note that clubbing in cystic fibrosis patients disappears after heart and lung or lung transplant.

The eyes. The eyes should be examined for pallor (anaemia), plethora (high haemoglobin) or jaundice (yellow colour due to liver or blood disturbances). Drooping of one eyelid with enlargement of that pupil suggests Horner's syndrome where there is a disturbance in the sympathetic nerve supply to that side of the head (sometimes seen in cancer of the lung).

Cyanosis. This is a bluish discolouration of the skin and mucous membranes. Central cyanosis, seen on examination of the tongue and mouth, is caused by hypoxaemia where there is an increase in the amount of haemoglobin not bound to oxygen. The degree of blueness is related to the quantity of unbound haemoglobin. Thus a greater degree of hypoxia is necessary to produce cyanosis in an anaemic patient (low haemoglobin), while a patient with polycythaemia (increased haemoglobin) may appear cyanosed with only a small drop in oxygen levels. Peripheral cyanosis, affecting the toes, fingers and earlobes, may also be due to poor peripheral circulation, especially in cold weather.

Jugular venous pressure. On the side of the neck the jugular venous pressure (JVP) is seen as a flickering impulse in the jugular vein. It is normally seen at the base of the neck when the patient is lying back at 45°. The JVP is usually measured in relation to the sternal angle as this point is relatively fixed in relation to the right atrium. A normal JVP at the base of the neck corresponds to a vertical height approximately 3–4 cm above the sternal angle. The JVP is generally expressed as the vertical height (in centimetres) above normal. The JVP provides a quick assessment of the volume of blood in the great vessels entering the heart. Most commonly it is elevated in right heart failure. This may occur in patients with chronic lung disease complicated by cor pulmonale. In contrast, dehydrated patients may only have a visible JVP when lying flat.

Peripheral oedema. This is an important sign of cardiac failure, but may also be found in patients with a low albumin level, impaired venous or lymphatic function, or those on high-dose steroids. When mild, it may only affect the ankles; with increasing severity, it may progress up the body. In bedbound patients, it is important to check the sacrum.

Observation of the chest

When examining the chest it is important to remember the surface landmarks of the thoracic contents (Fig. 1.3). Some important points are:

- The oblique fissure, dividing the upper and middle lobes from the lower lobes, runs underneath a line drawn from the spinous process of T2 around the chest to the sixth costochondral junction anteriorly.

- The horizontal fissure on the right, dividing the upper lobe from the middle lobe, runs from the

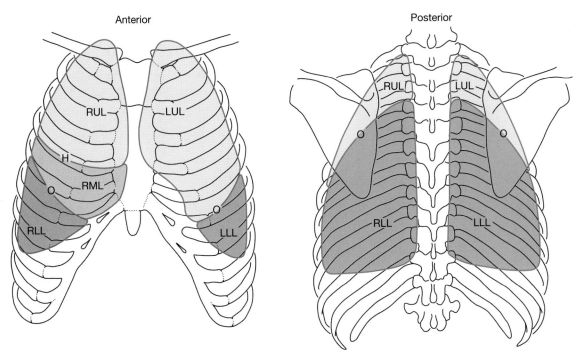

Figure 1.3 Surface markings of the lungs: H, horizontal fissure; O, oblique fissure; RUL, right upper lobe; LUL, left upper lobe; RML, right middle lobe; LLL, left lower lobe; RLL, right lower lobe.

fourth intercostal space at the right sternal edge horizontally to the midaxillary line, where it joins the oblique fissure.

■ The diaphragm sits at approximately the sixth rib anteriorly, the eighth rib in the midaxillary line and the 10th rib posteriorly.

■ The trachea bifurcates just below the level of the manubriosternal junction.

■ The apical segment of both upper lobes extends 2.5 cm above the clavicles.

Chest shape.   The chest should be symmetrical with the ribs, in adults, descending at approximately 45° from the spine. The transverse diameter should be greater than the anteroposterior (AP) diameter. The thoracic spine should have a slight kyphosis. Important common abnormalities include:

■ *kyphosis,* where the normal flexion of the thoracic spine is increased

■ *kyphoscoliosis,* which comprises both lateral curvature of the spine with vertebral rotation (scoliosis) and an element of kyphosis. This causes a restrictive lung defect which, when severe, may cause respiratory failure

■ *pectus excavatum,* or 'funnel' chest, is where part of the sternum is depressed inwards. This rarely causes significant changes in lung function but may be corrected surgically for cosmetic reasons

■ *pectus carinatum,* or 'pigeon' chest, is where the sternum protrudes anteriorly. This may be present in children with severe asthma and rarely causes significant lung function abnormalities

■ *hyperinflation,* where the ribs lose their normal 45° angle with the thoracic spine and become almost horizontal. The anteroposterior diameter of the chest increases to almost equal the transverse diameter. This is commonly seen in severe emphysema.

Breathing pattern.   Observation of the breathing pattern gives further information concerning the type and severity of respiratory disease.

Normal breathing should be regular with a rate of 12–16 breaths/min, as mentioned previously. Inspiration is active and expiration passive. The approximate ratio of inspiratory to expiratory time (I:E ratio) is 1:1.5 to 1:2.

Prolonged expiration may be seen in patients with obstructive lung disease, where expiratory airflow is severely limited by dynamic closure of the smaller airways. In severe obstruction the I:E ratio may increase to 1:3 or 1:4.

Pursed-lip breathing is often seen in patients with severe airways disease. By opposing the lips during expiration the airway pressure inside the chest is maintained, preventing the floppy airways from collapsing. Thus overall airflow is increased.

Tachypnoea refers to an increased respiratory rate, usually defined as >20 breaths/minute.

Bradypnoea, a rarely used term, refers to a respiratory rate of <10 breaths/minute.

Apnoea refers to a total cessation in breathing for >10 seconds.

Hypopnoea refers to shallow breathing (<50% of normal) for >10 seconds, usually recorded during the night as part of a sleep study.

Hypoventilation refers to reduced total ventilation (rate × volume) and usually increases arterial carbon dioxide. It is commonly seen with sedation or opiate analgesia. Severe obesity may also cause hypoventilation.

Hyperventilation refers to increased total ventilation (rate × volume) and usually lowers arterial carbon dioxide. It is commonly seen in anxiety/hyperventilation syndrome (Chapter 17).

Kussmaul's respiration is rapid, deep breathing with a high minute ventilation. It is usually seen in patients with metabolic acidosis.

Cheyne–Stokes respiration refers to irregular breathing with cycles consisting of a few relatively deep breaths, progressively shallower breaths (sometimes to the point of apnoea), and then slowly increasing depth of breaths. This is usually associated with heart failure, severe neurological disturbances or drugs (e.g. narcotics).

Ataxic breathing consists of haphazard, uncoordinated deep and shallow breaths. This may be found in patients with cerebellar disease.

Apneustic breathing is characterized by prolonged inspiration, and is usually the result of brain damage.

Chest movement. During normal inspiration, there are symmetrical increases in the anteroposterior, transverse and vertical diameters of the chest. The increase in vertical diameter is achieved by contraction of the diaphragm, causing the abdominal contents to descend. Sternal and rib movements are responsible for the increases in anteroposterior and transverse diameters of the chest. These movements can be divided into two components (Fig. 1.4). When elevated, the anterior ends of the ribs move forward and upwards with anterior movement of the sternum. This increase in anteroposterior diameter is likened to the movement of an old fashioned 'pump handle'. At the same time, rotation of the

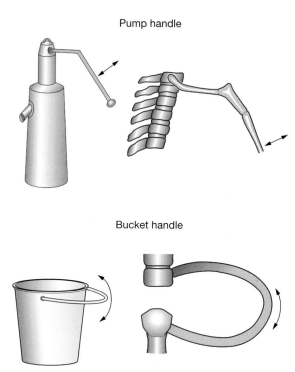

Figure 1.4 Chest wall movement.

ribs causes an increase in the transverse diameter, likened to the movement of a 'bucket handle'.

During normal quiet breathing, the diaphragm is the main inspiratory muscle increasing the vertical diameter. There is also an increase in the lower thoracic transverse diameter due to external intercostal muscle contraction. Expiration is passive, caused by the elastic recoil of the lung and chest wall. When breathing is increased, all the accessory inspiratory muscles (sternomastoid, scalenes, trapezii) contract to increase the anteroposterior and transverse diameters, and the diaphragm activity increases, thus further increasing the vertical dimensions. Expiration may become active with contraction of the abdominal and internal intercostal muscles.

Intercostal indrawing occurs where the skin between the ribs is drawn inwards during inspiration. It may be seen in patients with severe inspiratory airflow resistance. Larger negative pressures during inspiration suck the soft tissues inwards. This is an important sign of respiratory distress in children, but is less often seen in adults.

Palpation of the chest

Trachea. Firstly, the trachea is palpated to assess its position in relation to the sternal notch. Tracheal deviation indicates underlying mediastinal shift. The trachea may be pulled towards a collapsed or fibrosed upper

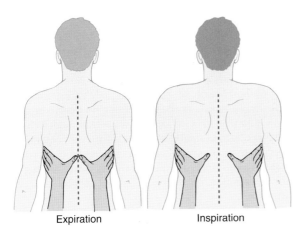

| Expiration | Inspiration |

Figure 1.5 Palpation of thoracic expansion.

lobe, or pushed away from a pneumothorax or large pleural effusion.

Chest expansion. This can be assessed by observation, but palpation is more accurate. The patient is instructed to expire slowly to residual volume. At residual volume the examiner's hands are placed spanning the postero-lateral segments of both bases, with the thumbs touching in the midline posteriorly, as shown in Figure 1.5. In obese patients, it helps if the skin of the anterior chest wall is slightly retracted by the fingertips. The patient is then instructed to inspire slowly and the movement of both thumbs is observed. Both sides should move equally, with 3–5 cm being the normal displacement.

A similar technique may be used anteriorly, again to measure basal movements. Measurement of apical movement is more difficult. By placing the hand over the upper chest anteriorly, a qualitative comparison of the two sides can be made. In all cases, diminished movement is abnormal.

Paradoxical breathing is where some or all of the chest wall moves inwards on inspiration and outwards on expiration. It can involve anything from a localized area to the entire chest wall. Localized paradox occurs when the integrity of the chest wall is disrupted. Fractures of multiple ribs with two or more breaks in each rib will result in the central section losing the support usually provided by the rest of the thoracic cage. Thus, during inspiration, this loose segment (often called a 'flail segment') is drawn inwards as the rest of the chest wall moves out. In expiration the reverse occurs.

Paradoxical movement of one hemithorax may be remarkably difficult to observe. It may be caused by unilateral diaphragm paralysis. Paradox of the entire chest wall occurs in bilateral diaphragm weakness or paralysis. It is most apparent when the patient is supine.

Paradoxical movement of the lower chest can occur in patients with severe chronic airflow limitation who are extremely hyperinflated. As the dome of the diaphragm cannot descend any further, diaphragm contraction during inspiration pulls the lower ribs inwards. This is called 'Hoover's sign'.

Surgical emphysema. Air in the subcutaneous tissues of the chest, neck or face should also be noted. On palpation there is a characteristic crackling in the skin. This occurs when a pneumomediastinum (air in the mediastinum) has tracked outwards. A chest radiograph must be performed immediately, as a pneumomediastinum may be associated with a pneumothorax.

Vocal fremitus. Vocal fremitus is the measure of speech vibrations transmitted through the chest wall to the examiner's hands. It is measured by asking the patient to repeatedly say 'ninety-nine' while the examiner's hands are placed flat on both sides of the chest. The hands are moved from apices to bases, anteriorly and posteriorly, comparing the vibration felt. Vocal fremitus is increased when the lung underneath is relatively solid (consolidated), as this transmits sound better. As sound transmission is decreased through any interface between lung and air or fluid, vocal fremitus is decreased in patients with a pneumothorax or a pleural effusion.

Percussion

Percussion of the chest provides further information that can help in the assessment and localization of lung disease. It is performed by placing the left hand firmly on the chest wall so that the fingers have good contact with the skin. The middle finger of the left hand is struck over the distal interphalangeal joint with the middle finger of the right hand. The right wrist should be relaxed so that the weight of the entire right hand is transmitted through the middle finger. Both sides of the chest from top to bottom should be percussed alternately, paying particular attention to the comparison between sides.

Resonance is generated by the chest wall vibrating over the underlying tissues. Normal resonance is heard over aerated lung, while consolidated lung sounds dull, and a pleural effusion sounds 'stony dull'. Increased resonance is heard when the chest wall is free to vibrate over an air-filled space, such as a pneumothorax or bulla. In situations where the chest wall is unable to move freely, as may occur in obese patients, the percussion note may sound dull, even if the underlying lung is normal.

Auscultation

Chest auscultation is the process of listening to and interpreting the sounds produced within the thorax. A stethoscope simplifies auscultation and facilitates localization of any abnormalities. It consists of a diaphragm and bell connected by tubing to two earpieces. The diaphragm is generally used for listening to breath sounds, while the bell is best for the very low frequencies generated by the heart (especially the third and fourth heart sounds). The diaphragm and bell must be intact for a sound to be heard properly, and the tubing relatively short to minimize absorption of the sound. The earpieces, made of plastic or rubber, should fit snugly within the ears, pointing slightly forward in order to maximize sound transmission into the auditory canal.

A teaching stethoscope (Fig. 1.6) is a useful tool to allow both the experienced and inexperienced physiotherapist to hear the same sounds simultaneously (Ellis 1985). More recently, a number of electronic stethoscopes have been produced, allowing teacher and students to listen together.

Chest auscultation should ideally be performed in a quiet room, with the chest exposed. The patient is instructed to take deep breaths through an open mouth, as turbulence within the nose can interfere with the breath sounds. There is a wide variation in the intensity of breath sounds depending on chest wall thickness. The terms used are described below.

Breath sounds

Normal breath sounds are generated by turbulent airflow in the trachea and large airways. These sounds, which can be heard directly over the trachea, comprise high, medium and low frequencies. The higher frequencies are attenuated by normal lung tissue so that breath sounds heard over the periphery are softer and lower pitched. Originally it was thought that the higher-pitched sounds were generated by the bronchi (bronchial breath sounds) and the lower ones by airflow into the alveoli (vesicular breath sounds). It is now known that normal breath sounds (previously called 'vesicular') simply represent filtering of the 'bronchial' breath sounds generated in the large airways. Although technically incorrect, normal breath sounds are still sometimes referred to as 'vesicular' or 'bronchovesicular'. Normal breath sounds are heard all over the chest wall throughout inspiration and for a short period during expiration.

Bronchial breath sounds are the normal tracheal and large airway sounds, transmitted through airless lung, which does not attenuate the higher frequencies. Thus, the sounds heard over an area of consolidated lung are similar to those heard over the trachea itself. Bronchial breath sounds are loud and high-pitched, with a harsh quality. They are heard equally throughout inspiration and expiration, with a short pause between the two. In all three respects, bronchial breath sounds differ from normal breath sounds which are faint, lower-pitched and absent during the latter half of expiration.

If the bronchus supplying an area of consolidated lung is obstructed (e.g. carcinoma, large sputum plug) bronchial breath sounds may not be heard as the obstruction blocks sound transmission.

Diminished sounds occur when there is a reduction in the initial generation of the sound or when there is an increase in sound attenuation. As the breath sounds are generated by flow-related turbulence, reduced flow

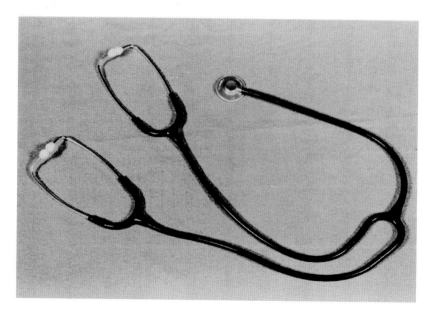

Figure 1.6 A Littmann teaching stethoscope.

causes less sound. Thus patients who will not (e.g. due to pain) or cannot (e.g. due to muscle weakness) breathe deeply will have globally diminished breath sounds. Similarly, diminished breath sounds are heard in some patients with emphysema where the combination of parenchymal destruction and hyperinflation causes greater attenuation of the normal breath sounds. In obese patients, breath sounds are diminished by attenuation through the fat over the chest wall.

Locally diminished breath sounds may represent obstruction of a bronchus by tumour or large sputum plugs. Localized accumulation of air or fluid in the pleural space will block sound transmission so that breath sounds are absent.

Added sounds

Wheezes, previously called 'rhonchi', are musical tones produced by airflow vibrating a narrowed or compressed airway. A fixed, monophonic wheeze is caused by a single obstructed airway, while polyphonic wheezes are due to widespread disease. Any cause of narrowing, for example, bronchospasm, mucosal oedema, sputum or foreign bodies, may cause wheezes. As the airways are normally compressed during expiration, wheezes are first heard at this time. When airway narrowing is more severe, wheezes may also be heard during inspiration. The pitch of the wheeze is directly related to the degree of narrowing, with high-pitched wheezes indicating near total obstruction. However, the volume of the wheeze may be misleading as the moderate asthmatic may have loud wheezes while the very severe asthmatic may have a 'quiet chest' because he is not generating sufficient airflow to cause wheezes.

Low-pitched, localized wheezes are caused by sputum retention and can change or clear after coughing.

Crackles, previously called 'crepitations' or 'râles', are clicking sounds heard during inspiration. They are caused by the opening of previously closed alveoli and small airways during inspiration. Crackles are described as 'early' or 'late', 'fine' or 'coarse', and 'localized' or 'widespread'. Coarse, early inspiratory crackles occur when bronchioles open (often heard in bronchiectasis and bronchitis), while fine, late inspiratory crackles occur when alveoli and respiratory bronchioles open (often heard in pulmonary oedema and pulmonary fibrosis). When severe, the late inspiratory crackles of pulmonary oedema and pulmonary fibrosis may become coarser and start earlier in inspiration.

Localized crackles may occur in dependent alveoli, which are gradually closed by compression from the lung above. This early feature of subsegmental lung collapse resolves when the patient breathes deeply or coughs. The crackles of pulmonary oedema are also more marked basally, but only clear transiently after coughing. The differentiation between subsegmental lung collapse and pulmonary oedema may be difficult, and sometimes auscultation will not clarify the situation. Elevation of the jugular venous pressure and peripheral oedema suggest pulmonary oedema, whereas ineffective cough, recent anaesthesia and pyrexia suggest sputum retention, which could lead to subsegmental lung collapse (Table 1.3). Postoperative and intensive care patients may have a combination of both pulmonary oedema and sputum retention.

Pleural rub is the creaking or rubbing sound that occurs with each breath when the pleural surfaces are roughened by inflammation, infection or neoplasm. Normally the visceral and parietal pleura slide silently. Pleural rubs range from being localized and soft to being loud and generalized, sometimes even palpable. In certain instances, they may be difficult to differentiate from crackles. An important distinguishing feature is that pleural rubs are heard equally during inspiration and expiration, with the sounds often recurring in reverse order during expiration.

Vocal resonance. Vocal resonance is the transmission of voice through the airways and lung tissue to the chest wall where it is heard through a stethoscope. It is usually tested by instructing the patient to say 'ninety-nine'

Table 1.3   Differentiation between pulmonary oedema and sputum retention

Chest sign	Pulmonary oedema	Sputum retention
Auscultation	Fine crackles, especially at bases, with or without wheezes	Scattered or localized crackles, with or without wheezes, may move with coughing
Sputum	Frothy white or pink	Thicker, more viscid, any colour
Other signs	Elevated JVP Peripheral oedema Increased weight, positive fluid balance History of previous cardiac disease	Pyrexia History of intercurrent chest disease, recent anaesthetic, aspiration, respiratory muscle weakness

JVP, jugular venous pressure

1

repeatedly (like vocal fremitus which is felt with the hands). As mentioned previously, normal lung attenuates the higher frequencies so that the lower frequencies dominate. Thus, speech normally becomes a low-pitched mumble. Consolidated lung transmits all sounds better, especially the high frequencies, so the transmitted sound is louder and higher pitched. In this situation speech can actually be understood. Whispered speech lacks the lower frequencies and is normally not transmitted to the chest wall. However, over areas of consolidation the whisper is clearly heard and intelligible – this is called 'whispering pectoriloquy'.

As with auscultation of breath sounds, vocal resonance is decreased when the transmission of sound through the lung or from the lung to chest wall is impeded. This occurs with emphysema, pneumothorax, pleural thickening or pleural effusion.

A summary of the chest examination in selected chest problems is given in Table 1.4.

Heart sounds. The normal heart sounds represent the closure of the four heart valves. The first heart sound is caused by closure of the mitral and tricuspid valves, while the second heart sound is due to closure of the aortic and pulmonary valves. A third heart sound indicates cardiac failure in adults, but may be normal in children. It is attributed to vibration of the ventricular walls caused by rapid filling in early diastole. The fourth heart sound is caused by vibration of the ventricular walls in late diastole as the atria contract. It may be heard in heart failure, hypertension and aortic valve disease.

A murmur is the sound generated by turbulent flow through a valve. The murmur of valvular incompetence is caused by back flow across the valve, while stenotic valves generate murmurs by turbulent forward flow.

Sputum

At the end of the respiratory examination, it is often worthwhile to instruct the patient to huff to a low lung volume to assess the presence of retained secretions. Any sputum produced should be examined for colour, consistency and quantity as previously described.

Physiotherapy techniques

In patients who have previously been taught physiotherapy, it is important to ascertain which techniques are used, how well they are performed, and their effectiveness. For example, patients who use huffing to clear retained secretions should have its effectiveness assessed. Suboptimal techniques need to be identified and their correction included in the treatment plan.

Exercise capacity

For a complete assessment of the respiratory system, exercise capacity should also be measured. Depending on the situation, this may vary from a full exercise test for measuring maximum oxygen uptake, to a simple assessment of breathlessness during normal activities. An exercise test provides the best measure of functional limitation, which may differ from that suggested by a patient's lung function. Two of the most common methods used to assess patients with respiratory disease are the 6-minute walking test (Butland et al 1982) and the shuttle walking tests (Bradley et al 1999, Revill et al 1999, Singh et al 1992).

Test results

The final stage of assessment of a respiratory or cardiac patient involves the use of tests, in particular spirometry, arterial blood gases and chest radiography. The following is a brief summary of the application of these tests. A full discussion is given in Chapters 2 and 3.

Spirometry

The forced expiratory volume in 1 second (FEV_1), the forced vital capacity (FVC) and peak expiratory flow (PEF) are important measures of ventilatory function. Normal values, based on population studies, depend on

Table 1.4 Summary of chest examination in selected chest problems

Disease	Breath sounds	PN	VF	VR
Consolidation:				
With open airway	Bronchial	Dull	↑	↑
With blocked airway	↓	Dull	↓	↓
Pneumothorax	↓ or absent	Hyperresonant	↓ or absent	↓ or absent
Pleural effusion	↓ or absent	Stony dull	↓ or absent	↓ or absent

PN, percussion note; VF, vocal fremitus; VR, vocal resonance; ↑, increased; ↓, decreased

age, height, sex and race. Weight is not an important determinant of lung function, except in the markedly obese or malnourished.

Although often expressed as absolute values, lung function should always be compared with predicted values and previous recordings for that patient. For example a 21-year-old, 6-foot-tall male asthmatic changing his spirometry (FEV_1/FVC) from 4.0/5.0 litres to 1.5/3.0 litres should cause concern, while a normal 81-year-old, 5-foot female may never manage to blow more than 1.3/1.8 litres!

Arterial blood gases

Arterial blood gases (ABGs) provide an accurate measure of oxygen uptake and carbon dioxide removal by the respiratory system as a whole. The arterial blood is usually sampled from the radial artery at the wrist, but arterialized capillary samples may be taken from the earlobe. Arterial blood gases are best used as a measure of steady-state gas exchange; thus it is imperative that the patient is resting quietly with a constant inspired oxygen level (FiO_2) and mode of ventilation for at least 30 minutes before sampling. When analysing the results, consideration must be given to all these factors. Normal values for arterial blood gases are given in Box 1.4.

Thoracic imaging

Chest radiographs and other imaging techniques (Chapter 2) are an important aid to physical examination as they provide a clear picture of the extent and severity of disease at that time. In some instances, chest radiographs or computed tomography (CT) may show more extensive disease than expected, while in others they may underestimate the pathology present. Comparison with previous images provides an excellent measure of improvement or deterioration over time, and an objective assessment of the response to treatment. It should be noted that chest radiograph may sometimes lag 1–2 days behind the clinical findings.

Electrocardiogram and echocardiograms

The electrocardiogram (ECG) and echocardiogram provide important information regarding cardiac electrical and mechanical function. An understanding of these is essential as abnormalities may alter the treatment plan. More detailed information about their measurement and implications are covered in Chapter 3.

PROBLEM LIST

The second part of the problem-oriented medical record (POMR) is the problem list (see Fig. 1.1). The information in the database, together with the subjective and objective assessment, are analysed as a whole, and integrated with the physiotherapist's knowledge of disease processes.

The problem list is then compiled. It consists of a simple, functional and specific list of the patient's problems at that time, not always listed in order of priority. Each problem is numbered and dated at the time of assessment. The problem list should not only include those problems amenable to physiotherapy (e.g. breathlessness on exertion) but should also include other problems for consideration when designing and implementing a treatment plan (e.g. anaemia). The problem list should not be a list of signs and symptoms, as this would provide the wrong emphasis for treatment. In the past, disease-based treatment tended to result in standardized treatment, ignoring the patient's individual problems. This meant that all chronic airflow limitation patients were given treatment for impaired airway clearance. All intubated patients also received standard treatment, irrespective of the presence or absence of excess secretions and the patient's ability to clear them. The best system is one that is individualized to each patient.

Problems once resolved should be signed off and dated. Any subsequent problems are added and dated appropriately.

INITIAL PLANS

For each of the physiotherapy problems listed, long- and short-term goals are formulated. These should be Specific, Measurable, Achievable, Realistic and Timed (SMART). Prioritizing the problem list and developing the goals for each problem should be performed, where possible, in consultation with the patient. The importance of involving the patient himself cannot be overstressed, as cooperation is fundamental to nearly all physiotherapy treatment. The patient assessment will have identified important factors that must be considered when developing a plan and goals. Such factors may include coexisting conditions or disease (e.g. diabetes mellitus) or other factors such as age, motivation, cultural or social factors.

Box 1.4 Normal values for arterial blood gases	
pH	7.35–7.45
PaO_2	10.7–13.3 kPa (80–100 mmHg)
$PaCO_2$	4.7–6.0 kPa (35–45 mmHg)
HCO_3^-	22–26 mmol/l
Base excess	−2 to +2

1

Long-term goals are generally directed at returning the patient to his maximum functional capacity. Specifically, goals may be simplified to functions that are important to the patient, e.g. to be able to walk home from the shops carrying one bag of shopping. When setting goals for an inpatient, consideration must be given to his discharge. If the home situation includes two flights of stairs to the bedroom then the goal of exercise ability should reflect this. If physiotherapy is to be continued at home after discharge, one of the goals must be to teach the patient or a relative how to perform the treatment effectively.

Short-term goals are the steps taken to achieve the long-term goals. In general these are small, simple activities that are more easily achieved. All goals, both short- and long-term, should state expected outcomes and time frames. The goals, especially the short-term goals, should be reviewed regularly as some patients may improve faster than others. If goals are not met within the agreed time frame, then revision is necessary. The time frame may have been too short, the goal inappropriate, or other problems need attention before this goal can be met.

The treatment plan includes the specifics of treatment, together with its frequency and equipment requirements. Patient education must not be omitted from the treatment plan, as it is an important component of physiotherapy.

A summary, as a reminder of the key points of assessment, is given in Box 1.5.

Box 1.5   Key points of assessment

Database
- Medical records

Subjective assessment
- Breathlessness, cough, sputum, wheeze, chest pain
- Duration, severity, pattern, associations
- Functional ability, disease awareness

Objective assessment
- General observation from end of bed
- Chest – observation, palpation, percussion, auscultation
- Sputum
- Physiotherapy techniques, exercise capacity

Test results
- Spirometry
- Arterial blood gases
- Thoracic imaging

Problem list → Treatment plan

PROGRESS NOTES

These are written on a daily basis using the 'subjective, objective, analysis, plan' (SOAP) format:

- **S**ubjective – what the patient, doctors or nurses report
- **O**bjective – any change in physical examination or test, e.g. auscultation, chest radiograph
- **A**nalysis – the physiotherapist's professional opinion of the subjective and objective findings
- **P**lan – including changes in treatment and any further action.

Entries should be made for each physiotherapy problem, signed and dated. If there have been no changes, nothing further needs to be written.

Progress notes may also include a graph or flow chart. Graphs are particularly useful in displaying the change in a parameter with time, for example an asthmatic's peak expiratory flow rates. Flow chart displays are useful if multiple factors are changing over a period of time, as may occur in the intensive care patient.

Outcomes

The short- and long-term goals provide a basis for evaluating the effectiveness of treatment for each problem. One of the best indicators of outcome is the change in objective findings after treatment. Although changes that occur immediately after a single treatment are related to physiotherapy intervention alone, changes over longer periods of time reflect treatment by the entire health team. Chest auscultation before and after a treatment may provide a simple indication of the effectiveness of that treatment. Similarly, the chest radiograph can demonstrate the effectiveness of physiotherapy treatment by showing diminution in the area of collapsed/consolidated lung. On a long-term basis, changes in lung function or exercise tolerance provide the most valuable measures of treatment outcome. If there are discrepancies between the actual and expected outcomes, the plan (P) documents the changes to the goals and/or treatment, as required.

The selection and use of appropriate outcome measures is fundamental to the evaluation of any therapy. Demonstrating the effects of physiotherapy intervention, using instruments that have high reliability and validity, is increasingly being required by healthcare providers and physiotherapists themselves. Other people who may require outcome data include the patient, caregivers, community and patient support groups.

To standardize the measurement of outcomes, the World Health Organization (WHO) has developed a scale of functioning and disability, the International Classification of Functioning, Disability and Health (ICIDH-2) (WHO 2001). This scale focuses on human functioning at the level of body, the whole person and the person within the social/environmental context. It classifies functioning of the affected body part, and the whole person in terms of impairment to bodily function and structure, limitation of activity and restriction to participation. It is designed to measure the effectiveness of an intervention using a patient-focused measure rather than the more traditional medical focus. For example, a patient with bronchiectasis who has had three admissions to hospital for chest infections over the last year is taught an airway clearance technique to assist sputum clearance. Over the next 12 months the outcome measure important to the patient is the ability to maintain a full-time job; while the outcome measure important to the Area Health Service is the cost saving achieved by a reduction in hospital admissions. Thus when selecting an outcome measure it is important to take into account for whom the data is needed.

DISCHARGE SUMMARY

Upon discharge or transfer elsewhere, a summary should be written of the patient's initial problems, treatment and outcomes. Instruction for home programmes and any other relevant information should also be included. Discharge summaries are helpful to other physiotherapists who may treat the patient in the future. The summary should always contain adequate information for future audit and studies of patient care.

AUDIT

'Audit' refers to the systematic and critical analysis of the quality of care. There are three main forms of audit: structure, process and outcome.

1. *Structural audit* examines the organization of resources within a certain area. This may address the availability of human and/or equipment resources, e.g. a hospital's requirements for transcutaneous electrical nerve stimulation (TENS) machines, batteries and electrodes.
2. *Process audit* investigates the system of delivery of care, e.g. studying the methods of patient referral.
3. *Outcome audit* is the most clinically based audit. It examines the results of physiotherapy care, e.g. assessing whether the goals of treatment have been met within the stated time frames.

The audit process is cyclical. Firstly, a standard of care is defined. The actual practice is then audited in comparison with the agreed standard. Discrepancies provoke further discussion. Changes are then made to eliminate these discrepancies. After an appropriate length of time the cycle begins again.

EDUCATIONAL PROGRAMME

By using a structured system of problem-oriented medical records and audit, the problem-oriented medical system allows identification of areas where goals are not being met within an appropriate time frame. Audit may also reveal situations where the agreed standards are not met. In both instances staff education programmes will improve patient care.

CONCLUSION

Accurate assessment should reveal the exact nature of the patient's problems and identify those amenable to physiotherapy. Only then can the best treatment be chosen for that patient. Subsequent reassessment is essential to ensure that treatment is specific, effective and efficient. This process ensures high-quality patient care.

References

Aaronson NK 1989 Quality of life assessment in clinical trials: methodological issues. Controlled Clinical Trials 10: 195S–208S

Borg GA. 1982 Psychophysical bases of perceived exertion. Medicine and Science in Sports and Exercise 14(5): 377–381

Bradley J, Howard J, Wallace E et al 1999 Validity of a modified shuttle test in adult cystic fibrosis. Thorax 54: 437–439

Butland RJA, Pang J, Gross ER et al 1982 Two-, six-, and 12-minute walking tests in respiratory disease. British Medical Journal 284: 1607–1608

Criteria Committee of the New York Heart Association 1994 Nomenclature and criteria for diagnosis of diseases of the heart and great vessels (www. americanheart.org/presenter.jhtml? identifier=1712) (Accessed 25 July 2007)

Ellis E 1985 Making a teaching stethoscope. Australian Journal of Physiotherapy 31: 244

Juniper EF, Guyatt GH, Cox FM et al 1999 Development and validation of the mini asthma quality of life questionnaire. European Respiratory Journal 14(1): 32–38

Kinney MR, Burfitt SN, Stullenbarger E et al 1996 Quality of life in cardiac

patient research: a meta-analysis. Nursing Research 45(3): 173–180

Mahler DA 2000 How should health-related quality of life be assessed in patients with COPD? Chest 117(2) Suppl: 54S–57S

Manthous CA, Hall JB, Olson D et al 1995 Effect of cooling on oxygen consumption in febrile critically ill patients. American Journal of Respiratory and Critical Care Medicine 151: 10–14

Miller D L 1963 A study of techniques for the examination of sputum in a field survey of chronic bronchitis.

1

American Review of Respiratory Disease 88: 473–483

Orr A, McVean RJ, Webb AK et al 2001 Urinary incontinence in women with cystic firosis is a marginalized and undertreated problem: questionnaire survey. British Medical Journal 322: 1521

Pashkow P, Ades PA, Emery CF et al 1995 Outcome measurement in cardiac and pulmonary rehabilitation. Journal of Cardiopulmonary Rehabilitation 15(6): 394–405

Revill SM, Morgan MDL, Singh SJ et al 1999 The endurance shuttle walk: a new field test for the assessment of endurance capacity in chronic

obstructive pulmonary disease. Thorax 54: 213–222

Rubinstein I, Zamel N, DuBarry L et al 1990 Airflow limitation in morbidly obese, non-smoking men. Annals of Internal Medicine 112(11): 828–832

Scottish Intercollegiate Guidelines Network 2004 Management of urinary incontinence in primary care (*www.sign.ac.uk*)

Singh SJ, Morgan MDL, Scott S et al 1992 The development of the shuttle walking test of disability in patients with chronic airways obstruction. Thorax 47(12): 1019–1024

Teasdale G, Jennett B 1974 Assessment of coma and impaired consciousness.

A practical scale. Lancet 2(7872): 81–84

Thakar R, Stanton S 2000 Management of urinary incontinence in women. British Medical Journal 321: 1326–1331

Ware JE, Sherbourne CD 1992 The MOS-short-form health survey (SF-36). Medical Care 30:473–483

Weed LL 1968 Medical records that guide and teach. New England Journal of Medicine 278: 593–600, 652–657

World Health Organization 2001 International Classification of Functioning, Disability and Health (*www.who.int/icidh*)

Chapter 2

Thoracic imaging

Adults
Susan J Copley, Conor D Collins,
David M Hansell

Paediatrics
Christopher D George

ADULTS

CHEST RADIOGRAPHY AND OTHER TECHNIQUES

Different types of chest radiograph

Chest radiography has been used as the main radiological investigation of the chest since the discovery of X-rays by Röentgen in 1895 and chest radiographs constitute 25–40% of all radiological investigations.

Chest radiographs are indicated in almost any condition in which a pulmonary abnormality is suspected.

The majority of chest radiographs are obtained in the main radiology department. The radiograph is obtained with the patient standing erect. Patients who are immobile or too ill to come to the main department have a chest radiograph performed using a mobile machine (portable film); the resulting radiograph differs from a departmental film in terms of projection, positioning, exposure and film used and is therefore not strictly comparable with a conventional posteroanterior (PA) film. Other types of chest radiograph are the lateral, lordotic,

[1]Images reproduced with permission of Nelson Thornes Ltd from Paediatric Respiratory Care, ISBN 0 1425 5000 8 first published 1995.

2

apical and decubitus views; these are generally taken in the main department.

Departmental films are referred to as 'posteroanterior' (or PA) chest radiographs and describe the direction in which the X-ray beam traverses the patient. The patient is positioned with his anterior chest wall against the film cassette and his back to the X-ray tube. The arms are abducted to rotate the scapulae away from the posterior chest and the radiograph is taken during full inspiration. The tube is centred at the spinous process of the fourth thoracic vertebra. For portable films taken in an anteroposterior (AP) projection, the patient's back is against the film cassette and the X-ray tube is positioned at a variable distance from the patient. As the heart is placed anteriorly within the chest, it is further from the cassette and is therefore magnified in an AP radiograph. The degree of magnification depends on the distance between the patient and the X-ray tube.

For a lateral radiograph the patient is turned 90° and the side of interest placed against the film cassette. The arms are extended forwards and the radiograph is again taken in full inspiration.

Lateral decubitus views are sometimes useful for the demonstration of small pleural effusions. For this projection the patient lies horizontally with the side in question placed downwards. The film cassette is positioned at the back of the patient and the X-ray beam is horizontal centred at the midsternum. This provides a sensitive means of detecting small quantities of pleural fluid (50–100 ml) that cannot be identified on a frontal chest radiograph. However, ultrasonography is usually used as a reliable means of confirming the presence of small pleural effusions.

Lordotic films are sometimes used to confirm middle lobe collapse and for demonstrating a questionable apical opacity otherwise obscured by the clavicle and ribs. For this AP projection, the patient arches back so that the shoulders are touching the cassette with the centring point remaining the same. Linear tomography is another technique designed to reveal lesions otherwise hidden by the skeleton by blurring out everything overlying and underlying the lesion in question. This is achieved by having the X-ray tube and film cassette move at the same time but in opposite directions. These two techniques are less frequently used with the advent of computed tomography (CT).

Factors influencing the quality of a chest radiograph

The quality and thus diagnostic usefulness of a chest radiograph depend critically on the conditions under which it is obtained. Of particular importance are the radiographic exposure, the projection, the orientation of

the patient relative to the film cassette, the X-ray tube to film distance, the depth of inspiration of the patient and the type of film–screen combination used.

The ideal chest radiograph provides an image of structures within the chest while exposing the patient to the lowest possible dose of radiation. Most radiology departments have a policy of obtaining either high-kilovoltage (kVp) or low-kilovoltage chest radiographs. Radiographs performed at high kilovoltage (e.g. 140 kVp) have much to recommend them. Even at total lung capacity with the patient erect, nearly a third of the lungs is partially obscured by the mediastinal structures, diaphragm and ribs. With the low-kilovoltage technique (80 kVp or less) these areas are often poorly visualized. This problem is partially overcome by using films exposed at high kilovoltage. The normal vessel markings and subtle differences in soft tissue densities are better demonstrated and a further advantage is the better penetration of the mediastinum, which improves visualization of the trachea and main bronchi. The disadvantage of high-kilovoltage radiographs is the relatively poor demonstration of calcified structures so that rib fractures and calcified pulmonary nodules or pleural plaques are less conspicuous.

During exposure the X-ray beam is modified according to the structures through which it passes. The photons that have passed through the patient carry information which then must be converted into a visual form. Some of the photons emerging from the patient are aligned in a virtually parallel direction and other photons are scattered. These scattered photons degrade the final image but can be absorbed by using lead strips embedded in an aluminium sheet positioned in front of the cassette. This device is known as a grid. Photons that are travelling in parallel pass through the grid to form the image on the film.

The sensitivity of film to direct X-ray exposure is very low and if film were used alone as the image receptor, this would result in a prohibitively large X-ray dose to the patient. Intensifying screens made of phosphorescent material are positioned on the inside of the cassettes and they convert the incident X-ray photons into visible light, which is recorded by the adjacent film. These phosphor screens are composed of either calcium tungstate or a rare-earth-containing compound. Rare-earth phosphors emit more light in response to X-ray photons and therefore less radiation is necessary to produce the image. Similarly, improvements in the quality of X-ray film have also occurred over the years. Standard film emulsions tend to lack detail in the relatively under- or overexposed areas of the radiograph and newer emulsions have been developed so that detail is similar in all areas of the chest radiograph. The choice of film–screen combination has a crucial influence on the

2

quality and 'look' of the radiograph produced. Further variations may result from film-processing problems.

In the intensive care setting, portable chest radiographs are often taken in less than ideal conditions. Multiple tubes, lines and dressings in conjunction with an immobile, supine patient and the use of a mobile low-kilovoltage machine often result in suboptimal radiographs. One approach to this is the development of phosphor plate technology, which is ultimately expected to replace conventional film–screen radiography. The phosphor plate is placed inside a conventional cassette and stores some of the energy of the incident X-ray photons as a latent image (the image produced on a film or phosphor plate before development). The plate is scanned with a laser beam and the light emitted from the 'excited' latent image is detected by a photomultiplier. Thereafter this signal is processed in digital form. This digital image may be viewed either on a television monitor or on film (on which it has been laser printed). The great advantage of this system is that it can retrieve an image of diagnostic quality from a suboptimal exposure. Similar gross over- or underexposure would result in a non-diagnostic conventional radiograph. Manipulation of the digital image, particularly 'edge enhancement', aids the detection of linear structures such as the edge of a pneumothorax or central venous catheters (Fig. 2.1). With the advent of picture archiving and communication systems (PACS), which enable storage and transfer of digital images, many radiology departments are now 'filmless', with images available to view simultaneously on monitors throughout the hospital.

Other techniques

Fluoroscopy

The patient is positioned, either standing or lying, in a screening unit allowing 'real-time' visualization of the area in question on a television monitor. The patient can be turned in any direction and this technique can help to distinguish pulmonary from extrapulmonary opacities. One of the main uses of fluoroscopy is to 'screen' the diaphragm to demonstrate paralysis or abnormal movement. It is also useful in needle placement during biopsy of lung masses.

Ultrasonography

High-frequency sound waves do not traverse air and the use of this technique is therefore limited in the chest. It is mainly used for cardiac imaging (echocardiography) and has become an essential technique in the investigation of patients with valvular and ventricular function problems. Outside the heart, ultrasonography is very useful in distinguishing between fluid above the diaphragm (pleural effusion, Fig. 2.2), fluid below the

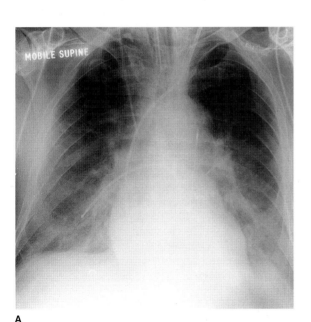

A

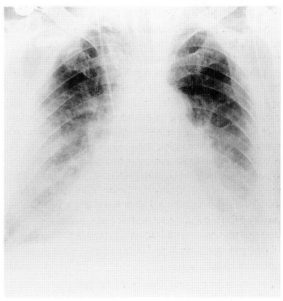

B

Figure 2.1 The same anteroposterior (AP) digital chest radiograph of a patient on the intensive care unit imaged on different settings. This technique has the advantage that the image can be made (**A**) darker or (**B**) lighter after it has been taken to allow better visualization of lines and tubes or lung parenchyma. Note the patient's endotracheal tube, right internal jugular central line, pulmonary artery catheter and intra-aortic balloon pump.

2

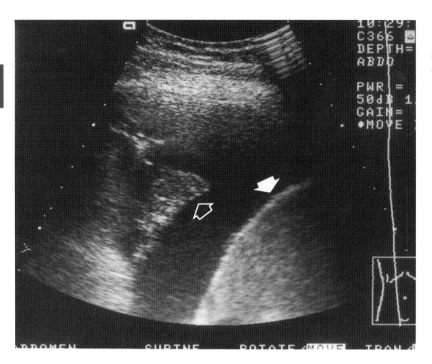

Figure 2.2 Ultrasound of lower right hemithorax/upper abdomen demonstrating a right basal effusion with fluid interposed between collapsed right lower lobe (open arrow) and diaphragm (closed arrow).

diaphragm (subphrenic) and pleural thickening. Chest radiography often cannot differentiate between pleural fluid and thickening with any certainty. Ultrasound can also be used to guide the placement of a percutaneous drain into a pleural effusion or biopsy peripheral lung lesions that are in contact with the pleura.

Computed tomography

Computed tomography (CT) scanning depends on the same basic physical principle as conventional radiography, namely the absorption of X-rays by tissues of different densities. The basic components of a CT machine are a table on which the patient lies and a gantry through which the table slides. An X-ray tube and a series of detectors are housed within the gantry. The X-ray tube and detectors rotate around the patient. A computer is used to reconstruct the signals received by the detectors into an image. The images acquired are transverse (axial) cross-sections of the patient. In orienting the patient's right and left sides, it is the convention to view all CT images as if from the patient's feet.

Because of the cross-sectional nature of CT, it can accurately localize lesions seen on only one view on plain chest radiographs. The superior contrast resolution of CT allows superb demonstration of mediastinal anatomy (e.g. lymph nodes and vessels) (Fig. 2.3) as well as calcification within a pulmonary nodule. Highly detailed thin sections of the lung parenchyma can also

be obtained, allowing the complex morphology of many interstitial lung diseases to be more accurately defined. The disadvantages of CT are its relatively high cost and increased radiation exposure to the patient compared with chest radiography.

Whereas conventional CT scanning involves alternating table movement through the gantry with exposure, helical or volumetric CT involves simultaneous table movement and X-ray exposure. The technique allows faster scan times and advantages are the elimination of respiratory artefacts, minimization of motion artefacts and production of overlapping images without additional radiation exposure. Helical (spiral) CT is so named because the X-ray can be thought of as tracing a helix or spiral curve on the patient's surface. Multiple rows of detectors are used in the newer helical CTs, so-called multidetector CT (MDCT). The technique allows viewing of images in multiple planes (Fig. 2.4) and, due to the very fast acquisition times, is increasingly used to evaluate cardiac structures such as the coronary arteries. Helical CT is also now commonly used to demonstrate pulmonary emboli, as accurate timing of a bolus of intravenous contrast allows optimal enhancement of the pulmonary arteries (Fig. 2.5).

Common indications for CT of the chest

1. CT scanning is used to further evaluate hilar or mediastinal masses seen or suspected on a chest radiograph.

2

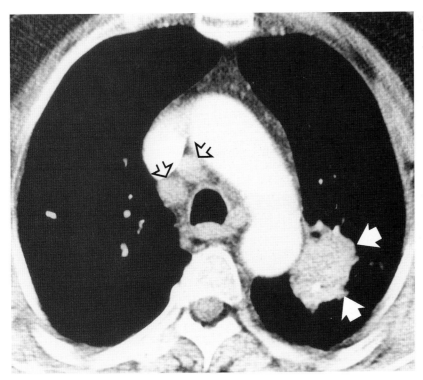

Figure 2.3 Computed tomography (CT) image post-intravenous contrast showing a lung tumour adjacent to the arch of the aorta (closed arrows). Lymph nodes are seen anterior to the trachea (open arrows), which were not visible on chest radiography.

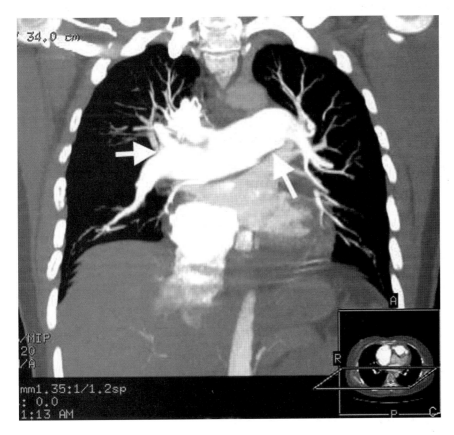

Figure 2.4 Example of coronal reconstruction of multidetector helical CT (MDCT) in a patient with primary pulmonary hypertension. Note the enlarged central pulmonary arteries (arrows).

2

2. Within the lungs it can be used to further define the nature of a mass or cavitating lesion not clearly seen on the plain film.
3. In patients with normal chest radiographs but abnormal pulmonary function tests, thin high-resolution computed tomography (HRCT) sections of the lung may provide the first radiological evidence of parenchymal disease. This type of scanning is also very useful for assessing patients with suspected bronchiectasis.
4. CT is useful in patients with neoplasms, in assessing both their operability and their response to treatment.
5. Detection of pulmonary embolism (spiral CT).
6. For guiding the percutaneous needle biopsy of lung lesions, mediastinal masses or chest wall abnormalities.

Magnetic resonance imaging

The physical principles of magnetic resonance imaging (MRI) are more complex and very different from those of CT scanning. The equipment consists of a sliding table on which the patient lies within the bore of a large magnet. A combination of the intense magnetic field and a series of radiofrequency waves produces an alteration in the alignment of protons (mostly in water) resulting in the emission of different signals which are detected and subsequently analysed for their intensity and position by a computer. The major advantages of MRI are that images may be obtained in any plane without the use of ionizing radiation. The disadvantages are its inability to produce detailed images of the lung, cost and reduced acceptability to patients because of the claustrophobic bore of the magnet. There are also important contraindications such as permanent cardiac pacemaker devices. Its application to chest imaging is limited at present but the technique is good for imaging chest wall lesions, the great vessels (Fig. 2.6) and the heart.

Radionuclide imaging

Ventilation–perfusion $(\dot{V}/\dot{Q})$ scanning is the commonest radionuclide study of the lungs. It is primarily used to investigate suspected pulmonary embolus. Perfusion is assessed by intravenous injection of minute particles labelled with technetium-99m, a radioactive tracer. These particles become temporarily lodged in a very small proportion of capillaries within the lung and the emitted radiation is detected by a so-called gamma camera. Ventilation is assessed by the inhalation of inert gases that have also been labelled with a radioactive tracer. The ventilation and perfusion images are then compared to see if there are any areas of mismatch (Fig. 2.7). Increasingly CT is used to investigate patients with

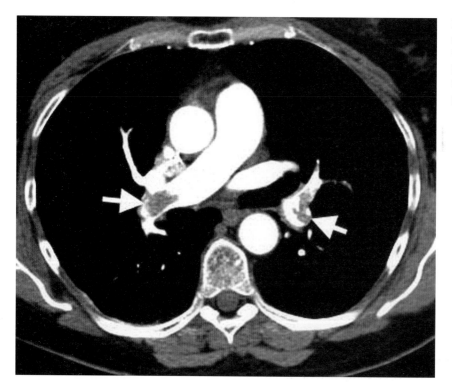

Figure 2.5 A CT pulmonary angiogram, showing bilateral filling defects of the pulmonary arteries (arrows) consistent with bilateral pulmonary emboli.

2

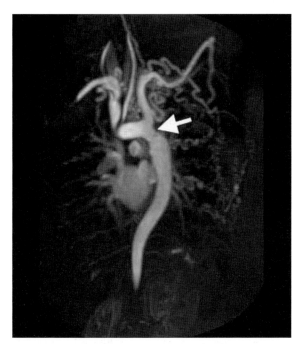

Figure 2.6 Magnetic resonance image (MRI) of the thorax. The image shows a MR angiogram (MRA) of a coarctation of the aorta (arrow). Note the extensive arterial collaterals.

possible pulmonary embolus, as $\dot{V}/\dot{Q}$ scanning is more difficult to interpret in patients with coexisting lung disease such as asthma. In addition, the tracers have a short period of radioactivity after they are produced of a few hours and therefore scanning late at night and at weekends may be difficult.

Positron emission tomography

Positron emission tomography (PET) is also a form of radionuclide imaging. A detector can pinpoint where there is uptake of tracer accurately within the body. PET highlights areas that are very metabolically active, such as cancers, but also infection and inflammation. Access to this type of costly scanner is becoming more widespread, and it is mainly used in the chest for assessment of disease spread of lung cancer to lymph nodes and sites outside the chest (Fig. 2.8). The images may be fused with CT images (PET/CT) to give a very precise location of tumour spread.

Interventional procedures

Percutaneous needle biopsy

Percutaneous needle biopsy of a pulmonary or mediastinal mass to provide a histological specimen is usually performed in patients in whom a bronchoscopic biopsy

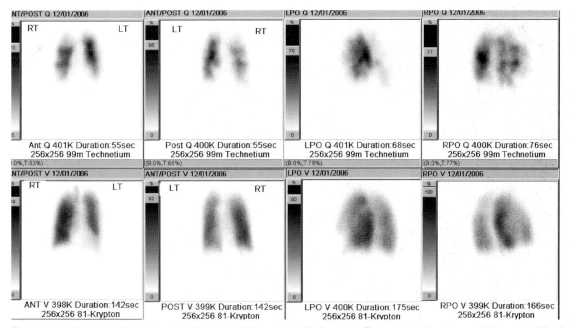

Figure 2.7 Example of a radionuclide lung ventilation and perfusion scan. The examination shows a high probability for multiple bilateral pulmonary emboli as there are multiple perfusion abnormalities (top row of images) with no matched ventilation defects (bottom row of images), so-called 'mismatched' defects.

2

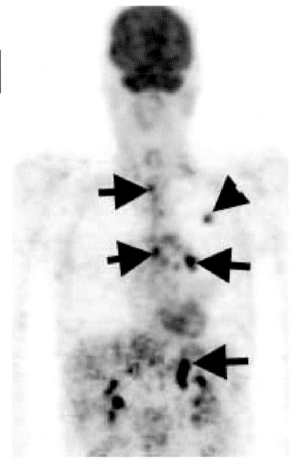

Figure 2.8 A PET scan showing metastatic spread of a lung cancer in the left lung (arrowhead) to hilar and mediastinal lymph nodes and the left adrenal (arrows). Note the normal increased metabolic activity in the brain, heart and gut.

has failed or a thoracotomy is inappropriate. Different types of needle are used and the complication rate (pneumothorax and haemoptysis) bears some relation to the site of the lesion, the size of the needle and the number of attempts to obtain tissue. Contraindications to the procedure include any patient with poor respiratory reserve unable to withstand a pneumothorax, pulmonary arterial hypertension and a previous contralateral pneumonectomy.

Pulmonary and bronchial arteriography, superior vena cavography

Pulmonary arteriography. This is usually undertaken in the investigation of suspected pulmonary arteriovenous malformations and, less commonly since the development of helical (spiral) CT, pulmonary embolism. It

requires puncture of either the femoral vein in the groin or the antecubital vein in the elbow and the guiding of a catheter through the right side of the heart under fluoroscopy. The tip of the catheter is positioned in the main pulmonary artery or selectively placed in a smaller pulmonary artery. Contrast is then injected. It is currently the most appropriate technique for the demonstration of pulmonary arteriovenous malformations. These can be treated at the time of the arteriogram by the injection of occlusive materials (embolization).

Bronchial arteriography. Demonstration of the bronchial arteries requires catheterization of the femoral artery and passage of a catheter into the midthoracic aorta from where the bronchial arteries are selectively catheterized. The major indication for this procedure is recurrent or life-threatening haemoptysis in patients with a chronic inflammatory disease, usually bronchiectasis. Accurate placement of the catheter not only allows demonstration of the bleeding vessel but also allows embolization to be performed simultaneously.

Superior vena cavography. This is performed for the evaluation of superior vena caval (SVC) obstruction and the investigation of anatomical variants. More recently, patients with SVC compression due to tumour have been palliated by the insertion of an expandable metallic mesh wire stent at the site of the SVC narrowing, thus restoring flow and relieving symptoms.

THE NORMAL CHEST

Anatomy

On the normal posteroanterior radiograph (Fig. 2.9) the following structures can be identified:

- outline of the mediastinum and heart
- the hila
- pulmonary vessels and main bronchi
- diaphragm
- soft tissues and bones of the thoracic cage.

The heart and mediastinum

The mediastinum consists of the organs and soft tissues in the central part of the chest. These comprise the trachea, aortic arch and great vessels, superior vena cava and oesophagus. In children the thymus gland is a prominent component. On the two-dimensional chest radiograph these structures are superimposed and cannot be clearly distinguished from each other. The mediastinum is conventionally divided into superior, anterior, middle and posterior compartments. While the boundaries of the latter three are arbitrary, it is usual to divide the mediastinum into equal thirds. The superior

2

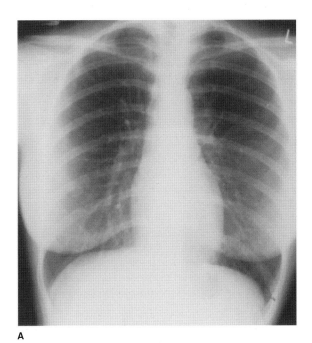

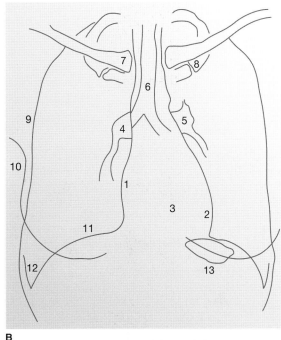

A   B

Figure 2.9 (A) Normal posteroanterior (PA) chest radiograph. (B) Normal structures visible on a PA chest radiograph: 1 right atrium; 2 left ventricle; 3 right ventricle; 4 right pulmonary artery; 5 left pulmonary artery; 6 air within trachea; 7 clavicle; 8 first rib; 9 lateral border of hemithorax; 10 breast shadow; 11 right hemidiaphragm; 12 costophrenic angle; 13 gastric air bubble.

mediastinum is that portion lying above the aortic arch and below the root of the neck.

The mediastinal border on the right is formed superiorly by the right brachiocephalic vein and superior vena cava. The mediastinal shadow to the left of the trachea above the aortic arch comprises the left carotid and left subclavian arteries together with the left brachiocephalic and jugular veins. On a correctly exposed chest radiograph, air in the trachea can be seen throughout its length as it descends downwards, deviating slightly to the right above the carina (where the trachea divides into the right and left main bronchi) due to displacement by the aortic arch.

The heart lies eccentrically in the chest, with one-third of the cardiac shadow to the right of the spine and two-thirds to the left. The density of the cardiac shadow on the left and right of the spine should be identical. The right cardiac border on a chest radiograph is formed by the right atrium. The left cardiac border is composed of the apex of the left ventricle and superiorly the left atrial appendage. The outline of the right ventricle, which is superimposed on the left ventricle, cannot be identified on a frontal radiograph. The maximum transverse diameter of the heart should be less than half the maximum transverse diameter of the thorax, as mea-sured from the inside border of the ribs (the so-called 'cardiothoracic ratio').

The hila

Hilar shadows are a complex summation of the pulmonary arteries and veins with minor contributions from other components (the main bronchi and lymph nodes). In general, the hila are of equal density and are approximately the same size. Adjacent to the left hilum, the main pulmonary artery forms a localized bulge just above the left atrial appendage and just below the aortic arch. The area between the aortic arch and the main pulmonary artery is known as the 'aortopulmonary window'.

The superior pulmonary veins run vertically and converge on the upper and mid-hilum on both sides. It is not possible to distinguish arteries from veins in the outer two-thirds of the lungs. The inferior pulmonary veins run obliquely in a near-horizontal plane below the lower lobe arteries to enter the left atrium beneath the carina. The hilar point is where the superior pulmonary vein on each side crosses the basal artery. This is more easily assessed on the right than on the left. Using this as an index point, the left hilum is normally 0.5–1.5 cm higher than the right one.

2

Abnormalities of the hilar shadows in the form of increased density or abnormal configuration are usually the result of lymph node or pulmonary artery enlargement. The detection of subtle hilar abnormalities is difficult and requires experience and knowledge of the many outlines that the hila may assume in normal individuals.

Fissures, vessels and segmental bronchi within the lungs

Each lung is divided into lobes surrounded by visceral pleura. There are two lobes on the left (the upper and lower, separated by the major (oblique) fissure) and three on the right (the upper, middle and lower lobes which are separated by the major (oblique) and minor (horizontal or transverse) fissures). In the majority of normal subjects some or all of the minor fissure is seen on a frontal radiograph. The major fissures are only identifiable on the lateral projection. Each lobe of the lung contains a number of segments, which have their own segmental bronchi. The walls of the segmental bronchi are invisible on the chest radiograph, except when seen end-on as ring shadows measuring up to 7 mm in diameter.

The pulmonary blood vessels are responsible for the branching and linear structures within the lungs. The diameter of the blood vessels beyond the hilum varies with the position of the patient and with haemodynamic factors. In the erect position there is a gradual increase in the diameter of the vessels, travelling from apex to base. This increase in size is seen in both the arteries and veins and is abolished if the patient lies supine.

The diaphragm

The interface between the lung and diaphragm should be sharp and, in general, the diaphragm is dome shaped with its highest point medial to the midclavicular line. The margin of the right hemidiaphragm at its highest point lies between the anterior ends of the fifth and seventh ribs. The right hemidiaphragm is usually higher than the left by up to 2 cm in the erect position. Laterally, the diaphragm dips downwards, forming a sharp angle with the chest wall known as the 'costophrenic angle'. Filling in or blunting of these angles reflects pleural disease, either fluid or thickening.

Thoracic cage

On a high-kilovoltage chest radiograph it should be possible to identify the edges of the vertebral bodies of the dorsal spine through the heart shadow. However, a high-kilovoltage radiograph may 'burn out' the ribs, particularly the posterior portions. Because of this the chest radiograph may be an insensitive means of demonstrating rib abnormalities, particularly fractures.

Common anatomical variants

The trachea lies centrally, but in the elderly may deviate markedly to the right in its lower portion due to unfolding and dilatation of the aortic arch. A small ovoid soft tissue shadow just above the origin of the right main bronchus represents the azygos vein. This may be enlarged as a result of posture (supine position) or haemodynamic factors. It may be indistinguishable from an azygos lymph node.

Occasionally, extra fissures are seen in the lungs. The most common of these is the azygos lobe fissure; this is seen as a fine white line running obliquely from the apex of the right lung to the azygos vein. Other accessory fissures are the superior and inferior accessory fissures, both of which are in the right lower lobe.

The surfaces of the two lungs abut each other anteriorly and posteriorly and give rise to two white lines projected over the vertebral column, known as the 'anterior and posterior junction lines', respectively. Both of these may be seen overlying the trachea – the anterior line extending from the clavicles to the left main bronchus and the posterior line lying more medially and extending above the clavicles. The azygo-oesophageal recess line is a curved line projected over the vertebral column and extending from the azygos vein to the diaphragm. It represents the interface between the right lung and right oesophageal wall.

A small 'nipple' may occasionally be seen projecting laterally from the aortic knuckle due to the left superior intercostal vein. The term 'paraspinal line' refers to the line that parallels the left and right margin of the thoracic spine. The left is thicker than the right because of the adjacent aorta.

The lateral view

It is conventional to read the lateral film (Fig. 2.10) with the heart to the viewer's left and the dorsal spine to the right, irrespective of whether the film is labelled 'right' or 'left'. The chamber of the heart that touches the sternum is the right ventricle. Behind and above the heart lies lung, the density of which should be the same both behind the heart and behind the sternum. As the eye travels down the spine, the vertebral column should appear increasingly transradiant or 'dark' (Fig. 2.10A); the loss of this phenomenon suggests the presence of disease in the posterobasal segments of the lower lobes. In the middle of the lateral film lie the hilar structures with the main pulmonary artery anteriorly. The aortic arch should be easily identified but only a variable proportion of the great vessels is visible depending on the degree of aortic unfolding. The brachiocephalic artery is most frequently identified arising anterior to the tracheal air column. The left and right brachiocephalic

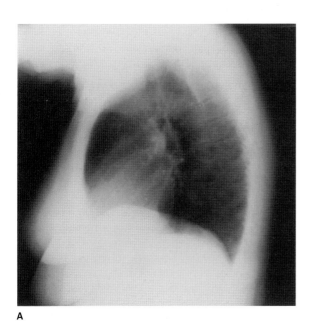

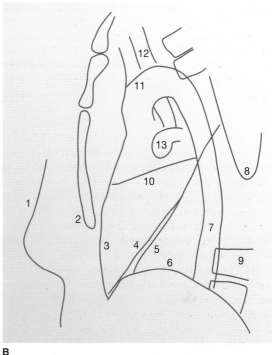

A   B

Figure 2.10   (A) Normal lateral chest radiograph. (B) Normal structures visible on a lateral chest radiograph: 1 breast shadow; 2 sternum; 3 position of right ventricle; 4 right oblique fissure; 5 left oblique fissure; 6 hemidiaphragm; 7 descending aorta; 8 inferior angle of scapula; 9 dorsal vertebrae; 10 horizontal fissure; 11 aortic arch; 12 trachea; 13 pulmonary artery.

veins form an extrapleural bulge behind the upper sternum in about a third of individuals.

The course of the trachea is straight with a slight posterior angulation but no visible indentation from adjacent vessels. The carina is not seen on the lateral view. The posterior wall of the trachea is always visible and is known as the 'posterior tracheal stripe'.

The oblique fissures are seen as fine diagonal lines running from the upper dorsal spine to the diaphragm anteriorly. The left is more vertically oriented and is visible just behind the right. The minor fissure extends forwards horizontally from the mid-right oblique fissure. Care must be taken not to confuse rib margins with fissure lines. As the fissures undulate, two distinct fissure lines may be generated by a single fissure. The fissures should be of no more than hairline width.

The scapulae are invariably seen in the lateral view and since they are incompletely visualized, lines formed by the edge of the scapula can easily be confused with intrathoracic structures. The arms are held outstretched in front of the patient on a lateral view and these give rise to soft tissue shadows projected over the anterior and superior mediastinum. A band-like opacity simulating pleural disease is often seen along the lower half of the anterior chest wall immediately behind the sternum. The left lung does not contact the most ante-

rior portion of the left thoracic cavity at these levels because the heart occupies the space. This band-like opacity is known as the 'retrosternal line'.

Useful points in interpreting a chest radiograph

Documentary information.   The name of the patient and the time and date on which the radiograph was taken, particularly in relation to other films in a series, should all be noted. Often the film is annotated with the patient's date of birth. Of particular importance is the presence of the side markers ('right' or 'left'). The radiograph should also be marked 'AP' if the anteroposterior projection was used; departmental posteroanterior (PA) films are generally not marked as such.

Radiographic projection.   A judgement as to whether a radiograph is AP or PA can be made from the following evidence:

1. The position of the label (this varies from department to department and is open to error).
2. The relationship of the scapulae to the lung margins (in the PA projection the scapulae are projected clear of the lungs and in AP projection they overlie the lungs).
3. The appearance of the vertebral bodies in the cervi-codorsal region. The vertebral endplates are seen

2

more clearly in the AP projection and the laminae are more clearly seen in the PA projection.

Supine versus erect position. It is important to know whether a chest radiograph was taken in the erect or supine position. In the supine position, blood flow is more evenly distributed throughout the lungs, making the upper zone vessels equal in size to those in the lower zones. This has implications in assessing the chest radiograph of a patient suspected of being in cardiac failure. In addition, fluid is distributed throughout the dependent part of the pleural space and any air–fluid levels that might be present on an erect film are impossible to detect. The position and contours of the heart, mediastinum and diaphragm are also different compared with an erect film. In the absence of any indication on the radiograph, one clue is the position of the gastric air bubble: if it is just under the left hemidiaphragm it is in the fundus and the patient is erect, whereas in the supine position air collects in the antrum of the stomach which lies centrally or slightly to the right of the vertebral column, well below the diaphragm.

Patient rotation. The patient may be rotated around one of three axes. Axial rotation is the most common cause of unilateral transradiancy (one lung appearing darker than the other). It also distorts the mediastinal outline. The degree of rotation can be assessed by relating the medial ends of the clavicles to the spinous process of the vertebral body at the same level – they should be equidistant from the spinous processes.

Rotation about the horizontal coronal axis results in a more kyphotic or lordotic projection than normal. The main pulmonary artery and subclavian vessels may appear unduly prominent. Rotation around the horizontal sagittal axis usually leads to obvious tilt of the chest in relation to the edge of the radiograph, which is assumed to be upright.

Physical attributes of the patient, such as a kyphoscoliosis or a depressed sternum (pectus excavatum), may also distort the appearance of the thoracic cage and its contents.

State of inspiration or expiration. The degree of inspiration is an important consideration for the correct interpretation of a chest radiograph. A poor inspiratory effort does not necessarily imply lack of patient cooperation and may as often be related to a pathological process. At full inspiration the midpoint of the right hemidiaphragm lies between the anterior end of ribs 5–7. A shallow inspiration affects the contour of the heart and mediastinum and may mimic the appearances of pulmonary congestion because the upper zone vessels will have the same diameter as the lower zone vessels.

Films taken deliberately with the patient in full expiration are invaluable in the investigation of air trapping. They are mandatory in any patient suspected of having inhaled a foreign body with consequent obstruction of a lobar bronchus. An expiratory film is also useful in accentuating a small pneumothorax.

Review areas. Several areas are difficult to assess on a frontal radiograph and should be scrutinized carefully. These review areas are:

- apices
- behind the heart
- hilar regions
- bones
- lung periphery just inside the chest wall.

Detection and description of radiographic abnormalities should then be undertaken and a differential diagnosis listed based on the abnormalities detected. With experience, the structured search gives way to the rapid identification of abnormalities and a search for confirmatory radiological signs and associated abnormalities.

COMMON RADIOLOGICAL SIGNS

Consolidation

'Consolidation' is the term used to describe lung in which the air-filled spaces are replaced by the products of disease, e.g. water, pus or blood. The two most important radiological signs of consolidation are (a) an air bronchogram and (b) the silhouette sign. The causes of widespread consolidation may be divided into four categories (Box 2.1).

An air bronchogram is present when the airways contain air and appear as radiolucent (black) branching structures against a now white background of airless lung. The silhouette sign is present when the border of a structure is lost because the normally air-filled lung outlining the border is replaced by radio-opaque fluid or tissue. Recognition of this sign can help localize the affected area of abnormality within the chest. Thus, loss of a clear right heart border is due to right middle lobe consolidation or collapse.

Localized areas of consolidation are usually due to infection. In some cases the borders of the consolidation are clearly demarcated. This usually corresponds to a fissure and the consolidation is confined to one lobe (lobar pneumonia) (Fig. 2.11). If consolidation is slow to clear with treatment, it may be secondary to partial obstruction of a lobar bronchus, such as carcinoma of the bronchus. Consolidation may also be widespread and affect both lungs (Figs. 2.12, 2.13).

Box 2.1   Causes of widespread pulmonary consolidation

Fluid transudation	Pulmonary oedema due to cardiac failure, renal failure, hepatic failure
Exudation	Infection, e.g. lobar pneumonia and bronchopneumonia, tuberculosis Acute respiratory distress syndrome (ARDS) Pulmonary haemorrhage due to contusion Pulmonary eosinophilia
Inhalation	Gastric contents Toxic fumes Oxygen toxicity
Infiltration	Lymphoma Alveolar cell carcinoma

Collapse (atelectasis)

'Collapse' (atelectasis) is the radiological term used when there is loss of aeration and, therefore, expansion in part or all of a lung. Collapse of a lobe or an entire lung is most frequently due to an endobronchial tumour, an inhaled foreign body or a mucus plug.

Although collapse is most often thought of as occurring at a lobar level, focal areas of pulmonary collapse at a subsegmental level occur very commonly in postoperative patients. There are many signs of lobar collapse but it is important to realize that not all these signs occur together. In addition, some non-specific signs may be present which indirectly point to the diagnosis and alert the observer to look for the more specific signs.

The most reliable and frequently present finding in lobar collapse is shift of the fissures, which invariably occurs to some extent. If air stays in the collapsed lobe, the contained blood vessels remain visible and appear crowded. If there is marked volume loss, the density of the collapsed and airless lobe increases. The hila may show two types of change consisting either of gross

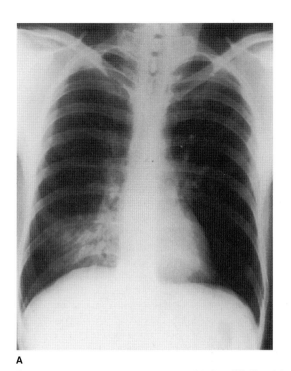

A

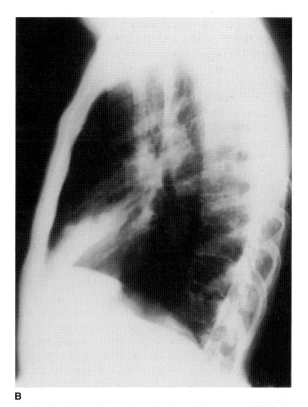

B

Figure 2.11   Right middle lobe consolidation. **(A)** The right heart border is not seen clearly, owing to adjacent consolidation. Note that the right hemidiaphragm is clearly visible as far as the vertebral column. **(B)** The lateral view confirms the presence of consolidation in the right middle lobe with the posterior aspect well demarcated by the oblique fissure.

2

displacement upwards or downwards, or of rearrangement of individual hilar components (i.e. vessels and airways) leading to changes in shape and prominence. Elevation of the hemidiaphragm, reflecting volume loss, is most marked in collapse of a lower lobe. 'Peaking' of the mid-portion of the hemidiaphragm occurs in upper lobe collapse due to displacement of the oblique fissure. The signs associated with collapse are listed in Box 2.2.

Collapse of individual lobes

Right upper lobe

On the PA radiograph there is elevation of the transverse fissure and the right hilum. If the collapse is complete the non-aerated lobe is seen as an increased density alongside the superior mediastinum adjacent to the trachea (Fig. 2.14). On the lateral view the minor fissure moves upwards and the major fissure moves forwards. The retrosternal area becomes progressively more opaque and the anterior margin of the ascending aorta becomes effaced.

Right middle lobe

On the PA radiograph the lateral part of the minor fissure moves down and there is blurring of the

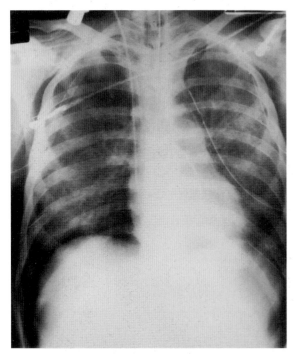

Figure 2.12 Widespread airspace consolidation in a patient with acute respiratory distress syndrome (ARDS). There are multiple chest drains for bilateral pneumothoraces.

Box 2.2   Signs associated with a collapsed lobe
■ Increased density of the collapsed lobe
■ Shift of fissures
■ Silhouette sign
■ Hilar shift and distortion
■ Crowding of vessels and airways
■ Mediastinal shift
■ Crowding of the ribs
■ Elevation of hemidiaphragm

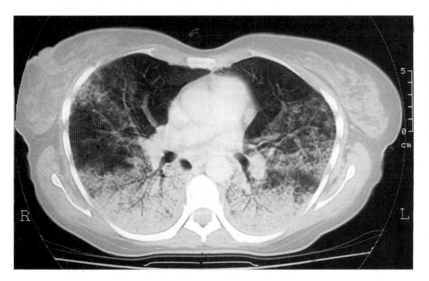

Figure 2.13 Diffuse consolidation within apical segments of both lower lobes. Note prominent bilateral air bronchograms within consolidated lung. Infection due to *Pneumocystis carinii* and cytomegalovirus in an immunocompromised patient.

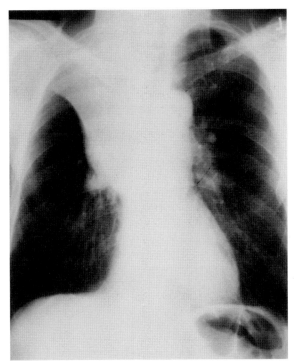

Figure 2.14 Right upper lobe collapse. There is increased density medial to the elevated horizontal fissure. The cause was a large central tumour obstructing the right upper lobe bronchus.

normally sharp right heart border. This may be a subtle abnormality that is easily overlooked. On the lateral view the minor fissure moves downwards and the lower half of the major fissure moves forwards, giving rise to a triangular shadow visible behind the lower sternum (Fig. 2.15).

Right lower lobe

On the PA view there is an increase in density overlying the medial portion of the right hemidiaphragm and the right hilum is displaced inferiorly. The right heart border usually remains sharply defined since this is in contact with the aerated right middle lobe. On the lateral view the oblique fissure moves backwards and, with increasing collapse, there is loss of definition of the right hemidiaphragm as well as increased density overlying the lower dorsal vertebrae. Right lower lobe collapse is a mirror image of left lower lobe collapse (Fig. 2.16).

Left upper lobe

The main finding on the PA radiograph is of a veil-like increase in density, without a sharp margin, spreading outwards and upwards from the left hilum, which is

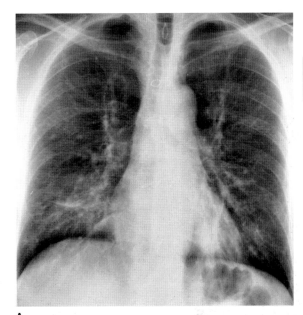

A

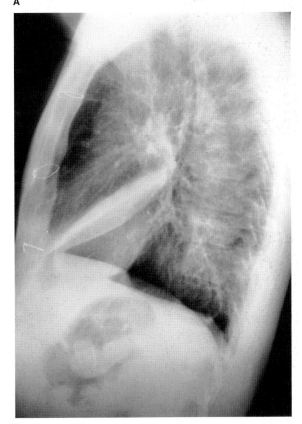

B

Figure 2.15 Right middle lobe collapse in a patient post-thoracotomy. **(A)** Loss of the right heart border may be subtle on the frontal film (note the patient also has some left lower lobe consolidation). **(B)** The lateral view shows the typical triangular opacity overlying the cardiac shadow.

2

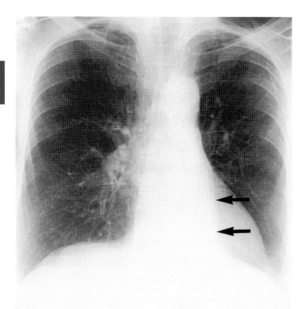

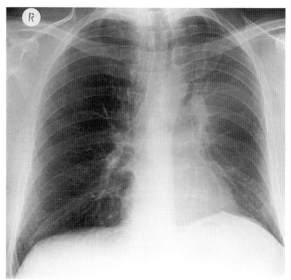

A

Figure 2.16 Left lower lobe collapse. A PA radiograph shows loss of the outline of the medial portion of the left hemidiaphragm and a triangular density behind the left side of the heart (arrows). There is also volume loss of the left hemithorax and the mediastinum is deviated to the left, allowing increased visibility of the thoracic spine.

elevated. The aortic knuckle, left hilum and left heart border may have ill-defined outlines. As volume loss increases, the collapsed lobe moves closer to the midline and the lung apex may become lucent due to hyperinflation of the apical segment of the left lower lobe. A sharp border may also return to the aortic arch. On the lateral view the oblique fissure moves upwards and forwards, remaining relatively straight and roughly parallel to the anterior chest wall (Fig. 2.17). On the PA projection, collapse (or consolidation) of the lingular segment of the left upper lobe should be suspected when the left cardiac border is ill defined.

Left lower lobe

This is most commonly seen in patients following cardiac surgery and a thoracotomy due to the retention of secretions in the left lower lobe bronchus. On the PA view there is a triangular density behind the heart with loss of the medial portion of the left hemidiaphragm (Fig. 2.16); if the PA radiograph is underexposed, it may be impossible to see this triangular opacity. On the lateral view there is backwards displacement of the oblique fissure and with increasing collapse there is increased density over the lower dorsal vertebrae.

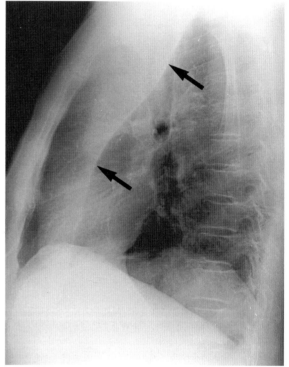

B

Figure 2.17 Left upper lobe collapse. (**A**) There is a veil-like density of the left hemithorax, which obscures the outline of the aortic knuckle and left heart border superiorly. There is also volume loss on the left (the trachea is deviated to the left and the left hemidiaphragm is raised with 'peaking' centrally). (**B**) The lateral radiograph shows increased density anterior to the oblique fissure (arrows).

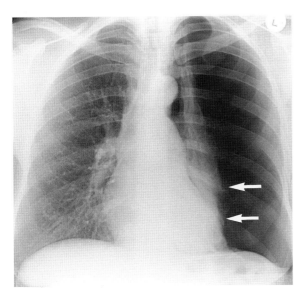

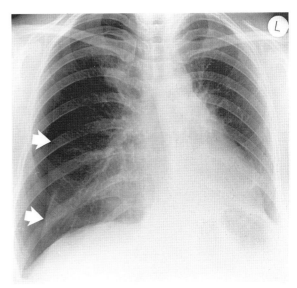

2

Figure 2.18 Spontaneous pneumothorax. There is a large left-sided pneumothorax with loss of vascular markings lateral to the edge of the collapsed lung. The visceral pleural edge is visible (arrows).

Figure 2.19 Tension pneumothorax post-thoracoscopic biopsy of a right upper zone lung nodule. The pneumothorax in Figure 2.18 involves more of the hemithorax but this pneumothorax is causing deviation of the mediastinum to the opposite side and is potentially life threatening unless treated promptly. The visceral pleural edge is visible (arrows).

Pneumothorax

When air is introduced into the pleural space, the resulting pneumothorax can be recognized radiographically. There are numerous causes of a pneumothorax but the most common include penetrating injuries (e.g. stab wound, placement of a subclavian line) and breaches of the visceral pleura (e.g. spontaneous rupture of a subpleural bulla or mechanical ventilation with high pressures). The cardinal radiographic sign is the visceral pleural edge: lateral to this edge no vascular shadows are visible and medial to it the collapsed lung is of higher density than the contralateral lung (Fig. 2.18). It is important to remember that in the supine position, the air of a small pneumothorax will collect anteriorly in the pleural space; thus on a portable supine chest radiograph, the pneumothorax will be visible as an area of relative translucency without a visceral pleural edge necessarily being identifiable.

If air enters the pleural space during inspiration but cannot leave on expiration (usually because of a check-valve effect of the torn flap of the visceral pleura), pressure increases rapidly and this results in a life-threatening tension pneumothorax. This can be recognized by a shift of the mediastinum to the opposite side (Fig. 2.19).

The opaque hemithorax

If one-half of a chest is completely opaque (a white-out) it is due either to collapse of a lung or a large pleural effusion. If there is a shift of the mediastinum to the affected side it implies that volume loss in the lung (i.e. collapse) on that side must have occurred. Where there is no shift of the mediastinum or it is shifted slightly to the side of the white-out, this is usually due to constricting pleural disease (including pleural tumour). A pleural effusion that is large enough to cause complete opacification of a hemithorax will displace the mediastinum away from the side of the white-out. While penetrated PA and lateral films may help, it is sometimes surprisingly difficult to differentiate between the causes of an opaque hemithorax. Ultrasound and computed tomography allow the distinction to be made with confidence and the latter may give further information about the underlying disease.

Decreased density of a hemithorax

The conditions outlined so far have all focused on increased density of the lungs on plain radiographs. However, there are a number of causes where one lung appears less dense than the other side. When a chest radiograph demonstrates greater radiolucency of one lung compared with the other, it is necessary first to determine whether this appearance is due to a pulmonary abnormality. The radiograph should be checked

2

for patient rotation and for soft tissue asymmetry, e.g. a mastectomy.

The pulmonary vessels are a helpful pointer to abnormalities causing a true decrease in density. In compensatory hyperinflation they are splayed apart. A search should also be made for a collapsed lobe. The vessels are considerably diminished or truncated in emphysema. Further radiological examination should include an expiration film if a pneumothorax is suspected. This will also demonstrate air trapping that occurs with bronchial obstruction. Computed tomography may also be useful in elucidating the cause of a hyperlucent lung. The lungs can be seen on computed tomography without the problem of overlying tissues and any decrease in density is more readily apparent.

Elevation of the diaphragm

The right or left dome of the diaphragm may be elevated because it is paralysed, pushed up or pulled up. However, there are a number of circumstances in which the diaphragm appears to be elevated without actually being so.

The radiographic evaluation of an apparently elevated diaphragm should begin with an assessment of the plain film, in particular evidence of previous surgery. Old radiographs are essential to determine whether the diaphragmatic elevation is of long standing. A decubitus film is particularly useful in ruling out a suspected subpulmonary effusion; in this instance the pleural effusion is confined to the space between the lung base and the superior surface of the diaphragm. The radiograph will show what appears to be an elevated hemidiaphragm. Ultrasound will assist in determining if fluid is present above and/or below the diaphragm.

If the hemidiaphragm is paralysed, fluoroscopic or ultrasound examination is useful as it may demonstrate paradoxical movement on vigorous sniffing (instead of the diaphragm moving down, it moves up). An important proviso is that a few normal individuals show this paradoxical movement of the diaphragm on sniffing. In congenital eventration part or all of the hemidiaphragm muscle is made up of a thin layer of fibrous tissue and it may be difficult to distinguish from paralysis even on fluoroscopy.

Pleural disease

Because the chest radiograph is a two-dimensional image, abnormalities of the pleura and chest wall are often difficult to assess. Gross pleural abnormalities are usually obvious on a chest radiograph (Fig. 2.20), but even when there is extensive pleural pathology it may be difficult to distinguish between pleural fluid, pleural thickening (e.g. secondary to a previous inflammatory

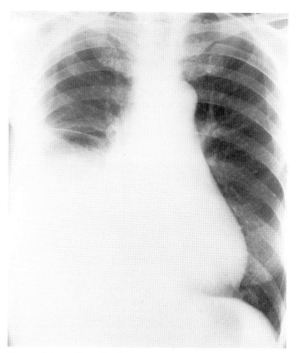

Figure 2.20 Pleural effusion. The right lower and mid zones are opaque due to a large right-sided pleural effusion.

process) and a neoplasm of the pleura. In such cases, a lateral decubitus film or ultrasound scan is useful in identifying the presence of fluid. Computed tomography can readily identify the encasing and constricting nature of a mesothelioma.

The pulmonary mass

Most pulmonary nodules or masses are discovered by plain chest radiography. It is important to obtain previous films if at all possible. If the mass was present on the previous films and has not changed over a number of years, it can be assumed that the lesion is benign and no further action needs to be taken. However, if the nodule was not previously present or has increased in size, further investigation is warranted.

Computed tomography (see Fig. 2.3) will detect or exclude the presence of other lesions within the lungs. The presence of calcification within the nodule, although often thought to be an indicator of benignity, will not exclude malignancy with complete certainty. In addition, computed tomography can be used to determine the presence of hilar or mediastinal lymph node enlargement as well as direct invasion of the adjacent mediastinum or chest wall. In patients in whom surgical resection of the pulmonary mass is not indicated, a cyto-

2

logical or histological specimen by percutaneous needle biopsy may be taken. This is usually reserved for small peripheral lesions that are not accessible by bronchoscopy. It can be performed under computed tomography guidance or fluoroscopy but complications include pneumothorax or pulmonary haemorrhage (see other interventional techniques).

Pulmonary nodules

A large number of conditions are characterized by multiple pulmonary nodules (Fig. 2.21). Combining the clinical information with an accurate description of the size and distribution of the nodules narrows down the list of differential diagnoses.

Metastatic deposits are by far the most common cause of multiple pulmonary nodules of varying sizes in adult patients in the United Kingdom (Fig. 2.21) but this is not the case worldwide. In some parts of the USA, histoplasmosis is endemic and multiple lesions due to this condition may be more common than those due to malignancy. Making this important distinction may be difficult and biopsy of one lesion may be the only reliable means of distinguishing a benign from a malignant cause for the multiple nodules.

Nodules are described as 'miliary' when they are less than 5 mm in diameter and are so numerous that they cannot be counted. The crucial diagnosis to consider, even if the patient is not particularly unwell, is miliary tuberculosis, since this life-threatening disease can be readily treated. If the patient is asymptomatic the differential diagnosis is more likely to lie between sarcoidosis, metastatic disease or a coal worker's pneumoconiosis. As ever, previous radiographs showing the rate of growth of the nodules may give valuable clues to the likely nature of the disease.

Cavitating pulmonary lesions

The radiological definition of cavitation is a lucency representing air within a mass or an area of consolidation. The cavity may or may not contain a fluid level and is surrounded by a wall of variable thickness (Fig. 2.22).

The two most likely diagnoses in an adult presenting with a cavitating pulmonary lesion on a chest radiograph are a cancer or a lung abscess. In children, infection is the most common cause. Cavitation secondary to necrosis is well recognized in a variety of bacterial pneumonias, particularly those associated with tuberculosis, *Staphylococcus aureus,* anaerobes and *Klebsiella*. Diagnosis is usually by plain chest radiograph in the first instance but computed tomography is also useful for localizing the abscess and sometimes to enable percutaneous aspiration to be undertaken. It also allows

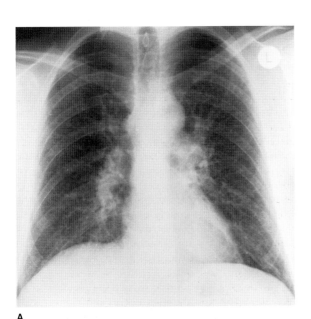
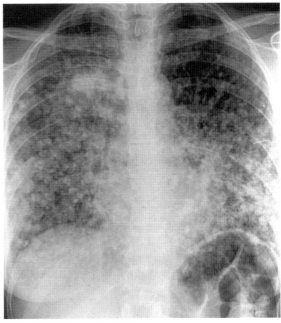

A　　　　　　　　　　　　　　**B**

Figure 2.21　Multiple pulmonary nodules. (A) Pulmonary sarcoidosis. These pulmonary nodules are small (2–3 mm) and subtle and there is bilateral hilar lymphadenopathy. (B) Multiple pulmonary metastases. These nodules are better defined, larger (most 0.5–1 cm in diameter) and are so numerous that they have coalesced in the right upper zone.

2

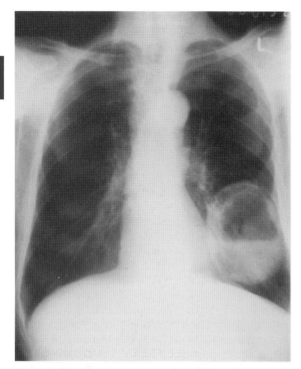

Figure 2.22 Lung abscess: there is a thick-walled cavity containing a fluid level in the left lower lobe.

assessment of the relationship of the abscess to adjacent airways so that appropriate postural drainage can be planned.

In all age groups it is important to consider tuberculosis, especially if the cavitating lesions are in the lung apices. Linear or computed tomography may be necessary if the presence of cavitation is questionable; in addition, computed tomography may show other features which help to narrow the differential diagnosis (e.g. pulmonary calcifications in tuberculosis, mediastinal lymph node enlargement in metastatic disease). In general, radiology alone cannot distinguish one cause of a cavitating mass from another.

SPECIFIC CONDITIONS

The postoperative and critically ill patient

In the context of intensive care medicine, the portable radiograph is one of the main means of monitoring critically ill patients. However, it is a far from perfect technique as the degree of inspiration is usually poor and may vary widely on serial radiographs. In addition, evaluation of cardiac size and the lung bases is, at best, difficult. This is often compounded by the rapidly changing haemodynamic state of the patient.

To some extent the advent of phosphor plate radiography has enabled more accurate assessments to be made because variations in exposure are not such a problem. Decubitus radiographs can be useful to evaluate the dependent side for fluid and the non-dependent side for small but clinically important pneumothoraces. For convenience it is useful to consider the various disease processes in the categories described below.

Support and monitoring apparatus

Careful radiographic monitoring of the position of various tubes and catheters used in the postoperative and critically ill patient is essential to decrease complications. Before evaluating the heart and lungs it is good practice to check each of these lines for proper positioning. The ideally placed central venous line ends in the superior vena cava (see Fig. 2.1). Catheters terminating in the right atrium or ventricle may cause arrhythmias or perforation. Swan–Ganz catheters used to monitor pulmonary capillary wedge pressure are ideally sited in a main or lobar pulmonary artery (see Fig. 2.1). Drugs inadvertently injected directly into the wedged catheter may cause lobar pulmonary oedema or necrosis. Both catheters (central venous pressure line and Swan–Ganz) are inserted percutaneously and therefore share certain complications. The most frequent is a pneumothorax due to puncture of the lung at the time of subclavian vein insertion. If the catheter is inserted into the mediastinum or perforates a vein or artery, there may be dramatic widening of the superior mediastinum due to haematoma. If the catheter enters the pleural space, infused fluid rapidly fills the pleural space. Catheter perforation of the right atrium or ventricle may lead to cardiac tamponade, which may result in progressive enlargement of the heart shadow on serial radiographs.

The intra-aortic balloon pump is usually inserted via the femoral artery and is used in patients with intractable heart failure or in weaning the patient from cardiopulmonary bypass. On the frontal radiograph the tip of the catheter should be seen lying just inferior to the aortic arch (see Fig. 2.1).

A cardiac pacemaker wire is usually inserted via the external jugular, the cephalic or femoral vein and passed under fluoroscopic control into the apex of the right ventricle. Kinks or coils of wire are undesirable and the wire should be examined carefully along its entire length.

The tip of a correctly positioned endotracheal tube (see Fig. 2.1) lies in the midtrachea, approximately 5–7 cm above the carina. This distance is needed to ensure that it does not descend into the right main stem bronchus with flexion of the head and neck or ascend into the pharynx when the head and neck are extended. If the endotracheal tube is inadvertently passed into the right main stem bronchus (the more vertical of the two main bronchi), the left lung may collapse, with a shift of the mediastinum to the left and hyperinflation of the right lung. If the endotracheal tube is positioned just below the vocal cords, the tube may retract into the pharynx, airway protection is lost and aspiration may occur. If the tube remains high in the trachea, inflation of the cuff may cause vocal cord damage. Delayed complications include focal tracheal necrosis leading ultimately to a localized stricture. It is worth noting that, even with correct positioning and cuff inflation, an endotracheal tube is not an absolute guarantee against aspiration of stomach contents into the airways.

Tracheostomy for long-term support has its own complications. A correctly placed tracheostomy tube should be parallel to the long axis of the trachea, approximately one-half to two-thirds the diameter of the trachea and end at least 5 cm from the carina. Marked subcutaneous or mediastinal emphysema may be due to tracheal injury or a large leak around the stoma. After prolonged intubation some tracheal scarring is inevitable. Symptomatic tracheal stenosis or collapse of a short length of the trachea is less common now owing to use of low-pressure occlusion cuffs on endotracheal tubes. When positive end-expiratory pressure (PEEP) is added, the patient's tidal volume and functional residual capacity increase. This is reflected in the radiograph as increased lung aeration. PEEP may open up areas of collapse and cause radiographic clearing. However, this may be spurious as any densities present will be less obvious owing to the increased lung volume. Similarly, when the patient is weaned off PEEP, the lung volume drops and the lungs may appear to be dramatically worse. Pulmonary barotrauma (air leakage due to elevated pressure) complicates approximately 10% of patients on positive pressure ventilation. If air continues to leak due to continued ventilation, a tension pneumothorax may develop. The chest radiograph is often the first indicator of this potentially fatal complication.

Collapse

Following laparotomy, at least half of all patients develop some postoperative pulmonary collapse. Volume loss is most often attributed to hypoventilation and retained secretions and it is most frequent in patients with chronic bronchitis, emphysema, obesity, prolonged anaesthesia or unusually heavy analgesia. The most common radiographic manifestation is of linear densities which appear in the lower lung zones soon after surgery. Patchy, segmental or complete lobar consolidation is less common. When due to hypoventilation or large airway secretions, marked volume loss rather than dense consolidation is the usual appearance. Careful

attention should be paid to unilateral elevation of the diaphragm and shifts of the minor fissure or hilar vessels. When collapse is due to multiple peripheral mucus plugs, the radiographic picture may be of pulmonary consolidation rather than volume loss. Areas of collapse tend to change rapidly and often clear with suction or physiotherapy. Postoperative collapse is not usually an infectious process, but, if not treated promptly, areas of collapse will usually become secondarily infected.

Aspiration pneumonia

Another postoperative complication is the aspiration of gastric contents. A depressed state of consciousness and the presence of a nasogastric tube that disables the protective oesophagogastric sphincter are the most frequent predisposing factors. An endotracheal or tracheostomy tube does not always protect the patient from aspiration. The radiographic appearance of patchy, often bilateral, consolidation appears any time within the first 24 hours of aspiration and then progresses rapidly. In an uncomplicated case there is usually evidence of stability or regression by 72 hours, with complete clearing within 1–2 weeks. The infiltrates are usually patchy and diffuse and are most often seen at the lung bases, more commonly on the right. Complications include progression to acute respiratory distress syndrome (ARDS). Any worsening of the radiograph on the third day or thereafter should suggest the diagnosis of secondary infection.

Acute respiratory distress syndrome

Acute respiratory distress syndrome (ARDS) consists of progressive respiratory insufficiency following a major bodily insult and can be due to a large number of factors. Over the years it has been known as 'shock lung', 'stiff lung syndrome' and 'adult hyaline membrane disease'.

At the pathophysiological level there is increased permeability of the pulmonary capillaries and the formation of platelet and fibrin microemboli. This results in alveolar oedema and haemorrhage, which can affect the entire lung. After several days, hyaline membranes form within the distal air spaces. As a general rule, symptoms occur on the second day after insult or injury, but the radiograph remains normal during the initial hours of clinical distress. Interstitial oedema is the first radiographic abnormality, which may be of a faint, hazy ground-glass appearance (Fig. 2.23), and this is followed rapidly by patchy air-space oedema. By 36–72 hours after insult, diffuse global air-space consolidation is evident. It is the timing of the radiographic changes relative to the insult and the onset of symptoms, rather than the radiological appearance alone, that suggest the diagnosis of ARDS.

2

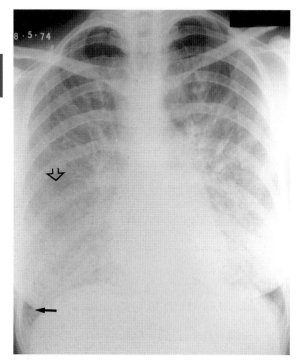

Figure 2.23 Pulmonary oedema due to mitral valve disease. There is increased opacity or 'haziness' throughout the lungs. There is fluid within the horizontal fissure (open arrow) and septal lines (closed arrow) corresponding with fluid in the interstitium of the lung.

Pneumonia

Pulmonary infection may occur several days after surgery. Pneumonia may complicate collapse but may result from aspiration or inhalation of infected secretions from the pharynx.

The features of consolidation have already been covered but the critically ill or postoperative patient may not show typical appearances of consolidation. Numerous factors, such as prior antibiotic therapy and coexistent heart or lung disease, may alter the radiographic features. The radiographic appearance may vary from a few ill-defined or discrete opacities to a pattern of coalescence and widespread patchy consolidation. Cavity or pneumatocele (a thin-walled air-filled space) formation is not infrequent.

Extrapulmonary air

The diagnosis of a pneumothorax is made by the identification of the thin line of the visceral pleura. Free air may also be found in the pulmonary interstitium, the mediastinum, the pericardial space and the subcutaneous tissues. In the intensive care setting, extrapulmo-

nary air is most often due to barotrauma from mechanical ventilation or secondary to surgery or other iatrogenic procedures. Pulmonary interstitial emphysema is difficult to recognize radiographically and is invariably due to ventilator-induced barotrauma. Unlike air bronchograms, the interstitial air is seen as black lines and streaks radiating from the hila; they do not branch or taper towards the periphery. Interstitial emphysema usually culminates in a pneumomediastinum and this is shown on a frontal radiograph as a radiolucent band against the mediastinum bordered by the reflected mediastinal pleura. Air may outline specific structures such as the aortic arch, the descending aorta or the thymus.

Cardiac failure

The radiographic diagnosis of early left ventricular failure is largely dependent on changes in the calibre of the pulmonary vessels in the erect patient. As the left atrial pressure rises, blood is shunted to the upper zones. This is the first and most important radiographic sign of elevated left ventricular pressure but it is important to remember that, because of redistribution of blood flow in the supine position, a supine radiograph does not allow this criterion to be used.

Interstitial pulmonary oedema then follows; this is manifested by blurring of the vessel margins, a perihilar haze and a vague increased density over the lower zones. When fluid fills and distends the interlobular septa, Kerley B lines (septal lines) may be visible (see Fig. 2.23). These are best visualized in the costophrenic angles as thin white lines arising from the lateral pleural surface. As the left ventricular pressure continues to rise, multiple small, ill-defined opacities occur in the lower half of the lungs. These represent alveoli filling with fluid. Alveolar oedema may also appear as poorly defined bilateral 'butterfly' perihilar opacification. Increasing cardiac size usually accompanies cardiac failure but, if it occurs following acute myocardial infarction or an acute arrhythmia, cardiac failure may be present without an increase in cardiac size. Bilateral pleural effusions often accompany cardiac failure.

Pulmonary embolism

The postoperative or critically ill patient has numerous risk factors for the development of deep venous thrombosis and thus pulmonary embolism. In this group, where respiratory distress is often multifactorial, the diagnosis of pulmonary embolism is extremely difficult.

Conventional radiographic findings are non-specific and include elevation of the diaphragm, collapse or segmental consolidation. A small pleural effusion may appear during the first 2 days following the embolus.

It is important to recognize that a normal chest radiograph does not exclude a major pulmonary embolus; indeed, a normal radiograph in a patient with acute respiratory distress is suggestive of the diagnosis. A radionuclide perfusion scan is of use because if it is normal a pulmonary embolus can be excluded; however, this is not a practical test for a patient in an intensive care unit and the decision to treat with anticoagulants is often made clinically.

The success of helical CT in the diagnosis of pulmonary embolism relates to its rapid scan time, volumetric data acquisition and high degree of vascular enhancement (see Fig. 2.5).

Kyphoscoliosis

Kyphoscoliosis makes assessment of the chest radiograph difficult and it is useful to reduce the distortion of thoracic contents due to the kyphoscoliosis by obtaining an oblique radiograph, positioning the patient in such a way that the spine appears at its straightest. Severe kyphoscoliosis may cause pulmonary arterial hypertension and cor pulmonale. Some congenital chest anomalies such as pulmonary agenesis (absence of a lung) and neurofibromatosis are associated with dorsal spine abnormalities. Because of the problems associated with getting a true posteroanterior and lateral view, computed tomography scanning is often the most satisfactory method of visualizing the lungs.

Bronchiectasis

Bronchiectasis is a chronic condition characterized by local, irreversible dilatation of the bronchi, usually associated with inflammation. On a chest radiograph (Fig. 2.24A) the findings include:

- the bronchial wall visible either as single thin lines or as parallel 'tram-lines'

- ring and curvilinear opacities which represent thickened airway walls seen end on. These tend to range in size from 8 to 20 mm, have thin (hairline) walls and may contain air–fluid levels

- dilated airways filled with secretions giving rise to broad-band shadows some 5–10 mm wide and several centimetres long (seen end on, these dilated fluid-filled airways produce rounded or oval nodular opacities)

- overinflation throughout both lungs (particularly in cystic fibrosis)

- volume loss where bronchiectasis is localized (this may give rise to crowding of bronchi or collapse due to mucus plugging that can be severe and result in complete collapse of a lobe)

- less specific signs including consolidation, scarring and pleural thickening.

The definitive diagnosis of bronchiectasis used to be made by bronchography (injection of contrast into the bronchial airway), but this is an invasive and

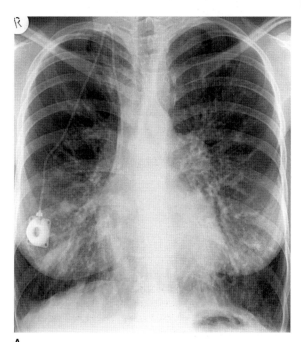

A

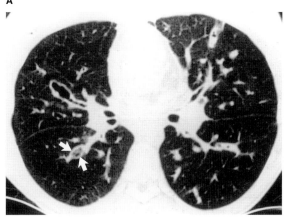

B

Figure 2.24 Cystic fibrosis. **(A)** The lungs are overinflated on the PA chest radiograph and there is widespread increased shadowing due to bronchial wall thickening and peribronchial consolidation. Note the prominent central pulmonary artery (pulmonary arterial hypertension may be a complication) and the catheter for long-term intravenous antibiotics. **(B)** A thin-section CT image of the same patient shows the dilated, bronchiectatic airways, some of which are plugged with mucus (arrows).

2

unpleasant procedure and a viable alternative is high-resolution computed tomography (Fig. 2.24B). With this technique, thin slices are taken throughout both lungs and the findings are similar to those on the plain film (thickened bronchial walls, bronchial dilatation, ring opacities containing air–fluid levels). Comparing the diameter of the bronchial wall with the adjacent vessel is helpful, as both should be approximately the same size. Computed tomography may also be helpful in determining the optimum position for postural drainage. Upper lobe predominance is present in early cystic fibrosis and after tubercle infection and allergic bronchopulmonary aspergillosis. The remaining causes of bronchiectasis (e.g. post-childhood infection) affect predominantly the middle and lower lobes.

Chronic airflow limitation

This comprises three conditions which are present simultaneously in a given patient to a greater or lesser degree: chronic bronchitis, asthma and emphysema. The first is diagnosed by the patient's history and, strictly speaking, does not have any characteristic radiological features. In asthma the chest radiograph is normal in the majority of patients between attacks, but as many as 40% reveal evidence of hyperinflation during an acute severe episode. In asthmatic children with recurrent infection, bronchial wall thickening occurs. Collapse of a lobe or an entire lung because of mucus plugging is another feature and may be recurrent, affecting different lobes. Complications include pneumomediastinum, which arises secondarily to pulmonary interstitial emphysema and pneumothorax due to rupture of a subpleural bulla. Expiratory radiographs may aid detection of a pneumothorax as well as demonstrating any air trapping secondary to bronchial occlusion.

Emphysema is a condition characterized by an increase in air spaces beyond the terminal bronchiole owing to destruction of alveolar walls. While it is strictly a pathological diagnosis, certain radiographic appearances are characteristic in more advanced cases. These include overinflation of the lungs, an alteration in the appearance of the pulmonary vessels and the presence of bullae. Overinflation results in flattening of the diaphragmatic dome (Fig. 2.25), resulting in an apparently small heart and a decreased cardiothoracic ratio. On the lateral chest radiograph the large retrosternal translu-

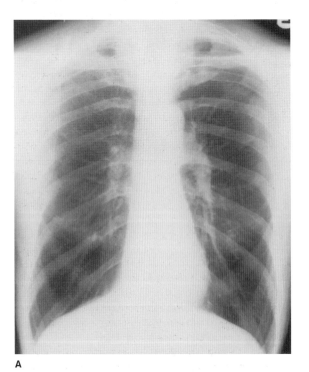

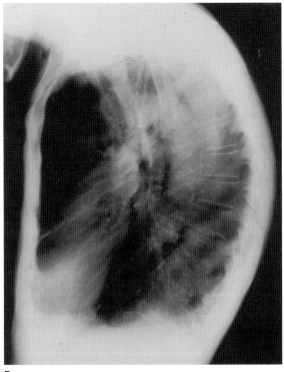

A   B

Figure 2.25 Emphysema. (A) Both lungs are hyperinflated. There is dilatation of the proximal pulmonary arteries with pruning of the peripheral vasculature. (B) The retrosternal and retrocardiac areas are strikingly transradiant.

cency caused by the hyperinflated lungs is particularly striking (Fig. 2.25B). The pulmonary vessels are abnormal: the smooth gradation in size of vessels from the hilum outwards is lost, with the hilar vessels being larger than normal and tapering abruptly, so-called 'pruning' of the vessels. However, the lungs are usually unevenly involved and this is mirrored by the uneven distribution of pulmonary vessels. When emphysema is predominantly basal in distribution, there is prominent upper lobe blood diversion which should not be mis-

taken for evidence of left heart failure. Bullae are recognized by their translucency, their hairline walls and a distortion of adjacent pulmonary vessels. They vary greatly in size and are occasionally big enough to occupy an entire hemithorax. When large they are an important cause of respiratory distress. Complications of bullae formation are infection and haemorrhage, which are usually manifested as the presence of an air–fluid level. Pneumothorax is another complication and occasionally may be difficult to distinguish from a large bulla.

PAEDIATRICS

INTRODUCTION

Despite the advent of new imaging modalities, such as ultrasound, computed tomography (CT), magnetic resonance imaging (MRI), ventilation/perfusion lung scans ($\dot{V}/\dot{Q}$ scans), positron emission tomography (PET) and CT–PET, the plain chest radiograph remains the mainstay of paediatric chest imaging. In most circumstances the clinical history and examination will be augmented by a chest radiograph before a working diagnosis is made and treatment or further investigations planned.

This section aims to provide a concise and practical introduction to imaging the paediatric chest, emphasizing the importance of the plain chest radiograph but also indicating where other modalities provide additional information or allow the same information to be acquired with less use of ionizing radiation. The first part provides an overview of imaging modalities currently available, the second reviews important radiological signs commonly seen in paediatric chest radiographs and the final part discusses common paediatric chest problems and their radiological signs.

The text has not been referenced extensively but a number of general references and review articles suitable for further reading are given at the end of the chapter.

MODALITIES IN PAEDIATRIC CHEST IMAGING

Plain chest radiographs and fluoroscopy

Chest radiographs may be taken in the erect posteroanterior (PA) or anteroposterior (AP) position or in the supine AP position. In some circumstances, such as on the neonatal unit (NNU) where patient handling is minimized, all films are obtained in the supine AP projection. Up to the age of 3 any of the projections may be used depending on the policy of the department. For patients over the age of 3, most units obtain erect PA films. It is important that within any given unit techniques are standardized and films clearly labelled,

as the appearances of some radiological signs, particularly those of pleural fluid and pneumothorax, are profoundly different in the erect and supine positions. These changes will be discussed in greater detail below. Chest radiographs should be obtained in inspiration, using a short exposure time and with attention to technical factors so as to minimize the radiation exposure to the patient and attendants.

The lateral chest radiograph necessitates a significantly higher exposure than the frontal and is not required routinely. It is usually obtained during the follow-up of patients with malignant disease likely to metastasize to the chest and sometimes in the assessment of recurrent chest infections and cystic fibrosis. A lateral view may also be performed to clarify an abnormality seen on the frontal projection.

Coned, AP plain radiographs using a high kVp technique and filtration to give an optimal exposure are used to demonstrate the anatomy and calibre of the major airways.

One of the disadvantages of conventional radiographs is that it is difficult to adequately demonstrate all soft tissue and bony structures using the same exposure factors. Two major developments have attempted to overcome these disadvantages. The first is digital chest radiography, in which a phosphor plate is used for the exposure. The plate is then scanned with a laser beam, which reads the information and stores it in digital form. The information can then be reconstructed as the 'chest X-ray' on a computer screen and manipulated to allow optimal visualization of areas of interest. Hard copies of the images can be printed on a laser imager. The advantages of this technique in paediatric radiology are the uniformity of image that can be maintained from day to day, the facility for image manipulation and a reduction in radiation dose.

The second technique, scanning equalization radiography (SER), uses a beam of X-rays to scan the patient. The exposure is continuously changing according to the tissues within the beam at any given time.

This results in a more even exposure and a more uniform image.

Fluoroscopy remains a useful technique for assessing diaphragmatic movements.

Bronchography and tomography

Since CT and MRI have become widely available, conventional tomography is no longer used. Bronchography is rarely undertaken to demonstrate focal bronchial narrowing; such cases are now investigated using multi-slice CT scans with three-dimensional reconstructions and virtual bronchoscopy software.

Ultrasound

Ultrasound is useful for examining the pleural space for fluid (Fig. 2.26). Effusions and empyemas can be located, measured and drained under ultrasound control. Because the ultrasound beam is strongly reflected by aerated lung, ultrasound is less useful for assessing lung lesions unless they are peripheral, lie against the chest wall and consist of either solid or fluid. The movement and integrity of the hemidiaphragms can be assessed using ultrasound. The disadvantage is that each hemidiaphragm can only be assessed independently and not in relationship to each other. This is important in mild hemidiaphragm paresis. Cardiac ultrasound is an extremely accurate non-invasive way of assessing congenital heart disease.

Computed tomography and magnetic resonance imaging

In many ways these techniques are complementary and will be discussed together. Both techniques require the patient to remain still for the duration of the scan and this is particularly important in MRI. Neonates and young infants may be examined if asleep after a feed, but older infants and children usually require sedation or general anaesthesia.

Computed tomography and high-resolution computed tomography

CT uses a narrow beam of X-rays to image the patient in 'slices'. The thickness of the slice may be varied from 1.5 mm to 1 cm and slices may be taken with or without gaps between them, depending on the region being examined and the likely pathology. Modern multislice scanners are very fast and allow the whole chest to be scanned in one breath hold. Assessment of the mediastinum and of vascular structures is facilitated by using intravascular contrast medium.

Lung pathology is best evaluated on CT, using high-resolution computed tomography (HRCT) if necessary. HRCT uses a thin slice thickness and special software to demonstrate the lung parenchyma. HRCT is used in the diagnosis of diffuse parenchymal disease and bronchiectasis.

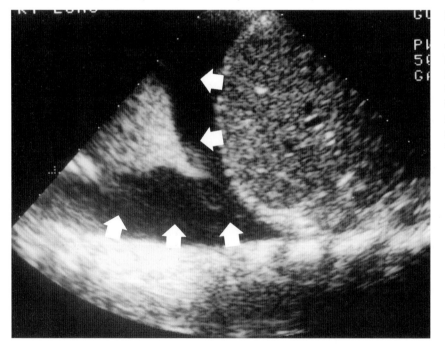

Figure 2.26 Sagittal ultrasound of a large pleural effusion, which is poorly echogenic and appears black (white arrows). The patient's back is seen to the bottom and the liver lies to the right of the image. The effusion surrounds the partly collapsed, triangular lower lobe.

CT has better spatial resolution and can detect fine calcification, which affords it an advantage over MRI in evaluating mediastinal masses and lymphadenopathy. Bone structure, and in particular cortical change, are better imaged on CT.

Vascular structures are well demonstrated on CT if an intravascular contrast agent containing iodine is used. Fast multislice CT scanners, which enable the entire chest to be scanned in a matter of seconds, facilitate the investigation of congenital vascular and cardiac abnormalities.

Magnetic resonance imaging

In MRI the patient lies within a strong magnetic field and is exposed to pulses of radiofrequency energy. This energy is absorbed by protons within the body. When the radiofrequency pulses are stopped, the protons return to their normal state but as they do they release energy, the magnetic resonance signal, which can be detected by coils placed around the body. Magnetic resonance signals are different for different tissues and may be altered by disease. Intravascular contrast medium for MRI is available.

MRI of the chest is complicated by cardiac and respiratory movements. These effects can be minimized by only taking images at the same point in each cardiac and respiratory cycle, a technique known as gating.

MRI has three major advantages over CT: its superior soft tissue contrast, its ability to acquire images in any plane and the fact that it does not use ionizing radiation. Sagittal, coronal and oblique images are of immense value in assessing mediastinal masses and in evaluating whether a paraspinal mass extends into the spinal canal.

One of the most exciting branches of MRI is magnetic resonance angiography (MRA), which allows blood vessels and the heart to be imaged without the need for arterial puncture. Optimal MRA images are obtained after intravenous injection of a contrast agent containing gadolinium and using oblique scan planes.

Angiography and cardiac catheterization

Cardiac ultrasound and MRI/MRA have reduced the need for diagnostic conventional angiography and cardiac catheterization to assess congenital anomalies of the aorta and pulmonary vessels and congenital arteriovenous malformations. Most conventional angiography or cardiac catheterization is now performed as part of a therapeutic interventional procedure.

Barium studies

These studies have a limited but very important place in the assessment of chest problems, specifically the barium swallow to evaluate extrinsic oesophageal compression by aberrant vessels or masses and the swallow/meal to assess intrinsic abnormalities such as uncoordinated swallowing, abnormal oesophageal peristalsis or gastro-oesophageal reflux that can cause aspiration. If a tracheo-oesophageal fistula is suspected, a tube oesophagram must be performed in the prone position.

There is no reliable technique for the positive diagnosis of aspiration; this includes the barium swallow/meal as well as the isotope milk scan. Recurrent aspiration may be inferred when there is severe gastro-oesophageal reflux.

Radionuclide studies

Radionuclide studies provide quantifiable functional information which complements the anatomical information provided by other imaging modalities. The ventilation/perfusion scan ($\dot{V}/\dot{Q}$ scan) uses krypton (^{81m}Kr) gas for ventilation and technetium (^{99m}Tc) labelled macroaggregates for perfusion. The $\dot{V}/\dot{Q}$ scan is the only method which will provide information on regional lung function. The radiation burden from the $\dot{V}$ scan is less than one-fifth of a chest radiograph while the $\dot{Q}$ scan has a dose equal to less than 60 seconds of fluoroscopy.

Most ventilatory disturbances result in a corresponding reduction in perfusion whereas if the pulmonary artery to a region is occluded (pulmonary embolus, sequestrated segment or pulmonary artery disease) that region remains ventilated. Occasionally other radionuclide studies such as bone scans or milk scans are indicated in the assessment of chest pathology.

Positron emission tomography and computed tomography–positron emission tomography

Positron emission tomography (PET) is a functional nuclear medicine technique that uses radioactive isotopes that have a short half-life and decay by emitting a positron. The emitted positrons collide with surrounding electrons producing a pair of photons, which can be detected by the scanner. The isotope most commonly used is ^{18}F and this is incorporated with glucose to form the tracer [^{18}F]fluorodeoxyglucose (FDG). Many malignant tumours have an altered glucose metabolism that results in FDG accumulating within their cells; this increased uptake allows them to be detected.

PET provides good information on tumour activity but very poor anatomical information on the location of the tumour, whereas CT provides excellent anatomical information but no functional information. The hybrid CT–PET scanners perform both scans and integrate the information to provide information on tumour activity (PET) superimposed on the fine anatomical CT images.

2

In paediatric chest imaging, PET and CT–PET have been used to stage and monitor malignant disease, particularly Hodgkin's lymphoma, bone sarcoma and neuroblastoma. Nonetheless their exact place in the management of these and other paediatric malignancies has yet to be determined.

Radiation and patient safety

Neonates, infants and children are more susceptible to the harmful effects of ionizing radiation than adults and their exposure to it should be kept to a minimum. Exposure can be minimized by using techniques like ultrasound and MRI, which do not use ionizing radiation, whenever possible. If plain radiographs are needed the dose can be minimized by using optimal radiographic techniques and modern dose-reducing equipment. High-dose investigations such as nuclear medicine studies, CT and CT–PET should be performed only after careful consideration of the potential benefits of the investigation weighed against the potential risks. This benefit–risk analysis may be best undertaken within a multidisciplinary team where the viewpoints of patient, parents and all of the professional groups involved in the patient's care can be considered.

BASIC SIGNS ON THE PLAIN CHEST RADIOGRAPH

Consolidation

Replacement of air in the very distal airways and alveoli by fluid or solid is called consolidation. The cardinal signs of consolidation are an area of increased opacity, which may have an irregular shape, irregular margins, a non-segmental distribution and contains an air bronchogram (Fig. 2.27). The volume of the affected lung remains unchanged and consequently there are no signs of loss of volume. If an area of consolidation abuts the mediastinum, heart or diaphragm their clear silhouette, which is dependent upon the sharp radiological contrast between normally aerated lung (black) and solid structures (white), is lost (Fig. 2.27). Similarly the presence of air bronchograms within an area of consolidation can be explained by the sharp contrast between air in the medium and large bronchi (black) and the surrounding non-aerated and 'solid' lung (white) (Figs 2.27, 2.28).

A variant of infective consolidation frequently seen in infants and children is the 'round pneumonia'. This may mimic a mass lesion radiologically since it has well-defined borders, but the clinical picture points to an infective aetiology. While infection is the most common cause, consolidation is also caused by any pathological process in which the alveoli are filled by fluid or solid.

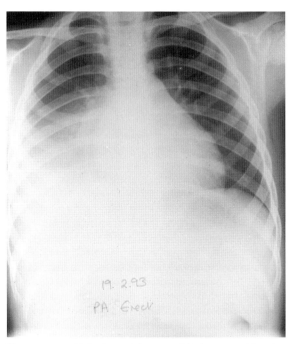

Figure 2.27 Right lower lobe consolidation caused by the bacterium *Streptococcus pneumoniae*. There is increased opacity in the right lower and mid zones, loss of the clear outline of the right hemidiaphragm and a proximal air bronchogram.

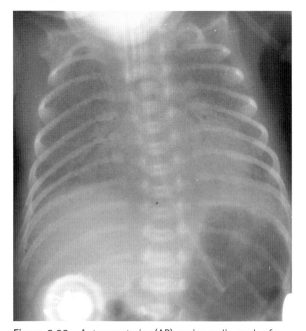

Figure 2.28 Anteroposterior (AP) supine radiograph of a premature neonate with respiratory distress syndrome (RDS). The lungs show generalized opacity due to consolidation and a prominent air bronchogram.

Box 2.3 Common causes of consolidation	
Pulmonary oedema	Cardiogenic
	Non-cardiogenic
	Respiratory distress syndrome
	Aspiration
Pulmonary exudate	Infection
Blood	Traumatic contusion
	Infarction
	Aspiration
Other causes	Alveolar proteinosis
	Alveolar microlithiasis
	Lymphoma
	Sarcoidosis

The most common causes of consolidation in paediatric practice are listed in Box 2.3.

Collapse

In collapse, air within the alveoli and distal airways is absorbed, resulting in loss of lung volume. This may affect a lung, lobe or segment. This is manifest on the radiograph by shift of the normal fissures and crowding of airways in the collapsed lung (Figs. 2.29, 2.30). If the volume loss is large there may also be mediastinal shift towards the affected side, elevation of the ipsilateral hemidiaphragm, ipsilateral rib crowding and alteration in hilar position. The collapsed lobe may or may not cause increased radio-opacity and there may be compensatory hyperinflation of unaffected lobes. If the collapsed lobe abuts on part of the diaphragm or cardiomediastinal silhouette, the clear outline of these may be lost on the radiograph, as in consolidation (Figs 2.29, 2.30). Collapse is most often due to obstruction of a large airway by foreign body, mucus plug, tumour or extrinsic compression. Less commonly it occurs secondary to poor ventilation.

Pleural fluid

The radiological appearance of pleural fluid is largely determined by the position of the patient. In the erect position the fluid collects at the bases and initially causes blunting of the costophrenic angles. Larger effusions cause a homogeneous opacity with a concave upper border higher laterally than medially – the meniscus. Very large effusions may cause mediastinal shift to the opposite side.

In the supine position, often used for neonatal and infant radiographs, an effusion causes reduced transradiancy (whiter hemithorax) of the affected side and may

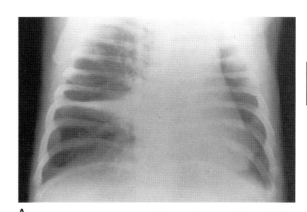

A

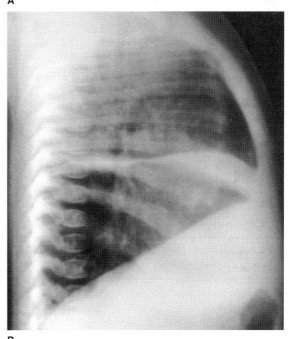

B

Figure 2.29   (A) Anteroposterior (AP) radiograph taken in a lordotic projection to show the band-like opacity of middle lobe collapse. Part of the right heart silhouette is lost where the collapsed lobe abuts the heart. (B) Lateral radiograph showing the collapsed middle lobe and displaced fissures. In addition, the lungs show generalized overinflation with some flattening of the diaphragm.

collect around the apex of the lung. In larger effusions a peripheral band of soft tissue density appears between the chest wall and the lung; on the right this band has a characteristic step at the position of the horizontal fissure (Figs 2.26, 2.31). Pleural fluid may collect and loculate within fissures or between the inferior surface of the lung and the diaphragm, the 'subpulmonic' effusion.

2

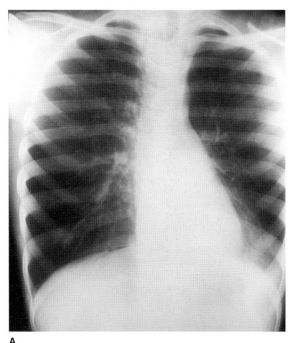

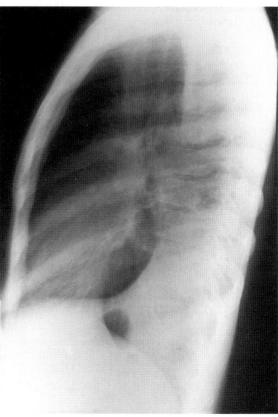

A   **B**

Figure 2.30   (A) Frontal radiograph of a patient with asthma and a left lower lobe collapse caused by a mucus plug. Generalized overinflation, increased opacity in the left cardiac region and loss of clarity of the outline of the medial left hemidiaphragm. (B) The lateral radiograph shows the collapsed left lower lobe as a wedge-shaped opacity in the lower chest posteriorly.

Pneumothorax

In the erect position pleural air collects at the apex, causing increased apical transradiancy (darker apex) and absent lung markings beyond a visible lung edge. In the supine position air collects initially in the antero-inferior chest, causing quite different and often subtle signs. These include small slivers of air at the apex, around the heart and between the lung and the diaphragm. Where free air as opposed to aerated lung abuts part of the cardiomediastinal or diaphragmatic silhouette, the clarity of that border is especially sharp, this being the opposite of the effect seen in consolidation. A large pneumothorax in neonates and infants when supine may collect anteriorly and cause an increased ipsilateral transradiancy (darker hemithorax) and increased sharpness of the cardiomediastinal silhouette (Fig. 2.32).

A tension pneumothorax occurs when a pleural tear acts as a one-way flap valve, allowing air into the pleural

space but preventing egress. The pressure within the hemithorax rises and may remain positive for much of the respiratory cycle, causing mediastinal shift to the contralateral side and flattening, or even eversion, of the ipsilateral hemidiaphragm (Fig. 2.33).

COMMON PAEDIATRIC CHEST PROBLEMS

Congenital abnormalities of the chest

Congenital diaphragmatic hernia

Large congenital diaphragmatic hernias frequently present as neonatal respiratory distress although many are now diagnosed antenatally on routine antenatal ultrasound examination. Many are associated with other congenital anomalies. Most hernias are left-sided, situated posteriorly and large. Abdominal organs are sited in the chest and appear on the radiograph as a cystic/solid mass. The mediastinum is shifted to the

2

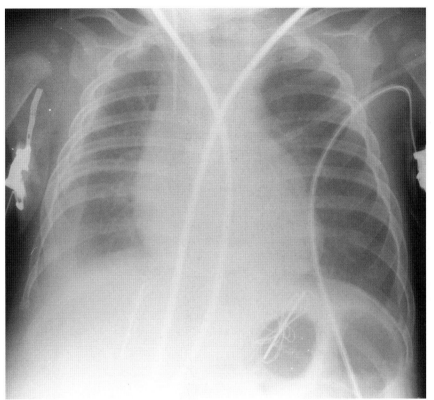

Figure 2.31 Supine radiograph showing a pleural effusion. There is reduced transradiancy on the right and a peripheral band of soft tissue density paralleling the chest wall with a 'step' at the position of the horizontal fissure.

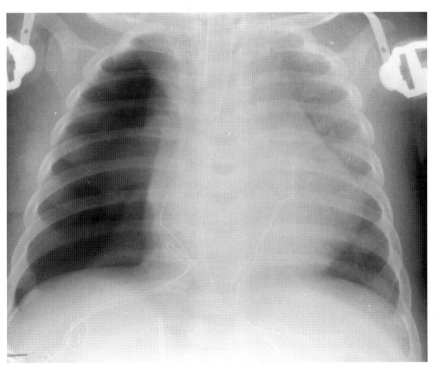

Figure 2.32 Supine radiograph showing a postoperative right pneumothorax. There is increased transradiancy of the right hemithorax. The right heart border is very clearly defined and the right lung edge is visible.

2

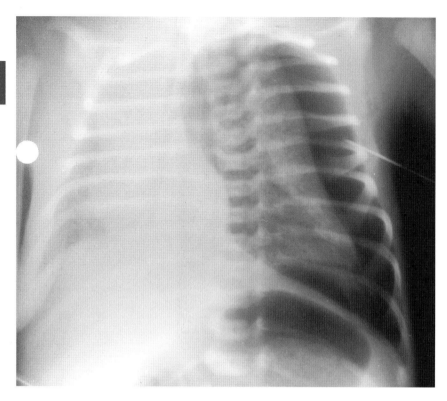

Figure 2.33 Supine radiograph of a patient with respiratory distress syndrome (RDS). There is a left tension pneumothorax causing flattening of the hemidiaphragm and mediastinal shift to the right. The pneumothorax is seen surrounding a consolidated left lung. A needle drain has been inserted.

contralateral side and one or both lungs may be hypoplastic (Fig. 2.34). When large, the condition carries a high mortality.

Hiatus hernia

A sliding hiatus hernia exists when the lower oesophageal sphincter and part of the stomach are situated in the thorax, above the diaphragm. This condition is usually associated with incompetence of the sphincter and may result in feeding problems, gastro-oesophageal reflux and aspiration. Gastro-oesophageal reflux may trigger episodes of reactive wheezing or of asthma. These episodes may be caused by microaspiration or be vagally mediated.

Congenital lobar emphysema

A focal abnormality of a lobar bronchus leads to a ball valve effect, causing air trapping and overinflation of the affected lobe. The left upper, right middle and right upper lobes are most frequently affected. Initial radiographs in the first few hours of life may show an opaque mass in the region of the affected lobe. As fluid clears, the appearances are those of an overinflated lobe with compression of normal surrounding lung and mediastinal shift to the contralateral side (Fig. 2.35). Treatment is surgical excision of the affected lobe if the neonate is

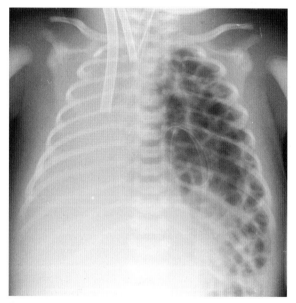

Figure 2.34 A large left diaphragmatic hernia. The left hemithorax contains the stomach (nasogastric tube) and loops of small bowel. The mediastinum is shifted to the right. The right lung is airless and opaque because the patient is on an extracorporeal membrane oxygenator (ECMO).

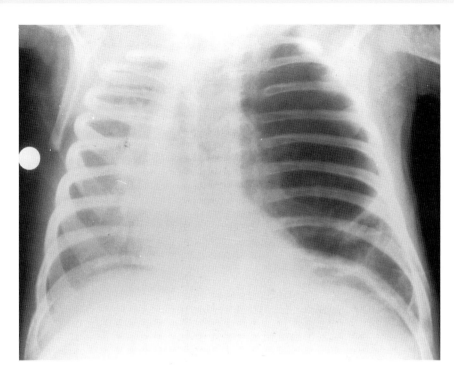

Figure 2.35 Congenital lobar emphysema of the left upper lobe. The lower lobe is compressed and the mediastinum is shifted to the right.

2

in respiratory distress; if found in the older infant, conservative management is advocated.

Congenital cystic adenomatoid malformation

This condition, caused by a disorganized and usually cystic mass of pulmonary tissue, can mimic both congenital diaphragmatic hernia and congenital lobar emphysema. The hamartomatous mass can affect any lobe, although the middle lobe is rarely affected, and in one-fifth of cases more than one lobe is affected. The radiograph shows a well-defined cystic mass, which may be large, compress adjacent lung and cause mediastinal shift.

Neonatal chest problems

Respiratory distress syndrome

Immature surfactant production in premature infants, infants of diabetic mothers and infants who experience perinatal asphyxia fail to reduce the alveolar surface tension sufficiently to prevent alveolar collapse. This is the most common cause of respiratory distress in premature neonates and causes tachypnoea, cyanosis, expiratory grunting and chest wall retraction. The radiograph shows bilateral symmetrical hypo-aeration, small volume lungs, ground-glass granularity of the pulmonary parenchyma and well-defined air bronchograms

extending from the hilum into the peripheral lung (see Fig. 2.28).

These neonates frequently require intermittent positive pressure ventilation which may give rise to specific complications of pulmonary interstitial emphysema (PIE) (Fig. 2.36), bronchopulmonary dysplasia (BPD) (Fig. 2.37), pneumothorax (Fig. 2.32) and pneumomediastinum.

Pulmonary interstitial emphysema is caused by gas leaking from overdistended alveoli and tracking along bronchovascular sheaths. The radiographic appearance is that of a branching pattern of gas with associated bubbles affecting all or part of the lung (see Fig. 2.36).

Bronchopulmonary dysplasia or chronic lung disease of prematurity (CLD) is seen exclusively in infants who have been on positive pressure ventilation, usually for RDS. The combination of high-pressure trauma and oxygen toxicity results in lung damage. The lung may pass through a number of radiological stages during the evolution of BPD. Initially there is an RDS pattern which progresses to almost complete opacification and then to a coarse pattern of linear opacities and cystic lucencies (Fig. 2.37). The lack of adequate oxygenation in RDS may result in failure of the ductus arteriosus to close. The consequent left-to-right shunt may progress to frank plethora and heart failure.

2

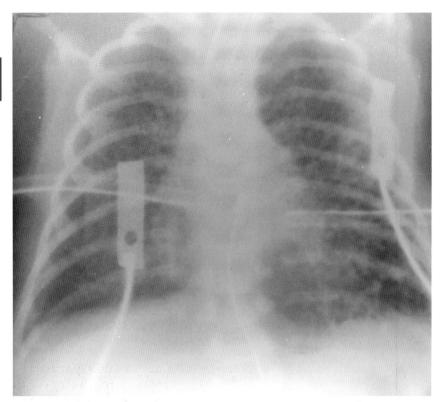

Figure 2.36 Pulmonary interstitial emphysema (PIE) complicating respiratory distress syndrome (RDS). There is a branching pattern of gas with associated small bubbles. Bilateral chest drains and persistent right pneumothorax.

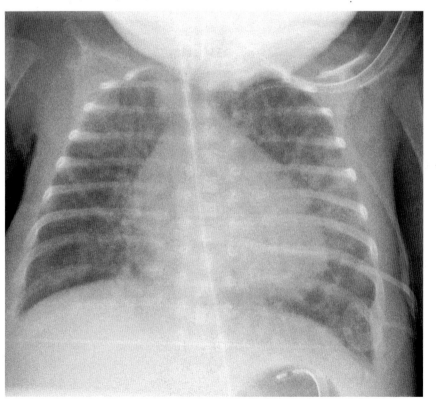

Figure 2.37 Bronchopulmonary dysplasia. A coarse pattern of linear opacities and cystic lucencies.

Meconium aspiration syndrome

This is the most common cause of respiratory distress in full- or post-term neonates. The aspirated meconium causes a chemical pneumonitis and bronchial obstruction. The radiographic picture is of bilateral diffuse patchy collapse with other areas of overinflation (Fig. 2.38). Spontaneous pneumothorax, pneumomediastinum and small effusions are common but air bronchograms are rare.

Respiratory tract infections

Viral infections

Viral infections generally affect the bronchi and peribronchial tissues and this is reflected in the radiological signs: symmetrical parahilar, peribronchial streaky shadowing radiating for a variable distance into the lung periphery, hilar lymphadenopathy, occasionally reticulonodular shadowing, segmental/lobar collapse and generalized overinflation secondary to narrowing of the bronchi (Fig. 2.39). Effusions are rare. Organisms commonly encountered are the respiratory syncytial virus (RSV), influenza and parainfluenza viruses, adenovirus and rhinovirus.

Bacterial and Mycoplasma infections

In the neonatal period the most common organisms are non-haemolytic streptococci, *Staphylococcus aureus* and *Escherichia coli*. Lobar consolidation is rare and more often the following signs are seen: radiating perihilar streakiness, coarse patchy parenchymal infiltrates, nodular or reticulonodular shadowing, or diffuse hazy shadowing, most often basal. One important pattern to recognize is the diffuse bilateral granularity of group B haemolytic streptococcal pneumonia, which so closely mimics RDS.

In infants bacterial infection is more often seen as lobar or patchy consolidations (Fig. 2.27). The organisms are most commonly *Haemophilus influenzae*, *Streptococcus pneumoniae*, *Staphylococcus aureus* and *Mycoplasma pneumoniae*. Pleural effusions, empyemas, abscesses and pneumatoceles are well-recognized complications. The 'round pneumonia' is an area of infective consolidation which transiently has a rounded configuration and mimics a mass lesion. *Mycoplasma pneumoniae* infection can mimic the radiographic appearances of both bacterial and viral pneumonia. However, one pattern that is highly specific is unilobar reticulonodular infiltration, especially if associated with hilar lymphadenopathy and a small pleural effusion.

Tuberculosis

Tuberculosis acquired in infancy is usually manifest by unilateral hilar or paratracheal lymphadenopathy and occasionally the primary or Ghon focus is seen as an area of consolidation in the periphery of the ipsilateral

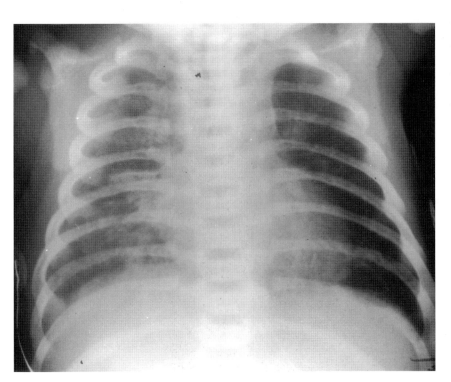

Figure 2.38 Meconium aspiration syndrome. Areas of patchy collapse with other areas of overinflation. The right lung is most severely affected.

2

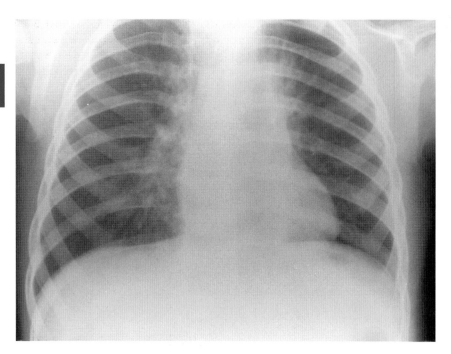

Figure 2.39 Viral pneumonia caused by the respiratory syncytial virus (RSV). There is symmetrical perihilar and peribronchial streaky shadowing and mild hilar lymphadenopathy.

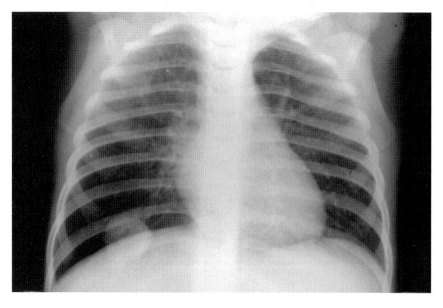

Figure 2.40 Primary tuberculous infection. Unilateral right hilar lymphadenopathy and an area of consolidation (Ghon focus) in the ipsilateral lower zone.

lung (Fig. 2.40). Collapse is seen, usually due to compression of a bronchus by lymph nodes. Bronchopneumonic spread, with widespread areas of consolidation, occurs if either an infected node discharges into a bronchus or when host resistance is very low, facilitating spread through the airways. Miliary tuberculosis, with multiple small nodules, is caused by the haematogenous spread that occurs when an infected node discharges

into the bloodstream. Cavitation is unusual in children.

Airway disease

Asthma

The radiological features are rarely seen before the age of 3 years. In chronic asthma there is generalized overinflation of the lungs with parahilar, peribronchial infiltrates but hilar lymphadenopathy is rare. Plugs of viscid mucus obstruct the airways and cause recurrent segmental or lobar collapse (Fig. 2.30). Pneumomediastinum is a common complication but rarely requires specific treatment; pneumothorax is seen less frequently. Asthma may be triggered by gastro-oesophageal reflux and barium studies may be useful in assessing the patient.

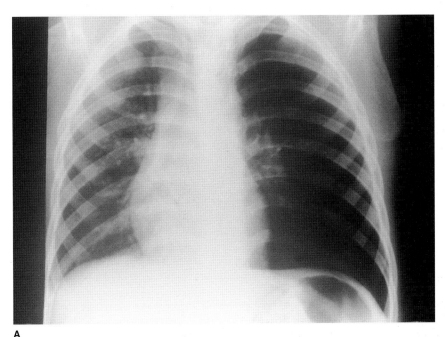

A

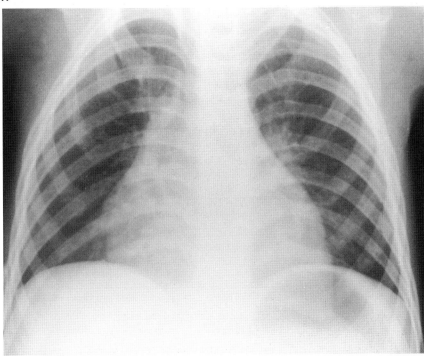

B

Figure 2.41 (A) Aspirated foreign body lodged in the left main stem bronchus. Marked air trapping in the affected lung causing overinflation, increased transradiancy and mediastinal shift. (B) Same patient after bronchoscopic removal of the obstruction.

2

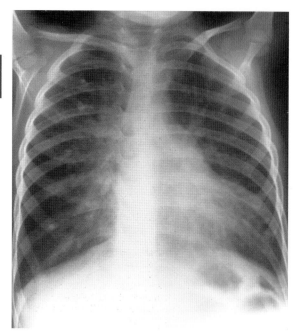

Figure 2.42 Cystic fibrosis: overinflation, focal collapse and parahilar, peribronchial infiltrates.

Obstruction by foreign bodies

Aspirated foreign bodies most commonly lodge in the major bronchi and act like a ball valve, causing a distal obstructive emphysema (Fig. 2.41). Radiographs are taken in inspiration and expiration to demonstrate the air trapping. Less commonly, the lung distal to the obstruction collapses and may become infected.

Cystic fibrosis and bronchiectasis

This autosomal recessive condition causes excessively thick and viscid mucus. In the neonatal period, bowel obstruction due to meconium ileus may draw attention to the condition. In the chest the earliest signs are very similar to those of viral bronchiolitis: overinflation, focal collapse and parahilar, peribronchial infiltrates (Fig. 2.42). Recurrent infections lead to bronchiectasis, fibrosis and generalized overinflation with segmental areas of collapse. Bronchial collaterals are recruited and when

these become large, haemoptysis may be a problem. HRCT is more accurate than radiographs in demonstrating early bronchiectasis and the involvement of small airways.

CT is also useful in identifying and accurately positioning small pneumothoraces facilitating accurate drainage.

Small airway disease

Inflammatory disease of the smaller airways is common and may occur following viral infection and as part of other conditions, including cystic fibrosis, asthma, recurrent aspiration, post-transplantation and post-chemotherapy. Inflammatory tissue narrows and obstructs the airways causing air trapping. Plain radiograph changes are variable and often underestimate the extent of the disease. Constrictive obliterative bronchiolitis (bronchiolitis obliterans) is best assessed using HRCT. The combination of areas of air trapping and inhomogeneous perfusion gives rise to the mosaic attenuation pattern with a mixed pattern of high- and low-density areas in the lung parenchyma. There may be associated abnormalities of the larger airways.

Swyer–James or Macleod's syndrome is an unusual form of post-infection constrictive obliterative bronchiolitis in which the lung changes are unilateral. In these cases the plain radiograph may show the characteristic feature of unilateral hypertransradiancy caused by air trapping.

Acknowledgements

I wish to acknowledge the huge contribution made to the paediatric section by Professor Isky Gordon of Great Ormond Street Hospital for Sick Children, an inspiring teacher and mentor who co-authored previous editions of this chapter. I also wish to thank Dr BJ Loveday at the Royal Surrey County Hospital, Guildford, and Dr DB Reiff at Ashford and St Peter's Hospital, for allowing us to use their radiographs as illustrations and Mrs Hazel Cook, Mrs Mary Shoesmith and Mrs Susan Ranson of the Department of Diagnostic Radiology at the Royal Surrey County Hospital, Guildford, and the Department of Medical Illustration at Great Ormond Street Hospital for Children, for their help in preparing the illustrations.

Further reading

Arthur R 2001 The neonatal chest X-ray. Paediatric Respiratory Reviews 2: 311–323

Copley SJ 2002 Application of computed tomography in childhood respiratory infections. British Medical Bulletin 61: 263–279

Copley SJ, Bush A 2000 HRCT of paediatric lung disease. Paediatric Respiratory Reviews 1: 141–147

De Bruyn R 1993 Paediatric chest. In: Cosgrove D, Meire H, Dewbury K (eds) Clinical ultrasound: abdominal and general ultrasound, vol. 2. Churchill Livingstone, London, pp 983–988

Frush DP 2005 Paediatric chest imaging. Radiologic Clinics of North America 43: 253–457

Gibson AT, Steiner GM 1997 Imaging the neonatal chest. Clinical Radiology 52: 172–186

Goodman LR 1999 Felson's principles of chest roentgenology: a programmed text, 2nd edn. WB Saunders, Philadelphia

Goodman LR, Putman CE 1991 Intensive care radiology: imaging of the critically ill, 3rd edn. WB Saunders, Philadelphia

Gordon I, Helms P, Fazio F 1981 Clinical applications of radionuclide lung scanning. British Journal of Radiology 54: 576–585

Gordon I, Matthew DJ, Dinwiddie R 1987 Respiratory system. In: Gordon I (ed) Diagnostic imaging in paediatrics. Chapman and Hall, London, pp 27–57

Grainger RG, Allison DJ, Dixon AK 2001 Grainger and Allison's diagnostic radiology. A textbook of medical imaging, 4th edn. Churchill Livingstone, Edinburgh

Hansell DM, Armstrong P, Lynch DA, McAdams HP 2005 Imaging of diseases of the chest, 4th edn. Elsevier Mosby, London

Hayden CK, Swischuk LE (eds) 1992 Pediatric ultrasonography, 2nd edn. Williams and Wilkins, Baltimore

Heitzmann ER 1988 The mediastinum: radiologic correlations with anatomy and pathology, 2nd edn. Springer-Verlag, Berlin

Hendry GMA 2000 Magnetic resonance imaging of the paediatric chest. Pae-diatric Respiratory Reviews 1: 249–258

Keats TE, Anderson MW 2001 Atlas of normal roentgen variants that may simulate disease, 7th edn. Mosby, St Louis

Kim OH, Kim WS, Kim MJ et al 2000 US (ultrasound) in the diagnosis of pediatric chest diseases. RadioGraphics 20: 653–671

Lipscombe DJ, Flower CDR, Hadfield JW 1981 Ultrasound of the pleura: an assessment of its clinical value. Clinical Radiology 32: 289–290

Newman B 1993 The pediatric chest. Radiologic Clinics of North America. 31: 453–719

Piepsz A, Gordon I, Hahn K 1991 Paediatric nuclear medicine. European Journal of Nuclear Medicine 18: 41–66

Reed JC 2003 Chest radiology: plain film patterns and differential diagnoses, 5th edn. Mosby, St Louis

Rossi UG, Owens CM 2005 The radiology of chronic lung disease in children. Archives of Disease in Childhood 90: 601–607

Simon G 1975 The anterior view chest radiograph – criteria for normality derived from a basic analysis of the shadows. Clinical Radiology 26: 429–437

Swischuk LE 1989 Imaging of the newborn, infant and young child, 3rd edn. Williams and Wilkins, Baltimore

Vix VA, Klatte EC 1970 The lateral chest radiograph in the diagnosis of hilar and mediastinal masses. Radiology 96: 307–316

Webb RW, Müller NL, Naidich DP 2001 High-resolution CT of the lung, 3rd edn. Lippincott Williams & Wilkins, Philadelphia

Chapter **3**

Cardiopulmonary function testing

Adults
Sally J Singh, Ian Hudson

The electrocardiogram[1]
Anne Ballinger, Stephen Patchett

Paediatrics
Indra Narang, Ian Balfour-Lynn

ADULTS

ASSESSMENT OF PULMONARY FUNCTION

Introduction

In health the human cardiorespiratory system has enormous reserve capacity to cope with the demands of exercise or illness. We are not normally aware of breathlessness or fatigue as a feature of resting activity. Furthermore, unless we harbour athletic ambitions, we are unlikely to explore the boundaries of our physiological limitations and assure ourselves that spare capacity would be present if it ever became necessary. The measurement of physiological capacity in health is, therefore, a matter of relevance only to the curious or the

[1]Reproduced from Ballinger & Patchett 2003 Saunders Pocket Essentials of Clinical Medicine, 3rd edn. WB Saunders, with permission.

serious competitor who wishes to improve his performance. In patients with heart or lung disease the erosion of physiological reserve eventually imposes limitations upon the activities of daily life. Under these circumstances the measurement of cardiopulmonary function allows the accurate assessment of disability and of the effect of therapeutic intervention. This chapter examines the scientific basis of clinical measurement and its relevance to physiotherapy.

It is reasonable and conventional to consider the function of the cardiovascular system in three compartments. First the lungs themselves, second the effectiveness of the integrated activity of gas exchange and acid–base balance, and finally the capacity of the circulatory system to deliver.

Lung function

The apparently simple function of the lung is to deliver oxygen to the gas-exchanging surface and exhaust carbon dioxide to the atmosphere. To achieve this, air is drawn by conductive flow into the alveoli and presented to the gas-exchanging surface where diffusion effects the process of exchange. The carriage of air through the airways depends on the patency of the tubes as well as on the consistency of the lung and the power of the respiratory muscles. These aspects of pulmonary function are commonly measured in lung function laboratories.

General principles of measurement

Lung function measurements are made to describe the lung for diagnostic purposes and subsequently in monitoring change. Accuracy and consistency are therefore very important and conventions exist for the procedures of measurement and expression of results. In general, a measurement will only be accepted after multiple attempts have been scrutinized and expressed under standard conditions. These are usually body temperature and atmospheric pressure (BTPS). To guarantee accuracy, laboratory practice should include regular physical and biological calibration of the equipment. Standards for good laboratory conduct have been described (British Thoracic Society/Association of Respiratory Technologists and Physiologists 1994). In health there are several factors that influence the magnitude of lung function. These include height, sex and age and to a lesser degree weight and ethnic origin (Anthonisen 1986, Cotes 1993). As a result, assessment of normality can only be made by comparison with reference values. The latter are obtained from the study of large numbers of normal people from the relevant population (European Community for Coal and Steel 1983). Once obtained, results can be expressed as percentage

predicted or, more correctly, by comparison with the 95% confidence interval for that value.

Airway function

For the purposes of measurement the lung has only one portal of entry and exit, i.e. through the mouth, and airway function is assessed by quantification of gas flow or volume. The calibre of the airways reduces through their generations and the major resistance to gas flow is normally in the upper airway. The larger airways are supported by cartilage, while the smaller airways are held patent by the radial traction of the surrounding lung so that their calibre increases with the volume of the lung. The diameter of these airways is also controlled by neural tone, which is predominantly parasympathetic.

The disruption of airway function can occur through physical or rigid obstruction to a large airway by, for example, a tracheal tumour. It may also occur because of more widespread disease in asthma, when large numbers of smaller airways are affected by episodic alteration of their calibre by smooth muscle contraction, mucosal oedema and intraluminal secretions. In chronic bronchitis, obstruction occurs by mucosal thickening and mucus secretion but in emphysema the mechanism is different. Though seldom occurring in isolation from other forms of airway obstruction, the result of parenchymal emphysema is to weaken the elastic structure which maintains radial traction on the airways and allows them to close too early in expiration.

Tests of airway function measure airway calibre and are now well established in clinical practice. Most tests of airway patency examine expiratory function. There are three common methods:

- spirometry (FEV_1 and FVC)
- flow–volume curves
- peak expiratory flow (PEF).

Production of the spirogram from a maximal forced expiration following a full inspiration is reliable and provides the forced expiratory volume in 1 second (FEV_1) and the forced vital capacity (FVC) (Fig. 3.1). The measurement is usually made using a spirometer, which measures volume, or is derived from a flow signal obtained from a pneumotachograph or turbine. Most commonly, the FEV_1 and FVC are measured during the same manoeuvre, but a greater vital capacity may be obtained in patients with airway disease if it is performed slowly. Reduction in FEV_1 with relative preservation of FVC or vital capacity (VC) is known as an 'obstructive' pattern, which indicates and grades airway obstruction: $FEV_1/FVC <75\%$ is graded as mild, $<60\%$ as moderate and $<40\%$ as severe impairment (American Thoracic Society 1986). Simultaneous reduction in both

3

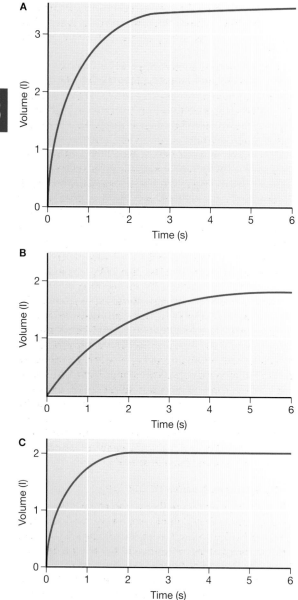

Figure 3.1   (A) In the normal spirogram the major part of the vital capacity (FVC) is expelled in 1 s (FEV₁). (B) In patients with airway obstruction the FEV₁ is reduced to a greater degree than the FVC. This pattern is known as 'obstructive'. (C) When the lungs are small and empty quickly the pattern is known as 'restrictive'.

FEV_1 and FVC with an increase in the FEV_1/FVC ratio is called a 'restrictive' defect and is usually associated with a reduction in lung volume. Abnormal values are defined as those recognized to be outside the normal range of two standard deviations for sex, height and age. This usually requires a reduction of about 15% from predicted values. Thus simple spirometry can detect and quantify airway obstruction, but gives no indication of the cause.

Measurement of the flow–volume curve is now commonplace and can provide information about the nature of airway obstruction. In this test, the gas flow from a full maximum expiration is plotted against the expired volume as the lung empties (Fig. 3.2). The flow of gas from the lung reaches a peak expiratory flow (PEF) after about 100 milliseconds and then declines linearly as the lung empties. If the measurement is continued into the subsequent full inspiration, a flow–volume 'loop' is produced and inspiratory flow rates can be measured. The shape of the expiratory and inspiratory portions are different, since in expiration the active expulsion is assisted by the elastic recoil of the lung while inspiratory flow rates are a reflection of airway calibre and inspiratory muscle strength only. Something of the nature of the airway obstruction can be learnt from consideration of the actual and relative values of PEF, peak inspiratory flow (PIF) and the values of expiratory flow at 50% and 75% vital capacity (MEF_{50} and MEF_{75}). Simple inspection of the loop is often sufficient to distinguish between rigid upper airway obstruction, intraluminal obstruction in chronic bronchitis and asthma, and the 'pressure-dependent' collapse seen in pure emphysema with relative preservation of inspiratory flow rates.

The PEF is one component of the flow–volume manoeuvre that is widely used owing to the availability of simple devices for its measurement. Provided that the patient does not have weak respiratory muscles and has made a maximum effort, the PEF will reflect airway calibre. The absolute values obtained are not particularly helpful unless they are extremely low but the easily repeated measurements can be used to obtain valuable insight into the mechanisms of variable airway obstruction in asthma. There is a normal diurnal variation in airway calibre of about 50 ml/min, which is exaggerated in patients with poorly controlled asthma (Benson 1983). Wider variation will be seen approaching or recovering from an attack and following exposure to trigger factors.

The real value of the PEF lies in its repeatability and its portability. The issue of meters to patients with asthma allows domiciliary and occupational investigation of asthma. PEF also provides an objective measurement for patients to use to monitor their asthma as part of a self-management plan and it can be used during hospital admissions to record the progress and predict the discharge of patients with airway disease. Although this is valuable in asthma where the airway obstruction is variable, it can show no change at all in patients with chronic airflow limitation in spite of a clinical improve-

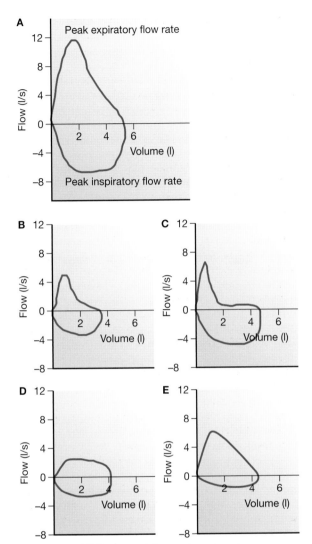

Figure 3.2 **(A)** The normal flow–volume loop has a characteristic shape. **(B)** Airway obstruction from asthma or chronic bronchitis appears as a concave expiratory limb and reduced inspiratory flows. **(C)** In emphysema the expiratory flows are suddenly attenuated but the inspiratory flows are relatively well preserved. **(D)** A rigid obstruction to a major airway can produce an oval loop. **(E)** Inspiratory flows are reduced in diaphragm weakness or extrathoracic tracheal obstruction.

3

ment. In this case the twice-weekly measurement of FEV_1 and FVC is more likely to mirror progress than will the slavish recording of the PEF chart (Gibson 1995).

Changes in spirometry are poorly related to clinical improvements after bronchodilator therapy in chronic obstructive pulmonary disease (COPD). O'Donnell et al (1999) have suggested that an increase in inspiratory capacity (a reflection of resting lung hyperinflation) may reflect improvements in exercise endurance capacity and dyspnoea more accurately than FEV_1 or FVC measures. Airway responsiveness is a measure of the degree of airway narrowing to specific and non-specific stimuli. Histamine and methacholine are the most widely used non-specific stimuli in challenge tests. Using the tidal breathing method (Juniper et al 1994), doubling concentrations of methacholine (0.03 to 16 mg/ml) are nebulized via a Wright nebulizer. Airway hyperresponsiveness is defined as a >20% fall in FEV_1 with a concentration of <8 mg/ml ($PC_{20}FEV_1$ <8 mg/ml).

Most asthmatics have a combination of eosinophilic airway, airway responsiveness and variable airflow obstruction to the extent that many definitions of asthma now include these three features. There is evidence that directing treatment at improving airway responsiveness reduces mild exacerbations of asthma. Elevated exhaled nitric oxide concentration due to increased inducible nitric oxide synthetase (INOS) expression and activity in the bronchial epithelium is a feature of untreated asthma (Kharitonov et al 1994). The relationship between nitric oxide (NO) and asthma severity or response to treatment is unclear (Sont et al 1999).

The physical properties of the lung

The two lungs contain millions of alveoli within a fibroelastic matrix. They do not have a very rigid structure and are held in contact with the rib cage by surface tension forces at the apposition of the two pleural surfaces. The resting volume of the lung (the functional residual capacity (FRC)) is thus determined by the outward spring of the rib cage and the inward elastic recoil of the lung matrix. Expansion and contraction of the lung therefore involves the controlled stretching or relaxation of the lung by the respiratory muscles away from FRC. The position of FRC can be influenced if the lung is stiffer than usual (as in interstitial disease) or if it is more compliant (as when damaged by emphysema). The measurement of the lung's volume can therefore give some insight into these conditions.

For obvious reasons direct measures of lung volume cannot be made. The most familiar method is helium dilution, which involves rebreathing through a closed circuit a mixture of gases containing a known concentration of helium, which is not absorbed into the circulation. The measurement of the final concentration of helium is used to calculate the gas dilution, or the 'accessible' volume, of the lung. An alternative method uses the Boyle's law principle: gas in the chest is compressed and the change in pressure is used to calculate the volume of gas within the chest. This method requires a large airtight box or plethysmograph. In both the actual volume that is estimated is the FRC, and total lung capacity (TLC) and residual volume (RV) are obtained from an additional spirometric trace. A further method involves the calculation of the total volume of the lung from the dimensions of a chest radiograph. This volume includes the total volume of gas, tissue and blood. Since the techniques do measure different aspects of volume, consistency in sequential measurements is important. In normal lungs the results are very similar, but where there is airway obstruction the values may be disparate. Such disparity can be used to advantage, e.g. in calculating the degree of trapped gas as the difference between the plethysmographic and helium dilution lung volumes.

The chest wall and the respiratory muscles

To maintain their shape the lungs depend on the support of the rib cage and the patency of the airways and alveoli. The expansion of the rib cage by the respiratory muscles is responsible for the tidal flow of gas into and out of the lungs. Over the past few years there has been increasing awareness of the importance of dysfunction of the respiratory muscles and the bony rib cage in contributing to respiratory failure. Such conditions include myopathies and polio as well as skeletal malformations such as scoliosis, which decrease rib cage compliance and reduce the effectiveness of the musculature.

The respiratory muscles include the diaphragm as the major muscle of inspiration and the intercostal muscles and scalenes. The latter, together with the sternomastoids, are known as the 'accessory muscles', but actually have a stabilizing role in tidal breathing. The combination of the respiratory muscles and the bony rib cage is called the 'chest wall' and conceptually is considered as the organ which inflates the lungs. Weakness of the respiratory muscles will eventually lead to ventilatory failure which may first become apparent during the night as an exaggeration of the normal nocturnal hypoventilation (Shneerson 1988).

The function of the respiratory muscles is difficult to study directly since the muscles have complex origins and insertions. Furthermore, their product, which is the pressure generated within the thoracic cavity, depends on the coordinated action of many muscles, the individual functions of which may be difficult to distinguish in life. It is possible to make some assessment of both the strength and endurance of the muscles and also to separate the diaphragm from the other muscles. The simple strength that the inspiratory and expiratory muscles can generate as pressure is easy to measure. The maximum inspiratory pressure ($P_i$max) and expiratory pressure ($P_e$max) are easy to measure with a manometer or electronic gauge. The normal values of approximately -100 cmH$_2$O and $+120$ cmH$_2$O (Black & Hyatt 1971) are well in excess of that needed to inflate the lungs (5–10 cmH$_2$O) and therefore provide a sensitive measure of developing muscle weakness. These measurements do have a learning requirement and are not suitable for monitoring of patients with rapidly developing muscle weakness, such as in Guillain–Barré syndrome. Under these circumstances the sequential measurement of the vital capacity is much more reliable, since a failure to maintain it will predict ventilatory failure.

The strength of the diaphragm can be separated from the other muscles by measuring the pressure gradient across it. This is achieved by using balloons attached to pressure transducers to estimate the pressure in the oesophagus and the stomach. The gradient across the diaphragm during a maximum inspiration or sniff is an indirect measure of the strength of the diaphragm. Normal values for sniff pressures have now been published (Uldry & Fitting 1995). If required, a value free of volition can be obtained by electrical stimulation of the phrenic nerve in the neck or even by magnetic stimulation of the cerebral cortex.

Fortunately, measurements of separate diaphragm strength are seldom required in clinical practice. A simple guide to diaphragm function can be obtained by observation of the change in vital capacity with posture. When supine, the vital capacity normally falls by 8–10%, but when diaphragm weakness is present it may fall by more than 30%. The measurement of the supine vital capacity is therefore a good screening test of diaphragm function (Green & Laroche 1990) and the measurement of sniff pressures at the mouth or nose is a reflection of pure diaphragmatic activity.

Gas exchange and oxygen delivery

The requirements of the average cell for oxygen are quite modest and a mitochondrion may need a PO_2 of as little as 1 kPa (7.5 mmHg) to function effectively. At sea level the atmospheric PO_2 is 20 kPa (150 mmHg) (FiO$_2$ = 0.21) and in the process of delivering oxygen to the cell, there is a loss along this gradient. The first step is the dilution of inspired air with expired air within the alveolus. Each tidal breath V_T contains a portion of gas which will remain within the airways and not come into contact with the alveoli. This is known as the 'dead-

3

space ventilation' V_D and must be achieved before any effective alveolar ventilation V_A can take place:

$$V_T = V_D + V_A$$

Alveolar gas therefore contains a mixture of fresh gas and some expired CO_2 and the alveolar PO_2 is reduced to about 16 kPa (120 mmHg) before gas exchange begins.

At the alveolar level, gas exchange involves the transfer across the alveolar–capillary membrane of oxygen molecules to the blood and the reverse transfer of carbon dioxide. This is achieved by simple diffusion, which is amplified in the case of oxygen by the affinity of haemoglobin. It normally takes mixed venous blood about 300 milliseconds (ms) to traverse a capillary and complete equilibrium usually occurs in about 100 ms. This aspect of oxygen transfer from the lung to the blood can be tested using carbon monoxide. Carbon monoxide has a very strong affinity for haemoglobin, follows the same path into the blood and can be measured easily. This principle forms the basis of the carbon monoxide transfer test, which measures the amount of carbon monoxide that can be transferred to the blood in the course of a single breath (TLCO). This gives a rough indication of the gas-transferring ability of the lung as a whole and is reduced in conditions such as fibrosing alveolitis, emphysema and pneumonectomy where the quality or quantity of the gas-exchanging surface is reduced. If the total TLCO is corrected for lung volume then the subsequent value is known as the 'coefficient of gas transfer' (KCO) and describes the gas-exchanging quality of the lung that is available for ventilation. For example, a very large normal man and a small child should have different TLCOs but their KCO values should be identical.

The carbon monoxide transfer test can give some information about the ability of the lung to transfer gas, but there is not a direct relationship between the TLCO and arterial oxygenation. The lung contains millions of alveolar–capillary units and adequate oxygenation depends on the coordinated, satisfactory function of the whole unit. The pulmonary causes of arterial hypoxaemia have four major origins:

- hypoventilation
- interference with pulmonary diffusion
- ventilation/perfusion imbalance
- true shunt.

Hypoventilation is fairly easy to recognize because the fall in arterial PO_2 is associated with a rise in arterial PCO_2. This occurs in ventilatory failure associated with airway obstruction, chest wall disease and drug intoxication. Interference with pulmonary diffusion is quite rare because the process is very efficient. However, the

system may be stretched at altitude or in the presence of disease such as fibrosing alveolitis. Even in this disease the hypoxia is related to increased pulmonary capillary transit time rather than to diffusion failure. The most common contribution to hypoxaemia in many diseases is ventilation/perfusion ($\dot{V}/\dot{Q}$) imbalance. Since effective lung function depends on the coordination of equivalent ventilation and perfusion to all units, it is not surprising that failure of the local matching mechanisms can cause trouble. The most extreme example would be a pulmonary embolus where ventilation continues in an area with no circulation. In other conditions such as asthma, the patchy distribution of airway obstruction will have similar but less dramatic effects. Some blood passes through the lung without coming into contact with the gas-exchanging surface. Normally this is a very small quantity (<5%), but effective shunts can be considerable in pneumonia and other conditions where the alveoli are blocked by inflammatory exudate although the circulation continues through the ineffective portion of the lung. This results in extreme hypoxia, which cannot easily be corrected by additional oxygen.

Oxygen carriage and arterial blood gases

Oxygen and carbon dioxide are carried in the blood in different ways. Oxygen is immediately bound to haemoglobin and released in the tissues under conditions of low oxygen tension or acidosis. Very little oxygen is carried in solution in the blood under conditions of normal pressure, although this can be increased in a hyperbaric chamber. By contrast, carbon dioxide is carried in the blood entirely in solution, mostly as bicarbonate. The difference between the two forms of carriage of the metabolic gases is fundamental to the interpretation of the measurement of arterial blood gases. The individual cell requires oxygen to survive, but the carriage of oxygen in the blood will have no effect on the body other than the delivery. By contrast, the chemistry involved in the carriage of carbon dioxide controls the short-term acid–base state of the body. When considering blood gas measurements, it is best to examine these functions separately.

The normal atmospheric PO_2 is approximately 20 kPa (150 mmHg) falling to 16 kPa (120 mmHg) within the alveolus. The arterial PO_2 (PaO_2) is usually about 14 kPa (105 mmHg) in a healthy subject. Although we are used to these values, they are only true at sea level and really only have relevance because the partial pressure is easy to measure. What matters to the individual cell is the quantity of oxygen that it receives, not the partial pressure. Oxygen delivery to the tissues depends on other factors, including the amount of haemoglobin, the degree of saturation of haemoglobin with oxygen and the rate at which oxygenated blood is delivered to the tissues. Assuming that the haemoglobin and the cardiac output are normal, then the measurement of oxygen saturation of haemoglobin is more relevant to oxygen delivery than is the PaO_2. The PaO_2 is related to oxygen saturation in a complex manner determined by the properties of haemoglobin and known as the 'oxygen dissociation curve' (Fig. 3.3). This relationship demonstrates that, under most conditions, once PaO_2 reaches 8 kPa (60 mmHg), haemoglobin is fully saturated and cannot carry more oxygen. Thus an arterial PO_2 above that value is only an insurance measure.

The availability of pulse oximeters has made the non-invasive measurement of oxygen saturation (SpO_2) com-

monplace. Pulse oximeters work by transcutaneous examination of the colour spectrum of haemoglobin, which changes with its degree of saturation. These instruments are reasonably accurate over the top range of saturation, but become unreliable below about 50% (Tremper & Barker 1989). The measurement of SpO_2 is an extremely valuable tool for monitoring patients' safety. There are, however, some important aspects of interpretation of its use that may be potentially hazardous. Oximetry provides information about oxygen saturation and this will relate to ventilation only if the inspired oxygen level is normal. Monitoring oxygen saturation will not detect underventilation and a rising $PaCO_2$. In patients who are breathing additional oxygen, a false sense of security can be given by a normal SpO_2 even though the $PaCO_2$ is rising. Furthermore, accurate recording of SaO_2 requires a good peripheral circulation which may often be compromised in patients who are hypovolaemic.

The assessment of acid–base status requires the measurement of arterial blood gas tensions. The average blood gas analyser measures PO_2, PCO_2 and pH. It subsequently calculates from the Henderson–Hasselbalch equation the values of bicarbonate, standard bicarbonate and base excess. The appreciation of the acid–base state requires examination of $PaCO_2$ and pH. Abnormalities are usually described in terms of their generation (Fig. 3.4). For example, a respiratory acidosis resulting from underventilation will display a low pH and an elevated $PaCO_2$. If this has been present for any length of time the serum bicarbonate will have become elevated and acid is excreted by the kidneys to compensate. In cases of nocturnal hypoventilation the daytime

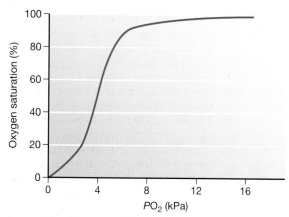

Figure 3.3 The oxygen dissociation curve relates oxygen saturation to ambient PO_2. In lung disease it is important to recognize that oxygen delivery is assured if PaO_2 is in excess of 8 kPa.

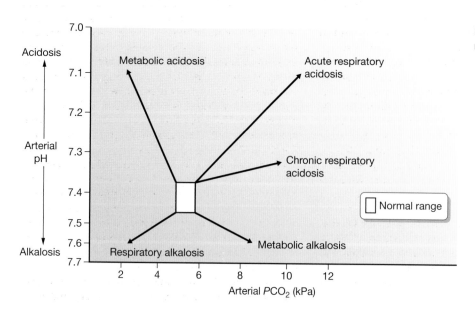

Figure 3.4 Acid–base relationships.

PaO_2 may be normal, but the elevation of the base excess gives a clue to the ventilatory history. If an alkalosis (high pH) is associated with a low $PaCO_2$, then this could be due to voluntary hyperventilation and is termed a 'respiratory alkalosis'. The build-up of acid products in diabetes or renal failure will result in a low pH and bicarbonate together with a low $PaCO_2$ in an attempt to compensate for a metabolic acidosis. Finally, the loss of acid from the stomach in prolonged vomiting can produce a metabolic alkalosis, which is characterized by high pH, high bicarbonate and normal $PaCO_2$. These sketches of blood gas disturbance are superficial interpretations, but they provide a useful framework for clinical management under most circumstances.

Respiratory failure

Respiratory failure is defined as inadequate oxygen delivery. As we have seen, this can be due to a variety of circumstances and may or may not be accompanied by a disturbance of the CO_2 level. The critical PaO_2 level is approximately 8kPa (60 mmHg), since a lower pressure than this will prejudice oxygen saturation and delivery. Therefore, respiratory failure is defined by convention as $PaO_2 < 7.3$ kPa (54.8 mmHg). If the $PaCO_2$ is elevated above 6.5 kPa (48.8 mmHg), this is termed 'ventilatory failure' and is associated with chronic airflow limitation or other forms of hypoventilation.

The understanding of respiratory failure has changed in recent years with the recognition that it is seldom due to a single malfunction of the respiratory system. For example, the rise in $PaCO_2$ and hyperinflation associated with worsening airway obstruction may adversely affect the respiratory muscles and introduce a chest wall contribution to failure. Conversely, the loss of lung volume associated with muscle weakness may lead to atelectasis and decreased pulmonary compliance, which will in turn put a greater load on the lung. Understanding of the complexities of chronic respiratory failure has helped to improve the outlook for some groups of patients, e.g. those with ventilatory failure due to chest wall disease or obstructive sleep apnoea. In these conditions there are abnormalities of breathing during sleep, which may result in nocturnal hypoventilation or transient apnoea that produce periods of oxygen desaturation which may spill over to the daytime. Recognition of this by oximetry and other more detailed somnography may result in effective treatment by nocturnal nasal intermittent positive pressure ventilation or continuous positive airway pressure (CPAP). By extension these techniques may also have a place in the acute management of selected patients with COPD who have diminished respiratory drive (Wedzicha 1996).

Oxygen prescription

The prescription of oxygen for patients with COPD is well defined for long-term (more than 15 hours/day) use. An indication for long-term oxygen therapy (LTOT) is a PaO_2 less than 7.3 kPa, when breathing room air during a period of clinical stability. Clinical stability is defined as the absence of exacerbation of COPD and of peripheral oedema for the last 4 weeks. Ambulatory oxygen is defined as 'oxygen delivered by equipment that can be carried by most patients during exercise and activities of daily living' (Ram & Wedzicha 2004). It should be provided to individuals who are on LTOT, need to be mobile and to leave the house. Patients without chronic hypoxaemia and LTOT should be considered for ambulatory oxygen if they have demonstrable desaturation on exercise. It is suggested that the level of desaturation should be at least 4%, to a saturation below 90%, on a standard exercise test while breathing room air. An improvement of at least 10% in distance and/or breathlessness score on repeat testing with supplemental oxygen warrants the prescription of an ambulatory system. Lacasse et al (2005) found that ambulatory oxygen had no effect on the Chronic Respiratory Questionnaire or the 6-minute walk test (6MWT) distance completed after a trial of domiciliary ambulatory oxygen. A second study did, however, report modest improvements in quality of life with domiciliary ambulatory oxygen (Eaton et al 2002). The prescription of short-burst oxygen is less well defined. There is no evidence to support firm recommendation and further research is required to establish its place.

Posture and thoracic surgery

Knowledge of the effect of posture and thoracic surgery on pulmonary function is obviously very important to the physiotherapist. The circumstances of treatment make this knowledge of practical benefit. Lung function measurements are usually made sitting or standing, but the major postural effect occurs due to gravity in the supine position. There is a small fall in VC (8%) and a reduction in FRC while lying down, which results from repositioning of the diaphragm and pooling of blood in the chest. This change can be used to advantage to identify patients with covert diaphragm weakness where the VC may drop by more than 30%. Gravity also produces a change in the distribution of ventilation and perfusion within the lungs. In the supine posture, ventilation and perfusion are preferentially directed to the dependent zones (Kaneko et al 1966). This is important in adults if the lung disease is unilateral, since oxygenation will be better if the good lung is dependent.

Physiotherapists are often involved in the assessment of patients for cardiothoracic surgery and their subsequent management. Some thoracic surgery, such as lung volume reduction surgery (American Thoracic Society 1996), bullectomy or decortication, improves lung function but most procedures impair the lung. The mechanisms of impairment include the anaesthetic, the thoracotomy and pulmonary resection. Following anaesthesia there is an immediate loss of FRC and subsequently VC, which reaches a trough of about 40% at 24 hours and may take up to 2 weeks to recover (Jenkins et al 1988). This immediate loss of volume is associated with a widened gradient across the lung (A–aDO$_2$) and potential hypoxia which is worsened by obesity, age and smoking. Thoracotomy itself, without pulmonary surgery, will reduce the VC by approximately 10%, which recovers over a period of 3 months. There are no strong arguments for the benefit of median sternotomy over thoracotomy as far as recovery of long-term lung function is concerned. In the short term the physiotherapist should be cautious during treatment as gas exchange will be impaired if the patient is lying on the thoracotomy side.

The surgical removal of lung tissue does not necessarily have the predictable effects on function that might be imagined. Following pneumonectomy the functional state of the patient is remarkably stable and in the long term the VC and total lung capacity (TLC) become slightly larger than expected for one lung. The TLCO eventually settles to 80% predicted and the KCO may be high since the whole pulmonary blood flow now travels through one lung. The changes after lobectomy are surprisingly different. The long-term effects may be small but in the postoperative phase the disruption may be unexpectedly large. The contusion of lung adjacent to the lobectomy sets up $\dot{V}/\dot{Q}$ disturbances which may in the short term be as significant as removal of the whole lung.

The physiological assessment of patients for thoracic surgery is not straightforward. There is no single test that allows a distinction to be made between success and failure. It is important to consider the nature of the operation and the preoperative function as well as general health, weight and smoking habit. If there is any doubt about the suitability of a candidate from spirometry, full lung function and oxygen saturation at rest, then some assessment of exercise capacity is advisable (British Thoracic Society and Society of Cardiothoracic Surgeons 2001).

Lung volume reduction surgery

There has been a recent resurgence of interest in this technique, which can potentially make a dramatic improvement to the function of patients with more diffuse pulmonary emphysema. The technique is a development of bullectomy, which removes approxi-

mately 30% of the substance of the lung, resulting in deflation of the chest wall. Surprisingly this operation can produce improvements in FEV$_1$ and elastic recoil pressure while reducing hyperinflation. There appear to be promising results in selected patients with more heterogeneous emphysema who have marked symptomatic hyperinflation (Criner et al 1999, Geddes et al 2000). Selection of patients for this procedure has yet to be well defined but preliminary data suggest that exercise capacity as measured by a SWT distance >150 m (Geddes et al 2000), or a 6MWD >200 m and a resting $PaCO_2$ <45 mmHg (Szekely et al 1997) were associated with a successful surgical outcome. A multicentre randomized controlled trial, conducted in North America, further refined the selection of patients for this procedure and suggested that upper lobe emphysema and a low baseline exercise tolerance was associated with a favorable outcome compared with other groups of patients. (Fishman et al 2003)

The effect of growth and ageing on lung function

The respiratory system reaches its peak in the third decade of life. Development of the lung continues from birth until the end of adolescence and starts to deteriorate after the age of 25 years. Fortunately, in the absence of disease there is sufficient reserve capacity to see out old age without discomfort!

The actual measurement of pulmonary function in childhood is problematic because of the obvious lack of cooperation. It is possible to measure lung volume and partial flow–volume curves in infancy by using an adapted plethysmograph. This is possible in the sedated child by producing a pneumatic 'hug' as an alternative to active expiration. In older children it is difficult to obtain cooperation for measurements until they are about 8 years old. After this age lung function can be measured easily, but there are difficulties in interpretation and production of reference values (see paediatric section of this chapter). The inconsistency of the timing of puberty and rapid growth spurts make comparisons difficult, but normal ranges have been produced for these age groups (Polgar & Promadhat 1971, Rosenthal et al 1993a).

The most obvious differences between children and adults lie in the development of airway function. The airways develop faster than the alveoli, which may not reach maturity until about the seventh year. As the lung matrix develops, the airway walls remain strong and relatively patent. As a result expiratory flow rates, although lower than in adulthood, are relatively high. For example, the FEV$_1$/FVC ratio may be greater than 90% and the expiratory flow–volume curve may have a flat or convex appearance. In addition to airway patency there are also developments in the behaviour of the chest wall with growth. In childhood the musculoskeletal structures are immature and flexible. Rib cage distortion is often seen in childhood during illness, but disappears with growth and muscularization. The combination of airway patency and plasticity of the chest wall allows an interesting experiment. In childhood the residual volume (RV) is not determined by airway closure but by the strength of the expiratory muscles. Thus if children or young adults are hugged at the end of a forced expiration more air can be expelled. After the age of 25 years, RV is determined by premature airway closure and the lungs cannot be emptied further.

Life after 25 years is all downhill for the respiratory system. As with general ageing, the tissues become less elastic and the lung elastic recoil diminishes. TLC tends to remain static but RV rises as the FEV_1 and FVC fall with age. Arterial PO_2 and A-aDO_2 worsen but do not reach critically low values. Exercise capacity, as judged by oxygen consumption, shows a decline with age but it can be retarded by regular activity. As general levels of activity reduce with age, these effects are not usually important, but smoking or disease may accelerate the changes.

Interpretation of lung function tests

Once a baseline has been established, changes in function can be used to assess progress with natural history or treatment. Although there may be some investigations that are specific to various diseases, it is seldom possible to rely on a single investigation for the purpose. The usual description of disease requires the combination of spirometry, lung volume and gas transfer measurement. The addition of bronchodilator response, a flow–volume loop and blood gases would provide further information, while additional specific tests are requested as indicated. The additional tests may include an exercise study or respiratory muscle function test to examine the relevant aspect. Interpretation of the tests involves the comparison of the values to the reference population and a description of the pattern of abnormality, if present. A helpful report will also give some guidance on the accuracy of the clinical diagnosis and suggest confirmatory investigations if the diagnosis is unclear. Some examples of clinical cases and the patterns of abnormal lung function are given in Table 3.1.

The measurement of disability and exercise testing

Static lung function tests can describe the physical properties of the lungs, but do not always reflect the perfor-

mance of the cardiopulmonary system in action. The relationship between disability and spirometry is poor. To assess disability, it must be measured by an exercise test or inferred from questioning. Exercise tests are valuable in making an objective assessment of disability and in observing the physiological response to exercise in order to assist diagnosis. Tests of exercise performance can either be performed in a complex manner in the laboratory or simply by observation of walking achievement down a hospital corridor. The former generally examines the detailed physiological response, while walking tests can give a useful and reproducible assessment of disability. A further value of exercise testing is to use the stimulus to provoke bronchoconstriction where exercise-induced asthma is suspected. In this context the exercise should be performed in an environment as close as possible to that which produces the symptoms.

Questionnaires

Most people do not ordinarily stress the lungs to their physiological limit. Furthermore, patients with exercise limitation adopt a restricted lifestyle, which may hide their disability. Sometimes simple questions can identify the disruption of normal activity. An overall picture of disability can be judged by application of a detailed questionnaire designed to cover either general features of disability or those that relate to specific examples. There are several disease-specific questionnaires available for chronic lung disease. The Chronic Respiratory Questionnaire (CRQ) (Guyatt et al 1987) and St George's Respiratory Questionnaire (Jones 1991) have been validated for use in patients with COPD and asthma. Until recently the CRQ was an operator-led questionnaire and therefore quite time consuming. A self-reported CRQ has been described, and tested for repeatability and sensitivity (Williams et al 2001, 2003)

These questionnaires are quite good at distinguishing change after an intervention (Griffiths et al 2000, Sewell et al 2005) but not as sensitive when making comparisons between patients. This is particularly true of the CRQ, which uses individualized questions to obtain sensitivity. The Breathing Problems Questionnaire (BPQ) (Hyland et al 1994) is another self-administered, disease-specific instrument that can provide a good comparative description of disability. More recent developments include the shortened BPQ (Hyland et al 1998) developed specifically for rehabilitation and the AQ-20 (Hajiro et al 1999). The Medical Research Council (MRC) dyspnoea scale has been shown to relate reasonably well to shuttle walk test performance (Bestall et al 1999) and may give a quick and simple yet reasonably accurate measure of function in a clinical setting.

3

Table 3.1 Conclusions from pulmonary function tests are best derived from the examination of several measurements

a A 66 year old man with chronic airflow limitation. There is an increase in lung volumes or hyperinflation of TLC and RV. The spirometry is obstructive but there is good bronchodilator reversibility, especially in the vital capacity. TLCO is slightly reduced but not as low as would be found in severe emphysema. The picture is one of smoking-related airflow obstruction, with the potential for some improvement.

b A 49 year old man with cryptogenic fibrosing alveolitis. There is a 'restrictive' defect with loss of lung volumes. Spirometry is not restrictive because of coexisting smoking-related airway obstruction. After treatment with prednisolone (10 March 1992) all values improved.

c A 40 year old woman with severe muscle weakness. There is a 'restrictive' picture, but the KCO is elevated because gas exchange is relatively normal. Respiratory muscle strength is reduced.

a	Predicted	Observed	Post-bronchodilator
FEV_1 (l)	2.86	1.15	1.30
FVC (l)	4.11	2.80	3.55
FEV_1/FVC (%)	70.00	41.00	37.00
TLC (l)	6.98	7.47	
RV (l)	2.54	4.24	
TLCO (mmol/min/kPa)	8.80	6.72	
KCO (mmol/min/kPa/l)	1.33	1.06	
VA (l)		6.33	

b	Predicted	23 April 1991	10 March 1992
FEV_1 (l)	3.75	1.70	2.45
FVC (l)	4.94	2.40	3.30
FEV_1/FVC (%)	75.00	71.00	74.00
TLC (l)	7.59	4.34	5.55
RV (l)	2.41	1.67	2.10
TLCO (mmol/min/kPa)	10.95	5.82	7.36
KCO (mmol/min/kPa/l)	1.57	1.38	1.77
VA (l)		4.06	4.20

c	Predicted	Observed
FEV_1 (l)	2.27	0.8
FVC (l)	2.83	1.10
FEV_1/FVC (%)	77.00	73.00
TLC (l)	4.25	1.89
RV (l)	1.22	0.85
TLCO (mmol/min/kPa)	7.49	3.84
KCO (mmol/min/kPa/l)	1.79	2.44
VA (l)	4.15	1.58
$P_e$max (cmH$_2$O)	59–127	50.00
$P_i$max (cmH$_2$O)	29–117	40.00

Laboratory estimation of exercise capacity

Observation of the physiological response to exercise in the laboratory is the gold standard measurement of disability. This is usually performed during a progressive maximal test, which is completed when the subject is unable to continue on either a treadmill or a cycle ergometer. The latter provides a stable platform and more accurate assessment of workload, while the walking action on the treadmill will be more familiar to most patients. In health a greater $\dot{V}O_2$ is achieved on the treadmill, but this is not necessarily the case in severe COPD where the cycle may be a greater exercise stimulus (Mathur et al 1995).

While the exercise is progressing, the basic physiological response is observed by measuring ventilation, heart rate and oxygen uptake and carbon dioxide production. Other measurements such as oxygen saturation or cardiac output can be made if necessary. The test is conducted in such a fashion as to obtain a symptom-limited duration of about 10 minutes with the increments of workload increased every minute by about 50 watts (W) for healthy subjects (10 W or less for patients with COPD). During this period the heart rate will rise linearly with workload. Ventilation also rises linearly until about 60% of maximum workload when it increases disproportionately. Oxygen uptake ($\dot{V}O_2$) will also rise linearly until the same point above which the rate of uptake slows and eventually reaches a plateau at the maximum oxygen uptake ($\dot{V}O_2$max) (Fig. 3.5). The $\dot{V}O_2$max is determined in health by the cardiovascular delivery of oxygen to the muscles and is a crude estimate of capacity and cardiopulmonary fitness. The point of inflection of pulmonary ventilation on the $\dot{V}_E$ vs $\dot{V}O_2$ slope is known as the 'anaerobic threshold'. It is usually measured by the gas exchange method ($\dot{V}O_2$ vs $\dot{V}CO_2$ plot) or lactate accumulation. In patients with lung disease the limits to maximal exercise may be different. For example, maximal performance may be limited by low muscle mass, ventilation, respiratory muscle impairment and gas exchange. For this reason patients with COPD do not demonstrate a true $\dot{V}O_2$max because performance is terminated prematurely by the ventilatory limit imposed by airway obstruction. Fatigue from limb muscle weakness may also be a significant factor in these patients.

The value of exercise testing in lung disease lies in the measurement of the degree of functional impairment by assessment of the maximal workload and $\dot{V}O_2$max in comparison with reference values. If a patient fails to achieve his predicted performance the mode of failure can help to identify the mechanism. For example, in patients with lung disease the early rise of $\dot{V}_E$ may be characteristically in excess of expectations, but reach a premature limit imposed by the physical constraints of damaged lungs. Concurrently the heart rate response may be attenuated, in contrast to patients with cardiac disease where the test may have to be terminated because of early attainment of maximum predicted heart rate or chest pain. It is always important to determine why the subject stops at the end of a test.

The value of exercise testing

- Differential diagnosis of dyspnoea
- Objective assessment of disability
- Assessment of therapeutic intervention
- Identification of exercise-induced asthma
- Prescription of an exercise training programme.

Field exercise tests

Laboratory tests of performance are the most accurate but are not always available and require expensive equipment. As an alternative, several field tests have been developed which can measure performance, and their results relate quite well to laboratory estimates. There are two main categories of field test – those which are unpaced and those where the speed of activity is imposed.

One of the first unpaced tests was the 12-minute running test, which was developed to assess the fitness of military personnel. This concept was adapted to the needs of the respiratory patient by downgrading the activity to a walk along a hospital corridor. Later, a reduction of the time to 6 minutes appeared to have no disadvantages. The 12- and 6-minute walks have become familiar forms of assessment for respiratory patients (Butland et al 1982, McGavin et al 1976). The test procedure is extremely simple, with a course marked out

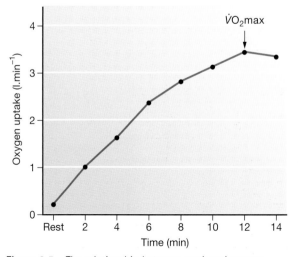

Figure 3.5 The relationship between work and oxygen uptake during progressive exercise.

along the corridor and the patient given the simple instruction to cover as much ground as possible in the time permitted. These tests have proven value but also have some limitations. There is quite a large learning effect and the reproducibility only becomes acceptable after two or more attempts (Knox et al 1988, Mungall & Hainsworth 1979). In addition, no two patients will attack the test in the same way and the relative stresses may not allow direct comparison. Lastly, the lack of pace constraint makes the test performance vulnerable to mood and encouragement (Guyatt et al 1984). Nevertheless, these simple tests require no equipment and, within their limitations, provide valuable information about general exercise capacity and major therapeutic changes. The minimal clinically important difference (MCID) for the 6MWT has been defined within the context of a rehabilitation programme. Redelmeier et al (1997) suggested that for a patient to notice an improvement the increase must be at least 54 metres.

The second type of field exercise test imposes a pace on the patient, which reduces the effect of motivation and encouragement. An endurance walking test instructs the patient to walk at a constant fast pace for an unlimited distance and measures the time and distance travelled. Another form of constrained exercise is the step test where the subject steps up and down a couple of steps in time to a metronome signal. Inability to continue signals the end of the test and could be due to fatigue or breathlessness. This test has the capacity for incremental progression by increasing the pacing rate, but is a rather unnatural form of exercise.

An attempt to combine the comprehensive nature of incremental laboratory tests and the flexibility of the 6MWT walk has been made in the shuttle walk test. This is an adaptation of the 20-metre shuttle running test where a subject runs between two cones 20 metres apart with the pace determined by a series of audio signals (Léger & Lambert 1982). At intervals the pace increases until the subject can continue no longer. For patients with lung disease the shuttle distance is reduced to 10 metres and the pace increments altered to provide a comfortable start and reasonable range (Singh et al 1992) (Fig. 3.6). Under these circumstances the test provides a similar physiological stimulus to an incremental tread-

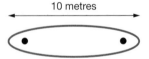

10 metres

Level	Shuttles/level	Speed (mph)
1	3	1.12
2	4	1.50
3	5	1.88
4	6	2.26
5	7	2.64
6	8	3.02
7	9	3.40
8	10	3.78
9	11	4.16
10	12	4.54
11	13	4.92
12	14	5.30

A

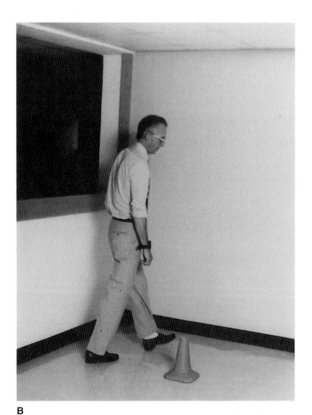

B

Figure 3.6 **(A)** The shuttle walk test involves the perambulation of an oval 10 m course. The walking speeds are increased every minute and thereby increase the number of shuttles per level. **(B)** The subject turns around the cone in the shuttle walk in time with an audio signal. This subject is wearing a heart rate telemeter on his wrist.

mill test and can be combined with measurements of heart rate and breathlessness to obtain almost as much information as provided by the laboratory standard. The standard shuttle walking test has been applied successfully in defining disability in patients with chronic respiratory disease and chronic heart failure (Keell et al 1998). The MCID for the shuttle has been explored, and for patients to notice some improvement an increase of at least 48 metres should be reported (Singh et al 2002).

A modification of the shuttle walking test has been described by Bradley et al (1999). This modified test allows the subject to run when required and includes an additional two levels. It has been validated in patients with cystic fibrosis, who were previously unchallenged by the standard test.

The endurance shuttle walking test (Revill et al 1999) complements the incremental test; patients are required to walk around an identical course for as long as possible at a constant speed (after a short warm-up) and the test result is recorded as time.

These functional walking tests are very useful in the context of pulmonary rehabilitation where mass laboratory testing is impractical; they provide a baseline measure of disability and have been shown to be sensitive to change (Griffiths et al 2000). Rehabilitation provokes significant changes in both incremental and endurance performance (Revill et al 1999). The magnitude of change reported was far greater for the endurance shuttle walking test than the incremental, reflecting the mode of training employed in this study (Fig. 3.7).

Muscle function and strength

Peripheral muscle dysfunction makes an important contribution to disability in patients with chronic respiratory disease (American Thoracic Society 1999). There is increasing evidence of reduced size and strength of muscles of the lower limb compared with healthy controls (Gosselink et al 1996, Gosselink & Decramer 1998). Others have shown an altered metabolic response to exercise (Maltais et al 1996). The sampling of peripheral muscle (biopsies) in healthy individuals has been undertaken both at rest and during exercise. In COPD patients, sampling at rest has been described by Maltais et al (1996). This technique may provide useful information for future therapies (Steiner & Morgan 2001).

The reduction in muscle mass (Schols et al 1993) is observed in approximately 30% of an outpatient population. The causes are thought to include inactivity, systemic inflammation, corticosteroid use and oxidative stress. Measures of muscle strength are most frequently reported as reductions in quadriceps force. This can be measured in a number of ways. A maximum volitional contraction can be measured on a sophisticated

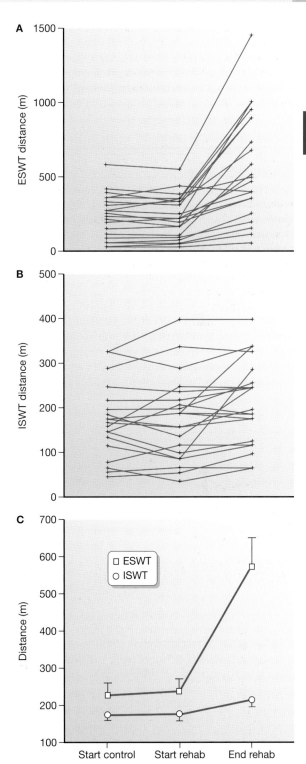

Figure 3.7 Changes observed in the endurance shuttle walking test (ESWT) (**A**), incremental shuttle walking test (ISWT) (**B**) and the mean (SE) distances for both tests after a short course of rehabilitation (**C**). (Reproduced with permission from Revill et al 1999)

isokinetic dynameter, where a number of variables are recorded. Alternatively a measure of peak torque can be obtained from a simple hand held dynamometer or a strain gauge attached to the patient's lower limb. A non-volitional contraction can be measured with magnetic stimulation (Pepin et al 2005).

3 ASSESSMENT OF CARDIAC FUNCTION

Introduction

The heart is a more straightforward organ compared with the lungs, and assessment of cardiac function can be made employing a variety of reliable and repro-ducible techniques. It is, however, a less forgiving organ and minor abnormalities of the coronary arteries or cardiac muscle function may have dramatic consequences.

The heart is composed of specialized muscle cells (myocytes) which together act as a coordinated pump to eject blood through the two major vascular circuits: the systemic vasculature and the pulmonary vascula-ture. Within the myocardium are electrical pathways, which are responsible for the coordinated and rhythmi-cal contraction of the heart, starting with the atria and followed by the ventricles. Within the four cardiac chambers are the heart valves, which prevent the ejec-tion of blood in the wrong direction. On the surface of the heart are the coronary arteries, which supply the myocardium with blood. Apart from congenital defects in the structure of the heart, disease processes can affect any of these components.

The symptomatic response to disease or malfunction depends very much on the individual structures affected. Angina pectoris and myocardial infarction are caused by disturbances of myocardial blood supply and usually result in the development of retrosternal chest tightness, heaviness and pain. Distinction between the two conditions can be difficult. Stable angina pectoris is more usually characterized by pain and/or dyspnoea on effort, whereas unstable angina and myocardial infarction tend to be more severe and may occur at any time, including at rest.

When left ventricular function is impaired, such as with myocardial cell death following myocardial infarc-tion, symptoms may include breathlessness. When severe enough to cause pulmonary oedema, severe breathlessness at rest associated with sweating and severe distress may ensue. If both ventricles are damaged or impaired (congestive cardiac failure), or if there is right ventricular dysfunction in isolation – in addition to breathlessness, significant peripheral oedema or ascites may be present along with elevated pressures in the neck veins.

Rhythm disturbances of the heart (arrhythmias) can manifest in a variety of ways. The presentation depends partly on the rhythm concerned, and partly on whether there is underlying cardiac disease. Atrial fibrillation is a rhythm characterized by an irregularly irregular pulse and can produce symptoms of fatigue and breathless-ness in the absence of a cardiac abnormality, but is much more likely to produce symptoms if myocardial func-tion is already impaired. It may also be characterized by an inappropriately fast pulse with a rapid increase in rate associated with exertion. This makes assessment of function more difficult in patients with this arrhythmia. Severe slowing of the heart (bradycardia) or accelera-tion (tachycardia) may present with dizziness or syncope.

The chest radiograph

The simple chest radiograph can provide valuable infor-mation about the presence of heart failure and is prob-ably the most useful clinical tool for monitoring its progress. Enlargement of the heart can be measured if the radiograph is taken in the posteroanterior (PA) pro-jection, and the cardiothoracic ratio (CTR) documented. This is the width of the cardiac border divided by the width of the thorax and should be less than 0·5. Enlarge-ment of the heart either represents increased muscle bulk or, more commonly, dilatation of the ventricular cavities. Pulmonary venous pooling will fill the upper lobe vessels followed by the engorgement of the inter-lobular lymphatics, which become visible as horizontal lines at the costophrenic angles (Kerley B lines) (Chapter 2). If the pulmonary venous pressure rises above 25 mmHg there is the risk of interstitial oedema. This is first visible as loss of definition of the hilum, but subse-quently may produce widespread shadowing (bat's wing appearance). If congestive cardiac failure is present the picture may be complicated by pleural effusions.

The electrocardiograph

The electrocardiograph (ECG) records the electrical activity of the heart (Fig. 3.8). Normally the ECG is recorded employing 12 different leads that record the activity over various aspects of the heart so that areas of abnormality can be anatomically located. For instance, if there are signs consistent with abnormality over the anterior leads (V2 to V6), then it is probable that there is a problem with the anterior wall of the heart that is composed predominantly of the left ventricle. Similarly, changes confined to the inferior leads (II, III and aVF) suggest a problem with the inferior surface of the heart that consists of both right and left ventricles.

The ECG is a well-established cardiological investi-gation and can provide a whole variety of information.

3

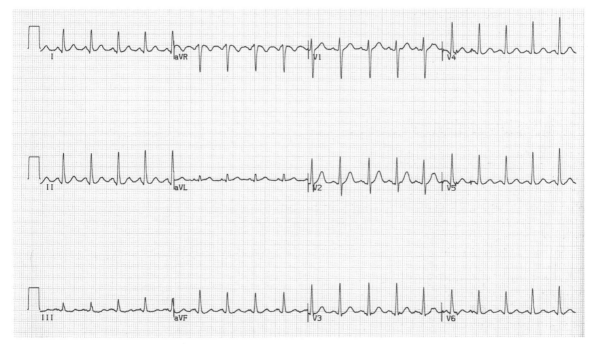

Figure 3.8   Normal 12-lead ECG.

Firstly it allows the reliable identification of the underlying cardiac rhythm. Normal rhythm is regular and called sinus rhythm. Other abnormal rhythms (arrhythmias) such as atrial flutter may also be regular but the ECG will allow ready identification. For intermittent arrhythmias a 24- or 48-hour ECG recording may be helpful. For patients with persistent symptoms of cardiac arrhythmia, but in whom no abnormality can be recorded, other techniques are available. Devices can be loaned to patients for several days that allow them to record their episodes and transmit them to a local centre via the telephone for analysis (cardiac memo recorders). For patients in whom more serious arrhythmias are suspected, devices can be implanted under the skin and activated by means of an external magnet (Reveal® device). This will automatically store the ECG for a predetermined period. This allows patients to store the event even following recovery from attacks that may have induced syncope. The device can then be interrogated via an external analyser and any abnormality of rhythm documented.

Some cardiac conditions produce characteristic abnormalities of the ECG waveform. For example myocardial infarction tends to produce elevation in the 'ST segment' of the waveform. In addition to helping diagnose the condition, the ECG also give the clinician an indication of the territory involved and the potential consequences of the episode (Figs 3.9, 3.10). Often

the presence of a previous myocardial infarction can be determined. Episodes of ischaemia such as angina tend to produce classical appearances on the ECG such as 'ST depression' or 'T wave inversion'. These appearances are looked for during exercise testing (see below). A normal ECG, however, does not exclude angina, especially if the patient was not symptomatic during the recording.

The presence of heart failure cannot be determined from the ECG but it can be said that a completely normal ECG makes the diagnosis of heart failure very unlikely.

Exercise testing

The exercise ECG is the first-line investigation in the assessment of patients with known or suspected ischaemic heart disease. In this investigation the 12-lead ECG is recorded during a progressive exercise test. This is usually by means of a treadmill, but cycle and step tests have been used for patients who cannot use a treadmill. A popular treadmill protocol is the Bruce protocol. In this test the difficulty increases in 3-minute stages:

- Stage 1 is at 1·7 mph on an incline of 10%
- Stage 2 is at 2·5 mph and 12%
- Stage 3 is at 3·4 mph and 14%
- Stage 4 is at 4·2 mph and 16%.

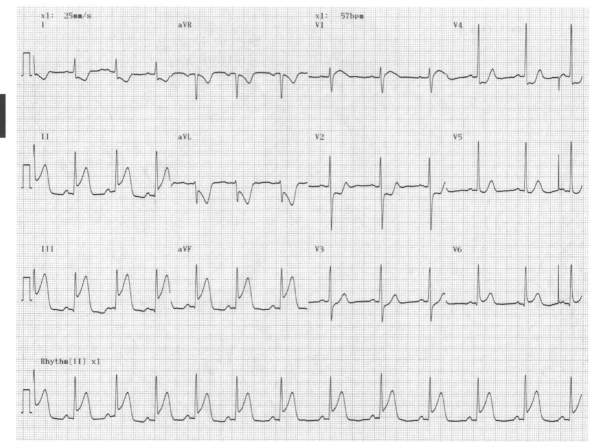

Figure 3.9 Inferior myocardial infarction. There is elevation in the ST segment of the ECG in leads II, III and aVF, which look at the inferior surface of the heart.

This is a difficult protocol, especially for elderly patients or individuals of short stature. Other gentler protocols are available, such as the Sheffield, Modified Bruce, Balke, and Northwick Park protocols (Table 3.2).

The normal response to exercise is a steady increase in heart rate. This is accompanied by a gradual rise in systolic blood pressure and a small (if any) rise in diastolic pressure. A lack of rise or a fall in the systolic pressure raises the possibility of multivessel coronary disease or left ventricular dysfunction.

The exercise ECG is deliberately provocative compared with those used to assess respiratory function. The aim is to place demands on the heart and achieve an adequate level of work accompanied by a rise in heart rate. In general, achievement of 85% or greater of the target heart rate provides an adequate level of stress for diagnostic purposes. Target heart rate can be calculated by the equation:

$$220 - \text{patient's age}$$

The main indication for exercise testing is for the assessment of myocardial ischaemia and coronary artery disease, in particular the diagnosis of chest pain, assessment of ischaemic risk, prognosis and residual ischaemia following myocardial infarction, evaluation of medical or surgical therapy, evaluation of cardiac function and exercise capacity and detection of exercise-induced arrhythmias.

False-positive tests can occur, as can false-negative tests, but overall the exercise test is an extremely useful guide to the presence or absence of ischaemic heart disease, and a good predictor of prognosis. Patients who cannot exceed 3 minutes of the Bruce protocol and who have ECG changes consistent with ischaemia (Fig. 3.11) have a mortality at 1 year in excess of 5%, whereas those who exceed 9 minutes (with no ECG changes) have a mortality of less than 1%. Similarly, patients who exercise for less than 3 minutes have a 3·5 times greater risk of dying than patients who exercise for more than 6 minutes.

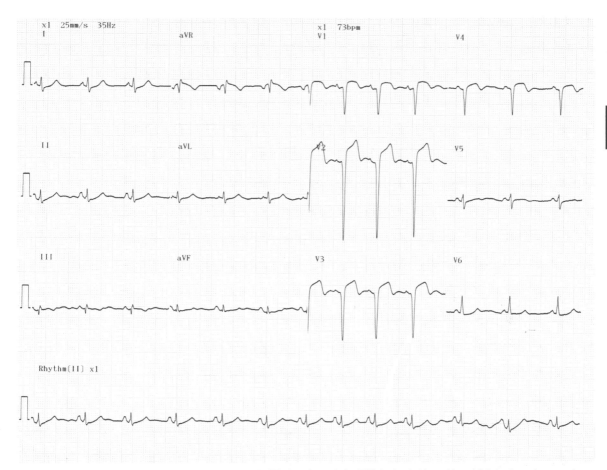

Figure 3.10 Anterior myocardial infarction. There is ST elevation of the ECG in leads V1 to V4, which look at the anterior surface of the heart.

Table 3.2 Examples of exercise testing protocols

	Bruce		Sheffield or Mod. Bruce		Northwick Park		Mod. Sheffield	
	Speed mph	*Incline %*	*Speed mph*	*Incline %*	*Speed mph*	*Incline %*	*Speed mph*	*Incline %*
Stage 1	1.7	10	1.7	0	2.0	0	1.7	0
Stage 2	2.5	12	1.7	5	3.0	4	1.7	5
Stage 3	3.4	14	1.7	10	3.0	8	1.7	10
Stage 4	4.2	16	2.5	12	3.0	12	2.5	10
Stage 5	5.0	18	3.4	14	3.0	16	2.5	12
Stage 6	5.5	20	4.2	16	3.0	20	3.4	12
Stage 7	–	–	5.0	18	4.5	20	–	–
Stage 8	–	–	5.5	20	–	–	–	–

3

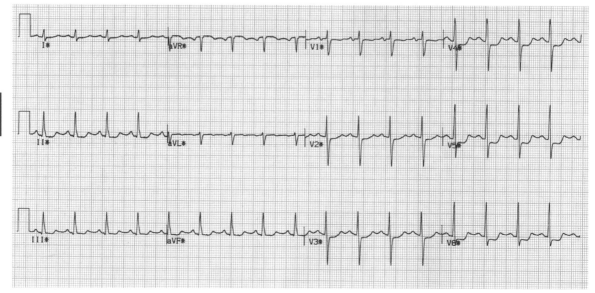

Figure 3.11 Example of a positive stress test with ST segment depression (consistent with ischaemia) in leads V4 to V6 during stage 2 of the Bruce protocol.

Electrophysiological studies

For patients with more complex cardiac arrhythmias, more invasive ECG assessment is possible. Electrophysiological studies involve the positioning of a number of electrodes within the cardiac chambers (usually via the femoral artery and/or vein) under radiological guidance. Intracardiac recordings of electrical activity can then be made. The appearance of the ECG is very different from that obtained by the standard 12-lead ECG. The procedure allows for the more accurate assessment and diagnosis of arrhythmias, and particularly allows identification of extra cardiac circuits (so-called 'accessory pathways'), which may predispose the individual to inappropriately fast rhythms. Ultimately this may allow therapeutic procedures to be offered whereby these extra circuits can be destroyed (radiofrequency ablation).

Radioisotope studies

A variety of radioisotope investigations are available in the assessment of cardiac function. Overall myocardial function can be accurately measured using isotope studies – for example multigated acquisition (MUGA) scans – so that a reliable assessment of the ejection fraction can be made. The ejection fraction is the amount of blood ejected by the heart in each cycle and in normal individuals is in excess of 50%. In patients with left

ventricular dysfunction, the ejection fraction may be anywhere between 10 and 45%. Obviously the lower the ejection fraction, the more severe the problem. The MUGA scan also allows for measurement of right ventricular function separately.

Radioisotope studies can also be used to assess myocardial perfusion (Fig. 3.12). This is particularly useful if the exercise ECG test fails to give an adequate assessment or answer. Pre-existing ECG abnormalities (such as left bundle branch block) do not allow for identification of the development of ischaemia. In some there may be a suspicion that the test was a false negative and the isotope study is more sensitive and specific for the identification of ischaemia.

Radioisotope studies also give the opportunity to assess patients who cannot walk on the treadmill, as the heart can be stressed pharmacologically using agents such as dobutamine or adenosine. Scanning patients before and after stress (be it exercise or pharmacological) allows a comparison to be made between images. Gamma cameras are employed to detect uptake of the isotope by the myocardium and areas of underperfusion can be seen. The test also allows for the identification of areas of fixed ischaemia which do not improve with rest. These often suggest the presence of scar tissue, which would not benefit from a revascularization procedure (such as bypass surgery or angioplasty). Another potential use is to assess the physiological significance

3

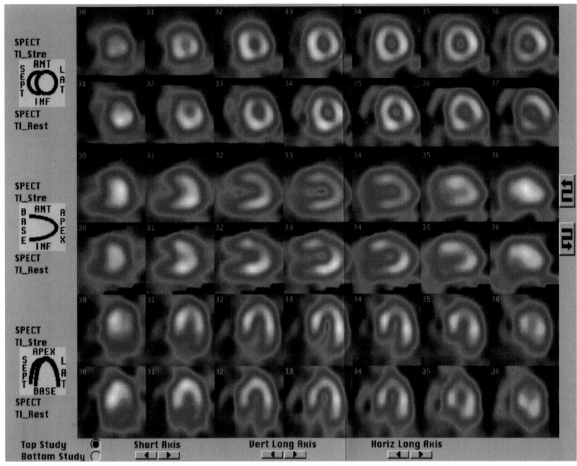

Figure 3.12 Images obtained following a stress radioisotope study comparing images taken during rest (rows 2, 4 and 6) and stress (rows 1, 3 and 5). The brighter the image, the better the blood supply to that region. This is a normal scan with no evidence of ischaemia.

of coronary artery stenoses detected by angiography (see later), and allow the clinician to determine whether revascularization is required.

Echocardiography

Ultrasound examination of the heart has become an invaluable asset to cardiac investigation and has superseded many invasive techniques. Standard transthoracic echocardiography provides an ultrasound image of the structure of the heart, while Doppler studies allow the assessment of flow patterns and pressure gradients within the chambers.

M-mode echocardiography involves a one-dimensional view of structures in the path of the ultrasound beam. This technique allows for the assessment of movement and the quantification of chamber size and a rough

estimate of cardiac function. Two-dimensional echocardiography produces more anatomically pleasing images that allow the direct visualization of the myocardium, heart valves and associated structures (Fig. 3.13). Doppler echocardiography records direction and velocity of blood flow within the heart and great vessels. Superimposing colour flow Doppler on two-dimensional images (Fig. 3.14) produces clear images of flow across structures and illustrates the presence or absence of abnormal flow such as valve regurgitation and turbulence.

Transoesophageal echocardiography is a technique that utilizes all of the features of transthoracic echocardiography, but involves the passage of an ultrasound transducer mounted at the end of an endoscope into the oesophagus. Extremely clear images of the heart and great vessels can be obtained because the oesophagus is

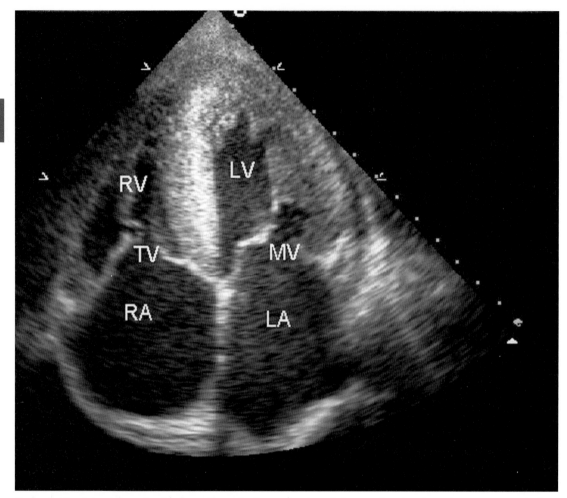

Figure 3.13 A two-dimensional echocardiography image showing all four cardiac chambers, the right atrium (RA), right ventricle (RV), the left atrium (LA) and the left ventricle (LV). The mitral (MV) and tricuspid (TV) valves are clearly seen.

in such close proximity to the relevant structures and there is little air or tissue interface. It is useful when transthoracic images are inconclusive because of poor image quality or when more detailed assessment is desirable (such as in mitral valve morphology or the diagnosis of endocarditis).

Stress echocardiography is a technique that involves the visualization of myocardial performance during infusion of various pharmacological stressing agents such as dobutamine. This allows the determination of ventricular performance and can give an indication of areas of underperfusion and of irreversible left ventricular damage.

Contrast echocardiography is a technique that involves the injection of microbubbles that appear as clouds of echoes on the ultrasound image. This is helpful to accurately determine the outline of the myocardium, particularly when measuring movement of the ven-

tricle. Precise areas of impaired movement can be visualized.

Cardiac catheterization

Cardiac catheterization allows the accurate assessment of coronary artery anatomy. The procedure involves the insertion of catheters into the arterial circulation (usually via the femoral artery) and the selective intubation of each of the coronary arteries. The presence of narrowings (stenoses) or blockages can be determined by the injection of dye to outline the vessels (Fig. 3.15). Images are acquired in various planes because of the three-dimensional nature of the heart. In addition, the procedure allows for a variety of other assessments to be made.

Continuous pressure monitoring gives the opportunity to measure pressures within the cardiac chambers, particularly the left ventricle during left heart catheter-

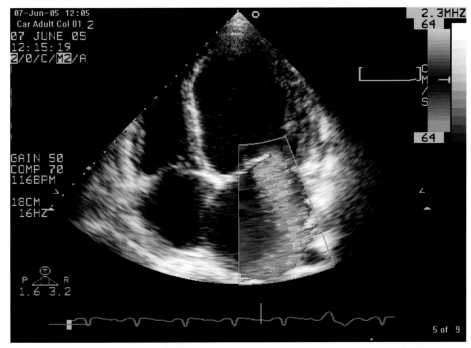

Figure 3.14 A 2D echocardiograph image with colour flow Doppler showing severe mitral regurgitation into a dilated left atrium in a patient with dilated cardiomyopathy.

ization. Elevation in the left ventricular end-diastolic pressure over 12 mmHg (the pressure trough immediately before ventricular contraction) suggests left ventricular dysfunction. Withdrawal of the catheter across the aortic valve also allows pressure gradients across the valve to be determined and the severity of any stenosis to be made.

Quantification of coronary stenoses is made visually and with the aid of computer programs. Other methods include the passage of tiny ultrasound probes mounted over flexible guidewires into the arteries themselves. This technique is called intravascular ultrasound (IVUS) and images of the inside of the coronary arteries and arterial wall are obtained. Recently the development of guidewires with pressure sensors has allowed the pressure within the arteries to be measured before and after a stenosis and an assessment of the severity of any given stenosis made.

Right heart catheterization (access being gained via the femoral vein) can measure pressures in the right heart chambers (right atrium and ventricle) and also the pulmonary arteries. Wedging of catheters or employing balloon-tipped catheters in the pulmonary arterial tree also enables the measurement of wedge pressure, which is an indirect measurement of left atrial pressure. Once left atrial pressure rises above 20 mmHg, pulmonary oedema can ensue, and therefore wedge pressure allows further assessment of left ventricular function.

A variety of other parameters can be assessed by the sampling of blood in various chambers and vessels which can ultimately allow very accurate measurements of cardiac output, intracardiac shunts and vascular resistance.

The major drawback of cardiac catheterization is the invasive nature of the procedure and the potential risks.

Magnetic resonance imaging

Magnetic resonance imaging (MRI) is a rapidly developing non-invasive technique for cardiac investigation. Previously, cardiac motion from patient respiration and the cyclic motion of the heart hampered imaging with this modality. However, the advent of ultrafast imaging sequences has enabled MRI to become the gold standard for evaluation of cardiac anatomy and function. The high resolution of MRI and the ability to image in any plane allows three-dimensional measurement of ejection fraction without need for geometrical assumptions. Studies have shown excellent intra- and inter-observer variability and so small changes in function over time can be estimated reliably. No ionizing radiation is required and so longitudinal (serial) patient studies are safe. First-pass contrast-enhanced imaging can be used to evaluate myocardial perfusion.

Both qualitative and quantitative parameters of myocardial blood flow can be obtained. MRI is now consid-

3

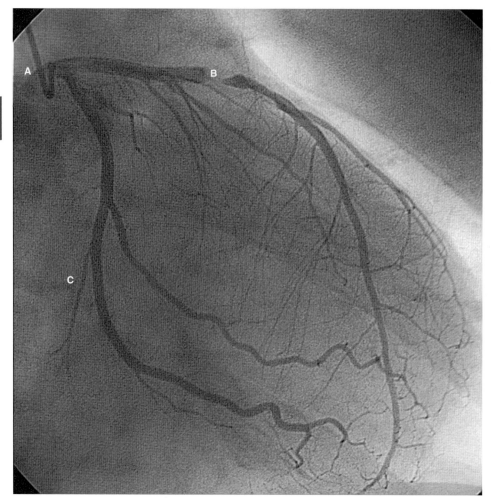

Figure 3.15 Example of cardiac catheterization of the left coronary artery. The catheter is illustrated (**A**), situated in the origin of the left coronary artery. A severe stenosis (narrowing) of the left anterior descending branch is seen (**B**). The circumflex branch is relatively healthy (**C**).

ered the best imaging technique for the detection of myocardial infarction and assessing myocardial viability in dysfunctional myocardium. Pharmacological stress protocols can be applied in a manner analogous to echocardiography and radioisotope studies so that regional abnormalities in function and/or perfusion can be assessed at rest and during stress.

MRI also has an increasing place in the investigation of patients with congenital heart disease. Due to a large field of view, MRI has the ability to image major vessels and quantify ventricular function and shunts. Not all patients are suitable for magnetic resonance. Contraindications include patients with permanent pacing systems, metallic implants and severe claustrophobia. As scanners with cardiac specifications and trained personnel become increasingly available in the workplace, MRI is likely to become a cardiac investigation of increasing usefulness.

THE ELECTROCARDIOGRAM

The electrocardiogram (ECG) is a recording from the body surface of the electrical activity of the heart. The standard ECG has 12 leads:

- Chest leads V_1–V_6 look at the heart in a *horizontal plane* (Fig. 3.16)

A

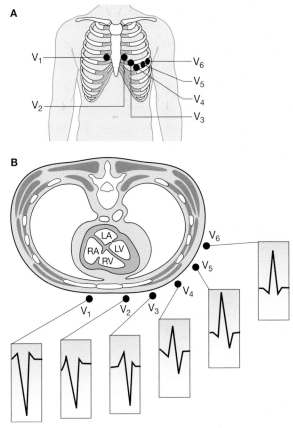

Figure 3.16 ECG chest leads. **A** The V leads are attached to the chest wall overlying the intercostal spaces as shown: V_4 in the mid-clavicular line, V_5 in the anterior axillary line, V_6 in the mid-axillary line. **B** Leads V_1 and V_2 look at the right ventricle, V_3 and V_4 at the interventricular septum, and V_5 and V_6 at the left ventricle. The normal QRS complex in each lead is shown. The R wave in the chest (precordial) leads steadily increases in amplitude from lead V_1 to V_6 with a corresponding decrease in S wave depth, culminating in a predominantly positive complex in V_6. (Reproduced with permission from Ballinger and Patchett 2003)

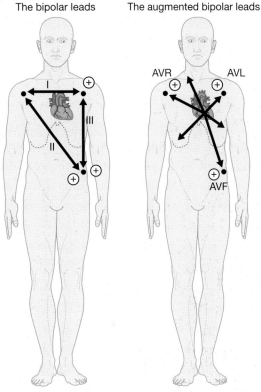

Figure 3.17 ECG limb leads. Lead I is derived from electrodes on the right arm (negative pole) and left arm (positive pole), lead II is derived from electrodes on the right arm (negative pole) and left leg (positive pole), and lead III from electrodes on the left arm (negative pole) and the left leg (positive pole). (Reproduced with permission from Ballinger and Patchett 2003)

- Limb leads look at the heart in a *vertical plane* (Fig. 3.17). Limb leads are unipolar (AVR, AVL and AVF) or bipolar (I, II, III).

The ECG machine is arranged so that when a depolarization wave spreads towards a lead the needle moves upwards on the trace, and when it spreads away from the lead the needle moves downwards.

ECG waveform and definitions (Fig. 3.18)

The *heart rate*. At normal paper speed (usually 25 mm/s) each 'big square' measures 5 mm wide and is equivalent to 0.2 s. The heart rate (if the rhythm is regular) is calculated by counting the number of big squares between two consecutive R waves and dividing into 300.

The *P wave* is the first deflection and is caused by atrial depolarization. When abnormal it may be:

- Broad and notched (>0.12 s, i.e. 3 small squares) in left atrial enlargement ('P mitrale', e.g. mitral stenosis)

- Tall and peaked (>2.5 mm) in right atrial enlargement ('P pulmonale', e.g. pulmonary hypertension)

- Replaced by flutter or fibrillation waves

- Absent in sinoatrial block.

The *QRS complex* represents ventricular depolarization:

- A negative (downward) deflection preceding an R wave is called a Q wave. Normal Q waves are small

3

and narrow; deep (>2 mm), wide (>1 mm) Q waves (except in AVR and V_1) indicate myocardial infarction.

- A deflection upwards is called an R wave whether or not it is preceded by a Q wave.

- A negative deflection following an R wave is termed an S wave.

Ventricular depolarization starts in the septum and spreads from left to right (Fig. 3.19). Subsequently the

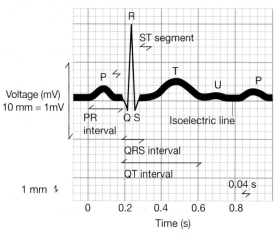

Figure 3.18   The waves and elaboration of the normal ECG. (Modified from Goldman (1976), reproduced with permission from Ballinger and Patchett 2003)

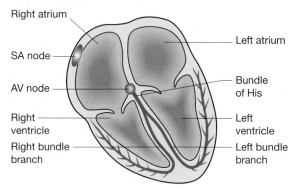

Figure 3.19   The normal cardiac conduction system. In normal circumstances only the specialized conducting tissues of the heart undergo spontaneous depolarization (automaticity), which initiates an action potential. The sinus (SA) node discharges more rapidly than the other cells and is the normal pacemaker of the heart. The impulse generated by the sinus node spreads first through the atria, producing atrial systole, and then through the atrioventricular (AV) node to the His–Purkinje system, producing ventricular systole. (Reproduced with permission from Ballinger and Patchett 2003)

main free walls of the ventricles are depolarized. Thus, in the right ventricular leads (V_1 and V_2) the first deflection is upwards (R wave) as the septal depolarization wave spreads towards those leads. The second deflection is downwards (S wave) as the bigger left ventricle (in which depolarization is spreading away) outweighs the effect of the right ventricle (see Fig. 3.16). The opposite pattern is seen in the left ventricular leads (V_5 and V_6), with an initial downward deflection (small Q wave reflecting septal depolarization) followed by a large R wave caused by left ventricular depolarization.

Left ventricular hypertrophy. The increased bulk of the left ventricular myocardium in left ventricular hypertrophy (e.g. with systemic hypertension) increases the voltage-induced depolarization of the free wall of the left ventricle. This gives rise to tall R waves (>25 mm) in the left ventricular leads (V_5, V_6) and/or deep S waves (>30 mm) in the right ventricular leads (V_1, V_2). The sum of the R wave in the left ventricular leads and the S wave in the right ventricular leads exceeds 40 mm. In addition to these changes there may be ST-segment depression and T wave flattening or inversion in the left ventricular leads.

Right ventricular hypertrophy (e.g. in pulmonary hypertension) causes tall R waves in the right ventricular leads.

The QRS duration reflects the time that excitation takes to spread through the ventricle. A wide QRS complex (>0.10 s, 2.5 small squares) occurs if conduction is delayed, e.g. with right or left bundle branch block, or if conduction is through abnormal pathways, e.g. ventricular ectopic.

T waves result from ventricular repolarization. In general the direction of the T wave is the same as that of the QRS complex. Inverted T waves occur in many conditions and, although usually abnormal, they are a non-specific finding.

The *PR interval* is measured from the start of the P wave to the start of the QRS complex whether this is a Q wave or an R wave. It is the time taken for excitation to pass from the sinus node, through the atrium, atrioventricular node and His–Purkinje system to the ventricle. A prolonged PR interval (>0.22 s) indicates heart block.

The *ST segment* is the period between the end of the QRS complex and the start of the T wave. ST elevation (>1 mm above the isoelectric line) occurs in the early stages of myocardial infarction and with acute pericarditis. ST segment depression (>0.5 mm below the isoelectric line) indicates myocardial ischaemia.

Exercise electrocardiography

Exercise electrocardiography is an ECG recording made during standard graded exercise treadmill testing (e.g.

the Bruce protocol) and is used in the investigation of patients with known or suspected ischaemic heart disease. Contraindications include recent myocardial infarction (within 6 days), unstable angina, severe hypertrophic cardiomyopathy, severe aortic stenosis and malignant hypertension. A positive test and indications for stopping the test are:

- Chest pain

- ST segment depression >1 mm

- ST segment elevation >1 mm

- Fall in systolic blood pressure >20 mmHg; a sustained fall in blood pressure usually indicates severe coronary artery disease

- Fall in heart rate despite an increase in workload

- BP > 240/110

- Significant arrhythmias or increased frequency of ventricular ectopics.

CARDIAC ARRHYTHMIAS

An abnormality of the cardiac rhythm is called a cardiac arrhythmia. Such a disturbance may cause sudden death, syncope, dizziness, palpitations or no symptoms at all. Paroxysmal arrhythmias may not be detected on a single ECG recording. Twenty-four-hour ambulatory ECG monitoring (continuous recording for 24 hours) and event recorders (a portable device activated by the patient to record the ECG when symptoms occur) are outpatient investigations often used to detect arrhythmias causing intermittent symptoms.

There are two main types of arrhythmia:

- *Bradycardia,* where the heart rate is slow (<60 beats/min). The slower the heart rate, the more probable that the arrhythmia will be symptomatic.

- *Tachycardia,* where the heart rate is fast (>100 beats/min). Tachycardias are more likely to be symptomatic when the arrhythmia is fast and sustained. They are subdivided into *supraventricular tachycardias,* which arise from the atrium or the atrioventricular junction, and *ventricular tachycardias,* which arise from the ventricles.

Sinus rhythms

Sinus arrhythmia.   Fluctuations of autonomic tone result in phasic changes in the sinus discharge rate. Thus, during inspiration parasympathetic tone falls and the heart rate quickens, and on expiration the heart rate falls. This variation is normal, particularly in children and young adults.

Sinus bradycardia.   Sinus bradycardia is normal during sleep and in well-trained athletes. During the acute phase of a myocardial infarction it often reflects ischaemia of the sinus node. Other causes include hypothermia, hypothyroidism, cholestatic jaundice, raised intracranial pressure, and drug therapy with beta-blockers, digitalis and other antiarrhythmic drugs. Patients with persistent symptomatic bradycardia are treated with a permanent cardiac pacemaker. Intravenous atropine is used in the acute situation.

Sinus tachycardia.   Sinus tachycardia is a physiological response during exercise and excitement. It may also occur with fever, anaemia, cardiac failure, thyrotoxicosis and drugs (e.g. catecholamines and atropine). Treatment is aimed at correction of the underlying cause. If necessary, beta-blockers may be used to slow the sinus rate, but not in uncontrolled heart failure.

Pathological bradycardias

There are two main forms of severe bradycardia: sinus node dysfunction and atrioventricular block.

Sinus node dysfunction (sick sinus syndrome).   Most cases of chronic sinus node dysfunction are the result of idiopathic fibrosis occurring in elderly people. Bradycardia is caused by intermittent failure of sinus node depolarization (sinus arrest) or failure of the sinus impulse to propagate through the perinodal tissue to the atria (sinoatrial block). This is seen on the ECG as intermittent long pauses between consecutive P waves (>2 s). The slow heart rate predisposes to ectopic pacemaker activity and tachyarrhythmias are common (tachy-brady syndrome).

Insertion of a permanent pacemaker is only indicated in symptomatic patients to prevent dizzy spells and blackouts. Antiarrhythmic drugs are used to treat tachycardias. Thromboembolism is common in sinus node dysfunction and patients should be anticoagulated unless there is a contraindication.

Atrioventricular block.   There are three forms: first-degree heart block, second-degree (partial) block and third-degree (complete) block. The common causes are coronary artery disease, cardiomyopathy and, particularly in elderly people, fibrosis of the conducting tissue.

- *First-degree atrioventricular (AV) block* is the result of delayed atrioventricular conduction and reflected by a prolonged PR interval (>0.22 s) on the ECG. No change in heart rate occurs and treatment is unnecessary.

3

■ *Second-degree (partial) AV block* occurs when some atrial impulses fail to reach the ventricles. There are three forms (Fig. 3.20):
— Mobitz type 1 block (Wenckebach's phenomenon), in which the PR interval gradually increases, culminating in a dropped beat, i.e. absent QRS after the P wave. The PR interval then returns to normal and the cycle repeats itself.
— Mobitz type II block occurs when a dropped QRS complex is not preceded by progressive PR prolongation.
— A 2:1 or 3:1 block occurs when only every second or third P wave conducts to the ventricles. A 4:1 or 5:1 block can also occur.

Progression to complete heart block occurs more frequently following anterior myocardial infarction and in Mobitz type II block, and treatment with pacing is usually indicated. Patients with Wenckebach AV block or those with second-degree block following inferior infarction are usually monitored.

A

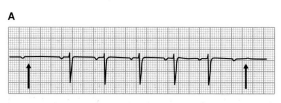

B

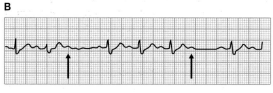

C

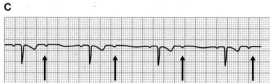

Figure 3.20   Three varieties of second-degree atrioventricular (AV) block. **(A)** Wenckebach (Mobitz type I) AV block. The PR interval gradually prolongs until the P wave does not conduct to the ventricles (arrows). **(B)** Mobitz type II AV block. The P waves that do not conduct to the ventricles (arrows) are not preceded by gradual PR interval prolongation. **(C)** Two P waves to each QRS complex. The PR interval prior to the dropped P wave is always the same. It is not possible to define this type of AV block as type I or type II Mobitz block and it is, therefore, a third variety of second-degree AV block (arrows show P waves), not conducted to the ventricles. (Reproduced with permission from Ballinger and Patchett 2003)

■ *Third-degree AV block (complete heart block).* There is no association between atrial and ventricular activity and ventricular contractions are maintained by a spontaneous escape rhythm (usually about 40/min) from an automatic centre below the site of the block. The ECG shows regular P waves and QRS complexes, which occur independently of one another. The usual symptoms are dizziness and blackouts (Stokes–Adams attacks). If the ventricular rate is very slow, cardiac failure may occur. Insertion of a permanent pacemaker is always required for sustained complete heart block. In the acute situation, e.g. myocardial infarction, recovery may be expected and intravenous atropine or a temporary pacemaker may be all that is necessary.

Intraventricular conduction disturbances.   The intraventricular conduction system consists of the His bundle, the right and left bundle branches and the anterosuperior and posteroinferior divisions of the left bundle branch block (see Fig. 3.19). Complete block of a bundle branch is associated with a wider QRS complex (0.12 s or more). The shape of the QRS depends on whether the right or the left bundle is blocked.

Pathological tachycardias

The mechanisms responsible for most tachyarrhythmias are abnormal automaticity and re-entry mechanisms.

Abnormal automaticity.   Arrhythmias arise if there is enhanced automaticity of the normal conducting tissue or automaticity is acquired by damaged cells of the atria or ventricles; this causes ectopic beats and, if sustained, tachyarrhythmias.

Re-entry.   Re-entry may occur if there are two separate pathways for impulse conduction (Fig. 3.21).

Atrial tachyarrhythmias.   Ectopic beats, tachycardia, flutter and fibrillation may all arise from the atrial myocardium. They share common aetiologies, which are listed in Table 3.3.

Atrial ectopic beats.   These are caused by premature discharge of an ectopic atrial focus. On the ECG this produces an early and abnormal P wave, usually followed by a normal QRS complex. Treatment is not usually required unless they cause troublesome palpitations or are responsible for provoking more significant arrhythmias when beta-blockade may be effective.

Atrial flutter.   Atrial flutter is almost always associated with organic disease of the heart. The atrial rate is usually about 300 beats/min. The AV node usually conducts every second flutter beat, giving a ventricular rate of 150 beats/min. The ECG (Fig. 3.22A) characteristically shows 'saw-tooth' flutter waves (F waves), which

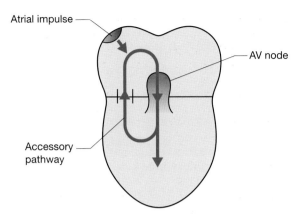

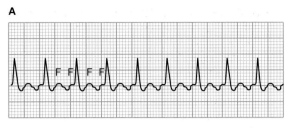

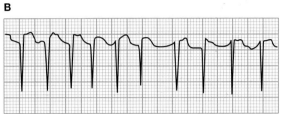

3

Figure 3.21 A re-entry circuit. The impulse is conducted normally through the AV node and initiates ventricular depolarization. In certain circumstances the accessory pathway is able to transmit the impulse retrogradely back into the atria, thus completing a circuit and initiating a self-sustaining re-entry tachycardia. (Reproduced with permission from Ballinger and Patchett 2003)

Figure 3.22 **(A)** Atrial flutter. The flutter waves are marked with an F, only half of which are transmitted to the ventricles. **(B)** Atrial fibrillation. There are no P waves; the ventricular response is fast and irregular. (Reproduced with permission from Ballinger and Patchett 2003)

Table 3.3   Causes of atrial arrhythmias
Ischaemic heart disease
Rheumatic heart disease
Thyrotoxicosis
Cardiomyopathy
Lone atrial fibrillation (i.e. no cause discovered)
Wollf–Parkinson–White syndrome
Pneumonia
Atrial septal defect
Carcinoma of the bronchus
Pericarditis
Pulmonary embolus
Acute and chronic alcohol abuse

(Ballinger and Patchett 2003)

are most clearly seen when AV conduction is transiently impaired by carotid sinus massage or drugs. Treatment of an acute paroxysm is electrical cardioversion. Prophylaxis is achieved with class Ia, Ic or III drugs (Table 3.4). Rate control of a chronic arrhythmia is with AV nodal blocking drugs, e.g. digoxin. Recurrent atrial flutter is best treated with radiofrequency catheter ablation of focal arrhythmogenic sites.

Atrial fibrillation (AF).   This is a common arrhythmia, occurring in 5–10% of patients over 65 years of age. It also occurs, particularly in a paroxysmal form, in younger patients. Atrial activity is chaotic and mechanically ineffective. The AV node conducts a proportion of the atrial impulses to produce an irregular ventricular response. Symptoms range from palpitations and fatigue to acute pulmonary oedema. There are no clear P waves on the ECG (Fig. 3.22B), only a fine oscillation of the baseline (so-called fibrillation or f waves).

When AF arises in an apparently normal heart it is sometimes possible to convert to sinus rhythm, either electrically (by cardioversion) or chemically (with class Ia, Ic or III drugs, see Table 3.4). When AF is caused by an acute precipitating event, such as alcohol toxicity, chest infection or thyrotoxicosis, the underlying cause should be treated initially.

Strategies for the long-term management of atrial fibrillation include:

- Maintenance of sinus rhythm with antiarrhythmic drugs after DC cardioversion
- Rate control and consideration of anticoagulation (e.g. digoxin and warfarin).

Atrial fibrillation is associated with an increased risk of thromboembolism, and anticoagulation with warfarin should be given for at least 3 weeks before (with the exception of those who require emergency cardioversion) and 4 weeks after cardioversion. Most patients with chronic AF should also be anticoagulated (INR

3

Table 3.4   Vaughan Williams' classification of antiarrhythmic drug therapy

Class	Mechanism of action	Individual drugs
Ia		Quinine, procainamide, disopyramide
Ib	Membrane stabilizing action	Lidocaine, mexiletine
Ic		Flecainide, propafenone
II	β-Adrenergic blockers	Metoprolol, atenolol, propranolol
III	Increases refractory period of conducting system	Amiodarone, sotalol, bretylium
IV	Calcium-channel blocking agents	Verapamil, diltiazem

Adenosine and digoxin are other antiarrhythmic drugs that do not fit into this classification. These drugs all have proarrhythmic effect (among others) and should be used with caution. All except amiodarone are negatively inotropic and may exacerbate heart failure. (Ballinger and Patchett 2003)

2.0–3.0). The exception is young patients (<65 years) with lone AF, i.e. in the absence of demonstrable cardiac disease, diabetes or hypertension. This group has a low incidence of thromboembolism and is treated with aspirin alone.

Junctional tachycardia. Junctional tachycardias are paroxysmal in nature and usually occur in the absence of structural heart disease. They are re-entrant arrhythmias caused by an abnormal pathway in the AV node or by an accessory pathway (bundle of Kent), as in the Wolff–Parkinson–White syndrome (Fig. 3.23). The usual history is of a sudden onset of fast (140–280/min) regular palpitations. On the ECG the P waves may be seen very close to the QRS complex, or are not seen at all. The QRS complex is usually of normal shape because, as with other supraventricular arrhythmias, the ventricles are activated in the normal way, down the bundle of His. Occasionally the QRS complex is wide, because of a rate-related bundle branch block, and it may be difficult to distinguish from ventricular tachycardia.

Termination of an attack
- Manoeuvres that increase vagal stimulation of the sinus node: carotid sinus massage, ocular pressure or the Valsalva manoeuvre.

- Drug treatment: adenosine is a very short-acting AV nodal blocking drug given as a 3 mg bolus dose intravenously. It will terminate most junctional tachycardias. If there is no response after 1–2 minutes, a further bolus of 6 mg is given. A third bolus of 12 mg may be given if there is still no response. Transient side effects include complete heart block, hypotension, nausea and bronchospasm. Asthma and second- or third-degree AV block are contraindications to adenosine. An alternative treatment is intravenous

verapamil 10 mg i.v. over 5–10 minutes (contraindicated if the QRS complex is wide and therefore differentiation from ventricular tachycardia difficult).

- Rapid atrial pacing or DC cardioversion is used if adenosine fails.

Prophylaxis
- Radiofrequency ablation of the accessory pathway via a cardiac catheter
- Flecainide, disopyramide, amiodarone and β-blockers are the drugs most commonly used.

Ventricular arrhythmias

Ventricular ectopic beats (extrasystoles, premature beats). Ventricular ectopic beats may be asymptomatic or patients may complain of extra beats, missed beats or heavy beats. The ectopic electrical activity is not conducted to the ventricles through the normal conducting tissue and thus the QRS complex on the ECG is widened, with a bizarre configuration (Fig. 3.24). In normal individuals ectopic beats are of no significance, but treatment is sometimes given for symptoms. In patients with heart disease they are associated with an increased risk of sudden death. Prophylaxis with amiodarone may reduce mortality by preventing arrhythmias and sudden death.

Ventricular tachycardia. Ventricular tachycardia and ventricular fibrillation are usually associated with underlying heart disease, e.g. ischaemia, cardiomyopathy and hypertensive heart disease. Ventricular tachycardia is defined as three or more consecutive ventricular beats occurring at a rate of 120/min or more. The ECG shows a rapid ventricular rhythm with broad abnormal QRS complexes, which can sometimes be confused with

A

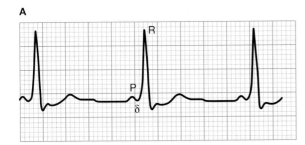

B

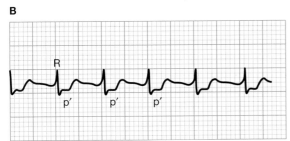

Figure 3.23   **(A)** An ECG showing Wolff–Parkinson–White syndrome. There is an abnormal connection, termed an accessory pathway, between the atria and ventricles. The accessory pathway has a more rapid rate of conduction from the atria to the ventricles than does the normal AV node and ventricular depolarization occurs sooner than expected. Such pre-excitation is apparent on the ECG during sinus rhythm as a short PR interval and wide QRS complex with a 'slurred' upstroke (δ wave). **(B)** A trace demonstrating the paroxysmal tachycardia that may result from this syndrome. Note the tachycardia p wave visible between QRS and T wave complexes. (Reproduced with permission from Ballinger and Patchett 2003)

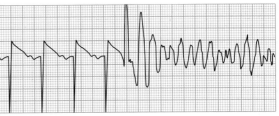

Figure 3.24   A rhythm strip demonstrating four beats of sinus rhythm followed by a ventricular ectopic beat that initiates ventricular fibrillation. The ST segment is elevated owing to acute myocardial infarction. (Reproduced with permission from Ballinger and Patchett 2003)

3

a broad complex junctional tachycardia. Ventricular tachycardia may produce severe hypotension, when urgent DC cardioversion is necessary. If there is no haemodynamic compromise, treatment is usually with intravenous lidocaine (50–100 mg i.v. over 5 minutes followed by an intravenous infusion of 2–4 mg/min). Prophylaxis is with mexiletine, disopyramide, flecainide or amiodarone. Patients who are refractory to all medical treatment may need an implantable defibrillator. This is a small device implanted behind the rectus abdominis and connected to the heart; it recognizes ventricular tachycardia or ventricular fibrillation and automatically delivers a defibrillation shock to the heart.

Ventricular fibrillation.   This is a very rapid and irregular ventricular activation (see Fig. 3.24) with no mechanical effect and hence no cardiac output. Ventricular fibrillation rarely reverts spontaneously and management is immediate cardioversion.

PAEDIATRICS

MEASUREMENT OF LUNG FUNCTION

History and examination

Taking a history is the starting place when assessing a child's lung function. Questions need to reflect the child's age and must take into account symptoms at rest, and when the child is running around playing or taking part in school games or sport. For example can a baby drink a full bottle of milk or does it become breathless and start spluttering? Does a boy keep up during a game of football or is he always put in goal? Can a

schoolgirl carry her books up several flights of stairs to lessons or does she have to rest at each floor? Questions are easier to answer if they relate to normal activities and information is then obtained about how the child functions in everyday life. When discussing noisy breathing, it is well to remember that many parents do not understand what is meant by terms such as wheezing (Cane et al 2000) and an ability to demonstrate these sounds may be helpful.

Physical examination is critical, although it will only give information about the child at rest. Nevertheless, inspection will soon reveal whether the patient is in respiratory distress with, for example, tachypnoea and/ or dyspnoea. The normal respiratory rate is age dependent, and decreases with age (Table 3.5). It is important to determine whether the child can speak sentences without becoming breathless and whether accessory muscles are being used leading to intercostal or subcostal recession. Cyanosis, if present, ought to be fairly obvious. When reviewing a child with cystic fibrosis (CF) or bronchiectasis, it is important to inspect the sputum (colour, consistency). Palpation is good for assessing chest expansion and placing the hands on the chest will indicate, by a feeling of vibration, whether the chest is full of sputum – a method used by many parents of children with cystic fibrosis. Percussion is most useful for determining the presence of a pleural effusion (parapneumonic or empyema) indicated by dullness. Before auscultating with a stethoscope, it is worth simply listening to the child's breathing for wheeze (an expiratory sound), stridor (an inspiratory sound) or upper respiratory tract secretions heard in the throat (harsh expiratory and inspiratory sounds that are transmitted throughout the chest). The presence of a cough and its nature (dry, moist, productive, spasmodic) should be listened for. A forceful huff may also reveal abnormal sounds not obvious with quiet breathing. Finally, listening with the stethoscope may indicate abnormal sounds that can then be located to a particular area or lobe. It is always worth asking the patient to cough before listening again, as often some of the added sounds will have disappeared.

Dynamic lung function

In clinical practice, lung function tests may help with the management of a child with respiratory disease, for example in assessing severity, time trends, response to

Table 3.5 Respiratory rate by age

Age (years)	Respiratory rate (per minute)	mean ± 2 SD
1	30	18–42
2	29	19–39
4	26	16–36
8	23	13–33
12	21	13–29
16	20	12–28

(Adapted from Hooker et al 1992)

treatment and sometimes prognosis (Silverman & Stocks 1999). They are also useful in helping with diagnoses: for example, distinguishing between obstructive and restrictive lung disease. Further, the demonstration of obstructive lung disease that responds to a bronchodilator or worsens with exercise is an important diagnostic aid for asthma. Key abbreviations and definitions can be found in Table 3.6.

Peak expiratory flow rate (PEFR)

Peak expiratory flow is defined as the maximal flow achieved during an expiration delivered with a maximal force starting from maximal lung inflation. In normal subjects, PEFR is determined by:

- the size of the lungs
- lung elasticity
- the dimensions and compliance of the central intrathoracic airways
- the strength and speed of the contraction of the respiratory muscles.

The normal values relate to the height and gender of the child (Rosenthal et al 1993a). A child over 5–6 years ought to be able to use a peak flow meter after appropriate training and practice, but the test is very effort-dependent and easy to fake. For this reason, PEFR must be ascertained separately using a peak flow meter rather than using the value calculated by a spirometer. It is most often used in the management of asthmatic children, and inexpensive cheap peak flow meters are available on prescription for home use. It may be valuable when assessing a new therapy, but regular use with a peak flow diary is of limited value due to the poor compliance with such a regimen (Redline et al 1996). Many children simply make up the results and fill in the diary the day before their clinic appointment. However, knowledge of a child's personal best and usual PEFR can help with asthma management, as a gradual drop in PEFR tends to precede an exacerbation and may sometimes occur before symptoms are recognized. Self-management plans can be in place whereby PEFR results can guide when to take bronchodilators, start oral corticosteroids or seek medical help. Poor control is also indicated by an increase in day-to-day variability of PEFR measurements.

Spirometry

Spirometry, which can be performed in a clinic or at the bedside, is the most valuable and reproducible lung function test used in children. A normal spirogram is shown in Fig 3.1. Most 6 year olds can perform the technique reliably, with some 5 year olds also managing it. Normal values take into account the child's gender and height (Polgar & Weng 1979, Rosenthal

Table 3.6 Variables, abbreviations and definitions

Variable	Abbreviation	Definition
Peak expiratory flow rate	PEFR	The maximal expiratory flow rate achieved during a forced expiratory manoeuvre
Forced expired volume in one second	FEV_1	The volume expired in the first second of maximal expiration after a maximal inspiration
Forced vital capacity	FVC	The maximum volume of air which can be exhaled after a maximal inspiration
Maximum mid-expiratory flow	MEF_{25-75}	The average expired flow over the middle half of the FVC manoeuvre
Maximum oxygen consumption	$\dot{V}O_2max$	During maximal exercise, a point is reached where further increases in workload do not cause further increases in the maximum volume of oxygen that the body can consume
Peak oxygen consumption	$\dot{V}O_2peak$	This is highest volume of oxygen that an individual consumes during exercise when they have not reached $\dot{V}O_2max$ (for whatever reason)
Maximum minute ventilation	$\dot{V}_Emax$	The maximum ventilatory capacity that can be achieved during maximal exercise
Anaerobic threshold	AT	This is the point at which anaerobic metabolism (marked by lactate production) supplements aerobic metabolism
Diffusing capacity of the lung for carbon monoxide	DL_{CO}	This is a measure of the surface area of the lung available for gas exchange

3

et al 1993a). Results are usually expressed as a 'percent predicted', but it is better to use standard deviation (SD) scores (z-scores) – even though these are more difficult for parents to understand. First, the SD scores are able to reflect accurately how far an individual's spirometry result deviates from the expected norm and, secondly, SD scores will provide valuable tracking data over time. Generally, FEV_1 (forced expiratory volume in one second) and FVC (forced vital capacity) >80% of the predicted mean are considered normal, while a cut-off of 60% is used for MEF_{25-75} (maximal expiratory flow at 25% to 75% vital capacity), as these correspond roughly to values that lie within 2 SD of the mean (Pattishall 1990). FEV_1 values of 60–79% are considered to represent mild, 40–59% moderate and <40% severe dysfunction, particularly when related to CF lung disease. Puberty has a dramatic effect on lung function in that both before and after there is a linear increase of lung function with height, while during puberty the relationship is more complex (Rosenthal et al 1993a).

Spirometry is effort-dependent and it is important to watch the child's technique; the flow–volume and volume–time curves will also indicate whether a proper effort was made. The child inhales maximally then exhales as hard as possible and for as long as possible. Expiratory flow–volume loops are obtained, along with data such as FVC and FEV_1. Flow rates at smaller lung volumes e.g. maximal expiratory flow at 25% vital capacity (MEF_{25}) or mean flows across the mid-portion can also be obtained (MEF_{25-75}). Although these give more sensitive information about flow in the small airways, the measurements are less reliable due to their greater variability. It is best to view trends over time and FVC and FEV_1 are the two measurements most often followed. The shape of the flow–volume loop can indicate the presence of airway obstruction (a scooped-out concave appearance) and is particularly useful in children when assessing for the possible diagnosis of asthma. The ratio of FEV_1 to FVC, used in adult practice to differentiate restrictive from obstructive disease, is less important in children where this differentiation is usually more obvious. However, children have relatively higher flows for their size than adults, so the FEV_1 / FVC ratio tends to be higher at around 90% (compared with 75–85% in adults). Inspiratory flow–volume curves can also be obtained and may be useful when considering extrathoracic obstruction, e.g. from a vascular ring. Infection control is important when using spirometers, particularly in a CF clinic.

Bronchodilator responsiveness

Evidence of airway reversibility is useful both for the diagnosis of asthma and its further management. Bronchodilators should ideally be withheld for 4 hours before assessing reversibility and long-acting β_2-agonists are withheld that morning. Baseline FEV_1 should be measured, followed by the administration of a short-acting bronchodilator. In an effort to demonstrate reversibility, a large dose should be used, such as 1000 µg (10 puffs) of salbutamol via a metered dose inhaler with a spacer device or 5 mg via a nebulizer. FEV_1 should then be measured 15 minutes later. Bronchodilator reversibility is commonly expressed as a calculated increase in FEV_1 >15% of the baseline value, but this is not the best statistical method. In adults, change in FEV_1 should be expressed in absolute terms with an increase of >190 ml indicating reversibility (Editorial 1992). However, in children it has been suggested that an absolute increase >9% of the predicted value (e.g. from 60% predicted to >69%) is the most appropriate way of defining reversibility (Waalkens et al 1993). In some children with genuine asthma, it may not be possible to document reversibility because they have near-normal lung function at the time of testing. In children with CF, the variability of spirometric testing is greater than in normal children, so a larger response is needed to be confident that bronchodilator responsiveness is present (Nickerson et al 1980).

Bronchial challenge

Tests of bronchial hyperreactivity (BHR) involve challenging the airway with cold air or pharmacological agents such as methacholine or histamine. Although commonly performed in adults, bronchial challenge in children tends to be reserved for research protocols and clinical studies. The principal outcome is PC_{20}, which is the provocative concentration of bronchoconstricting agent that produces a 20% fall in FEV_1 from baseline sustained for 3 minutes. Methacholine or histamine produce similar results and may be more sensitive than an exercise test at diagnosing non-specific BHR. These challenges do not produce a late-phase response. Using American Thoracic Society (ATS) guidelines (Crapo et al 2000), spirometry is performed at baseline (and the test should not proceed if FEV_1 is <60% predicted), then the subject inhales the agent (diluted in 3 ml 0.9% saline) via a nebulizer. The starting dose of methacholine is 0.03 mg/ml, and it is doubled each time to a maximum of 16 mg/ml. After 2 minutes of nebulization with a mouthpiece, spirometry is performed 30 seconds and

then 90 seconds after the finish. If the FEV_1 falls less than 20%, the subject proceeds to the next challenge dose. If the FEV_1 falls more than 20% from baseline, no further methacholine should be given. The test should be terminated and signs and symptoms should be noted. A bronchodilator should be given and spirometry repeated 10 minutes later. The subject is monitored until spirometry has returned to baseline. The dose that produced the fall in FEV_1 is calculated and recorded as the PC_{20}. This value can be used to categorize a normal, mild, moderate or severe response to the challenge (Crapo et al 2000).

Static lung volume measurements

Plethysmography or gas dilution are employed to measure static absolute lung volumes and have been discussed in the adult section. The principal difference between the two methods is that gas dilution techniques measure gas communicating with the airways while plethysmography measures all intrathoracic gas. Using these techniques, data on total lung capacity (TLC), residual volume (RV) and functional residual capacity (FRC) can be obtained in children usually over the age of 5 years although some of the younger ones are not keen on getting inside the plethysmographic box. Normative data have been published for UK children aged 4–19 years and male puberty leads to a profound change in lung function, mostly related to size of the thoracic cage, an effect not observed in girls (Rosenthal et al 1993b). The use of these techniques, however, tends to be limited to tertiary care; for example, during annual review in children with CF or as part of investigations for children with complex respiratory disorders.

Resistance and compliance

Measurements of airway resistance and conductance in children are usually measured by plethysmography, but the measurements can be quite variable. Their greatest use in children is to help in the assessment of difficult asthma as they are non-volitional, unlike spirometry, which is easy to fake. Measurements of compliance in spontaneously breathing subjects either requires the subject to relax their respiratory muscles against an occluded airway at various points during tidal breathing, or depends on the insertion of an oesophageal balloon to measure changes in intrathoracic pressure. Changes in resistance and compliance may occur in asthma.

Diffusing capacity of the lungs

Carbon monoxide diffusing capacity or transfer factor of the lung (DL_{CO}) is a measurement of carbon monoxide transfer from inspired gas to pulmonary capillary blood. A correction is used to take into account the patient's size (K_{CO}). The approaches to measuring DL_{CO} include rebreathing, steady state and a variety of single breath techniques. In a single breath method, children need to be able to hold their breath for 10 seconds (this is usually possible over the age of 5 years) and need a minimum vital capacity of 800 ml, although rebreathing techniques can be used in smaller children. DL_{CO} has its greatest place in assessment of lung abnormalities that impair alveolar capillary gas transport as seen in interstitial lung disease, sarcoidosis and sickle cell anaemia. Normal data have been published for UK children aged 4–19 years (Rosenthal et al 1993b). DL_{CO} using the rebreathing technique can also be used during exercise to measure DL_{CO} in children as young as 7 years of age (Rosenthal et al 1995, 1997, Rosenthal & Bush 1998). It is utilized as a surrogate marker of alveolar–capillary growth. Essentially DL_{CO} may be normal at rest but may not increase appropriately during exercise, suggesting a failure of recruitment and distension of the alveolar–capillary bed as observed in chronic lung disease of prematurity (Mitchell & Teague 1998).

Preschool children

Measurement of lung function in this age group is problematic due to lack of coordination and cooperation. Over the last 10 years, studies have shown that it is possible to measure lung function in many preschool children (3–6 years) using incentive spirometry (Bridge et al 1999) or the interrupter technique (Bridge et al 1996). Other methods for assessing peripheral airway function include the multiple-breath inert gas washout (Gustafsson et al 2003).

Incentive spirometry

This method involves teaching the child the forced expired manoeuvre in a manner that is appropriate for the child's development, with plenty of encouragement and positive reinforcement. One such method is the use of breath-activated computer animation programs showing lit candles. The procedure is explained to the child and the child is encouraged to 'blow' the candles out and in doing so, performs a forceful expiration. During a test, it is important to watch the child. Blows should be rejected if the tester feels the child has not tried maximally.

Resistance measured by the interruptor technique (R_{int})

R_{int} is a method, recently applied to young children, whereby airways resistance and bronchodilator respon-

siveness can be measured in children as young as 2–3 years (Bridge et al 1996, 1999). The child, wearing a nose-clip, breathes quietly (tidal breathing) into the mask. Then, in response to a trigger during expiration, at the peak of a tidal flow, a shutter closes off airflow automatically for 100 milliseconds (ms). This gives a measure for airways resistance, which can then be repeated after administration of a bronchodilator or even a bronchial challenge. Normal data are becoming available and this technique may find a place in clinical practice, particularly as this is an ambulatory test that can be carried out anywhere. R_{int} can differentiate individual children (aged 2–5 years) with a history of wheezing, from those with recurrent cough and those with no history of respiratory symptoms (McKenzie et al 2000). Overall, the most useful application of R_{int} appears to be in the assessment of short-term bronchodilator responsiveness where it has been shown to be as sensitive as spirometry in asthmatic children aged 5–15 years (Bridge et al 1996, 1999).

Multiple–breath inert gas washout (MBW)

The MBW method is used to measure the efficiency of ventilation distribution in the lungs and to measure functional residual capacity (FRC). Hardware for this method includes a gas analyser (typically a respiratory mass spectrometer), flow meter, a suitable inert gas marker such as sulphur hexafluoride (SF_6) and a computer for analyzing the data. Typically, a preschool child will wear a facemask with a tight seal, connected to a pneumotachometer. The child will then breathe a 4% SF_6 gas mixture until this gas has equilibrated in the lung. This is called the wash-in phase. At the end of this phase, the inert gas supply is disconnected and the subject breathes room air. The cumulative expired volume for the SF_6 concentration in the lung to reach less than 1/40th of the starting concentration is recorded. This is called the washout phase. The value obtained from these measurements is called the lung clearance index (LCI). This value is the cumulative expired volume to clear an inert gas from the lungs, divided by the FRC. An elevated LCI (>7.8) indicates uneven ventilation distribution, which can be the result of generalized peripheral airway obstruction. In preschool children with CF, the MBW is a more sensitive method than both airway resistance measurements and spirometry in detecting lung function abnormalities (Aurora et al 2005). Little is yet known about the usefulness of the MBW in preschool children with asthma.

Infant lung function

Infant lung function measurements are usually carried out under sedation in specialist centres, and in general are much less standardized than those in older, more cooperative children. This has made obtaining reference data difficult, although recently a multicentre group have collated data on over 400 healthy infants using similar methods in the first 2 years of life and reference data have been derived (Hoo et al 2002).

The techniques employed include the rapid thoracoabdominal compression (RTC) technique, which is used to generate partial forced expiratory manoeuvres and determine maximal flow at functional residual capacity ($\dot{V}_{max}$FRC), a measure of peripheral airway function. The sleeping child breathes quietly until a jacket, placed around the chest, is suddenly inflated (squeeze technique). This produces a sharp expiration, resulting in a recorded flow–volume curve and a measurement of maximal flow at FRC.

In a variation, called raised volume RTC, the chest is passively inflated prior to the squeeze. This gives $FEV_{0.4}$, which is similar to the information provided by the FEV_1 in an older child. Normal data are available, although ideally each infant lung function laboratory will have generated its own data. Standards for infant respiratory function testing have been produced jointly by the European Respiratory Society and American Thoracic Society and published as a series of six articles (Bates et al 2000, Frey et al 2000a, 2000b, Gappa et al 2001, Sly et al 2000, Stocks et al 2001). Infant lung function testing may also include MBW techniques to measure lung clearance index, described earlier.

OXYGEN AND CARBON DIOXIDE MONITORING

Pulse oximetry

Pulse oximeters measure arterial oxygen saturation (SaO_2) non-invasively, which is physiologically related to oxygen partial pressure according to the oxygen dissociation curve (see Fig. 3.3). It is immensely useful, but its shortcomings must be recognized, particularly the lack of accuracy at $SaO_2 <70\%$ (Gaskin & Thomas 1995, Schnapp & Cohen 1990). Further, severe hypotension, low cardiac output, vasoconstriction and hypothermia reduce the pulsatile volume of blood in any given tissue. This reduces the signal strength and quality and causes inaccurate readings. With children, it is important that the correct-sized probe is used otherwise poor contact with the skin may result in an inaccurate reading. Finger clubbing does not seem to cause problems with finger probes.

Particular caution must be used when a pulse oximeter is the only measure of oxygenation available in a sick premature baby where too much oxygen is positively harmful. Due to the shape of the oxyhaemoglobin dissociation curve, pulse oximetry is unreliable at diagnosing hyperoxia due to the flat part of the curve. This means for example, that although a $SaO_2 >97\%$ might at first sight be fine, the PaO_2 may be so high as to cause toxicity (Table 3.7). Furthermore, the shape and variability of the oxyhaemoglobin dissociation curve in critically ill children means that a given SaO_2 is compatible with a range of arterial oxygen tensions (Clark et al 1992). In these situations, direct measurement of the PaO_2 is more appropriate. An alternative non-invasive method is transcutaneous PaO_2 monitoring, although this tends to be restricted to use in neonatal units (Clark et al 1992). Particular care must be taken in the newborn not to overheat the skin, and the electrode needs changing every 3–4 hours.

Overnight continuous SaO_2 monitoring is also an important technique to assess nocturnal hypoxia. However, it is important to state that currently there is no consistent agreed definition of what constitutes nocturnal hypoxia and this appears to be institution dependent. Monitoring is useful when assessing whether a child with CF requires nocturnal oxygen during a chest exacerbation, or when evaluating a child with difficult asthma. It is important that a continuous paper recording is produced that can be analysed the next morning, although these need to be looked at manually rather than simply relying on the computer-generated data summaries. These summaries inevitably include periods when movement artefact produces a falsely low reading which gets included in the summary data. This form of monitoring has been used in certain circumstances as a screening procedure for deciding on the need for full polysomnography in suspected cases of obstructive sleep apnoea (OSA), although a negative oximetry result will not necessarily rule out the diagnosis (Brouillette et al 2000). Although it is true that a normal overnight SaO_2 is encouraging, significant hypercarbia can sometimes accompany normal oxygen levels so caution must be exercised. In addition, arousal may be so rapid in

Table 3.7 Arterial PO_2 with corresponding SaO_2 from oxyhaemoglobin dissociation curve

Arterial PO_2 (kPa)	O_2 saturation (%)
13	97
9	93
8	89
6	80
5	75
4	57

some children with OSA that there is not enough time for hypoxaemia to develop, and the diagnosis can be missed with oximetry alone. Domiciliary pulse oximetry in infants with chronic lung disease receiving home oxygen is supported by the American Thoracic Society (Allen et al 2003). However, in the UK there is no evidence that the provision of oximeters improves the outcome of babies on home oxygen, and in practice may lead to excessive adjustments of the flow rate (Balfour-Lynn et al 2005).

Non-invasive CO_2 monitoring

As mentioned above, measurement of SaO_2 alone gives only half the picture. This is particularly true in children with neuromuscular disease and occasionally so in cases of OSA. Ideally, continuous CO_2 levels should be measured to detect alveolar hypoventilation. This is usually done using a transcutaneous monitor with an electrode that can be left on the skin for up to 8 hours. These measurements correlate reasonably well with the arterial PCO_2, although the response time is too slow to pick up changes secondary to brief apnoeas or hypopnoeas (Clark et al 1992). If a transcutaneous monitor is not available, then a compromise is to measure a capillary PCO_2 immediately the child awakes. Another method for continuous CO_2 monitoring is measurement of airway end-tidal CO_2, but usually this can only be accurately carried out on an intubated patient as ambient air dilutes the measurements if used with mask ventilation (Clark et al 1992).

Capillary blood gases

Measurement of 'capillary gases', i.e. pH, PO_2, PCO_2, bicarbonate and base excess, is very useful, especially in infancy, an age at which arterial sampling is difficult. Up to 12 months, blood is obtained by a heel prick, and in older children a finger prick is used. Although the capillary PO_2 is unrepresentative of arterial levels (normally reading only about 4–5 kPa), the rest of the measurements give a reasonable guide to the child's respiratory status. It is important that the child's heel is warmed to ensure sufficient blood flow, and after a heel prick with a sterile lancet, 150 microlitres of free-flowing blood is collected into a heparinized capillary tube and the blood should be put into the blood gas analyser promptly. It is important that air bubbles are not sucked up into the capillary tube, otherwise the sample is spoiled.

Arterial blood gases

For a complete picture of blood gas analysis, an arterial blood sample is required. In practice, this tends to be routinely available only in neonatal and paediatric intensive care units, where an indwelling arterial or umbilical catheter has been placed. A single arterial stab is painful and difficult in a child who understandably will not cooperate. This means that the resultant analysis may not be valid, as a screaming child will have a reduced $PaCO_2$ and possibly an altered PaO_2.

EXERCISE TESTING

3

Exercise testing has become an important tool in the evaluation and treatment of adult and paediatric disorders. Exercise stresses many aspects of normal physiology, including ventilation and gas exchange, cardiovascular, neuromuscular and thermoregulatory functions. Cardiopulmonary limitation may not be clinically evident at rest, but exercise testing may unmask dysfunction of gas exchange and consequent functional abnormalities.

Exercise capacity

There are three major influences of exercise capacity in a normal individual:

- anatomical
- oxygen transport
- psychological.

Anatomical. This really refers to body size. Body size influences muscle mass and the mechanical conditions under which the muscle operates. Body size is influenced by genetic and environmental factors such as diet and levels of habitual activity.

Oxygen transport. Oxygen is transported from the atmosphere and incorporated into mitochondria of the muscle. The stages involved include ventilation of the lung, diffusion from lungs to the blood, circulation of oxyhaemoglobin, diffusion of oxygen across the capillary muscle membrane, diffusion within the muscle and finally transport to the oxidative pathways of the mitochondria. The principal limiting factor in normal circumstances is the rate of diffusion of oxygen across the capillary muscle membrane. This is greatly influenced by the mean capillary oxygen tension, which is determined by the ability of the circulation to deliver blood to the muscle capillaries.

Psychological. The psychological factors should never be undervalued. Motivation and confidence are key players in exercise ability.

Physiological response to exercise in children

Understanding the physiological response to exercise is necessary in order to understand the concepts of exercise testing and which exercise test is most appropriate for the situation.

3

During exercise cardiac output may increase five times, as a result of increases in both heart rate (HR) and stroke volume (SV), and minute ventilation ($\dot{V}_E$) may increase 25-fold in healthy individuals. As a result of these changes, DL_{CO} increases by approximately 50% during exercise (Manier et al 1993) due to recruitment and distension of the pulmonary capillaries (particularly in the upper parts of the lung), which improve any ventilation–perfusion inequality. The red cell pulmonary capillary transit time (the time taken for a red blood cell to traverse a pulmonary capillary) falls from one second (s) at rest to 0.3 s during exercise. Additionally, during exercise, oxygen consumption ($\dot{V}O_2$) will also increase linearly with increases in workload but will eventually reach a plateau whereby any further increase in workload will not increase $\dot{V}O_2$. This is known as the maximum oxygen consumption ($\dot{V}O_2$max) (Editorial 2003). $\dot{V}O_2$max is the best index for aerobic capacity and is the gold standard marker for cardiopulmonary fitness (Editorial 2003). It is related to oxygen availability and provides information regarding aerobic metabolism in response to exercise stress. However, when $\dot{V}O_2$max is not reached, an individual's peak oxygen consumption ($\dot{V}O_2$peak) can also used as a marker of aerobic capacity. $\dot{V}O_2$max increases with age until puberty, after which the rate of increase accelerates in adolescent boys and levels off in girls. $\dot{V}O_2$max will be affected by age, gender, physical fitness, genetics, population characteristics and mode of testing.

$\dot{V}_E$ increases linearly initially through an increase in the tidal volume (V_T). During exercise, lactic acid is produced and this increases the ventilatory drive, which causes an increase in respiratory frequency. $\dot{V}_E$ will eventually reach a plateau with increased workload and this is termed maximum minute ventilation ($\dot{V}_E$max). Anaerobic threshold (AT) is considered an estimator of the onset of metabolic acidosis secondary to this rise in lactic acid during exercise (Editorial 2003). AT appears to be a good indicator of physical performance capacity in that it correlates well with endurance capacity (Sullivan et al 1995, Wasserman et al 1973) and is relatively independent of maximal effort (Editorial 2003). Physical training increases the numbers of capillaries and mitochondria in muscle and will increase both $\dot{V}O_2$ and AT.

Maximal cardiac output increases with increasing body size mainly due to the increase in ventricular size and stroke volume. The maximal HR is fairly stable through childhood, then begins to decline in late teens towards adult values, whereas resting HR progressively decreases throughout childhood. A commonly used formula for predicting the maximal expected HR in children is (Nixon & Orenstein 1988):

220 − age (in years) ± 10 beats per minute

Gender differences are present throughout childhood but are more marked after puberty: for example boys have a greater $\dot{V}O_2$max and maximal cardiac output, whereas girls have higher HR values.

Indications for exercise testing

Exercise testing is valuable because clinical examination and static cardiopulmonary tests are poor at predicting exercise capacity. Guidelines have been produced by the American College of Cardiology and American Heart Association to make recommendations on the appropriate use of exercise testing in the diagnosis or treatment of patients with known or suspected cardiovascular disease, which includes a section on children (Gibbons et al 2002). The indications for exercise testing are:

- diagnostic tool
- determine severity and functional effects of known disease
- determine prognosis
- outcome measures for therapeutic interventions
- outcome measure in clinical trials
- aid to improving fitness in health and disease.

Diagnostic tool

Dyspnoea assessment. Dyspnoea is the uncomfortable sensation that breathing is difficult. Exercise can assess true dyspnoea from perceived dyspnoea (for example, due to poor fitness) by assessing appropriate physiological responses during exercise.

Diagnostic differentiation. Exercise tests are useful for making a specific diagnosis such as exercise-induced bronchospasm and differentiating it from psychological causes. It is also useful for differentiating between cardiac and muscular pain. Further, an exercise test may identify a deficiency in a specific component of fitness: for example, differentiate a problem of muscle endurance and strength from aerobic capacity (Tomassoni 1996a).

Objective assessment of disability. Exercise testing may help identify abnormal cardiovascular, respiratory or metabolic responses to exercise: for example, cardiac arrhythmias, hypertension, hypoxaemia or hypoglycaemia (Nixon & Orenstein 1988). The test may amplify pathophysiological changes and trigger changes not seen at rest. Similarly, exercise tests can be used to provide objective evidence that there are no functional deficits or that exercise limitation is not secondary to organic disease.

Determine severity and functional effects of known disease

An inability to perform daily physical activities can severely affect quality of life. Exercise testing can provide objective information on any reduction in physical activity. This information is often only partially obtainable from standard lung function testing performed with the child essentially at rest. Further, repeated exercise testing using reproducible outcome measures can help chart disease progression. This may be useful as part of the annual review of children with CF, or for children affected by neuromuscular disorders such as Duchenne muscular dystrophy. It can also help determine the severity of cardiac dysrhythmias, especially those that are precipitated by exercise.

Determine prognosis

In some circumstances, it may be possible to estimate prognosis from exercise ability; for example cycle ergometry in CF (Nixon et al 1992) or 6-minute walking test in severe left ventricular dysfunction (Bittner et al 1993).

Outcome measure for therapeutic interventions

Exercise testing may help in deciding the appropriateness of medical and surgical interventions. Having established a baseline, repeat testing can then be used as a measure of the effectiveness of the particular intervention. Studies in children with pulmonary hypertension treated with sildenafil were assessed by monitoring exercise performance (Humpl et al 2005, Karatza et al 2004). Exercise testing revealed an increase in exercise capacity, specifically the distance walked over this time period. Another example would be its use as one of the criteria for deciding both suitability and appropriate timing of a heart-lung transplant. Further, the functional success of surgical correction of congenital heart lesions can be monitored non-invasively with laboratory-based exercise tests (Derrick et al 2000, Rosenthal & Bush 1999, Rosenthal et al 1995).

Outcome measure in clinical trials

Exercise tests are a useful outcome measure for clinical trials (Ramsey & Boat 1994). If the test is simple and portable it may have a place in phase III multicentre trials (Pike et al 2001).

Aid to improving fitness in health and disease

Many children and their parents are anxious about allowing the child to exercise if the child has an underlying cardiac or respiratory disorder. Exercise testing, conducted with the reassurance of the supervising staff, in the protective environment of the laboratory, can be used to provide evidence that it is safe for the child to exercise. Children can then be encouraged to adopt an active lifestyle to increase their exercise tolerance and improve their level of fitness.

Types of tests available and their application in children

There are many types of exercise tests available, and choosing the appropriate test depends on the question being asked and the aspect of exercise tolerance that needs elucidating. The questions may focus on cardio-ventilatory variables or muscle strength. Tests may be categorized as either maximal or submaximal and their relative merits have been recently reviewed (Noonan & Dean 2000). These include:

- walking tests
- stepping tests
- cycle ergometry and treadmill running.

Walking tests

Self-paced walking tests were initially developed for adults with chronic obstructive pulmonary disease and the techniques have been reviewed (Noonan & Dean 2000). The advantages of such tests are that they are cheap, easy to learn and can be used in an ambulatory setting by children as young as 5 years. However, they require adequate space and are effort-dependent so that the patient's attitude and motivation are a major factor in determining the distance walked. One such test, the 6-minute walk test is designed such that the distance walked in 6 minutes is measured (usually walking up and down a known length of corridor). No verbal or other encouragement is given. It has been shown to be a reliable assessment of exercise performance in healthy children (Li et al 2005) and in severely ill children, the distance walked in 6 minutes correlated with $\dot{V}O_2$peak, physical work capacity and the minimum SaO_2 (Nixon et al 1996). The effects of exercise training in children with congenital heart disease were monitored using a 6-minute walk test, the results of which demonstrated an increase in walking distance (Moalla et al 2005). The 6-minute walk has been further validated in children with mild and moderate CF lung disease, being compared with cycle ergometry (Gulmans et al 1996) and the 3-minute step test (Balfour-Lynn et al 1998). The 6-minute walk test is used as part of the assessment for lung transplantation in children (Aurora et al 2001).

Stepping tests

The 3-minute step test was developed for use in children over 6 years of age as a means of assessing submaximal

3

exercise tolerance by a simple method (Balfour-Lynn et al 1998). Adapted from an adult cardiac test used since the 1920s, it consists of stepping up and down a commercially available aerobic step for 3 minutes (Fig. 3.25).

The step test has been compared with the 6-minute walk in 54 children with cystic fibrosis; the step produced significantly greater changes in heart rate and breathlessness than the walk, with a comparable fall in SaO_2 (Balfour-Lynn et al 1998). A fall in SaO_2 >4% was felt to be clinically significant and could not always have been predicted from the baseline FEV_1. The test was found to be simple to learn, quick to perform and required little space or expense. Importantly, motivation is excluded as a possible variable, and although patients can stop if they wish, in practice this rarely happens. The ambulatory nature of the test means it has even been used in outdoors high-altitude exercise testing of children with cystic fibrosis (Dinwiddie et al 1999). The step test has also been studied in children

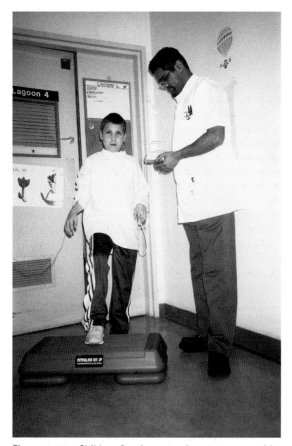

Figure 3.25 Child performing a 3-minute step test with pulse oximeter which measures oxygen saturations and heart rate.

with severe cystic fibrosis lung disease being assessed for heart-lung transplantation (Aurora et al 2001). In this patient group it produced a greater fall in SaO_2 and rise in heart rate than the 6-minute walk.

The step test has also been used to assess the effects of intravenous antibiotics on exercise tolerance in 36 children with cystic fibrosis, and all exercise outcomes were shown to improve (Pike et al 2001). It was found that it complemented spirometry and simple SaO_2 monitoring, and importantly it was demonstrated that the step test was sensitive to changes after a therapeutic intervention. A modified incremental version of the original test has also been used in the evaluation of breathlessness in both normal children and children with cystic fibrosis. In this test the stepping rate rises at 2-minute intervals using rates of 20/min, 30/min and then 40/min and, although incremental, this test still remains submaximal (Prasad et al 2000). A criticism of the step test is that the workload varies with each subject. This is because the work performed in the test is a product of the stepping height and rate (both fixed) as well as the subject's weight and height (particularly leg length). In order to keep the amount of work constant between subjects, the height or rate could be adjusted to account for differences in patient size. However, in practice this is neither feasible nor important in the context of the way the test is used, although the pubertal growth spurt might affect interpretation of longitudinal results from annual testing through puberty. A further factor to consider is that it is not shown to be a sensitive test in children with mild cystic fibrosis lung disease (Narang et al 2003).

The recommended protocol is outlined below:

- It is best for children to practise the test first with sufficient resting time before the test begins.

- Comfortable shoes should be worn (not high heels, preferably trainers) and ideally there should be a cushioned mat on the floor to lessen impact on knee joints.

- A pulse oximeter is used with the probe attached to the patient's finger and the lead taped to the forearm to ensure minimal trace interference during stepping.

- Subjects step up and down a single 15 cm (6 inch) aerobic step.

- Stepping rate is 30 steps per minute, regulated by a metronome.

- Test duration is 3 minutes and a stopwatch is used.

- Subjects are shown how to change the lead leg while stepping (i.e. the leg placed on the step first) so that one leg does not get overtired (muscle fatigue).

■ Standard encouragement at 1 and 2 minutes is given. This should state how far into the test the patient is and that they are doing well.

Outcome measures used are:

■ Baseline and lowest SaO_2 during the test. This may occur at any time within the 3 minutes. A fall in SaO_2 over 4% should be considered abnormal.

■ Baseline and highest pulse rate during the test. This usually occurs towards the end of the test.

■ Breathlessness determined at the start and end of the test using a subjective score (10 cm visual analogue) and the objective 15-count breathlessness score (Prasad et al 2000) or ease of breathing score (Orenstein et al 2002).

The patients are told that they can stop the test at any time if they feel unable to continue for any reason. The investigator should stop the test if the SaO_2 falls below 75%, the patient is unduly breathless or is struggling to keep pace and rhythm. If the patient stops stepping within 3 minutes, the reason why they felt unable to continue should be recorded as well as the time they stopped.

Shuttle tests

There are various forms of the shuttle test (Noonan & Dean 2000). The shuttle walk test is an incremental test of maximal capacity which is achieved by walking the subject around two cones 10 metres apart and increasing the paced walking speed every minute (see adult section). The pace is provided by an audiotape, which 'beeps' at progressively shorter time intervals. The result is expressed in metres. The shuttle test is akin to the standard incremental laboratory test of maximal performance. It has been used to study the effects of training on a group of asthmatic children aged 12–17 years and when compared with standard cycle ergometry, it had sufficient validity to register training effects (Ahmaidi et al 1993). The modified shuttle test has been validated in children and adolescents with cystic fibrosis (Cox et al 2006).

Maximal tests – cycle ergometry and the treadmill

The maximal exercise tests in which subjects are encouraged to reach their maximal level of tolerance remain the cornerstone of most exercise tests in adults and children.

Despite much discussion and debate over protocols, there has yet to emerge a common, standardized approach for assessing exercise capacity in children (Hebestreit 2004).

Nixon & Orenstein (1988) have reviewed the different maximal exercise protocols suitable for children. Briefly, these tests utilize a cycle ergometer or treadmill and the workload is increased progressively (usually at preset time intervals) until the subject reaches their maximal level of tolerance, with online analysis of inspired and expired gases. These tests are considered the gold standard exercise tests, with oxygen consumption, $\dot{V}O_2$peak or $\dot{V}O_2$max as the principal outcome measures. One such gas analyser is the respiratory mass spectrometer (RMS), which allows measurements of both cardiac and ventilatory variables (Fig. 3.26). Normal reference ranges and ventilatory variables for children undergoing cycle ergometry using an RMS have been published (Rosenthal & Bush 1998, 2000). These data have been used to assess cardioventilatory variables during exercise in children following repair of congenital heart disease (Derrick et al 2000, Rosenthal & Bush 1999, Rosenthal et al 1995, 1997). Similar techniques have shown normal exercise capacity following congenital diaphragmatic hernia repair (Trachsel et al 2006) and abnormal ventilatory response to exercise in children with chronic lung disease following preterm birth (Jacob et al 1997, Trachsel et al 2006).

Children over 6 years of age can perform these tests although a degree of coordination and motivation are required (Fig 3.27 shows a subject attached to an RMS). Children are required to pedal or run at a particular workload for a specific period of time while simultaneously wearing a facemask connected to a gas analyser. At specific time intervals, the workload is increased again and this process will continue until the child reaches exhaustion or refuses to carry on. Gas analysis continues during the time of exercise and recovery.

Although the cycle ergometer is familiar as most children ride bicycles, some children find it easier to run than pedal and prefer the treadmill. Some children also find it difficult to maintain a constant pedalling rate. For smaller children, the speed of the treadmill must be adjusted to account for their shorter strides. Also, both cycling and running are more difficult when a tightly fitting facemask is worn. Such tests are time consuming and require significant laboratory space with highly skilled personnel needed to supervise and analyse the exercise test. The equipment is also expensive to buy, use and service.

Peak or maximal exercise tests in children do not necessarily represent their normal daily activities (Cooper 1995). Children tend to engage in very short bursts of high-intensity physical activity interspersed with variable periods of low and moderate intensity. They do not tend to perform sustained heavy exercise, which is the format of most maximal tests. Furthermore, the tests are highly effort-dependent and healthy control

3

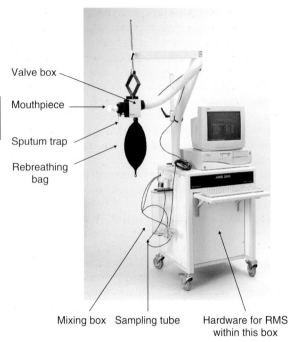

Valve box

Mouthpiece

Sputum trap

Rebreathing bag

Mixing box   Sampling tube   Hardware for RMS within this box

Figure 3.26 Respiratory mass spectrometer, with gas analyser and components.

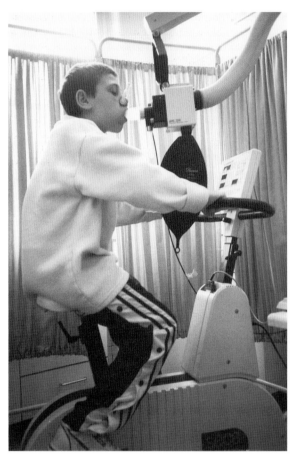

Figure 3.27 Child undergoing cycle ergometry with online respiratory gas analysis.

children can be strongly encouraged, even cajoled, to make a maximal effort. In contrast, children who have an underlying cardiorespiratory disorder may not be pushed so hard, making comparison with normal values less valid (Cooper 1995). In addition, these tests are physiologically stressful and there may be concerns over taking unnecessary risks in children with moderate to severe cardiorespiratory compromise.

Wingate Anaerobic Test (WAnT)

While some children's daily activities are predominantly aerobic, most activities rely on both aerobic and anaerobic energy (Boas et al 1996). The intensity and duration of the activity, as well as the child's level of fitness, determine the relative contribution of these energy sources: for example, high-intensity exercise of short duration is principally anaerobic in nature. As discussed above, this form of exercise is typical of children; hence the relevance of this form of exercise testing in paediatric practice. Anaerobic capacity is determined by the muscles' ability to produce energy quickly from anaerobic sources, and to test this, the subject performs a 30-second all-out sprint at the highest tolerable workload on a cycle ergometer. This is designed to test anaerobic

performance only and the indices of performance are peak power and mean power. A version also exists, using arm cranking, that has been used in children with neuromuscular disorders (Bar-Or 1996). Studies in children and adolescents with cystic fibrosis have shown that anaerobic exercise capacity is reduced and this mainly reflects decreased nutritional status, with pulmonary function playing a smaller part (Boas et al 1996). There is conflicting data as to whether anaerobic capacity is reduced in asthma (Welsh et al 2004).

Exercise testing and muscle strength

The main type of exercise tests performed are those assessing cardioventilatory variables. However, there is also a place for exercise tests to assess muscle strength and these usually involve lifting simple weights or measuring isometric muscle force using a dynamometer or myometer. Muscle strength has been shown to improve with age (Ioakimidis et al 2004) and this must be taken into consideration. These tests are particularly relevant in neuromuscular disorders where maximal aerobic power is less important, because it is seldom the limiting factor in the child's ability to perform daily physical activities (Bar-Or 1996). However, peripheral muscle force is impaired in children with cystic fibrosis, even in the absence of reduced pulmonary or nutritional status (de Meer et al 1999). It is also possible to measure inspiratory muscle strength non-invasively, and in children with cystic fibrosis, it has been found to be impaired, even in those with good nutritional status (Hayot et al 1997). However, in one study, children with CF, admitted to hospital for treatment of chest exacerbations with intravenous antibiotics, were randomized to receive supervised exercise training (Selvadurai et al 2002). The first group received 30 minutes of aerobic exercise 5 times per week; the second group received 30 minutes of weight training (upper and lower limbs) for 30 minutes 5 times per week and the third group were encouraged to undertake their usual physical activity. An exercise test was performed on admission, discharge and 1 month post-discharge. The results showed that the group randomized to muscle training improved their FEV_1 to a greater extent than the other groups. There are little data in children with cystic fibrosis that have examined the effects of both aerobic and anaerobic training on the impact on lung disease.

Outcome measures

There are many useful outcome measures during an exercise test and those employed for a specific individual really depend on the question to be answered. In children, it has been suggested that the cardiopulmonary data collected during the submaximal phases, rather than from the final single data point at peak or maximal power, should be utilized as they more likely equate to daily physical activity (Cooper 1995).

O_2 consumption ($\dot{V}O_2$)

As discussed earlier, $\dot{V}O_2$ is the principal outcome measure from maximal exercise testing such as cycle ergometry or a treadmill test, and it is the single measure most commonly used to represent overall aerobic fitness in children (Nixon & Orenstein 1988). During progressively increasing exercise, $\dot{V}O_2$ increases linearly with increases in work level. However, $\dot{V}O_2$max is observed in less than a third of children and adolescents (unlike adults) (Cooper 1995), so $\dot{V}O_2$max cannot be precisely determined in many paediatric studies. However, the value often recorded is $\dot{V}O_2$peak, which is the highest oxygen consumption of an individual during a specific exercise test (Washington et al 1994). Part of the reason for this is that the test is effort-dependent so many children feel tired and stop before the true $\dot{V}O_2$max is reached. Typical $\dot{V}O_2$max values in healthy children are 40–50 ml O_2/kg/min, while children with cardiorespiratory disease may have values as low as 10 ml O_2/kg/min (Nixon & Orenstein 1988). The intra-individual day-to-day variation in $\dot{V}O_2$max is around 4–6% in fit subjects, although this figure is higher in those with pulmonary disease (Noonan & Dean 2000).

As well as O_2, the CO_2 is measured in the inspired and expired gas collected during formal maximal testing. This gives the full picture of ventilation and pulmonary gas exchange. In addition to $\dot{V}O_2$, CO_2 excretion ($\dot{V}CO_2$), $\dot{V}_E$, respiratory gas exchange ratio ($\dot{V}CO_2/\dot{V}O_2$), and the oxygen ventilatory equivalent ($\dot{V}_E/\dot{V}O_2$) can be calculated. With the addition of flow measurements (by turbine or pneumotachograph) the average respiratory rate and tidal volume can also be measured.

Anaerobic threshold (AT)

Above a certain work rate threshold, the AT is the point when the oxygen demand of the exercising muscle exceeds the oxygen supply, and anaerobic metabolism is required to enable the subject to continue further exercise (Washington et al 1994). At this point, the lactate concentration of the blood increases. During the process of buffering the blood lactate levels there is an increased production of bicarbonate. This leads to a rise in $PaCO_2$, and this in turn results in reflex compensatory hyperventilation. The AT is usually expressed as a percentage of $\dot{V}O_2$max and may vary from 40 to 60%, depending on the degree of physical conditioning. Measurement of the AT is one of the better ways of determining aerobic fitness, as the fitter the person, the higher the $\dot{V}O_2$ before the blood lactate starts to rise. An AT less than 40% may indicate cardiac disease but also may indicate moderate deconditioning (due to lack of fitness).

AT has advantages over $\dot{V}O_2$max as a primary outcome as it is more easily reproducible between occasions and between patients. The reason for this is because $\dot{V}O_2$max requires the patient to get up to maximal exercise capacity whereas AT is a submaximal measure and is relatively independent of effort. The onset of hyperventilation beyond the anaerobic threshold is known as the ventilatory anaerobic threshold, and it can be seen as the point of inflexion on the minute ventilation / $\dot{V}O_2$ curve (Washington et al 1994).

Minute ventilation ($\dot{V}_E$) and ventilatory limit

In healthy subjects, $\dot{V}_E$ increases with oxygen uptake and is not usually limiting. The increase in $\dot{V}_E$ is first achieved by a rise in tidal volume (V_T), due to both a reduction in the end-expiratory lung volume and an increase an increase in end-inspired volume, until V_T reaches a plateau at approximately two-thirds of vital capacity. Further increases in $\dot{V}_E$ are achieved by an increase in respiratory rate. The maximum minute ventilation ($\dot{V}_E$max) during exercise is the highest ventilation that can be achieved and further increases in workload or effort do not give rise to further increases in $\dot{V}_E$. When $\dot{V}_E$ is compromised by lung disease, the subject's predicted $\dot{V}_E$max is reached at a time when the heart rate is considerably less than its maximum; i.e. heart rate reserves greatly exceed ventilatory reserves. The predicted $\dot{V}_E$max on exercise can be calculated from measurements of maximum voluntary ventilation (MVV) or indirectly using (Hansen et al 1984):

$$\text{FEV}_1 \; (\dot{V}_E\text{max} = \text{FEV}_1 \times 40)$$

However, the latter method may underestimate exercise ventilation in subjects with airflow obstruction and a severely reduced FEV_1.

Respiratory exchange ratio (RER)

The ratio of $\dot{V}CO_2 / \dot{V}O_2$ is called the respiratory exchange ratio. RER is usually measured by gas exchange at the mouth. An RER >1.0 suggests the production of lactic acidosis but it may also represent hyperventilation. An RER >1.2 usually indicates maximum effort.

Oxygen saturation (SaO$_2$)

A useful measure of gas exchange that is readily available and accessible is the SaO_2 determined by pulse oximetry, and desaturation <90% during exercise is an abnormal response in children. In practice, even dramatic falls in SaO_2 have no untoward results, and most children gain pre-exercise levels within 5 minutes and all by 15 minutes (Henke & Orenstein 1984).

It is particularly important that movement artefact is eliminated during exercise, otherwise measurements are invalid. In our experience, a flexi-probe taped to the index finger with the lead strapped to the forearm overcomes this problem (Balfour-Lynn et al 1998). The use of a supraorbital probe (placed on the supraorbital artery) during maximal exercise has shown to be less prone to artefact (Derrick et al 2000). Ideally, traces are also recorded on to a computer program alongside the numbers, for later review. This allows elimination of false reading due to low-quality signals. The type of test may also affect the frequency of movement artefact; for example, fewer occur during the step test compared with the walking test, as the children's arms can be kept relatively still while stepping, whereas they tend to swing their arms when walking (Balfour-Lynn et al 1998). In addition, the oximeter and its lead are kept stationary during the step test rather than being wheeled or carried up and down a corridor.

Heart rate

Measurement of heart rate is mandatory for all exercise testing. The dynamics of the heart rate response to exercise are proving to be increasingly useful to identify abnormalities in a variety of disease states. Heart rate monitoring is usually done by a pulse oximeter or cardiorater with electrodes attached to the chest; potential problems of using the former method have been discussed above. During dynamic exercise, the heart rate increases in a linear fashion with the rate of work, and increases up to 3 to 5 times from resting can be seen. Variables that affect heart rate during exercise include the type of exercise, body position during testing, gender, state of health and fitness of the subject, and environmental conditions (temperature, humidity, altitude) (Washington et al 1994). Young children compensate for their relatively small heart size (with lower stroke volume) by an increased heart rate for a given amount of work, so they attain higher maximal heart rates than adults. In pulmonary disease, the patients may not attain the expected maximal heart rate, as their exercise is ventilation-limited. Resting heart rate is also a useful measure in children with lung disease, and was shown to be significantly reduced after treatment of a chest exacerbation in children with cystic fibrosis (Pike et al 2001). Presumably, this was due to a reduction in the high metabolic rate and increased work of breathing associated with a chest infection. In addition, a high resting age-adjusted heart rate was associated with a poorer prognosis in children with cystic fibrosis (Aurora et al 2001).

Work

Maximal work capacity is the highest workload achievable on a progressive test, and is influenced by age, body size and gender. Older and larger children have a greater work capacity, as do boys (Nixon & Orenstein 1988). Obviously children with higher levels of aerobic fitness can do more work. Estimates of the amount of exercise performed are made using the following definitions (Washington et al 1994):

- *Work* is force expressed by distance irrelevant of time (joules)

- *Total work* is the total amount of work performed until exhaustion or another predetermined endpoint

3

lessness, or the intensity of the 'unpleasantness' of the breathlessness, something only the patient can know, and are therefore best used together with one of the subjective scores.

Fatigue

A muscle is considered to fatigue when its force output decreases for a given stimulus and fatigue can be quantified formally (Fulco et al 1995). However, in practical terms, it is simply a feeling of tiredness, which is more difficult to quantify. Like breathlessness, it is somewhat subjective and motivation plays a large part in its perception. It can be a generalized body fatigue or localized leg muscle fatigue, and levels of fitness tend to determine its onset. There are measures such as the Fatigue Severity Scale and the Fatigue Scale but these are best applied to everyday fatigue. For measuring exercise-induced fatigue, a visual analogue score can be used.

Chest pain

Non-specific chest pain is not that uncommon a symptom, particularly in adolescents, and exercise testing may offer reassurance to the child and family. Often no specific diagnosis is made, but exercise testing can certainly indicate whether the pain is due to chest tightness from exercise-induced bronchospasm. The inclusion of an ECG monitor will help distinguish true cardiac pain secondary to ischaemia from non-cardiac pain, such as muscular pain. Ratings of pain measurement exist but are not relevant here, as the exercise test should be terminated if chest pain occurs.

Safety of exercise testing in children

The safety of exercise testing in children, particularly in those with chronic disease, must be considered. There is little specific work with regard to this. However, Alpert and colleagues (1983) reviewed over 1500 studies performed in their laboratory over a 9-year period in which children, including those with congenital heart disease performed cycle ergometry testing to the point of fatigue. There were no deaths, and the total complication rate was 1.8%, which included chest pain, dizziness, syncope and hypotension. Hazardous arrhythmias occurred in only 0.46% of the population. In the authors' laboratory, where more than 500 children have undergone progressive exercise tests using the cycle ergometer and the respiratory mass spectrometer, there have been no reported major complications.

When to stop an exercise test

In general, the test can be stopped when the diagnosis is made or a predetermined endpoint is reached. Certain signs and symptoms should make the investigator terminate the test prematurely:

- Subject feels unable to continue for *any* reason
- Chest pain, muscle cramps, headache, dizziness, syncope, lightheadedness
- Excessive breathlessness or fatigue
- Significant desaturation, usually SaO_2 <75% (but check probe!)
- Abnormalities on ECG
- ST segment depression or elevation greater than 3 mm
- Premature ventricular contractions with increasing frequency
- Supraventricular tachycardia
- Ventricular tachycardia
- Atrioventricular conduction block
- Blood pressure signs
  — Fall in BP >20 mmHg from rest
  — Hypertension (systolic >250 mmHg, diastolic >120 mmHg).

Exercise testing in clinical situations

Asthma

Exercise-induced asthma (EIA) or bronchospasm (EIB) is a common manifestation of asthma in children and adolescents. Unfortunately, pre-exercise spirometry cannot predict response to physical activity and asthmatic subjects with normal lung function at rest may have severe exercise-induced airflow limitation. EIA has been used as an epidemiological measure of asthma in many countries and it is thought that between 40 and 95% of asthmatic patients experience a degree of EIA (McFadden Jr. & Gilbert 1994). It is likely that both the increased water loss from the respiratory tract and the cooling of the airways that occur by increased ventilation during exercise contribute to EIA and EIB (Anderson et al 1985, Gilbert & McFadden Jr. 1992, McFadden Jr. & Gilbert 1994).

EIA or EIB onset is within 5–10 minutes of starting exercise, which usually results in a variable combination of wheeze, cough, breathlessness, and chest pain or tightness. After the normal transient bronchodilation, asthmatic children experience progressive bronchoconstriction, which is usually at its worst 5–10 minutes after stopping the exercise (when symptoms are also usually at their worst). Symptoms have usually gone within 15–30 minutes of stopping, and lung function is back to normal within 30–60 minutes (Cypcar & Lemanske Jr. 1994). The response is of course variable, with some patients able to continue the exercise with spontaneous resolution of their symptoms. Rarely, a late response can be elicited with symptoms reported 4–12 hours after exercise. The severity of the response is determined by exercise intensity, climate (worst in cold dry air) and baseline airway reactivity and function. Some sports are more likely to cause problems, e.g. long-distance running, cycling, soccer, rugby and cross-country skiing, while less provoking sports include swimming, tennis and gymnastics. In fact, the incidence of EIB, as diagnosed by exercise tests, among American Olympic athletes in the 1998 Winter Olympics was reported to be 23% (Wilber et al 2000).

Exercise testing therefore has an important place in the evaluation of asthmatic children, particularly those who only develop symptoms with exercise or in whom standard treatment is not helping these exercise-induced symptoms. Further, supervised exercise testing may reassure the child and their parents that they can actually perform exercise without adverse effects, particularly if bronchodilators are taken 15–20 minutes before the start. The optimal method is to employ a standardized exercise test and measure lung function before and after the exercise. Standardization is particularly important in the follow up of EIA over time when comparing individuals and in the comparison of epidemiological studies. FEV_1 or peak flow are the main outcome measures for determining EIB. There are various regimens for formally testing known or suspected asthmatic children. One example involves the child running on a treadmill to elicit a heart rate of approximately 85% of age-predicted maximum, which in practice is usually up to 8 minutes of exercise. The speed and angle of the treadmill is adjusted to ensure adequate rise in heart rate. Peak flow is measured at baseline, then every 2 minutes until completion of exercise. Measurements then continue every 1 minute for 5 minutes (to ensure an early dip is not missed), then every 5 minutes for 30 minutes. A bronchodilator is then given to demonstrate reversibility using standard methods for testing bronchodilator responsiveness (see above). SaO_2 and heart rate are monitored throughout the procedure. There are two main medical treatment principles for managing EIA: prophylactic treatment (anti-inflammatory) and premedication with bronchodilators prior to physical activity.

Cystic fibrosis

In the 36 years since Godfrey and Mearns (1971) showed that exercise was limited by pulmonary mechanics in children with cystic fibrosis (CF), these children have been subjected to all forms of exercise testing and there is now a wealth of publications in this area (Orenstein & Higgins 2005). The importance lies in the fact that patients with mild disease have a normal exercise toler-

ance. As the disease progresses, exercise tolerance diminishes but cannot be predicted from standard spirometry (Britto et al 2000). Maximal exercise testing has been shown to predict mortality in this disease, with those with higher aerobic fitness having a three times greater increase in 8-year survival compared with those with lower fitness, even after controlling for lung function and nutritional status (Nixon et al 1992). For these reasons, it is a recommended standard of care set by the Cystic Fibrosis Trust (United Kingdom) (2001) to perform exercise testing yearly to assess disease progression. In practice, this is difficult to achieve.

CF patients tend to have high respiratory rates and low tidal volumes during exercise, with a large proportion of each breath moving in and out of an increased dead space and not participating in gas exchange. In healthy children, some ventilatory reserve remains at peak exercise, with minute ventilation remaining less than two-thirds of their maximum voluntary ventilation (MVV). In patients with CF, it is not unusual for $\dot{V}_E$ to reach or even exceed MVV at peak exercise; hence exercise is restricted by a mechanical ventilatory limitation. Other limiting factors include breathlessness, muscle fatigue, nutritional status and psychological parameters. In those with severe disease, ventilation–perfusion mismatching results in O_2 desaturation and even CO_2 retention; however, significant desaturation is unusual in those with an FEV >50% predicted (Henke & Orenstein 1984). Anaerobic performance is also limited in CF, principally due to nutritional factors (Boas et al 1996). Cardiovascular responses to exercise are normal in CF patients with mild disease. Those with moderate to severe disease may not attain expected peak heart rates and cardiac output, since non-cardiac factors, such as those already discussed, limit their ability to exercise before their cardiovascular systems are maximally stressed.

Numerous studies have suggested that exercise training improves aerobic fitness, contains the decline in pulmonary function and may even extend longevity in children with CF, suggesting an improved prognosis and quality of life in physically active CF patients (Orenstein & Higgins 2005). This benefit was more likely when the exercise programmes were supervised, included activities such as running or swimming, lasted for at least 8 weeks and patient adherence was good. Exercise has also been shown to aid airway clearance (Zach & Oberwaldner 1987), but generally it is not recommended as a substitute for the usual physiotherapy techniques. In practice, however, it is sometimes difficult to persuade those children who play regular sport and are fit, to carry out regular chest physiotherapy.

Heart–lung transplant

Measurement of exercise tolerance is an important part of heart-lung transplant assessment Severe exercise intolerance may predict life expectancy and provide information about the patient's quality of life. Various exercise tests have been employed, including the 6-minute walk test (Nixon et al 1996) and the 3-minute step test (Aurora et al 2001). Further, exercise testing has been used to assess change in cardiopulmonary performance in a group of patients both before and after heart and lung transplantation (Schwaiblmair et al 1999).

Congenital heart disease

Exercise testing is an important part of evaluation of children with cardiac disease and the American Heart Association has produced comprehensive guidelines for paediatric testing (Washington et al 1994). Exercise testing is rarely diagnostic in congenital heart disease but has its greatest value in evaluating severity. In particular, it may reveal abnormalities that are not present at rest. Tomassoni (1996b) has outlined common reasons for exercise testing in the evaluation of cardiovascular disease:

- Objective assessment of exercise-induced symptoms, e.g. chest pain, palpitations, dizziness or syncope. In particular, dysrhythmias or ischaemia can be determined.

- Evaluation of cardiac arrhythmia to see whether exercise has an effect.

- Establishment of severity of obstructive heart disease such as aortic stenosis or coarctation of the aorta. The onset of exercise-induced ischaemia can be determined.

- Determination of exercise tolerance and production of recommendations on what exercise it is safe for the child to take part in.

- Evaluation of responses to medical therapy or cardiac pacing.

In addition, the American Heart Association suggests that exercise testing should be *avoided* if there is evidence of:

- Severe pulmonary vascular disease
- Poorly compensated congestive heart failure
- Recent myocardial infarction
- Active rheumatic fever with carditis
- Acute myocarditis or pericarditis
- Severe aortic stenosis
- Severe mitral stenosis
- Unstable arrhythmia

- Marfan's syndrome with suspected aortic dissection
- Uncontrolled severe hypertension
- Hypertrophic cardiomyopathy with a history of syncope.

Musculoskeletal disorders

A recent systematic review looking at aerobic fitness in children with juvenile arthritis showed that overall, there was evidence of reduced oxygen consumption during exercise when compared with controls (Takken et al 2002). Furthermore, a more recent study showed there was impairment in peak and mean power during the WAnT test (Takken et al 2005). These results may suggest that there is a degree of deconditioning in such patients as a result of functional limitations.

Neuromuscular disease

Children with neuromuscular diseases may lead a sedentary lifestyle compared with their peers, causing secondary detrainment and markedly reduced exercise tolerance. A recent Cochrane review suggests that these subjects benefit from both targeted aerobic and muscle training exercise programmes (van der Kooi et al 2005). Muscle function, for example muscle strength and endurance, peak mechanical power and effect on oxygen status of physical movement are most commonly tested. It is important to test several muscle groups, as depending on the condition, certain muscles are affected more than others. For more severe conditions, the arm-cranking version of the Wingate Anaerobic Test may be the only test that the patients can perform, as they are too weak to walk or cycle. Children with conditions such as spastic cerebral palsy may have reasonable muscle strength, but the difficulties of incoordination make testing difficult. In addition, the inefficiency of movement means that for a given task, $\dot{V}O_2$ is much higher in these children (Nixon & Orenstein 1988). At the advanced stage of diseases such as Duchenne muscular dystrophy, the heart muscles are also affected, further limiting the severely weakened movement ability.

Exercise testing in children with neuromuscular diseases can be useful for (Bar-Or 1996):

- Monitoring progression of the disease, e.g. the rate of decline in thigh muscle strength, can be useful in patients with Duchenne or Becker's muscular dystrophy.

- Measuring effect of treatment, e.g. improvement in movement seen after a child with cerebral palsy has had a procedure such as surgical release of hip adductors or lengthening of Achilles tendons.

- Assessing functional effect of exercise, e.g. a child with severe scoliosis who has ventilatory limitation

3

3

may have a normal SaO_2 at rest but desaturate during exercise.

- Monitoring levels of fitness during training programmes or rehabilitation.

Scoliosis

Children with a marked scoliosis have a deformed thoracic cage that leads to a restrictive lung disorder, often accompanied by ventilation–perfusion mismatch. They may be able to perform spirometry, and arm span is substituted for height to calculate predicted values. If a scoliosis is secondary to neuromuscular disease, the child will have the additional burden of severe muscle weakness, which may make even spirometry impossible. Although patients with mild or moderate scoliosis do not exhibit cardiopulmonary restrictions in basal static conditions, they do show a significantly lower tolerance to maximal exercise (Barrios et al 2005). Respiratory inefficiency together with lower ventilation capacity and lower $\dot{V}O_2$max may be responsible for reduced exercise tolerance in adolescents with idiopathic scoliosis. Exercise deconditioning in scoliotic patients may also contribute to exercise intolerance. With severe scoliosis, exertional dyspnoea is common (Nixon & Orenstein 1988).

Chronic lung disease of prematurity (CLD)

Advances in neonatal care have led to an increasing number of extremely premature neonates surviving. Since preterm birth occurs during a vulnerable period of lung maturation, the clinical outcome is determined by the circulatory and gas exchange capacity of the lungs, as well as the medical interventions required (these include oxygen therapy and intermittent positive pressure ventilation). This may lead to considerable respiratory morbidity and preterm subjects with persistent oxygen dependency after 36 weeks corrected gestational age are defined as having CLD (Jobe & Bancalari 2001). Because cardiopulmonary limitations may not be clinically evident while the child is at rest, exercise testing may be useful in schoolage children born preterm and who developed CLD, to determine the presence and extent of any dysfunction of gas exchange secondary to alveolar growth impairment.

There are no longitudinal studies examining exercise performance in children who were preterm and had a low birthweight. In one cross-sectional study (Mitchell & Teague 1998), during treadmill exercise, the CLD and ex-preterm groups had increased wheezing and coughing. Although lung function did not change significantly during exercise, recovery was accompanied by a significant reduction in FEV_1, both in the CLD and ex-preterm

groups compared with the controls. The DL_{CO} increased significantly above pre-exercise in the control and ex-preterm groups but not in CLD group, suggesting problems with recruitment and/or distension of the alveolar capillary bed. The cardiac output was also significantly lower in the CLD group during exercise. In contrast, two other groups have shown normal cardiac responses to exercise (Jacob et al 1997, Pianosi & Fisk 2000). Pianosi & Fisk (2000) showed that cardiac output was normal in CLD subjects but found that these subjects had a higher respiratory rate and maintained a lower end-tidal CO_2 during submaximal exercise when compared with ex-preterm healthy term control groups. Santuz et al (1995) used an incremental protocol on a treadmill and exercised CLD subjects until exhaustion and measured expired gases throughout. The CLD group had exercise-induced bronchospasm, and a lower $\dot{V}O_2$max, $\dot{V}_E$max and a higher respiratory rate compared with controls, indicating both reduced aerobic capacity and ventilatory adaptation. There was no correlation between exercise performance and resting pulmonary function. Using the same exercise protocol, Bader and colleagues (1987) observed a significantly lower $\dot{V}_E$max with a normal $\dot{V}O_2$max in the CLD group than in the control group.

In summary, there does appear to be sufficient evidence to suggest exercise impairment and ventilatory adaptation during exercise in subjects with CLD. The conflicting results may be in part due to the different techniques employed during exercise testing. A detailed review of this topic has been published (Narang et al 2006).

Obesity

Obesity is becoming a serious problem among an ever-increasing number of children, due to poor eating habits and a sedentary lifestyle, with approximately 15% of children in the UK being classified as obese (Owens & Gutin 1999). Paediatric obesity commonly precedes adult obesity and is associated with the development of weight-related co-morbid conditions and increased morbidity (Must 1996, Must et al 1992). Exercise is said to be a cornerstone of treating paediatric obesity along with dietary and behaviour modification. One study showed that, of 20 obese children who attended a 'camp' to help with weight reduction which incorporated exercise prescription, 16 showed a significant reduction in their body mass index (Deforche et al 2003); however, not all the research on the benefits gained by training has been conclusive (Epstein et al 1996). Exercise testing may be a useful way of monitoring progress, and may also be used to alter the exercise prescription with ongoing weight loss. The cardiopulmonary response of the obese child to exercise has recently been reviewed (Owens & Gutin 1999), and it was concluded that the physiological changes are similar to non-obese children. Graded exercise tests on the treadmill produced similar maximum heart rates in obese and non-obese children (Maffeis et al 1994). Similarly, cardiac output values were not different at 33% and 66% of maximal work capacity in obese and non-obese children (Davies et al 1975). However, they may have a higher oxygen demand during submaximal exercise due to the increased metabolic demand of having to move their excess weight (Norman et al 2005). Cardiac constraints may also play a role and this warrants closer, more detailed evaluation (Norman et al 2005). The current literature suggests that exercise testing can be successfully accomplished with most obese children and that the key is to be sensitive and instil confidence in these children at the time of testing as these factors alone can affect exercise performance (Owens & Gutin 1999).

References

Ahmaidi SB, Varray AL, Savy-Pacaux AM, Prefaut CG 1993 Cardiorespiratory fitness evaluation by the shuttle test in asthmatic subjects during aerobic training. Chest 103: 1135–1141

Allen J, Zwerdling R, Ehrenkranz R et al 2003 Statement on the care of the child with chronic lung disease of infancy and childhood. American Journal of Respiratory and Critical Care Medicine 168(3): 356–396

Alpert BS, Verrill DE, Flood NL, Boineau JP, Strong WB 1983 Complications of ergometer exercise in children. Pediatric Cardiology 4(2): 91–96

American Thoracic Society 1986 Evaluation of impairment/ disability secondary to respiratory disorders. American Review of Respiratory Disease 133: 1205–1209

American Thoracic Society 1996 Lung volume reduction surgery. American Journal of Respiratory and Critical Care Medicine 154: 1151–1152

American Thoracic Society 1999 Skeletal muscle dysfunction in chronic obstructive pulmonary disease. A statement of the American Thoracic Society and European Respiratory Society. American Journal of Respiratory and Critical Care Medicine 159: s1–40

Anderson SD, Schoeffel RE, Black JL, Daviskas E 1985 Airway cooling as the stimulus to exercise-induced asthma – a re-evaluation. European Journal of Respiratory Diseases 67(1): 20–30

Anthonisen NR 1986 Tests of mechanical function. In: Fishman AP (ed) Handbook of respiratory physiology: the respiratory system III. American Physiological Society, Bethesda

Aurora P, Bush A, Gustafsson P et al 2005 Multiple-breath washout as a marker of lung disease in preschool children with cystic fibrosis. American Journal of Respiratory and Critical Care Medicine 171(3): 249–256

Aurora P, Prasad SA, Balfour-Lynn IM et al 2001 Exercise tolerance in children with cystic fibrosis undergoing lung transplantation assessment. European Respiratory Journal 18: 293–297

Aurora P, Wade A, Whitmore P, Whitehead B 2000 A model for predicting life expectancy of children with cystic fibrosis. European Respiratory Journal 16: 1056–1060

Bader D, Ramos AD, Lew CD et al 1987 Childhood sequelae of infant lung disease: exercise and pulmonary function abnormalities after bronchopulmonary dysplasia. Journal of Pediatrics 110(5): 693–699

Balfour-Lynn IM, Prasad SA, Laverty A, Whitehead BF, Dinwiddie R 1998 A step in the right direction: assessing exercise tolerance in cystic fibrosis. Pediatric Pulmonology 25: 278–284

Balfour-Lynn IM, Primhak RA, Shaw BN 2005 Home oxygen for children: who, how and when? Thorax 60(1): 76–81

Bar-Or O 1996 Role of exercise in the assessment and management of neuromuscular disease in children. Medicine and Science in Sports and Exercise 28: 421–427

Barrios C, Perez-Encinas C, Maruenda JI, Laguia M 2005 Significant ventilatory functional restriction in adolescents with mild or moderate scoliosis during maximal exercise tolerance test. Spine 30(14): 1610–1615

Bates JH, Schmalisch G, Filbrun D, Stocks J 2000 Tidal breath analysis for infant pulmonary function

testing. ERS/ATS Task Force on Standards for Infant Respiratory Function Testing. European Respiratory Society/American Thoracic Society. European Respiratory Journal 16(6): 1180–1192

Benson MK 1983 Diseases of the airways. In: Weatherall DJ, Ledingham JGG, Warrel DA (eds) Oxford textbook of medicine, Vol 2. Oxford University Press, Oxford, pp 15.60–15.70

Bestall JC, Paul EA, Garrod R et al 1999 Usefulness of the MRC dyspnoea scale as a measure of disability in patients with chronic obstructive pulmonary disease. Thorax 54 (7): 581–586

Bittner V, Weiner DH, Yusuf S et al 1993 Prediction of mortality and morbidity with a 6-minute walk test in patients with left ventricular dysfunction. SOLVD Investigators. Journal of the American Medical Association 270(14): 1702–1707

Black LF, Hyatt RE 1971 Maximal static respiratory pressures in generalised neuromuscular disease. American Review of Respiratory Disease 103: 641–650

Boas SR, Joswiak ML, Nixon PA, Fulton JA, Orenstein DM 1996 Factors limiting anaerobic performance in adolescent males with cystic fibrosis. Medicine and Science in Sports and Exercise 28: 291–298

Borg GA 1982 Psychophysical bases of perceived exertion. Medicine and Science in Sports and Exercise 14(5): 377–381

Bradley J, Howard J, Wallace E, Elborn S 1999 Validity of a modified shuttle test in adult cystic fibrosis. Thorax 54: 437–439

Bridge PD, Lee H, Silverman M 1996 A portable device based on the interrupter technique to measure bronchodilator response in schoolchildren. European Respiratory Journal 9(7): 1368–1373

Bridge PD, Ranganathan S, McKenzie SA 1999 Measurement of airway resistance using the interrupter technique in preschool children in the ambulatory setting. European Respiratory Journal 13: 792–796

British Thoracic Society/Association of Respiratory Technologists and Physiologists 1994 Guidelines for the measurement of respiratory function. Respiratory Medicine 88: 165–194

British Thoracic Society and Society of Cardiothoracic Surgeons of Great Britain and Ireland Working Party 2001 Guidelines on the selection of patients with lung cancer for surgery. Thorax 56: 89–108

Britto MT, Garrett JM, Konrad TR, Majure JM, Leigh MW 2000 Comparison of physical activity in adolescents with cystic fibrosis versus age-matched controls. Pediatric Pulmonology 30: 86–91

Brouillette RT, Morielli A, Leimanis A et al 2000 Nocturnal pulse oximetry as an abbreviated testing modality for pediatric obstructive sleep apnea. Pediatrics 105(2): 405–412

Burdon GW, Juniper EF, Killian KJ, Hargreave FE, Campbell EJM 1982 The perception of breathlessness in asthma. American Review of Respiratory Disease 126: 825–828

Butland RJA, Pang J, Gross ER et al 1982 Two-, six-, and 12-minute walking tests in respiratory disease. British Medical Journal 284: 1607–1608

Cane RS, Ranganathan SC, McKenzie SA 2000 What do parents of wheezy children understand by 'wheeze'? Archives of Disease in Childhood 82: 327–332

Clark JS, Votteri B, Ariagno RL et al 1992 Noninvasive assessment of blood gases. American Review of Respiratory Disease 145(1): 220–232

Cooper DM 1995 Rethinking exercise testing in children: a challenge. American Journal of Respiratory and Critical Care Medicine 152: 1154–1157

Cotes JE 1993 Lung function: assessment and application in medicine, 5th edn. Blackwell Science, Oxford

Cox NS, Follet J, McKay KO 2006 Modified shuttle test performance in hospitalized children and adolescents with cystic fibrosis. Journal of Cystic Fibrosis 5(3): 165–170

Crapo RO, Casaburi R, Coates AL et al 2000 Guidelines for methacholine and exercise

challenge testing, 1999. This official statement of the American Thoracic Society was adopted by the ATS Board of Directors, July 1999. American Journal of Respiratory and Critical Care Medicine 161(1): 309–329

Criner GJ, Cordova FC, Furukawa S et al 1999 Prospective randomized controlled trial comparing bilateral lung volume reduction surgery to pulmonary rehabilitation in severe chronic obstructive pulmonary disease. American Journal of Respiratory and Critical Care Medicine 160: 2018–2027

Cypcar D, Lemanske Jr RF 1994 Asthma and exercise. Clinics in Chest Medicine 15: 351–368

Cystic Fibrosis Trust 2001 Standards for the clinical care of children and adults with cystic fibrosis in the UK 2001. Cystic Fibrosis Trust, Bromley

Davies CT, Godfrey S, Light M, Sargeant AJ, Zeidifard E 1975 Cardiopulmonary responses to exercise in obese girls and young women. Journal of Applied Physiology 38(3): 373–376

de Meer K, Gulmans VAM, Van Der Laag J 1999 Peripheral muscle weakness and exercise capacity in children with cystic fibrosis. American Journal of Respiratory and Critical Care Medicine 159: 748–754

Deforche B, De Bourdeaudhuij I, Debode P et al 2003 Changes in fat mass, fat-free mass and aerobic fitness in severely obese children and adolescents following a residential treatment programme. European Journal of Pediatrics 162(9): 616–622

Derrick GP, Narang I, White PA et al 2000 Failure of stroke volume augmentation during exercise and dobutamine stress is unrelated to load-independent indexes of right ventricular performance after the Mustard operation. Circulation 102(19 Suppl 3): III154–III159

Dinwiddie R, Madge S, Prasad SA, Balfour-Lynn IM 1999 Oxygen therapy for cystic fibrosis. Journal of the Royal Society of Medicine 92(Suppl 37): 19–22

Eaton T, Garrett JE, Young P et al 2002 Ambulatory oxygen improves quality of life of COPD patients: a randomised controlled study. European Respiratory Journal 20(2): 306–312

Editorial 1992 Reversibility of airflow obstruction: FEV$_1$ vs peak flow. Lancet 340: 85–86

Editorial 2003 ATS/ACCP Statement on cardiopulmonary exercise testing. American Journal of Respiratory and

Critical Care Medicine 167(2): 211–277

Epstein LH, Coleman KJ, Myers MD 1996 Exercise in treating obesity in children and adolescents. Medicine and Science in Sports and Exercise 28: 428–435

European Community for Coal and Steel 1983 Standardized lung function testing. Bulletin Europeén de Physiopathologie Respiratoire 19 (Suppl 5): 1–95

Fishman A, Martinez F, Naunheim K, et al 2003 A randomized trial comparing lung-volume-reduction surgery with medical therapy for severe emphysema. New England Journal of Medicine 348: 2059–2073

Frey U, Stocks J, Coates A, Sly P, Bates J 2000a Specifications for equipment used for infant pulmonary function testing. ERS/ATS Task Force on Standards for Infant Respiratory Function Testing. European Respiratory Society/ American Thoracic Society. European Respiratory Journal 16(4): 731–740

Frey U, Stocks J, Sly P, Bates J 2000b Specification for signal processing and data handling used for infant pulmonary function testing. ERS/ ATS Task Force on Standards for Infant Respiratory Function Testing. European Respiratory Society/ American Thoracic Society. European Respiratory Journal 16(5): 1016–1022

Fulco CS, Lewis SF, Frykman PN et al 1995 Quantitation of progressive muscle fatigue during dynamic leg exercise in humans. Journal of Applied Physiology 79: 2154–2162

Gappa M, Colin AA, Goetz I, Stocks J 2001 Passive respiratory mechanics: the occlusion techniques. European Respiratory Journal 17(1): 141–148

Gaskin L, Thomas J 1995 Pulse oximetry and exercise. Physiotherapy 81: 254–261

Geddes D, Davies M, Koyama H et al 2000 Effect of lung volume reduction surgery in patients with severe emphysema. New England Journal of Medicine 343: 239–245

Gibbons RJ, Balady GJ, Bricker JT et al 2002 ACC/AHA 2002 guideline update for exercise testing: summary article: a report of the American College of Cardiology/American Heart Association Task Force on Practice Guidelines (Committee to Update the 1997 Exercise Testing Guidelines). Circulation 106(14): 1883–1892

Gibson GJ 1995 Respiratory function tests. In: Brewis RAL, Corrin B, Geddes DM, Gibson GJ (eds)

Respiratory medicine, 2nd edn. WB Saunders, London, pp 229–243

Gilbert IA, McFadden ER, Jr 1992 Airway cooling and rewarming. The second reaction sequence in exercise-induced asthma. Journal of Clinical Investigation 90(3): 699–704

Godfrey S, Mearns M 1971 Pulmonary function and response to exercise in cystic fibrosis. Archives of Disease in Childhood 46: 144–151

Gosselink R, Decramer M 1998 Peripheral skeletal muscle and exercise performance in patients with chronic obstructive pulmonary disease. Monaldi Archives for Chest Disease 53: 419–423

Gosselink R, Troosters T, Decramer M 1996 Peripheral muscle weakness contributes to exercise limitation in COPD. American Journal of Respiratory and Critical Care Medicine 153: 976–980

Green M, Laroche CM 1990 Respiratory muscle weakness. In: Brewis RAL, Corrin B, Geddes DM, Gibson GJ (eds) Respiratory medicine. WB Saunders, London, pp 1373–1387

Griffiths TL, Burr ML, Campbell IA et al 2000 Results at 1 year of outpatient multi-disciplinary pulmonary rehabilitation: a randomised controlled trial. Lancet 335: 362–368

Gulmans VAM, Van Veldhoven NHMJ, De Meer K, Helders PJM 1996 The six-minute walking test in children with cystic fibrosis: reliability and validity. Pediatric Pulmonology 22: 85–89

Gustafsson PM, Aurora P, Lindblad A 2003 Evaluation of ventilation maldistribution as an early indicator of lung disease in children with cystic fibrosis. European Respiratory Journal 22(6): 972–979

Guyatt GH, Berman LB, Townsend M et al 1987 A measure of the quality of life for clinical trials in chronic lung disease. Thorax 42: 773–778

Guyatt GH, Pugsley SO, Sullivan MJ et al 1984 Effect of encouragement on walking test performance. Thorax 39: 818–822

Hajiro T, Nishimura K, Jones PW et al 1999 A novel, short, and simple questionnaire to measure health related quality of life in patients with chronic obstructive pulmonary disease. American Journal of Respiratory and Critical Care Medicine 159: 1874–1878

Hansen JE, Sue DY, Wasserman K 1984 Predicted values for clinical exercise testing. American Review of Respiratory Disease 129(2 Pt 2): S49–S55

Hayot M, Guillaumont S, Ramonatxo M, Voisin M, Préfaut C 1997

Determinants of the tension-time index of inspiratory muscles in children with cystic fibrosis. Pediatric Pulmonology 23: 336–343

Hebestreit H 2004 Exercise testing in children – what works, what doesn't, and where to go? Paediatric Respiratory Reviews 5 Suppl A: S11–S14

Henke KG, Orenstein DM 1984 Oxygen saturation during exercise in cystic fibrosis. American Review of Respiratory Disease 129: 708–711

Hoo AF, Dezateux C, Hanrahan JP et al 2002 Sex-specific prediction equations for Vmax(FRC) in infancy: a multicenter collaborative study. American Journal of Respiratory and Critical Care Medicine 165(8): 1084–1092

Hooker EA, Danzl DF, Brueggmeyer M, Harper E 1992 Respiratory rates in pediatric emergency patients. Journal of Emergency Medicine 10: 407–410

Humpl T, Reyes JT, Holtby H, Stephens D, Adatia I 2005 Beneficial effect of oral sildenafil therapy on childhood pulmonary arterial hypertension: twelve-month clinical trial of a single-drug, open-label, pilot study. Circulation 111(24): 3274–3280

Hyland ME, Bott J, Singh SJ, Kenyon CAP 1994 Domains, constructs and the development of the breathing. Quality of Life Research 3: 245–256

Hyland ME, Singh SJ, Sodergren SC, Morgan MD 1998 Development of a shortened version of the Breathing Problems Questionnaire suitable for use in a pulmonary rehabilitation clinic: a purpose specific, disease specific questionnaire. Quality of Life Research 7: 227–233

Ioakimidis P, Gerodimos V, Kellis E, Alexandris N, Kellis S 2004 Combined effects of age and maturation on maximum isometric leg press strength in young basketball players. Journal of Sports Medicine and Physical Fitness 44(4): 389–397

Jacob SV, Lands LC, Coates AL et al 1997 Exercise ability in survivors of severe bronchopulmonary dysplasia. American Journal of Respiratory and Critical Care Medicine 155(6): 1925–1929

Jenkins SC, Soutar SA, Moxham J 1988 The effects of posture on lung volumes in normal subjects and in patients pre- and post-coronary artery surgery. Physiotherapy 74: 492–496

Jobe AH, Bancalari E 2001 Bronchopulmonary dysplasia. American Journal of Respiratory and Critical Care Medicine 163(7): 1723–1729

Jones PW 1991 Quality of life measurement for patients with disease of the airway. Thorax 46: 676–682

Juniper EF, Cockcroft DW, Hargreave FE 1994 Histamine and methacholine inhalation tests: a laboratory tidal breathing protocol, 2nd edn. Astra Draco AB, Lund, Sweden

Kadikar A, Maurer J, Kesten S 1997 The six-minute walk test: a guide to assessment for lung transplantation. Journal of Heart and Lung Transplantation 16: 313–319

Kaneko KM, Milic-Emili J, Dolovich MB et al 1966 Regional distribution of ventilation and perfusion as a function of body position. Journal of Applied Physiology 21: 767–777

Karatza AA, Narang I, Rosenthal M, Bush A, Magee AG 2004 Treatment of primary pulmonary hypertension with oral sildenafil. Respiration 71(2): 192–194

Keell SD, Chambers JS, Francis DP, Edwards DF, Stables RH 1998 Shuttle walk test to assess chronic heart failure (letter). Lancet 352: 705

Kharitonov SA, Yates D, Robins RA et al 1994 Increased nitric oxide in exhaled air of asthmatic patients. Lancet 343: 133–135

Knox AJ, Morrison JFJ, Muers MF 1988 Reproducibility of walking test results in chronic obstructive airways disease. Thorax 43: 388–392

Lacasse Y, Lecours R, Pelletier C, Begin R, Maltais F 2005 Randomised trial of ambulatory oxygen in oxygen-dependent COPD. European Respiratory Journal 25(6): 1032–1038

Léger LA, Lambert J 1982 A multi-stage 20-m shuttle run test to predict $\dot{V}O_2$ max. European Journal of Applied Physiology 49: 1–12

Li AM, Yin J, Yu CC et al 2005 The six-minute walk test in healthy children: reliability and validity. European Respiratory Journal 25(6): 1057–1060

Maffeis C, Schena F, Zaffanello M et al 1994 Maximal aerobic power during running and cycling in obese and non-obese children. Acta Paediatrica 83(1): 113–116

Maltais F, Simard AA, Simard C et al 1996 Oxidative capacity of the skeletal muscle and lactic acid kinetics during exercise in normal subjects and in patients with COPD. American Journal of Respiratory and Critical Care Medicine 153: 288–293

Manier G, Moinard J, Stoicheff H 1993 Pulmonary diffusing capacity after maximal exercise. Journal of Applied Physiology 75(6): 2580–2585

Mathur RS, Revill SM, Vara DD et al 1995 Comparison of peak oxygen consumption during cycle and treadmill exercise in severe chronic airflow obstruction. Thorax 50: 829–833

McFadden ER, Jr, Gilbert IA 1994 Exercise-induced asthma. New England Journal of Medicine 330(19): 1362–1367

McGavin CR, Gupta SP, McHardy GJR 1976 Twelve-minute walking test for assessing disability in chronic bronchitis. British Medical Journal 1: 822–823

McKenzie SA, Bridge PD, Healy MJR 2000 Airway resistance and atopy in preschool children with wheeze and cough. European Respiratory Journal 15: 833–838

Mitchell SH, Teague WG 1998 Reduced gas transfer at rest and during exercise in school-age survivors of bronchopulmonary dysplasia. American Journal of Respiratory and Critical Care Medicine 157(5 Pt 1): 1406–1412

Moalla W, Gauthier R, Maingourd Y, Ahmaidi S 2005 Six-minute walking test to assess exercise tolerance and cardiorespiratory responses during training program in children with congenital heart disease. International Journal of Sports Medicine 26(9): 756–762

Mungall IPF, Hainsworth R 1979 Assessment of respiratory function in patients with chronic obstructive airways disease. Thorax 34: 254–258

Must A 1996 Morbidity and mortality associated with elevated body weight in children and adolescents. American Journal of Clinical Nutrition 63(3 Suppl): 445S–447S

Must A, Jacques PF, Dallal GE, Bajema CJ, Dietz WH 1992 Long-term morbidity and mortality of overweight adolescents. A follow-up of the Harvard Growth Study of 1922 to 1935. New England Journal of Medicine 327(19): 1350–1355

Narang I, Baraldi E, Silverman M, Bush A 2006 Airway function measurements and the long-term follow-up of survivors of preterm birth with and without chronic lung disease. Pediatric Pulmonology 41(6): 497–508

Narang I, Pike S, Rosenthal M, Balfour-Lynn IM, Bush A 2003 Three-minute step test to assess exercise capacity in children with cystic fibrosis with mild lung disease. Pediatric Pulmonology 35(2): 108–113

Nickerson BG, Lemen RJ, Gerdes CB, Wegmann MJ, Robertson G 1980 Within-subject variability and per cent change for significance of spirometry in normal subjects and patients with cystic fibrosis. American Review of Respiratory Disease 122: 859–866

Nixon PA, Joswiak ML, Fricker FJ 1996 A six-minute walk test for assessing exercise tolerance in severely ill children. Journal of Pediatrics 129: 362–366

Nixon PA, Orenstein DM 1988 Exercise testing in children. Pediatric Pulmonology 5: 107–122

Nixon PA, Orenstein DM, Kelsey SF, Doershuk CF 1992 The prognostic value of exercise testing in patients with cystic fibrosis. New England Journal of Medicine 327: 1785–1788

Noonan V, Dean E 2000 Submaximal exercise testing: clinical application and interpretation. Physical Therapy 80: 782–807

Norman AC, Drinkard B, McDuffie JR et al 2005 Influence of excess adiposity on exercise fitness and performance in overweight children and adolescents. Pediatrics 115(6): e690–e696

O'Donnell DE, Lam M, Webb KA 1999 Spirometric correlates of improvement in exercise performance after anticholinergic therapy in chronic obstructive pulmonary disease. American Journal of Respiratory and Critical Care Medicine 160: 542–549

Orenstein DM, Higgins LW 2005 Update on the role of exercise in cystic fibrosis. Current Opinion in Pulmonary Medicine 11(6): 519–523

Orenstein DM, Holt LS, Rebovich P et al 2002 Measuring ease of breathing in young patients with cystic fibrosis. Pediatric Pulmonology 34: 473–477

Owens S, Gutin B 1999 Exercise testing of the child with obesity. Pediatric Cardiology 20: 79–83

Pattishall EN 1990 Pulmonary function testing references values and interpretations in pediatric training programs. Pediatrics 85: 768–773

Pepin V, Saey D, Whittom F, Leblanc P, Maltais F 2005 Walking versus cycling: sensitivity to bronchodilation in chronic obstructive pulmonary disease. American Journal of Respiratory and Critical Care Medicine 172(12): 1517–1522

Pianosi PT, Fisk M 2000 Cardiopulmonary exercise performance in prematurely born children. Pediatric Research 47: 653–658

Pike SE, Prasad SA, Balfour-Lynn IM 2001 Effect of intravenous antibiotics on exercise tolerance (3-minute step test) in cystic fibrosis. Pediatric Pulmonology 32: 38–43

Polgar G, Promadhat V 1971 Pulmonary function testing in children: techniques and standards. WB Saunders, Philadelphia

Polgar G, Weng TR 1979 The functional development of the respiratory system from the period of gestation to adulthood. American Review of Respiratory Disease 120: 625–695

Prasad SA, Randall SD, Balfour-Lynn IM 2000 Fifteen-count breathlessness score: an objective measure for children. Pediatric Pulmonology 30: 56–62

Ram FSF, Wedzicha JA 2004 Ambulatory oxygen for chronic obstructive pulmonary disease (Cochrane Review). In: The Cochrane Library, Issue 2, 2004. John Wiley & Sons, Chichester, UK

Ramsey BW, Boat TF 1994 Outcome measures for clinical trials in cystic fibrosis. Summary of a cystic fibrosis foundation consensus conference. Journal of Pediatrics 124: 177–192

Redelmeier DA, Bayoumi AM, Goldstein RS, Guyatt GH 1997 Interpreting small differences in functional status: the Six Minute Walk test in chronic lung disease patients. American Journal of Respiratory and Critical Care Medicine 155(4): 1278–1282

Redline S, Wright EC, Kattan M, Kercsmar C, Weiss K 1996 Short-term compliance with peak-flow monitoring: results from a study of inner city children with asthma. Pediatric Pulmonology 21: 203–210

Revill SM, Morgan MDL, Singh SJ, Williams J, Hardman AE 1999 The endurance shuttle walk: a new field test for the assessment of endurance capacity in chronic obstructive pulmonary disease. Thorax 54: 213–222

Rosenthal M, Bain SH, Cramer D et al 1993a Lung function in white children aged 4 to 19 years: I - spirometry. Thorax 48: 794–802

Rosenthal M, Bush A 1998 Haemodynamics in children during rest and exercise: methods and normal values. European Respiratory Journal 11(4): 854–865

Rosenthal M, Bush A 1999 The effects of surgically treated pulmonary stenosis on lung growth and cardiopulmonary function in children during rest and exercise. European Respiratory Journal 13(3): 590–596

Rosenthal M, Bush A 2000 Ventilatory variables in normal children during rest and exercise. European Respiratory Journal 16: 1075–1083

Rosenthal M, Bush A, Deanfield J, Redington A 1995 Comparison of cardiopulmonary adaptation during exercise in children after the atriopulmonary and total cavopulmonary connection Fontan procedures. Circulation 91(2): 372–378

Rosenthal M, Cramer D, Bain SH et al 1993b Lung function in white children aged 4 to 19 years: II – single

3

breath analysis and plethysmography. Thorax 48: 803–808

Rosenthal M, Redington A, Bush A 1997 Cardiopulmonary physiology after surgical closure of asymptomatic secundum atrial septal defects in childhood. Exercise performance is unaffected by age at repair. European Heart Journal 18(11): 1816–1822

Santuz P, Baraldi E, Zaramella P, Filippone M, Zacchello F 1995 Factors limiting exercise performance in long-term survivors of bronchopulmonary dysplasia. American Journal of Respiratory and Critical Care Medicine 152(4 Pt 1): 1284–1289

Schnapp LM, Cohen NH 1990 Pulse oximetry. Uses and abuses. Chest 98: 1244–1249

Schols AM, Soeters PB, Dingemans AM et al 1993 Prevalence and characteristics of nutritional depletion in patients with stable COPD eligible for pulmonary rehabilitation. American Review of Respiratory Disease 147(5): 1151–1156

Schwaiblmair M, Reichenspurner H, Muller C et al 1999 Cardiopulmonary exercise testing before and after lung and heart-lung transplantation. American Journal of Respiratory and Critical Care Medicine 159(4 Pt 1): 1277–1283

Selvadurai HC, Blimkie CJ, Meyers N et al 2002 Randomized controlled study of in-hospital exercise training programs in children with cystic fibrosis. Pediatric Pulmonology 33(3): 194–200

Sewell L, Singh SJ, Williams JE, Collier R, Morgan MD 2005 Can individualized rehabilitation improve functional independence in elderly patients with COPD? Chest 128(3): 1194–1200

Shneerson J 1988 Disorders of ventilation. Blackwell Science, Oxford, pp 78–85

Silverman M, Stocks J 1999 Pediatric pulmonary function. In: Hughes JMB, Pride NB (eds) Lung function tests. Physiological principles and clinical applications. WB Saunders, London, pp 163–183

Singh SJ, Jones, PJ, Sewell L, Williams JE, Morgan MD 2002 What is the minimum clinically important difference in the incremental shuttle walking test (ISWT) observed in pulmonary rehabilitation? European Respiratory Journal 20(Suppl 38): 67s

Singh SJ, Morgan MDL, Scott S et al 1992 The development of the shuttle walking test of disability in patients with chronic obstructive airways obstruction. Thorax 47: 1019–1024

Sly PD, Tepper R, Henschen M, Gappa M, Stocks J 2000 Tidal forced expirations. ERS/ATS Task Force on Standards for Infant Respiratory Function Testing. European Respiratory Society/American Thoracic Society. European Respiratory Journal 16(4): 741–748

Sont JK, Willems LN, Bel EH et al 1999 Clinical control and histopathologic outcome of asthma when using airway responsiveness as an additional guide to long-term treatment. American Journal of Respiratory and Critical Care Medicine 159: 1043–1051

Steiner MC, Morgan MDL 2001 Enhancing physical performance in chronic obstructive pulmonary disease Thorax 56: 73–77

Stocks J, Godfrey S, Beardsmore C, Bar-Yishay E, Castile R 2001 Plethysmographic measurements of lung volume and airway resistance. ERS/ATS Task Force on Standards for Infant Respiratory Function Testing. European Respiratory Society/American Thoracic Society. European Respiratory Journal 17(2): 302–312

Sullivan CS, Casaburi R, Storer TW, Wasserman K 1995 Non-invasive prediction of blood lactate response to constant power outputs from incremental exercise tests. European Journal of Applied Physiology and Occupational Physiology 71(4): 349–354.

Szekely LA, Oelberg DA, Wright C et al 1997 Pre-operative predictors of operative morbidity and mortality in COPD patients undergoing bilateral lung volume reduction surgery. Chest 111: 550–558

Takken T, Hemel A, van der NJ, Helders PJ 2002 Aerobic fitness in children with juvenile idiopathic arthritis: a systematic review. Journal of Rheumatology 29(12): 2643–2647

Takken T, van der NJ, Helders PJ 2005 Anaerobic exercise capacity in patients with juvenile-onset idiopathic inflammatory myopathies. Arthritis and Rheumatism 53(2): 173–177

Tomassoni TL 1996a Introduction: the role of exercise in the diagnosis and management of chronic disease in children and youth. Medicine and Science in Sports and Exercise 28: 403–405

Tomassoni TL 1996b Role of exercise in the management of cardiovascular disease in children and youth. Medicine and Science in Sports and Exercise 28: 406–413

Trachsel D, Selvadurai H, Adatia I et al 2006 Resting and exercise cardiorespiratory function in survivors of congenital diaphragmatic hernia. Pediatric Pulmonology 41(6): 522–529

Tremper KK, Barker S 1989 Pulse oximetry. Anesthesiology 70: 98–108

Uldry C, Fitting JW 1995 Maximal values of sniff nasal inspiratory pressures in healthy subjects. Thorax 50: 371–375

van der Kooi EL, Lindeman E, Riphagen I 2005 Strength training and aerobic exercise training for muscle disease. Cochrane Database of Systematic Reviews (1): CD003907

Waalkens HJ, Merkus PJFM, Van Essen-Zandvliet EE et al 1993 Assessment of bronchodilator response in children with asthma. Dutch CNSLD Study Group. European Respiratory Journal 6: 645–651

Washington RL, Bricker JT, Alpert BS et al 1994 Guidelines for exercise testing in the pediatric age group. From the Committee on Atherosclerosis and Hypertension in Children, Council on Cardiovascular Disease in the Young, the American Heart Association. Circulation 90(4): 2166–2179

Wasserman K, Whipp BJ, Koyl SN, Beaver WL 1973 Anaerobic threshold and respiratory gas exchange during exercise. Journal of Applied Physiology 35(2): 236–243

Wedzicha JA 1996 Domiciliary ventilation in chronic obstructive pulmonary disease: where are we? Thorax 51: 455–457

Welsh L, Roberts RG, Kemp JG 2004 Fitness and physical activity in children with asthma. Sports Medicine 34(13): 861–870

Wilber RL, Rundell KW, Szmedra L et al 2000 Incidence of exercise-induced bronchospasm in Olympic winter sport athletes. Medicine and Science in Sports and Exercise 32(4): 732–737

Williams JE, Singh SJ, Sewell L, Guyatt GH, Morgan MD 2001 Development of a self-reported Chronic Respiratory Questionnaire (CRQ–SR). Thorax 56(12): 954–959

Williams JE, Singh SJ, Sewell L, Morgan MD 2003 Health status measurement: sensitivity of the self-reported Chronic Respiratory Questionnaire (CRQ–SR) in pulmonary rehabilitation. Thorax 58(6): 515–518

Zach MS, Oberwaldner B 1987 Chest physiotherapy – the mechanical approach to antiinfective therapy in cystic fibrosis. Infection 15(5): 381–384

Further reading

American College of Sports Medicine 2000 Guidelines for exercise testing and prescription, 6th edn. Lea and Febiger, Philadelphia

Borg GAV 1982 Psychophysical bases of perceived exertion. Medicine and Science in Sports and Exercise 14: 377–381

Braunwald E, Zipes DP, Libby P, Bonow R (eds) 2004 Heart disease: a textbook of cardiovascular medicine, 7th edn. WB Saunders, Philadelphia

British Thoracic Society/Association of Respiratory Technologists and Physiologists 1994 Guidelines for the measurement of respiratory function. Respiratory Medicine 88: 165–194

Burdon GW, Juniper EF, Killian KJ, Hargreave FE Campbell EJM 1982 The perception of breathlessness in asthma. America Review of Respiratory Disease 126: 825–826

Castile RG 1998 Pulmonary function testing in children. In: Chernick V, Boat TF (eds) Kendig's disorders of the respiratory tract in children. WB Saunders, Philadelphia, pp 196–214

Cooper C, Storer T 2001 Exercise testing and interpretation: a practical approach. Cambridge University Press, Cambridge

ERS Task Force 1997 Clinical testing with reference to lung diseases: indications, standardisation and interpretation strategies. European Respiratory Journal 10: 2662–2689

Houghton AR, Gray D 1997 Making sense of the ECG. Edward Arnold, London

Hyatt RE, Scanlon PD, Nakamura M 1997 Interpretation of pulmonary function tests. A practical guide. Lippincott–Raven, Philadelphia

Jones NL 1997 Clinical exercise testing, 4th edn. WB Saunders, Philadelphia

Julian DG, Cowan JC, McLenachan JM 2005 Cardiology, 8th edn. WB Saunders, Philadelphia

Stocks J, Sly PD, Tepper RS, Morgan WJ 1996 Infant respiratory function testing. John Wiley, New York

Sutton P 1999 Measurements in cardiology. Parthenon, London

West JB 2003 Pulmonary pathophysiology, 4th edn. Williams and Wilkins, Baltimore

West JB 2004 Respiratory physiology, 7th edn. Williams and Wilkins, Baltimore

Wilson RC, Jones PW 1989 A comparison of the visual analogue scale and modified Borg scale for the measurement of dyspnoea during exercise. Clinical Science 76: 277–282

Chapter **4**

Effects of positioning and mobilization

Elizabeth Dean, Christiane Perme

INTRODUCTION

The purpose of this chapter is to provide a framework for clinical decision-making in the management of patients with cardiopulmonary dysfunction, with special emphasis on positioning and mobilization. 'Cardiopulmonary dysfunction' refers to impairment of one or more steps in the oxygen transport pathway. First, the oxygen transport pathway and the factors that contribute to impairment of oxygen transport are described. Second, three clinically significant effects of positioning and mobilization are distinguished:

- to improve oxygen transport in acute cardiopulmonary dysfunction

- to improve oxygen transport in the post-acute and chronic stages of cardiopulmonary dysfunction

- to prevent the negative effects of restricted mobility, particularly those that adversely affect oxygen transport.

In addition, the physiological and scientific rationale for use of positioning and mobilization for each of the above effects is described. Conceptualizing cardiopulmonary dysfunction as impairment of the steps in the oxygen transport pathway and exploiting positioning and mobilization as primary interventions in remediating this impairment will maximize physiotherapy efficacy. Emphasis is placed on impairment of oxygen transport given that such impairment in large part determines disability and handicap (Verbrugge & Lette 1993), as defined by the World Health Organization (1980), secondary to cardiopulmonary dysfunction.

The following terms (Ross & Dean 1989) have been adopted in this chapter:

4

1. *Positioning* refers to the application of body positioning to optimize oxygen transport, primarily by manipulating the effect of gravity on cardiopulmonary and cardiovascular function.
2. *Mobilization and exercise* refer to the application of progressive exercise to elicit acute cardiopulmonary and cardiovascular responses to enhance oxygen transport. In the context of cardiopulmonary physiotherapy, 'mobilization' refers to low-intensity exercise for typically acutely ill patients or those with severely compromised functional work capacity.
3. *Optimizing oxygen transport* is the goal of positioning and mobilization. The 'adaptation' or 'training-sensitive' zone defines the upper and lower limits of the various indices of oxygen transport needed to elicit the optimal adaptation of the steps in the oxygen transport pathway. This zone is based on an analysis of the factors that contribute to cardiopulmonary dysfunction and thus is specific for each patient.

CONCEPTUAL FRAMEWORK FOR CLINICAL DECISION-MAKING

The oxygen transport pathway

Optimal cardiopulmonary function and gas exchange reflect the optimal matching of oxygen demand and supply (Dantzker 1983, Weber et al 1983). Oxygen delivery and oxygen consumption based on demand are essential components of the oxygen transport system. Figure 4.1 shows the components of oxygen delivery ($\dot{D}O_2$), namely arterial oxygen content and cardiac output (CO), and the components of oxygen consumption ($\dot{V}O_2$), namely the arteriovenous oxygen content difference and CO. In health, $\dot{D}O_2$ is approximately four times greater than $\dot{V}O_2$ at rest so there is considerable oxygen reserve that is drawn upon during times of increased metabolic demand such as exercise, stress, illness and repair. Because of the large reserve, $\dot{V}O_2$ is thought to be normally supply-independent. This reserve capacity, however, becomes compromised secondary to acute and chronic pathological conditions. In patients who are critically ill and $\dot{D}O_2$ is severely compromised, $\dot{V}O_2$ may be supply-dependent until $\dot{D}O_2$ reaches a critical threshold, i.e. the level at which metabolic demands are met (Phang & Russell 1993). Below this critical threshold, patients are increasingly dependent on anaerobic metabolism reflected by increased minute ventilation, respiratory exchange ratio and serum lactate levels.

The efficiency with which oxygen is transported from the atmosphere along the steps of the oxygen transport pathway to the tissues determines the efficiency of oxygen transport overall (Fig. 4.2). The steps

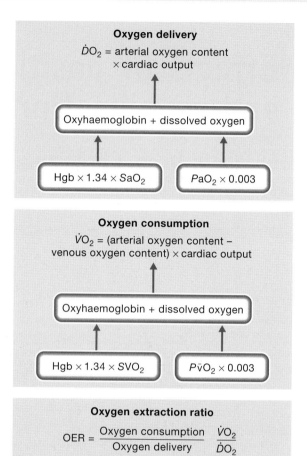

Oxygen delivery

$\dot{D}O_2$ = arterial oxygen content × cardiac output

Oxyhaemoglobin + dissolved oxygen

Hgb × 1.34 × SaO_2 PaO_2 × 0.003

Oxygen consumption

$\dot{V}O_2$ = (arterial oxygen content − venous oxygen content) × cardiac output

Oxyhaemoglobin + dissolved oxygen

Hgb × 1.34 × SVO_2 $P\bar{v}O_2$ × 0.003

Oxygen extraction ratio

$$OER = \frac{\text{Oxygen consumption}}{\text{Oxygen delivery}} \quad \frac{\dot{V}O_2}{\dot{D}O_2}$$

Figure 4.1 The components of oxygen delivery ($\dot{D}O_2$) and oxygen consumption ($\dot{V}O_2$).

in the oxygen transport pathway include ventilation of the alveoli, diffusion of oxygen across the alveolar capillary membrane, perfusion of the lungs, biochemical reaction of oxygen with the blood, affinity of oxygen with haemoglobin, cardiac output, integrity of the peripheral circulation and oxygen extraction at the tissue level (Wasserman et al 1987). At rest, the demand for oxygen reflects basal metabolic requirements. Metabolic demand changes normally in response to gravitational (positional), exercise and psychological stressors. When one or more steps in the oxygen transport pathway are impaired secondary to cardiopulmonary dysfunction, oxygen demand at rest and in response to stressors can be increased significantly. Impairment of one step in the pathway may be compensated by other steps, thereby maintaining normal gas exchange and arterial oxygenation. With severe impairment involving several steps, arterial oxygenation may be reduced, the work of the heart and lungs increased, tissue oxygenation impaired and, in the most extreme situation, multiorgan system failure may ensue.

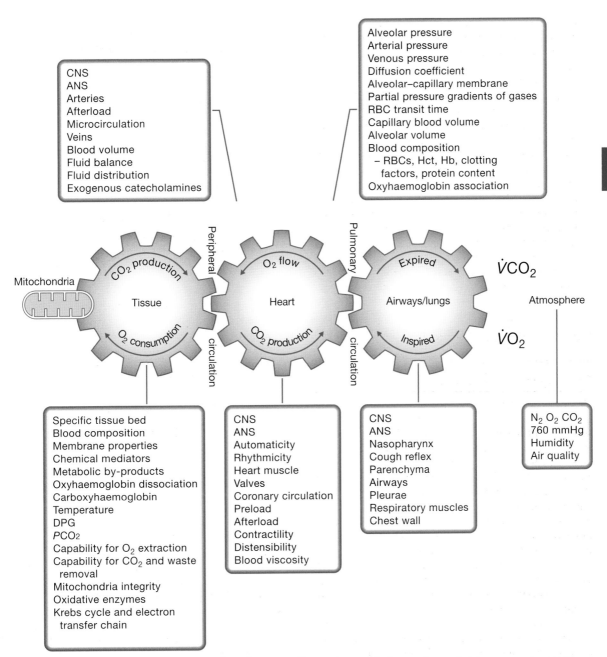

Figure 4.2 A scheme of the components of ventilatory–cardiovascular–metabolic coupling underlying oxygen transport. CNS, central nervous system; ANS, autonomic nervous system; DPG, diphosphoglycerate; RBC, red blood cell; Hct, haematocrit; Hb, haemoglobin. (Modified from Wasserman et al 1987)

While the oxygen transport pathway ensures that an adequate supply of oxygen meets the demands of the working tissues, the carbon dioxide pathway ensures that carbon dioxide, a primary by-product of metabolism, is eliminated. This pathway is basically the reverse of the oxygen transport pathway in that carbon dioxide is transported from the tissues, via the circulation, to the lungs for elimination. Carbon dioxide is a highly diffusible gas and is readily eliminated from the body. However, carbon dioxide retention is a hallmark of diseases in which the ventilatory muscle pump is operating inefficiently or the normal elastic recoil of the lung parenchyma is lost.

4

Factors contributing to cardiopulmonary dysfunction

Cardiopulmonary dysfunction, in which oxygen transport is threatened or impaired, results from four principal factors:

- the underlying disease pathophysiology
- bed rest/recumbency and restricted mobility
- extrinsic factors imposed by the patient's medical care
- intrinsic factors relating to the patient (Box 4.1) (Dean 1994a, Dean & Ross 1992a).

An analysis of the factors that contribute to cardiopulmonary dysfunction provides the basis for assessment and prescribing the parameters of positioning and mobilization, to enhance oxygen transport for a given patient. The treatment is directed at the specific underlying contributing factors. In some cases, e.g. low haemoglobin, the underlying impairment of oxygen transport cannot be affected directly by physical intervention. However, mobilization and exercise can improve aerobic capacity in patients with anaemia, a factor not directly modifiable by non-invasive physiotherapy interventions, by increasing the efficiency of other steps in the oxygen transport pathway (Williams 1995). Further, even though some factors are not directly modifiable by non-invasive physiotherapy interventions, they influence treatment outcome, and thus need to be considered when planning, modifying and progressing treatment. Fluid imbalance for example is the result of many factors, including reduced muscle activity (Koomans & Boer 1997). Physiotherapy that incorporates body position and exercise challenges may have a profound effect on fluid balance by maintaining fluid balance between the intra- and extravascular compartments. Research is needed to address this compelling proposition.

Ageing and weight deserve special consideration. Patients who are older have progressively lower lung function, and oxygen transport reserve capacity overall (Rossi et al 1996). These changes predispose this population, who tend to constitute the majority of patients in the intensive care unit (ICU), to complications. In addition, obesity often complicates the clinical picture of patients in the ICU: the heavier the patient, the greater the risk. Body positioning and mobilization are particularly important is offsetting the deleterious effects of being recumbent with the added physical burden of adipose tissue surrounding the chest wall (Beck 1998).

Multisystem organ dysfunction and failure may lead to or result from cardiopulmonary dysfunction; thus they are associated with significant mortality and mor-

> **Box 4.1 Factors contributing to cardiopulmonary dysfunction, i.e. factors that compromise or threaten oxygen transport**
>
> - **Cardiopulmonary pathophysiology**
>   Acute
>   Chronic – primary
>   – secondary
>   Acute and chronic
> - **Bed rest/recumbency and restricted mobility**
> - **Extrinsic factors**
>   Reduced arousal
>   Surgical procedures
>   Incisions
>   Dressings and bindings
>   Casts/splinting devices/traction
>   Invasive lines/catheters
>   Monitoring equipment
>   Medications
>   Intubation
>   Mechanical ventilation
>   Suctioning
>   Pain
>   Anxiety
>   Hospital admission
> - **Intrinsic factors**
>   Age
>   Gender
>   Ethnicity
>   Congenital abnormalities
>   Smoking history
>   Occupation
>   Air quality
>   Obesity
>   Nutritional deficits
>   Deformity
>   Fluid and electrolyte balance
>   Conditioning level
>   Impaired immunity
>   Anaemia/polycythaemia
>   Thyroid abnormalities
>   Multisystem complications
>   Previous medical and surgical history
>
> (Adapted from Dean 1993, Dean and Ross 1992a and Ross and Dean 1992)

bidity. In these conditions, multiple factors impair multiple steps in the oxygen transport pathway, so identifying which steps are affected and amenable to physiotherapy interventions is central to optimal treatment outcome (Dean 1994b, 2006a).

Consultation with the ICU team, including a nutritionist, is critical to enhancing physiotherapy outcomes (Dean & Perme 2006). Increased metabolic demands of patients in the ICU, coupled with the demands of interventions, necessitate appropriate nutritional support to prevent or address malnutrition. Such screening has been shown to lead to better outcomes from ICU in terms of reduced complications, reduced hospital stays and reduced costs (Reid & Allard-Gould 2004).

Anaemia associated with critical illness (Shander 2004) is a concern for the physiotherapist whose goal is to optimize $\dot{D}O_2$. Haemoglobin is fundamental to optimal $\dot{D}O_2$, however, optimal management of anaemia is not performed universally. Special attention should be paid to haemoglobin status and its remediation should be a focus of discussion by the multidisciplinary team.

Assessment and monitoring

The physiotherapist needs to be particularly skilled at assessment and monitoring in the ICU both for safety reasons and when monitoring treatment response. Response to treatment can vary from minute to minute. The intervention is prescribed and progressed, and modified as needed during a treatment. Assessment has been addressed in Chapter 1 and includes a range of measures and indices of each step in the oxygen transport pathway (Dean 1999). Further, the physiotherapist needs to recognize that oxygen transport deficits and threats are mediated through impairments of virtually all organ systems not only the lungs and heart (Dean 1997). Consistent with the World Health Organization's Definition of Health (World Health Organization 2006) and the International Classification of Function (World Health Organization 2002), consideration is also given to assessing activity and health-related quality of life measures even for patients in the ICU setting. Central to prescription and progression of treatment is the patient's response. For safe and optimal outcomes, response-driven treatment progression is paramount, rather than blind adherence to a protocol-driven intervention. This approach helps to provide seamless care from the ICU back to the community with reduced risk of re-admission to the hospital, in the interest of lifelong health.

THERAPEUTIC EFFECTS OF POSITIONING AND MOBILIZATION

To improve oxygen transport in acute cardiopulmonary dysfunction

Positioning and mobilization have profound acute effects on cardiovascular and cardiopulmonary function and hence on the up-regulation of oxygen transport capacity (Table 4.1). These effects translate into improved gas exchange overall: reduction in the fraction of inspired oxygen, pharmacological and ventilatory support (Burns & Jones 1975, Dean 2006b, 2006c, Svanberg 1957). Such effects need to be exploited in the management of acute cardiopulmonary dysfunction with the use of positioning and mobilization as *primary* treatment interventions to enhance oxygen transport and as between-treatment interventions (Dean & Ross 1992b). The physiotherapist's role is to prescribe these interventions judiciously, to optimize gas exchange and oxygen transport overall. This role is distinct from *routine* positioning and mobilization often performed jointly by the physiotherapy and nursing staff. The aim of routine positioning and mobilization is primarily to reduce the adverse effects of restricted mobility, including pulmonary complications, bedsores and contractures. Critical-illness neuropathies and myopathies can lead to irreversible consequences and need to be prevented or at least detected early and managed.

To simulate the normal 'physiologic' body position, the primary goal of physiotherapy is to get the patient upright and moving. Mobilization and exercise are the most physiologic and potent interventions to optimize oxygen transport and aerobic capacity and so need to be exploited with every patient. Body positioning, however, is discussed in this chapter first because a patient cannot be in a position uninfluenced by gravity. Furthermore, a patient's oxygen transport status reflects the body position assumed regardless of whether the position is part of a treatment regimen, a routine positioning regimen or assumed randomly by the patient.

Non-invasive care in the form of physiotherapy has a particularly important place in the contemporary ICU unit. Advances in medical management have contributed to the avoidance of ICU admissions in patients who would have been admitted to the ICU a couple of decades ago. Similar advances have also contributed to patient survival; many of those who survive today may not have survived a couple of decades ago. Furthermore, advances in ventilatory support including non-invasive mechanical ventilation have helped to titrate ventilatory support more effectively to each patient, and in turn, reduce the need for intubation and invasive ventilation, and the iatrogenic effects of invasive ventilatory support. These advances have increased the demand on physiotherapy to optimize $\dot{D}O_2$, and minimize undue $\dot{V}O_2$. Priming the oxygen transport system with progressive gravitational and exercise stress is the primary responsibility of the physiotherapist in the ICU. This requires a high level of expertise in monitoring and judiciously challenging the oxygen transport system through prescriptively challenging the patient, while

4

4

Table 4.1 Acute effects of upright positioning and mobilization on oxygen transport

Systemic response	Stimulus	
	Positioning (supine to upright)	Mobilization
Cardiopulmonary	↑ Total lung capacity	↑ Alveolar ventilation
	↑ Tidal volume	↑ Tidal volume
	↑ Vital capacity	↑ Breathing frequency
	↑ Functioning residual capacity	↑ A–aO_2 gradient
	↑ Residual volume	↑ Pulmonary arteriovenous shunt
	↑ Expiratory reserve volume	↓ $\dot{V}_A/\dot{Q}$ matching
	↑ Forced expiratory volume	↑ Distension and recruitment of lung units with low
	↑ Forced expiratory flow	ventilation and low perfusion
	↑ Lung compliance	↑ Mobilization of secretions
	↓ Airway resistance	↑ Pulmonary lymphatic drainage
	↓ Airway closure	↑ Surfactant production and distribution
	↑ PaO_2	
	↑ AP diameter of chest	
	↓ Lateral diameter of rib cage and abdomen	
	Altered pulmonary blood flow distribution	
	↓ Work of breathing	
	↑ Diaphragmatic excursion	
	↑ Mobilization of secretions	
Cardiovascular	↑ Total blood volume	↑ Cardiac output
	↓ Central blood volume	↑ Stroke volume and heart rate
	↓ Central venous pressure	↑ Oxygen binding in blood
	↓ Pulmonary vascular congestion	↑ Oxygen dissociation and extraction at the tissue
	↑ Lymphatic drainage	level
	↓ Work of the heart	

(Adapted from Dean and Ross (1992a) and Imle and Klemic (1989))
AP, anteroposterior; ↑, increases; ↓, decreases; A-aO_2, alveolar–arterial oxygen gradient; $\dot{V}_A/\dot{Q}$, alveolar-ventilation perfusion; PaO_2, partial pressure of oxygen in arterial blood

minimizing risk to haemodynamic and ventilatory status. As patient survival has improved, the severity of the illness of patients in the ICU has increased, and patients can be kept alive longer. Thus, the physiotherapist needs to assess patients early, in order to establish the appropriate timing for intervention. Weaning or freeing patients from mechanical ventilation is a priority from the beginning. Weaning failure is not uncommon given the severity of the patients' status, and warrants careful consideration by the team as a whole in helping to prevent failure in both those patients who are non-invasively and invasively ventilated, and contributing to weaning success (Moretti et al 2000, Squadrone et al 2004). However, the physiotherapist needs to do everything possible to optimize $\dot{D}O_2$ through intervention, and minimize the need for mechanical ventilation, particularly invasive ventilation because it is associated with poorer clinical outcomes (Bernieh et al 2004).

Mechanical ventilation, both non-invasive and invasive, needs to be thoroughly understood by the physio-

therapist in terms of advantages and disadvantages, and these may differ depending on the patient's status and needs (Brochard 2003). The physiotherapist should be particularly interested in promoting non-invasive ventilation as it facilitates body positioning and mobilization. These interventions have evidence-based support for optimizing oxygen delivery when prescribed appropriately. When a patient is intubated and receiving invasive mechanical ventilation, this in no way precludes the prescription of these interventions. Patients decondition rapidly when gravitational and exercise stressors are removed. It is particularly important to offset these effects in patients with a history of prolonged debility before admission, and elderly patients (Sevransky & Haponik 2003).

Extubation success is a primary concern of the physiotherapist. Failure to extubate is associated with prolonged hospital stay and, in turn, healthcare cost (Seymour et al 2004). Body positioning and mobilization maintain or increase general body conditioning, which may be argued is fundamental to successful weaning from mechanical ventilation. This may be particularly important for patients with neuromuscular conditions who are weak and at high risk of aspiration (Vianello et al 2000). While the objective of optimizing conditioning may initially appear a premature priority given the status of patients who are severely ill in the ICU, cough strength that can be correlated to general body strength, or the converse, a weak cough related to general debility, can be predictive of extubation outcome (Khamiees et al 2001). Being able to tolerate a spontaneous breathing trial is key to eventual weaning. Furthermore, maintaining spontaneous breathing may help minimize sedation and improve cardiopulmonary function in some patients, for example patients with acute lung injury and receiving airway pressure-released ventilation (Putensen et al 2001). Weaning needs to be tailored to each patient and should not be unnecessarily prolonged (Nevins & Epstein 2001).

Figure 4.3 illustrates positioning upright and mobilization of a patient in the ICU. The progression is based on ongoing assessment and monitoring, with a gravitational challenge followed by progressive movement. The rationale and the details of ongoing monitoring follow.

Positioning

Physiological and scientific rationale.   The distributions of ventilation ($\dot{V}_A$), perfusion ($\dot{Q}$) and ventilation and perfusion matching in the lungs are primarily influenced by gravity and therefore body position (Clauss et al 1968, West 1962, 1977). The goal is to reduce closing volume and optimize functional residual capacity (Manning et al 1999). The intrapleural pressure becomes less negative down the upright lung. Thus, the apices have a greater initial volume and reduced compliance than the bases. Because the bases are more compliant in this position, they exhibit greater volume changes during ventilation. In addition to these gravity-dependent inter-regional differences in lung volume, ventilation is influenced by intra-regional differences, which are dependent on regional mechanical differences in the compliance of the lung parenchyma and the resistance to airflow in the airways. Perfusion increases down the upright lung such that the $\dot{V}_A/\dot{Q}$ ratio in the apices is disproportionately high compared with that in the bases. Ventilation and perfusion matching is optimal in the mid-lung region. Manipulating body position alters both inter-regional and intra-regional determinants of ventilation and perfusion and their matching. When choosing specific positions to enhance arterial oxygenation for a given patient, the underlying pathophysiology impairing cardiopulmonary function, the effects of bed rest/recumbency and restricted mobility, extrinsic

factors related to the patient's care and intrinsic factors related to the patient need to be considered.

Although the negative effects of the supine position have been well documented for several decades (Dean & Ross 1992b, Dripps & Waters 1941), supine or recumbent positions are frequently assumed by patients in hospital. These positions are non-physiologic and are associated with significant reductions in lung volumes and flow rates and increased work of breathing (Craig et al 1971, Hsu & Hickey 1976). The decrease in functional residual capacity (FRC) contributes to closure of the dependent airways and reduced arterial oxygenation (Ray et al 1974). This effect has long been known to be accentuated in older persons (Leblanc et al 1970), patients with cardiopulmonary disease (Fowler 1949), patients with abdominal pathology, smokers and individuals who are obese.

The haemodynamic consequences of the supine position are also remarkable. The gravity-dependent increase in central blood volume may precipitate vascular congestion, reduced compliance and pulmonary oedema (Blomqvist & Stone 1983, Sjostrand 1951). The commensurate increase in stroke volume increases the work of the heart (Levine & Lown 1952). Within 6 hours, a compensatory diuresis can lead to a loss of circulating blood volume and orthostatic intolerance: i.e. haemodynamic intolerance to the upright position. Bed rest deconditioning has been attributed to this reduction in blood volume and the impairment of the volume-regulating mechanisms rather than physical deconditioning per se (Hahn-Winslow 1985). Thus, the upright position is essential to maximize lung volumes and flow rates and this position is the only means of optimizing fluid shifts such that the circulating blood volume and the volume-regulating mechanisms are maintained. The upright position coupled with movement is necessary to promote normal fluid regulation and balance (Lamb et al 1964).

The upright position is a potent stimulus to the sympathetic nervous system. This is an important clinical effect, which offsets impaired blood volume and pressure-regulating mechanisms secondary to recumbency (Hahn-Winslow 1985). Stimulation of the sympathetic nervous system has been reported to augment the effects of potent sympathomimetic pharmacological agents such that the dosages of these drugs can be reduced (Warren et al 1983). The reduction or elimination of sympathomimetic drugs is an important outcome of non-invasive physiotherapy interventions.

Side-to-side positioning is frequently used in the clinical setting. If applied in response to assessment rather than routinely (Chuley et al 1982), the benefits derived from such positioning can be enhanced. Adult patients with unilateral lung disease may derive greater

4

4

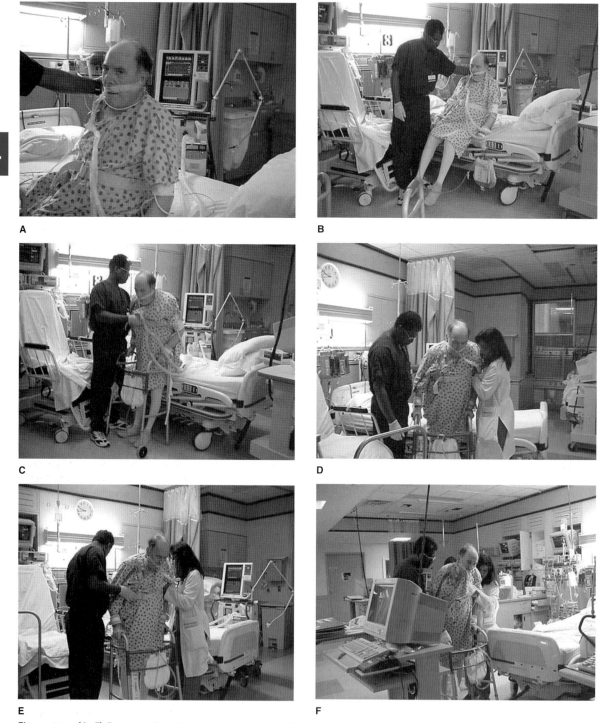

A

B

C

D

E

F

Figure 4.3   (A–F) Example of mobilizing a patient to a self-supported upright sitting position. Mobilizing a critically ill patient needs to be a priority whenever possible. Short frequent sessions to the erect position (sitting or standing if possible) with continual monitoring of the patient's response should be the goal. As the patient progresses, sessions increase in intensity and duration and reduce in frequency.

benefit when the affected lung is uppermost (Remolina et al 1981). Markedly improved gas exchange without deleterious haemodynamic effects has been reported for patients with severe hypoxaemia secondary to pneumonia (Dreyfuss et al 1992). Arterial oxygen tension is increased secondary to improved ventilation of the unaffected lung when this lung is dependent, in the adult patient. Patients with uniformly distributed bilateral lung disease may derive greater benefit when the right lung is lowermost (Zack et al 1974). In this case, arterial oxygen tension is increased secondary to improved ventilation of the right lung, which may reflect the increased size of the right lung compared with the left and that, in this position, the heart and adjacent lung tissue are subjected to less compression. Improved gas exchange through non-invasive interventions can reduce or eliminate the need for supplemental oxygen, both of which are primary treatment outcomes. Although various studies have shown beneficial effects of side lying, body positioning should be based on multiple considerations including the distribution of disease if optimal results are to be obtained.

The prone position has long been known to have considerable physiological justification in patients with cardiopulmonary compromise (Douglas et al 1977), even those who are critically ill with acute respiratory failure (Bittner et al 1996, Chatte et al 1997, Mure et al 1997), those with acute respiratory distress syndrome (Vollman 2004), and patients with trauma-induced adult respiratory distress syndrome (Fridrich et al 1996). The beneficial effects of the prone position on arterial oxygenation may reflect improved lung compliance secondary to stabilization of the anterior chest wall, tidal ventilation, diaphragmatic excursion, functional residual capacity (FRC) and reduced airway closure (Dean 1985, Pelosi et al 1998). In a dog model of acute lung injury, however, improved PaO_2 in prone has been attributed to a reduced shunt fraction (Albert et al 1987). A variant of the prone position, prone abdomen-free, has shown additional benefits over prone abdomen-restricted. In the prone abdomen-free position, the patient is positioned such that the movement of the abdomen is unencumbered by the bed. This can be achieved either by raising the patient's body in relation to the bed so that the abdomen falls free or by using a bed with a hole cut out at the level of the abdomen. Despite compelling evidence to support the prone position, it may be poorly tolerated in some patients or may be contraindicated in patients who are haemodynamically unstable. In these situations, intermediate positions approximating prone may produce many of the beneficial effects and minimize any potential hazard.

The use of the prone position, like other body positions, needs to be prescribed based on the patient's presentation as well as underlying pathophysiology. The response to prone positioning may differ, for example in early adult respiratory distress syndrome the effect of prone positioning may depend on whether the primary insult is of a pulmonary or non-pulmonary nature (Lim et al 2001). The benefits of the prone position in respiratory distress syndrome have been reported to be additive to invasive medical interventions (Jolliet et al 1997). Prone positioners that passively change the patient's body position to prone have been reported to have comparable benefit (Vollman & Bander 1996).

Extreme body position changes can be beneficial in patients who are unable to participate actively in mobilization. Although the literature to date has been mostly related to children in the ICU, the results with respect to improving oxygenation are compelling (Casadro-Flores et al 2002). Such positioning includes dramatic shifts from supine to prone, and prone to supine, as opposed to supine to side lying. Abdomen-free prone positioning has been shown to have greater benefit than abdomen-restricted prone positioning in infants. The half prone position in adults, which displaces the viscera forward, allowing greater caudal displacement of the diaphragm, may elicit comparable benefits in adults.

Positioning for drainage of pulmonary secretions may be indicated in some patients (Kirilloff et al 1985). Historically, these positions have been based on the anatomical arrangement of the bronchopulmonary segments to facilitate drainage of a particular segment (Chapter 5). The bronchiole to the segment of interest is positioned perpendicular to facilitate drainage with the use of gravity. The efficacy of postural drainage compared with deep breathing and coughing induced with mobilization/exercise and repositioning of the patient has not been established. The fact that mobilization impacts on more steps in the oxygen transport pathway including the airways, to effect secretion clearance, supports the exploitation of mobilization coupled with deep breathing manoeuvres and coughing as a *primary* treatment intervention.

Physiotherapists need to consider two aspects of body positioning when the goal is to optimize oxygen transport. One is to select and apply specific body positions based on the patient's presentation, laboratory test results and radiographic imaging. The other is to elicit physiologic 'stir-up' with the use of extreme body positions (Dean 2006c, Dripps & Waters 1941). The purpose is to effect the normal gravitational stress on cardiopulmonary and cardiovascular function that is experienced in health. This is best simulated if patients are changed from one extreme position to another, for example supine to prone or upright, rather than from half to full side lying which is associated with a lesser 'stir-up' effect. Patients who are haemodynamically unstable

4

require greater monitoring during extreme position changes and may not tolerate some position changes well or for too long a period. Thus, based on assessment and patient response, frequent extreme position changes may be preferable to minimal shifts in body position in order to optimize cardiovascular, pulmonary and haemodynamic function. Ongoing monitoring is essential to ensure responses are optimal and adverse responses averted.

Assessment and treatment planning. Body positioning – the specific positions selected, the duration of time spent in each position and the frequency with which the position is assumed – is based on a consideration of the factors that contribute to cardiopulmonary dysfunction and treatment response. Understanding of the physiology of cardiopulmonary and cardiovascular function and the effects of disease highlights certain positions that are theoretically ideal. However, these positions need to be modified or may be contraindicated for a given patient, based on other considerations (see Box 4.1). For example, if extreme positional changes are contraindicated, small degrees of positional rotation, performed frequently, can have significant benefit on gas exchange and arterial oxygenation. A three-quarters prone position may produce favourable results when the full prone position is contraindicated or is not feasible. This modification may simulate the prone abdomen-free position, which has been shown to augment the effect of the traditional prone abdomen-restricted position (Douglas et al 1977). Furthermore, a three-quarters prone position may be particularly beneficial in patients with obese or swollen abdomens who may not tolerate other variations of the prone position. With attention to the patient's condition, invasive lines and leads and appropriate monitoring, a patient can be aggressively positioned.

The time that a patient spends in a position and the frequency with which that position is assumed, over a period of time, are based on the indications for the position and treatment outcome. Objective measures of the various steps that are compromised in the oxygen transport pathway, as well as indices of oxygen transport overall, are used in making these decisions. Subjective evaluation based on clinical judgement is also important. A specific position can be justified, provided there is objective and subjective evidence of improvement. Signs and symptoms of deterioration need to be monitored so that deleterious positions can be avoided and deterioration secondary to excessive time in any one position can be detected. Prolonged duration in any single position will inevitably lead to compromise of the function of dependent lung zones and impaired gas exchange.

The ratio of treatment to between-treatment time is low. Typically, between-treatment time consists of some combination of positioning and mobilization. Positioning and mobilizing patients between treatments may be incorporated as an extension of treatment. Patients require monitoring and observation during these periods, as well as during treatment. Between-treatment time may include the use of maximally restful positions that do not compromise oxygen transport. Lastly, patients are positioned and mobilized between treatments to prevent the negative effects of restricted mobility and recumbency.

Special consideration (for example, with respect to specific positioning and the use of supports) needs to be given to positioning patients who are comatose or paralysed because their joints and muscles are relatively unprotected and prone to trauma. Positions need to be selected that avoid injury to unprotected head, neck and limbs.

Progression. Progression of positioning involves new positions or modification of previous positions and modification of the duration spent in each position and the frequency with which each position is assumed over a period of time. These clinical decisions are based on the factors that contribute to cardiopulmonary dysfunction and objective and subjective indices of change in the patient's cardiopulmonary status. With improvement in cardiopulmonary status, the patient spends more time in erect positions and is mobilized more frequently and independently.

Mobilization

Physiological and scientific rationale. The negative effects of recumbency during critical illness, combined with the patient's life-threatening pathology, are compounded by progressive deconditioning. These problems need to be anticipated by the physiotherapist. A patient for whom short-term mechanical ventilation is anticipated may be one who eventually requires long-term ventilation. Thus, a whole-body rehabilitation approach warrants being considered from the start (Martin et al 2005) to prevent as well as address recumbency and deconditioning effects and their compounded effects on the patient's other problems.

Compared with long-term exercise, the mechanisms underlying adaptation of the oxygen transport system to acute exercise, from session to session and day to day, are less well understood. Although these mechanisms have yet to be elucidated, the responses to acute exercise are well documented. The acute response to mobilization/exercise reflects a commensurate increase in oxygen transport to provide oxygen to the working muscles and other organs. The increase is dependent on the intensity of the mobilization/exercise stimulus. The demand for oxygen and oxygen consumption ($\dot{V}O_2$)

increases as exercise continues, with commensurate increases in minute ventilation ($\dot{V}_E$), that is, the amount of air inhaled per minute, cardiac output and oxygen extraction at the tissue level. Relatively low intensities of mobilization can have a direct and profound effect on oxygen transport in patients with acute cardiopulmonary dysfunction (Dean 2006a, Dull & Dull 1983, Lewis 1980) and need to be instituted early after the initial pathological insult or surgery (Orlava 1959, Wenger 1982). The resulting exercise hyperpnoea, the increase in $\dot{V}_E$, is effected by an increase in tidal volume and breathing frequency (Zafiropoulos et al 2004). In addition, ventilation and perfusion matching is augmented by the distension and recruitment of lung zones with low ventilation and low perfusion. Spontaneous exercise-induced deep breaths are associated with improved flow rates and mobilization of pulmonary secretions (Wolff et al 1977). In clinical populations, these effects elicit spontaneous coughing. When mobilization is performed in the upright position, the anteroposterior diameter of the chest wall assumes a normal configuration compared with the recumbent position in which the anteroposterior diameter is reduced and the transverse diameter is increased. In addition, diaphragmatic excursion is favoured, flow rates augmented and coughing is mechanically facilitated. The work of breathing may be reduced with caudal displacement of the diaphragm and the work of the heart is minimized by the displacement of fluid away from the central circulation to the legs. Thus, despite increased metabolic demands of mobilization and exercise, the goal is to ensure that this increased demand is not wasteful and the demand can be met by the supply.

With respect to cardiovascular effects, acute mobilization/exercise increases cardiac output (CO) by increasing stroke volume and heart rate. This is associated with increased blood pressure and increased coronary and peripheral muscle perfusion. Despite their energetic demands, mobilization and exercise may augment outcomes even in acute respiratory failure (Wong 2000, 2004), and patients requiring left ventricular assist devices (Perme 2006). When titrated carefully, based on the patient's response, mobilization can be performed safely with potential benefit, including avoidance of mechanical ventilation.

Passive movement of the limbs may stimulate deep breaths and heart function; however, this effect is considered minimal compared with active movement (West 2004). In addition, there is little scientific evidence to support any additional benefit from various facilitation techniques (Bethune 1975). Thus, time allocated to the use of passive manoeuvres may compete with time for positioning and mobilization, that is, interventions with demonstrated clinical efficacy. Although passive movements have a relatively small effect on cardiopulmonary function, they have several important benefits for neuromuscular and musculoskeletal function which support their use, provided they do not replace active movement.

Current medical research has been focusing on protection of the heart in patients in the ICU. Such measures include new inotropic agents, supporting the metabolic activity of the heart which has a high $\dot{V}O_2/\dot{D}O_2$ ratio, conservative administration of blood products and greater use of mechanical support devices (Bosenberg & Royston 2002). Irrespective of these advances, the place of physiotherapy is to exploit the person's capacity for $\dot{D}O_2$ through priming the oxygen transport system and optimizing aerobic conditioning regardless of how small an effect may result.

Assessment and treatment planning. For practical and ethical considerations, the mobilization plan for the patient with acute cardiopulmonary dysfunction cannot be based on a standardized exercise test, as is the case for patients with chronic conditions. However, response to a mobilization/exercise stimulus can be assessed during a mobilization challenge test, that is, during the patient's routine activities such as turning or moving in bed, activities of daily living or responding to routine nursing and medical procedures. Comparable to prescribing exercise for the patient with chronic cardiopulmonary dysfunction, the parameters are specifically defined so that the stimulus is optimally therapeutic. The optimal stimulus is that which stresses the oxygen transport capacity of the patient and effects the greatest adaptation without deterioration or distress.

To promote adaptation of the steps in the oxygen transport pathway to the stimulation of acute mobilization in patients who are acutely ill, the stimulus is administered in a comparable manner to that in an exercise programme prescribed for patients with chronic cardiopulmonary dysfunction and who are medically stable. The components include a pre-exercise period, a warm-up period, a steady-state period, a cool-down period and a recovery period (Blair et al 2005). These components optimize the response to exercise by preparing the cardiopulmonary and cardiovascular systems for steady-state exercise and by permitting these systems to re-establish resting conditions following exercise. The cool-down period, in conjunction with the recovery period, ensures that exercise does not stop abruptly, and allows for biochemical degradation and removal of the by-products of metabolism. Mobilization consists of discrete warm-up, steady-state and cool-down periods; the components need to be identified, even in the patient with a very low functional capacity; for example, a patient who is critically ill and may be only able to sit

4

4

up over the edge of the bed. In such cases, preparing to sit up constitutes a warm-up period for the patient; the stimulus of sitting unsupported for several minutes while being aroused and encouraged to talk or be interactive non-verbally, if mechanically ventilated, constitutes a steady-state period; returning to bed constitutes the cool-down period. In the recovery period, observation of the patient continues to ensure that mobilization is tolerated well and that the indices of oxygen transport return to resting levels. This information is then used as the basis for mobilization in the next treatment.

Monitoring. As clinical exercise physiologists, physiotherapists can benefit from the use of metabolic measures in monitoring and evaluating mobilization and exercise as interventions. Although these measures are mostly used in exercise laboratories, indirect calorimetry is a tool used by nutritionists in the ICU to estimate dietary needs. The concept that the metabolic demands of patients in the ICU can vary considerably from day to day has been well established (Vermeij et al 1989). Physiotherapists can benefit greatly from knowledge of the metabolic demands of their interventions when superimposed on such daily variation; thus, these measures should be used routinely by physiotherapists who may stress the patient energetically more than any other team member (Brandi et al 1997).

Valid and reliable monitoring practices provide the basis for defining the parameters of mobilization, assessing the need for progression and defining the adaptation or training-sensitive zone. In the case of patients who are acutely ill and particularly those who are critically ill, the training-sensitive zone refers to the physiologic zone where conditioning of the oxygen transport system is stimulated. This zone will be based on many more variables than for the patient who is medically stable, and will be at a markedly reduced intensity. Sessions will be shorter in duration as well as less intense. This ensures that the oxygen transport system and aerobic conditioning are progressively challenged commensurate with the patient's responses and within the margins of safety. Ongoing monitoring is essential given that subjecting patients to mobilization/exercise stimulation is inherently risky, particularly for patients with cardiopulmonary dysfunction. Indices of overall oxygen transport in addition to indices of the function of the individual steps in the oxygen transport pathway provide a detailed profile of the patient's cardiopulmonary status. In critical care settings, the physiotherapist has access to a wide range of measures to assess the adequacy of gas exchange. Minimally, in the general ward setting, measures of breathing frequency, arterial blood gases, arterial saturation, heart rate, blood pressure and clinical observation provide the basis for ongoing assessment, mobilization/exercise and pro-

gression. With appropriate attention to the patient's condition, invasive lines and leads and appropriate monitoring, a patient can be aggressively mobilized and ambulated (see Fig. 4.3).

A fundamental requirement in defining the parameters for mobilization is that the patient's oxygen transport system is capable of increasing the oxygen supply to meet an increasing metabolic demand. If not, mobilization is absolutely contraindicated and the treatment of choice to optimize oxygen transport is body positioning. However, in the case of a patient being severely haemodynamically unstable or at risk of being so, for example hypotensive or on a high FiO_2, even the stress of positioning may be excessive. Thus, although patients who are critically ill may be treated aggressively, every patient has to be considered individually and in conjunction with the team's goals as a whole, otherwise the patient may deteriorate or be seriously endangered. Physiotherapy interventions including mobilization alter metabolic demand. This has particular implications for the patient with blood sugar abnormalities, as the stress of illness and hospital admission can compound this abnormality. Discussion of sliding-scale insulin with the team may be warranted in a patient whose blood sugars fluctuate widely (Kee et al 2006). Monitoring of glycaemic control is important in that poor control is associated with poor outcomes in patients who have diabetes and those who are not known to have diabetes (Laver & Padkin 2005, Rady et al 2005).

Progression. Progression and modification of the mobilization stimulus usually occur more rapidly in the management of the patient with acute cardiopulmonary dysfunction compared with the progression of the exercise stimulus for the patient with chronic illness. The status of patients who are acutely ill can vary considerably within minutes or hours. Whether the mobilization stimulus is increased or decreased in intensity depends on the patient's status and altered responses to mobilization. The mobilization stimulus is adjusted to remain optimal despite the patient's changing metabolic needs. Capitalizing on narrow windows of opportunity for therapeutic intervention must be exploited 24 hours a day with respect to the type of mobilization stimulus, its intensity, duration and frequency, particularly in the critically ill patient. At times, the intensity and duration of the intervention may be quite minimal, yet cumulatively produce a marked improvement in oxygen transport efficiency.

Fluctuations in blood gases should correct with appropriate treatment pacing, and the provision of supplemental oxygen during treatment. However, if the PaO_2/FiO_2 remains below 250, or the alveolar–arterial (A-a) gradient remains widened, these signs may portend deterioration including acute renal failure

(Chawla et al 2005). Acute renal failure is associated with a high mortality rate (Ympa et al 2005).

The 'immovable' patient.   Given the well-documented negative effects of restricted mobility, the 'immovable' patient deserves special consideration. Although bed rest or activity restriction is ordered for patients frequently without reservation, the risks need to be weighed against the benefits (Allen et al 1999). Restricted mobility coupled with recumbency constitutes a death knell for many patients who are severely compromised. Thus, an order for bed rest needs to be evaluated and challenged to ensure that this order is physiologically justified. For many years, chair nursing has been advocated based on solid physiologic evidence, yet this knowledge has lagged behind integration into practice.

There are some instances where a patient cannot be moved, for example with an open chest, with intra-aortic balloon pumps, on neuromuscular blockade, or hypotensive. Patients receive neuromuscular blockade to facilitate mechanical ventilation. The effects of prolonged blockade are being better documented, for example neuropathies and myopathies (Gehr & Sessler 2001, Hund 1999). Periodic peripheral nerve stimulation may need to be conducted to offset these effects. However, body positioning needs to be exploited to relieve the effect of prolonged pressure on muscles and nerve, in addition to skin, that can complicate this clinical picture.

Kinetic beds and chairs.   Advances in furniture technology to facilitate positioning and mobilizing patients have lagged behind advances in clinical medicine, particularly in the critical care area. Conventional hospital beds are designed to be stationary and their widths and heights are often non-adjustable, making it difficult for the patient to get in and out of bed. Kinetic beds and chairs have become increasingly available over the past decade but they are not widely used clinically. These devices were originally designed to facilitate positioning and moving heavy and comatose patients. Some beds are designed to rotate on their long axis from side to side over several minutes. Other beds simulate a side-to-side movement with inflation and deflation of the two sides of an air-filled mattress. Although these beds have potential cardiopulmonary benefit (Powers & Daniels 2004), they do not replace active positioning and movement.

Mechanically adjustable bedside chairs and stretcher chairs constitute an important advance. These chairs adjust to a flat horizontal surface that can be matched to bed height and positioned beneath the patient lying on the bed. The device with the patient on top is then wheeled parallel to the bed where it can be adjusted back into a chair and thus the patient assumes a seated position. The degree of recline can be altered to meet the patient's needs – for example those who are very weak but capable of bearing some weight and some transferring activities – safety considerations and for comfort. This chair also facilitates returning the patient to bed. Comparable to these chairs are beds that can be converted into a chair while the patient is lying down. These avoid the negative effects of using tilt tables where the fluid shifts caudally are extreme and more risky by comparison.

Kinetic beds have a place in the management of some patients. Patients who are immobile because of induced coma or marked haemodynamic instability may benefit. Patients with multiple injuries have also been shown to benefit substantially from the continual movement of kinetic beds (Stiletto et al 2000). In addition, kinetic beds may increase safety to physiotherapists and nurses in obviating the need for shifting and moving heavy patients. The disadvantages of kinetic beds and chairs include the expense and the potential for over-reliance on them. Without these devices, a heavy patient may require several people and several minutes to position in a chair that may be tolerated only for a few minutes. However, the cardiopulmonary benefits of the stimulation of preparing to be moved, the reflex attempts of the patient to assist and adjust to changing position, as well as actually sitting upright in a chair are not reproduced by bed positioning alone or by a kinetic bed. Each case, in terms of therapeutic benefit and safety, needs to be evaluated individually. Research is needed to determine the indications and potential benefits of kinetic beds and chairs so that they can be used judiciously in the clinical setting as an integral therapeutic intervention.

To improve oxygen transport in post–acute and chronic cardiopulmonary dysfunction

In post-acute and chronic cardiopulmonary dysfunction, a primary consequence of impaired oxygen transport is reduced functional work capacity (Belman & Wasserman 1981, Wasserman & Whipp 1975). Work capacity can be improved with long-term exercise which improves the efficiency of the steps in the oxygen transport pathway and promotes compensation within the pathway as well as by other mechanisms. To optimize the patient's response, exercise can be carried out in judicious body positions in which oxygen transport is favoured.

Exercise is the treatment of choice for patients whose impaired oxygen transport has resulted from chronic cardiopulmonary dysfunction. Body positioning may have a place in severely ill patients by optimizing oxygen transport at rest. Barach & Beck (1954) reported that emphysematous patients were less breathless, had reduced accessory muscle activity and had a significant reduction in ventilation when positioned in a 16° head-

4

down position. Some patients exhibited greater symptomatic improvement than in the upright position with supplemental oxygen. Classic relaxation positions, for example leaning forward with the forearms supported, can also be supported physiologically. Coupling such physiologically justifiable positions with mobilization/exercise will augment the benefits of exercise.

Physiological and scientific rationale. Although the physiological responses to long-term exercise in patients with chronic cardiopulmonary disease may differ from those in healthy persons, patients can significantly improve their functional work capacity (Table 4.2). In healthy people, an improvement in aerobic capacity reflects improved efficiency of the steps in the oxygen transport pathway to adapt to the increased oxygen demands imposed by exercise stress. This adaptation is effected by both central (cardiopulmonary) and peripheral (at the tissue level) changes (Dean 2006b, Wasserman & Whipp 1975). Such aerobic conditioning is characterized by a training-induced bradycardia secondary to an increased stroke volume and increased oxygen extraction capacity of the working muscle. These adaptation or training responses result in an increased maximal oxygen uptake and maximal voluntary ventilation and reduced submaximal $\dot{V}_E$, cardiac output,

heart rate, blood pressure and perceived exertion. However, patients with chronic lung disease are often unable to exercise at the intensity required to elicit an aerobic training response. Their functional work capacity may be improved by other mechanisms, for example desensitization to breathlessness, improved motivation, improved biomechanical efficiency, increased ventilatory muscle strength and endurance or some combination (Belman & Wasserman 1981, Bernard et al 1999). Aerobic capacity can be increased through peripheral adaptations (Gosselin et al 2003), but peripheral myopathies in patients with primary lung and heart disease have been reported (Storer 2001). Patients with chronic heart disease, such as those with severe infarcts, may be able to train aerobically; however, training adaptation primarily results from peripheral rather than central factors commensurate with the level of impairment (Bydgman & Wahren 1974, Larsen et al 2001, 2002). Most patients in the ICU have oxygen transport dysfunction or threat to this life-preserving system. Patients with ventilatory failure secondary to neuromuscular and musculoskeletal conditions also constitute a significant proportion of patients in the ICU. These patients may not have primary heart or lung disease, yet their lives may be threatened due to secondary effects of neuromuscular or musculoskeletal dysfunction.

Planning an exercise programme. The exercise programme is based on the principle that oxygen delivery and uptake are enhanced in response to an exercise stimulus which is precisely defined for an individual in terms of the type of exercise, its intensity, duration, frequency and the course of the training programme. These parameters are based on an exercise test in conjunction with assessment findings. Exercise tests are performed on a cycle ergometer, treadmill or with a walk test (Noonan & Dean 2000). The general procedures and protocols are standardized to maximize the validity and reliability of the results (Blair et al 2005, Dean et al 1989). The principles of, and guidelines for, exercise testing and training patients with chronic lung and heart disease have been well documented (Dean 2006d). The training-sensitive zone is defined by objective and subjective measures of oxygen transport determined from the exercise test. The components of each exercise training session include baseline, warm-up, steady-state portion, cool-down and recovery period (Blair et al 2005, Dean 1993). The cardiopulmonary and cardiovascular systems are gradually primed for sustaining a given level of exercise stress, while in addition the musculoskeletal system adapts correspondingly. Following the steady-state portion of the training session, the cool-down period permits a return to the resting physiological state. Cool-down and recovery periods are essential for

Table 4.2 Chronic effects of mobilization/exercise on oxygen transport

Systemic response	Effect
Cardiopulmonary	↑ Capacity for gas exchange ↑ Cardiopulmonary efficiency ↓ Submaximal minute ventilation ↓ Work of breathing
Cardiovascular	Exercise-induced bradycardia ↑ Maximum $\dot{V}O_2$ ↓ Submaximal heart rate, blood pressure, myocardial oxygen demand, stroke volume, cardiac output ↓ Work of the heart ↓ Perceived exertion ↑ Plasma volume Cardiac hypertrophy ↑ Vascularity of the myocardium
Tissue level	↑ Vascularity of working muscle ↑ Myoglobin content and oxidative enzymes in muscle ↑ Oxygen extraction capacity

↑, increases; ↓, decreases; $\dot{V}O_2$, oxygen consumption

the biochemical degradation and elimination of the metabolic by-products of exercise.

Progression. Progression of the exercise programme is based on a repeated exercise test. This is indicated when the exercise prescription no longer elicits the desired physiological responses – specifically when the steady-state work rate consistently elicits responses at the low end or below the lower limit of the training-sensitive zone for the given indices of oxygen transport. This reflects maximal adaptation of the steps in the oxygen transport pathway to the given exercise stimulus. The degree of conditioning achieved is precisely matched to the demands of the exercise stimulus imposed.

To prevent the negative effects of restricted mobility

Although physiologically distinct, the effects of immobility are frequently confounded by the effects of recumbency in the hospitalized patient. Patients with restricted mobility include those under sedation, those with acute spinal cord injury, and critically ill patients who are unable to be mobilized because of haemodynamic instability due to other causes. Restricted mobility and the concomitant reduction in exercise stress affect virtually every organ system in the body, with profound effects on the cardiovascular and neuromuscular systems. Patients who are recumbent but rousable warrant vigilant monitoring. Recumbency and the elimination of the vertical gravitational stress exert effects primarily on the cardiovascular and cardiopulmonary systems (Blomqvist & Stone 1983, Dock 1944, Harrison 1944). The most serious consequences of restricted mobility and recumbency are those resulting from the effects on the cardiopulmonary and cardiovascular systems and hence on oxygen transport. Although other consequences of restricted mobility, e.g. increased risk of infection, skin breakdown and deformity, may not constitute the same immediate threat to oxygen transport and tissue oxygenation, they can have significant implications with respect to morbidity and mortality. Thus, restricted mobility and recumbency need to be minimized. Mobility and the upright position should be maximized to avert the negative consequences of restricted mobility, the risk of morbidity associated with these effects and the direct and indirect cardiopulmonary and cardiovascular effects. These negative consequences are preventable with frequent repositioning and mobilizing of the patient (Table 4.3). The prevention of these effects is a primary goal of positioning and mobilizing patients between treatments.

Education of the patient, family and ICU staff regarding early mobilization and frequent body position

Table 4.3 Effects of positioning and mobilization that prevent the negative effects of restricted mobility and recumbency*

Systemic response	Effect
Cardiopulmonary	↑ Alveolar ventilation
	↓ Airway closure
	Alters the distributions of ventilation, perfusion and ventilation and perfusion matching
	Alters pulmonary blood volume
	Alters distending forces on uppermost lung fields
	↓ Secretion pooling
	Secretion mobilization and redistribution
	Alters chest wall configuration and pulmonary mechanics
	Varies work of breathing
Cardiovascular	Alters cardiac compression (positioning), wall tensions, filling pressures
	Alters preload, afterload and myocardial contraction
	Alters lymphatic drainage
	Varies work of the heart
	Promotes fluid shifts
	Stimulates pressure- and volume-regulating mechanisms of the circulation
	Stimulates vasomotor activity
	Maintains normal fluid balance and distribution
Tissue level	Alters hydrostatic pressure and tissue perfusion
	Maintains oxygen extraction capacity (mobilization)

*Some of the preventative effects of body positioning and mobilization are comparable; however, the magnitude of these effects in response to mobilization tends to be greater than with body positioning

changes is key. Physiotherapists should work closely with other ICU team members, as well as with the patient and family. Client-focused care including extensive education has become increasingly important and given attention to health-related quality of life even in patients who are critically ill. Loved ones may provide important information about a patient's quality of life, when that individual is unable to speak for himself.

SUMMARY AND CONCLUSION

Cardiopulmonary dysfunction refers to impairment of one or more steps in the oxygen transport pathway that can impair oxygen transport overall. Thus, a conceptual framework for clinical problem-solving in the management of patients with cardiopulmonary dysfunction, based on oxygen transport, can facilitate the identification of deficits and the directing of treatment to each specific deficit. Factors that can impair the transport of oxygen from the atmosphere to the tissues include cardiopulmonary pathology, bed rest, recumbency and restricted mobility, extrinsic factors related to the patient's medical care, intrinsic factors related to the patient or a combination of these. Positioning and mobilization are two interventions that have potent and direct effects on several of the steps in the oxygen transport pathway. These interventions have a *primary* role in improving oxygen transport in acute and chronic cardiopulmonary dysfunction and in averting the negative effects of restricted mobility and recumbency, particularly those related to cardiopulmonary and cardiovascular function.

The principal goal of physiotherapy in the management of cardiopulmonary dysfunction is to optimize oxygen transport. A systematic approach to achieving this goal consists of:

1. Distinguishing the specific steps in the oxygen transport pathway that are impaired or threatened.
2. Establishing factors which contribute to this impairment.
3. Distinguishing the factors that are (a) amenable to positioning and mobilization and (b) not directly amenable to positioning and mobilization, as these will modify treatment.
4. Specifying the parameters for positioning and mobilization to directly address the factors responsible for the cardiopulmonary dysfunction wherever possible, either to elicit the acute effects of these interventions to enhance oxygen transport or to elicit the long-term effects on oxygen transport, i.e. training responses and improved functional work capacity.
5. Avoiding the multisystem consequences of restricted mobility and recumbency, particularly those that impair or threaten oxygen transport.
6. Recognizing when positioning or mobilizing a patient needs to be modified to avoid a deleterious outcome.
7. Educating the patient, the family and healthcare colleagues about the place of physiotherapy, and coordination of interventions and care overall.
8. Considering patients in the overall context of their activities and social participation that contribute to their health-related quality of life.

Conceptualizing cardiopulmonary dysfunction as deficits in the steps in the oxygen transport pathway and identifying the factors responsible for each impaired step provides a systematic, evidence-based approach to clinical decision-making in cardiopulmonary physiotherapy. Positioning and mobilization can then be specifically directed at the mechanisms underlying cardiopulmonary dysfunction wherever possible. Such an approach will maximize the efficacy of positioning and mobilizing patients with cardiopulmonary dysfunction and enhance the outcome of medical management overall.

References

Albert RK, Leasa D, Sanderson M, Robertson HT, Hlastala MP 1987 The prone position improves arterial oxygenation and reduced shunt in oleic-acid-induced acute lung injury. American Review of Respiratory Diseases 138: 828–833

Allen C, Glasziou P, Delman C 1999 Bedrest: a potentially harmful treatment needing more careful evaluation. The Lancet 354: 1229–1233

Barach AL, Beck GJ 1954 Ventilatory effect of head-down position in pulmonary emphysema. American Journal of Medicine 16: 55–60

Beck LA 1998 Morbid obesity and spinal cord injury: a case study. Spinal Cord Injury Nurse 15: 3–5

Belman MJ, Wasserman K 1981 Exercise training and testing in patients with chronic obstructive pulmonary

disease. Basics of Respiratory Disease 10: 1–6

Bernard S, Whittom F, Leblanc P et al 1999 Aerobic and strength training in patients with chronic obstructive lung disease. American Journal of Respiratory and Critical Care Medicine 159: 896–901

Bernieh B, Al Hakim M, Boobes Y, Siemkovics E, El Jack H 2004 Outcome and predictive factors of acute renal failure in the intensive care unit. Transplantation Proceedings 36: 1784–1787

Bethune DD 1975 Neurophysiological facilitation of respiration in the unconscious patient. Physiotherapy Canada 27: 241–245

Bittner E, Chendrasekhar A, Pillai S 1996 Changes in oxygenation and compliance as related to body

position in acute lung injury. American Journal of Surgery 62: 1038–1041

Blair SN, Painter P, Pate RR et al 2005 Resource manual for guidelines for exercise testing and prescription, 5th edn. Lea and Febiger, Philadelphia

Blomqvist CG, Stone HL 1983 Cardiovascular adjustments to gravitational stress. In: Shepherd JT, Abboud FM (eds) Handbook of physiology. Section 2: circulation, vol 2. American Physiological Society, Bethesda, pp 1025–1063

Bosenberg C, Royston D 2002 Protect the heart in the intensive care unit – but how? Current Opinions in Critical Care 8: 417–420

Brandi LS, Bertolini R, Calafa M 1997 Indirect calorimetry in critically ill patients: clinical applications and

4

practical advice. Nutrition 13: 349–358

Brochard L 2003 Mechanical ventilation: invasive versus non invasive. European Respiratory Journal Supplement 47: 31s–37s

Burns JR, Jones FL 1975 Early ambulation of patients requiring ventilatory assistance. Chest 68: 608

Bydgman S, Wahren J 1974 Influence of body position on the anginal threshold during leg exercise. European Journal of Clinical Investigation 4: 201–206

Casadro-Flores J, Martinez de Azagra A, Ruiz-Lopez MJ, Ruiz M, Serrano A 2002 Pediatric ARDS: effect of supine-prone postural changes on oxygenation. Intensive Care Medicine 28: 1792–1796

Chatte G, Sab J-M, Dubois J-M 1997 Prone position in mechanically ventilated patients with severe acute respiratory failure. American Journal of Critical Care Medicine 155: 473–478

Chawla LS, Abell L, Mazhari R et al 2005 Identifying critically ill patients at high risk for developing acute renal failure: a pilot study. Kidney International 68: 2274–2280

Chuley M, Brown J, Summer W 1982 Effect of postoperative immobilization after coronary artery bypass surgery. Critical Care Medicine 10: 176–178

Clauss RH, Scalabrini BY, Ray RF, Reed GE 1968 Effects of changing body position upon improved ventilation–perfusion relationships. Circulation 37(Suppl 2): 214–217

Craig DB, Wahba WM, Don HF 1971 'Closing volume' and its relationship to gas exchange in seated and supine positions. Journal of Applied Physiology 31: 717–721

Dantzker DR 1983 The influence of cardiovascular function on gas exchange. Clinics in Chest Medicine 4: 149–159

Dean E 1985 Effect of body position on pulmonary function. Physical Therapy 65: 613–618

Dean E 1993 Bedrest and deconditioning. Neurology Report 17: 6–9

Dean E 1994a Oxygen transport: a physiologically-based conceptual framework for the practice of cardiopulmonary physiotherapy. Physiotherapy 80: 347–359

Dean E 1994b Invited commentary on 'Are incentive spirometry, intermittent positive pressure breathing, and deep breathing exercises effective in the prevention of postoperative pulmonary complications after upper abdominal surgery? a systematic overview and meta-analysis.' Physical Therapy 74: 10–15

Dean E 1997 Oxygen transport deficits in systemic disease and implications for physical therapy. Physical Therapy 77: 187–202

Dean E 1999 Preferred practice patterns in cardiopulmonary physical therapy: a guide to physiologic measures. Cardiopulmonary Physical Therapy Journal 10: 124–134

Dean E 2006a Optimizing outcomes: relating interventions to an individual's needs. In: Frownfelter D, Dean E (eds) Cardiovascular and pulmonary physical therapy: evidence and practice, 4th edn. Mosby, St Louis

Dean E 2006b Mobilization and exercise. In: Frownfelter D, Dean E (eds) Cardiovascular and pulmonary physical therapy: evidence and practice, 4th edn. Mosby, St Louis

Dean E 2006c Body positioning. In: Frownfelter D, Dean E (eds) Cardiovascular and pulmonary physical therapy: evidence and practice, 4th edn. Mosby, St Louis

Dean E 2006d Exercise testing and training for individuals with primary cardiopulmonary dysfunction. In: Frownfelter D, Dean E (eds) Cardiovascular and pulmonary physical therapy: evidence and practice, 4th edn. Mosby, St Louis

Dean E, Perme C 2006 Comprehensive management of individuals in the intensive care unit. In: Frownfelter D, Dean E (eds) Cardiovascular and pulmonary physical therapy: evidence and practice, 4th edn. Mosby, St Louis

Dean E, Ross J 1992a Oxygen transport: The basis for contemporary cardiopulmonary physical therapy and its optimization with body positioning and mobilization. Physical Therapy Practice 1:34–44

Dean E, Ross J 1992b Discordance between cardiopulmonary physiology and physical therapy: toward a rational basis for practice. Chest 101: 1694–1698

Dean E, Ross J, Bartz J, Purves S 1989 Improving the validity of exercise testing: the effect of practice on performance. Archives of Physical Medicine and Rehabilitation 70: 599–604

Dock W 1944 The evil sequelae of complete bed rest. Journal of the American Medical Association 125: 1083–1085

Douglas WW, Rehder K, Froukje BM 1977 Improved oxygenation in patients with acute respiratory failure: the prone position. American Review of Respiratory Disease 115: 559–566

Dreyfuss D, Djedaini K, Lanore J-J et al 1992 A comparative study of the effects of almitrine bismesylate and lateral position during unilateral bacterial pneumonia with severe hypoxemia. American Review of Respiratory Disease 148: 295–299

Dripps RD, Waters RM 1941 Nursing care of surgical patients. I. The 'stir-up'. American Journal of Nursing 41: 530–534

Dull JL, Dull WL 1983 Are maximal inspiratory breathing exercises or incentive spirometry better than early mobilization after cardiopulmonary bypass? Physical Therapy 63: 655–659

Fowler WS 1949 Lung function studies. III. Uneven pulmonary ventilation in normal subjects and patients with pulmonary disease. Journal of Applied Physiology 2: 283–299

Fridrich P, Krafft P, Hochleuthner H 1996 The effects of long-term prone positioning in patients with trauma-induced adult respiratory distress syndrome. Anesthesia and Analgesia 83: 1206–1211

Gehr LC, Sessler CN 2001 Neuromuscular blockade in the intensive care unit. Seminars in Respiratory and Critical Care Medicine 22: 175–188

Gosselin N, Lambert K, Poulain M et al 2003 Endurance training improves skeletal muscle electrical activity in active COPD patients. Muscle Nerve 28: 744–753

Hahn-Winslow E 1985 Cardiovascular consequences of bed rest. Heart and Lung 14: 236–246

Harrison TR 1944 The abuse of rest as a therapeutic measure for patients with cardiovascular disease. Journal of the American Medical Association 125: 1075–1078

Hsu HO, Hickey RF 1976 Effect of posture on functional residual capacity postoperatively. Anesthesiology 44: 520–521

Hund E 1999 Myopathy in critically-ill patients. Critical Care Medicine 27: 2544–2547

Imle PC, Klemic N 1989 Changes with immobility and methods of mobilization. In: Mackenzie CF (ed) Chest physiotherapy in the intensive care unit, 2nd edn. Williams and Wilkins, Baltimore, pp 188–214

Jolliet P, Bulpa P, Ritz M et al 1997 Additive beneficial effects of the prone position, nitric oxide, and almitrine bismesylate on gas exchange and oxygen transport in acute respiratory distress syndrome. Critical Care Medicine 25: 786–794

Kee CA, Tomalty JA, Cline J, Novick RJ, Stitt L 2006 Change in practice

4

patterns in the management of diabetic cardiac surgery patients. Canadian Journal of Cardiovascular Nursing 16: 20–27

Khamiees M, Raju P, DeGirolamo A, Amoateng-Adjepong Y, Manthous CA 2001 Predictors of extubation outcome in patients who have successfully completed a spontaneous breathing trial. Chest 120: 1262–1270

Kirilloff LH, Owens HR, Rogers RM, Mazzocco MC 1985 Does chest physical therapy work? Chest 88: 436–444

Koomans HA, Boer WH 1997 Causes of edema in the intensive care unit. Kidney International Supplement 59: S105–S110

Lamb LE, Johnson RL, Stevens PM 1964 Cardiovascular deconditioning during chair rest. Aerospace Medicine 23: 646–649

Larsen AI, Lindal S, Aukrust P et al 2002 Effect of exercise training on skeletal muscle fibre characteristics in men with chronic heart failure. Correlation between muscle alterations, cytokines, and exercise capacity. International Journal of Cardiology 83: 25–32

Larsen AI, Aarsland T, Kristiansen M, Haugland A, Dickstein K 2001 Assessing the effect of exercise training in men with heart failure; comparison of maximal, submaximal and endurance exercise protocols. European Heart Journal 22: 684–692

Laver SR, Padkin A 2005 Does hyperglycaemia precede the clinical onset of myocardial ischemia? Resuscitation 66: 237–239

Leblanc P, Ruff F, Milic-Emili J 1970 Effects of age and body position on airway closure in man. Journal of Applied Physiology 28: 448–451

Levine SA, Lown B 1952 'Armchair' treatment of acute coronary thrombosis. Journal of the American Medical Association 148: 1365–1369

Lewis FR 1980 Management of atelectasis and pneumonia. Surgical Clinics of North America 60: 1391–1401

Lim CM, Kim EK, Lee JS et al 2001 Comparison of the response to the prone position between pulmonary and extrapulmonary acute respiratory distress syndrome. Intensive Care Medicine 27: 477–485

Manning F, Dean E, Ross J, Abboud RAT 1999 Lung function in side lying positions compared with supine in older healthy individuals. Physical Therapy 79: 456–466

Martin V, Hincapie L, Nimbuck M, Gaugham J, Criner G 2005 Impact of

whole-body rehabilitation in patients receiving chronic mechanical ventilation. Critical Care Medicine 33: 2255–2265

Moretti M, Cilione C, Tampieri A et al 2000 Incidence and causes of non-invasive mechanical ventilation failure after initial success. Thorax 55: 819–825

Mure M, Martling C-R, Lindahl SGE 1997 Dramatic effect on oxygenation in patients with severe acute lung insufficiency treated in the prone position. Critical Care Medicine 25: 1539–1544

Nevins ML, Epstein SK 2001 Weaning from prolonged mechanical ventilation. Clinics in Chest Medicine 22: 13–33

Noonan V, Dean E 2000 Submaximal exercise testing: clinical application and interpretation. Physical Therapy 80: 782–807

Orlava OE 1959 Therapeutic physical culture in the complex treatment of pneumonia. Physical Therapy Review 39: 153–160

Pelosi P, Tubiolo D, Mascheroni D 1998 Effects of the prone position on respiratory mechanics and gas exchange during acute lung injury. American Journal of Critical Care Medicine 157: 387–393

Perme C 2006 Early mobilization of LVAD recipients who require prolonged mechanical ventilation. Texas Heart Institute Journal 33: 130–134

Phang PT, Russell JA 1993. When does $\dot{V}O_2$ depend on $\dot{V}O_2$? Respiratory Care 38: 618–630

Powers J, Daniels D 2004 Turning points: implementing kinetic therapy in the ICU. Nursing Management 35(Suppl): 1–7

Putensen C, Zech S, Wrigge H et al 2001 Long-term effects of spontaneous breathing during ventilatory support in patients with acute lung injury. American Journal of Respiratory Care Medicine 164: 43–49

Rady MY, Johnson DJ, Patel BM, Larson JS, Helmers RA 2005 Influence of individual characteristics on outcome of glycemic control in intensive care unit patients with or without diabetes mellitus. Mayo Clinic Proceedings 80: 1558–1567

Ray JF, Yost L, Moallem S et al 1974 Immobility, hypoxemia and pulmonary arteriovenous shunting. Archives of Surgery 109: 537–541

Reid MB, Allard-Gould P 2004 Malnutrition and the critically ill elderly patient. Critical Care Nursing Clinics of North America 16: 531–536

Remolina C, Khan AV, Santiago TV, Edelman NH 1981 Positional hypoxemia in unilateral lung disease. New England Journal of Medicine 304: 523–525

Ross J, Dean E 1989 Integrating physiological principles into the comprehensive management of cardiopulmonary dysfunction. Physical Therapy 69: 255–259

Ross J, Dean E 1992 Body positioning. In Zadai C (ed) Pulmonary management in physical therapy. Churchill Livingstone, New York

Rossi A, Ganassini A, Tantucci C, Grassi V 1996 Aging and the respiratory system. Aging (Milano) 8: 143–161 (English abstract)

Sevransky JF, Haponik EF 2003 Respiratory failure in elderly patients. Clinics in Geriatric Medicine 19: 205–224

Seymour CW, Martinez A, Christie JD, Fuchs BD 2004 The outcome of extubation failure in a community hospital intensive care unit: a cohort study. Critical Care 8: R322–R327

Shander A 2004 Anemia in the critically ill. Critical Care Clinics 20: 159–178

Sjostrand T 1951 Determination of changes in the intrathoracic blood volume in man. Acta Physiologica Scandinavica 22: 116–128

Squadrone E, Frigerio P, Fogliati C et al 2004 Non invasive vs invasive ventilation in COPD patients with severe acute respiratory failure deemed to require ventilatory assistance. Intensive Care Medicine 30: 1303–1310

Stiletto R, Gotzen L, Goubeaud S 2000 Kinetic therapy for therapy and prevention of post-traumatic lung failure. Results of a prospective study of 111 polytrauma patients. Unfallchirurgie 103: 1057–64 (English abstract)

Storer TW 2001 Exercise in chronic pulmonary disease: resistance exercise prescription. Medicine and Science in Sport and Exercise 33(7 Suppl): S680–692

Svanberg L 1957 Influence of position on the lung volumes, ventilation and circulation in normals. Scandinavian Journal of Laboratory Investigation 25(Suppl): 7–175

Verbrugge LM, Jette AM 1993 The disablement process. Social Sciences and Medicine 38: 1–14

Vermeij CG, Feenstra BW, van Lanschot JJ, Bruining HA 1989 Day-to-day variation of energy expenditure in critically ill surgical patients. Critical Care Medicine 17: 623–626

Vianello A, Bevilacqua M, Arcaro G, Gallan F, Serra F 2000 Non-invasive ventilatory approach to treatment of acute respiratory failure in neuromuscular disorders. A comparison with endotracheal intubation. Intensive Care Medicine 26: 384–390

Vollman KM 2004 Prone positioning in the patient who has acute respiratory distress syndrome: the art and science. Critical Care Nursing Clinics of North America 16: 319–336

Vollman KM, Bander JJ 1996 Improved oxygenation utilizing a prone positioner in patients with acute respiratory distress syndrome. Intensive Care Medicine 22: 1105–1111

Warren JB, Turner C, Dalton N et al 1983 The effect of posture on the sympathoadrenal response to theophylline infusion. British Journal of Clinical Pharmacology 16: 405–411

Wasserman K, Hansen JE, Sue DY, Whipp BJ 1987 Principles of exercise testing and interpretation. Lea and Febiger, Philadelphia

Wasserman K, Whipp BJ 1975 Exercise physiology in health and disease. American Review of Respiratory Disease 112: 219–249

Weber KT, Janicki JS, Shroff SG, Likoff MJ 1983 The cardiopulmonary unit: the body's gas transport system. Clinics in Chest Medicine 4: 101–110

Wenger NK 1982 Early ambulation: the physiologic basis revisited. Advances in Cardiology 31: 138–141

West JB 1962 Regional differences in gas exchange in the lung of erect man. Journal of Applied Physiology 17: 893–898

West JB 1977 Ventilation and perfusion relationships. American Review of Respiratory Disease 116: 919–943

West JB 2004 Respiratory physiology – the essentials, 6th edn. Williams and Wilkins, Baltimore

Williams C 1995 Haemoglobin – is more better? Nephrology Dialysis and Transplant 2(Suppl): 48–55

Wolff RK, Dolovich MB, Obminski G, Newhouse MT 1977 Effects of exercise and eucapnic hyperventilation on bronchial clearance in man. Journal of Applied Physiology 43: 46–50

Wong WP 2000 Physical therapy for a patient in acute respiratory failure. Physical Therapy 80: 662–670

Wong WP 2004 Use of body positioning in the mechanically ventilated patient with acute respiratory failure: Application of the Sackett's rules of evidence. Physiotherapy Theory and Practice 15:25–41

World Health Organization 1980 International classification of impairments, disabilities and handicaps. A manual for classification relating to the consequences of disease. World Health Organization, Geneva

World Health Organization 2002 International classification of functioning, disability and health. *www.sustainable-design.ie/arch/ICIDH-2PFDec-2000.pdf* Retrieved July 2007

World Health Organization 2006 Definition of health. *www.who.int/about/definition* Retrieved July 2007

Ympa YP, Sakr Y, Reinhart K, Vincent JL 2005 Has mortality from acute renal failure decreased? A systematic review of the literature. American Journal of Medicine 118: 827–832

Zack MB, Pontoppidan H, Kazemi H 1974 The effect of lateral positions on gas exchange in pulmonary disease. American Review of Respiratory Disease 110: 49–55

Zafiropoulos B, Alison J, McCarren B. 2004 Physiological responses to the early mobilization of the intubated, ventilated abdominal surgery patient. Australian Journal of Physiotherapy 50 95–100

Further reading

American College of Sports Medicine 2005 Guidelines for exercise testing and prescription, 7th edn. Lea and Febiger, Philadelphia

Dean E, Frownfelter D 1996 Clinical case study guide to accompany principles and practice of cardiopulmonary physical therapy, 3rd edn. Mosby, St Louis

Dean E, Perme C 2006 Intensive care unit management of individuals with primary cardiopulmonary dysfunction. In: Frownfelter D, Dean E (eds) Cardiovascular and pulmonary physical therapy: evidence and practice, 4th edn. Mosby, St Louis

Dean E, Perme C 2006 Complications, adult respiratory distress syndrome, shock, sepsis and multiorgan system failure. In: Frownfelter D, Dean E (eds) Cardiovascular and pulmonary physical therapy: evidence and practice, 4th edn. Mosby, St Louis

McArdle WD, Katch FI, Katch VL 1996 Exercise physiology. Energy, nutrition and human performance, 4th edn. Lea and Febiger, Philadelphia

West JB 1990 Ventilation, blood flow and gas exchange, 5th edn. Blackwell Science, Oxford

4

Chapter **5**

Physiotherapy techniques

Jennifer A Pryor, S Ammani Prasad

with contributions from

Delva Bethune
(Neurophysiological facilitation of respiration)

Michelle Chatwin
(Insufflation/exsufflation-assisted cough, intrapulmonary percussive ventilation)

Stephanie Enright
(Inspiratory muscle training)

Leyla P Osman
(High frequency chest wall oscillation)

Helen M Potter
(Manual therapy techniques)

Linda Tagg
(Acupuncture)

Barbara A Webber
(Glossopharyngeal breathing)

Physiotherapy techniques are discussed throughout the book, but some are described in more detail in this chapter.

ACUPUNCTURE

What can be treated with acupuncture?

Acupuncture is recognized by the World Health Organization (WHO) in the treatment of respiratory conditions (Hopwood 1993) and acupuncture techniques can also be used to treat associated symptoms: acute and chronic pain, panic attacks and stress, which are so often a contributing or causative factor. Acupuncture has been found to be safe and potentially effective for bronchial asthma and chronic obstructive pulmonary disease (COPD) (Jobst 1995). It has been reported to help control disabling breathlessness (Linde et al 1986), asthma (Blackwell 2004) and improve lung function and quality of life in COPD (Neumeister et al 1999). Acupuncture used pre- and postoperatively may reduce postoperative pain, the risk of infection and improve recovery rate.

The techniques used and the evidence base

Needling is the biggest cause of adverse effects in acupuncture (Halvorsen et al 1995, Rampes & James 1995). Many respiratory patients have contraindications to needling and to the use of certain body acupuncture points (acupoints). Therefore a combination of non-invasive body and ear acupuncture (auriculotherapy) is used to overcome these limitations. Each can be used on its own, but they are more effective if used together or with another treatment modality. Acupuncture treatment is based on evidence from different levels of research, from systematic reviews (Ezzo 2000) to clinical opinion.

   Non-invasive options include acupressure, laser, magnetic and electrical stimulation (Baxter 1994, Kenyon 1983, 1988, Lawrence et al 1998) and have been found to be as effective as needling in the body (Vickers 1986). In auriculotherapy, electrical stimulation was more effective than needling for pain relief (Oleson 1998). Acupressure, where no equipment is required, is an invaluable tool for both therapist and patient, and it can be used as a home treatment to enhance and maintain the effect of treatment. Acupressure was found to reduce dyspnoea and be a useful adjunct for patients undergoing a pulmonary rehabilitation programme (Man et al 1997). Laser acupuncture was of benefit in the treatment of sinusitis, asthma and pnuemonia (Rindge 2005). Unpublished case studies have also shown that non-invasive methods can be as effective as needling and in some cases, more effective.

How do acupuncture techniques work?

Stimulation of an acupoint activates A-delta, A-beta and C afferents, which inhibit the sensory and affective components of pain via gating and descending inhibitory pathways (Lund et al 2006). Endorphins and serotonin are released which, as well as having an analgesic effect, have been shown to effect cell growth and healing. (Kishi et al 1996, Pakala & Benedict 1998). Stimulation of certain acupoints activates cortical areas of the brain that have controlling effects on symptoms being treated (Zhang 1986). The traditional concept is one of energy flowing within meridians. The energy becomes imbalanced by disease and acupoints are chosen to create a re-balance. Active points that require treatment are detectable by electrical skin resistance measurement and by palpation for tenderness. Acupoints and meridians have a high concentration of gap junctions (Mashanskii et al 1983), facilitating intercellular communication and thereby mediating the effects of acupuncture.

Auriculotherapy (ear acupuncture)

Auriculotherapy (Fig. 5.1) is safer than body acupuncture, quicker and access is easier. It is therefore useful in situations such as critical care. Patients contraindicated to body acupuncture, for example those with

5

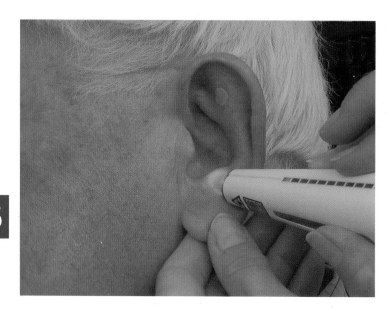

Figure 5.1   Laser therapy to the ear.

heart conditions, can be safely treated via the ear. Certain drugs will reduce the effectiveness of body acupuncture, for example corticosteroids acting as a partial opiate antagonist, but these same drugs do not reduce the effectiveness of auriculotherapy. Every anatomical structure and physiological function of the body is represented by an acupoint on the ear (Nogier 1981, Oleson 1998, Practical Ear Needling Therapy 1980). These points become active when disease is present and are detected by palpation for tenderness, ideal when treating pain; and electrical resistance measurement, ideal for non-painful conditions. Stimulation of these points has an effect on the corresponding body area or function. An electromagnetic balancing is achieved, internal opiates are released and there can be an immediate reflex effect on, for example, pain. Tiny gold-plated magnets can be placed over selected points between treatments, creating constant pressure and a magnetic field to prolong the effectiveness of treatment. The patient can apply additional pressure to obtain further relief of symptoms, thus reducing the frequency and number of visits required. Auriculotherapy is one of the safest and most effective ways of dealing with conditions more complicated than pain. In addition to treatment, it can also be used for prevention and diagnosis (Lichstein et al 1974).

Some useful body points

The following acupoints may be useful for certain respiratory symptoms, *but these techniques are contraindicated in pregnant women and people with pacemakers or heart conditions.* The points are found by palpating for a tender

spot and acupressure is given using gentle circular massage over the point for about a minute.

CV 17 On the sternum roughly midway between the nipples. Useful for shortness of breath and in conjunction with breathing exercises, works well by applying straight pressure to the point on exhalation.

PC 6 In the centre of the anterior aspect of the forearm, three fingers' breadth from the anterior wrist crease. Effective for hyperventilation, stress reduction and relief of nausea and vomiting (Stainton & Neff 1994).

LI 4 Adduct the thumb, find the high point of the interosseus muscle and press towards the second metacarpal. One of the most useful points in the body. Useful for pain relief and stress reduction.

Acupuncture used appropriately as part of a team approach, whether by needle or non-invasive means, can act as a very effective complementary therapy to help to improve quality of life and reduce potential side effects from drug therapy. It works wells alongside the conventional treatment of respiratory diseases and concomitant symptoms, to enhance the outcome of treatment.

AIRWAY CLEARANCE TECHNIQUES

Airway clearance techniques are used to facilitate mucociliary clearance. Under normal circumstances the mucociliary clearance mechanism is extremely effective and efficient but in the presence of many respiratory diseases and following anaesthesia and surgical procedures, airway clearance techniques may be required to enhance mucociliary clearance. There is as yet no evidence to support the use of any one airway clearance technique over any other (Accurso et al 2004, Prasad & Main 1998, Pryor 2005, Pryor et al 2006). Practice tends to be influenced by culture and patient preference. The airway clearance techniques available to patients may be determined by the skills of the therapist (Hardy et al 1994) and the financing of healthcare provision. When a device, for example positive expiratory pressure (PEP) or oscillating PEP (Acapella®, Flutter® or RC-Cornet®), is included in an airway clearance regimen, meticulous cleaning and thorough drying of the equipment after use is essential to prevent the possibility of infection from the device. Other techniques, for example intermittent positive pressure breathing and glossopharyngeal breathing, may also assist in the clearance of secretions and have additional effects.

If an airway clearance technique is required in the long term, it is important to negotiate rather than prescribe a physiotherapy home programme to increase adherence to treatment (Carr et al 1996). Programmes must be realistic and appropriate general physical activities should be encouraged. Revision of techniques at intervals is important to assess the effectiveness of the regimen and to correct and update techniques as necessary. Currie et al (1986) recognized the importance of reassessment in maintaining adherence to treatment.

Traditionally airway clearance techniques have been associated with head-down tipped positioning, but this is now used only if individual patient benefit is identified on assessment. Several systematic reviews have been undertaken looking at airway clearance in people with cystic fibrosis (Elkins et al 2006a, Main et al 2005, van der Schans et al 2000). Chest physiotherapy (postural drainage and percussion) was compared with no chest physiotherapy (van der Schans et al 2000). It was concluded that airway clearance techniques may have short-term effects in the context of increasing mucus transport, but no evidence was found on which to draw conclusions concerning the long-term effects. Elkins et al (2006a) studied PEP and Main et al (2005) compared 'conventional' chest physiotherapy (postural drainage and percussion) with other contemporary airway clearance techniques (active cycle of breathing techniques, autogenic drainage, PEP, oscillating PEP and high-frequency chest wall oscillation). There appeared to be no advantage of 'conventional' chest physiotherapy over the other airway clearance techniques, in the primary outcome measure of lung function. In the review by Elkins et al (2006a), there was an indication

that individuals prefer regimens that can be self-administered.

Holland & Button (2006) reviewed the place of airway clearance techniques in chronic respiratory disease and proposed a physiological rationale for the use of airway clearance techniques in chronic obstructive pulmonary disease taking into consideration the presence of bronchiectasis, amount of sputum expectorated, degree of airflow obstruction and presence of decreased lung elastic recoil.

Active cycle of breathing techniques

The active cycle of breathing techniques (ACBT) has been shown to be effective in the clearance of bronchial secretions (Pryor et al 1979, Wilson et al 1995) and to improve lung function (Webber et al 1986) without increasing hypoxaemia (Pryor et al 1990) or airflow obstruction (Pryor & Webber 1979, Pryor et al 1994, Thompson & Thompson 1968).

The ACBT is a flexible regimen that can be adapted for any patient in whom there is a problem of excess bronchial secretions and can be used with or without an assistant. It is a cycle of breathing control, thoracic expansion exercises and the forced expiration technique (FET) (Fig. 5.2). The original studies of 'the forced expiration technique' (Hofmeyr et al 1986, Pryor et al 1979, Webber et al 1986) used this cycle of techniques, but people began to use a regimen of huffing alone or other variations on the FET (Falk et al 1984, Reisman et al 1988) and the literature became confusing. In order to emphasize the use of thoracic expansion exercises and the periods of breathing control, in addition to the FET, the whole regimen was renamed the active cycle of breathing techniques (ACBT) (Webber 1990). The regimen did not change in practice and the early studies on the FET were controlled clinical trials on the ACBT.

Breathing control

Breathing control is the resting period between the more active parts of the cycle. It is tidal breathing, at the patient's own rate and depth. The person is encouraged to relax the upper chest and shoulders and to use the lower chest, diaphragmatic, pattern of breathing as much as they are able. It allows the lungs and chest wall to revert to their resting position. This period should be continued until the person is ready to use either the thoracic expansion exercises or the huffing of the forced expiration technique.

Thoracic expansion exercises

Thoracic expansion exercises are deep breathing exercises emphasizing inspiration. Inspiration is active and is usually combined with a 3-second end-

5

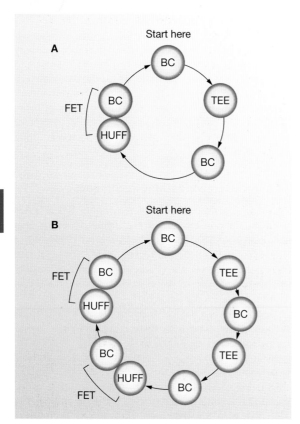

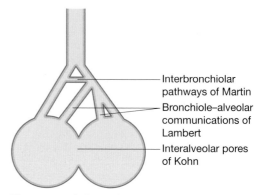

Figure 5.3 Collateral ventilation pathways.

Interbronchiolar pathways of Martin

Bronchiole–alveolar communications of Lambert

Interalveolar pores of Kohn

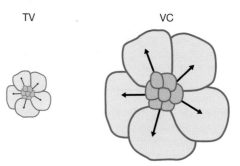

Figure 5.4 Interdependence. The effect of expanding alveoli at tidal volume (TV) and vital capacity (VC).

Figure 5.2 Diagrammatic representation of two examples of the active cycle of breathing techniques, demonstrating the flexibility of the technique: BC, breathing control; TEE, thoracic expansion exercises; FET, forced expiration technique.

inspiratory hold before passive relaxed expiration. The postoperative manoeuvre of a 3-second hold at full inspiration has been shown to decrease collapse of lung tissue (Ward et al 1966). This 'hold' may also be of value in patients with medical chest conditions to allow for asynchronous ventilation as air flows more quickly into healthy, unobstructed areas than into diseased and obstructed regions. *Pendelluft* flow is that which takes place between parallel respiratory units with different time constants (Mead et al 1970).

> *'Airflow is essential for airway clearance'*
> (Lapin 2002)

In the normal lung, the resistance to airflow via the collateral ventilatory system is high and there is little movement of gas through these channels. With increasing lung volume and in the presence of lung pathology, resistance decreases allowing air to flow via the collateral channels – the interalveolar pores of Kohn, bronchiole–alveolar communications of Lambert and

interbronchiolar pathways of Martin (Menkes & Traystman 1977) (Fig. 5.3) and to come in behind secretions. These collateral channels are not present in infants and young children and it is unknown when, in the developmental process, they become patent.

The effectiveness of thoracic expansion exercises, in re-expanding lung tissue and in mobilizing and clearing excess bronchial secretions, can also be explained by the phenomenon of interdependence (Mead et al 1970). This is the effect of expanding forces exerted between adjacent alveoli. At high lung volumes the expanding forces between alveoli are greater than at tidal volume and may assist in re-expansion of lung tissue (Fig. 5.4). About three expansion exercises are usually appropriate before pausing for a few seconds for a period of breathing control. Too many deep breaths may produce the effects of hyperventilation, are tiring and reduce the number of huffs undertaken within the time period. The thoracic expansion exercises may be undertaken consecutively or patients may like to take a normal-sized breath in between.

Thoracic expansion exercises can be facilitated with proprioceptive stimulation by placing a hand, either the patient's or the physiotherapist's, over the part of the chest wall where movement of the chest is to be encouraged (Fig. 5.5). There may be an initial increase in ven-

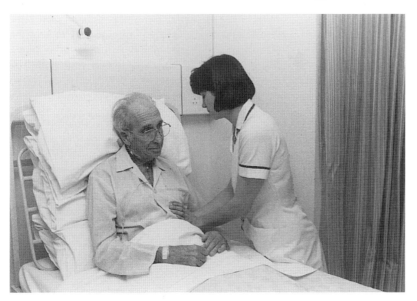

Figure 5.5 Thoracic expansion exercises.

tilation to this part of the lung (Tucker et al 1999) and there should be an increase in chest wall movement.

Sometimes an additional increase in lung volume can be achieved by using a 'sniff' manoeuvre at the end of a deep inspiration. This manoeuvre may not be appropriate in patients who are hyperinflated, but for surgical patients who need further motivation to increase their lung volume, it may be a useful technique.

Thoracic expansion exercises may be combined with chest shaking, vibrations and/or chest clapping, if there is an indication that the inclusion of these techniques may assist further the clearance of secretions.

Forced expiration technique (FET)

The forced expiration technique is a combination of one or two forced expirations (huffs) and periods of breathing control. Huffing to low lung volumes should assist the movement of the more peripherally situated secretions and when secretions have reached the larger more proximal upper airways, a huff or cough from a high lung volume can be used to clear them.

> *'Forced expiratory manoeuvres are probably the most effective part of chest physiotherapy'*
> (van der Schans 1997)

With any forced expiratory manoeuvre there is dynamic compression and collapse of the airways downstream (towards the mouth) of the equal pressure point (West 2004). This is an important part of the clearance mechanism of either a huff or cough. At lung volumes above functional residual capacity, the equal pressure points are located in lobar or segmental bronchi (Macklem 1974). As lung volume decreases, during a

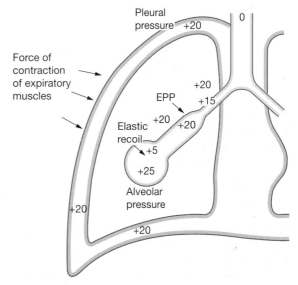

Figure 5.6 Forced expiratory manoeuvre: huff or cough. (Pryor 1991. In Pryor JA (ed) Respiratory care, p 84. Reproduced with permission of Elsevier, Edinburgh)

forced expiratory manoeuvre, the equal pressure points move distally into the smaller more peripheral airways. Figure 5.6 is a static representation of the dynamic state of a forced expiratory manoeuvre (huff or cough). The pleural pressure at this instance is +20 cmH$_2$O, the elastic recoil pressure of the lungs is +5 cmH$_2$O and consequently the peripheral pressure is +25 cmH$_2$O. There is a downward gradient from +25 cmH$_2$O at the alveolus to zero at the mouth and, somewhere along the airway, the pressure within the airway will equal

5

the pleural pressure. Proximal to this, dynamic collapse and compression of the airway takes place. The dynamic collapse and compression during a forced expiratory manoeuvre is effective from points, choke points (Dawson & Elliott 1977), downstream of the equal pressure point.

A series of coughs without intervening inspirations was advocated by Mead et al (1967) to clear bronchial secretions, but clinically a single continuous huff down to the same lung volume is as effective and less exhausting. Hasani et al (1994) compared cough with the FET and concluded that both were equally effective in clearing lung secretions, but that the FET required less effort.

The mean transpulmonary pressure during voluntary coughing is greater than during a forced expiration. This results in greater compression and narrowing of the airways, which limits airflow and reduces the efficiency of bronchial clearance (Langlands 1967). In 1989 Freitag et al demonstrated an oscillatory movement, 'hidden' vibrations, of the airway walls in addition to the squeezing action produced by the forced expiratory manoeuvre.

The viscosity of mucus is shear-dependent (Lopez-Vidriero & Reid 1978) and the shear forces generated during a huff should reduce mucus viscosity (Selsby & Jones 1990). This, together with the high flow of a forced expiratory manoeuvre, would also be expected to aid mucus clearance and the expectoration of sputum.

When mobilizing and clearing peripheral secretions, it is an unnecessary expenditure of energy to start the huff from a high lung volume. A huff from mid-lung volume is more efficient and probably more effective. To huff from mid-lung volume a medium-sized breath should be taken in and, with the mouth and glottis open, the air is squeezed out using the chest wall and abdominal muscles. It should be long enough to loosen secretions from the more peripherally situated airways and should not be just a clearing noise in the back of the throat. However, if the huff is continued for too long it may lead to unnecessary paroxysmal coughing. Too short a huff may be ineffective (Partridge et al 1989) but when secretions have reached the upper airways, a shorter huff or a cough from a high lung volume is used to clear them.

The huff is a forced but not violent manoeuvre. To be maximally effective, the length of the huff and force of contraction of the expiratory muscles should be altered to maximize airflow and to minimize airway collapse. A peak flow mouthpiece, or similar piece of tubing, may improve the effectiveness of the huff as it should help to keep the glottis open. Some people find huffing through a tube, at a tissue or a cotton wool ball, helpful in perfecting the technique. The huff can be introduced to children as blowing games (Thompson 1978) and from about the age of 2 years they are usually able to copy others huffing (Fig. 5.7).

An essential part of the forced expiration technique is the pause for breathing control after one or two huffs,

Figure 5.7   Huffing games.

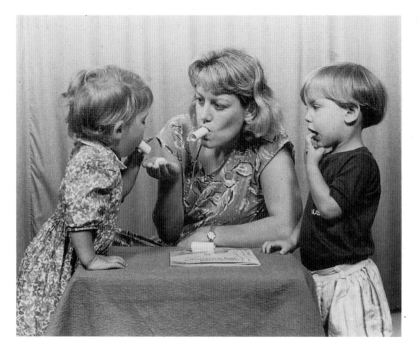

to prevent any increase in airflow obstruction. The length of the pause will vary from patient to patient. In a patient with bronchospasm or unstable airways or in one who is debilitated and fatigues easily, longer pauses (perhaps 10–20 seconds) may be appropriate. In patients with no bronchospasm the periods of breathing control may be considerably shorter (perhaps two or three breaths or 5–10 seconds).

In the tetraplegic patient, clearance of secretions from the upper airways is difficult because maximum lung volume cannot be achieved and the equal pressure points will therefore never reach the largest airways (Morgan et al 1986). Secretions can be cleared from the smaller airways, but accumulate in the larger upper airways. The use of glossopharyngeal breathing may assist clearance from the upper airways.

The techniques of breathing control, thoracic expansion exercises and the forced expiration technique should be used flexibly and adapted for, and by, each patient during each treatment session. One set of thoracic expansion exercises may be followed by the forced expiration technique (see Fig. 5.2A) but if secretions loosen slowly, it may be more appropriate to use two sets of thoracic expansion exercises (see Fig. 5.2B) interspersed with a period of breathing control. Most surgical patients will benefit from the 3-second hold with the thoracic expansion exercises and there is rarely an indication, in the surgical patient, for the use of chest clapping. Wound support may be more suitable than chest compression during huffing and coughing (Fig. 5.8).

In many patients, medical and surgical, secretions can be cleared effectively using the ACBT in the sitting position, but on occasions gravity-assisted positions may be indicated, for example a lung abscess. Cecins et al (1999) studied the effects of gravity (positions with and without a head-down tilt) in a group of patients with cystic fibrosis, bronchiectasis and immotile cilia syndrome, using the ACBT. There were no significant differences in lung function or in the weight of sputum expectorated during treatment. Most of the patients preferred the horizontal position and felt less breathless without a head-down tilt.

The 'endpoint' of a treatment session can be recognized, either by the physiotherapist or the patient self-treating, when an effective huff to low lung volume has become dry sounding and non-productive (for example two cycles). The sicker patient may not reach this endpoint before tiring and should stop before becoming exhausted with any airway clearance technique.

Autogenic drainage

Autogenic drainage (AD) aims to maximize airflow within the airways, to improve ventilation and the clearance of mucus (Chevaillier 2002). Chevaillier developed this concept in Belgium in the late 1960s but little was published until 1979 (Dab & Alexander 1979). Autogenic drainage utilizes gentle breathing at different lung volumes to loosen, mobilize and clear bronchial secretions.

In people with pressure-dependent airway collapse the increase in airflow, with an unforced compared with a forced expiratory manoeuvre, can be demonstrated using the flow–volume loop (Fig. 5.9). Many people with chronic respiratory disease will have a degree of

5

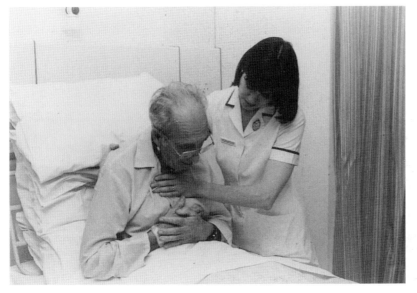

Figure 5.8   Huffing with wound support.

pressure-dependent airway collapse, but in the absence of pressure-dependent collapse it is not possible to move outside the flow–volume loop, i.e. to increase airflow with an unforced expiratory manoeuvre.

Chevaillier originally described three phrases: 'unstick', 'collect' and 'evacuate' (Schöni 1989) (Fig. 5.10). The breathing technique is that of a slow breath in, keeping the upper airways (mouth and glottis) open.

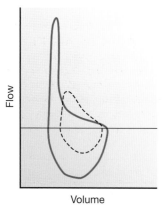

Figure 5.9 Flow–volume loop demonstrating pressure-dependent collapse (concave shape of expiratory loop). The continuous line represents a forced manoeuvre and the broken line, an unforced manoeuvre. There is an increase in expiratory airflow, from the small airways, with the forced expiratory manoeuvre.

It is recommended that the breath in be held for 2–4 seconds. This 'hold' facilitates more equal filling of lung segments, by allowing for the variation in time constants within different lung regions (collateral ventilation). Expiration is performed keeping the upper airways open, as if sighing. The expiratory force is balanced so that the expiratory flow reaches the highest rate possible without causing airway compression. Air flow at a high velocity enhances shear forces. As mucus is mobilized it can be both heard and felt (by placing the hands on the chest) (Fig. 5.11). This cycle is repeated through varying lung volumes.

Breathing at low lung volumes is said to mobilize peripheral mucus. This is the first or 'unstick' phase. It is followed by a period of breathing around the individual's tidal volume which is said to 'collect' mucus from the middle airways. Then, by breathing around high lung volumes, the 'evacuate' phase, expectoration of secretions from the central airways is promoted. When sufficient mucus has been collected in the large airways it may be cleared by coughing or huffing. Coughing before this point is discouraged (Chevaillier 2001 personal communication, Chevaillier 2002). Autogenic drainage is usually undertaken in the sitting or supine lying positions.

A short-term study compared AD with the ACBT (Miller et al 1995), but this was not the ACBT as outlined above. In a long-term study of patients with cystic fibrosis, AD was compared with postural drainage and per-

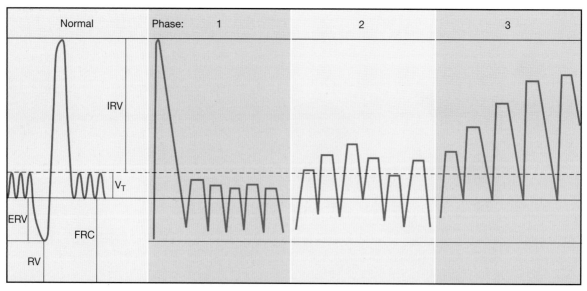

Figure 5.10   Autogenic drainage: Belgian method. Phases of autogenic drainage shown on a spirogram of a normal person. Phase 1: unstick; Phase 2: collect; Phase 3: evacuate. (V_T = tidal volume, ERV = expiratory reserve volume, RV = reserve volume, FRC = functional residual capacity, IRV = inspiratory reserve volume, IRV + V_T + ERV = vital capacity). (Schöni 1989. Reproduced with permission of the Journal of the Royal Society of Medicine)

cussion, with an assistant (Davidson et al 1992). AD was found to be at least as effective as the conventional treatment and the patients expressed a marked preference for AD.

For infants and young children (under the age of about 5 years), 'passive' AD is used in some countries. The goals of AD are achieved by the therapist using their hands to guide the thorax and respiratory movements. The treatment is passive, gentle and effective.

In Germany the practice of AD was modified (David 1991, Kieselmann 1995) and not split into the three phases, as the patients found breathing at low lung volumes uncomfortable. This technique is known as modified autogenic drainage (M AD) (Fig. 5.12). The patient breathes around tidal volume while breath holding for 2–3 seconds at the end of each inspiration. Coughing is used to clear mucus from the larynx (Kieselmann 1995).

Chest clapping

Chest clapping is performed using a cupped hand with a rhythmical flexion and extension action of the wrist. The technique is often performed with two hands but, depending on the area of the chest, it may be more appropriate to use one hand. For the infant, chest clapping is performed using two or three fingers of one hand or using a soft rubber facemask (Chapter 10). Single-handed chest clapping is probably the technique

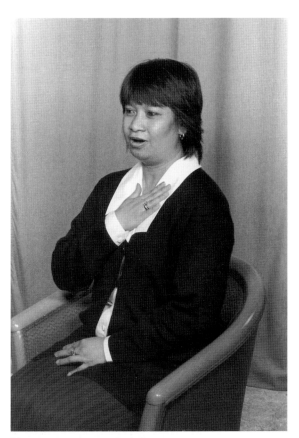

Figure 5.11 Autogenic drainage.

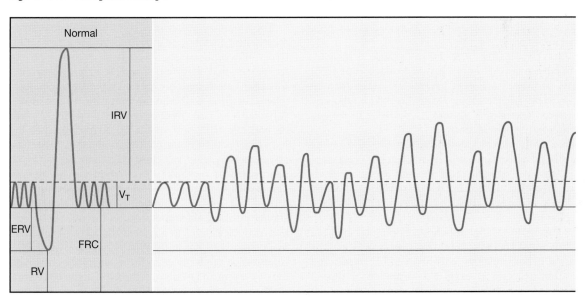

Figure 5.12 Autogenic drainage: German method. Autogenic drainage shown on a spirogram of a normal person. The method is not divided into separate phases. (V_T = tidal volume, ERV = expiratory reserve volume, RV = reserve volume, FRC = functional residual capacity, IRV = inspiratory reserve volume, IRV + V_T + ERV = vital capacity). (David 1991. In: Pryor JA (ed) Respiratory care, p 69. Reproduced with permission of Elsevier, Edinburgh)

of choice for self-chest clapping as it is difficult to coordinate two-handed clapping at the same time as using thoracic expansion exercises.

Chest clapping should never be uncomfortable and should be performed over a layer of clothing to avoid sensory stimulation of the skin. It should not be necessary to use extra layers of clothing or towelling, as the force of the chest clapping should be adapted to suit the individual.

Mechanical percussion has been shown to increase intrathoracic pressure (Flower et al 1979) and chest clapping may have a similar effect, but this change in intrathoracic pressure has not been correlated with an increase in the clearance of bronchial secretions. Andersen (1987, personal communication) hypothesized that the air-filled alveoli would buffer increases in intrathoracic pressure and markedly reduce the mechanical effect of chest clapping.

Some studies (Campbell et al 1975, Wollmer et al 1985) have demonstrated an increase in airflow obstruction when chest clapping is included in an airway clearance regimen, but other studies (Gallon 1991, Pryor & Webber 1979) have shown no increase in airflow obstruction with chest clapping.

In infants and small children who are not yet old enough to cooperate with voluntary breathing techniques, in patients with neuromuscular weakness or paralysis and in the intellectually impaired, chest clapping may be a useful technique to stimulate coughing. The cough is probably stimulated by the mobilization of secretions; however, other methods such as physical activity or other airway clearance modalities may be more appropriate.

Chest clapping has been shown to cause an increase in hypoxaemia (Falk et al 1984, McDonnell et al 1986) when performed for short periods only (less than 30 seconds) but when combined with three to four thoracic expansion exercises there was no decrease in oxygen saturation (Pryor et al 1990).

In a group of clinically stable patients with cystic fibrosis, no advantage was shown when self-chest clapping was used in addition to thoracic expansion exercises (Webber et al 1985), but this cannot be extrapolated to either all medical chest conditions or to acute chest problems.

If a patient feels that self-chest clapping is beneficial but the physiotherapist thinks it is tiring and may be causing hypoxaemia, the patient should be monitored using an oximeter. If oxygen desaturation of clinical significance occurs during the self-chest clapping, the patient should be encouraged to omit the clapping but to continue with the thoracic expansion exercises. Patients studied by Carr et al (1995) felt that self-chest clapping was useful when they were clinically stable, but more particularly when they were unwell. The benefits of chest clapping remain uncertain, but if chest clapping is considered to be clinically beneficial for an individual it should be continued, provided there are no adverse effects.

There is probably no indication for chest clapping in postoperative patients and in patients following chest trauma. Severe osteoporosis and frank haemoptysis are contraindications, although chest clapping is unlikely to increase bleeding when bronchial secretions are lightly streaked with blood.

Vigorous and rapid chest clapping may lead to breath holding and may induce bronchospasm in a patient with hyper-reactive airways. There is no evidence that alteration in the rate of chest clapping increases or decreases the mobilization of bronchial secretions. A rhythmical rate that is comfortable for both patient and physiotherapist is probably the most appropriate.

Chest shaking, vibrations and compression

The therapist's hands are placed on the chest wall and, during expiration, a vibratory action in the direction of the normal movement of the ribs is transmitted through the chest using body weight. This action augments expiratory flow (McCarren & Alison 2006) and may help to mobilize secretions. It is unknown whether airway closure will be increased if the vibratory action is continued into the expiratory reserve volume, but these techniques are frequently combined with thoracic expansion exercises, which would be likely to counteract any resulting airway closure.

The vibratory action may be either a coarse movement (chest shaking) or a fine movement (chest vibrations). Physiotherapists have tended to adopt the techniques that they find the most helpful clinically. Vibrations are commonly used in infants and children, where the chest wall is more compliant than in adults (Chapter 10). Chest vibrations and shaking should never be uncomfortable and should be adapted to suit the individual patient. Some patients, doing their own chest physiotherapy, find self-chest vibrations helpful. One hand is placed on top of the other on the appropriate part of the chest wall and vibrations or shaking are carried out during expiration. With the hands in a similar position, chest compression throughout expiration may be helpful to augment the forced expiratory manoeuvre of the huff. When in side lying, self-compression can be given over the side of the chest with the upper arm and elbow and the hand of the other arm.

The physiotherapist or the patient's carer may give compression during huffing or coughing. Some patients find this helpful, but others prefer to be unsupported. Postoperative patients usually find that supporting the wound facilitates both huffing and coughing (Fig. 5.8).

With fractured ribs and other chest injuries, shaking of the chest wall would be inappropriate but compressive support may assist the clearance of secretions.

In the paralysed patient the technique of rib springing may be used, where compression of the chest wall is continued throughout expiration and overpressure is applied at the end of the breath out. By releasing the hands quickly, inspiration is encouraged. This technique is inappropriate in the non-paralysed patient and may be harmful as compression against a reflexly splinted chest wall may produce rib fractures. Assisted coughing for the paralysed patient is described in Chapter 16.

In the drowsy, semicomatose patient (for example, the chronic bronchitic in respiratory failure with sputum retention), chest compression similar to, but less vigorous than, rib springing may stimulate a deeper inspiration. Chest shaking or chest vibrations are often used during the expiratory phase of a manual hyperinflation treatment to assist the clearance of secretions (Chapters 8 and 10). Care must be taken when using the techniques of chest shaking, vibrations and compression if there are signs of osteoporosis or metastatic deposits affecting the ribs or vertebral column.

A study by McCarren & Alison (2006) of people with cystic fibrosis compared the expiratory flow rates and frequencies of airflow oscillation of vibration and percussion (chest clapping) with positive expiratory pressure and the oscillating positive expiratory pressure of the Flutter® and Acapella®. They concluded that vibration produced greater expiratory flow rates and a higher peak expiratory/peak inspiratory flow ratio, although the Flutter® and Acapella® had higher oscillation frequencies. Their clinical recommendation was that if patients were unable to cough or huff effectively, vibration could be used.

High-frequency chest wall oscillation

High-frequency chest wall oscillation (HFCWO) (also known as high-frequency chest wall compression (HFCWC) or high-frequency chest compression (HFCC)) commonly provides compression of the chest wall at frequencies of 5–20 Hz. Usually this compressive force is created using an inflatable jacket adjusted to fit snugly over the thorax. This is linked to an air-pulse generator, which delivers intermittent positive pressure airflow into the jacket. As a result the jacket rapidly expands, compressing the chest wall, producing a transient (hence oscillatory) increase in airflow in the airways (Fig. 5.13).

It is hypothesized that mucus clearance is enhanced as a consequence of this airflow oscillation and vibration of the airway walls. The proposed mechanism is that increased mucus / airflow interaction leads to increased cough-like shear forces and decreased mucus viscoelasticity (King et al 1983, Tomkiewicz et al 1994). Furthermore, HFCWO creates an expiratory bias to airflow and it is hypothesized that this promotes movement of mucus downstream toward the mouth. It has also been suggested that HFCWO may enhance ciliary activity (Chang et al 1988, Freitag et al 1989, Hansen et al 1994, King et al 1984, 1990).

There is short-term evidence to support increased mucociliary clearance with HFCWO in patients with cystic fibrosis. Some studies have demonstrated a significant increase in sputum clearance after HFCWO in comparison with baseline or control, but no significant difference in efficacy between HFCWO and other airway

5

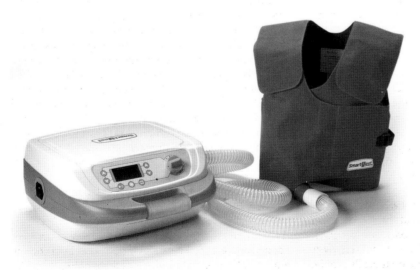

Figure 5.13 The SmartVest®. (Electromed Inc)

5

clearance techniques including postural drainage and percussion (PD&P), positive expiratory pressure (PEP) and high-frequency oral oscillation (HFOO) (Braggion et al 1995, Scherer et al 1998). Other studies, comparing HFCWO with PD&P, have demonstrated significantly more sputum clearance with HFCWO over PD&P (Hansen & Warwick 1990, Kluft et al 1996). Benefits in airway clearance with HFCWO have also been reported in other conditions including asthma, chronic obstructive pulmonary disease, neuromuscular disease, postoperative patients and those requiring long-term ventilatory support (Allan et al 2003, Chiappetta & Beckerman 1995, Perry et al 1998, Wen et al 1996, Whitman et al 1993).

Different studies have used different protocols in the application of HFCWO (Arens et al 1994, Braggion et al 1995, Darbee et al 2005, Kluft et al 1996, Oermann et al 2001, Stites et al 2006, Varekojis et al 2003, Warwick & Hansen 1991, Warwick et al 2004). Most commonly, a total treatment time of 30 minutes covering six frequencies between 6–25Hz has been used and standard manufacturers' guidelines suggest 10–30 minutes of total treatment time (Electromed 2006, Hill-Rom

2006). Early animal studies found 13 Hz to be an optimum treatment frequency (Gross et al 1985, King et al 1983) and some manufacturers suggest 10 minutes each at 10, 12 and 14 Hz (Electromed 2006). However, more recently it has been recommended that an individual 'tuning' method should be used to identify optimum treatment frequencies, which vary among individuals and according to the waveform of the machine used (Milla et al 2006).

HFCWO is widely used in the USA where it is an attractive alternative to PD&P with an assistant, with cost benefit. However, in the UK and Europe where other independently performed techniques are the mainstay of care for airway clearance, HFCWO is not used as extensively and has cost implications.

Infants and young children

For infants and young children regular physical activity is important, not just for airway clearance but for the many other benefits it provides. Physical activity is possible even in the infant, for example, playing on a gym ball (Fig. 5.14). In babies who have a chronic respiratory disorder (with increased airway secretions) an additional airway clearance technique may be necessary (e.g. modified postural drainage and percussion, positive expiratory pressure (PEP) or assisted autogenic drainage (AD)). For young children, trampolining (Fig. 5.15) and, when they are able to cooperate, bubble PEP (Fig. 5.24) are fun. At an older age, other airway clearance techniques can be added.

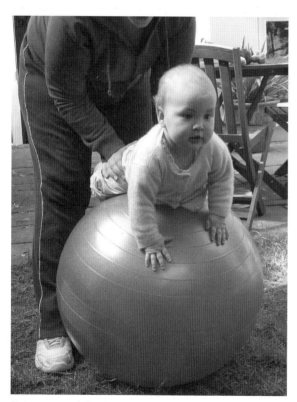

Figure 5.14 Infant on a gym ball.

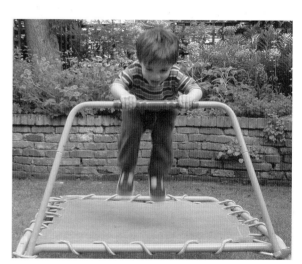

Figure 5.15 Child on a trampoline.

Insufflation/exsufflation–assisted cough

A mechanical insufflator/exsufflator uses positive pressure to deliver, to the upper airway, a maximal lung inhalation followed by an abrupt switch to negative pressure. The rapid change from positive to negative pressure is aimed at simulating the airflow changes that occur during a cough, thereby assisting sputum clearance. In 1953 various portable devices were manufactured to deliver mechanical insufflation/exsufflation (e.g. OEM Cof-flater portable cough machine, St Louis). The most commonly used mechanical insufflator/exsufflator today is the CoughAssist™ (Emerson, Massachusetts) (Fig. 5.16). Initial investigations showed mechanical insufflation/exsufflation to be effective at removing foreign bodies from anaesthetized dogs (Bickerman 1954).

Beck & Barach (1954) demonstrated clinical and radiographic improvements in 92 of 103 acutely ill patients with respiratory tract infections, with the use of mechanical insufflation/exsufflation. Seventy-two patients had bronchopulmonary lung disease and 27 had chest wall or neuromuscular disease. Improvement was more evident in patients with neuromuscular disease. The cardiovascular effects of mechanical insufflation/exsufflation were evaluated by Beck & Scarrone (1956) who found that patients demonstrated an increase in mean heart rate of 17 beats per minute and an increase in systolic blood pressure of 8 mmHg. There was also

an increase in cardiac output of 2.1 litres per minute and echocardiograph changes reflective of rotation of the heart during normal coughing.

Mechanical insufflation/exsufflation has been shown to increase peak cough flow (PCF) in patients with neuromuscular disease (Bach 2003, Chatwin et al 2003, Mustfa et al 2003, Sancho et al 2004, Sivasothy et al 2001). An increase in PCF is thought to improve the efficacy of the cough and thus assist in secretion removal. Mustfa et al (2003) and Sancho et al (2004) found a significant improvement from baseline PCF with mechanical insufflation/exsufflation for both bulbar and non-bulbar motor neuron disease patients, although non-bulbar patients had the greatest change in PCF. Mechanical insufflation/exsufflation has not been shown to increase PCF in patients with chronic obstructive pulmonary disease (Sivasothy et al 2001, Winck et al 2004).

Patients who are novices to the device may not tolerate high pressure changes initially and very high pressures cause leakage around the mask. Several authors (Chatwin et al 2003, Miske et al 2004, Sivasothy et al 2001, Vianello et al 2005) have reported a good outcome with low pressures. One study (Miske et al 2004) (age range 3 months to 28.6 years) used median pressures of +30 to −30 cmH$_2$O with a range from +15 to +40 cmH$_2$O (insufflation) and −20 to −50 cmH$_2$O (exsufflation). Other researchers however, advocate higher pressure spans of +40 to −40/−60 (Bach 1993, 1994; Bach et al 1993, 2000, 2003, Tzeng & Bach 2000). The CoughAssist™ (Emerson, Massachusetts) is often used in automatic mode (Bach 1993, 1994, Bach et al 1993, 2000, 2003, Tzeng & Bach 2000) enabling the device to be used in the domiciliary environment without a trained professional. In this mode the device swings between a set negative and positive pressure, and will hold in insufflation for a set period before switching to exsufflation for a set time and then providing a pause. The movement in manual mode should be one sweeping movement with no pauses between insufflation and exsufflation.

Patients learn to coordinate their cough when the device switches to exsufflation and initial instructions should indicate that a deep breath will be coming and they should cough when they feel the negative pressure. Mechanical insufflation/exsufflation can be combined with a manually assisted cough (Chapter 16). Initially the patient acclimatizes to the device in manual mode and usually with a full-face mask. The insufflation (positive) pressure should be set between 15 and 20 cmH$_2$O and increased to give an inspiration to total lung capacity. Initially the exsufflation (negative) pressure should be the same as the insufflation pressure, but when appropriate the negative pressure should be increased

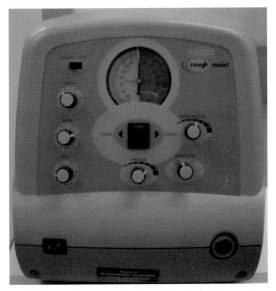

Figure 5.16 A mechanical insufflator/exsufflator device. (CoughAssist™, Emerson, Massachusetts)

to 10–20 cmH$_2$O above the positive pressure. The best indicator of efficacy is an increase in the audible sound of the cough.

Intrapulmonary percussive ventilation

Intrapulmonary percussive ventilation (IPV) has been used as a method of airway clearance, both within hospitals and in the home. The IPV device was developed in 1979 by Forrest M Bird (Percussionaire®, Idaho). It consists of a high-pressure flow generator, a valve for flow interruption and a breathing circuit with a nebulizer that can be attached to a face mask, mouthpiece or catheter mount (Fig. 5.17). IPV is a modified method of intermittent positive pressure breathing (IPPB) which superimposes high-frequency mini bursts of air (50 to 550 cycles per minute) on the individual's intrinsic breathing pattern to create an internal vibration (percussion) within the airways. It is hypothesized that internal or external vibration of the chest may promote clearance of mucus from the peripheral bronchial tree (Fink & Mahlmeister 2002). IPV may provide ventilatory support in patients with neuromuscular disease (Chatwin et al 2004) and in patients with chronic obstructive pulmonary disease (Nava et al 2006). IPV devices include: IMPULSATOR®-F00012, IPV1C®-F00001-C, IPV2C®-F00002-C, Percussionaire® (Idaho) and IMP II (Percussionaire, Breas, Sweden).

In tracheostomized patients with Duchenne muscular dystrophy (DMD), IPV has been compared with physiotherapy consisting of the forced expiration technique and manually assisted coughing (Toussaint et al 2003) using sputum weight as the primary outcome measure. The subjects were divided into a hypersecretive group and a normosecretive group. It was concluded that IPV enhanced peripheral bronchial secretion clearance in the hypersecretive DMD patients compared with conventional physiotherapy. Clini et al (2006) investigated the effects of IPV ICU patients in the intensive care unit with a tracheostomy, who were weaning from mechanical ventilation. The patient group ($n = 46$) received 15 days of two, 1-hour physiotherapy sessions per day with one group ($n = 24$) receiving IPV for 10 minutes before physiotherapy sessions. The subjects were assessed every 5 days, over a 15-day period, using the outcome measurements of arterial blood gases, PaO_2/FiO_2 ratio and maximal expiratory pressure. At 15 days the IPV group had a significantly improved PaO_2/FiO_2 ratio and a higher maximal expiratory pressure. At follow-up the IPV group also had a lower incidence of pneumonia, indicating that IPV may have a place in decreasing atelectasis in long-term weaning patients.

Vargas et al (2005) investigated patients with chronic obstructive pulmonary disease during an acute respiratory exacerbation and mild respiratory acidosis. In this study, one group received standard treatment (including oxygen, bronchodilators, steroids and antibiotics) and the other standard treatment with the addition of IPV (30 minutes twice a day). The patients who received IPV were discharged home significantly earlier 6.8 ± 1

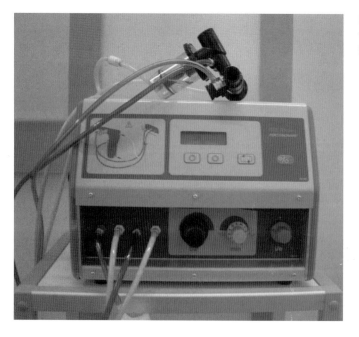

Figure 5.17   The intrapulmonary percussive ventilation device. (IMP II Percussionaire, Breas, Sweden)

days versus 7.9 ± 1.3 days (p <0.05). IPV also helped to prevent further deterioration, that of pH <7.35 requiring non-invasive ventilation (IPV and standard treatment 0/16 patients, standard treatment alone 6/17 patients ($p < 0.05$)). The authors hypothesized that the IPV group may have benefited from improved secretion removal; however, they do state that this cannot be confirmed as sputum weight was not measured. Previous studies investigated sputum mobilization, in people with cystic fibrosis, by comparing the use of IPV to other airway clearance techniques e.g. postural drainage and percussion, high-frequency chest wall oscillation and the Flutter (Newhouse et al 1998, Scherer et al 1998, Varekojis et al 2003). These studies demonstrated IPV to be equal in efficacy to the other methods of airway clearance in sputum mobilization, when the amount of sputum expectorated was assessed by dry weight. IPV can also be used in conjunction with other airway clearance techniques, for example autogenic drainage and the active cycle of breathing techniques, to assist in clearance of secretions.

IPV has a place in the clearance of secretions in both restrictive and obstructive patients. Following preliminary safety studies investigating the physiogical affects of IPV (Chatwin et al 2004, Nava et al 2006) and sputum clearance (Toussaint et al 2003), guidelines for starting settings have been suggested.

1. Patients who need increased ventilatory support: start with a higher working pressure of 1.2–1.4 millibar and low frequency (100–200 cycles/min) and increase the pressure rapidly until vibrations can be felt when palpating the chest wall. Starting with a low frequency should ensure adequate ventilatory support.
2. Patients with the ability to breathe spontaneously: start with a lower pressure of 1.0 millibar and higher frequency (200–350 cycles/min) and increase the pressure rapidly until vibrations can be felt when palpating the chest wall.

When the patient has acclimatized to IPV, the pressure and frequency should be adjusted to optimize secretion clearance. Inverting the I : E ratio, to 2 : 1, will assist ventilatory support (Toussaint et al 2003). When treating patients with neuromuscular weakness, manually assisted coughs may be required to clear secretions from the large airways (Chapter 16).

Oscillating positive expiratory pressure

These devices combine an oscillation of the air within the airways during expiration and a variable positive expiratory pressure. Three commonly used ones are described below.

The *Flutter®* (Flutter) is a small, portable device (Fig. 5.18). It is pipe-shaped with a single opening at the mouthpiece and a series of small outlet holes at the top of the bowl. The bowl contains a high-density stainless steel ball enclosed in a small cone. During expiration the movement of the ball along the surface of the cone creates a positive expiratory pressure (PEP) and an oscillatory vibration of the air within the airways. In addition, intermittent airflow accelerations are produced by the same movements of the ball. The device is held horizontally and tilted slightly either downwards or upwards until a maximal oscillatory effect can be felt. It is usually used either sitting or in supine lying, but may be used in other positions provided an effective oscillation can be maintained. Sputum viscoelasticity has been shown to be reduced following the use of the Flutter (App et al 1998).

The Flutter is placed in the mouth and inspiration is either through the nose or through the mouth by breathing around the Flutter mouthpiece (it is not possible to breathe in through the Flutter device). A slow breath in, only slightly deeper than normal, with a breath hold of 3–5 seconds is followed by a breath out, through the Flutter, at a slightly faster rate than normal. This is known as the 'mucus loosening and mobilization' stage. After four to eight of these breaths, a deep breath with a 'hold' at full inspiration is followed by a forced expiration through the Flutter. This may be repeated a second time and is the 'mucus elimination' stage. It may precipitate expectoration and should be followed by a

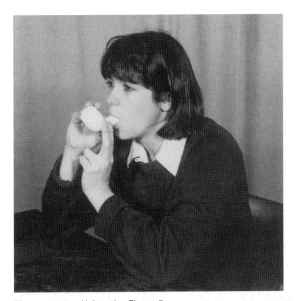

Figure 5.18   Using the Flutter®.

5

5

pause for breathing control following a huff or cough. In some parts of Europe this forced expiratory manoeuvre, down to a low lung volume, is not used as a part of the regimen.

Konstan et al (1994) compared three regimens: the Flutter, voluntary coughing and a regimen of postural drainage and percussion, which included up to ten positions in the treatment session. Each session lasted 15 minutes. The Flutter regimen was the most effective as measured by the weight of sputum expectorated. Ambrosino et al (1995) and Homnick et al (1998) compared the Flutter with 'standard' chest physiotherapy and showed the Flutter to be as effective.

Originally the recommended technique for the Flutter was a gentle exhalation through the device. Treatment was continued for a period of 10 minutes and secretions were expectorated by spontaneous coughing. It was this regimen that was shown by Pryor et al (1994) to be less effective than the ACBT. The inclusion of a forced expiratory manoeuvre or huffing, in the regimen, would be likely to increase the effectiveness of airway clearance and this was demonstrated, in the short term, by Pike et al (1999).

When autogenic drainage was compared with the Flutter it was concluded that both regimens were equally effective, but the Flutter was easier to teach (Lindemann 1992). A clinical trial was undertaken using the Flutter in patients following thoracotomy, but no advantage was found in its inclusion (Chatham et al 1993). Two studies including the Flutter were published in 2001, both in people with cystic fibrosis. Oermann et al (2001) compared high-frequency chest wall oscillation and the Flutter, and McIlwaine et al (2001) compared the Flutter with PEP. In the 4-week study by Oermann et al, there were no significant differences between the regimens, but the authors stated that patient preference varied and patient satisfaction and preference should be considered. In the longer-term (1 year) study by McIlwaine et al there were significant rates of decline in lung function (forced vital capacity) in the Flutter group during this period. The authors hypothesized that the differences between the two regimens may be a consequence of the continuation of expiration into the expiratory reserve volume with the Flutter. This was likely to enter closing volume, with consequent airway closure. With the positive expiratory pressure regimen, end expiration remains above resting lung volume. Pryor et al (2006) did not observe deterioration in lung function with the Flutter but this study was in adults, whereas the McIlwaine study used a much younger population.

The *Shaker®* (NCS, Sao Paulo, Brazil) (Fig. 5.19) is similar to the Flutter. It also contains a high-density stainless steel ball enclosed in a small cone, but has a detachable mouthpiece making it easier to use in positions other than sitting.

The *R-C Cornet®* (Cornet) (Fig. 5.20) consists of a curved hard plastic outer tube, mouthpiece and flexible latex-free inner tube (valve-hose). The Cornet is placed in the mouth and inspiration is either through the nose or through the mouth, by breathing around the Cornet mouthpiece (it is not possible to breathe in through the Cornet). During expiration through the Cornet, a positive expiratory pressure and an oscillatory vibration of the air within the airways are generated. The flow, pressure and frequency of the oscillations can be adjusted to suit the individual and it can be used in any position (e.g. sitting, side lying, head-down tilt) as it is independent of gravitational forces. It is used in a similar way

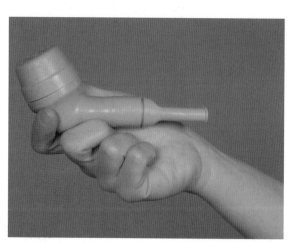

Figure 5.19 The Shaker®. (NCS, Sao Paulo, Brazil)

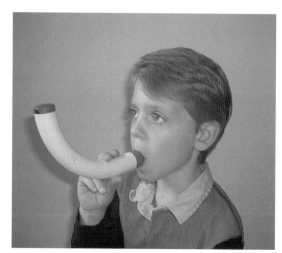

Figure 5.20 Using the R-C Cornet®.

to the Flutter with initial breaths (five to eight) being only slightly deeper than normal and these breaths may be interspersed with one or two deeper and more forceful ones. A breath hold of 2–3 seconds at the end of inspiration is usually included. Huffing or coughing is used to clear secretions mobilized to the upper airways and is followed by breathing control. It is recommended that the Cornet be used for 10–15 minutes (Cegla 1999, personal communication). The Cornet has been shown to be as effective as the Flutter in airway clearance (Cegla et al 1997), to be beneficial in the management of people with chronic obstructive pulmonary disease (Cegla et al 2002) and to be equivalent, in the long term, to the ACBT, AD, Flutter and PEP in people with cystic fibrosis (Pryor et al 2006). It has also been shown to decrease the cohesiveness and viscoelasticity of sputum from patients with bronchiectasis (Feng et al 1998, Nakamura et al 1998).

The *Acapella®* (Acapella) (Fig. 5.21) is another form of oscillating PEP which uses a counterweighted plug and magnet to create airflow oscillations. Again, following six to eight breaths (with inspiration through the nose or around the mouthpiece of the device and expiration through the device) one or two deeper breaths, with a more active expiration, are followed by huffing and coughing. A short end-inspiratory hold is usually included. As with the Cornet, it is gravity-independent. Patterson et al (2005) compared the Acapella with the ACBT and concluded that both were effective in airway clearance. Volsko et al (2003) undertook a physical comparison between the Acapella and the Flutter and con-

cluded that the devices have similar performance (pressure flow) characteristics.

Positive expiratory pressure

The delivery of positive expiratory pressure (PEP) via a face mask was described by Falk et al (1984) who found an increase in sputum yield and an improvement in transcutaneous oxygen tension when compared with postural drainage, percussion and breathing exercises. It was suggested that the increase in sputum yield was produced by the effect of PEP on peripheral airways and collateral channels. Falk & Andersen (1991) suggest that with the PEP treatment, the increase in lung volume may allow air to get behind secretions blocking small airways and assist in mobilizing them.

The original PEP apparatus, on which most of the clinical trials have been undertaken, consists of a face-mask and a one-way valve to which expiratory resistances can be attached. A small-sized mask is available for infants. A flanged mouthpiece and nose clip can be used in place of the mask if the patient will not tolerate a mask but the required pressure, in mid-expiration, must be achieved for this equipment to be equivalent to that of a mask. A manometer is inserted into the system between the valve and resistance to monitor the pressure, which should be between 10 and 20 cmH$_2$O during mid-expiration (Falk & Andersen 1991).

The patient sits leaning forward with the elbows supported on a table and holding the mask firmly over the nose and mouth (Fig. 5.22) while breathing at tidal

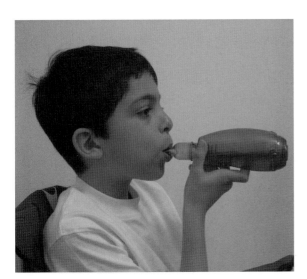

Figure 5.21 Using the Acapella®.

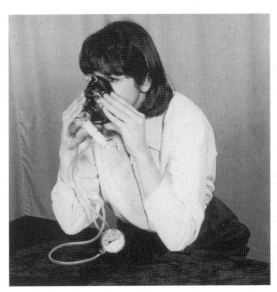

Figure 5.22 Using the PEP mask.

5

volume, with a slightly active expiration, for 6–10 breaths. The lung volume should be kept up by avoiding complete expiration. This is followed by the forced expiration technique to clear secretions that have been mobilized. The duration and frequency of treatment are adapted to each individual, but treatment is usually performed for approximately 15 minutes, twice a day, in patients with stable chest disease and excess bronchial secretions (Falk & Andersen 1991). This should be adjusted according to the patient's signs and symptoms. In postoperative patients, short periods of PEP used every hour as a prophylactic treatment have been described by Ricksten et al (1986).

The study by Falk et al (1984) in patients with cystic fibrosis compared an assisted 'conventional' postural drainage treatment with an unassisted PEP mask regimen and found that the PEP mask regimen was more effective and the one preferred by the patients. Hofmeyr et al (1986) compared the unassisted treatment of PEP combined with the forced expiration technique, with thoracic expansion exercises combined with the forced expiration technique (the active cycle of breathing techniques). In this study the ACBT was found to be advantageous in terms of the amount of sputum expectorated. van der Schans et al (1991) studied mucus clearance with PEP using a radio-aerosol technique in patients with cystic fibrosis. They showed that PEP temporarily increased lung volume, but did not lead to an improvement in mucus transport. Mortensen et al (1991) demonstrated improved central and peripheral radio-aerosol clearance with both PEP and the ACBT compared with controls. More recently Darbee et al (2004) studied the ventilation distribution and gas mixing with positive expiratory pressure breathing in adults with cystic fibrosis and demonstrated improved gas mixing associated with improvements in lung function, sputum expectoration and oxygen saturation.

Falk and Andersen (1991) have demonstrated collateral flow in experiments in postmortem human lungs (Fig. 5.23). In this experiment, a 3 mm airway was completely blocked and the pressures across the obstruction monitored during normal breathing and during breathing with 10 cmH$_2$O PEP. In normal lungs and lungs affected by disease, acute respiratory failure and chronic airflow limitation, the obstruction pressure swings around zero during normal breathing. When PEP is applied at the airway opening, the pressure behind the obstruction becomes negative initially. This would tend to move the obstruction towards the periphery, but this is followed rapidly by a positive pressure tending to move the obstruction centrally. The duration of the positive obstruction period was far greater than the negative period and this culminated in movement towards the more central airways.

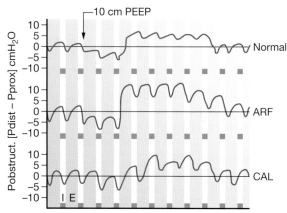

Figure 5.23   Pressure across a peripheral experimental airway obstruction (3 mm in diameter) during application of 10 cmH$_2$O PEP in different human pathology. Studies were performed in excised postmortem human lungs (Pobstruct: Obstruction pressure, positive if distal pressure exceeds proximal pressure; Pdistal: Pressure distal to obstruction; Pprox: Pressure proximal to obstruction; Normal: Normal lungs; ARF: Lungs affected by severe acute respiratory failure; CAL: Lungs affected by severe chronic airflow limitation; I: Inspiratory time; E: Expiratory time; PEP: positive expiratory pressure). (Falk and Andersen 1991. In: Pryor JA (ed) Respiratory care, p 55. Reproduced with permission of Elsevier, Edinburgh)

Lung function has been shown to improve with PEP in a long-term study (1 year) when compared with postural drainage and percussion (McIlwaine et al 1997). McIlwaine et al (2001) also compared the use of PEP and the Flutter in the long term (1 year). They concluded that PEP was more effective than Flutter in maintaining lung function, but Pryor et al (2006) did not identify any significant deterioration in lung function with the Flutter, compared with other airway clearance techniques, and this was also over a period of 1 year. Elkins et al (2006a) in a Cochrane review concluded that there was no clear evidence that PEP was a more or less effective intervention than other forms of physiotherapy.

Inspiratory resistance–positive expiratory pressure (IR-PEP) is obtained by placing a resistor into the inspiratory port of the PEP mask which provides resistance to both inspiration and expiration. The patient breathes in and out against a resistance and this has the effect of slowing down the flow rate and making the inspiratory breath more even. IR-PEP has been studied in patients undergoing abdominal surgery (Olsen et al 1999) and coronary artery bypass graft surgery (Westerdahl et al

5

2001) and its effects are said to be similar to PEP and bubble PEP.

Bubble PEP is an alternative way to administer PEP to young children, using a system that incorporates a column of water (to the level of PEP required: 10–12 cmH$_2$O) and asking the child to blow through the column of water via a flexible straw or tubing (Fig. 5.24). By adding a little liquid detergent to the water, exhalations produce a stream of bubbles and the addition of a drop or two of food colouring to the water adds to the novelty of the treatment.

The equipment for bubble PEP is outlined in Fig. 5.25. When using bubble PEP, it is imperative that all the equipment is kept thoroughly clean. The water should be discarded immediately following treatment and the equipment cleaned. Fresh water should be used for each treatment session and the carton and tubing should be changed regularly. It is also important that the child is instructed only to exhale through the tubing and never to inhale (suck).

High-pressure PEP is a modified form of PEP mask treatment described by Oberwaldner et al (1986) for the treatment of patients with cystic fibrosis. The mask is used during tidal volume breaths and also for a full forced expiratory manoeuvre. By applying a positive expiratory pressure during forced expiration, secretions may be mobilized more easily in patients with unstable airways. Assessment for the technique involves forced

vital capacity manoeuvres with the mask attached to a spirometer (Oberwaldner et al 1986). The resultant expiratory flow volume curves are used to determine the appropriate resistor for the PEP mask. The appropriate resistance is one that obtains a good flow plateau, achieves an expiration in excess of the patient's normal forced vital capacity and eliminates any curvilinearity or scooping (indicating airway obstruction) (Fig. 5.26). The technique should be used only if full lung function equipment is available for regular reassessment of the appropriate expiratory resistance for each individual. Meticulous care must be taken, as an incorrect resistance may lead to deterioration in lung function and ineffective airway clearance.

For treatment, the patient sits upright holding the mask firmly against the face. Six to ten rhythmical breaths, at tidal volume, are followed by an inspiration to total lung capacity and then a forced expiratory manoeuvre against the resistance to low lung volume. The pressure generated during this manoeuvre ranges from 50 to 120 cmH$_2$O and usually results in the expectoration of sputum (Oberwaldner et al 1991).

Pfleger et al (1992) compared high-pressure PEP and autogenic drainage. More sputum was cleared with high-

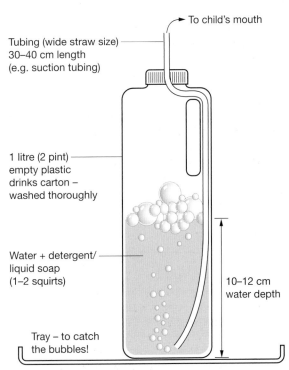

Figure 5.25 Equipment required for bubble PEP. (Reproduced with permission from Great Ormond Street Hospital for Children, London, UK)

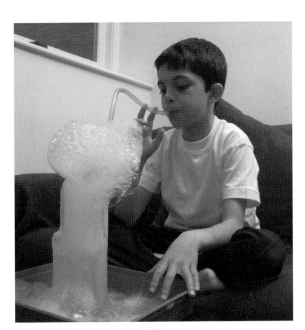

Figure 5.24   Using bubble PEP.

5

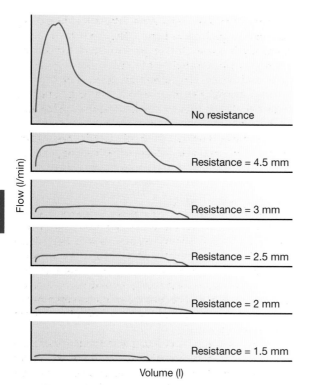

Figure 5.26 High-pressure PEP. Maximum expiratory flow–volume curves obtained without resistance (top) and with each of the PEP mask expiratory resistors. In this example, the resistor of choice for treatment is the 2 mm aperture as it demonstrates a maximal forced vital capacity, good plateau formation and no curvilinearity at the end of flow.

pressure PEP than with AD or with a combination of PEP and AD. Using this technique there is no evidence of any increase in incidence in pneumothorax (Zach & Oberwaldner 1992).

Physical activity

Physical activity will augment airway clearance (Sahl et al 1989), but may often not be as effective as other airway clearance techniques, particularly in people who produce moderate to large amounts of sputum. In people with cystic fibrosis, the combination of an airway clearance technique and exercise programme led to a reduction in the decline in lung function when compared with airway clearance and usual physicial activities (Schneiderman-Walker et al 2000). In addition to airway clearance there are many other benefits of physical activity (Chapters 13, 14 and 18).

Resistive inspiratory manoeuvres

The technique of resistive inspiratory manoeuvres is that of repeated maximal inspiratory vital capacity manoeuvres against a fixed resistance. Chatham et al (2004) reported an increase in sputum expectorated, using resistive inspiratory manoeuvres, when compared with the ACBT in a group of people with cystic fibrosis. In contrast, Patterson et al (2004) found that more sputum was expectorated with the ACBT than with resistive inspiratory manoeuvres in people with bronchiectasis.

With this technique the subject is required to carry out a full inspiratory vital capacity manoeuvre at 80% of maximal pressure by breathing against a fixed resistance. The maximum pressure is that developed between residual volume and total lung capacity. More research is required in this field, but it is hypothesized that the resistance results in an increased inspiratory time and that resistive inspiratory manoeuvres may increase inspiratory airflow to more peripheral airways with consequent shearing forces acting on airway secretions during the inspiratory phase. This may in turn reduce the need for higher expiratory flows (Chatham et al 2004).

AIRWAY SUCTION

Airway suction for intubated adults is described in Chapter 8 and for children, including the non-intubated infant and small child, see Chapter 10. Suction is required occasionally in the *non-intubated* adult who has retained secretions, usually via the nasopharynx.

Nasotracheal suction is a means of stimulating a cough, but is an unpleasant procedure for the patient and should be performed only when absolutely necessary. The indication for suction is the inability to cough effectively and expectorate, when airway secretions are retained. It may be necessary, for example, when an acute exacerbation of chronic bronchitis has led to carbon dioxide narcosis and respiratory failure, in neurological disorders, postoperative complications or laryngeal dysfunction. Before airway suction is undertaken it is very important that the procedure is explained carefully to the patient.

It is important to be aware of the possibility of causing laryngeal spasm (Sykes et al 1976) or vagal nerve stimulation, which may lead to cardiac arrhythmias (Jacob 1990). Nasopharyngeal suction is contraindicated when there is stridor or severe bronchospasm, and in patients with head injuries when there is a leak of cerebrospinal fluid into the nasal passages. Retention of secretions may be a problem in patients with respiratory muscle paralysis, but there is usually no benefit in using airway suction in an attempt to stimulate an effective cough. It is the lack of volume of air that prevents clearance of secretions in these patients and techniques such as mechanical insufflation/exsufflation, assisted cough, intermittent positive pressure breathing, glossopharyngeal breathing and gravity-assisted positioning should be considered.

Airway suction causes damage to the tracheal epithelium and this can be minimized by the appropriate choice of catheter and careful technique (Brazier 1999). A flexible catheter of suitable size, usually 12 FG in adults, should be lubricated with a water-soluble jelly and gently passed through the nasal passage so that it curves down into the pharynx. Occasionally a cough may be stimulated when the catheter reaches the pharynx and suction can then be applied, the secretions aspirated and the catheter withdrawn. More often it is necessary to pass the catheter between the vocal cords and into the trachea to stimulate coughing. The catheter is less likely to enter the oesophagus if the neck is extended, and if the patient is able to cooperate it is often helpful if they can put their tongue out. The catheter should be inserted during the inspiratory phase and if it passes into the trachea, will stimulate vigorous coughing. When suction is applied the vacuum pressure should be kept as low as possible, usually in the range 60–150 mmHg (8.0–20 kPa), although this will vary depending on the viscosity of the mucus. A built-in fingertip control or Y-connector is recommended to allow a more gradual build-up of suction pressure than is possible by the release of a kinked catheter tube.

Oxygen should always be available during the suction procedure and the patient observed for signs of hypoxia. If it has been difficult to insert the catheter and the patient looks cyanosed, instead of withdrawing the catheter from the trachea, suction should be stopped and oxygen administered until the patient's colour has improved. Suction can then be restarted.

Suction can be performed in adults who are being nursed in the sitting position, but comatosed patients should be suctioned in side lying to avoid the possibility of aspiration if vomiting occurs.

The nasopharyngeal suctioning clinical practice guidelines of the American Association for Respiratory Care (2004) provide useful evidence-based points on the technique.

Oropharyngeal suction through an airway is an alternative method, if suction is necessary. An oropharyngeal airway is a plastic tube shaped to fit the curved palate. It is inserted with its tip directed towards the roof of the mouth and is then rotated so that the tip lies over the back of the tongue.

Portable suction units are available for domiciliary use and for patients in transit. They may be powered manually, by mains electricity or by battery, for example from a car cigarette lighter adapter.

Provided suction is carried out carefully and oxygen is always available, it is a valuable technique and may avoid the need for more invasive procedures such as bronchoscopy, endotracheal intubation or minitracheotomy. However, it should not be undertaken until every attempt to achieve effective coughing has failed.

BREATHING CONTROL

Breathing techniques can be divided into normal breathing, known as 'breathing control', where the pattern of breathing is maximally efficient for the individual with minimal effort expended, and breathing exercises, where either inspiration is emphasized (as in thoracic expansion exercises and inspiratory muscle training) or expiration is emphasized (as in the huff of the forced expiration technique).

Breathing control is normal tidal breathing using the lower chest and encouraging relaxation of the upper chest and shoulders. This used to be known as 'diaphragmatic breathing', but the term is a misnomer as during normal tidal breathing there is activity not only in the diaphragm but also in the internal and external intercostal muscles, the abdominal and scalene muscles (Green & Moxham 1985). This pattern of breathing is not appropriate for everyone. Dyspnoea has been shown to increase in some people with chronic obstructive pulmonary disease using 'diaphragmatic breathing' owing to an increase in asynchronous and paradoxical breathing movements (Gosselink 2004, Gosselink et al 1995 and Chapter 13).

To be taught breathing control, the patient should be in a comfortable well-supported position either sitting (Fig. 5.27) or in high side lying (Fig. 5.28). The patient is encouraged to relax the upper chest, shoulders and arms. One hand, which may be either the patient's or the physiotherapist's or one hand of each, can be positioned lightly on the upper abdomen. As the patient breathes in, the hand should be felt to rise up and out; as the patient breathes out, the hand sinks down and in. Inspiration using the lower chest in this way is the active phase. Expiration should be relaxed and passive, and both inspiration and expiration should be barely audible. Inspiration through the nose allows the air to be warmed, humidified and filtered before it reaches the upper airways. If the nose is blocked, breathing through the mouth will reduce the resistance to the flow of air and reduce the work of breathing. If the patient is very

5

5

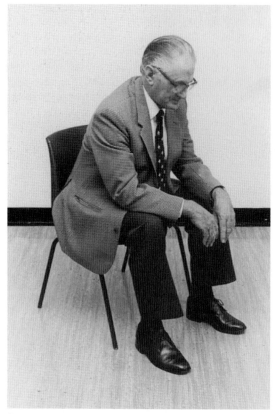

A

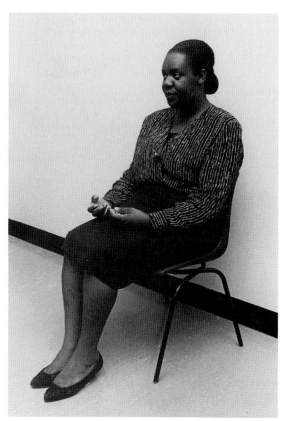

B

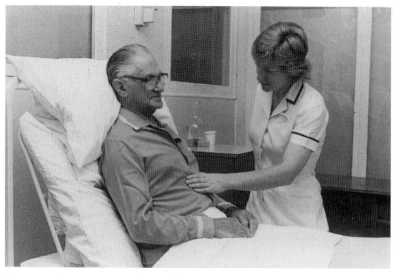

C

Figure 5.27   (A, B, C) Breathing control in sitting.

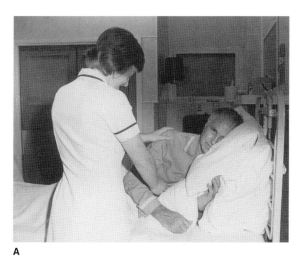
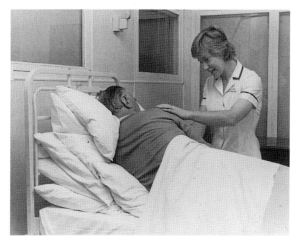

A   B

Figure 5.28   (A, B) Breathing control in high side lying.

breathless, breathing through the mouth will reduce the anatomical dead space.

Many breathless patients, for example those with emphysema, asthma, pulmonary fibrosis or lung cancer, may benefit from using breathing control in positions that encourage relaxation of the upper chest and shoulders and allow movement of the lower chest and abdomen. These positions also optimize, by lengthening, the length tension status of the diaphragm (American Thoracic Society 1999, Dean 1985, O'Neill & McCarthy 1983, Sharp et al 1980). When the patient is sitting or standing leaning forward, the abdominal contents raise the anterior part of the diaphragm, probably facilitating its contraction during inspiration. A similar effect can be seen in the side lying and high side lying positions where the curvature of the dependent part of the diaphragm is increased. This effect, combined with relaxation of the head, neck and shoulders, promotes the pattern of breathing control.

Useful positions are:

- high side lying (see Fig. 5.28) – for maximal relaxation of the head, neck and upper chest, the neck should be slightly flexed and the top pillow should be above the shoulder, supporting only the head and neck.

- relaxed sitting (see Fig. 5.27)

- forward lean standing (Fig. 5.29)

- relaxed standing (Fig. 5.30)

- kneeling position (Fig. 5.31) – this may be preferred by children.

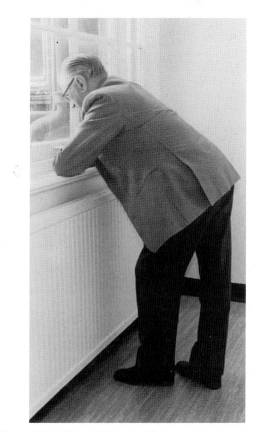

Figure 5.29   Forward lean standing.

5

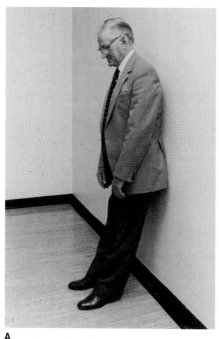
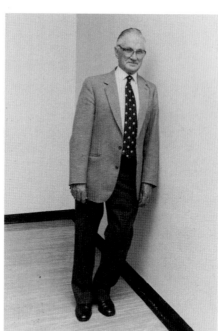

A   B

Figure 5.30 (A, B) Relaxed standing.

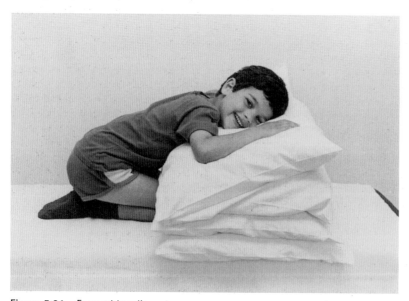

Figure 5.31 Forward kneeling.

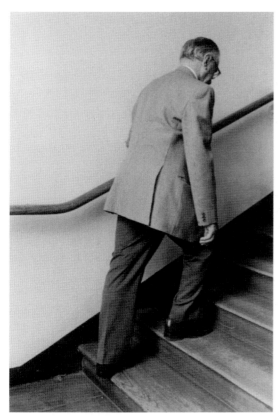

Figure 5.32   Breathing control while stair climbing.

These positions discourage the tendency of breathless patients to push down or grip with their hands, which causes elevation of the shoulders and overuse of the accessory muscles of breathing, and may result in a more effective length tension status of the diaphragm.

Breathing control may also be used to improve exercise capacity in breathless patients when walking up slopes, hills and stairs (Fig. 5.32). Breathless patients tend to hold their breath on exertion and rush, for example, up a flight of stairs arriving at the top extremely breathless and unable to speak. The simple technique of relaxing the arms and shoulders, reducing the walking speed a little and using the pattern of breathing *in* on climbing up one step and breathing *out* on climbing up the next step may lead to a marked reduction in breathlessness (Webber 1991). When this technique has been mastered some patients, on days when they are less breathless, may find breathing *in* for *one* step and out for

two steps more comfortable. The severely breathless patient may also find the combination of breathing control with walking helpful when walking on level ground. A respiratory walking frame (see Fig. 13.4) with or without portable oxygen can be used to assist ambulation in the severely breathless patient.

Breathing control can also be used to control a bout or paroxysm of coughing.

Some people with chronic respiratory disease automatically use *pursed-lip breathing*. Breathing through pursed lips has the effect of generating a small positive pressure during expiration, which may to some extent reduce the collapse of unstable airways.

CONTINENCE

Management of stress incontinence

Many people with chronic respiratory disease who require airway clearance techniques have stress incontinence of urine, and sometimes faeces. Urinary incontinence, the involuntary loss of urine, is associated with adverse effects on quality of life (National Institute for Health and Clinical Excellence 2006). The prevalence of urinary incontinence in the population as a whole increases with increasing age up to 46% in women and 34% in men aged over 80 years (Scottish Intercollegiate Guidelines Network 2004). The prevalence associated with chronic lung disease is known to be higher and at an earlier age, for example in people with cystic fibrosis incontinence in women ranges from 38–68% (Cornacchia et al 2001, Orr et al 2001, White et al 2000); in men 16% (Gumery et al 2005); and in children 14–33% (Moraes et al 2002, Prasad et al 2006).

Urinary incontinence frequently reduces adherence to an airway clearance technique and often causes embarrassment. During assessment (Chapter 1) the physiotherapist should include questions to identify this problem, even in young girls with chronic respiratory disorders. Voluntary contraction of the pelvic floor muscles just before and throughout a cough or huff, known as 'The Knack', can be used to reduce stress-related leakage of urine (Miller et al 1998). If this technique does not lead to a clinically significant reduction in leakage, referral to a physiotherapist specializing in continence therapy should be considered.

GLOSSOPHARYNGEAL BREATHING

Glossopharyngeal breathing (GPB) is a technique useful in patients with a reduced vital capacity resulting from respiratory muscle weakness or paralysis. Although its original use was in rehabilitation of patients with polio-

5

myelitis, it can be invaluable when taught to people with tetraplegia (Alvarez et al 1981, Bach & Alba 1990, Bianchi et al 2004, Warren 2002) and in some people with neuromuscular diseases (Bach 1995, Baydur et al 1990).

GPB was first described by Dail (1951) when patients with poliomyelitis were observed to be gulping air into their lungs. It was this gulping action that gave the technique the name 'frog breathing'. GPB is a form of positive pressure ventilation produced by the patient's voluntary muscles where boluses of air are forced into the lungs. It is essential to understand that GPB is *not* swallowing air into the stomach, but gulping air into the lungs.

Paralysed patients dependent on a mechanical ventilator are sometimes able to use GPB continuously, other than during sleep, to substitute the mechanical ventilation. GPB is very useful in patients who are able to breathe spontaneously but whose power to cough and clear secretions is inadequate. The technique also enables these patients to shout to attract attention and to help to maintain or improve lung and chest wall compliance (Bach et al 1987, Dail et al 1955). For patients dependent on a ventilator, either non-invasively or via a tracheostomy, GPB can be life saving (Bach 1995) in an emergency if the ventilator becomes disconnected or if there should be a power failure, and can increase the feeling of independence (Make et al 1998). The uses of GPB are summarized in Box 5.1.

To breathe in, a series of pumping strokes is produced by action of the lips, tongue, soft palate, pharynx and larynx. Air is held in the chest by the larynx, which acts as a valve as the mouth is opened for the next gulp. Expiration occurs by normal elastic recoil of the lungs and rib cage.

Before starting to teach GPB it may be helpful for the patient to experience the feeling of inflating the chest by using an intermittent positive pressure ventilator with a mouthpiece. After inflating the lungs, the mouthpiece is removed and the patient should try and hold all the air in the lungs with the mouth open, avoiding escape of air through the larynx or nose. A teaching video is available that may help both patient and physiotherapist when learning or teaching GPB (Webber & Higgens 1999).

Box 5.2 Three stages of glossopharyngeal breathing

1. Enlarge throat cavity
2. Hold throat open – close lips
3. Let floor of mouth rise to normal position while air is pumped through larynx

---

Each gulp of air is made up of three stages (Box 5.2). The first and most important stage (Box 5.3 & Fig. 5.33A) in learning GPB is the enlargement of the mouth and throat cavity by depressing the tracheal and laryngeal cartilages. The tongue should remain flat with the tip touching the inside of the lower teeth. Using a torch, the physiotherapist should be able to see the uvula when this is correct. The patient may find it helpful to watch the movement in a mirror and possibly by feeling the cartilages with their fingers. An exercise that often helps to initiate movement of the cartilages is for the physiotherapist to place a finger horizontally under the chin back against the trachea and give pressure in an upwards direction resisting downward movement of the base of the tongue. To emphasize the downward cartilage movement, practice should progress to holding the throat in this open position for 3–5 seconds.

When this movement has been achieved, stages 2 and 3 are added to complete the cycle (Box 5.4 & Fig. 5.33B, Box 5.5 & Fig. 5.33C). The cycle should be practised slowly at first and then gradually speeded up until the movement flows. It is important to avoid stages 2 and 3 being done simultaneously. The air has to be trapped in the throat in stage 2 before the jaw and cartilages are allowed to rise in stage 3. It is *essential* to maintain the lowered jaw during stage 2.

The next stage is to take a maximum breath in and, while holding this breath, to add several glossopharyngeal gulps, to augment the vital capacity. A 'normal' breath must not be taken before each gulp.

When correct, the patient will feel the chest filling with air and the physiotherapist can test the 'GPB vital capacity' by putting a mouthpiece attached to the expiratory limb of a Wright's respirometer in the patient's mouth before exhalation.

Box 5.1 Uses of glossopharyngeal breathing

Where the lungs are normal, but the respiratory muscles are weak or paralysed:

- to produce a more effective cough
  - to avoid chest infections
  - treat chest infections
  - to assist in weaning from a tracheostomy
- to make the voice louder
- to maintain or improve lung and chest wall compliance
- to be a substitute for mechanical ventilation
- to provide security if ventilator dependent

Box 5.3   Stage 1 (Fig. 5.33A)

(a) Enlargement of throat cavity
  ■ Depress cartilages
  ■ Tongue flat
  ■ Uvula visible
(b) Hold this open position for 3–5 seconds
(c) Progress to starting with closed mouth – open mouth, jaw and throat at the same time – hold open
(d) Take deep breath – hold it – open mouth, jaw and throat

Box 5.4   Stage 2 (Fig. 5.33B)

(a) With throat open – close lips to trap air in throat
(b) Check that tongue position and open throat are maintained while opening and closing lips. Do not let jaw rise

Box 5.5   Stage 3 (Fig. 5.33C)

After opening throat (stage 1) and trapping air with lips (stage 2):
  Let floor of mouth, tongue and cartilages rise to the normal position while air is pumped through the larynx

The respirometer can be used to measure the volume per gulp; the patient will require less effort and reach maximum capacity more quickly if a large volume gulp is achieved. The volume per gulp is directly related to the amount of downward movement of the cartilages. A study by Kelleher & Parida (1957) reported a group of patients in whom the average volume per gulp varied from 25 to 120 ml and when teaching GPB an attempt should be made to achieve at least 80 ml per gulp.

If GPB were being used continuously as a substitute for normal tidal breathing, approximately 6–8 gulps would be taken before breathing out. When used for clearance of secretions, 10–25 gulps may be required to obtain a maximal vital capacity. Volumes of 2.5–3.0 litres can be achieved and the expiratory flow produced is sufficient to mobilize secretions (Make et al 1998).

GPB would normally be taught with the patient in a comfortable sitting position, but for patients with postural hypotension following spinal cord injury, a reclined position would be more appropriate at first. When mastered, GPB should be practised in positions

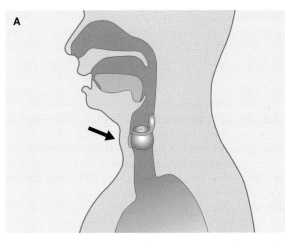

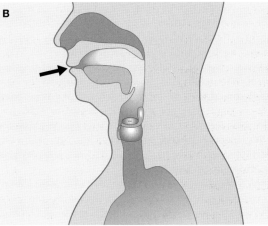

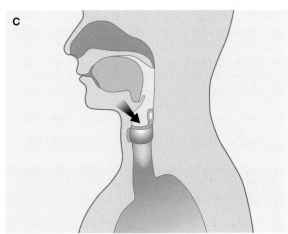

Figure 5.33   (A, B, C) The stages of glossopharyngeal breathing.

5

useful for the patient to clear bronchial secretions. After filling the chest to capacity the patient signals to the physiotherapist who compresses the chest as the air is let out. The patient may have sufficient muscle power to apply compression, or carers can be taught to give assistance.

GPB is learnt easily by some patients, but others need time and patience to acquire this skill. Although frequent self-practice can be helpful in the learning stages it is recommended to ensure correct opening of the throat (stage 1) before letting the patient proceed to stages 2 and 3. It can be tiring to learn GPB and therefore short frequent sessions are most effective. Once learnt, it is *not* tiring to use the technique.

There are reasons why a person may fail to achieve GPB initially. The soft palate may not be closing, so air passes out through the nose instead of into the trachea. This can often be corrected by asking the patient to take several gulps while the nose is alternately pinched closed for two gulps and released for two gulps. When the nose is held closed, the patient will feel pressure inside the mouth and throat and possibly in the ears. GPB should then be repeated without the nose being pinched and the patient should attempt to reproduce the same feeling of pressure with every gulp. Occasionally patients have very poor soft palate control and will need to wear a nose clip. Exercises to improve soft palate control may be helpful.

A few patients who find it difficult to stop air leaking through the nose achieve GPB by taking the gulps through the nose, while keeping the mouth shut. Other people prefer to do nasal GPB as it is less obtrusive and the gulps of air are humidified. It is important initially to teach the stages using the mouth technique in order to observe the tongue position. The stages for nasal GPB are shown in Box 5.6.

Another problem that may be found during the learning stages of GPB is weakness of the vocal cords. If the cords are unable to hold the air in the lungs, the vital capacity is decreased after attempting some gulps.

Box 5.6   Stages with nasal glossopharyngeal breathing

1. Take a deep breath through the nose, flaring the nostrils and hold the air in the lungs
2. Depress cartilages and tongue and try to flare nostrils at the same time
3. Let cartilages rise to normal position as air is forced through the larynx
4. Repeat 2 and 3 until lungs are full

This can be tested by asking the patient to take a very deep breath using intermittent positive pressure by mouthpiece and then, with the mouthpiece removed, he should say 'Ah, ah, ah . . .' in short staccato bursts during expiration. If all the 'Ahs' run into a continuous sound, the cords are failing to shut off the flow of air under pressure. To strengthen the cords, the patient can start to take a volume of air just greater than his vital capacity and practise the 'Ah, ah' sounds. When this is achieved, the volume of air can be gradually increased and the expiration exercises repeated.

GPB is a valuable technique to consider when treating tetraplegics with a vital capacity of less than 2 litres. Instruction can begin when the patient has reached a stable condition, but it is inappropriate in the acute phase or during an acute chest infection. When successfully learnt, it is invaluable during a period of chest infection to assist in the clearance of secretions. In patients with Duchenne muscular dystrophy and other neuromuscular diseases it would often be easiest to teach GPB as a 'normal' part of treatment, before deterioration in respiratory muscle function and difficulty in clearing secretions occurs. GPB has been of benefit to patients with motor neurone disease (Bereiter 2001) by making the voice more audible and providing an effective cough; and in multiple sclerosis (Aldridge 2005), allowing effective clearance of secretions.

It is possible to teach GPB to patients with an uncuffed tracheostomy tube, if there is a dressing providing an effective seal around the tube to avoid air leaks and some form of plug to the tube. A one-way valve, for example a Passy–Muir valve, fitted between the tracheostomy tube and the ventilator tubing acts as a plug preventing air escaping into the ventilator tubing, but allowing it to enter the lungs. If a ventilator-dependent patient has a one-way valve in situ and can do GPB, it gives a great sense of security should a ventilator tube become kinked or disconnected. Before starting to learn GPB, it is essential that patients who are entirely ventilator-dependent learn to use intermittent positive pressure by mouthpiece. It gives them a reliable respiratory support during the learning stages. While increasing the period of time using GPB, it is important to ensure that normal blood gases are maintained. Patients usually take 6–8 gulps per breath, 10–12 times per minute, to provide a normal minute volume. When learning to build up their endurance they may experience a sense of desperate need for air but by taking a larger number of gulps (perhaps 20 or 25) at high speed, this feeling can be relieved and the normal pattern resumed.

Weakness of the oropharyngeal muscles may make it impossible to do GPB, but it can be successful with mild weakness. The technique is contraindicated in patients with obstructive airways disease where the positive pressure could increase air trapping. It is also contraindicated in cardiac failure, where the long inspiratory period with high intrathoracic pressure could decrease venous return, causing a fall in blood pressure.

To learn GPB requires commitment from both patient and physiotherapist and, if taught as an outpatient, tuition sessions at least weekly are recommended to maintain motivation. Filming the patient on video to give visual feedback is sometimes a useful teaching tool. GPB can be a much more versatile breathing technique than using a mechanical insufflator/exsufflator. It requires no equipment and in addition to making coughing more effective, for many patients it gives confidence when away from the home ventilator allowing greater independence and improved quality of life. When taught successfully a physiotherapist gains confidence and sees the benefits it can give to patients. Bach (1992) wrote that although potentially extremely useful, GPB is rarely used because there are few healthcare professionals familiar with the technique. Many patients would benefit if physiotherapists familiarized themselves with the technique and included it as a treatment option when indicated.

GRAVITY-ASSISTED POSITIONING

Gravity-assisted positions can be used to:

- assist clearance of bronchial secretions
- improve ventilation and perfusion.

Clearance of bronchial secretions. Gravity has been shown to assist clearance of bronchial secretions (Eaton et al 2007, Ewart 1901, Hofmeyr et al 1986, Sutton et al 1983). Nelson (1934) described the use of positioning for draining secretions based on the anatomy of the bronchial tree. The recognized positions (Thoracic Society 1950) (Fig. 5.34) are shown in Figures 5.35–5.45 and described in Table 5.1.

The effects of gravity on airway clearance are likely to be a consequence of both drainage and the increase in ventilation (Lannefors & Wollmer 1992) and specific positioning is likely to be of significance only, for example, in the drainage of an identified lung abscess or specific areas of atelectasis. Cecins et al (1999) demonstrated that the side lying position was as effective as the head-down tipped position for people with excess bronchial secretions as a consequence of chronic respiratory disease (non-cystic fibrosis bronchiectasis and cystic fibrosis). Eaton et al (2007) demonstrated that the inclusion of gravity-assisted positioning increased the wet weight of sputum expectorated in patients with non-cystic fibrosis bronchiectasis. In patients with cystic fibrosis the upper lobes are frequently the most severely

affected, although the cause is unknown (Tomashefski et al 1986) and positions other than sitting may be indicated only occasionally.

Individual assessment will indicate whether gravity-assisted drainage positions are of clinical benefit. In some patients with very tenacious secretions, gravity is unlikely to help and a comfortable position in which effective breathing techniques can be carried out is likely to be the most beneficial. It is inappropriate to use the head-down tipped positions immediately following meals and in the following conditions: cardiac failure, severe hypertension, cerebral oedema, aortic and cerebral aneurysms, severe haemoptysis, abdominal distension, gastro-oesophageal reflux and after recent surgery or trauma to the head or neck.

Ventilation/perfusion. In the adult, both ventilation and perfusion are preferentially distributed to the dependent parts of the lung (West 2004). In children this differs and there is a preferential distribution of ventilation to the uppermost lung and perfusion to the dependent lung (Chapter 10). In adults with unilateral lung disease, gas exchange may be improved by using the side lying position with the unaffected lung dependent (Zack et al 1974). Postoperatively the easiest method of increasing functional residual capacity (FRC) and preventing lung collapse is appropriate positioning and early ambulation (Jenkins et al 1988). Most patients can sit out of bed the day of or the day after surgery (Fig. 5.46A). If they cannot sit in a chair, they should be encouraged to sit either upright in bed or to adopt a side-lying position, but they should not be in a slumped sitting position as this will reduce lung volumes (Fig. 5.46B). See also Chapter 4, *Effects of positioning and mobilization*.

INCENTIVE SPIROMETRY

Incentive spirometers are mechanical devices that were originally introduced in surgical patients in an attempt to reduce postoperative pulmonary complications, by increasing inspiratory capacity. The device is activated by the patient's inspiratory effort. When a slow deep inspiration is performed, with the lips sealed around the mouthpiece (Fig. 5.47), the ongoing inspiration is motivated by visual feedback, for example a ball rising to a preset marker. The patient aims to generate a predetermined flow or to achieve a preset volume and is encouraged to hold at full inspiration for 2–3 seconds. A short, sharp inspiration can activate the flow-generated incentive spirometry devices with little increase in tidal volume, but with a volume-dependent device an increase in tidal volume must be achieved before the preset level can be reached. The increased work of

5

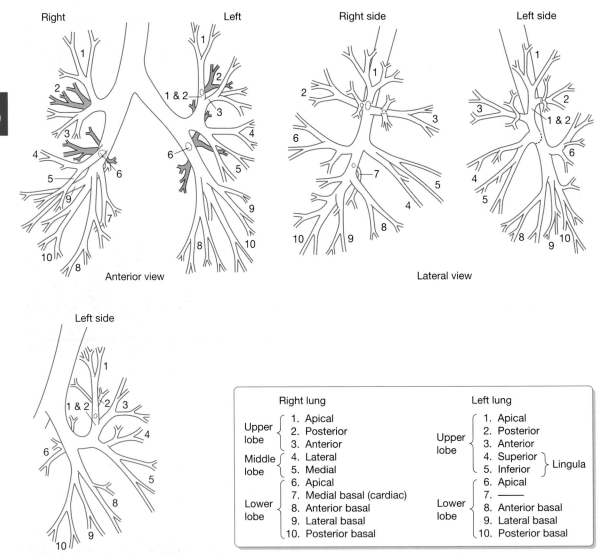

Right   Left   Right side   Left side

Anterior view   Lateral view

Left side

Left oblique view

	Right lung		Left lung
Upper lobe	1. Apical 2. Posterior 3. Anterior	Upper lobe	1. Apical 2. Posterior 3. Anterior
Middle lobe	4. Lateral 5. Medial		4. Superior ⎤ Lingula 5. Inferior ⎦
Lower lobe	6. Apical 7. Medial basal (cardiac) 8. Anterior basal 9. Lateral basal 10. Posterior basal	Lower lobe	6. Apical 7. —— 8. Anterior basal 9. Lateral basal 10. Posterior basal

Figure 5.34   Diagram illustrating the bronchopulmonary nomenclature approved by the Thoracic Society (1950). (Reproduced with permission of the Editor of *Thorax*)

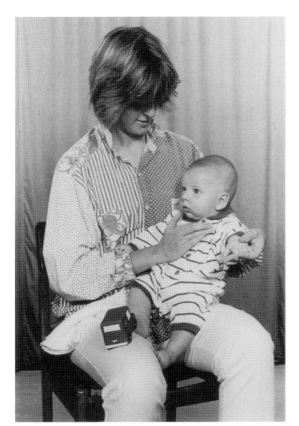

Figure 5.35   Apical segments upper lobes.

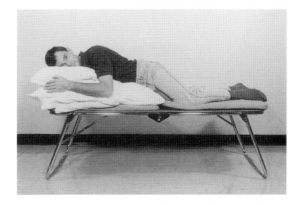

Figure 5.37   Posterior segment left upper lobe.

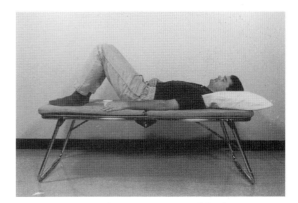

Figure 5.38   Anterior segments upper lobes.

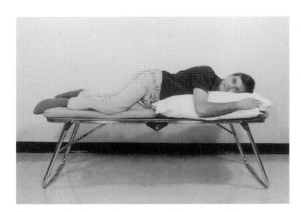

Figure 5.36   Posterior segment right upper lobe.

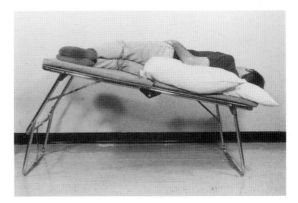

Figure 5.39   Lingula.

5

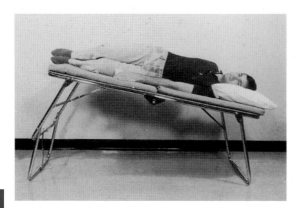

Figure 5.40   Right middle lobe.

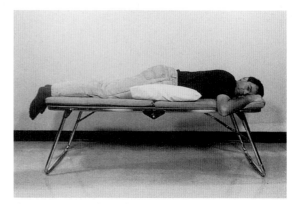

Figure 5.41   Apical segments lower lobes.

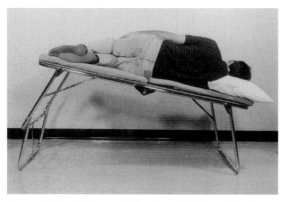

Figure 5.42   Right medial basal and left lateral basal segments lower lobes.

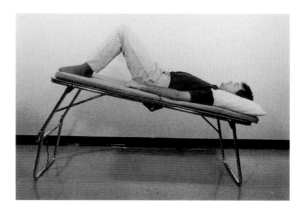

Figure 5.43   Anterior basal segments.

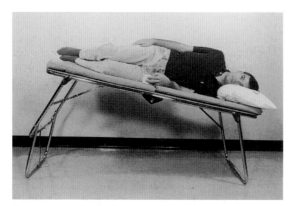

Figure 5.44   Lateral basal segment right lower lobe.

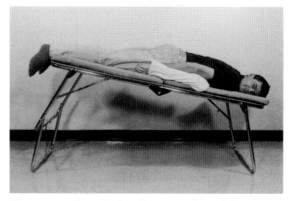

Figure 5.45   Posterior basal segments lower lobes.

Table 5.1 Gravity-assisted drainage positions (numbers refer to Fig. 5.34 and patient position is shown in Figs 5.35–5.45)

	Lobe			Position	
Upper lobe	1	Apical bronchus	1	Sitting upright	
	2	Posterior bronchus			
		(a) Right	2a	Lying on the left side horizontally turned 45° on to the face, resting against a pillow, with another supporting the head	
		(b) Left	2b	Lying on the right side turned 45° on to the face, with three pillows arranged to lift the shoulders 30 cm from the horizontal	
	3	Anterior bronchus	3	Lying supine with the knees flexed	
Lingula	4	Superior bronchus	4 and 5	Lying supine with the body a quarter turned to the right maintained by a pillow under the left side from shoulder to hip. The chest is tilted downwards to an angle of 15°	
	5	Inferior bronchus			
Middle lobe	4	Lateral bronchus	4 and 5	Lying supine with the body a quarter turned to the left maintained by a pillow under the right side from shoulder to hip. The chest is tilted downwards to an angle of 15°	
	5	Medial bronchus			
Lower lobe	6	Apical bronchus	6	Lying prone with a pillow under the abdomen	
	7	Medial basal (cardiac) bronchus	7	Lying on the right side with the chest tilted downwards to an angle of 20°	
	8	Anterior basal bronchus	8	Lying supine with the knees flexed and the chest tilted downwards to an angle of 20°	
	9	Lateral basal bronchus	9	Lying on the opposite side with the chest tilted downwards to an angle of 20°	
	10	Posterior basal bronchus	10	Lying prone with a pillow under the hips and the chest tilted downwards to an angle of 20°	

5

breathing required should be considered in patients at risk of inspiratory muscle fatigue and in patients with severely impaired respiratory muscle function. Spirometers with a low imposed work of breathing should be considered, if appropriate for these groups, and in some postoperative patients (Weindler & Kiefer 2001).

The pattern of breathing while using an incentive spirometer is important. Expansion of the lower chest should be emphasized rather than the use of the accessory muscles of respiration, which would encourage expansion of the upper chest. Diaphragmatic movement (Chuter et al 1990) is thought to be an important factor in the prevention of postoperative pulmonary complications. Incentive spirometry has been shown to increase abdominal movement in normal subjects, but not in subjects following abdominal surgery (Chuter et al 1989). Postoperatively, an increase in diaphragmatic move-

ment has been observed by encouraging an increase in lung volume while using the pattern of breathing control without the resistive loading of an incentive spirometer (Chuter et al 1990). This may help to reduce postoperative pulmonary complications by increasing ventilation to the dependent parts of the lungs.

A systematic review by Overend et al (2001) examined the use of incentive spirometry for the prevention of postoperative pulmonary complications (PPCs). The authors concluded that the evidence does not support the use of incentive spirometry for decreasing the incidence of PPCs following cardiac or upper abdominal surgery. Gosselink et al (2000) undertook a randomized controlled trial to investigate the additional effect of incentive spirometry to chest physiotherapy in the prevention of PPCs following thoracic surgery for lung and oesophageal resections. The addition of incentive

5

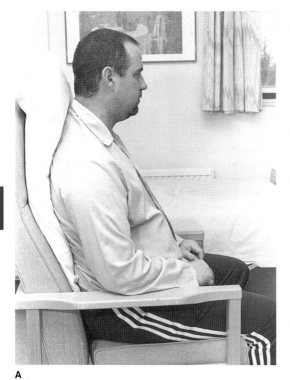

A

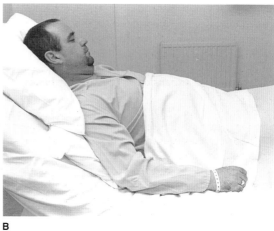

B

Figure 5.46 Positioning: (**A**) sitting upright; (**B**) Slumped sitting.

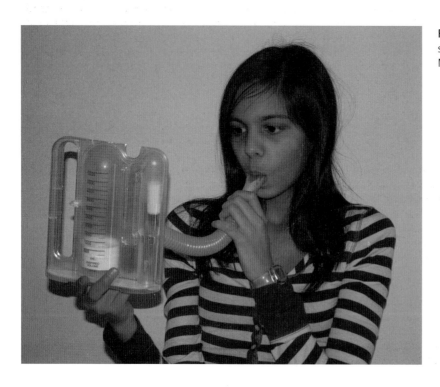

Figure 5.47 Using an incentive spirometer. (Voldyne®, Sherwood Medical)

spirometry to physiotherapy did not further reduce either pulmonary complications or hospital stay. However, a systematic review for the American College of Physicians on strategies to reduce PPCs following non-cardiothoracic surgery (Lawrence et al 2006) concluded that any type of lung expansion intervention is better than no prophylaxis.

There may be a place for the use of incentive spirometry, to increase lung volume following surgery, in children and in some adolescents to provide motivation and in patients who are immobilized, but with significant advances in anaesthesia and surgery (including the increasing use of minimally invasive surgery) ambulation may be the 'treatment' of choice for the majority of patients who are able to mobilize postoperatively.

INHALATION: DRUGS AND HUMIDIFICATION

Inhalation therapy has progressed significantly over the past two decades. 'Intelligent' nebulizers have reduced inhalation time and improved the efficacy of drug delivery. However, an understanding of the aerosol particle and its pattern of deposition within the airways remains essential when considering the delivery of drugs by the inhaled route and many 'conventional' systems are still in use.

A suspension of fine liquid or solid particles in air is known as an 'aerosol'. The pattern of deposition of aerosol particles within the bronchial tree depends on particle size, method of inhalation and on the degree of airflow obstruction (Newman et al 1986). Large particles in the size range 5–10 μm deposit by impaction in the oropharynx and upper airways where the cross-sectional diameter of the airway is small and the airflow high. The total cross-section of the airway increases rapidly beyond the 10th generation of bronchi, airflow slows significantly and particles of 0.5–5 μm, known as the 'respirable particles', deposit in the small airways and alveoli by gravitational sedimentation. It is the particles of less than 2 μm that reach the alveoli. Gravitational sedimentation is time dependent and enhanced by breath holding. A more central patchy deposition is seen in patients with airflow obstruction (Clarke 1988).

The topical deposition of a drug by inhalation allows a smaller dose to be given than when other routes are used, the onset of action is often more rapid and with minimal systemic absorption the side effects are reduced.

Metered dose inhaler (MDI) and dry powder inhaler (DPI)

Numerous devices are available for the inhalation of drugs, ranging from the simple MDI or powder inhalers

to breath-actuated inhalers and a variety of nebulizers. The physiotherapist should be aware of the range of possibilities to enable the patient to gain maximum benefit from the prescribed drugs. The choice of device will depend on the patient's age, coordination and dexterity, severity of the respiratory condition and patient preference.

Practice with placebo inhalers may be necessary to perfect the technique. Even if a patient has been using an inhalation device for a long time, it is important to observe and review the technique, as it may not be effective.

To gain maximum effect from a pressurized MDI (pMDI), the device should first be shaken to ensure that the drug is evenly distributed in the propellant gases. The inhaler is held upright and the cap is removed. The patient breathes out gently but not fully and then, with the mouth around the mouthpiece of the inhaler, the device is pressed to release the drug as soon as inspiration has begun. The breath in should be slow and deep and inspiration should be held for 10 seconds if possible, before breathing out gently through the nose (Burge 1986, Clarke 1988). Effective technique is essential as it has been shown that as little as 10% of the drug actually reaches the lungs (Clarke 1988).

Frequently, the prescribed dose will involve the inhalation of more than one 'puff'. It is recommended that puffs be taken one after the other. If the inhalation technique described above is used, the length of time between inhalations is likely to be 15–20 seconds, which allows sufficient time to overcome the problem of cooling of the metering chamber (pMDI) as the gas evaporates. Compliance is improved when doses are taken one after the other (Burge 1986).

Spacers can be used to improve the deposition of the drug in the lungs. Large volume spacers (Fig. 5.48) have been shown to improve this by approximately 15% (Clarke 1988) and to reduce the deposition in the oropharynx, as the larger particles drop out in the spacer rather than the oropharynx. The patient is encouraged to take a slow deep breath with a hold, but if this is difficult, tidal breathing can be used. Gleeson & Price (1988) showed that a bronchodilator was equally effective when a child breathed several times at tidal volume through a spacer when compared with a deep breath and inspiratory hold.

For people with poor coordination a breath-actuated inhaler may be considered (Newman et al 1991) or a dry powder device. The dry powder inhalers may also be breath-actuated, releasing the drugs on inspiration, but require a faster inspiratory flow rate than a pMDI. The inspiratory flow required depends on the resistance within the device. It is not only important that the patient can use the device effectively but also that

5

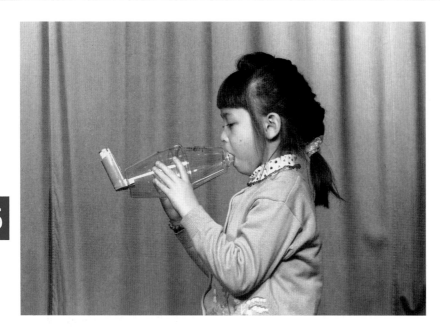

Figure 5.48   Spacer device. (Volumatic®, Allen and Hanbury)

the patient or parent can easily recall whether a dose of the drug has been taken and many devices incorporate a monitoring system.

The British Guideline on the Management of Asthma (British Thoracic Society & Scottish Intercollegiate Guidelines Network 2004) outlines current evidence for the inhalation of β_2-agonists (short- and long-acting), anticholinergics and steroids in adults and children and the recommended device. Oral candidiasis can be minimized by rinsing the mouth thoroughly following inhalation of steroids.

Nebulizers

A nebulizer may be used for the inhalation of drugs, if a more simple method is not optimally effective or if the drug cannot be administered by other means. Lannefors (2006) has reviewed the practical considerations for nebulizer therapy. A nebulizer converts a solution into aerosol particles (fine droplets), which are suspended in a stream of gas. It delivers a therapeutic dose of a prescribed drug as an aerosol in the form of respirable particles (particles <5 µm in diameter) and may be 'continuously running' or 'breath actuated'. There are several types of nebulizers.

Jet nebulizers

With the jet nebulizer, a driving gas (electric air compressor or compressed air or oxygen from a hospital line or cylinder) is forced through a narrow orifice. The negative pressure created around the orifice draws the drug solution up the feed tube from the liquid reservoir and the jet of gas fragments the liquid into droplets. A screening baffle allows the smaller particles in the form of a mist to be available for inhalation by the patient and the larger particles to drop back into the reservoir to be recycled (Medic-Aid Ltd 1996).

Ultrasonic nebulizers

An aerosol can also be created by high-frequency (1–2 MHz) sound waves. An electric current applied to a piezo-electric crystal causes ultrasonic vibrations. The sound waves will travel through a liquid to the surface where they produce an aerosol. The particle size is influenced by the frequency of oscillation of the crystal. Ultrasonic nebulizers can produce a higher output than jet nebulizers and operate quietly.

Vibrating mesh technology systems

Vibrating mesh systems employ a vibrating mesh or plate with multiple apertures to generate a fine-particle, low-velocity aerosol (Dhand 2002). This development has led to shorter treatment times together with improved efficiency and efficacy of drug delivery (Fig. 5.49). *Adaptive aerosol delivery systems* use mesh technology in the generation of aerosol particles. They identify and adapt to the patient's breathing pattern and deliver a preset volume of the drug during the first part of each inspiratory breath. They are programmed to deliver a total preset dose of a particular drug and give feedback on completion of administration of the dose (McGuire 2006). With an adaptive aerosol delivery system almost

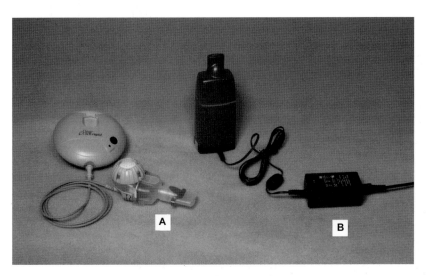

Figure 5.49 The smaller more efficient nebulizer systems using vibrating mesh technology. **(A)** eFlow by PARI. **(B)** I-neb adaptive aerosol delivery system by Profile Pharma.

5

no drug is lost during expiration, obviating the need for the use of filters or wide-bore tube systems and minimizing 'wasted' medication. The residual volume is about 0.1 ml (McGuire 2006).

Nebulizer performance

The performance of a nebulizer can be measured by its respirable output. The *respirable output* is the mass of *respirable particles* (particles less than 5 μm in diameter) produced per minute, that is:

aerosol output (mg/min) × respirable fraction

The *respirable fraction* is the percentage of respirable particles within the aerosol output. It is recommended that a nebulizer should provide a respirable fraction of at least 50% at its recommended driving gas flow (British Standards Institution 1994) and a number of nebulizers exceed this level. The performance of an individual nebulizer has often been described by the mass median aerodynamic diameter (MMAD) of the particles. The MMAD indicates the range of size of particles leaving the nebulizer. Half of the aerosol mass from the nebulizer is of particles smaller than the MMAD and half of the aerosol mass is of particles larger than the MMAD. This is a less useful measurement of nebulizer performance, as it is not related to the mass of drug. It is important to consider an air compressor and nebulizer system as a unit and they should be matched to provide an acceptable output (Kendrick et al 1995). Factors that affect individual nebulizer performance include the following (Nebuliser Project Group 1997):

Driving gas. Most jet nebulizers operate efficiently with a flow rate of 6–8 l/min. For patients in hospital it is often convenient to use the piped oxygen supply and in hypoxic patients without carbon dioxide retention, oxygen should be used. For patients retaining carbon dioxide who are dependent on their hypoxic drive to stimulate breathing, compressed air should be the driving gas (Gunawardena et al 1984). Occasionally it may be appropriate to increase the inspired oxygen concentration by entraining a low flow of oxygen.

Nebulizer chamber design. With a 'conventional' nebulizer the output flow (from the nebulizer, towards the patient) is equal to the input flow (from the driving gas source) and nebulization is continuous. With a 'Venturi' nebulizer the output flow is greater than the input flow due to the presence of an open vent, but the output flow does not change with the patient's breathing pattern. With an 'active Venturi' nebulizer the output flow is breath assisted and is increased during inspiration. There is therefore less wastage of the drug during expiration. When selecting a nebulizer the age of the patient must be considered. The inspiratory flow of an infant will probably be less than the output from a Venturi nebulizer. The concentration of the aerosolized drug may therefore be increased as there will be little or no air entrainment, but the total dose of the drug may be reduced (Collis et al 1990). Consideration should also be given to the optimal particle size of the drug to be delivered. Inhaled pentamidine or antibiotics need to be delivered to the more peripheral airways (requiring a high percentage of particles of less than 2 μm), whereas bronchodilator drugs probably have their effect in the more central airways.

Residual volume. This is the volume of solution that remains in the nebulizer after nebulization has stopped.

5

The Nebuliser Project Group of the British Thoracic Society (1997) recommends that a fill volume of 2–2.5 ml may be adequate if the residual volume is less than 1 ml, but nebulizers with a higher residual volume will probably require a fill volume of 4 ml. The patient should be encouraged to tap the side of the nebulizer to allow as much as possible to be delivered (Everard et al 1994).

Fill volume. For effective nebulization, it is important not to exceed the manufacturer's recommended fill volume.

Physical properties of drug solution or suspension. Most bronchodilator solutions when nebulized have a similar volume output to normal (0.9%) sodium chloride, but solutions with a higher viscosity or a high surface tension (e.g. carbenicillin) are slow to nebulize, and other characteristics of the aerosol output may change.

Breathing pattern of the patient. The optimal pattern of breathing using a nebulizer other than an adaptive aerosol delivery device has not yet been ascertained, but a recommended one is to intersperse one or two slow deep breaths with breathing at tidal volume. The deep breathing may increase peripheral deposition of the drug and the periods of breathing control will prevent hyperventilation. When inhaling from a nebulizer, the patient should be in a comfortable and well-supported position.

Drug delivery

A range of drugs often administered via a nebulizer include bronchodilators, corticosteroids, antibiotics, pentamidine, antifungals, local anaesthetics, rhDNase and surfactant. The nebulizer system used must be appropriate for the drug that has been prescribed. The evidence for drug device matching is outlined in the European Respiratory Society nebulizer guidelines: clinical aspects (2000). It is important to remember that the relative proportions of the airway and the anatomy and structure of the lung will alter during childhood. This will affect the deposition of inhaled drugs (Barry et al 2000).

Other points for consideration

- The dose of a prescribed nebulized bronchodilator may seem large compared with that from a pressurized aerosol, but only 10–20% of the initial dose, using a conventional jet nebulizer, is received by the patient and only 50% of this reaches the lungs. The drug that does not reach the patient is lost in the equipment and exhaled gas (Lewis & Fleming 1985).

- A facemask is necessary for an infant or small child (Fig. 5.50), but as soon as the child is able to cooper-

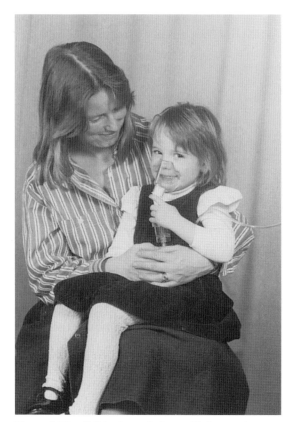

Figure 5.50 Child using nebulizer with facemask.

ate, a mouthpiece should be used to minimize deposition of the drug on the face and in the nasal passages (Wolfsdorf et al 1969). Other disadvantages of a mask are facial skin irritation from nebulized antibiotics and steroids and nebulized ipratropium bromide and salbutamol by mask have been associated with glaucoma in a group of adults with chronic airflow limitation (Shah et al 1992).

- For infants and children, parents should be given written instruction, in addition to verbal instruction, to improve adherence to treatment (Barry et al 2000).

- For nebulized antibiotics and pentamidine a one-way valve system is recommended (Wilson et al 2000). This can be achieved either with an effective filter on the exhalation port (Fig. 5.51) or wide-bore tubing to allow the exhaled gas to be vented out through a window. This is to prevent small quantities of antibiotics remaining in the atmosphere, which could lead to patients, family members and medical personnel in the vicinity receiving a subtherapeutic

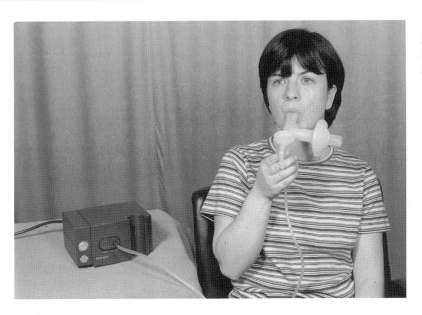

Figure 5.51 Inhalation of antibiotics using an active Venturi nebulizer (PARI LC STAR), filter and air compressor (PARI TurboBOY).

dose (Smaldone et al 1991) and environmental organisms becoming resistant to the antibiotic (Sanderson 1984). A nose clip is necessary if the patient is breathing partially through the nose. A bronchoconstriction test should be undertaken at the time of the first inhalation of an antibiotic or pentamidine.

- If inhaled antibiotics are prescribed for a pseudomonal infection in the upper respiratory tract, for example a patient with cystic fibrosis following lung transplantation, a nebulizer producing large particles is necessary (Webb et al 1996). A mask should be used and the patient encouraged to breathe through the nose.

- More than one antibiotic may be prescribed. A few antibiotics are compatible when mixed, but others must be inhaled separately. Either normal saline or sterile water is used to reconstitute a powdered antibiotic or to make a prescribed solution up to the necessary volume for nebulization. Information on the advisability of mixing drugs should be obtained from a pharmacist.

- Hypertonic saline (3–7%) has been shown to assist in the clearance of secretions (Elkins et al 2006b, Eng et al 1996). It may cause an increase in airflow obstruction (Schoeffel et al 1981) and a bronchoconstriction test should be undertaken at the time of the first inhalation.

- Sputum induction, commonly using a hypertonic solution of saline and an ultrasonic nebulizer, is a technique that can be used to obtain sputum from

people who do not produce it spontaneously. A Task Force set up by the European Respiratory Society details a standardized methodology of sputum induction and processing (European Respiratory Society Task Force 2002). Airway clearance techniques have often been used in conjunction with the inhalation, but there is no evidence to support any increase in the volume of sputum expectorated or quality of the sample obtained when these techniques are included (Elkins et al 2005).

- The mucolytic rhDNase should not be mixed with any other inhaled medication and it is recommended that where possible a separate nebulizing chamber should be used. Ultrasonic nebulizers are not recommended to deliver rhDNase (Suri et al 2002) as the drug composition may be denatured by this technology.

- The inhaled mucolytic acetylcysteine should be used with caution. A reduction in sputum viscosity does not necessarily produce an increase in expectoration of sputum and bronchospasm may be induced. A bronchoconstriction test should be undertaken at the time of the first inhalation. Acetylcysteine is inactivated by oxygen and, if nebulized, the driving gas should be air (Reynolds 1996).

Domiciliary nebulization

If there is an indication for domiciliary nebulization, it is essential that the appropriate equipment is selected and careful instructions provided (both verbal and written). Instructions in the care and cleaning of the

5

equipment must be given in accordance with local infection control policies.

A spare jet nebulizer and an inlet filter for the air compressor (if necessary) should be available. The nebulizer must be washed and dried thoroughly after each treatment to reduce the possibility of bacterial infection (Hutchinson et al 1996) and to keep the jets clear. The transducer of an ultrasonic nebulizer should be cleaned regularly with acetic acid (white vinegar) to maintain its efficiency. An annual check of output and general and electrical safety should be undertaken and there should be provision for servicing as required (Dodd et al 1995).

Some patients may benefit from a compressor that can be used when travelling, either by using a 12-volt adaptor in a socket in the car, 'crocodile clips' fitted on to a battery or, more conveniently, a compact battery pack supplied with the compressor. Those travelling to a country using a different voltage may require a transformer or a dual-voltage compressor. Some compressors incorporate a universal power pack that adapts to voltages throughout the world. An international travel plug adaptor is an accessory required for all who travel abroad. A foot pump may be useful to power a nebulizer where no electricity is available, but it requires considerable energy to operate. When travelling abroad, it is advisable to take a letter from a doctor explaining the need to travel with drugs and possibly syringes and needles.

Bronchodilator and bronchoconstriction testing

Bronchodilator testing

'The efficacy of bronchodilator therapy should not be assessed by lung function alone but should include a variety of other measures such as improvement in symptoms, activities of daily living, exercise capacity, and rapidity of symptom relief'
(National Institute for Clinical Excellence 2004).

Short-term responses may not reflect long-term responses and there is known variability (National Institute for Clinical Excellence 2004).

A peak flow meter (Miller 2000) is often used to assess bronchodilator response. This may be suitable in a patient with asthma, but will not detect the more subtle response of a change in forced vital capacity (FVC), which can occur in those with more irreversible airflow obstruction (Fig. 5.52). For these patients the response to a bronchodilator, detected by a change in FVC, may lead to an increase in exercise ability and improved quality of life. The unnecessary use of nebulized bronchodilators can restrict activities of daily living. A nebulizer and air compressor system should

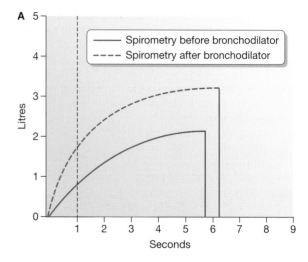

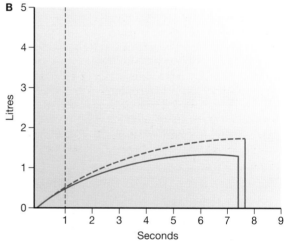

Figure 5.52 (A) Increase in FEV_1 and FVC. (B) Increase in FVC only. —, Spirometry before bronchodilator; ---- spirometry after bronchodilator.

be prescribed only when a more simple delivery device, used correctly, is ineffective.

The Thoracic Society of Australia and New Zealand and The Australian Lung Foundation (McKenzie et al 2003) have outlined a bronchodilator response test:

Short-acting bronchodilators should be withheld for the previous 6 hours, long acting β-agonists for 12 hours and sustained release theophyllines for 24 hours. Baseline spirometry should be measured and repeated 15–30 minutes following administration of medication. An increase in FEV_1 of >12% and 200 ml is greater than the average day-to-day variability and unlikely to occur by chance.

O'Driscoll et al (1990), in their study on home nebulizers, could not demonstrate a correlation between formal lung function testing and the domiciliary use of a nebulizer system. They recommended that patients who are referred for consideration of home nebulizer therapy be given the equipment to try under supervision for several weeks at home and that the patient's subjective assessment should be considered. In assessing bronchodilator treatment Vora et al (1995) concluded that a quality of life measure and shuttle walking test appeared to be sensitive outcome measures. 'Clinical thresholds' using health-related quality of life instruments, for example the Chronic Respiratory Questionnaire, St George's Respiratory Questionnaire and Asthma Quality of Life Questionnaire, have been identified and may be useful in assessing responsiveness to bronchodilator therapy (Jones 2002). Demonstrating a positive response to a simple inhalation device in a clinical setting and showing that nebulized therapy provides no further benefit is often sufficient to reassure a patient who is anxious that sufficient benefit may not be achieved from an inhaler compared with a compressor system.

Many patients with asthma keep a diary card at home, which will include recordings of peak expiratory flow before and after bronchodilator drugs. These will be valid only if the technique of performing a peak flow manoeuvre through the flow meter (Fig. 5.53) is correct. In terms of technique, it is important to emphasize the following points:

- A maximal inspiration is essential (in their haste to perform the test, the patient may not take a full deep breath)

- Expiration should be short and sharp

- The best of three 'blows' is usually recommended

- Sufficient rests (of at least 15 seconds) should be allowed between 'blows' to prevent any increase in airflow obstruction with the forced expiratory manoeuvre

- The same position, sitting or standing, should be used each time a reading is taken.

Bronchoconstriction testing

If a patient is to be started on inhaled antibiotics, pentamidine and/or hypertonic saline, an initial test dose should be given. Nebulized antibiotics may be isotonic, hypo- or hypertonic solutions and may cause airflow obstruction (Cunningham et al 2001, Dodd et al 1997). The first dose of a nebulized antibiotic should be monitored by recording the FEV_1 and FVC before, immediately after, 15 minutes after and, if evidence of airflow obstruction persists, 30 minutes after the inhalation (Maddison et al 1994).

Individual patients respond differently and this response may vary with different drugs and over time. If airflow obstruction occurs, it can usually be controlled

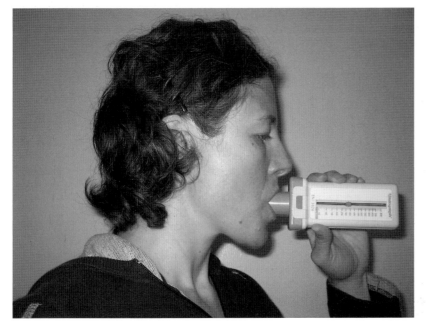

Figure 5.53 Using a peak flow meter. (Vitalograph®)

by the inhalation of a bronchodilator taken before physiotherapy for the clearance of secretions, preceding the inhalation of the antibiotic.

Heliox

A mixture of helium and oxygen (80:20 or 70:30) is sometimes used on a temporary basis to relieve respiratory distress in patients with upper airways obstruction, for example a tumour causing partial obstruction of the trachea. Helium is of lower density than air and may pass more easily through a narrowed airway, requiring less effort from the patient (Vater et al 1983). A side-effect of heliox is an alteration in the pitch of the voice, due to its effect on the vocal cords. This is only temporary, but should be explained to the patient before use of heliox to avoid unnecessary concern. Heliox has not been shown to be of benefit in patients with an exacerbation of chronic obstructive pulmonary disease (Rodrigo et al 2001) or in the treatment of acute asthma (Rodrigo et al 2006).

Humidification

A device to provide humidification of the airways may be considered if either the normal means of humidifying the airways or the mucociliary escalator is not functioning effectively. Inspired gas is adequately humidified in the normal situation but additional humidification may be required (Bersten 2003) during an episode of respiratory infection, in those with existing respiratory disease and in the acute situation. Humidification of inspired gases may be indicated to assist clearance of secretions when the clearance mechanism is not optimally effective or when the normal heat and moisture exchange system of the upper airways is bypassed by an endotracheal or tracheostomy tube. Patients with a long-term tracheostomy may develop metaplasia of the tracheal epithelium.

Ambient air is normally about 22°C with a relative humidity of 50%. Alveolar air usually presents a temperature of 37°C with a relative humidity of 100% (Chiumello et al 2002). During inspiration the inspired gases are progressively heated and humidified along the nose and upper airways, normally reaching the isothermic saturation boundary (ISB) of 37°C and 100% relative humidity at about 5–6 cm below the carina (Chiumello et al 2002). The volume, temperature and absolute humidity of the inspired gases can change the point of the ISB.

The epithelial lining of the airways, from the trachea to the respiratory bronchioles, contains ciliated cells that are responsible for moving mucus and particulate matter proximally to the level of the larynx. The optimal temperature for cilial activity is normal body temperature with reduced activity occurring below 20°C and above 40°C (Wanner 1977). The cilia beat within a watery fluid, the 'periciliary' or 'sol' layer. A mucus layer 'gel' covers the periciliary layer and interacts with the tips of the cilia.

The efficiency of mucus transport is dependent on correctly functioning cilia and the composition of the periciliary and mucus layers. If the periciliary layer becomes too shallow, as with dehydration, the cilia become enmeshed in the viscous mucus layer and cannot function effectively. If the periciliary layer is too deep, the tips of the cilia are not in contact with the mucus layer and propulsion of the mucus is inefficient.

The viscosity of mucus is increased during bacterial infection owing to an increase in the DNA content of the mucus (Wilson & Cole 1988). With hypersecretory disorders of, for example, bronchiectasis and chronic airflow limitation, there is an increase in both quantity and viscosity of mucus secretions. Bacteria directly affect cilial beating and coordination, disrupt the epithelium, stimulate mucus secretion and alter periciliary fluid composition (Cole 1995). Humidification has been shown to enhance tracheobronchial clearance when used as an adjunct to physiotherapy in a group of patients with bronchiectasis (Conway et al 1992).

Clarke (1995) has suggested that the efficiency of cough increases with a decrease in viscosity of mucus and an increase in the periciliary layer of the airway. Conway (1992) hypothesized that humidification by water or saline aerosol produces an increase in depth of the periciliary and mucus layers, thereby decreasing viscosity and enhancing the shearing of secretions by huffing or coughing.

Methods of humidification

Systemic hydration

Adequate humidification may be obtained by increasing the oral or intravenous fluid intake of a patient. Breathless patients find drinking fluids an effort, but need encouragement to avoid dehydration. Patients should be reminded to maintain an adequate fluid intake as this may help to prevent airway secretions from becoming more tenacious. During periods of infection and fever a higher fluid intake is required.

Heated water bath humidifiers

Gas is blown over a reservoir of heated sterile water and absorbs water vapour, which is then inhaled by the patient (Fig. 5.54). If the delivery tube is cold there is a temperature drop as the gas passes along the tube and condensation occurs. The humidifier should be positioned below the level of the patient's airway to avoid flooding of the airway by condensed water. Sealed

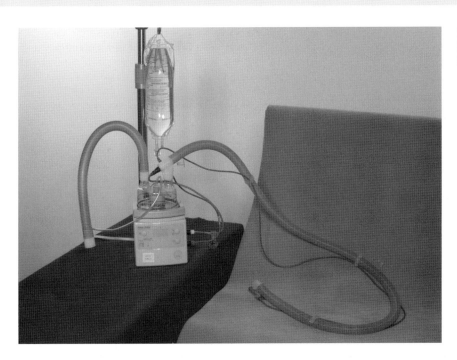

Figure 5.54 Heated humidifier. (Fisher and Paykel Healthcare)

water traps (to prevent contamination) should be included in the circuit to allow regular emptying without interrupting ventilation. A heated delivery tube eliminates the problem of condensation and allows the gas to be delivered at a desired temperature of 32–36°C with a water content of 33–43 g/m³ (Hinds & Watson 1996). Sterile water must be used in these devices. If saline is used, only the water vaporizes and the sodium chloride crystallizes out.

Humidifiers can be used for the spontaneously breathing patient or can be incorporated into ventilator circuits including continuous positive airway pressure and non-invasive ventilation. If using a low output humidifier, it may be necessary to use two devices in series in order to achieve adequate humidification (Harrison et al 1993).

Heat and moisture exchangers

A heat and moisture exchanger (HME) or the 'Swedish nose' is a lightweight disposable device and may be used in the intubated patient either mechanically ventilated or breathing spontaneously. In patients receiving pressure support ventilation (Pelosi et al 1996) and in spontaneously breathing patients, it is important to be aware of the slight resistance that may increase the work of breathing. The HME acts in a similar way to the nasopharynx. The heat and moisture of the exhaled gas are retained either by condensation (condenser humidifier) or by absorption and returned in the inhaled gas as it passes through the device. A variety of hygroscopic

materials and chemicals are used for absorption within heat and moisture exchangers.

HMEs are inefficient if there is a large air leak around an uncuffed tracheostomy tube (Tilling & Hayes 1987) and generally do not provide adequate humidification for infants. In children with an increased work of breathing, the additional resistance from a heat and moisture exchanger may further compromise breathing. If the secretions of a patient using an HME become tenacious, a more effective form of humidification will be required (Bransen et al 1993). The HME should be changed every 24 (Boots et al 2006) to 48 hours (Djedaini et al 1995) and immediately if it becomes soiled with secretions.

Large-volume jet nebulizers

A large-volume jet nebulizer which uses the same principle as a small-volume jet nebulizer (used for inhalation of medication) may be used for humidification of inspired gas and may include a heater within the circuit. However, the droplets can carry bacteria, thus increasing the risk of respiratory infection (Bersten 2003).

Ultrasonic

Many ultrasonic humidifiers (Fig. 5.55) do not have a heater, but the mist is at ambient temperature and warmer than that produced from a jet nebulizer powered from compressed piped gas. There is often an airflow control valve in addition to a control for the density of the mist. By regulating these two controls the density of mist can be adjusted to the patient's comfort.

5

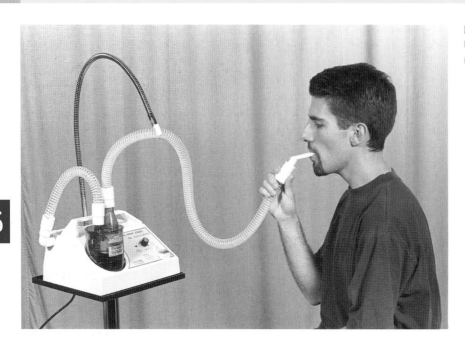

Figure 5.55 DeVilbiss Ultra-neb 2000 ultrasonic nebulizer.

Sterile normal saline (0.9%) is isotonic and probably the most appropriate solution, although sterile water can be used if saline is unavailable, but has been shown to cause bronchoconstriction in patients with hyperreactive airways (Schoeffel et al 1981).

Bubble-through humidifiers

A device containing cold water, through which the inspired gas is bubbled, has not been shown to be an effective means of humidification. No objective benefits were identified when a bubble-through humidifier was attached to nasal cannulae (Campbell et al 1988). Many patients do, however, report subjective benefits from these devices. When bubble-through humidifiers are connected to nasal cannulae or an oxygen mask with narrow-bore tubing, care must be taken to ensure that water does not condense in the tubing, as this may alter the inspired oxygen concentration by partially blocking the passage of gas through the tubing. A bubble-through humidifier attached to the narrow-bore tubing of a Venturi mask is inappropriate, as the flow of oxygen is likely to be reduced by the back pressure from the humidifier device and by condensation blocking the narrow-bore tubing.

Delivery to the patient

Patients with retained secretions postoperatively or those with excess viscous secretions due to a chronic bronchopulmonary infection may benefit from a period of 10–20 minutes' humidification before physiotherapy to assist the clearance of secretions. If the concentration of oxygen required by the patient is not critical, a *mouthpiece* with a hole for entrainment of additional air is simple and comfortable to use. Deep breathing, interspersed with tidal volume breathing, may encourage peripheral deposition of an aerosol, while avoiding hyperventilation.

Patients requiring an inspired oxygen concentration of 24% will probably wear a Venturi mask connected to the oxygen by narrow-bore tubing. It is impossible to give high humidification through a narrow-bore tube owing to condensation within the tubing. Effective humidification can be obtained by using a *humidity adaptor,* which allows the air entrained by the mask to be humidified. It is a cuff fitted over the air-entraining holes of the mask and connected by wide-bore humidity tubing to a humidifier powered by an air source. A humidity adaptor can be used to give humidification to Venturi masks delivering accurate higher concentrations of oxygen (e.g. 28% or 35%), but is unsatisfactory with a 60% Venturi mask because the air-entraining holes are too small to entrain the humidity. An ultrasonic nebulizer, set at a high flow, can be used and is quieter than a jet nebulizer system. If a patient is breathing spontaneously through a tracheostomy, a *tracheostomy mask* may be attached to a humidifier or nebulizer via wide-bore tubing. Alternatively a heat moisture exchanger or a 'laryngectomy-permanent tracheostomy protector' (tracheostomy 'bib') may be used.

Humidification through a *head box* (Chapter 10) is often used in the treatment of spontaneously breathing infants. With the narrow airways of an infant the risk of mucus plugging is higher than in adults. Humidity to a head box may be either from a heated water bath humidifier or a heated nebulizer system.

Hazards of humidification

Inhalation of cold mist or water (a hypotonic solution) may cause bronchoconstriction in patients with hyper-reactive airways (Schoeffel et al 1981). Heated humidi-fication and normal saline solution are less likely to cause this problem. It may be appropriate to take peak flow or spirometry recordings before and immediately after the first treatment.

Water reservoirs had been considered good culture mediums for bacteria, but there is little evidence to support humidification as an important factor in noso-comial respiratory tract infections (Bersten 2003). A par-ticularly vulnerable site is the catheter mount of the ventilator circuit in the intubated patient. Regular dis-posal, disinfection or sterilization of all equipment is essential to prevent infection and local infection control policies must be observed.

INSPIRATORY MUSCLE TRAINING

Individuals with chronic respiratory disease, for example COPD, experience inspiratory muscle dysfunc-tion due to a combination of problems, which include hyperinflation, increased work of breathing, hypox-aemia, and hypercapnia (Laghi & Tobin 2003). Other problems that may reduce inspiratory muscle strength and endurance include corticosteroid-induced myopa-thy, chronic inflammation and chronic gas exchange abnormalities (Maltais et al 2000). Factors that lead to inspiratory muscle dysfunction contribute to the devel-opment of dyspnoea and to limitation of exercise toler-ance (Solcher & Dechman 1998). Optimizing function through a reduction in dyspnoea is a key aim of therapy and there is now unequivocal evidence that pulmonary rehabilitation is the only treatment shown convincingly to reduce dyspnoea in chronic respiratory disease. A contributory factor in this is through training-induced improvements in aerobic capacity of the skeletal muscles, achieved through increasing mechanical effi-ciency and lowering blood lactate concentrations (Casaburi et al 1991, O'Donnell et al 1995). However, it is also established that whole-body exercise condition-ing fails to improve respiratory muscle strength and endurance (Weiner et al 1992). As inspiratory muscle dysfunction contributes to dyspnoea in COPD, it is evident that specifically targeting the inspiratory muscles may lead to further reductions in dyspnoea (Hill et al 2004).

The inspiratory muscles, like other skeletal muscles, undergo physiological adaptations in response to train-ing. Despite this being evident, the early literature on the use of inspiratory muscle training (IMT) in patients with COPD presented a rather mixed picture. In part this was due to the paucity of controlled clinical trials, but more importantly due to the nature of the training adopted. In general the trials were confounded by the methodology of the training in which the frequency, duration and intensity of training were less than that required to achieve a true training response, as high-lighted in an early meta-analysis (Smith et al 1992). Ten years later Lotters et al (2002) published a second meta-analysis, which included only studies in which IMT was controlled in terms of fixing the intensity of IMT in order to achieve a training response. This review con-cluded that IMT improved respiratory muscle strength and endurance although the effects of IMT on exercise capacity remained to be determined. More recently Geddes et al (2005) published a systematic review in which IMT was shown to be effective, not only in terms of increasing inspiratory muscle strength and endur-ance but also in improving exercise capacity in adults with COPD. However, this review emphasized that the method of IMT employed is important if clinical benefits are to be obtained and that training of the ventilatory muscles must follow the basic principles of training for any striated muscle with regard to the intensity and duration of the stimulus, the specificity of training and the reversibility of training.

The principle of specificity of training states that the effects of training are very specific to the neural and muscular elements of overload. The overload principle states that overload must be applied to a muscle for a training response to occur (Kennedy 1995). Overload may be applied by increasing the frequency or duration of training or the intensity of the loading, or a combina-tion of these factors. Generally, training theory suggests that inspiratory muscle strength gains can be achieved at intensities of 80–90% of maximal inspiratory pres-sure. Strength-endurance gains (maximal effective force that can be maintained) can be achieved at 60–80%, and endurance (the ability to continue a dynamic task for a prolonged period) at approximately 60% of peak, which equates with high-intensity training regimens used in systemic exercise (Kraemer et al 2002).

Overload may also include the concept of incremen-tal loading. This involves decreasing the rest periods between muscle contractions (Komi & Hakkinen 1991), which has been shown to recruit a larger proportion of muscle fibres and, hence, a larger pool of fibres are trained for subsequent lower but potentially fatiguing loads (Reid & Samrai 1995, Reid et al 1994). In studies that have used the principle of high-intensity incremen-tal IMT improvements in lung volumes, diaphragm thickness and exercise capacity have been obtained in

5

healthy subjects and in patients with cystic fibrosis (Enright et al 2004, 2006).

In many previous investigations training methodologies have varied to include loads imposed on the respiratory muscles which can be characterized as flow, pressure and volume loads (McCool 1992). A low-pressure high-flow load was first described in 1976 by Leith & Bradley which involves training the respiratory muscles by voluntarily ventilating at high levels for a prolonged period (usually 15 minutes). It is therefore analogous to the high ventilatory demands imposed on the inspiratory muscles during high-intensity exercise (Belman 1993). The load imposed on the inspiratory muscles requires a high flow rate at low pressure, although it is generally impractical, as it requires the assembly of complex breathing circuits in order to ensure that the individual remains normocapnic. In addition, breathless patients find this method of IMT uncomfortable to maintain and hence this method of IMT tends to be reserved for laboratory-based investigations rather than being used in a clinical setting (Scherer et al 2000). In contrast to a flow load, a high-pressure low-flow load occurs with any process that increases the transpulmonary pressure required to breathe in. These loads can be experimentally imposed by inhaling from a rigid chamber or by breathing through an external resistance. Such loads can be achieved by either resistive or threshold devices. Resistive training devices incorporate a range of apertures, which vary in size in order to apply the prescribed resistive load. Threshold devices impose a threshold or a critical inspiratory opening pressure that the subject is required to overcome before the start of an inspiratory flow. The efficacy of both these modes of IMT have been the subject of some debate, although recently it has been shown that targeted resistive IMT is as effective as threshold IMT for adults with COPD (Hsiao et al 2003). On a practical level some issues require consideration, for example targeted resistive devices provide visual feedback which enhances motivation, although ensuring that the patient is maintaining the required training intensity can be problematic. Conversely, threshold trainers provide a more constant resistance although the loss of visual feedback may result in loss of motivation.

In addition to the mode of training adopted, the frequency of training in IMT interventions, the duration of the training intervention and the issue of reversibility of training requires consideration. Standard guidelines of the American College of Sports Medicine (Kennedy 1995) suggest a training frequency of one to two times per day for a total duration of 20–30 minutes, three to five times per week for 6 weeks. However, functional improvements and adaptive cellular changes in the inspiratory muscles have been shown to occur following 5 weeks of training (Ramirez-Sarmiento et al 2002) although training must be maintained for the cellular training effects to be sustained (McArdle et al 2001). In summary, the optimal frequency of training is thought to be three times weekly, to continue beyond 4 weeks and with maintenance achieved by continuing training at one or two times weekly (Fleck 1994).

In conclusion, although there is much conflicting evidence in the literature, which has cast doubt on the place of IMT in patients with respiratory muscle dysfunction, more recent data that have incorporated the appropriate physiological training principles during IMT look promising (Geddes et al 2005). The use of targeted inspiratory resistive or threshold modes of IMT as opposed to non-targeted inspiratory resistive modes ensures that the training intensity is achieved and maintained. Thus with effective IMT regimens, exercise intolerance, dyspnoea and hypercapnic ventilatory failure may be prevented or alleviated. In addition, another indication for IMT is that weakness of the inspiratory muscles may lead to an inability to generate an adequate flow to assure lung deposition when using dry powder inhalers. Hence strengthening the inspiratory muscles may improve the efficacy of inhaled drug therapy (Weiner & Weiner 2006). These considerations are vital if IMT is to find a proven place in pulmonary rehabilitation programmes (Hill & Eastwood 2005).

INTERMITTENT POSITIVE PRESSURE BREATHING

Intermittent positive pressure breathing (IPPB) is the maintenance of a positive airway pressure throughout inspiration, with airway pressure returning to atmospheric pressure during expiration. The American Association for Respiratory Care (AARC) has developed clinical practice guidelines for the use of IPPB as a hyperinflation and aerosol delivery technique (American Association for Respiratory Care 2003). The literature on IPPB has been reviewed by Bott et al (1992) and Denehy & Berney (2001). Denehy & Berney concluded that although the use of IPPB has declined, it may still have a place in the management of patients with reduced lung volumes. They also state that the rationale for using IPPB should be based on its known physiological effects, the availability of other treatment modalities, the condition of the patient and the current research knowledge base. The Bird ventilator (Fig. 5.56) is a pressure-cycled device convenient to use for providing IPPB as an adjunct to physiotherapy in the spontaneously breathing patient.

IPPB has been shown to augment tidal volume (Stiller et al 1992, Sukumalchantra et al 1965) and using an IPPB device in the completely relaxed subject, the work of

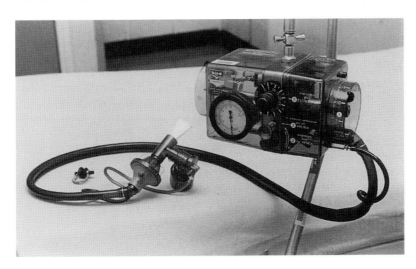

Figure 5.56 The Bird Mark 7 ventilator.

breathing during inspiration approaches zero (Ayres et al 1963). These two effects support the use of IPPB to help in the clearance of bronchial secretions when more simple airway clearance techniques alone are not maximally effective, for example in the semi-comatosed patient with chronic bronchitis and sputum retention (Pavia et al 1988), the postoperative patient or in a patient with neuromuscular disease and a chest infection. The reduction in the work of breathing can be used with effect in the exhausted patient with acute severe asthma, but there is no evidence that the effect of bronchodilators delivered by IPPB is greater than from a nebulizer alone (Webber et al 1974).

An ideal IPPB device for use with physiotherapy should be portable and have simple controls. Other important features are as follows:

Positive pressure.   The range of pressures is likely to be from 0 to 35 cmH$_2$O.

Sensitivity.   The patient should be able to 'trigger' the inspiratory phase with minimal effort. Fully automatic control is unpleasant for most patients and unnecessary for physiotherapy. A hand triggering device is useful to test the ventilator and nebulizer.

Flow control.   With ventilators such as the Bird Mark 7, the inspiratory gas is delivered at a flow rate that can be preset by means of a control dial. Optimal distribution of gas to the more peripheral airways is achieved at relatively slow flow rates, but if the patient is very short of breath and has a fast respiratory rate, a slow inspiratory phase may be unacceptable. It is often useful to alter the flow control several times during a single treatment session, providing slow breaths during the periods attempting to mobilize peripheral secretions and a faster flow rate when a patient is recovering his

breath after expectoration. Some Bennett positive pressure ventilators do not require flow rate adjustment because automatic variable flow is provided with each breath. This feature is known as 'flow sensitivity' and means that the flow of the inspired gas adapts to the resistance of the individual's airways.

Nebulizer.   An efficient nebulizer in the circuit is necessary to humidify the driving gas and, when appropriate, to deliver bronchodilator drugs.

Air-mix control.   When driven by oxygen, air must be entrained by the apparatus to provide an air/oxygen mixture for the patient. Some Bird ventilator devices have a control that should be set to give a mixture, while others have no control but automatically entrain air. The use of 100% oxygen for a patient is very rare and when it is indicated, an IPPB device with an air-mix control will be needed. When air is not entrained through the apparatus, the flow rate control must be regulated to provide an adequate flow to the patient.

When IPPB (a Bird ventilator) is driven by oxygen and the air-mix control is in use, the percentage of oxygen delivered to the patient is approximately 45% (Starke et al 1979). This percentage will be considerably higher than the controlled percentage delivered by an appropriate Venturi mask, for example to a patient with chronic bronchitis. This higher percentage is rarely dangerous during treatment because the patient's ventilation is assisted and the removal of secretions as a result of treatment is likely to lead subsequently to an improvement in arterial blood gas tensions (Gormezano & Branthwaite 1972).

It has been suggested that a few patients become more drowsy during or after IPPB as a result of the high percentage of oxygen received. Starke et al (1979) showed that increased drowsiness caused by hypercapnia occurred whether oxygen or air was the driving gas for IPPB and that the deterioration was dependent on inappropriate settings of the ventilator. The pressure and flow controls must be set to provide an adequate tidal volume, this being particularly important when treating patients with a rigid thoracic cage (Starke et al 1979).

Occasionally, IPPB may be powered by Entonox and in this case the air-mix control would need to be in the position to provide 100% of the driving gas with no additional air entrained.

Breathing circuit. To prevent cross-infection it is essential for each patient to have his own breathing circuit, which consists of tubing, nebulizer, exhalation valve and a mouthpiece or mask. The majority of patients prefer to use a mouthpiece, but a facemask is required when treating confused patients. A flange mouthpiece (Fig. 5.57) is useful for patients who have difficulty making an airtight seal around the mouthpiece.

The type of breathing circuit used will depend on local infection control guidelines. The circuits can be autoclavable, non-disposable but non-autoclavable, or disposable. Many countries use single patient disposable circuits.

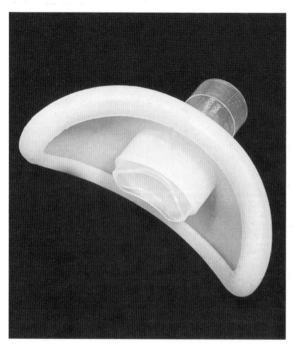

Figure 5.57 Flange mouthpiece for use with IPPB.

Preparation of the apparatus

1. Normal saline solution or the drug to be nebulized (3–4 ml in total) is inserted into the nebulizer chamber.
2. The breathing circuit is connected to the IPPB ventilator and the ventilator connected to the driving gas source. It can be used from an oxygen or air cylinder if piped compressed gas is unavailable.
3. If there is an air-mix control, this should be in the position for entrainment of air.
4. If there is an automatic control (expiratory timer) this should be turned off to allow the patient to 'trigger' the machine at his desired rate.
5. The sensitivity, flow and pressure controls are set appropriately for the individual. With the Bird Mark 7 the sensitivity control is usually adjusted to a low number (5–7) where minimal inspiratory effort is required. The pressure and flow controls are adjusted to provide regular assisted ventilation without discomfort. A patient with a rigid rib cage will require a higher pressure setting to obtain an adequate tidal volume than someone with a more mobile rib cage. When adjusting the settings for a new patient, it may be easiest to start with a pressure at approximately 12 cmH$_2$O and the flow at about '10', then gradually increase the pressure and reduce the flow until the pattern of breathing is the most appropriate for the individual. Some IPPB devices do not have numbered markings, but after finding the most effective settings for a patient during one treatment, it is useful to note the positions of the controls in order to use these as a starting point at the next treatment. The controls to be set on the Bennett PR-1 are the nebulizer, sensitivity and pressure.
6. Before starting a treatment, the hand triggering device is operated to check that there are no leaks in the breathing circuit and that the nebulizer is functioning well.

Treatment of the patient

The position in which IPPB is used depends on the indication for treatment. It may be used in side lying, high side lying or in the sitting position. The patient should be positioned comfortably and encouraged to relax the upper chest and shoulder girdle.

After the purpose of the IPPB treatment has been explained, the patient is asked to close his lips firmly around the mouthpiece and then to make a slight inspiratory effort, which will trigger the device into inspiratory flow. The patient should then relax throughout inspiration, allowing his lungs to be inflated. When the preset pressure is reached at the mouth the ventilator cycles into expiration; the patient should remain relaxed and let the air out quietly.

If the patient attempts to assist inspiration there will be a delay in reaching the cycling pressure. A delay will also occur if there is a leak around the mouthpiece, at any of the circuit connections or from the patient's nose. A nose clip may be required until the patient becomes familiar with the technique.

Observation of the manometer on the ventilator should allow detection of any faults in the patient's technique. At the start of inspiration the needle should swing minimally to a negative pressure and then swing smoothly up to the positive pressure set, before cutting out into expiration and returning to zero. A larger negative swing at the beginning of inspiration shows that the patient is making an unnecessary effort in triggering the device. If the patient makes an active effort throughout inspiration, the needle will rise very slowly to the inspiratory set pressure and if they attempt to start expiration before the preset pressure is reached, the needle will rise sharply above the set pressure and then cut out into expiration.

When IPPB is taught correctly the work of breathing is relieved, but if the patient is allowed to assist either inspiration or expiration there may be an increase in the work of breathing.

A short pause between completion of expiration and the next inspiration avoids hyperventilation and possible dizziness. Occasionally children using IPPB tend to swallow air during treatment. It is important to observe the size of the abdomen before and during IPPB to rec-ognize signs of abdominal distension and discontinue treatment if this occurs.

When IPPB is used to relieve the work of breathing while delivering bronchodilator therapy, for example in the acute severe asthmatic patient, it is often helpful for the physiotherapist to hold the breathing circuit to allow the patient to relax the shoulders and arms as much as possible (Fig. 5.58).

A facemask for IPPB is used in the drowsy or confused patient and in those with facial weakness unable to make an airtight seal at the mouth. When using IPPB to assist in mobilizing secretions, the patient should be appropriately positioned to assist loosening and mobilization of secretions, for example in side lying. The patient's jaw should be elevated and the mask held firmly over the face, ensuring an airtight fit. Chest shaking during the expiratory phase may be used to assist in mobilizing secretions. In a drowsy patient it may be necessary to stimulate coughing using nasotracheal suction if spontaneous coughing is not stimulated by IPPB and chest shaking.

In medical patients with retained secretions and poor respiratory reserve, IPPB may be useful both to mobilize secretions and to relieve the effort of breathing following expectoration. The flow control on a Bird ventilator should be adjusted to give a slow, comfortable breath to mobilize secretions, but following the exertion of expectoration there may be an increase in respiratory requirements, which may necessitate increasing the flow and possibly reducing the pressure until the breathing effort and pattern return to normal or baseline.

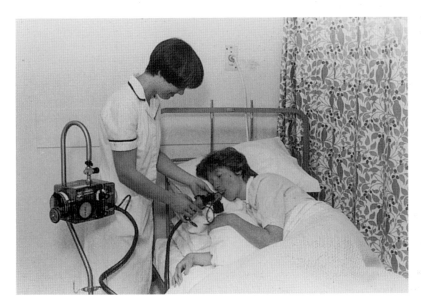

Figure 5.58 IPPB to reduce the work of breathing during inhalation of nebulized bronchodilator.

5

IPPB may be used in patients with chest wall deformity, for example kyphoscoliosis (Sinha & Bergofsky 1972), when there is difficulty with clearing secretions during an infective episode. To achieve an adequate increase in ventilation in patients with a rigid rib cage, the pressure setting needs to be higher than for a more mobile rib cage.

Occasionally, in postoperative patients, IPPB is the adjunct of choice when the patient is unable to augment tidal volume adequately during treatment. In these patients, in contrast to the relaxed technique normally used with IPPB, thoracic expansion may be actively encouraged during the inspiratory phase.

Contraindications for IPPB

- Pneumothorax.

- Large bullae.

- Lung abscess, as the size of the air space may increase.

- Severe haemoptysis, as treatment is inappropriate until the bleeding has lessened.

- Postoperative air leak, unless the advantages of IPPB would outweigh the possibility of increasing the air leak during treatment.

- Bronchial tumour in the proximal airways. Air may flow past the tumour during inspiration and may be trapped on expiration as the airways narrow. There would be no contraindication if the tumour were situated peripherally.

MANUAL HYPERINFLATION

The technique of manual hyperinflation may be indicated to mobilize and assist clearance of excess bronchial secretions and to reinflate areas of lung collapse in the intubated patient. It is described in Chapter 8.

MANUAL THERAPY TECHNIQUES

Musculoskeletal dysfunction is common in people with respiratory disease. People with chronic cardiorespiratory disease may often demonstrate skeletal, musculoskeletal and nervous systems adaptations over time, related to the severity and management of their disease. As age increases the incidence of musculoskeletal deterioration will also increase (Parasa & Maffulli 1999). Any postural or degenerative changes are likely to have implications for physical function and quality of life as well as influencing the cardiorespiratory system.

Postural and skeletal changes occurring over time relate to the overuse of upper chest breathing patterns,

lack of lower rib expansion and reduction in the more efficient pattern of diaphragmatic breathing. Chronic hyperinflation typically leads to the development of a barrel-shaped chest with an increase in the anteroposterior diameter of the chest. Pain may limit rib expansion and abdominal breathing, particularly in patients following abdominal surgery.

Secondary malalignment of the scapulae is associated with prolonged coughing using trunk flexion and the increased outward pressure on the chest wall. More sputum may mean more pain and less efficient airway clearance (Massery 2005).

In a study of 143 young adults with cystic fibrosis, Henderson and Specter (1994) found 77% of females and 36% of males over 15 years of age had a kyphosis of more than 40° (the upper limit of normal). Kyphosis tends to worsen with age and disease severity (Massie et al 1998).

The neck and shoulder girdle structures adapt to counterbalance the flexed trunk sitting position. Neutral neck and head position is compromised as the neck and head are drawn forwards by the large superficial muscle groups and hyperactivity of the suboccipital extensors. The greater the thoracic kyphosis, the more likely it is that the middle and upper cervical regions will become lordotic, as the upper cervical spine hyperextends and tilts the head upward to maintain a vertical orientation of the face.

This upper cervical spine hyperextension and forward head posture combine, with a loss of endurance of the deep cervical flexor muscles, to increase the likelihood of cervicogenic headache (Jull et al 2002, Watson & Trott 1993). Chronic headaches may also be associated with medical causes in patients with cardiorespiratory disease (Festini et al 2004, Ravilly et al 1996).

The incidence of musculoskeletal chest pain in people with cystic fibrosis tends to increase as the disease progresses. Painful stiffness in the chest may inhibit airway clearance and increase the work of breathing (Massery 2005). A decrease in muscle strength and mobility in the trunk, chest and shoulders has been demonstrated in people with cystic fibrosis (Ross et al 1987).

In the presence of an inefficient, upper chest breathing pattern, the overactive scalene muscles elevate the first and second ribs while the levator scapulae depress and rotate the lateral shoulder girdle (Fig. 5.59). Shortening of upper trapezius and tightness of pectoralis minor and major elevate and anteriorly tilt the scapulae, respectively. At the same time the antagonist and stabilizing muscles, serratus anterior and the middle and lower fibres of trapezius, lengthen and weaken, causing winging and inferior rotation of the scapulae (Sahrmann 2005). Over time the long thoracic extensors and multifidus lose their segmental stabilizing capacity and

5

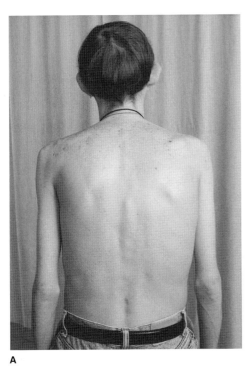
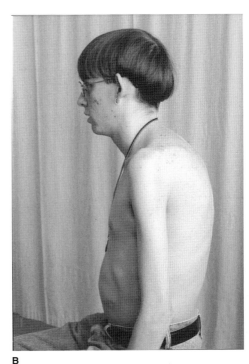

A   **B**

Figure 5.59   CJ, aged 16, cystic fibrosis. **(A)** Relaxed sitting posture (posterior view). **Note:** forward head position, tight suboccipital and mid-cervical extensors, tight upper and middle fibres of trapezius, asymmetry and abducted and protracted position of the scapulae, increased thoracic kyphosis, reduced upper lumbar lordosis, posterior rotation of pelvis. **(B)** Relaxed sitting posture (side view). **Note:** forward head position, increased sternocleidomastoid activity, increased low cervical lordosis and thoracic kyphosis, abducted and protracted scapulae, anterior position of humerus in glenoid fossa, internal rotation of humerus, lax abdominal muscles.

endurance, and become less able to sustain the upright sitting neutral posture.

The sternocleidomastoids are used excessively during coughing. Muscle fatigue related to the excess work of breathing may further accentuate poor posture in people with moderate to severe chronic lung disease. The existing kyphosis of the thoracic spine is increased due to prolonged bed rest and reductions in general exercise tolerance. Habitual slouching due to dyspnoea and feeling unwell will place more kyphotic strain on the thoracic and lumbar spines, and the lumbopelvic angle will be flexed instead of lordotic.

Vertebral intersegmental motion will be gradually lost as the chest becomes fixed in elevation and flexion. Reduced range of thoracic extension will contribute to loss of the final 30 degrees of shoulder flexion and abduction; while tightness in anterior deltoid, teres major and latissimus dorsi muscles and disturbance of normal scapulothoracic rhythm will decrease the free range of external rotation and flexion available at the glenohumeral joint. As a consequence the overstretch-

ing of infraspinatus and teres minor, associated with the internally rotated position of the humerus, may lead to poor stability of the humerus in the glenoid fossa (Fig. 5.60).

These muscular and skeletal aberrations are likely to have consequences on the range and quality of pelvic position in sitting, neck and shoulder motion, and both general and specific trunk and shoulder movement and function. In particular they cause a physical limit to the end range of shoulder elevation and an alteration in muscle recruitment likely to increase the risk of shoulder tendon impingement and wear.

Individuals with respiratory disease may complain of acute or chronic cervical, thoracic or rib joint pain, which may decrease chest expansion as measured by a reduction in vital capacity. Joint manifestations (mainly hypertrophic osteoarthropathy) are common in children with cystic fibrosis, affecting 2–8.5% of patients (Botton et al 2003, Parasa & Maffulli 1999). Back pain may be due to cystic fibrosis-related arthropy, arthritis due to coexistent conditions or drug reactions as well as the

5

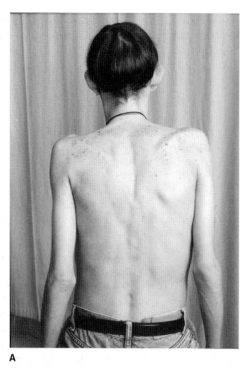
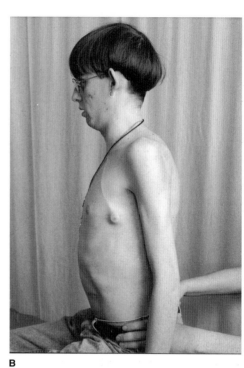

A   **B**

Figure 5.60   (**A**) Sitting posture (posterior view) following active assisted anterior rotation of pelvis. **Note:** decreased mid-cervical lordosis, improved position of scapulae, reduced thoracic kyphosis, neutral rotation of pelvis and improved lumbar lordosis. (**B**) Sitting posture (side view) following active assisted anterior rotation of pelvis. **Note:** less forward head position, activation of deep cervical flexors, reduced sternocleidomastoid activity, improved scapulae and humeral position and thoracic kyphosis.

more obvious mechanical reasons. Mechanical back pain in people with cystic fibrosis has been described in the literature, but the incidence and prevalence have not been reliably established for the different age groups.

With increasing longevity in people with cystic fibrosis, musculoskeletal changes will become more important. Decreased bone mineral density is common at all ages but further reduction tends to occur with time, increasing illness and adverse effects of medication. With an increased emphasis on encouraging general exercise to improve respiratory and general health and bone density, musculoskeletal problems may become more prevalent, requiring careful monitoring (Buntain et al 2004).

With chronic respiratory disease, fracture rates are reported to be approximately twice as high in women aged 16 to 32 years and the same increase is observed at a slightly later stage in men (Parasa & Maffulli 1999). Low bone mineral density is related to poor nutrition, reduced weight bearing, resistive muscle activity and the use of corticosteroids (Aris et al 1998, Bachrach et al 1994, Henderson & Madsen 1996). The combination of

vertebral wedging, soft tissue contractures, poor posture and coughing may also cause persistent back pain in these patients (Fok et al 2002).

There is a high prevalence of acute episodes of pain in adults with cystic fibrosis (Festini et al 2004). As children with chest pain and cystic fibrosis are more likely to have a lower FEV_1 per cent predicted and poorer quality of life, the assessment of musculoskeletal pain in this client group should be routine (Koh et al 2005).

Pain may restrict the ability to attain an upright posture and to use an efficient muscle pattern. Tensioning or compression of the neural tissues, as they exit from the cervical spine and proceed through the axilla, may also occur in some individuals (Butler 1991) associated with chronic overuse of the accessory muscles of respiration, elevated first rib and a depressed lateral shoulder girdle.

Subjective assessment

Assessment of those with chronic respiratory disease, or following heart or chest surgery, should include questioning regarding headache, neck, thoracic or lumbar pain and any upper limb pain or distal arm paraesthesia. The use of valid and reliable outcome measures improves evaluation of the effect of treatment. The area of pain can be recorded on a body chart and the intensity quantified using an absolute visual analogue scale (AVAS). The impact of any pain or movement restriction on activities of daily living may be assessed using a functional disability scale (e.g. Neck Disability Index (Vernon & Mior 1991), Shoulder, Arm and Hand Disability Index (Institute for Work & Health 1996) or headache questionnaire (Niere & Jerak 2004)). Individual involvement in the identification of treatment goals and expectations will enable clearer planning and prioritization. In those with dyspnoea, it will be helpful to quantify dyspnoea intensity using an AVAS or Borg scale (Pfeiffer et al 2002) before any postural correction or treatment. Questioning about the behaviour of musculoskeletal pain, during the night and in the morning, will help to clarify the degree of inflammation involved. Headache may be multifactorial in origin and may be related to upper cervical spine dysfunction or to various other physiological and biochemical changes.

Activities that aggravate the problem may include sustained end-range postures of the neck or thoracic spine, trunk movements which require a reversal of the thoracic kyphosis or activities involving shoulder elevation. Repetitive coughing will load the costotransverse joints and may result in localized pain. Additionally, the increased abdominal pressure related to persistent cough may result in increased lumbar disc pressure and rupture, while the repetitive flexion and extension of the spine during coughing may aggravate existing cervical pathology or dysfunction.

Physical assessment: posture

Musculoskeletal assessment should proceed in a systematic manner from evaluation of posture to assessment of joint mobility, muscle recruitment patterns, muscle length, strength and endurance, keeping in mind the specific function loss or pain area and type reported. Any change in symptoms during assessment should be noted. In particular any improvement in pain when posture is modified may assist motivation to change.

In the presence of chronic respiratory disease, the physiotherapist will need to keep in mind the possibility of reduced bone density and fragile skin tissue related to age or the long-term use of systemic steroids. Pain, dyspnoea and fatigue will also need to be monitored concurrently and the assessment adjusted as necessary. The presence of wound and drain sites in the postsurgical patient may require modified assessment positions. While the assessment is ideally performed in sitting,

supine and prone, examination of those with dyspnoea may need to be conducted in semi-supine, sitting or high side lying.

With the individual in relaxed sitting, the following should be noted:

1. The relaxed posture of the pelvis, lumbar, thoracic and cervical spines
2. The point of maximal curve of each of these segments
3. Whether the spinal posture is fixed or able to be corrected
4. The position of the scapulae and the location of the humeral head within the glenoid
5. The posture of the neck and head and alignment with the trunk and pelvis.

If it is possible to assist the pelvis to roll anteriorly to move the body weight on to the ischial tuberosities, note whether the thoracic kyphosis, cervical lordosis and head forward position all automatically improve (Fig. 5.60). Is the lumbosacral flexed position able to be reversed as the pelvis is assisted to roll forward? The cervical spine and the head may need to be guided to move the centre of gravity of the body over the pelvis and the head placed in a less protracted position to assess the reversibility of the resting posture. The inability to maintain this corrected position will indicate the extent of loss of endurance of the postural muscles.

Observe where the scapulae are resting and how the arms are hanging in standing and then in sitting. Usually if the position of the pelvis and spine is faulty, the scapulae will be elevated or dropped, protracted and winging with either upward or downward rotation. This 'weak' position of the scapulae means that stress will be transferred to the shoulder and neck joint structures during overhead activities. Arm elevation will also be weak. If the arms rest in an internally rotated position, this will interfere with smooth coordinated arm elevation and increase the risk of shoulder tendon impingement.

Physical assessment: range of motion

Total range of thoracic motion is dependent on the mobility of the apophyseal, costovertebral, costotransverse joints and ribs and in particular the extensibility of the intercostal, pectoralis and latissimus dorsi muscles. Stiffness in the upper thoracic spine may be indicated by an inability to reverse the kyphosis on request or during cervical extension and shoulder abduction. A flattened or lordotic area in the mid-thoracic region usually indicates hypomobility (Boyling & Palastanga 1994). People with chronic respiratory disease and breathlessness are often unable to lie flat during the night, due to difficulty breathing and/or

5

persistent coughing, and the spine is not rested in extension.

The major portion of thoracic rotation is expected to be in the middle thoracic spine (T6 to T8) (Gregersen & Lucas 1967) with lateral flexion occurring as a conjunct movement (White & Panjabi 1990). During lateral flexion the ribs should flare and spread on the contralateral side and approximate on the ipsilateral side (Boyling & Palastanga 1994).

The end-feel of normal thoracic rotation is springy due to limitation by ligamentous tissue and joint capsules. Age or postural changes at the costovertebral joints may restrict rib motion and lead to a harder end-feel (Nathan 1962). Gentle overpressure applied at end-range will assist determination of the quality of restriction, but overpressure should be used with caution if the risk of osteoporosis or existing fracture is suspected.

During spinal flexion, the inferior facets of the apophyseal joint of the superior vertebra normally glide superoanteriorly on the facets of the inferior vertebra. In extension the reverse movement occurs. Although the initial limitation to extension is from the anterior ligaments, the anterior annulus and the posterior longitudinal ligament, the normal end-feel is one of bony impingement as the inferior articular facets contact the lamina of the caudad vertebrae (White & Panjabi 1990). The mobility of the upper and middle ribs may be assessed by palpating bilaterally anteriorly and posteriorly during a deep inspiration; the lower ribs are assessed by palpating laterally during a full cycle of inspiration and expiration (Lee 2003).

The range of glenohumeral rotation will depend on the resting position of the humerus and tightness of the anterior and posterior shoulder capsule and muscles. During normal bilateral shoulder flexion and abduction the thoracic spine extends (particularly in the younger age group). Any restriction in the range of thoracic lateral flexion and rotation will limit the range of unilateral shoulder elevation (Boyling & Palastanga 1994). Shortened or overactive latissimus dorsi and teres major will add further limitation.

Observing posteriorly during shoulder elevation should enable assessment of any abnormal patterns of muscle recruitment. The upper trapezius and levator scapulae muscles, sternocleidomastoid and the scalenes tend to be overactive in people with respiratory disease while the deep upper cervical and scapular stabilizers will be underactive (Fig. 5.61). Abnormal scapulohumeral rhythm is usually most obvious as shoulder movement is initiated and then again towards the end of range. Assessing passive shoulder motion in supine (or half sitting in those with dyspnoea) will enable better differentiation between scapulohumeral and scapulo-

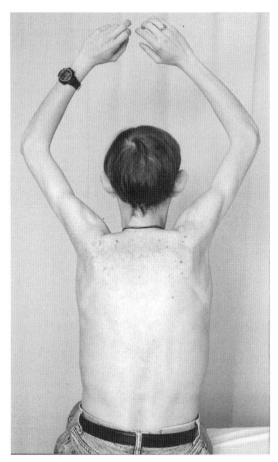

Figure 5.61 Shoulder abduction. **Note:** overactivity of upper trapezius, poor reversal of thoracic kyphosis, abducted, protracted and rotated scapulae, shortened teres major and latissimus dorsi and absence of lower trapezius activity.

thoracic motions. The excursion, strength and endurance of specific muscle groups identified as overactive or underactive need to be examined individually, in order to determine the relationship of movement impairment to pain and disability. Neural tissue provocation tests (Butler 1991) and tests for reflexes, power and sensation should be performed if any arm or hand pain or paraesthesia is reported. Thoracic outlet disorder may develop in the chronic respiratory disease due to the fixed and limited posture of the neck and upper body structures.

Physiotherapy management

Prioritization of the main problems needs to be identified before treatment is started; the severity of musculoskeletal and cardiorespiratory dysfunction and the chronicity of the pain and disability need to be assessed. The time available and ability to perform home treatment techniques need to be considered in the choice of technique and in estimated prognosis.

Postural correction and motor control training

Postural correction may change the breathing pattern and the intensity of dyspnoea. These factors need to be monitored carefully during treatment. As the individual becomes familiar with the gentle effort required to activate the correct muscles, oxygen consumption may be reduced. Adherence to a home exercise programme will be improved if a direct link can be demonstrated between improvement in posture and relief of pain or shortness of breath.

The 'ideal' posture is one where the body is positioned so that the spine, pelvic and shoulder girdle are in their neutral zone allowing the muscles to work in the most efficient manner. In the ideal posture the deep neck flexors, lower trapezius, transversus abdominus, gluteus medius and the pelvic floor will be softly activated milliseconds before the movement is begun.

Posture may be improved by educating awareness of positioning of the pelvis in sitting and the use of more efficient movement patterns using visual, auditory and sensory feedback. Postural correction utilizes motor learning with training of the holding ability of the postural stabilizers, while avoiding substitution by the stronger prime movers (White & Sahrmann 1994). The principles of motor control require frequent gentle repetition of the corrected movement or position. The initial focus should be on correcting any posterior pelvic rotation in sitting and on reducing the lumbar and thoracic kyphosis to bring the head back over the trunk. A small pillow or lumbar roll may then be used to maintain this position. If necessary, postural correction can be started in semi-supine or high side lying and then incorporated into maintenance of corrected posture during specific activities. The use of the diaphragm, abdominal and neck shoulder muscles will need to be monitored and changed if inappropriate.

Mobilization techniques

Physiotherapy management of joint restriction and pain may include passive mobilizations of cervical and thoracic apophyseal, costotransverse, costochondral and sternochondral joints and the glenohumeral joint (Bray 1994, Vibekk 1991). Manipulation is usually contraindicated. The focus of treatment will most commonly be on improving the range and quality of thoracic extension and rotation and on increasing the mobility of the ribs. Positioning during treatment will need to be carefully selected to minimize dyspnoea or pain. Specific joint restrictions may be treated with passive mobilization techniques in static positions or functional movements, and then optimally followed by active assisted or active exercises. General techniques to the upper, mid or lower regions of the spine or localized techniques to a specific vertebral level or rib can be performed in sitting, forward lean sitting or in high side lying (Lee 2003) (Figs 5.62, 5.63). Mobilization of the ribs may be performed in side lying, with the upper arm elevated to stretch the intercostal muscles or in sitting, using active shoulder abduction combined with lateral flexion. In forward lean sitting with the head and arms supported on pillows, the rib cage will be free to move during mobilization techniques.

Active or passive bilateral arm flexion and spine extension may be combined with deep inspiration and expiration to improve rib mobility. In sitting, the active extension or rotation can be performed while the therapist assists the movement to encourage an increase in range. Self-mobilizations can be performed over the back of a chair, in four-point kneel or leaning against a

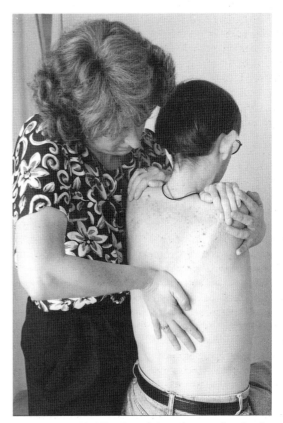

Figure 5.62 Mobilization of thoracic extension. Passive or active assisted, with fulcrum at T8.

5

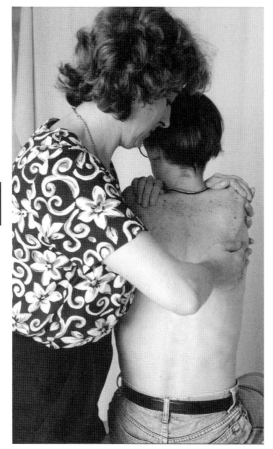

Figure 5.63 Mobilization of thoracic rotation. Passive or active assisted, with posteroanterior pressure on ribs 7 and 8.

wall using a rolled towel for localization (Fig. 5.64). Home mobilization exercises will be necessary if the respiratory condition is chronic and the musculoskeletal dysfunction long term. A mirror, or training a family member, will assist self-treatment and provide helpful feedback.

Following surgery via sternotomy or thoracotomy, specific gentle passive mobilizations of the sternocostal joints or costotransverse joints may be required, if localized painful limitation of shoulder or thoracic movement or pain on breathing are present. Following thoracotomy, patients may tend to immobilize the arm on the side of the incision and need to be encouraged to move within pain limits as early as possible to reduce the risk of frozen shoulder. The scapula may be taken through its range of protraction, retraction, elevation and depression while the patient is in side lying. Bilateral arm movements are preferred in the early stage

following surgery, initially avoiding abduction and external rotation to reduce stress on the scar.

The long-term ventilated patient may also develop musculoskeletal problems. Routine passive mobilization of the shoulder through its full range of flexion, external rotation and abduction should be mandatory. Lateral flexion and extension of the thoracic spine can be performed via arm elevation when in side lying. Gentle passive rotation of the thoracic spine can also be performed in this position with the upper arm resting on the lateral chest wall.

Muscle–lengthening techniques

Stretching of tight muscle groups may precede or accompany endurance training of the lengthened muscle groups (Janda 1994). Stretching of the anterior deltoid and pectoralis major muscles, using a proprioceptive neuromuscular facilitation hold–relax technique, has been shown to increase vital capacity and shoulder range of movement (Putt & Paratz 1996). Other muscles that may require careful stretching are: sternocleido-mastoid, the scalenes, upper and middle fibres of trapezius, levator scapulae, pectoralis minor, teres major, latissimus dorsi, subscapularis and the suboccipital extensors (Table 5.2). Sustained stretches may be facilitated by conscious or reflex relaxation of the muscle during exhalation. Hold–relax techniques using the agonist or contract-relax techniques using the antagonist of the shortened muscle (White & Sahrmann 1994) may augment sustained stretches and myofascial release massage along the line of the muscle fibres. Where possible, individuals should be taught to perform their own stretches and mobilizations as part of long-term maintenance.

Taping

Taping of the scapula in a more neutral position, or of the thoracic spine in a reduced kyphosis, may temporarily unload the affected tissue to gain pain relief and facilitate healing. It will also provide a feeling as to which posture will assist pain reduction of the thoracic kyphosis and what may need to be assisted until the holding capacity of the thoracic extensors and lower fibres of trapezius has been improved. Strapping tape (over anti-allergy tape), applied in the corrected sitting, may give proprioceptive feedback in the early stages of retraining. It is important to ensure comfort and that cervical motion is freer following taping. Appropriate warnings and instructions regarding removal of the tape should be given.

There are many different approaches to taping. A long piece of tape starting anteriorly above the clavicle and crossing the mid-fibres of trapezius may inhibit overactivity of this muscle. The tape is then crossed over

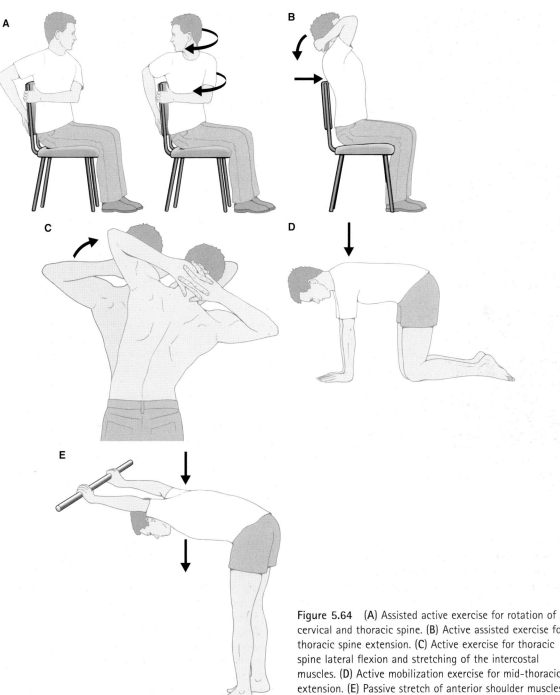

Figure 5.64   (**A**) Assisted active exercise for rotation of cervical and thoracic spine. (**B**) Active assisted exercise for thoracic spine extension. (**C**) Active exercise for thoracic spine lateral flexion and stretching of the intercostal muscles. (**D**) Active mobilization exercise for mid-thoracic extension. (**E**) Passive stretch of anterior shoulder muscles and mobilization of thoracic extension.

5

Table 5.2   Assessment of muscle length

Muscle	Observation if muscle tight	Length testing position
Pectoralis major	Internal rotation and anterior translation of the humerus	Horizontal extension and abduction to 140°
Pectoralis minor	Anterior and inferior position of coracoid process and elevation of ribs 3–5	Retraction and depression of scapula
Upper cervical extensors	Forward position of head on neck, increased upper cervical lordosis	Flexion of the head on the upper cervical spine
Upper trapezius	Elevation of scapula, palpable anterior border of trapezius (occiput to distal clavicle)	Cervical flexion with contralateral lateral flexion and ipsilateral rotation
Levator scapula	Increased muscle bulk anterior to upper trapezius and posterior to sternocleidomastoid from C2–4 to superior angle of scapula	Cervical flexion, contralateral lateral flexion and contralateral rotation, keeping the medial superior scapula border depressed
Sternocleidomastoid	Forward position of head on neck, elevated 1st rib and prominence at the clavicular insertion of sternocleidomastoid	Upper cervical flexion with lower cervical extension
Anterior scalenes	Elevation of ribs 1–3, ipsilateral lateral flexion of head on neck	Exhalation with depression of ribs 1–3 and upper cervical flexion
Latissimus dorsi	Internal rotation of humerus	Elevation of shoulder in external rotation with posterior pelvic tilt
Teres major	Medial rotation of humerus, protracted and upward rotation of scapula	Flex shoulder while sustaining scapular retraction and depression
Diaphragm	Flexed thorax and localized lordosis at the thoracolumbar junction	Relaxed diaphragmatic breathing

at the peak of the thoracic kyphosis and extended down to the lumbar spine if necessary. It should not be so firm that pain is produced or neural symptoms provoked. A horizontal tape to lift the lateral edge of the acromion and a tape around the inferior border of the scapula to facilitate serratus anterior action may both help. Tape under the axilla to lift the scapula and relieve neural tension may also assist pain reduction, but care needs to be taken with the sensitive skin of the axilla. All taping should be designed and applied related to the individual's specific and individual needs. Retesting range of motion and pain on aggravating movements will allow direct appraisal of the effectiveness of taping. Warnings regarding possible skin reaction and pain provocation should be given.

Muscle retraining (strength and endurance)

Training of scapular retraction and depression using middle and lower fibres of trapezius is important to complement any gain in range of thoracic extension and to improve scapular stability (Fig. 5.65). The holding capacity of the deep upper cervical flexors and cervico-thoracic extensors will need to be trained to reduce the degree of forward head posture and to assist relaxation of sternocleidomastoid and the scalene muscles (Table 5.3). The longus colli and rectus capitus anterior major may be trained initially in high sitting, then progressed to supine if shortness of breath allows (Fig. 5.66). Alternatively, gentle nodding of the head on neck against slight self-applied resistance using the thumb can be taught in sitting. The serratus anterior action of holding the scapula against the chest wall will be improved with training using a half push-up action against a wall (taking care that upper trapezius is not overactive) (O'Leary et al 2007).

A gym ball may be useful for encouraging a more upright sitting posture in younger clients. Prone positions over the ball may be used to stimulate

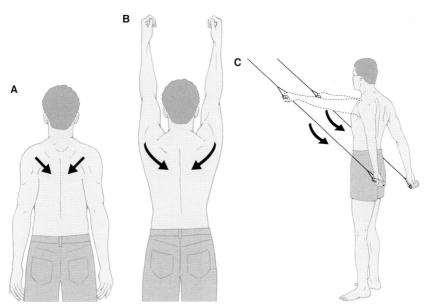

Figure 5.65 (A) Active scapulae retraction/depression (rhomboids, middle and lower trapezius). (B) Active scapulae retraction/depression in shoulder elevation. (C) Active scapulae retraction/depression in shoulder extension.

Table 5.3 Assessment of holding capacity of lengthened muscles	
Muscle	**Test position**
Deep upper cervical flexors	Half supine, nodding of head on neck. Test holding ability
Middle and lower trapezius	With patient prone (or sitting if short of breath), test holding ability by placing scapula in retraction and depression and asking patient to hold
Serratus anterior	Note ability to maintain scapula against chest wall during a partial push-up against a wall
Infraspinatus	Test strength of external rotation

the antigravity muscles. Side lying over the ball will assist with rib mobility and stretching of the intercostal muscles if mobility and shortness of breath allow. Thera-Band® can be used to apply resistance to weak motion and to give more specific directional feedback.

Neural tissue techniques

When neural tissue provocation tests reveal irritation or restriction, the primary aim of treatment will be to mobilize the tight adjacent structures and improve posture to reduce load on the sensitive tissues. The effect on the neural system should be monitored during and after treatment. If progress is inadequate, gentle mobilization (not stretching) of the neural tissues at the site of restriction may be required.

Summary

People with chronic respiratory disease may have postural dysfunction and musculoskeletal pathology in addition to their cardiothoracic disease. Early identification of disability and musculoskeletal limitations will provide the physiotherapist with the opportunity to teach preventative strategies and enable early, more effective intervention. Postural awareness and education with a home mobilizing and strengthening programme may be usefully included in a holistic home programme.

Clinical research is required to evaluate whether the musculoskeletal complications described in this section can be prevented or minimized by an early intervention programme, and whether improving the function of the

5

5

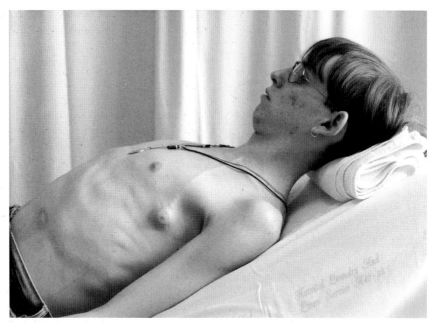

Figure 5.66 Position for training activation of deep upper cervical flexors and lower trapezius and for stretching of upper cervical extensors and pectoralis minor and major.

musculoskeletal system has a positive effect on respiratory function.

NEUROPHYSIOLOGICAL FACILITATION OF RESPIRATION

The respiration of mammals involves a ventilatory system in which the essential part, the lung, effects exchange between the surrounding air and the blood. Even though this organ is richly supplied with nerves, it does not have an autonomous function. It undertakes this task by the conjoint action of two elements, the rib cage and the diaphragm, which form the chamber enclosing it (Duron & Rose 1997).

Breathing is a complex behaviour. It is governed by a variety of regulating mechanisms under the control of large parts of the central nervous system. Ongoing research into the respiratory ventilatory system (rib cage and diaphragm) has dramatically altered traditional understanding of the respiratory muscles and their neural control. The motor synergy of respiration includes the major and accessory respiratory muscles and motoneuron pools from the level of the fifth cranial nerve down to the upper lumbar segments (Euler 1986).

Respiratory rhythmicity, as with other rhythmical repetitive motor actions (i.e. locomotion and mastica-

tion), is supported in the central nervous system by a central pattern generator (CPG). CPGs are neuronal networks capable of generating the characteristic rhythmic patterns in the complete absence of extrinsic reflexes and feedback loops (Atwood & MacKay 1989, Euler 1986, Gordon 1991). However, in order to adapt the ventilatory system to prevailing and anticipated needs and to achieve coordination with the cardiovascular system, breathing is regulated by a multitude of reflexes, negative feedback circuits and feedforward mechanisms (Ainsworth 1997, Euler 1986, Koepchen et al 1986).

The purpose of this discussion is to assist the integration of evidence from biological research with clinical practice and to consider the implications of models of respiratory neural control for clinical work. Much biological research now validates empirical practices of earlier years. For example, research into the function of the abdominal muscles now supports empirical practices of the 1940s and 1950s, when abdominal supports were used to assist those with emphysema (Alvarez et al 1981, De Troyer 1997, Grassino 1974). The present models of the neural control of respiration, with their emphasis on the roles of spinal neurons and on the importance of afferent (sensory) input, provide further biological support for neurophysiological facilitation procedures, i.e. clinical use of selective afferent input in respiratory care.

Neurophysiological facilitation of respiration is the use of selective external proprioceptive and tactile stimuli that produce reflexive movement responses in the ventilatory apparatus to assist respiration. The responses they elicit appear to alter the rate and depth of breathing and can be demonstrated to occur in other mammals (dogs) as well as in humans (Bethune 1975, 1976). These procedures are particularly useful in the chest care of the unconscious patient and of the conscious postsurgical patient who frequently find that the reflexive nature of the respiratory movements reduces the perception of pain (Bethune 1991).

Neural control

Research on ventilatory muscle control presently places considerable emphasis on spinal respiratory motoneurons and their controlling or modifying influence on central respiratory programmes. One of the newer theoretical models of the functional organization of the neural control of breathing identifies three major central nervous system levels: suprabulbar mechanisms, bulbar mechanisms and spinal motoneuron pools and integrating mechanisms (Euler 1986) (Fig. 5.67).

Based on a similar model, Miller et al (1997) have considered the many neural structures that can potentially modify the final output of the ventilatory muscles.

Input from peripheral sensory structures (proprioceptive, cutaneous, vagal and chemoceptive) and from a variety of brain regions (cerebral cortex, pons, cerebellum and others) is all integrated in the premotor bulbospinal respiratory neurons. Adjustments to the respiratory control of these multifunctional muscles occurs in order to support their many non-respiratory behaviours including speech, swallowing, coughing, vomiting. The motoneuron pools that drive these multifunctional ventilatory muscles are subjected to changes in activity pattern due to their control by the neuronal networks, recruited on the basis of the different incoming stimuli. The spinal respiratory motoneurons are the final common pathway. They determine the output of the major respiratory muscles including their 'rhythmic breath-by-breath respiratory drive'. The actions of the ventilatory apparatus only during eupneic respiration (normal easy breathing) will be discussed.

Breathing in all mammalian species depends on a bilateral neuronal respiratory network within the lower brainstem, which generates three neural phases: inspiration, post-inspiration and expiration. Inspiration involves augmenting activity in the inspiratory nerves and muscles. The post-inspiratory phase represents declining activity in the inspiratory nerves (early expiration). During late or active expiration the expiratory nerves and muscles exhibit augmenting activity which

5

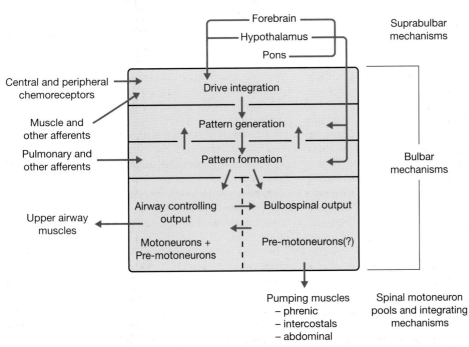

Figure 5.67   Functional organization of neural control of breathing. (Modified from Euler 1986)

5

ends abruptly at the next inspiration. All phase activities are generated without the need for peripheral feedback. Although classical studies proposed a hierarchical organization of various 'centres' in the pons and medulla, studies have revealed that supramedullary structures are not essential for the maintenance of respiratory rhythm. Respiratory neurons in the rostral pons, previously known as the 'pneumotaxic center' controlling respiratory rhythm, are not necessary for rhythm generation. These pontine neurons are now thought to stabilize the respiratory pattern, slow the rhythm and influence timing. Efferent axons from the medullary neurons project to the inspiratory neurons in the spinal cord (Atwood & MacKay 1989, Bianchi & Pasaro 1997, Richler et al 1997).

The origin of the respiratory rhythm remains unclear as precise knowledge of all possible interactions among neurons in the respiratory network is incomplete.

'Respiratory drive is regulated by information from sensory receptors within the airway, lungs and respiratory muscles, as well as central and peripheral chemoceptors'

(Frazier et al 1997)

Proprioceptive information arising from respiratory muscles may regulate the motor activity through long loop reflexes that include the medullary respiratory centres. Proprioceptive information through segmental and intersegmental loops at the spinal level may also influence the motor activity. Although complex spinal circuitry exists for modulating diaphragmatic activity through large and small phrenic afferents, proprioceptive regulation of phrenic motoneurons seems weak or absent. Afferent information from the lower intercostals and the abdominal muscles (T9–10) may facilitate phrenic motoneurons by a spinal reflex. Emerging evidence suggests that phrenic afferents are more involved in respiratory regulation during stressed breathing (Frazier et al 1997, Hilaire & Monteau 1997). There are apparent differences between the neural mechanisms controlling the diaphragm and those controlling the thoracic muscles. While phrenic motoneurons appear mainly under medullary control and seem insensitive to proprioception, thoracic respiratory neurons seem to receive respiratory drive mainly via a network of thoracic interneurons.

Respiratory muscles

The diaphragm

The diaphragm is the major inspiratory muscle in humans. Current understanding of its action suggests that it does not expand the entire chest wall, as previously proposed. Actions of the diaphragm are being investigated with more attention being paid to the direction of the muscle fibres that compose it and the insertional and 'appositional' forces that are generated. The insertional forces are the result of muscular attachments. The appositional force is that pleural pressure that develops on the inner aspect of the lower ribs between the ribs and the diaphragm where the diaphragmatic fibres, that are directed cranially, are in direct contact with the rib cage (De Troyer 1997).

Diaphragmatic muscle fibres originate from three major sites: the xiphisternal junction, the costal margin of the lower rib cage and the transverse processes of the lumbar vertebrae. All fibres insert into the central tendon. Thus, the orientation of these fibres differs. For example, midcostal diaphragmatic muscle fibres are perpendicular to midsternal and midcrural fibres. In humans, diaphragmatic muscle fibres have tendinous insertions within the muscle and do not traverse the full length of the muscle from origin to insertion, as in some smaller animals. Therefore, the mechanical action of these fibres is complex, depending on relationships imposed by the specific attachments and the loads imposed by the rib cage and abdominal wall.

Older literature raised the possibility that there might be motor innervation of some parts of the diaphragm from intercostal nerves. It is now clear that the only innervation is the phrenic nerve via the phrenic motoneurons originating in the third, fourth and fifth segments of the cervical cord in humans. Animal studies have demonstrated that the diaphragm is somatotopically innervated. In the cat, C5 innervates the ventral portions of both costal and crural diaphragmatic fibres, while their dorsal portions are innervated by C6. Studies in other animals have produced similar data. The compartmentalization related to these innervation patterns and the further sub-compartmentalization of motor unit territories within these areas 'provide the potential for differential control' of different regions of diaphragmatic muscle. The differences between the diaphragmatic fibres from the three sites of origin have prompted some investigators to suggest that the crural portion is a separate muscle, under separate neuromotor control (Sieck & Prakash 1997). The crural portion has no costal attachment. Crural fibres surrounding the oesophagus may be under separate neural control in order to act as a sphincter. Detailed histochemical studies have demonstrated other differences between fibres from the three originating sites. A recognized uniqueness of the diaphragm is that it has few muscle spindles. When they are present, they are found primarily in the crural portion (Agostoni & Sant' Ambrogio 1970, Sieck & Prakash 1997).

Studies of isolated diaphragmatic contractions, examined by electrical stimulation of the phrenic nerve in dogs, demonstrated that while the lower ribs moved cranially and the cross-sectional area of the lower rib cage increased, the upper ribs moved caudally and the cross-sectional area of the upper rib cage decreased. Similar results have been obtained in human subjects with phrenic nerve pacing following traumatic transaction of the upper cord and during spontaneous breathing in subjects with transaction of the lower cord, who use the diaphragm exclusively. In seated humans (as in the dog) the diaphragm has both an expiratory action on the upper rib cage and an inspiratory action on the lower rib cage, which increases in its transverse diameter.

It has been established that the inspiratory action of the diaphragm on the rib cage is due in part to the insertional force of its attachment to the lower ribs. During inspiration the muscle fibres of the diaphragm shorten and the dome descends relative to the costal insertions of the muscle. The descent of the dome, which remains relatively constant in size and shape during breathing, expands the thorax vertically, resulting in a fall in pleural pressure. The descent also displaces abdominal viscera caudally, increasing abdominal pressure, which pushes the abdominal wall outwards. The diaphragmatic fibres inserting on the upper borders of the lower six ribs also apply a force on these ribs when they contract. This force equals the force exerted on the central tendon. If the abdominal viscera effectively oppose the diaphragmatic descent, the lower ribs are lifted and rotated outwards.

The inspiratory force of the diaphragm is also related to its apposition to the rib cage. This is best explained in the words of De Troyer (1997):

> 'The zone of apposition makes the lower rib cage in effect part of the abdominal container and measurements in dogs have established that during breathing the changes in pressure in the pleural recess between the apposed diaphragm and the rib cage are almost equal to the changes in abdominal pressure. Pressure in the pleural recess rises, rather than falls during inspiration, thus indicating that the rise in abdominal pressure is truly transmitted through the apposed diaphragm to expand the lower rib cage'

The inspiratory efficiency of the insertional and appositional forces is largely dependent on the resistance the abdominal viscera provide to diaphragmatic descent. If the resistance of the abdominal contents was eliminated, the zone of apposition would disappear during inspiration and the contracting diaphragmatic muscle would become oriented transversely at their attachments onto the ribs. In this case, the insertional force would have an expiratory action on the lower ribs. These studies reinforce the view of Goldman (1974) that abdominal muscle contraction, commonly associated only with an expiratory action, appears to have an important role in defending diaphragmatic length during inspiration.

The intercostal muscles

The place of the intercostal muscles has been more difficult to establish. Conventional wisdom regards the external intercostals as inspiratory in function, elevating the ribs, and the internal intercostals as expiratory in function, depressing the ribs. This theory was based on geometric considerations proposed in 1848 (the Hamberger theory) and it has been challenged since 1867, when electrical stimulation of the intercostal muscles was undertaken for the first time. These latter studies suggested that the external and internal intercostal muscles were synergistic in action. The Hamberger theory is regarded as being incomplete. Its theoretical model is planar but real ribs are curved. Therefore, the changes in length of the intercostal muscles (i.e. their mechanical advantage) vary with respect to the position of the muscle fibres along the rib. Also, the Hamberger theory assumed that all ribs rotate by equal amounts around parallel axes. The radii of curvature of the different ribs are different (Duron & Rose 1997).

Histological and electrophysiological studies have disclosed that the rib cage is non-homogeneous. It has motor components that vary with their location in the upper or lower thorax. In addition, each intercostal can be functionally different depending on its position in the same intercostal space (Gray 1973). It is now generally accepted that most of the external intercostal muscles do not participate in the ventilatory process during quiet breathing (De Troyer 1997, Duron & Rose 1997). Unlike the diaphragm, the intercostal muscles also have a postural function. Detailed studies of the respiratory and postural actions of the intercostal muscles have revealed functional differences from segment to segment and between external and internal intercostal muscles within the same segment. The major place of each intercostal muscle in postural activity and/or respiratory cycles has yet to be established. Nevertheless, Duron & Rose (1997) reviewed extensive studies in animal and human subjects and report precise distributions of inspiratory and expiratory activity. A summary of their findings follows:

1. In addition to the diaphragm, the inspiratory muscles active during normal breathing are the ventral intercartilaginous part of the intercostal muscles and the dorsal levator costae muscle.

5

2. The lateral part of the external and internal intercostal muscles of the upper rib spaces are synergistic muscles. They often have a postural type of activity. Their motoneurons may be activated by the central inspiratory drive; thus they may participate in respiration.

3. In the four lowest intercostal spaces, the lateral parts of the external and internal intercostal muscles are also synergistic. The lateral part of the internal intercostal is active in expiration during quiet breathing. The lateral part of the external intercostal is also expiratory but only during dyspnoea, similar to abdominal expiratory action.

4. The lateral part of the intercostal muscles are antagonistic in the 5th–8th intercostal spaces. The external intercostals are inspiratory and the internal intercostals are expiratory.

5. In every intercostal space the dorsal part of the external (inspiratory) and the dorsal part of the internal (expiratory) muscles are antagonistic during quiet breathing.

6. All intercostal muscles of the lateral part of the rib cage participate in posture. There appears to be a clear distinction between the dorsal and ventral part of each intercostal space from which phasic respiratory activities are always recorded and the lateral part of each intercostal space where tonic postural activities are observed.

The insertions of both the external and internal intercostal muscles suggest that their orientation would assist rotation of the thorax. Indeed, electromyographical (EMG) studies on normal human subjects have demonstrated that external intercostals on the right were activated when the torso was rotated to the left, but silent when the torso was rotated to the right. On the other hand, the internal intercostals on the right were only active when the torso was rotated to the right. The abundance of muscle spindles and the preponderance of type I (slow) muscle fibres in intercostal muscles are consistent with postural activity. Eighty-five percent of external intercostal muscle fibres in dogs are type 1, a percentage that is higher than that of antigravity limb muscles.

Accessory muscles of inspiration

The scalene muscles in humans have traditionally been considered as accessory inspiratory muscles. However, EMG studies have established that scalene muscles invariably contract with the diaphragm and parasternal intercostals during inspiration. No clinical situation exists in which paralysis of all inspiratory muscles occurs without also affecting the scalene muscles, so it is impossible to accurately define the isolated action of these muscles on the human rib cage. Observations on quadriplegic patients have demonstrated that persistent inspiratory action in scalene muscles is observed in those subjects with a spinal transection at C7 or lower that preserves scalene innervation. In these situations the anteroposterior diameter of the rib cage remains constant or increases, as opposed to the inward displacement of the upper rib cage when the level of transection interferes with scalene innervation (De Troyer 1997). Accessory muscles of the neck assist thoracic respiration by stabilizing the upper rib cage. This is a minor function in normal persons at rest. These muscles become more active during exercise and in the presence of diseases such as asthma and chronic obstructive pulmonary disease. Generally, neck and upper airway muscles have a higher proportion of fast muscle fibres, faster isometric contraction times and lower fatigue resistance than the diaphragm (Lunteren & Dick 1997).

Many other muscles can elevate the ribs when they contract and are therefore truly 'accessory' muscles of inspiration. These are muscles running between the head and the rib cage, shoulder girdle and rib cage, spine and shoulder girdle. Such muscles as the sternocleidomastoid, pectoralis minor, trapezius, serrati and erector spinae are primarily postural in function. They are active in respiration in healthy humans only during increased respiratory effort. Of these accessory muscles, only the sternocleidomastoids have been extensively studied. In patients with transection of the upper cord causing paralysis of the diaphragm, intercostals, scalene and abdominal muscles, the sternocleidomastoids (innervation cranial nerve 11) contract forcefully during unassisted inspiration, causing a large increase in the expansion of the upper rib cage but an inspiratory decrease in the transverse diameter of the lower rib cage (De Troyer 1997).

The abdominal muscles

The four muscles of the ventrolateral wall of the abdomen, the rectus abdominis, the external oblique, the internal oblique and the transversus abdominis, have significant respiratory function in humans. The fibres in each of these muscles assume a direction different from each other; consequently, the mechanical action of an abdominal muscle contraction depends on fibre direction and the concurrent action of the other abdominal muscles. Added to this complexity is the fact that the force generated by the abdominal wall is applied to a load that is determined by viscous and non-linear elastic resistances. The capacity of the abdominal wall to function adequately varies markedly among individuals and correlates well with an individual's activity level, gender, corpulence and age.

Abdominal muscle fibres are similar to those of other skeletal muscle. Differences in fibre composition between them are minor. Generally speaking, type 1 (slow) muscle fibres predominate. Bishop (1997) reports that although details of the morphology of abdominal motor units are not known and information on the number and distribution of muscle proprioceptors (muscle spindles and tendon organs) in abdominal muscle is scarce, proprioceptive feedback is recognized as an important modulator of abdominal motoneuron excitability. Electrically evoked reflexes studied in cats under the conditions of bilateral rhizotomy of the lumbar segments or C6 spinal cord transection, demonstrated that both segmental feedback and supraspinal signals control abdominal motoneurons. Furthermore, studies on the phasic and tonic abdominal stretch reflexes suggest a special functional significance for the gamma-spindle loop. Normal individuals, when standing, develop tonic abdominal muscle activity unrelated to respiratory phases.

Many brain regions can modify abdominal motoneuron output via multiple descending pathways. Spinal abdominal motoneurons receive strong projections from the brainstem. However, brainstem and spinal abdominal motoneurons receive direct and indirect projections from the premotor cortex, the motor cortex, the cerebellum, the hypothalamus, the pons and many other regions of the brain. The voluntary control over the abdominal muscles via the motor cortex is very similar to control by the cortex over muscles of the limbs and digits.

The respiratory action of the abdominal muscles is first to contract and pull the abdominal wall inward and so increase abdominal pressure. This pressure causes the diaphragm to move upwards into the thoracic cavity, which in turn results in an increase in pleural pressure and a decrease in lung volume. The abdominal muscles also displace the rib cage. By virtue of their insertions on the ribs, it would appear that the action of the abdominal muscles is to pull the lower ribs caudally and thus deflate the rib cage in another expiratory action. However, experiments in dogs have shown that these muscles also have an inspiratory action. Because of the large zone where the diaphragm is directly apposed to the rib cage, the rise in abdominal pressure due to abdominal muscle contraction is transmitted to the lower rib cage. In addition, the rise in abdominal pressure forcing the diaphragm cranially and the consecutive increase in passive diaphragmatic tension also tend to raise the lower ribs and expand the lower rib cage (insertional force of the diaphragm). Regardless of

their actions on the ribs, the abdominal muscles are primarily expiratory muscles through their actions on the diaphragm and the lung.

Neurophysiological facilitatory stimuli

The proprioceptive and tactile stimuli selected produce remarkably consistent reflexive responses in the ventilatory muscles. Inspiratory expansion of the ribs, increased epigastric excursion, visibly increased and often palpably increased tone in the abdominal muscles and change in the respiratory rate (usually slower) are among the responses observed. In the clinical setting these responses are often accompanied by involuntary coughing, changes in breath sounds on auscultation, rapid return of mechanical chest wall stability, less necessity for suctioning, a more normal respiratory pattern and retention of the improved breathing pattern for some time after the treatment period. In some unconscious patients there is an apparent increase in the level of consciousness (more reaction to other stimuli). These effects appear to be cumulative. Successive application of the stimuli elicits faster responses and longer retention of the altered pattern. The changes noted during treatment application are frequently dramatic. The responses are most pronounced in the most deeply unconscious. The facilitatory stimuli are:

- intercostal stretch
- vertebral pressure to the upper thoracic spine
- vertebral pressure to the lower thoracic spine
- anterior-stretch lift of the posterior basal area
- moderate manual pressure
- perioral pressure
- abdominal co-contraction.

The foregoing discussion of neural control models, with the emphasis on the importance of afferent input and the place of spinal motoneurons, indicates that the majority of the responses to these stimuli are mediated by muscle stretch receptors via dorsal roots and intersegmental reflexes (Table 5.4).

Intercostal stretch (Fig. 5.68A)

Intercostal stretch is provided by applying pressure to the upper border of a rib in a direction that will widen the intercostal space above it. The pressure should be applied in a downward direction, not pushing inward into the patient. The application of the stretch is timed with an exhalation and the stretched position is then maintained as the patient continues to breathe in his usual manner. As the stretch is maintained, a gradual increase in inspiratory movements in and around the area being stretched occurs. This may be done as a uni-

Table 5.4   Neurophysiological facilitation for the chest

Procedure	Method	Observations	Suggested mechanism
Perioral stimulation	Pressure is applied to the patient's top lip by the therapist's finger – and maintained	• Increased epigastric excursion • 'Deep breathing' • Sighing • Mouth closure • Swallowing • 'Snout phenomena'	Primitive reflex response related to sucking
Vertebral pressure high	Manual pressure to thoracic vertebrae in region of T2–T5	• Increased epigastric excursions • 'Deep breathing'	Dorsal root-mediated intersegmental reflex
Vertebral pressure low	Manual pressure to thoracic vertebrae in region of T7–T10	Increased respiratory movements of apical thorax	
Anterior stretch – lifting posterior basal area	• Patient supine • Hands under lower ribs • Ribs lifted upward	• Expansion of posterior basal area • Increased epigastric movements	• Dorsal root as above • Stretch receptors in intercostals, back muscles
Co-contraction – abdomen	• Pressure laterally over lower ribs and pelvis • Alternate right and left sides	• Increased epigastric movements • Increased muscle contraction (rectus abdominus) • Decreased girth in obese • Increased firmness to palpation • Depression of umbilicus	Stretch receptors in abdominal muscles? intercostal to phrenic reflex
Intercostal stretch	Stretch on expiratory phase maintained	Increased movement of area being stretched	Intercostal stretch receptors
Moderate manual pressure	Moderate pressure open palm	Gradually increased excursion of area under contact	Cutaneous afferents

lateral or bilateral procedure. It should not be performed on fractured or floating ribs. Care must be exercised around sensitive mammary tissue in females. When performed over areas of instability, as in the presence of paradoxical movement of the upper rib cage or over areas of decreased mobility, this procedure is effective in restoring normal breathing patterns. Epigastric excursions can be observed if intercostal stretch is performed over the lower ribs, but above the floating ribs. This may represent the reflexive activation of the diaphragm by the intercostal afferents that innervate its margins.

Vertebral pressure (Fig. 5.68B)

Firm pressure applied directly over the vertebrae of the upper and lower thoracic cage activates the dorsal intercostal muscles. Pressure should be applied with an open

hand for comfort and must be firm enough to provide some (intrafusal) stretch. For this reason it is easier to apply when the patient is supine, as in the supine position it is not necessary to stabilize the body and one may also observe the patient's reactions. Afferent input that activates the dorsal intercostal muscles is consistent with the observations of Duron & Rose (1997) that in every intercostal space the dorsal part of the external (inspiratory) and the dorsal part of the internal (expiratory) intercostal muscles are antagonistic during quiet breathing.

Firm pressure over the uppermost thoracic vertebrae results in increased epigastric excursions in the presence of a relaxed abdominal wall. Pressure over the lower thoracic vertebrae results in increased inspiratory movements of the apical thorax. These responses correlate

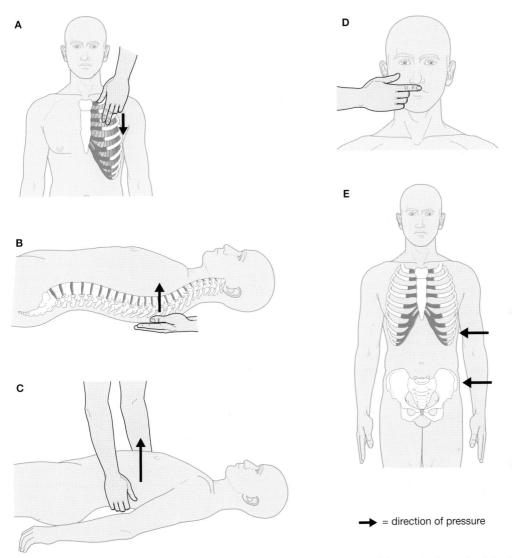

➡ = direction of pressure

Figure 5.68 (**A**) Intercostal stretch: pressure down towards the next rib, not 'in' towards the patient's back. (**B**) Vertebral pressure (i) over T2, 3, 4, (ii) T9, 10, 11. (**C**) Lifting posterior basal area. (**D**) Perioral stimulation: moderate pressure on top lip (the airway should not be occluded). (**E**) Co-contraction of abdominal muscles: pressure over lower ribs and pelvic bone.

with the observations of Helen Coombs (1918) who demonstrated that section of the thoracic roots diminished costal respiration. She stated:

> 'If the spinal roots are cut in the thoracic region alone there is diminution of costal respiration although abdominal respiration remains unaltered and the rate is very little changed: if the cervical dorsal roots are also involved, independent costal respiration disappears '

In 1930, in research with kittens, Coombs and Pike said:

> '. . . when dorsal roots of spinal nerves are divided in the thoracic region, costal respiration in kittens from birth to ten days old almost ceases . . . when dorsal roots of cervical nerves are sectioned, the thoracic nerves being intact, the movements of the diaphragm are much cut down and the respiratory rate is slower at no matter what age'

5

There is little to be found in the literature defining intersegmental respiratory reflexes. Sieck & Prakash (1997) noted that phrenic motoneurons do not receive a major excitatory input from muscle spindle afferents. However, they recognize that there are extrasegmental reflexes that affect phrenic motoneuron activation. Group I and II afferents from intercostal nerves have been shown to exert both inhibitory and facilitatory influences on phrenic nerve activity.

Anterior–stretch basal lift (Fig. 5.68C)

This procedure is performed by placing the hands under the ribs of the supine patient and lifting gently upwards. The lift is maintained and provides a maintained stretch and pressure posteriorly and an anterior stretch as well. This may be done bilaterally if the patient is small enough. If this is not possible or necessary, it should also be effective when performed unilaterally. As the lift is sustained, stretch is maintained and increasing movement of the ribs in a lateral and posterior direction can be seen and felt. Increased epigastric movements also often become obvious. The lift to the back places some stretch on the dorsal intercostal area and should also stretch the spaces between some of the mid-thoracic ribs (5–8). These are both areas where the intercostal muscles are considered to be antagonistic in action. The epigastric movements suggest that the diaphragm is being activated by intercostal afferents.

Maintained manual pressure

When firm contact of the open hand(s) is maintained over an area in which expansion is desired, gradual increasing excursion of the ribs under the contact will be felt. This is a useful procedure to obtain expansion in any situation where pain is present; for instance, when there are chest tubes or after cardiac surgery which may have required splitting of the sternum. Manual contact over the posterior chest wall is also useful and comfortable for persons with chronic obstructive pulmonary disease. The inspiratory response is thought to be due to cutaneous tactile receptors. The contact should be firm so that it does not tickle.

In 1963 Sumi studied hair, tactile and pressure receptors in the cat and reported thoracic cutaneous fields for both inspiratory and expiratory motoneurons. He proposed that since the excitatory skin fields for inspiratory motoneurons were more extensive than those for expiratory motoneurons, more inspiratory motoneurons could be excited by a single skin stimulus. Local cutaneous stimulation of the thoracic region would then tend to reflexly produce an inspiratory position of the rib cage. Duron & Bars (1986) also studied thoracic cutane-

ous stimulation in the cat. They directly electrically stimulated desheathed lateral cutaneous nerves in anaesthetized decerebrate cats and cats that were both decerebrate and spinal. Among their findings was widespread inhibition on both inspiratory and expiratory activity after stimulation of the cutaneous nerve. Their observations also suggested that responses from the upper and lower thoracic areas were different. They acknowledge that the place of each of the different cutaneous afferent components needs to be identified.

Perioral pressure (Fig. 5.68D)

Perioral stimulation is provided by applying firm maintained pressure to the patient's top lip, being careful not to occlude the nasal passage. (The use of surgical gloves is advised to avoid contamination.) The response to this stimulus is a brief (approximately 5 second) period of apnoea followed by increased epigastric excursions. The initial response may frequently be observed as a large maintained epigastric swell. Pressure is maintained for the length of time the therapist wishes the patient to breathe in the activated pattern. As the stimulus is maintained the epigastric excursions may increase so that movement is transmitted to the upper chest and the patient appears to be deep breathing. Respiratory rate is usually slower. The patient may sigh on initiation of the procedure or some time after the response has become established.

The paucity of muscle spindles in the diaphragm determines that phrenic motoneurons which provide its motor activation do not receive any significant excitatory input from muscle spindle afferents and there are few, if any, gamma motoneurons in the phrenic motor nucleus (Sieck & Prakash 1997). Information regarding afferent facilitation of phrenic motoneurons and/or other reflex interactions influencing their excitability is sparse. The responses that are observed on application of this stimulus correlate very well with the work of Peiper (1963).

When this perioral stimulus is applied to the unconscious patient if the mouth is open, it will close. Swallowing is noted and sucking movements are often evident even in the presence of oral airways. Swallowing and sucking may not be evident initially, but may appear in the more deeply unconscious after repeated stimulation. Occasionally such a patient has been observed to push pursed lips forward in a 'mouth phenomenon' or 'lip phenomenon' or 'snout phenomenon'. These observations are similar to observations made by Peiper (1963) while studying the neurology of respiration and the neurology of food intake and the relationship between sucking, swallowing and breathing in infants. The 'mouth' or 'lip' or 'snout phenomenon' has been reported by Peiper and other investigators, as a reflex response to gentle tapping on the upper lip noted in young normal infants and in adults with severe cerebral disorders. Movement of the lips, sucking, swallowing and chewing motions have been reported on stroking the lips of comatose adults and are thought to be related to infantile rooting reflexes.

Peiper observed that three centrally directed rhythmic movements arise during an infant's food intake: sucking, breathing and swallowing. Earlier experiments on young animals had established that there was a sucking centre located bilaterally in the medulla. Peiper established the dominance of the sucking centre over respiration. Infants can breathe while they nurse, partly due to the high position of the larynx. The initiation of sucking was observed to immediately disturb respiration. There was initial lowering of the diaphragm for 5 seconds or more before respirations began at a new rhythm led by the sucking centre. When the sucking movements ceased, the respiratory movements continued in the new pattern for a period (in this instance, faster rhythm). The similarity between the observations recorded by Peiper and those observed in response to the perioral stimulus suggests that these phenomena are related. The stimulus on the top lip is thought to imitate, in part, the pressure of the mother's breast against the lips of a nursing infant. The lack of recent recorded material would seem to indicate that the investigation into sucking centres per se has not been pursued much further. The related activity of swallowing has been investigated, especially with respect to its interactions with respiration.

Swallowing is a complex behaviour. Although it is one of the most elaborate of motor functions in humans, swallowing is a primitive reflex with implications of a stereotyped and fixed behaviour (Jean et al 1997). In most mammals, including humans, all the muscles concerned with swallowing are striated. Similar to respiration, swallowing is considered an autonomic function, but is governed by the same neural principles as those serving some somatic functions, such as locomotion. Great differences among species are observed concerning swallowing during the respiratory cycle. Most of the significant data were obtained from sheep. The oropharynx serves both deglutition and respiration. Several muscles in the mouth, pharynx and larynx are active to ensure the patency of the upper airways and to regulate the airflow during the respiratory cycle. In humans, swallows occur mainly during expiration. When the swallowing rhythm is regular, one swallow occurs for every one or few breaths. A brief minor inspiration called a 'swallow breath' ('Schluckatmung' by pioneer investigators) occurs at the onset of swallowing. The

functional significance of this brief inspiration is not known.

The central pattern generator (CPG) for swallowing is located in the medulla in two main groups of neurons in two regions that also contain respiratory neurons. The mechanisms that generate its rhythms are not understood. The factors regulating the functional interactions between swallowing and respiration have yet to be determined. Margaret Rood (1973) taught the use of perioral stimulation to reduce spastic muscle tone. She believed that it induced a parasympathetic bias (as opposed to a sympathetic bias) and that it promoted general relaxation. It was a prerequisite for her light, moving touch facilitation procedure to activate limb muscles. Rood's treatment focus and patient population probably accounts for her lack of awareness of the respiratory responses to this stimulus.

Co-contraction of the abdomen (Fig. 5.68E)

Rood (1973) taught co-contraction of the abdomen as a procedure to facilitate respiration. Pressure is applied simultaneously over the patient's lower lateral ribs and over the ilium in a direction at right angles to the patient. Moderate force is applied and maintained. Rood believed that this procedure increased tone in the abdominal muscles and also activated the diaphragm. She proposed that the pressure directed across the abdomen produced intrafusal stretch, thus activating the muscle spindles (mainly in the rectus). She thought that the side contralateral to the pressure reacted first. As those muscles responded to the stretch and shortened, they would stretch the intrafusal fibres of the opposite muscles, which in turn would activate their homonymous extrafusal muscles, which would contract, shorten and stretch the first set again and so the cycle would be repeated. A series of alternating contractions was thought to occur as long as the pressure was maintained. Co-contraction of the abdomen should be performed bilaterally with pressure applied alternately and maintained for some seconds on either side. The maintained pressure is repeated as necessary to obtain and maintain the response for the desired period.

In practice, activation of the abdominal muscles does not always occur in the contralateral side first. There can be considerable variation in individual responses. Preexisting muscle tone, corpulence, postoperative status and the integrity of the abdominal wall are some of the influencing factors. Lax abdominal muscles (for any reason) appear to respond more slowly. If activation is slow, it is often helpful to observe the umbilicus, which may exhibit changes in its movement pattern, becoming more depressed on exhalations before changes in the muscles can be detected.

This is an effective procedure. As pressure is maintained, increasing abdominal tone can be both seen and palpated. In the presence of retained secretions abdominal co-contractions may produce coughing more readily than the other procedures. As ventilation increases with any procedure, coughing may occur. In obese patients abdominal co-contraction has frequently resulted in decreased abdominal girth.

Clinical application

In the clinical setting auscultation and standard chest assessment should be undertaken before, during and after treatment. Ventilatory movement patterns should be noted. Is chest expansion simultaneous and equal? Are there paradoxical movements or any areas of indrawing on inspiration? The therapist must be aware of the patterns of ventilation and how they are changing. Since the patient's response determines the duration of treatment, assessment is critical. The procedure of choice is continued until the desired treatment effect has been achieved, whether increased breath sounds, cough or stabilized respiratory pattern. Many patients raise secretions and cough. (Advice given to therapists was frequently 'co-contract and duck'.) Unconscious patients need assistance to get rid of their secretions, but suctioning may not be required as often or as deeply. Some unconscious patients appear to become less obtunded. Eyelids may flutter, eyes may open or there may be spontaneous movements. Sometimes, such a patient will initially turn the head away or push the therapist's hand away. These are positive signs as these patients are often thought to be unresponsive.

Responses to the facilitatory procedures are individual reactions and therefore every patient will not demonstrate the same level of responsiveness to each procedure. It is not necessary to do each procedure with every patient, but it is imperative to observe the individual response and modify treatment accordingly. Treatment should not be continued in the presence of an undesirable response. Anecdotally a dramatic example of an undesirable response was observed in a decerebrate patient who was so hypertonic that abdominal co-contractions applied in the supine position began to elevate him into a sitting position. Such a response necessitates the use of other procedures. Conscious medical patients often appreciate the sense of relaxation and the lack of a sense of effort when facilitation procedures are used in their care. Many perform their own perioral stimulation. Acute and chronic neurological conditions such as amyotrophic lateral sclerosis, Guillain–Barré, cerebral vascular accidents and others may also be treated with these procedures and derive benefit.

OXYGEN THERAPY

Oxygen therapy is indicated for many patients with hypoxaemia. The physiotherapist frequently treats patients requiring added inspired oxygen and may be involved with the setting up of oxygen therapy equipment. Oxygen is a drug and should be prescribed. The delivery device, flow rate, concentration, frequency and duration should be documented on the patient's drug chart (Dodd et al 2000, Thiagamoorthy et al 2000). It should be monitored using arterial blood gas analysis or oxygen saturation (SpO_2) recordings. When measuring SpO_2 recordings only, it must be remembered that an increase in PaO_2 may be associated with an increase in $PaCO_2$, but any rise in $PaCO_2$ will be difficult to detect. If a patient is dependent on continuous oxygen therapy the mask should be removed only briefly for expectoration, eating and drinking and sometimes during these periods it may be appropriate to continue oxygen therapy using nasal cannulae.

Devices for administering oxygen therapy may be divided into fixed and variable performance devices (Hinds & Watson 1996):

A *variable performance device* supplies a flow of oxygen that is less than the patient's minute volume. The inspired oxygen concentration (FiO_2) will vary with the rate and volume of breath and considerable variations between and within subjects have been demonstrated (Bazuaye et al 1992). Commonly used variable performance devices are the simple facemask (Fig. 5.69A) and nasal cannulae (Fig. 5.69B). Nasal cannulae are often preferred as the patient can eat, drink and speak more comfortably and may find them less claustrophobic than a mask. Although high flows of oxygen can be delivered via nasal cannulae, 1–4 l/min (approximately 24–36%) is optimal in terms of patient comfort. Higher flows, up to 6 l/min, tend to irritate and dry the nasal mucosa, but this may be alleviated by including a bubble-through humidifier in the circuit. However, humidification via narrow-bore tubing is not the most effective means of humidifying dry inspired gas (Campbell et al 1988). Nasal cannulae should be used with caution with very breathless hypoxic patients, as they are likely to be breathing through the mouth and not benefiting from nasal oxygen. Wide variations in inspired oxygen concentration have been shown to be produced by variable performance devices, even with the recommended flows (Jeffrey & Warren 1992).

A *fixed performance device* should be used when accurate delivery of oxygen concentrations is required, especially at low concentrations. This will deliver a

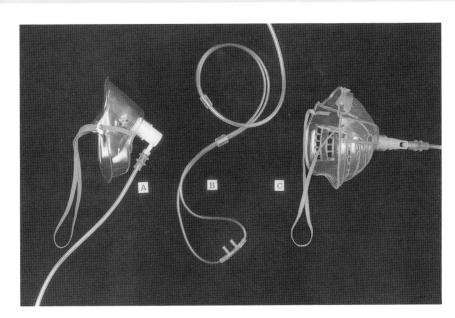

Figure 5.69   Oxygen delivery devices: (**A**) Variable performance mask. (**B**) Nasal cannulae. (**C**) Fixed performance Venturi mask. (Intersurgical)

5

known inspired oxygen concentration (FiO₂) by providing a sufficiently high flow of premixed gas that should exceed the patient's peak inspiratory flow rate. A Venturi system allows a relatively low flow of oxygen to entrain a large volume of air and the mixed gas is conveyed to the facemask (Fig. 5.69C). With a 24% Venturi mask the usual setting of 2 l/min flow of oxygen will entrain approximately 50 l/min of air, giving a total flow of approximately 52 l/min. An extremely breathless patient, with a greatly increased work of breathing and high peak inspiratory flow rate, may find this flow too low and then it is necessary to increase the flow to exceed the inspiratory flow of the patient (Hill et al 1984). The manufacturer should provide information for each mask (e.g. a 24% mask run at 3 l/min may augment the total flow to 78 l/min without changing the oxygen concentration). It is not easy to measure the critically ill patient's peak inspiratory flow, but by careful observation the physiotherapist should be able to tell if the total flow is sufficient. If gas can be felt flowing out through the holes and around the edges of the mask during inspiration, the flow will be exceeding the patient's requirements.

For most patients using a Venturi mask, the entrained room air provides sufficient humidification, but occasionally additional humidification is indicated. A bubble-through humidifier attached to the narrow-bore tubing of a Venturi mask is inappropriate as the flow of oxygen is likely to be reduced by the back pressure from the humidifier device and by condensation blocking the narrow-bore tubing.

When high concentrations of oxygen, at high flows, are required, a *high-flow variable FiO₂ generator* can be used. The gas flows along wide-bore tubing from the generator across an appropriate heated humidifier to the facemask. It is essential to have an oxygen analyser in the circuit. Oxygen concentrations between 35% and 100% can be delivered at flows of up to 130 l/min. High-flow oxygen should be considered when patients requiring oxygen concentrations greater than or equal to 40% are not responding to a fixed-performance device.

Nebulizers for the delivery of drugs in hospital are frequently powered by piped oxygen but in the patient dependent on his hypoxic drive to breathe, air should be used as the driving gas. Occasionally in the severely hypoxic patient, who is also hypercapnic and dependent on a controlled 24% oxygen mask, it is important not to deprive the patient of this added oxygen while using a nebulizer. The level of oxygen entrained to maintain the baseline oxygen saturation can be monitored using an oximeter.

For most patients an *intermittent positive pressure breathing device* (IPPB) should be driven by compressed oxygen. Starke et al (1979) demonstrated that in hypercapnic patients oxygen can be used as the driving gas. In hypoxic patients without hypercapnia, for example in acute asthma, oxygen is required and it may be dangerous to use air alone as the driving gas for IPPB.

Long-term oxygen therapy

Long-term oxygen therapy (LTOT) has been shown to improve the length and quality of life in selected patients with severe chronic airflow limitation (Medical Research Council Working Party 1981, Nocturnal Oxygen Therapy Trial Group 1980). Clinical guidelines for the prescribing of domiciliary oxygen have been established (Royal College of Physicians 1999) and three main forms of home oxygen services have developed (Wedzicha & Calverley 2006):

1. LTOT for patients with chronic hypoxaemia (PaO_2 = 7.3 kPa (55 mmHg) for continuous use at home.
2. Ambulatory oxygen therapy for oxygen therapy using a portable device during exercise and daily activities.
3. Short-burst oxygen therapy for the intermittent use of oxygen at home for periods of 10–20 minutes at a time, to relieve the symptom of breathlessness. There is little evidence for the benefit of short-burst oxygen therapy.

A Cochrane Review (Ram & Wedzicha 2002) looked at the effectiveness of long-term ambulatory oxygen therapy and concluded that it was not possible to determine whether patients on long-term oxygen therapy should be provided with ambulatory oxygen during exercise and for activities of daily living. Bradley & O'Neill (2005) looked at the effects of short-term ambulatory oxygen. They concluded that there was strong evidence that short-term ambulatory oxygen improves exercise capacity.

Ambulatory and training oxygen have been discussed in the review by Young (2005) and ambulatory oxygen, assessment and practical considerations for physiotherapists have been outlined by O'Neill & Dodd (2006).

Oxygen supply

For domiciliary provision, patients should be assessed to determine the flow rate and concentration for short-burst, ambulatory or long-term oxygen therapy use. There are three sources of oxygen: compressed gas cylinders, oxygen concentrators and liquid reservoirs.

Compressed gas cylinder (Weg & Haas 1998). Large cylinders can provide oxygen for up to 57 hours at a flow of 2 l/min and flows up to 15 l/min can be attained.

Small, portable *oxygen cylinders* can be used for short trips outside the home and either carried or transported on a lightweight trolley.

Oxygen concentrator. This is a convenient and efficient means of providing oxygen therapy in the home, in the presence of a reliable supply of electricity. The concentrator filters and concentrates oxygen molecules from ambient air, generating flows of 3 to 8 l/min, but the fraction of oxygen in the inspired gas (FiO_2) will decrease as the flow increases (Weg & Haas 1998). Oxygen tubing can be fitted in areas of the home to allow for mobility, but a maximum length of 50 feet (15.25 metres) has been recommended (DeVilbiss Oxygen Services 2000). A back-up compressed gas cylinder is necessary for emergency use. Humidifiers are sometimes fitted to oxygen concentrators, but care must be taken as these are a potential source of infection (Pendleton et al 1991).

Liquid oxygen reservoir. This will provide oxygen for 5 to 7 days at 2 l/min and can be used to fill small portable units (Weg & Haas 1998). The portable units are lightweight, convenient and may improve compliance with treatment (Lock et al 1992, Wurtemberger & Hutter 2000).

In an attempt to give patients, dependent on oxygen, greater mobility and the opportunity to participate in activities outside the home, an *inspiratory phased delivery system* or *oxygen by transtracheal catheter* may be considered (Shneerson 1992). A microcatheter inserted into the trachea will reduce the dead space and decrease the requirement for oxygen. Some patients find this more cosmetically acceptable than nasal cannulae, but there is the increased possibility of infection.

Acknowledgement

For many of the figures in this chapter, we are indebted to the Photographic Department of the Royal Marsden Hospital, Ella Thorpe-Beeston, Matthew Thorpe-Beeston, Daniel Wallis, Catherine Sandsund, Barbara Webber and the Intensive Care Unit, Royal Brompton Hospital. We are also grateful to Catherine Sandsund for her help with the section on incentive spirometry.

References

Accurso FJ, Sontag MK, Koenig M, Quittner AL 2004 Multi-center airway secretion clearance study in cystic fibrosis. Pediatric Pulmonology Supplement 27: 314

Agostoni E, Sant'Ambrogio G 1970 The diaphragm. In: Campbell EJM,

Agostoni E, Newsom Davies J (eds) The respiratory muscles, mechanics and neural control. WB Saunders, Philadelphia

Ainsworth D 1997 Respiratory muscle recruitment during exercise. In: Miller AD, Bianchi A, Bishop BP

(eds) Neural control of the respiratory muscles. CRC Press, New York

Aldridge A 2005 Glossopharyngeal breathing in multiple sclerosis. Personal communication (Lymington New Forest Hospital, Hampshire,

United Kingdom. Telephone (+44)1590-663212. Email: alison. aldridge@nfpct.nhs.uk)

Allan JS, Garrity JM, Donohue DM 2003 The utility of high frequency chest wall oscillation therapy in the post-operative management of thoracic surgical patients. Chest 124(Suppl 4): 235S

Alvarez SE, Peterson M, Lunsford BR 1981 Respiratory treatment of the adult patient with spinal cord injury. Physical Therapy 61(12): 1737–1745

Ambrosino N, Callegari G, Galloni C, Brega S, Pinna G 1995 Clinical evaluation of oscillating positive expiratory pressure for enhancing expectoration in diseases other than cystic fibrosis. Monaldi Archives of Chest Disease 50(4): 269–275

American Association for Respiratory Care 2003 AARC clinical practice guideline: intermittent positive pressure breathing. Respiratory Care 48(5): 540–546

American Association for Respiratory Care 2004 AARC clinical practice guideline: nasotracheal suctioning. Respiratory Care 49(9): 1080–1084

American Thoracic Society 1999 Dyspnea. Mechanisms, assessment and management: a consensus statement. American Journal of Respiratory and Critical Care Medicine 159: 321–340

App EM, Kieselmann R, Reinhardt D et al 1998 Sputum rheology changes in cystic fibrosis lung disease following two different types of physiotherapy. Flutter vs autogenic drainage. Chest 114: 171–177

Arens R, Gozal D, Omlin KJ et al 1994 Comparison of high frequency compression and conventional chest physiotherapy in hospitalized patients with cystic fibrosis. American Journal of Respiratory and Critical Care Medicine 150: 1154–1157

Aris RM, Renner JB, Winders AD et al 1998 Increased rate of fractures and severe kyphosis: sequelae of living into adulthood with cystic fibrosis. Annals of Internal Medicine 128:186–93

Atwood HL, MacKay WA 1989 Essentials of neurophysiology. Decker, Toronto

Ayres SM, Kozam RL, Lukas DS 1963 The effects of intermittent positive pressure breathing on intrathoracic pressure, pulmonary mechanics and the work of breathing. American Review of Respiratory Disease 87: 370–379

Bach JR 1992 Airway secretion management and general pulmonary rehabilitation considerations for patients with neuromuscular ventilatory failure. Journal of Neurological Rehabilitation 6(2): 75–80

Bach JR 1993 Mechanical insufflation-exsufflation: a comparison of peak expiratory flows with manually assisted coughing techniques. Chest 104: 1553–1562

Bach JR 1994 Update and perspective on noninvasive respiratory muscle aids. Part 2: The expiratory aids. Chest 105 1538–1544

Bach JR 1995 Respiratory muscle aids for the prevention of pulmonary morbidity and mortality. Seminars in Neurology 15(1): 72–83

Bach JR 2003 Mechanical insufflation/ exsufflation: has it come of age? A commentary. European Respiratory Journal 21: 385–386

Bach JR, Alba AS 1990 Noninvasive options for ventilatory support of the traumatic high level quadriplegic patient. Chest 98 (3): 613–619

Bach JR, Alba AS, Bodofsky E, Curran FJ, Schultheiss M 1987 Glossopharyngeal breathing and noninvasive aids in the management of post-polio respiratory insufficiency. Birth Defects 23: 99–113

Bach JR, Baird JS, Plosky D, Navado J, Weaver B 2002 Spinal muscular atrophy type 1: management and outcomes. Pediatric Pulmonology 34: 16–22

Bach JR, Smith WH, Michaels J et al 1993 Airway secretion clearance by mechanical exsufflation for post-poliomyelitis ventilator assisted individuals. Archives Physical Medical Rehabilitation 74: 170–177

Bach JR, Vis N, Weaver B 2000 Spinal muscular atrophy Type 1. A non-invasive management approach. Chest 117: 1100–1105

Bachrach LK, Loutit CW, Moss RB, Marcus R 1994 Osteopenia in adults with cystic fibrosis. American Journal of Medicine 96: 27–34

Barry PW, Fouroux B, Pedersen S, O'Callaghan C 2000 Nebulizers in childhood. European Respiratory Review 10(7): 527–535

Baxter GD 1994 Therapeutic lasers: theory and practice. Churchill Livingstone, Edinburgh

Baydur A, Gilgoff I, Prentice W et al 1990 Decline in respiratory function and experience with long-term assisted ventilation in advanced Duchenne's muscular dystrophy. Chest 97: 884–889

Bazuaye EA, Stone TN, Corris PA, Gibson GJ 1992 Variability of inspired oxygen concentration with nasal cannulas. Thorax 47: 609–611

Beck G, Barach A 1954 Value of mechanical aids in the management of a patient with poliomyelitis. Annals of Internal Medicine 40(6): 1081–1094

Beck GJ, Scarrone LA 1956 Physiological effects of exsufflation with negative pressure (EWNP). Chest 29: 80–95

Belman MJ 1993 Exercise in patients with chronic obstructive pulmonary disease. Thorax 48: 936–946

Bereiter M 2001 Glossopharyngeal breathing in motor neurone disease. Personal communication. Schweizer Paraplegiker Zentrum, Switzerland

Bersten AD 2003 Humidification and inhalation therapy. In: Bersten AD, Soni N (eds) Oh's intensive care manual, 5th edn. Butterworth-Heinemann, Edinburgh, pp 321–327

Bethune D 1975 Neurophysiological facilitation of respiration in the unconscious adult patient. Physiotherapy Canada 27(5): 241–245

Bethune D 1976 Facilitation of respiration in unconscious adult patients. Respiratory Technology 12(4): 18–21

Bethune D 1991 Neurophysiological facilitation of respiration. In: Pryor JA (ed) Respiratory care. Churchill Livingstone, Edinburgh

Bianchi AL, Pasaro R 1997 Organization of central respiratory neurons. In: Miller AD, Bianchi AL, Bishop BP (eds) Neural control of the respiratory muscles. CRC Press, New York

Bianchi C, Grandi M, Felisari G 2004 Efficacy of glossopharyngeal breathing for a ventilator-dependent, high-level tetraplegic patient after cervical cord tumor resection and tracheotomy. American Journal of Physical Medicine and Rehabilitation 83(3): 216–219

Bickerman H 1954 Exsufflation with negative pressure (EWNP); elimination of radiopaque material and foreign bodies from bronchi of anesthetized dogs. AMA Archives of Internal Medicine 93: 698–704

Bishop BP 1997 The abdominal muscles. In: Miller AD, Bianchi A, Bishop BP (eds) Neural control of the respiratory muscles. CRC Press, New York

Blackwell R 2004: Asthma – Evidence & tradition. Acupuncture Association of Chartered Physiotherapy Journal (United Kingdom) July, pp 33–40

Boots RJ, George N, Faoagali JL et al 2006 Double-heater-wire circuits and heat-and-moisture exchangers and the risk of ventilator-associated pneumonia. Critical Care Medicine 34(3): 687–693

Bott J, Keilty SEJ, Noone L 1992 Intermittent positive pressure breathing – a dying art? Physiotherapy 78: 656–660

Botton E, Saraux A, Laselve H, Jousse S, Le Goff P 2003 Musculoskeletal manifestations in cystic fibrosis. Joint Bone Spine 70(5): 327–335

Boyling JD, Palastanga N 1994 In: Grieve GP (ed) Modern manual therapy of the vertebral column, 2nd edn. Churchill Livingstone, Edinburgh

Bradley JM, O'Neill B 2005 Short-term ambulatory oxygen for chronic obstructive pulmonary disease. Cochrane Database of Systematic Reviews, Issue 4. Art. No.: CD004356 www.cochrane.org/reviews (accessed 5 July 2007)

Braggion C, Cappelletti LM, Cornacchia M, Zanolla L, Mastella G 1995 Short-term effects of three physiotherapy regimens in patients hospitalized for pulmonary exacerbations of cystic fibrosis: a cross-over randomized study. Pediatric Pulmonology 19: 16–22

Bransen RD, Davis K, Campbell RS, Johnson DJ, Porembka DT 1993 Humidification in the intensive care unit: prospective study of a new protocol utilizing heated humidification and a hygroscopic condenser humidifier. Chest 104: 1800–1805

Bray C 1994 Thoracic mobilisation in the management of respiratory and cardiac problems. In: The forgotten thoracic spine. Manipulative Physiotherapists Association of Australia Symposium, University of Sydney, Australia

Brazier D 1999 Endotracheal suction technique – putting research into practice. Journal of the Association of Chartered Physiotherapists in Respiratory Care 32: 13–17

British Standards Institution 1994 Specification for gas powered nebulisers for the delivery of drugs. BS7711 Part 3. British Standards Institution, London

British Thoracic Society & Scottish Intercollegiate Guidelines Network 2004 British guideline on the management of asthma www.enterpriseportal2.co.uk/filestore/bts/asthmafull.pdf (accessed 5 July 2007)

Buntain HM, Greer RM, Schluter PJ et al 2004 Bone mineral density in Australian children, adolescents and adults with cystic fibrosis: a controlled cross sectional study. Thorax 59: 149–155

Burge PS 1986 Getting the best out of bronchodilator therapy. Patient Management July: 155–185

Butler DS 1991 Mobilisation of the nervous system. Churchill Livingstone, Melbourne

Campbell AH, O'Connell JM, Wilson F 1975 The effect of chest physiotherapy upon the FEV_1 in chronic bronchitis. Medical Journal of Australia 1: 33–35

Campbell EJ, Baker D, Crites-Silver P 1988 Subjective effects of humidification of oxygen for delivery by nasal cannula. Chest 93: 289–293

Carr L, Pryor JA, Hodson ME 1995 Self-chest clapping: patients' views and the effects on oxygen saturation. Physiotherapy 81: 753–757

Carr L, Smith RE, Pryor JA, Partridge C 1996 Cystic fibrosis patients' views and beliefs about chest clearance and exercise – a pilot study. Physiotherapy 82: 621–626

Casaburi R, Patessio A, Loli F et al 1991 Reductions in exercise lactic acidosis and ventilation as a result of exercise training in patients with obstructive pulmonary disease. American Review of Respiratory Disease 143: 9–18

Cecins NM, Jenkins SC, Pengelley J, Ryan G 1999 The active cycle of breathing techniques – to tip or not to tip? Respiratory Medicine 93: 660–665

Cegla UH, Bautz M, Fröde G, Werner Th 1997 Physiotherapie bei patienten mit COAD und tracheobronchialer instabilität-verleich zweier oszillierender PEP-systeme (RC-CORNET®, VRP1 DESITIN). Pneumologie 51: 129–136

Cegla UH, Jost HJ, Harten A et al 2002 Course of severe COPD with and without physiotherapy with the RC-Cornet®. Pneumologie 56(7): 418–424

Chang HK, Weber ME, King M 1988 Mucus transport by high frequency non-symmetrical oscillatory flow. Journal of Applied Physiology 65: 1203–1209

Chatham K, Ionescus AA, Nixon LS, Shale DJ 2004 A short-term comparison of two methods of sputum expectoration in cystic fibrosis. European Respiratory Journal 23: 435–439

Chatham K, Marshall C, Campbell IA, Prescott RJ 1993 The Flutter VRP1 device in post-thoracotomy patients. Physiotherapy 79: 95–98

Chatwin M, O'Driscoll D, Corfield D, Morrell M, Simonds A 2004 Controlled trial of intrapulmonary percussion in adults and children with stable severe neuromuscular disease. American Journal of Critical Care Medicine 169: A438

Chatwin M, Ross E, Hart N et al 2003 Cough augmentation with

mechanical insufflation/exsufflation in patients with neuromuscular weakness. European Respiratory Journal 21: 502–508

Chevaillier J 2002 Autogenic drainage (AD). In: Physiotherapy in the treatment of cystic fibrosis (CF), 3rd edn. International Physiotherapy Group for Cystic Fibrosis (IPG/CF), pp 12–15 www.cfww.org/IPG-CF/index.asp (accessed 5 July 2007)

Chiappetta A, Beckerman R 1995 High frequency chest wall oscillation in spinal muscular atrophy (SMA). RT Journal for Respiratory Care Practitioners 8(4): 112–114

Chiumello D, Pelosi P, Gattinoni L 2002 Conditioning of inspired gases in mechanically ventilated patients. In: Vincent J-L (ed) Intensive Care Medicine. Springer (ISBN 0387916253)

Chuter TAM, Weissman C, Starker PM, Gump FE 1989 Effect of incentive spirometry on diaphragmatic function after surgery. Surgery 105: 488–493

Chuter TAM, Weissman C, Mathews DM, Starker PM 1990 Diaphragmatic breathing maneuvers and movement of the diaphragm after cholecystectomy. Chest 97: 1110–1114

Clarke SW 1988 Inhaler therapy. Quarterly Journal of Medicine 67(253): 355–368

Clarke SW 1995 Physical defences. In: Brewis RAL, Corrin B, Geddes DM, Gibson GJ (eds) Respiratory medicine, vol 1, 2nd edn. WB Saunders, London

Clini E, Antoni F, Vitacca M et al 2006 Intrapulmonary percussive ventilation in tracheostomized patients: a randomized controlled trial. Intensive Care Medicine, 32: 1994–2001

Cole P 1995 Bronchiectasis. In: Brewis RAL, Corrin B, Geddes DM, Gibson GJ (eds) Respiratory medicine, Vol 2, 2nd edn. WB Saunders, London

Collis GG, Cole CH, Le Souëf PN 1990 Dilution of nebulised aerosols by air entrainment in children. Lancet 336: 341–343

Conway JH 1992 The effects of humidification for patients with chronic airways disease. Physiotherapy 78: 97–101

Conway JH, Fleming JS, Perring S, Holgate ST 1992 Humidification as an adjunct to chest physiotherapy in aiding tracheo-bronchial clearance in patients with bronchiectasis. Respiratory Medicine 86: 109–114

Coombs HC 1918 The relation of the dorsal roots of the spinal nerves and the mesencephalon to the control of respiratory movements. American Journal of Physiology 46: 459–471

Coombs HC, Pike FH 1930 The nervous control of respiration in kittens. American Journal of Physiology 95: 681–693

Cornacchia M, Zenorini A, Perobelli S et al 2001 Prevalence of urinary incontinence in women with cystic fibrosis. British Journal Urology International 88: 44–48

Cunningham S, Prasad SA, Collyer L et al 2001 Bronchoconstriction following nebulised Colistin in cystic fibrosis. Archives of Disease in Childhood 84(5): 432–433

Currie DC, Munro C, Gaskell D, Cole PJ 1986 Practice, problems and compliance with postural drainage: a survey of chronic sputum producers. British Journal of Diseases of the Chest 80: 249–253

Dab I, Alexander F 1979 The mechanism of autogenic drainage studied with flow volume curves. Monographs of Paediatrics 10: 50–53

Dail CW 1951 'Glossopharyngeal breathing' by paralyzed patients. California Medicine 75: 217–218

Dail CW, Affeldt JE, Collier CR 1955 Clinical aspects of glossopharyngeal breathing. Journal of the American Medical Association 158: 445–449

Darbee JC, Kanga JF, Ohtake PJ 2005 Physiologic evidence for high-frequency chest wall oscillation and positive expiratory pressure breathing in hospitalized subjects with cystic fibrosis. Physical Therapy 85(12): 1278–1289

Darbee JC, Ohtake PJ, Grant BJ, Cerny FJ 2004 Physiologic evidence for the efficacy of positive expiratory pressure as an airway clearance technique in patients with cystic fibrosis. Physical Therapy 84(6): 524–537

David A 1991 Autogenic drainage – the German approach. In: Pryor JA (ed) Respiratory care. Churchill Livingstone, Edinburgh, pp 65–78

Davidson AGF, Wong LTK, Pirie GE, McIlwaine PM 1992 Long-term comparative trial of conventional percussion and drainage physiotherapy versus autogenic drainage in cystic fibrosis. Pediatric Pulmonology (Suppl) 8: 298

Dawson SV, Elliott, EA 1977 Wave-speed limitation on expiratory flow – a unifying concept. Journal of Applied Physiology 43(3): 498–515

Dean E 1985 Effect of body position on pulmonary function. Physical Therapy 65: 613–618

Denehy L, Berney S 2001 The use of positive pressure devices by physiotherapists. European Respiratory Journal 17: 821–829

De Troyer A 1997 Mechanics of the chest wall muscles In: Miller AD, Bianchi AL, Bishop BP (eds) Neural control of the respiratory muscles. CRC Press, New York

DeVilbiss Oxygen Services 2000 Manufacturer's guidelines for oxygen concentrators. Sunrise Medical Ltd, West Midlands DY8 4PS, England

Dhand R 2002 Nebulizers that use a vibrating mesh or plate with multiple apertures to generate aerosol. Respiratory Care 47(12): 1406–1416

Djedaini K, Billiard M, Mier L et al 1995 Changing heat and moisture exchangers every 48 hours rather than 24 hours does not affect their efficacy and the incidence of nosocomial pneumonia. American Journal of Respiratory and Critical Care Medicine 152: 1562–1569

Dodd ME, Abbott J, Maddison J, Moorcroft AJ, Webb AK 1997 Effect of tonicity of nebulised colistin on chest tightness and pulmonary function in adults with cystic fibrosis. Thorax 52: 656–658

Dodd ME, Hanley SP, Johnson SC, Webb AK 1995 District nebuliser compressor service: reliability and costs. Thorax 50: 82–84

Dodd ME, Kellet F, Davis A et al 2000 Audit of oxygen prescribing before and after the introduction of a prescription chart. British Medical Journal 321: 864–865

Duron B, Bars P 1986 Effect of thoracic cutaneous nerve stimulations on the activity of the intercostal muscles and motoneurons of the cat. In: Euler C, Lagercrantz A (eds) Neurobiology of the control of breathing (Nobel conference series). Raven Press, New York

Duron B, Rose D 1997 The intercostal muscles. In: Miller AD, Bianchi AL, Bishop BP (eds) Neural control of the respiratory muscles. CRC Press, New York

Eaton T, Young P, Zeng I, Kolbe J 2007 A randomized evaluation of the acute efficacy, acceptability and tolerability of flutter and active cycle of breathing with and without postural drainage in non–cystic fibrosis bronchiectasis. Chronic Respiratory Disease 4: 23–40

Electromed 2006 SmartVest® Airway Clearance System: prescribing protocols. Electromed, Minnesota, USA. *www.electromed–usa.com* (accessed 5 July 2007)

Elkins MR, Jones A, van der Schans C 2006a Positive expiratory pressure physiotherapy for airway clearance in people with cystic fibrosis. *Cochrane Database of Systematic Reviews* Issue 2. Art. No.: CD003147

Elkins MR, Lane T, Goldberg H et al 2005 Effect of airway clearance techniques on the efficacy of the sputum induction procedure. European Respiratory Journal 26: 904–908

Elkins MR, Robinson M, Rose BR et al 2006b National Hypertonic Saline in Cystic Fibrosis (NHSCF) Study Group. A controlled trial of long-term inhaled hypertonic saline in patients with cystic fibrosis. New England Journal of Medicine 354(3): 229–240

Eng PA, Morton J, Douglass JA et al 1996 Short-term efficacy of ultrasonically nebulized hypertonic saline in cystic fibrosis. Pediatric Pulmonology 21: 77–83

Enright S, Chatham K, Ionescu AA, Unnithan VB, Shale DJ 2004 Inspiratory muscle training improves lung function and exercise capacity in adults with cystic fibrosis. Chest 126: 406–411

Enright SJ, Unnithan VB, Heward C, Withnall L, Davies DH 2006 Effect of high-intensity inspiratory muscle training on lung volumes, diaphragm thickness, and exercise capacity in subjects who are healthy. Physical Therapy 86 (3): 345–354

Euler C 1986 Breathing behavior. In: Euler C, Lagercrantz A (eds) Neurobiology of the control of breathing (Nobel conference series). Raven Press, New York

European Respiratory Society 2000 European Respiratory Society nebulizer guidelines: clinical aspects. European Respiratory Review 10 (76)

European Respiratory Society Task Force 2002 Standardised methodology of sputum induction and processing. European Respiratory Journal 20; Supplement 37

Everard ML, Evans M, Milner AD 1994 Is tapping jet nebulisers worthwhile? Archives of Disease in Childhood 70: 538–539

Ewart W 1901 The treatment of bronchiectasis and of chronic bronchial affections by posture and by respiratory exercises. Lancet 2: 70–72

Ezzo J 2000 Is acupuncture effective for the treatment of chronic pain? A systematic review. Pain 86: 217–225

Falk M, Andersen JB 1991 Positive expiratory pressure (PEP) mask. In: Pryor JA (ed) Respiratory care. Churchill Livingstone, Edinburgh, pp 51–63

Falk M, Kelstrup M, Andersen JB, Kinoshita T, Falk P, Støvring S, Gøthgen I 1984 Improving the ketchup bottle method with positive expiratory pressure, PEP, in cystic

5

fibrosis. European Journal of Respiratory Diseases 65: 423–432

Feng W, Deng WW, Huang SG et al 1998 Short-term efficacy of RC-Cornet in improving pulmonary function and decreasing cohesiveness of sputum in bronchiectasis patients. Chest 114(4); Suppl, pp 320S

Festini F, Ballarin S, Codamo T, Doro R, Loganes C 2004 Prevalence of pain in adults with cystic fibrosis. J Cyst Fibrosis Mar; 3(1): 51–57

Fink JB, Mahlmeister MJ 2002 High-frequency oscillation of the airway and chest wall. Respiratory Care 47: 797–807

Fleck S 1994 Detraining: its effects on endurance and strength. National Strength and Conditioning Journal 2: 22–28

Flower KA, Eden RI, Lomax L, Mann NM, Burgess J 1979 New mechanical aid to physiotherapy in cystic fibrosis. British Medical Journal 2: 630–631

Fok J, Brown NE, Zuberbuhler P et al 2002 Low bone mineral density in cystic fibrosis patients. Canadian Journal of Dietetic Practice and Research 63: 192–197

Frazier DT, Xu Fadi, Lee L-Y 1997 Respiratory-related reflexes and the cerebellum. In: Miller AD, Bianchi AL, Bishop BP (eds) Neural control of the respiratory muscles. CRC Press, New York

Freitag L, Bremme J, Schroer M 1989 High frequency oscillation for respiratory physiotherapy. British Journal of Anaesthesia 63: 44S–46S

Gallon A 1991 Evaluation of chest percussion in the treatment of patients with copious sputum production. Respiratory Medicine 85: 45–51

Geddes EL, Reid DW, Crowe J, O'Brian K, Brooks D 2005 Inspiratory muscle training in adults with chronic obstructive pulmonary disease: a systematic review. Respiratory Medicine 99: 1440–1458

Gleeson JG, Price JF 1988 Nebuliser technique. British Journal of Diseases of the Chest 82: 172–174

Goldman M 1974 Mechanical coupling of the diaphragm and the rib cage. In: Pengelly LD, Rebuck AS, Campbell EJM (eds) Loaded breathing. Proceedings of an international symposium, 'The effects of mechanical loads on breathing'. Longman Canada, Don Mills, Ontario

Gordon J 1991 Spinal mechanisms of motor coordination. In: Kandel ER, Schwartz JH, Jessel JM (eds) Principles of neural science. Appleton & Lange, Connecticut

Gormezano J, Branthwaite MA 1972 Pulmonary physiotherapy with assisted ventilation. Anaesthesia 27: 249–257

Gosselink R 2004 Breathing techniques in patients with chronic obstructive pulmonary disease (COPD). Chronic Respiratory Disease 1: 163–172

Gosselink R, Schrever K, Cops P et al 2000 Incentive spirometry does not enhance recovery after thoracic surgery. Critical Care Medicine 28(3): 679–683

Gosselink RA, Wagenaar RC, Rijswijk H, Sargeant AJ, Decramer ML 1995 Diaphragmatic breathing reduces efficiency of breathing in patients with chronic obstructive pulmonary disease. American Journal of Respiratory and Critical Care Medicine 151(4): 1136–1142

Grassino A 1974 Influence of chest wall configuration on the static and dynamic characteristics of the contracting diaphragm. In: Pengelly LD, Rebuck AS, Campbell EJM (eds) Loaded breathing. Proceedings of an international symposium, 'The effects of mechanical loads on breathing'. Longman Canada, Don Mills, Ontario

Gray's Anatomy 1973. Longman, Edinburgh

Green M, Moxham J 1985 The respiratory muscles. Clinical Science 68: 1–10

Gregersen GG, Lucas DL 1967 An in vivo study of the axial rotation of the human thoraco-lumbar spine. Journal of Bone and Joint Surgery 49A: 247–262

Gross D, Zidulka A, O'Brien C et al 1985 Peripheral mucociliary clearance with high frequency chest wall compression. Journal of Applied Physiology 58: 1157–1163

Gumery L, Lee J, Whitehouse J, Honeybourne D 2005 The prevalence of urinary incontinence in adult cystic fibrosis males. Journal of Cystic Fibrosis 4(Suppl 1): S97

Gunawardena KA, Patel B, Campbell IA, Macdonald JB, Smith AP 1984 Oxygen as a driving gas for nebulisers: safe or dangerous? British Medical Journal 288: 272–274

Halvorsen TB, Anda SS, Naess AB, Levang OW 1995: Fatal cardiac tamponade after acupuncture through congenital sternal foramen. Lancet 345: 1175

Hansen LG, Warwick W 1990 High-frequency chest compression system to aid in clearance of mucus from the lung. Biomedical Instrumentation and Technology 24: 289–294

Hansen LG, Warwick WJ, Hansen KL 1994 Mucus transport mechanisms in

relation to the effect of high frequency chest compression (HFCC) on mucus clearance. Pediatric Pulmonology 17: 113–118

Hardy KA, Bach JR, Stoller JK et al 1994 A review of airway clearance: new techniques, indications, and recommendations. Respiratory Care 39(5): 440–445

Harrison DA, Breen DP, Harris ND, Gerrish SP 1993 The performance of two intensive care humidifiers at high gas flows. Anaesthesia 48: 902–905

Hasani A, Pavia D, Agnew JE, Clarke SW 1994 Regional lung clearance during cough and forced expiration technique (FET): effects of flow and viscoelasticity. Thorax 49: 557–561

Henderson RC, Madsen CD 1996 Bone density in children and adolescents with cystic fibrosis. Journal of Pediatrics 128: 28–34

Henderson RC, Specter BB 1994 Kyphosis and fractures in children and young adults with cystic fibrosis. Journal of Paediatrics 125: 208–212

Hilaire G, Monteau R 1997 Brainstem and spinal control of respiratory muscles during breathing. In: Miller AD, Bianchi AL, Bishop BP (eds) Neural control of the respiratory muscles. CRC Press, New York

Hill K, Eastwood PR 2005 Respiratory muscle training: the con argument. Chronic Respiratory Disease 2(4): 223–224

Hill K, Jenkins SC, Hillman Eastwood PR 2004 Dyspnoea in COPD: can inspiratory muscle training help? Australian Journal Physiotherapy 50: 169–180

Hill SL, Barnes PK, Hollway T, Tennant R 1984 Fixed performance oxygen masks: an evaluation. British Medical Journal 288: 1261–1263

Hill-Rom 2006 The Vest™ Airway Clearance System: information for physicians. Hill-Rom, Minnesota, USA. *www.hill-rom.com* (accessed 5 July 2007)

Hinds CJ, Watson D 1996 Intensive care, 2nd edn. WB Saunders, London, pp 33, 175

Hofmeyr JL, Webber BA, Hodson ME 1986 Evaluation of positive expiratory pressure as an adjunct to chest physiotherapy in the treatment of cystic fibrosis. Thorax 41: 951–954

Holland AE, Button BM 2006 Is there a role for airway clearance techniques in chronic obstructive pulmonary disease? Chronic Respiratory Disease 3: 83–91

Homnick DN, Anderson K, Marks JH 1998 Comparison of the flutter device to standard chest physiotherapy in hospitalized patients with cystic fibrosis: a pilot study. Chest 114(4): 993–997

Hopwood V 1993: Acupuncture in physiotherapy. Complementary Therapies in Medicine 1: 100–104

Hsiao SF, Wu YT, Wu HD, Wang TG 2003 Comparison of the effectivness of pressure threshold and targeted resistive muscle training in patients with chronic obstructive pulmonary disease. Journal of the Formosan Medical Association 102: 204–205

Hutchinson GR, Parker S, Pryor JA et al 1996 Home-use nebulizers: a potential source of *Burkholderia cepacia* and other colistin-resistant, gram-negative bacteria in patients with cystic fibrosis. Journal of Clinical Microbiology 34: 584–587

Institute for Work & Health 1996 DASH Index. The American Academy of Orthopaedic Surgeons (AAOS) *www.iwh.on.ca* (accessed 5 July 2007)

Jacob W 1990 Physiotherapy in the ICU. In: Oh TE (ed) Intensive care manual, 3rd edn. Butterworths, Sydney, Chapter 4, p 24

Janda V 1994 Muscles and motor control in cervicogenic disorders: assessment and management physical therapy for the cervical and thoracic spine. In: Grant R (ed) Clinics in physical therapy, 2nd edn. Churchill Livingstone, New York

Jean A, Car A, Kessler JP 1997 Brainstem organization of swallowing and its interaction with respiration. In: Miller AD, Bianchi AL, Bishop BP (eds) Neural control of the respiratory muscles. CRC Press, New York

Jeffrey AA, Warren PM 1992 Should we judge a mask by its cover? Thorax 47: 543–546

Jenkins SC, Soutar SA, Moxham J 1988 The effects of posture on lung volumes in normal subjects and in patients pre- and post-coronary artery surgery. Physiotherapy 74: 492–496

Jobst KA 1995 A critical analysis of acupuncture in pulmonary disease: efficacy and safety of acupuncture needle. Journal of Alternative and Complementary Medicine 1: 54–85

Jones PW 2002 Interpreting thresholds for a clinically significant change in health status in asthma and COPD European Respiratory Journal 19: 398–404

Jull G, Trott P, Potter H et al 2002 A randomized controlled trial of exercise and manipulative therapy for cervicogenic headache. Spine 27(17): 1835–1843

Kelleher WH, Parida RK 1957 Glossopharyngeal breathing. British Medical Journal 2: 740–743

Kendrick AH, Smith EC, Denyer J 1995 Nebulizers – fill volume, residual volume and matching of nebulizer to compressor. Respiratory Medicine 89: 157–159

Kennedy WL 1995 (ed) ACSM's Guidelines for Exercise Testing and Prescription. Williams & Willsins, Media, PA

Kenyon JN 1983 Modern techniques of acupuncture; Vol 1: A practical scientific guide to electro-acupuncture. Thorsons, Wellingborough

Kenyon JN 1988 Acupressure techniques. Healing Arts Press, Canada

Kieselmann R 2002 Modified AD. In: Physiotherapy in the treatment of cystic fibrosis (CF), 3rd edn. International Physiotherapy Group for Cystic Fibrosis (IPG/CF), pp 16–17 *www.cfww.org/IPG-CF/index.asp* (accessed 5 July 2007)

King M, Phillips DM, Gross D et al 1983 Enhanced tracheal mucus clearance with high frequency chest wall compression. American Review of Respiratory Disease 128: 511–515

King M, Phillips DM, Zidulka A, Chang HK 1984 Tracheal mucus clearance in high-frequency oscillation II. Chest wall versus mouth oscillation. American Review of Respiratory Disease 130: 703–706

King M, Zidulka A, Phillips DM et al 1990 Tracheal mucus clearance in high frequency oscillation Effect of peak flow rate bias. European Respiratory Journal 3: 6–13

Kishi H, Mishima HK, Sakamoto I, Yamashita U 1996 Stimulation of retinal pigment epithelial cell growth neuropeptides in vitro. Current Eye Research 15: 708–713

Kluft J, Beker L, Castagnino M et al 1996 A comparison of bronchial drainage treatments in cystic fibrosis. Pediatric Pulmonology 22: 271–274

Koepchen HP, Abel H-H, Klussendorf D, Lazar H 1986 Respiratory and cardiovascular rhythmicity. In: Euler C, Lagercrantz A (eds) Neurobiology of the control of breathing (Nobel conference series). Raven Press, New York

Koh JL, Harrison D, Palermo TM, Turner H, McGraw T 2005 Assessment of acute and chronic pain symptoms in children with cystic fibrosis. Pediatric Pulmonology 40(4): 330–335

Komi PV, Hakkinen K 1991 Strength and power. In: Dirix A Knuttgen HG, Tittel K (eds) The Olympic book of sports medicine. Blackwell, Oxford, pp 181–193

Konstan MW, Stern RC, Doershuk CF 1994 Efficacy of the Flutter device for airway mucus clearance in patients with cystic fibrosis. Journal of Pediatrics 124: 689–693

Kraemer W, Adams K, Cararelli E et al 2002 American College of Sports Medicine position stand. Progressive models in resistance training for healthy adults. Medicine and Science in Sports and Exercise 34: 364–380

Laghi F, Tobin MJ 2003 Disorders of the respiratory muscles. American Journal of Respiratory and Critical Care Medicine 168: 10–48

Langlands J 1967 The dynamics of cough in health and in chronic bronchitis. Thorax 22: 88–96

Lannefors L 2006 Inhalation therapy: practical considerations for nebulisation therapy. Physical Therapy Reviews 11: 21–27

Lannefors L, Wollmer P 1992 Mucus clearance with three chest physiotherapy regimes in cystic fibrosis: a comparison between postural drainage, PEP and physical exercise. European Respiratory Journal 5(6): 748–753

Lapin CD 2002 Airway physiology, autogenic drainage, and active cycle of breathing. Respiratory Care 47(7): 778–785

Lawrence RM, Rosch PJ, Plowden J 1998 Magnet therapy: the pain cure alternative. Prima Publishing, California

Lawrence VA, Cornell JE, Smetana GW 2006 Strategies to reduce postoperative pulmonary complications after noncardiothoracic surgery: systematic review for the American College of Physicians. Annals of Internal Medicine 144(8): 596–608

Lee D 2003 The thorax: an integrated approach, 2nd edn. Orthopaedic Physical Therapy, Minneapolis

Leith DE, Bradley M 1976 Ventilatory muscle strength and endurance training. Journal of Applied Physiology 41: 508–516

Lewis RA, Fleming JS 1985 Fractional deposition from a jet nebuliser: how it differs from a metered dose inhaler. British Journal of Diseases of the Chest 79: 361–367

Lichstein E, Chadda KD, Naik D, Gupta PK 1974 Diagonal ear lobe crease: relevance and implications as a coronary risk factor. New England Journal of Medicine 290; 615–616

Linde D, Jobst K, Panton J 1986 Controlled trial of acupuncture for disabling breathlessness. Lancet 2: 1417–1419

5

Lindemann H 1992 The value of physical therapy with VRP1 Desitin ('Flutter'). Pneumologie 46(12): 626–630

Lock SH, Blower G, Prynne M, Wedzicha JA 1992 Comparison of liquid and gaseous oxygen for domiciliary portable use. Thorax 47: 98–100

Lopez-Vidriero MT, Reid L 1978 Bronchial mucus in health and disease. British Medical Bulletin 34(1): 63–74

Lotters F, van Tol B, Kwakkel G, Gosselink R 2002 Effect of controlled inspiratory muscle training in patients with COPD: a meta-analysis. European Respiratory Journal 20: 570–576

Lund I, Lundberg T, Carleson J et al 2006 Are minimal, superficial or sham acupuncture procedures acceptable as inert placebo controls. Acupuncture in Medicine 24(1): 13–15

Lunteren E, Dick TE 1997 Muscles of the upper airway and accessory respiratory muscles. In: Miller AD, Bianchi AL, Bishop BP (eds) Neural control of the respiratory muscles. CRC Press, New York

Macklem PT 1974 Physiology of cough. Transactions of the American Broncho-Esophalogical Association 150–157

Maddison J, Dodd M, Webb AK 1994 Nebulised colistin causes chest tightness in adults with cystic fibrosis. Respiratory Medicine 88(2): 145–147

Main E, Prasad A, van der Schans C 2005 Conventional chest physiotherapy compared to other airway clearance techniques for cystic fibrosis. Cochrane Database of Systematic Reviews, Issue 1. Art. No.: CD002011

Maltais F, Le Blanc P, Jobin J, Caraburi R 2000 Peripheral muscle dysfunction in chronic obstructive pulmonary disease. Clinics in Chest Medicine 21: 665–677

Make BJ, Hill NS, Goldberg AL et al 1998 Mechanical ventilation beyond the intensive care unit. Report of a consensus conference of the American College of Chest Physicians. Chest 113 (Suppl 5): 289S–344S

Man SH, Gauthier D, Turner M 1997 Acupressure as an adjunct to a pulmonary rehabilitation program. J Cardiopulmonary Rehabilitation 17(4): 268–276

Mashanskii VF, Markov IuV, Shpunt VKh, Li SE, Mirkin AS 1983 Topography of the gap junctions in human skin and their possible role in the non-neural transmission of information [Article in Russian].

Arkhiv Anatomii, Gistologii i Émbriologii 84(3): 53–60

Massery M 2005 Musculoskeletal and neuromuscular interventions: a physical approach to cystic fibrosis. Journal of the Royal Society of Medicine 98 (Suppl 45): 55–66

Massie RJ, Towns SJ, Bernard E et al 1998 The musculoskeletal complications of cystic fibrosis. Journal of Paediatrics and Child Health 34(5): 467–470

McArdle WD, Katch FI, Katch VL 2001 Exercise physiology, energy, nutrition, and human performance, 5th edn. Lippincott, Williams & Wilkins, Philadelphia

McCarren B, Alison JA 2006 Physiological effects of vibration in subjects with cystic fibrosis. European Respiratory Journal 27(6): 1204–1209

McCool FD 1992 Inspiratory muscle weakness and fatigue. RT: The Journal for Respiratory Care Practitioners 5(6): 32–41

McDonnell T, McNicholas WT, FitzGerald MX 1986 Hypoxaemia during chest physiotherapy in patients with cystic fibrosis. Irish Journal of Medical Science 155: 345–348

McGuire S 2006 The I-neb™ adaptive aerosol delivery (AAD®) system – a holistic approach to inhaled drug delivery including regulatory approval. Drug Delivery Report Spring/Summer 68–71

McIlwaine PM, Wong LT, Peacock D, Davidson AG 1997 Long-term comparative trial of conventional postural drainage and percussion versus positive expiratory pressure physiotherapy in the treatment of cystic fibrosis. Journal of Pediatrics 131(4): 570–574

McIlwaine PM, Wong LT, Peacock D, Davidson AG 2001 Long-term comparative trial of positive expiratory pressure versus oscillating positive expiratory pressure (flutter) physiotherapy in the treatment of cystic fibrosis. Journal of Pediatrics 138(6): 845–850

McKenzie DK, Frith PA, Burdon JGW, Town GI 2003 The COPDX Plan: Australia and New Zealand Guidelines for the management of COPD. Medical Journal Australia 178 (6 Suppl): S1–S40

Mead J, Takishima T, Leith D 1970 Stress distribution in lungs: a model of pulmonary elasticity. Journal of Applied Physiology 28: 596–608

Mead J, Turner JM, Macklem PT, Little JB 1967 Significance of the relationship between lung recoil and maximum expiratory flow. Journal of Applied Physiology 22: 95–108

Medic-Aid Ltd 1996 Nebulizer therapy training pack. Medic-Aid Ltd, Heath Place, Bognor Regis, W Sussex, UK

Medical Research Council Working Party 1981 Long-term domiciliary oxygen therapy in chronic hypoxic cor pulmonale complicating chronic bronchitis and emphysema. Lancet 1: 681–686

Menkes HA, Traystman RJ 1977 Collateral ventilation. American Review of Respiratory Disease 116: 287–309

Milla CE, Hansen LG, Warwick W 2006 Different frequencies should be prescribed for different high frequency chest compression machines. Biomedical Instrumentation & Technology 40: 319–324

Miller AD, Bianchi AL, Bishop BP 1997 Overview of the neural control of the respiratory muscles. In: Miller AD, Bianchi AL, Bishop BP (eds) Neural control of the respiratory muscles. CRC Press, New York

Miller JM, Ashton-Miller JA, DeLancey JO 1998 A pelvic muscle precontraction can reduce cough-related urine loss in selected women with mild SUI. Journal of the American Geriatrics Society 46(7): 870–874

Miller MR 2000 Peak expiratory flow meters. European Respiratory Society: The Buyer's Guide 3: 12–14

Miller S, Hall DO, Clayton CB, Nelson R 1995 Chest physiotherapy in cystic fibrosis: a comparative study of autogenic drainage and the active cycle of breathing techniques with postural drainage. Thorax 50: 165–169

Miske LJ, Hickey EM, Kolb SM, Weiner DJ, Panitch HB 2004 Use of the mechanical in-exsufflator in pediatric patients with neuromuscular disease and impaired cough. Chest 125: 1406–1412

Moraes T, Carpenter S, Taylor L 2002 Cystic fibrosis incontinence in children. Pediatric Pulmonology Supplement 24: 315

Morgan MDL, Silver JR, Williams SJ 1986 The respiratory system of the spinal cord patient. In: Bloch RF, Basbaum M (eds) Management of spinal cord injuries. Williams and Wilkins, Baltimore, pp 78–115

Mortensen J, Falk M, Groth S, Jensen C 1991 The effects of postural drainage and positive expiratory pressure physiotherapy on tracheobronchial clearance in cystic fibrosis. Chest 100(5): 1350–1357

Mustfa N, Aiello M, Lyall RA et al 2003 Cough augmentation in amyotrophic lateral sclerosis. Neurology 61: 1285–1287

Nakamura S, Mikami M, Kawakami M et al 1998 Comparative evaluation of the flutter and the cornet in improving the cohesiveness of sputum from patients with bronchiectasis. European Respiratory Journal, 12 (Suppl 28): 212s–213s

National Institute for Health and Clinical Excellence 2004 Chronic obstructive pulmonary disease – management of chronic obstructive pulmonary disease in adults in primary and secondary care. Developed by the National Collaborating Centre for Chronic Conditions. NICE clinical guideline 12. www.nice.org.uk/ CG012NICEguideline (accessed 5 July 2007)

National Institute for Health and Clinical Excellence 2006 Urinary incontinence. The management of urinary incontinence in women. Developed by the National Collaborating Centre of Women's and Children's Health. NICE clinical guideline 40. www.nice.org.uk/ CG040NICEguideline (accessed 5 July 2007)

Nathan H 1962 Osteophytes of the vertebral column. An anatomical study of their development according to age, race and sex with considerations as to their aetiology and significance. Journal of Bone and Joint Surgery 44: A243

Nava S, Barbarito N, Piaggi G, De Mattia E, Cirio S 2006 Physiological response to intrapulmonary percussive ventilation in stable COPD patients. Respiratory Medicine 100: 1526–1533

Nebuliser Project Group of the British Thoracic Society Standards of Care Committee 1997 Current best practice for nebuliser treatment. Thorax 52 (Suppl 2): S1–S106

Nelson HP 1934 Postural drainage of the lungs. British Medical Journal 2: 251–255

Neumeister W, Kuhlemann H, Bauer T et al 1999 Effect of acupuncture on quality of life, mouth occlusion pressures and lung function in COPD. Medizinische Klinik 94: 106–109

Newhouse PA, White F, Marks JH, Homnick DN 1998 The intrapulmonary percussive ventilator and flutter device compared to standard chest physiotherapy in patients with cystic fibrosis. Clinical Pediatrics 37: 427–432

Newman SP, Pellow PGD, Clarke SW 1986 Droplet size distributions of nebulised aerosols for inhalation therapy. Clinical Physics and Physiological Measurement 7: 139–146

Newman SP, Weisz AWB, Talaee N, Clarke SW 1991 Improvement of drug delivery with a breath actuated pressurised aerosol for patients with poor inhaler technique. Thorax 46: 712–716

Niere K, Jerak A 2004 Measurement of headache frequency, intensity and duration: comparison of patient report by questionnaire and headache diary. Physiotherapy Research International 9(4): 149–156

Nocturnal Oxygen Therapy Trial Group 1980 Continuous or nocturnal oxygen therapy in hypoxemic chronic obstructive lung disease: a clinical trial. Annals of Internal Medicine 93: 391–398

Nogier PMF 1981 Handbook to auriculotherapy. Maisonneuve SA, France

Oberwaldner B, Evans JC, Zach MS 1986 Forced expirations against a variable resistance: a new chest physiotherapy method in cystic fibrosis. Pediatric Pulmonology 2: 358–367

Oberwaldner B, Theissl B, Rucker A, Zach MS 1991 Chest physiotherapy in hospitalized patients with cystic fibrosis: a study of lung function effects and sputum production. European Respiratory Journal 4: 152–158

O'Donnell DE, McGuire M, Samis L, Webb KA 1995 The impact of exercise reconditioning on breathlessness in severe chronic airflow limitation. American Journal of Respiratory and Critical Care Medicine 152: 2005–2013

O'Driscoll BR, Kay EA, Taylor RJ, Bernstein A 1990 Home nebulizers: can optimal therapy be predicted by laboratory studies? Respiratory Medicine 84: 471–477

Oermann CM, Sockrider MM, Giles D et al 2001 Comparison of high-frequency chest wall oscillation and oscillating positive expiratory pressure in the home management of cystic fibrosis: a pilot study. Pediatric Pulmonology 32: 372–377

O'Leary S, Jull G, Kim M, Vicenzino B 2007 Cranio-cervical flexor muscle impairment at maximal, moderate, and low loads is a feature of neck pain. Manual Therapy 12(1): 34–39

Oleson T 1998 Auriculotherapy manual. ISBN 0-9629-415-5-7, p 7

Olsen MF, Lonroth H, Bake B 1999 Effects of breathing exercises on breathing patterns in obese and non-obese subjects. Clinical Physiology 19(3): 251–257

O'Neill B, Dodd ME 2006 Oxygen on the move: practical considerations for physiotherapists. Physical Therapy Reviews 11: 28–36

O'Neill SO, McCarthy DS 1983 Postural relief of dyspnoea in severe chronic airflow limitation: relationship to respiratory muscle strength. Thorax 38: 595–600

Orr A, McVean RJ, Web AK, Dodd ME 2001 Questionnaire survey of urinary incontinence in women with cystic fibrosis. British Medical Journal 322: 1521

Overend TJ, Anderson CM, Lucy SD et al 2001 The effect of incentive spirometry on postoperative pulmonary complications. Chest 120: 971–978

Pakala R, Benedict CR 1998 Effect of serotonin and thromboxane A_2 on endothelial cell proliferation: effect of specific receptor antagonists. Journal of Laboratory and Clinical Medicine 131(6): 527–537

Parasa RB, Maffulli N 1999 Musculoskeletal involvement in cystic fibrosis. Bulletin of the Hospital for Joint Diseases 58(1): 37–44

Partridge C, Pryor J, Webber B 1989 Characteristics of the forced expiration technique. Physiotherapy 75: 193–194

Patterson JE, Bradley JM, Elborn JS 2004 Airway clearance in bronchiectasis: a randomized crossover trial of active cycle of breathing techniques (incorporating postural drainage and vibration) versus test of incremental respiratory endurance. Chronic Respiratory Disease 1: 127–130

Patterson JE, Bradley JM, Hewitt O et al 2005 Airway clearance in bronchiectasis: a randomized crossover trial of active cycle of breathing techniques versus Acapella. Respiration 72(3): 239–242

Pavia D, Webber B, Agnew JE et al 1988 The role of intermittent positive pressure breathing (IPPB) in bronchial toilet. European Respiratory Journal 1 (Suppl 2): 250S

Peiper A 1963 Cerebral function in infancy and childhood. Consultants Bureau, New York

Pelosi P, Solca M, Ravagnan I et al 1996 Effects of heat and moisture exchangers on minute ventilation, ventilatory drive, and work of breathing during pressure-support ventilation in acute respiratory failure. Critical Care Medicine 24(7): 1184–1188

Pendleton N, Cheesbrough JS, Walshaw MJ, Hind CRK 1991 Bacterial colonisation of humidifier attachments on oxygen concentrators prescribed for long-term oxygen therapy: a district review. Thorax 46: 257–258

Perry RJ, Man CGW, Jones RL 1998 Effects of positive end-expiratory pressure on oscillated flow rate during high frequency chest compression. Chest 113: 1028–1033

Pfeiffer KA, Pivarnik JM, Womack CJ, Reeves MJ, Malina RM 2002 Reliability and validity of the Borg and OMNI rating of perceived exertion scales in adolescent girls. Medicine and Science in Sports and Exercise 34(12): 2057–2061

Pfleger A, Theissl B, Oberwaldner B, Zach MS 1992 Self-administered chest physiotherapy in cystic fibrosis: a comparative study of high-pressure PEP and autogenic drainage. Lung 170: 323–330

Pike SE, Machin AC, Dix KJ, Pryor JA, Hodson ME 1999 Comparison of flutter VRP1 and forced expirations (FE) with active cycle of breathing techniques (ACBT) in subjects with cystic fibrosis. Netherlands Journal of Medicine 54: S55–56

Practical Ear Needling Therapy 1980 Medicine & Health Publishing Co, Hong Kong

Prasad SA, Balfour-Lynn IM, Carr SB, Madge SL 2006 A comparison of the prevalence of urinary incontinence in girls with cystic fibrosis, asthma, and healthy controls. Pediatric Pulmonology 41(11): 1065–1068

Prasad SA, Main E 1998 Finding evidence to support airway clearance techniques in cystic fibrosis. Disability and Rehabilitation 20 (6/7): 235–246

Pryor JA 1991 The forced expiration technique. In: Pryor JA (ed) Respiratory care. Churchill Livingstone, Edinburgh, pp 79–100

Pryor JA 2005 A comparison of five airway clearance techniques in the treatment of people with cystic fibrosis. Thesis submitted for the degree of Doctor of Philosophy, Imperial College London

Pryor JA, Tannenbaum E, Cramer D et al 2006 A comparison of five airway clearance techniques in the treatment of people with cystic fibrosis Journal of Cystic Fibrosis 5 (Suppl 1): S76; 347

Pryor JA, Webber BA 1979 An evaluation of the forced expiration technique as an adjunct to postural drainage. Physiotherapy 65: 304–307

Pryor JA, Webber BA, Hodson ME, Batten JC 1979 Evaluation of the forced expiration technique as an adjunct to postural drainage in treatment of cystic fibrosis. British Medical Journal 2: 417–418

Pryor JA, Webber BA, Hodson ME 1990 Effect of chest physiotherapy on oxygen saturation in patients with cystic fibrosis. Thorax 45: 77

Pryor JA, Webber BA, Hodson ME, Warner JO 1994 The Flutter VRPI as an adjunct to chest physiotherapy in cystic fibrosis. Respiratory Medicine 88: 677–681

Putt MT, Paratz JD 1996 The effect of stretching pectoralis major and anterior deltoid muscles on the restrictive component of chronic airflow limitation. In: Proceedings of the National Physiotherapy Conference, Brisbane, Queensland. Australian Physiotherapy Association, Brisbane, Queensland

Ram FSF, Wedzicha JA 2002 Ambulatory oxygen for chronic obstructive pulmonary disease. Cochrane Database of Systematic Reviews, Issue 1. Art. No.: CD000238

Ramirez-Sarmiento A, Orozco-Levi M, Guell R et al 2002 Inspiratory muscle training in patients with chronic obstructive pulmonary disease: structural adaptations and physiological outcomes. American Journal of Respiratory and Critical Care Medicine 166: 1491–1797

Rampes H, James R 1995 Complications of acupuncture. Acupuncture Medicine 13(1): 26–33

Ravilly S, Robinson W, Suresh S, Wohl ME, Berde CB 1996 Chronic pain in cystic fibrosis. Paediatrics 98 (4 Pt 1): 741–747

Reid WD, Huang J, Bryson S 1994 Diaphragm injury and myofibrillar structure induced by resistive loading. Journal of Applied Physiology 76: 176–184

Reid WD, Samrai B 1995 Respiratory muscle training for patients with chronic obstructive pulmonary disease. Physical Therapy 75 (11): 996–1005

Reisman JJ, Rivington-Law B, Corey M et al 1988 Role of conventional physiotherapy in cystic fibrosis. Journal of Pediatrics 113: 632–636

Reynolds JEF (ed) 1996 Martindale. The extra pharmacopoeia, 31st edn. Royal Pharmaceutical Society, London, pp 1060–1063

Richler DW, Ballanyi K, Ramirez J-M 1997 Respiratory rhythm generation. In: Miller AD, Bianchi AL, Bishop BP (eds) Neural control of the respiratory muscles. CRC Press, New York

Ricksten SE, Bengtsson A, Soderberg C, Thorden M, Kvist H 1986 Effects of periodic positive airway pressure by mask on postoperative pulmonary function. Chest 89: 774–781

Rindge D 2005 Laser acupuncture and respiratory disease. Acupuncture Today 6(2)

Rodrigo G, Pollack C, Rodrigo C, Rowe B, Walters EH 2001 Heliox for treatment of exacerbations of chronic obstructive pulmonary disease. Cochrane Database of Systematic Reviews 2001, Issue 1. Art. No.: CD003571

Rodrigo G, Pollack C, Rodrigo C, Rowe BH 2006 Heliox for non-intubated acute asthma patients. Cochrane Database of Systematic Reviews, Issue 4. Art. No.: CD002884

Rood M 1973 Unpublished lectures given at the University of Western Ontario, London, Ontario

Ross J, Gamble J, Schultz A, Lewiston N 1987 Back pain and spinal deformity in cystic fibrosis. American Journal of Diseases in Children 141(12): 1313–1316

Royal College of Physicians 1999 Domiciliary oxygen therapy services. Clinical guidelines and advice for prescribers. Royal College of Physicians, London

Sahl W, Bilton D, Dodd M, Webb AK 1989 Effect of exercise and physiotherapy in aiding sputum expectoration in adults with cystic fibrosis. Thorax 44: 1006–1008

Sahrmann SA 2005 Diagnosis and treatment of movement impairment syndromes. Mosby, St Louis

Sanderson PJ 1984 Common bacterial pathogens and resistance to antibiotics. British Medical Journal 289: 638–639

Sancho J, Servera E, Diaz J, Marin J 2004 Efficacy of mechanical insufflation-exsufflation in medically stable patients with amyotrophic lateral sclerosis. Chest 125: 1400–1405

Scherer TA, Barandun J, Martinez E, Wanner A, Rubin EM 1998 Effect of high-frequency oral airway and chest wall oscillation and conventional chest physical therapy on expectoration in patients with stable cystic fibrosis. Chest 113: 1019–1027

Scherer TA, Spengler CM, Owassapian D, Imhof E, Boutellier U 2000 Respiratory muscle endurance training in chronic obstructive lung disease. American Journal of Respiratory and Critical Care Medicine 162: 1709–1714

Schneiderman-Walker J, Pollock SL, Corey et al 2000 A randomized controlled trial of a 3-year home exercise program in cystic fibrosis. Journal of Pediatrics 136(3): 304–310

Schoeffel RE, Anderson SD, Altounyan REC 1981 Bronchial hyperreactivity in response to inhalation of ultrasonically nebulised solutions of distilled water and saline. British Medical Journal 283: 1285–1287

Schöni MH 1989 Autogenic drainage: a modern approach to physiotherapy in cystic fibrosis. Journal of the Royal Society of Medicine 82(Suppl 16): 32–37

Scottish Intercollegiate Guidelines Network 2004 Management of urinary incontinence in primary care, p 79 www.sign.ac.uk/pdf/sign (accessed 5 July 2007)

Selsby D, Jones JG 1990 Some physiological and clinical aspects of chest physiotherapy. British Journal of Anaesthesia 64(5): 621–631

Shah P, Dhurjon L, Metcalfe T, Gibson JM 1992 Acute angle closure glaucoma associated with nebulised ipratropium bromide and salbutamol. British Medical Journal 304: 40–41

Sharp JT, Drutz WS, Moisan T, Forster J, Machnach W 1980 Postural relief of dyspnea in severe chronic obstructive pulmonary disease. American Review of Respiratory Disease 122: 201–211

Shneerson J 1992 Transtracheal oxygen delivery. Thorax 47: 57–59

Sieck GC, Prakash YS 1997 The diaphragm muscle. In: Miller AD, Bianchi AL, Bishop BP (eds) Neural control of the respiratory muscles. CRC Press, New York

Sinha R, Bergofsky E 1972 Prolonged alteration of lung mechanics in kyphoscoliosis by positive pressure hyperinflation. American Review Respiratory Disease 106: 47–57

Sivasothy P, Brown L, Smith IE, Shneerson JM 2001 Effects of manually assisted cough and insufflation on cough flow in normal subjects, patients with chronic obstructive pulmonary disease (COPD), and patients with respiratory muscle weakness. Thorax 56: 438–444

Smaldone GC, Vinciguerra C, Marchese J 1991 Detection of inhaled pentamidine in health care workers. New England Journal of Medicine 325: 891–892

Smith K, Cook D, Guyatt GH, Madhavan J, Oxman AD 1992 Respiratory muscle training in chronic airflow limitation: a meta-analysis. American Review of Respiratory Disease 145: 533–539

Solcher J, Dechman G 1998 Inspiratory muscle function in chronic obstructive pulmonary disease (COPD). Phy Ther Rev 3: 31–39

Stainton MC, Neff EJ 1994 The efficacy of Seabands for the control of nausea and vomiting in pregnancy. Health Care for Women International 15 (6): 563–575

Starke ID, Webber BA, Branthwaite MA 1979 IPP Band hypercapnia in respiratory failure: the effect of different concentrations of inspired oxygen on arterial blood gas tensions. Anaesthesia 34: 283–287

Stiller K, Simionato R, Rice K, Hall B 1992 The effect of intermittent positive pressure breathing on lung volumes in acute quadriparesis. Paraplegia 30(2): 121–126

Stites SW, Perry GV, Peddicord T, Cox G, Becker B 2006 Effect of high frequency chest wall oscillation on the central and peripheral distribution of aerosolized diethylene triamine penta-acetic acid as compared to standard chest physiotherapy in cystic fibrosis. Chest 129: 712–717

Sukumalchantra Y, Park SS, Williams MH 1965 The effect of intermittent positive pressure breathing (IPPB) in acute ventilatory failure. American Review of Respiratory Disease 92: 885–893

Sumi T 1963 The segmental reflex relations of cutaneous afferent inflow to thoracic respiratory motoneurons. Journal of Neurophysiology 26: 478–493

Suri R, Wallis C, Bush A et al 2002 A comparative study of hypertonic saline, daily and alternate-day rhDNase in children with cystic fibrosis. Health Technology Assessment 6(34): 1–60

Sutton PP, Parker RA, Webber BA et al 1983 Assessment of the forced expiration technique, postural drainage and directed coughing in chest physiotherapy. European Journal of Respiratory Diseases 64: 62–68

Sykes MK, McNicol MW, Campbell EJM 1976 Respiratory failure, 2nd edn. Blackwell Science, Oxford, p 153

Thiagamoorthy S, Carter M, Merchant S et al 2000 Administering, monitoring and withdrawing oxygen therapy (letter). Respiratory Medicine 94: 1253

Thompson B 1978 Asthma and your child, 5th edn. Pegasus Press, Christchurch, New Zealand

Thompson B, Thompson HT 1968 Forced expiration exercises in asthma and their effect on FEV1. New Zealand Journal of Physiotherapy 3: 19–21

Thoracic Society 1950 The nomenclature of bronchopulmonary anatomy. Thorax 5: 222–228

Tilling SE, Hayes B 1987 Heat and moisture exchangers in artificial ventilation. British Journal of Anaesthesia 59: 1181–1188

Tomashefski JF, Bruce M, Goldberg HI, Dearborn DG 1986 Regional distribution of macroscopic lung disease in cystic fibrosis. American Review of Respiratory Disease 133: 535–540

Tomkiewicz RP, Biviji A, King M 1994 Effects of oscillating airflow on the rheological properties and clearability of mucous gel simulants. Biorheology 31: 511–520

Toussaint M, De Win H, Steens M, Soudon P 2003 Effect of intrapulmonary percussive ventilation on mucus clearance in Duchenne muscular dystrophy patients: a preliminary report. Respiratory Care 48: 940–947

Tucker B, Jenkins S, Cheong D, Robinson P 1999 Effect of unilateral breathing exercises on regional lung ventilation. Nuclear Medicine Communications 20: 815–821

Tzeng AC, Bach JR 2000 Prevention of pulmonary morbidity for patients with neuromuscular disease. Chest 118: 1390–1396

van der Schans CP 1997 Forced expiratory manoeuvres to increase transport of bronchial mucus: a mechanistic approach. Monaldi Archives of Chest Disease 52: 367–370

van der Schans C, Prasad A, Main E 2000 Chest physiotherapy compared to no chest physiotherapy for cystic fibrosis. Cochrane Database of Systematic Reviews, Issue 2. Art. No: CD001401

van der Schans CP, van der Mark Th W, de Vries G et al 1991 Effect of positive expiratory pressure breathing in patients with cystic fibrosis. Thorax 46: 252–256

Varekojis SM, Douce FH, Flucke RL et al 2003 A comparison of the therapeutic effectiveness of and preference for postural drainage and percussion, intrapulmonary percussive ventilation, and high frequency chest wall compression in hospitalized cystic fibrosis patients. Respiratory Care 48(1): 24–28

Vargas F, Bui H, Boyer A et al 2005 Intrapulmonary percussive ventilation in acute exacerbations of COPD patients with mild respiratory acidosis: a randomized controlled trial. Critical Care 9: R382–R389

Vater M, Hurt PG, Aitkenhead AR 1983 Quantitative effects of respired helium and oxygen mixtures on gas flow using conventional oxygen masks. Anaesthesia 38: 879–882

Vernon H, Mior S 1991 The Neck Disability Index: a study of reliability and validity. Journal of Manipulative and Physiological Therapeutics 14: 409–415

Vianello A, Corrado A, Arcaro G et al 2005 Mechanical insufflation-exsufflation improves outcomes for neuromuscular disease patients with respiratory tract infections. American

5

Journal of Physical Medicine and Rehabilitation 84: 83–88

Vibekk P 1991 Chest mobilisation and respiratory function. In: Pryor JA (ed) Respiratory care. Churchill Livingstone, Edinburgh, pp 103–119

Vickers AJ 1986 Systematic review of acupuncture anti-emesis trials. Journal of the Royal Society of Medicine 89: 303–311

Volsko TA, DiFiore JM, Chatburn RL 2003 Performance comparison of two oscillating positive expiratory pressure devices: Acapella versus Flutter. Respiratory Care 4892: 124–130

Vora VA, Vara DD, Walton R, Morgan MDL 1995 The assessment of nebulised bronchodilator treatment in COPD by shuttle walk test and breathing problems questionnaire. Thorax 50 (Suppl 2): A29

Wanner A 1977 Clinical aspects of mucociliary transport. American Review of Respiratory Disease 116: 73–125

Ward RJ, Danziger F, Bonica JJ, Allen GD, Bowes J 1966 An evaluation of postoperative respiratory maneuvers. Surgery, Gynecology and Obstetrics 123: 51–54

Warren VC 2002 Glossopharyngeal and neck accessory muscle breathing in a young adult with C2 complete tetraplegia resulting in ventilator dependency. Physical Therapy 82(6): 590–600

Warwick WJ, Hansen LG 1991 Vest (HFCC) bronchial drainage therapy: two year follow-up. Pediatric Pulmonology 11(3): 265–271

Warwick WJ, Wielinski CL, Hansen LG 2004 Comparison of expectorated sputum after manual chest physical therapy and high-frequency chest compression. Biomedical Instrumentation & Technology 38: 470–475

Watson D, Trott P 1993 Cervical headache – an investigation of natural head posture and upper cervical flexor muscle performance. Cephalgia 13: 272–284

Webb AK, Egan JJ, Dodd ME 1996 Clinical management of cystic fibrosis patients awaiting and immediately following lung transplantation. In: Dodge JA, Brock DJH, Widdicombe JH (eds) Cystic fibrosis – current topics, vol 3. John Wiley, Chichester, p 332

Webber BA 1990 The active cycle of breathing techniques. Cystic Fibrosis News Aug/Sep: 10–11

Webber BA 1991 The role of the physiotherapist in medical chest problems. Respiratory Disease in Practice Feb/Mar: 12–15

Webber BA, Higgens JM 1999 Glossopharyngeal ('frog') breathing – what, when and how? Video or DVD available: telephone +44 (0)1494 725724

Webber BA, Hofmeyr JL, Morgan MDL, Hodson ME 1986 Effects of postural drainage, incorporating the forced expiration technique, on pulmonary function in cystic fibrosis. British Journal of Diseases of the Chest 80: 353–359

Webber BA, Parker R, Hofmeyr J, Hodson M 1985 Evaluation of self-percussion during postural drainage using the forced expiration technique. Physiotherapy Practice 1: 42–45

Webber BA, Shenfield GM, Paterson JW 1974 A comparison of three different techniques for giving nebulized albuterol to asthmatic patients. American Review of Respiratory Disease 109: 293–295

Wedzicha JA, Calverley PMA 2006 All change for home oxygen services in England and Wales. Thorax 61: 7–9

Weg JG, Haas CF 1998 Long-term oxygen therapy for COPD. Improving longevity and quality of life in hypoxemic patients Postgraduate Medicine 103(4): 143–144, 147–148, 153–155

Weindler J, Kiefer RT 2001 The efficacy of postoperative incentive spirometry is influenced by the device-specific imposed work of breathing. Chest 119: 1858–1864

Weiner P, Azgad Y, Garnam R 1992 Inspiratory muscle training combined with general exercise training in COPD. Chest 102: 1351–1356

Weiner P, Weiner M 2006 Inspiratory muscle training may increase peak inspiratory flow in chronic obstructive pulmonary disease. Respiration 73: 151–156

Wen AS, Woo MS, Keens TG 1996 Safety of chest physiotherapy in asthma. American Journal of Respiratory and Critical Care Medicine 153: A77

West JB 2004 Respiratory physiology – the essentials, 7th edn. Williams and Wilkins, Baltimore

Westerdahl E, Lindmark B, Almgren S-O, Tenling A 2001 Chest physiotherapy after coronary artery bypass graft surgery – a comparison of three different deep breathing techniques. Journal of Rehabilitation Medicine 33(2): 79–86

White AA, Panjabi MM 1990 Clinical biomechanics of the spine, 2nd edn. Lippincott, Philadelphia

White D, Stiller K, Roney F 2000 The prevalence and severity of symptoms of incontinence in adult cystic fibrosis patients. Physiotherapy Theory Practice 16: 35–42

White S, Sahrmann S 1994 Physical therapy for the cervical and thoracic spine. In: Grant R (ed) Clinics in physical therapy, 2nd edn. Churchill Livingstone, New York

Whitman J, van Beusekom R, Olson S, Worm M, Indihar F 1993 Preliminary evaluation of high frequency chest compression for secretion clearance in mechanically ventilated patients. Respiratory Care 38(10): 1081–1087

Wilson AM, Nikander K, Brown PH 2000 Drug device matching. European Respiratory Review 10(76): 558–566

Wilson GE, Baldwin AL, Walshaw MJ 1995 A comparison of traditional chest physiotherapy with the active cycle of breathing in patients with chronic suppurative lung disease. European Respiratory Journal 8 (Suppl 19): 171S

Wilson R, Cole PJ 1988 The effect of bacterial products on ciliary function. American Review of Respiratory Disease 138: S49–S53

Winck JC, Goncalves MR, Lourenco C, Viana P, Almeida J, Bach JR 2004 Effects of mechanical insufflation-exsufflation on respiratory parameters for patients with chronic airway secretion encumbrance. Chest 126: 774–780

Wolfsdorf J, Swift DL, Avery ME 1969 Mist therapy reconsidered: an evaluation of the respiratory deposition of labelled water aerosols produced by jet and ultrasonic nebulizers. Pediatrics 43: 799–808

Wollmer P, Ursing K, Midgren B, Eriksson L 1985 Inefficiency of chest percussion in the physical therapy of chronic bronchitis. European Journal of Respiratory Diseases 66: 233–239

Wurtemberger G, Hutter BO 2000 Health-related quality of life, psychological adjustment and compliance to treatment in patients on domiciliary liquid oxygen. Monaldi Archives for Chest Disease 55(3): 216–214

Young P 2005 Ambulatory and training oxygen: a review of the evidence and guidelines for prescription New Zealand Journal of Physiotherapy 33(1): 7–12

Zach MS, Oberwaldner B 1992 Effect of positive expiratory pressure breathing in patients with cystic fibrosis. Thorax 47: 66–67

Zack MB, Pontoppidan H, Kazemi H 1974 The effect of lateral positions on gas exchange in pulmonary disease. American Review of Respiratory Disease 110: 49–55

Zhang X 1986 Relationship between cerebral cortex and acupuncture: inhibition of visceral pain. In: Zhang X (ed) Research on acupuncture, moxibustion and acupuncture anaesthesia. Science Press, Beijing and Springer-Verlag, Berlin, p 227

5

Chapter **6**

Patients' problems, physiotherapy management and outcome measures

Sue Jenkins, Beatrice Tucker, Nola Cecins

INTRODUCTION

This chapter discusses the problems commonly encountered by the physiotherapist when working with patients who have respiratory or cardiovascular dysfunction. The patient problems identified in this chapter are those developed following assessment of the patient and are most likely to respond to physiotherapy treatment. This chapter will assist the physiotherapist to utilize clinical reasoning skills by linking and interpreting information (subjective and objective findings) to develop an analysis that is based on the patient's problems (Chapter 1). The presence of pathology affecting the respiratory and cardiovascular systems affects normal physiological functioning and the signs and symptoms produced are the clinical manifestations of this pathophysiology. The physiotherapist therefore requires a thorough knowledge of normal physiology as well as the pathology and pathophysiology of the respiratory and cardiovascular systems. In addition, an understanding is required of the possible sequelae of the pathological process, the clinical presentations of the disorder(s), the likely impairments, activity limitations and participation restrictions, impact on quality of life (QoL) and the anticipated prognosis for the patient.

Patient assessment, problem solving and physiotherapy management should be tailored to the individual. Individuals with common problems, such as dyspnoea and reduced exercise tolerance, resulting from respiratory or cardiovascular disease may be managed in groups, for example, in cardiopulmonary rehabilitation programmes.

PROBLEM SOLVING

The key to the effective physiotherapy management of a patient is the accurate identification of the patient's problems. The assessment will reveal clinical features that the physiotherapist considers important and these are used to determine the patient's main problem(s). The problems commonly encountered are:

- impaired airway clearance
- dyspnoea
- decreased exercise tolerance
- reduced lung volume
- impaired gas exchange
- airflow limitation
- respiratory muscle dysfunction
- dysfunctional breathing
- pain
- musculoskeletal dysfunction – postural abnormalities, decreased compliance or deformity of the chest wall.

The patient problems identified in this chapter are particular to the physiotherapist and are not based on pathologies or derived in the same manner as the medical problem list. For example, a patient may be admitted to hospital with a diagnosis of chest infection associated with excess sputum production, cough and fever. The physiotherapist is not able to treat infection per se but is able to manage the problem of impaired airway clearance. In order to determine the patient's

problem(s) it is essential to identify the significant information gained from the subjective and objective examination. For example, increased production of sputum may be reported by the patient or objectively inspected and measured. Colonization of mucus, evident from microculture, and coarse inspiratory crackles on auscultation are common clinical features that indicate impaired airway clearance.

Some clinical features may provide evidence for a number of patient problems; for example, reduced chest expansion may be a feature of airflow limitation as a result of lung hyperinflation or reduced lung volume (e.g. resulting from significant atelectasis or interstitial lung disease (ILD)). It is necessary to make a judgement about the clinical features collectively to determine which problem(s) they provide evidence for. Once the problem(s) has been identified, the physiotherapist needs to consider the likely pathophysiological basis for the problem(s) so that an appropriate intervention plan can be determined. Patients often present with more than one problem that is amenable to physiotherapy. In this situation, the intervention plan should focus on strategies that address as many patient problems as possible, using best evidence and practice, and should be determined in collaboration with the individual and with a focus on self-management where appropriate.

Some of the clinical features revealed during the assessment may not be features of any of the cardiopulmonary problems listed in this chapter (e.g. poor self-management skills, the presence of risk factors for postoperative pulmonary complications (PPCs) such as cigarette smoking, incorrect use of an inhaler or immobility in the early postoperative period). Patient assessment will also identify the presence of any important factors that must be considered when applying the principles of physiotherapy management for a particular problem to an individual patient. Examples of such factors include the presence of co-morbid conditions (e.g. diabetes mellitus, osteoporosis), psychosocial barriers or special communication needs (e.g. language or cultural requirements).

Case studies

The following case studies provide examples of how to formulate a patient problem list. The reasoning for identifying each problem and the considerations for patient intervention are given. Assessment of the patient may reveal many features. The clinical features reported in these case studies include only those considered to be important in formulating the problem list for each case.

6

6

CASE STUDY 6.1

A 57-year-old woman is admitted to a tertiary hospital via the emergency department.

History of presenting condition
Has been feeling unwell for 4 days with increasing cough and breathlessness and difficulty clearing her sputum.

Previous medical history
Chronic obstructive pulmonary disease (COPD)
Hypertension
Gastro-oesphageal reflux disorder (GORD)
Osteoarthritis affecting both knees.

Medications
Long-acting anticholinergic and combination therapy (long-acting β_2-agonist and corticosteroid) administered via a dry powder inhaler
Angiotensin-converting enzyme (ACE) inhibitor for hypertension
Proton pump inhibitor for GORD
Statin for raised cholesterol.

Personal history
Lives at home with her husband but is finding it increasingly difficult to manage
Independent in self-care when her condition is stable (e.g. showering, dressing), but now requires significant help from her husband.

Previous investigations
Pulmonary function tests were performed at a recent clinic visit at a time when her condition was stable Table 6.1.

Current medical investigations
Temperature 38.5°C
Blood pressure 140/90 mmHg
Pulse 110 beats/min
Respiratory rate 28 breaths/min
Chest radiograph reveals hyperinflation of lungs with an increase in the retrosternal space; low, flattened diaphragms; hyperlucent lung fields with paucity of vascular markings in the periphery but prominent hilar markings and narrow heart silhouette
Arterial blood gas results on admission: pH 7.28, PaO_2 8.7 kPa (65 mmHg), $PaCO_2$ 9.3 kPa (70 mmHg), HCO_3^- 29mmol/l, base excess −1 and SaO_2 92% on 28% oxygen via a Venturi oxygen mask
Sputum microculture result – *Pseudomonas aeruginosa.*

Physiotherapy subjective examination
Normally has a productive cough. Presently coughing throughout the day especially in the morning and when moving about the bed
Sputum is usually scant and clear. Over last week sputum has become yellow and cough is productive all day
Reports being progressively more short of breath over the last 5 years and now reports being breathless when mobilizing around the bed. Sleeps with two pillows at night to relieve breathlessness and symptoms of heartburn
Although limited by breathlessness, patient normally able to walk about 150 metres and is independent in self-care when condition is stable (e.g. showering, dressing) but now requires significant help and is breathless walking to the toilet
Smoked 25 cigarettes per day for 30 years (ceased 10 years ago).

Physiotherapy objective examination
Patient appears thin and frail
Barrel-shaped chest with increased anteroposterior diameter and thoracic kyphosis
Obvious respiratory distress with prominent use of accessory muscles, elevated shoulder girdle and intercostal recession. Increased inspiratory : expiratory (I : E) ratio (prolonged expiration)
Increased use of abdominal muscles during expiration
Using pursed-lip breathing (PLB) during conversation
Chest expansion symmetrical and poor in all zones
Auscultation reveals decreased breath sounds with coarse inspiratory crackles in lower lobes and a prolonged expiratory phase and generalized expiratory wheeze
Sputum – productive of 20 ml thick, purulent mucus (P2) expectorated in past 12 hours
Cough – effective and tight but having significant difficulty expectorating sputum
Table 6.2.

Table 6.1	Pulmonary function tests, case study 1	
Test	Observed	Predicted
FVC (l)	2.76	2.90
FEV$_1$ (l)	1.04	2.30
FEV$_1$/FVC (%)	38.00	77.00
FRC (l)	4.67	2.62
RV (l)	3.24	1.96
TLC (l)	6.16	5.02
TLCO (mmol/min/kPa)	4.16	7.59

FVC, forced vital capacity; FEV$_1$, forced expiratory volume in 1 second; FRC, functional residual capacity; RV, residual volume; TLC, total lung capacity; TLCO, transfer factor of the lung for carbon monoxide

Table 6.2 Analysis of problems from case study 1

Current cardiopulmonary problems	Evidence for each problem based on clinical features	Most likely pathophysiological basis for each problem
Impaired airway clearance	Increased sputum production which has changed in colour and is now purulent; coarse inspiratory crackles in lower lobes Significant difficulty expectorating sputum Patient is febrile Sputum culture grew *Pseudomonas aeruginosa*	Increased production of mucus with altered composition due to colonization with pathogen
Dyspnoea	On conversation, on lying flat, mobilizing to toilet and around the bed	Increased work of breathing due to an increase in airways resistance: increased expiratory muscle work to effect airflow through narrow airways and increased inspiratory muscle work due to lung hyperinflation Increase in ventilatory requirements due to fever and hypoxaemia
Airflow limitation	FEV_1/FVC indicates airflow obstruction, FEV_1 indicates severe airflow obstruction Evidence of hyperinflation: chest X-ray findings, chest shape (barrel), poor chest expansion, increased TLC and FRC Adaptive breathing pattern: increased expiratory phase, PLB, increased abdominal effort, intercostal recession Expiratory wheeze on auscultation Tight cough	Loss of radial traction to airways due to a decrease in elastic recoil Mucus causing partial occlusion of airway lumen
Impaired gas exchange	Respiratory acidosis with CO_2 retention. 28% oxygen required to maintain adequate PaO_2 Reduced TLCO	Mixed causes for hypoxaemia, including $\dot{V}/\dot{Q}$ mismatch, diffusion limitation, wasted perfusion (intrapulmonary shunt) and hypoventilation Mixed causes for hypercapnia, including added load on the mechanics of breathing resulting in hypoventilation, increased $\dot{V}CO_2$ and increased dead space as a fraction of V_T
Decreased exercise tolerance	Reports needing significant help going to the toilet. Further assessment is recommended	
Considerations for treatment	GORD and orthopnoea – a head-up position should be maintained during all interventions Patient thin and frail – consideration required in selection of intervention and implementation of treatment (e.g. care with patient handling) Patient acutely unwell – treatments should be short and interspersed with sufficient rest periods	

Note: respiratory muscle dysfunction may be present (clinical features include orthopnoea, CO_2 retention and altered breathing pattern) and further assessment may be warranted

FEV_1, forced expiratory volume in 1 second; FVC, forced vital capacity; TLC, total lung capacity; FRC, functional residual capacity; PLB, pursed-lip breathing; TLCO, transfer factor of the lung for carbon monoxide; GORD, gastro-oesophageal reflux disorder; $\dot{V}/\dot{Q}$, ventilation/perfusion ratio; V_T, tidal volume

6

CASE STUDY 6.2

A 65-year-old man was admitted to hospital for emergency surgery to treat an acute perforated duodenal ulcer. A suture and omentoplasty were performed via a midline upper abdominal incision. On the third postoperative day the patient's condition deteriorated and assessment revealed the following features.

History of presenting condition
Sudden onset of abdominal pain and vomiting.

Previous medical history
Diabetes mellitus controlled with diet
Hypertension
Ischaemic heart disease (IHD).

Medications
Home medications: aspirin, nitrate, ACE inhibitor, β-adrenoreceptor blocker, statin and diuretic
Current medications: postoperative pain managed with an opioid (morphine) administered via patient-controlled analgesia (PCA), antiemetic for nausea.

Personal history
Lives at home with wife and is independent
Smoked 20 cigarettes a day for 40 years (ceased 2 years ago).

Current medical investigations
Temperature 38.0°C
Blood pressure 140/90 mmHg
Pulse 92 beats/min
Respiratory rate 28 breaths/min
Nasogastric tube aspirate 300 ml over 24 hours.

Urine output 1700 ml over 24 hours
White blood cell count (WCC) $14 \times 10^9/l$
Absent bowel sounds
Chest radiograph revealed right middle and lower lobe infiltrate consistent with collapse and consolidation
Arterial blood gas results: pH 7.48, PaO_2 7.8 kPa (59 mmHg), $PaCO_2$ 4.5 kPa (34 mmHg) and SaO_2 91% on room air.

Physiotherapy subjective examination
Slept poorly overnight
Reports that he has coughed very little overnight and today
No sputum produced either overnight or today
Only ambulating with assistance, as a result of persistent nausea
Reports that he forgets to use the PCA.

Physiotherapy objective examination
Oriented and obeying commands
Appears ill and is pale and clammy
Pain – 6 out of 10 at rest
Shallow breathing pattern
Chest expansion poor lower zones: right < left
Abdominal splinting on inspiration
Cough is painful, weak, moist and ineffective
Auscultation reveals decreased breath sounds left lower lobe, right middle and lower lobes
Sputum – nil produced
Nil calf tenderness, warmth or redness
Table 6.3.

Table 6.3 Analysis of problems from case study 2

Current cardiopulmonary problems	Evidence for each problem based on clinical features	Most likely pathophysiological basis for each problem
Reduced lung volume	Chest radiograph reveals collapse and consolidation Decreased breath sounds on auscultation Reduced chest expansion Abnormal breathing pattern – rapid shallow breathing	Atelectasis resulting from marked decrease in FRC, postoperative diaphragmatic dysfunction, reduced function of surfactant, airway obstruction from mucus plugging and abdominal incisional pain
Impaired gas exchange	Acute hypoxaemia: PaO_2 7.8 kPa (59 mmHg) and SaO_2 91% on room air	Mixed causes for hypoxaemia including $\dot{V}/\dot{Q}$ mismatch caused by a decrease in FRC
Impaired airway clearance	Patient is febrile, elevated WCC, moist cough	Possible colonization of sputum, possible systemic dehydration, impaired MCC from opioid, ineffective cough

Table 6.3	Analysis of problems from case study 2 — *cont'd*
Considerations for treatment	Reduced mobility further increases risk factors for PPC, a reduction of oxygen transport and risk of a deep vein thrombosis – mobilization of patient is a major goal of treatment IHD, hypertension and diabetes – careful monitoring required during treatment Incisional pain – patient needing encouragement to use PCA Patient feeling ill – consideration required during treatments (e.g. ensure optimal use of anti-emetic medication before treatment, short treatments)

FRC, functional residual capacity; MCC, mucociliary clearance; WCC, white blood cell count; PPC, postoperative pulmonary complication; IHD, ischaemic heart disease; PCA, patient-controlled analgesia, $\dot{V}/\dot{Q}$, ventilation/perfusion ratio; PaO_2, partial pressure of oxygen in arterial blood; SaO_2, arterial oxygen saturation

The problem-solving approach to determining patient management not only assists with the identification of existing problems but also enables recognition of potential patient problems. For example, a high-risk surgical patient will develop reduced lung volume and has the added potential to develop problems of impaired airway clearance but if active treatment, such as early ambulation, is started during the at-risk period, these problems may be prevented. Some problems are not amenable to physiotherapy intervention or physiotherapy intervention may be detrimental.

For the patient with more than one problem, it is essential to prioritize the problem list and to establish the short- and long-term goals of the patient and, where appropriate, their relatives and/or caregiver and any other service providers (e.g. other allied health professionals, nurses and medical practitioners). Some problems may only be short term, for example, reduced lung volume in the immediate postoperative period. Developing and prioritizing the problem list and developing the intervention should, whenever possible, take place in consultation with the patient. Some interventions may be determined by taking into consideration other factors such as the availability of resources and the model of service delivery.

Once the short- and long-term goals of the patient and, where appropriate, their relatives and/or caregiver and any other service providers have been established, the next stage is to identify the means of achieving these goals through physiotherapy intervention and the time frame over which they are to be achieved. The appropriate intervention requires selecting the optimal physiotherapy management strategy and this should be evidence based where possible. When a patient has several physiotherapy problems, the physiotherapy techniques selected should ideally address more than one of the high-priority problems. When selecting a treatment approach, the potential risks to the patient (e.g. the possibility of causing adverse physiological responses) and methods to minimize such risks must be taken into consideration. Other factors to be considered include ensuring that the intervention is appropriate for the patient's age, occupation, ability to communicate, cultural beliefs, level of understanding and motivation and the presence of any psychosocial factors which may interfere with the treatment approach (e.g. fear, anxiety or depression). It is important also to determine the patient's likes and dislikes; for example, patient preferences for types of activities are vital considerations when developing an exercise programme.

Common to the management of most problems is the education of the patient by the physiotherapist. This is essential to ensure that the patient takes responsibility for their own management and becomes actively involved in the management of their problem and the prevention of associated problems. If the problem is amenable to physiotherapy, treatment should be started. Conditions that are not amenable to physiotherapy intervention or that require the expertise of a specialist physiotherapist (e.g. a physiotherapist specializing in continence problems) should be referred appropriately. With some problems, a stage will be reached when the natural rate of recovery will no longer be augmented by physiotherapy intervention and treatment should then be discontinued.

The selection and use of appropriate outcome measures are fundamental to the evaluation of physiotherapy intervention. Healthcare fundholders increasingly require data demonstrating the effects of physiotherapy intervention, using instruments that are reliable and valid. Other parties requiring outcome data include the patient, the patient's relatives and caregivers, employers of physiotherapists, clinicians, patient support groups and associations of patients with particular conditions (e.g. cystic fibrosis, heart failure), members of

6

other healthcare professions and insurers. Thus, when selecting which outcome data to monitor it is important to consider the relevant stakeholders.

In this chapter the problems commonly encountered by the physiotherapist when managing patients with respiratory or cardiovascular dysfunction are discussed. The underlying pathophysiology for each problem is outlined and the clinical features that assist in the identification of the problem are described. The physiotherapy management is listed alongside each problem and discussed in greater detail in other chapters. The discussion of each problem concludes with guidelines for the choice of clinical outcome measures to be used to evaluate physiotherapy intervention.

PROBLEM – IMPAIRED AIRWAY CLEARANCE

6

Impaired airway clearance is an important physiotherapy problem because of the potential for the patient to develop an overwhelming infection, major atelectasis and other associated problems such as impaired gas exchange and airflow limitation. Further, untreated persistent infections may predispose to the development of chronic lung disease such as bronchiectasis.

Normal airway clearance depends upon two mechanisms – mucociliary clearance (MCC) and effective cough. Alveolar clearance may also contribute to the clearance of secretions from the peripheral airways (Houtmeyers et al 1999a).

Secretions and debris in the small airways are transported toward the large airways by the mucociliary blanket or escalator and eventually swallowed or cleared by a cough. The mucociliary escalator consists of cilia and a mucus layer. Impurities are caught in the mucus layer and the cilia beat synchronously to move the mucus towards the upper airway. In health, airway mucus is composed mostly of water and the daily volume of mucus in a healthy adult is up to 100 ml (Clarke 1990).

When the volume of secretions reaching the larynx and pharynx has increased to the extent that an individual becomes conscious of the presence of secretions on coughing or 'clearing the throat' the mucus is defined as sputum; the presence of sputum is abnormal.

While mucociliary transport is the major mechanism for clearing secretions in healthy subjects, cough is an important mechanism, especially in people with lung disease. The effectiveness of a cough is related to the volume and viscosity of secretions and the velocity of airflow through the airway lumen. An effective cough requires a high flow rate and a small cross-sectional area of the airway. Dynamic compression of the airways starts downstream from the equal pressure point (Chapter 5) where intraluminal and extraluminal pressures around the bronchial wall are equal (Irwin & Widdicombe 2000). This compression will increase airflow velocity by decreasing the cross-sectional diameter of the airways.

Vigorous coughing can cause a number of adverse effects including abnormal cardiovascular responses (e.g. systemic hypotension and hypertension, rhythm disturbances), abnormalities of the genitourinary tract (e.g. urinary incontinence), gastrointestinal symptoms (e.g. gastro-oesophageal reflux, inguinal hernia), musculoskeletal problems (e.g. rupture of rectus abdominis, rib fractures), neurologic features (e.g. cough syncope, headache, stroke, seizures) and respiratory complications (e.g. airflow limitation, laryngeal trauma, pneumothorax, tracheobronchial trauma). These effects are largely due to the high intrathoracic pressures and expiratory velocities associated with vigorous coughing (Irwin & Widdicombe 2000).

Abnormalities in the normal airway clearance system (i.e. MCC and cough) will result in an accumulation of secretions causing airway obstruction and possibly lead to atelectasis. The subsequent inhomogeneity of ventilation may adversely affect gas exchange. Airway obstruction and the presence of excess secretions also increase the risk of infection. Inflammatory responses to infection cause the release of chemical mediators such as proteases and elastases that can destroy the airway epithelium. This leads to unstable, overcompliant airways that contribute to impaired airway clearance (Barker 2002).

Table 6.4 lists the pathophysiological basis of impaired airway clearance and includes clinical examples (Clarke 1990, Houtmeyers et al 1999a, Irwin & Widdicombe 2000).

Special case – postoperative patient with impaired airway clearance

Many factors either present preoperatively or arising in the peri- or postoperative period increase mucus secretion and/or impair MCC and may be responsible for the development of PPC. It is therefore important for the physiotherapist to identify patients who have an increased risk of developing PPCs (Chapter 12).

Clinical features

The clinical features of impaired airway clearance are usually those resulting from excess or retained secretions. The history of usual daily sputum production obtained from the patient may reveal a chronic productive cough. Changes in the normal pattern of sputum production, such as an increase in the amount or a change in the colour or consistency of the sputum, are likely. Some patients report difficulty expectorating secretions. Further questioning may reveal an increase in the number of chest infections or hospitalizations for

Table 6.4 Pathological basis of impaired airway clearance and clinical examples

Pathophysiological basis		Comment and clinical examples
Increased or altered composition of mucus	1. Increase in production	Bronchiectasis, chronic bronchitis, cystic fibrosis, asthma, pneumonia Presence of an artificial airway increases mucus secretion
	2. Colonization of mucus, e.g. viral, bacterial and fungal organisms	Changes viscosity and increases amount of secretions, thereby slowing MCC
	3. Systemic dehydration	Leads to viscous secretions which are difficult to mobilize and expectorate May occur postoperatively if fluid restriction imposed Excess fluid loss due to prolonged very high respiratory rate
Abnormalities in cilial structure or function		Primary ciliary dyskinesia Damage to ciliated epithelium from excessive endotracheal suctioning
Impaired MCC	1. Age	Rate of MCC decreases with age
	2. Sleep	Decreases MCC
	3. Environmental pollutants	e.g. Tobacco smoke, NO_x – may decrease MCC
	4. Drugs	Some general anaesthetics and narcotics depress MCC
	5. High flow gases	May cause a loss of ciliated epithelium causing mucus retention and slowing MCC
	6. Hypoxaemia and hypercapnia	Slows MCC
	7. Social factors	Coughing and expectoration may be avoided due to embarrassment
Abnormal cough reflex	1. Decreased	Decreased level of consciousness, general anaesthesia, narcotic analgesics Inhibition due to pain, e.g. postoperatively, chest trauma, pleurisy Damage to vagal or glossopharyngeal nerves Laryngectomy Paralysed vocal cords Denervated lungs (heart-lung or lung transplantation)
	2. Increased	Bronchial hyperreactivity Poorly controlled asthma Viral infections may increase sensitivity
Ineffective cough due to the inability to generate sufficient expiratory flow		Severe reduction in VC Respiratory muscle weakness Airflow limitation may cause cough to be weak and/or ineffective Decreased airflow through dilated bronchiectatic airways
Abnormal cough	1. Post-nasal drip	Stimulates the cough reflex
	2. GORD	May lead to chronic cough and microaspirations of gastric contents

MCC, mucociliary clearance; NO_x nitrogen oxides; VC, vital capacity; GORD, gastro-oesophageal reflux disorder

their illness compared with previous years. Patients with chronic lung disease may report signs of stress incontinence on coughing.

Examination of the patient may reveal an altered breathing pattern due to increased work of breathing (WOB). The presence of infection may produce fever and tachycardia. When the secretions cause marked airflow limitation, wheezing may be audible (see *Problem – airflow limitation*). Auscultatory findings include diminished or absent breath sounds, bronchial breath

6

sounds, crackles or wheezes. The cough may be moist or dry and hacking, effective and productive or ineffective and weak. Some patients have a paroxysmal cough with associated adverse effects such as dizziness, syncope or exhaustion. The examination of any sputum expectorated may reveal an increase in the volume or weight compared with the patient's normal expectorant. The colour of the sputum may have changed to yellow, green or brown and there may be blood present (haemoptysis). Also the consistency of the sputum may have altered and microculture may reveal colonization (e.g. with bacteria) (Chapter 1).

Chest radiographs sometimes show signs of lung collapse and/or consolidation or abnormalities reflecting the underlying disease process; for example bronchiectatic changes.

The clinical features of impaired airway clearance in the postoperative patient may include an increased volume of sputum expectorated compared with the patient's usual expectorant; a weak, ineffective moist cough; possible bacterial contamination of expectorated sputum; fever; and chest radiographic changes consistent with atelectasis or pneumonia (Chapter 12).

Physiotherapy management

Physiotherapy is an integral part of the management of patients with impaired airway clearance but bronchial secretions only become a physiotherapy problem when they are excessive, retained or difficult to eliminate. Some patients expectorate a small amount of foul-smelling, tenacious sputum postoperatively but this is not a problem if the patient is conscious, able to cough effectively and self-ambulating.

Airway clearance techniques comprise a range of physiotherapy interventions used for the management of impaired airway clearance (Chapter 5). These techniques aim to promote clearance of excessive secretions from the distal airways and thereby prevent the consequences of obstruction and thus improve ventilation homogeneity and gas exchange. Airway clearance techniques may incorporate positive pressure or oscillation applied at the mouth or chest wall (manual or mechanical) and/or breathing strategies to aid the movement of secretions to the central airways. From the central airways, forced expiratory manoeuvres such as coughing or huffing are used to facilitate expectoration. Such manoeuvres aim to use high expiratory flow rates to shear secretions from the airway walls.

The physiotherapy management of impaired airway clearance is influenced by the underlying cause and acuity of the patient's condition. For patients with chronic hypersecretory lung disease who regularly produce excess bronchial secretions, the use of daily

airway clearance techniques is recommended (Jones & Rowe 1998, van der Schans et al 2000). The rationale for daily treatment is to reduce stagnation of secretions in an attempt to avoid contamination with pathogens and thereby reduce the destruction of airway walls caused by the inflammatory response. This may slow the cycle of progressive tissue damage. The physiotherapist's role in this case is to prescribe and teach a daily airway clearance regimen that is individually tailored and acceptable to the patient. Factors to be considered when choosing an airway clearance technique include:

- evidence supporting the technique
- patient age and ability to learn the technique
- patient motivation
- patient preference and comfort
- physiotherapist's skill in teaching the technique.

The physiotherapist's role may change in a patient with hypersecretory lung disease when the patient experiences a worsening of their condition such as during a chest infection. During a hospital admission for an acute illness the physiotherapist may take a more active role and the frequency and duration of treatments may increase. It may be that a change of technique is indicated and it is the physiotherapist's role, in consultation with the patient, to select a technique that addresses the changing condition.

A number of additional measures are available that have been shown to enhance or improve airway clearance. Table 6.5 outlines these measures (Conway et al 1992, Elkins et al 2006, Houtmeyers et al 1999b, Jones et al 2003, Wark et al 2005, Wills & Greenstone 2006).

In the postoperative patient it is essential to establish whether the patient has excess secretions and whether they have difficulty managing their own airway clearance. This is one of the factors influencing the risk of the patient developing PPCs. The techniques to assist sputum clearance in the postoperative patient aim to increase alveolar ventilation and expiratory flow rates using, for example, upright positioning and ambulation at an adequate intensity with encouragement to take deep breaths. Expectoration of secretions can be facilitated by supported coughing or huffing (Chapter 12). If the patient has large amounts of secretions, techniques such as the active cycle of breathing techniques (ACBT) and vibrations may be used.

For patients who are reluctant or unable to cough, a spontaneous cough may be elicited by physical activity or a change of position. The cough reflex may be elicited using a tracheal rub or suctioning. Strengthening of the abdominal muscles and assisted cough techniques (e.g. abdominal support with an upward pressure) or a mechanical insufflation-

Table 6.5   Additional measures to enhance airway clearance

Measure	Examples and uses
Humidification	Patients with thick, tenacious secretions For some patients receiving high-flow gases, e.g. oxygen therapy or NIV When the normal heat and exchange system of the upper airways is bypassed by endotracheal or tracheostomy tube
Nebulization	MCC may be improved by hypertonic saline, amiloride, recombinant human deoxyribonuclease and β-adrenergic agonists
Analgesia	Patients in whom pain is inhibiting an effective cough
Physical activity	Increased respiratory rate and V_T increase expiratory flow rates and sputum clearance

NIV, non-invasive ventilation; MCC, mucociliary clearance; V_T, tidal volume

exsufflation device may be helpful for patients with impaired cough due to weakness of the abdominal muscles (Chapter 16). For the intubated and ventilated patient, improved alveolar ventilation and increased expiratory flow rates can be achieved by positioning and manual hyperinflation, and secretions cleared by suctioning (Chapter 8).

Outcome measures

Short-term outcomes can be monitored by a change in sputum expectorated, as measured by weight, volume or rate of expectoration. Ease of sputum expectoration can be measured using a categorical scale or visual analogue scale (VAS). In acute conditions, chest radiographs and auscultatory findings may provide evidence for a change in the patient's condition. Radio-aerosol clearance may be used as an outcome measure in studies of airway clearance techniques (van der Schans et al 1999).

Long-term outcomes in patients with hypersecretory lung disease may be assessed by the number of exacerbations, courses of antibiotics, hospitalizations and days lost from work/study per year. Quality of life scales, such as the St George's Respiratory Disease Questionnaire (SGRQ), include a section that quantifies symptoms of cough and sputum (Jones et al 1992). Pulmonary function, in particular spirometry, has been used to evaluate the effects of airway clearance techniques but may be relatively insensitive to the intervention (van der Schans et al 1999).

In the high-risk postoperative patient with excess bronchial secretions, outcomes from physiotherapy intervention may be measured by the prevention of PPCs.

Improved cough or huff technique may be associated with a reduction in associated problems such as fatigue, dyspnoea, syncope, airflow limitation, arterial oxygen desaturation or stress incontinence.

PROBLEM – DYSPNOEA

Dyspnoea is the term generally applied to the sensations experienced by individuals complaining of unpleasant or uncomfortable respiration (Ambrosino & Scano 2001). In clinical practice, the terms breathlessness and dyspnoea are used interchangeably. However 'breathlessness' is one of many descriptors used by patients to convey their experience of dyspnoea. Other common terms used by patients suggest unrewarded inspiration (i.e. 'can't get the air in') and chest tightness. It is possible these different descriptors originate from different pathological processes. For example, individuals with COPD frequently use terms that reflect an increase in the effort of breathing or WOB (Scano et al 2005).

Dyspnoea is a common and distressing symptom experienced by patients with respiratory and cardiovascular disease and is frequently the symptom that causes the patient to seek medical care. On occasions, it may be difficult to distinguish from the patient's account whether the symptoms are of respiratory or cardiovascular origin as in both the patient may report breathlessness on exertion, when lying supine, causing waking during the night and acute episodes of breathlessness at rest.

Many healthy individuals become aware of their breathing when exercising at a moderate or high intensity and report that their breathing is rapid and that they are puffing. These changes in breathing reflect the increased ventilation required during exercise and are appropriate for the situation. In contrast, individuals with respiratory or cardiovascular disease may become aware of unpleasant breathing sensations at very low levels of physical activity and even at rest or in response to emotional or stressful situations. In such situations the appropriate term for these respiratory sensations is dyspnoea. Dyspnoea is not tachypnoea, hyperventilation or hyperpnoea. These three terms all describe

6

ventilation in response to different stimuli and may represent normal physiological responses. Although hypoxaemia and hypercapnia increase ventilatory response, the severity of hypoxaemia and hypercapnia are not directly linked to the perception of dyspnoea. The sensation of dyspnoea appears to originate with the activation of sensory systems within the lung, chest wall and respiratory muscles that give rise to an awareness of breathing discomfort (American Thoracic Society (ATS) 1999, Schwartzstein & Parker 2006).

The sensation of dyspnoea is influenced by many factors including the patient's psychological status and their experience and memory. The presence of fear, anxiety, depression and anger heighten the perception of dyspnoea (ATS 1999). In some patients, dyspnoea may be perceived as life threatening. A patient's ability to describe and quantify the unpleasant sensation of dyspnoea is also very variable. This is not unlike the variability seen when patients report pain. These factors may in part explain why the intensity of dyspnoea for a given level of impairment in lung function, or exercise capacity, can vary greatly among individuals.

Although it is generally contended that dyspnoea arises as a consequence of multiple complex and varied interactions, the precise mechanisms responsible for the sensation of dyspnoea are poorly understood and the management of dyspnoea poses considerable difficulties. Clinically, dyspnoea results from several different pathophysiological mechanisms and in some patients more than one mechanism will be responsible (Table 6.6) (ATS 1999, Scano et al 2005, Schwartzstein & Parker 2006).

Special case – chronic lung disease

There are several pathophysiological causes of dyspnoea in patients with chronic lung disease. In patients with moderate to severe COPD, the increase in airway resistance is associated with lung hyperinflation and gives rise to an increase in the WOB (see *Problem – airflow limitation*). In patients with ILD, a greater than normal inspiratory effort is required to overcome the increased lung elastic recoil and may give rise to dyspnoea. Peripheral muscle dysfunction and deconditioning are common in patients with chronic lung disease and the associated increase in lactic acid accumulation during submaximal levels of exercise stimulates ventilation. Respiratory muscle dysfunction may also be a contributory factor to dyspnoea especially in patients with COPD (see *Problem – respiratory muscle dysfunction*). The presence of hypoxaemia may contribute to the WOB by stimulating ventilation. Psychosocial factors (e.g. anxiety) may heighten the perception of dyspnoea.

Some patients with moderate or severe disease, especially those with COPD, report marked dyspnoea when performing activities of daily living (ADL) that involve the use of the upper limbs, especially when the upper limbs are unsupported. Performing activities that involve unsupported upper limb movements leads to a loss of these arm trunk muscles as elevators of the rib cage, thereby reducing their contribution to the generation of the intrapleural pressure needed for inspiration. The breathing pattern during unsupported upper limb exercise in patients who report dyspnoea with upper limb movements is often rapid and irregular, and dyssynchronous thoraco-abdominal movements and breath holding may occur (Celli 1994). A further workload is imposed when activities involve raising the arms above the head. This arm position gives rise to the early onset of lactate accumulation in the upper limbs leading to an increase in carbon dioxide (CO_2) production, which stimulates ventilation.

Clinical features

The time course for the onset of dyspnoea (e.g. acute vs insidious) gives important information as to the likely aetiology and is obtained from the subjective assessment. Most commonly, the patient's account will reveal that dyspnoea is elicited by physical activity, for example during ADL or when walking on the flat or up inclines. The patient may also report that adopting certain body positions causes dyspnoea, for example, when attempting to lie flat to sleep. Many patients with chronic lung disease will report day-to-day variability in dyspnoea intensity and this may include variation depending on the time of day and climatic conditions. Extremes of temperature and humidity and high levels of atmospheric pollution tend to heighten the perception of dyspnoea in most individuals. In chronic hyperventilation disorder, dyspnoea may occur at rest and is often accompanied by an excessive frequency of sighs (Chapter 17).

Some patients may seek medical care when they become very breathless playing sports, for example golf or bowls, but many individuals attribute breathlessness to ageing or a poor level of fitness and fail to seek help until breathlessness occurs during ADL. Patients with respiratory disease or heart failure may also report feeling fatigued; this may be a generalized symptom or felt predominantly in the legs during physical activity.

On examination, the patient may display an altered breathing pattern. Abnormalities in the rate and depth of breathing, inspiratory to expiratory ratio and symmetry of chest movements are often observed. Clinical features indicative of an increase in the WOB associated with airflow limitation include the adoption of an upper chest breathing pattern with shoulder girdle fixation to enable the accessory muscles to assist with inspiration. Other signs commonly seen in patients with severe airflow limitation who report dyspnoea include an

Table 6.6 Pathophysiological basis for dyspnoea in respiratory and cardiovascular disease and clinical examples

Pathophysiological basis		Clinical examples
1. Increase in elastic load due to:	a. Decrease in lung compliance	Increases the inspiratory muscle work required to overcome the elastic recoil of the lungs. Increases in $\dot{V}_E$ are achieved mainly by increasing respiratory rate, e.g. ILD, breathing at low lung volumes, pulmonary congestion. Hyperinflation (e.g. COPD, cystic fibrosis, asthma) increases the WOB
	b. Decrease in chest wall compliance and /or compliance of the abdominal compartment	Obesity, kyphoscoliosis, ankylosing spondylitis
2. Increase in airways resistance		Increases expiratory muscle work to effect airflow through narrowed airways (e.g. COPD, asthma)
3. Weakness or fatigue of the respiratory muscles		See *Problem – respiratory muscle dysfunction*
4. Increase in metabolic rate		Increases ventilatory requirements, e.g. fever, exercise
5. Low cardiac output / ischaemia		Inadequate cardiac output causes reflex medullary ventilatory stimulation when the oxygen supply to the exercising muscle is inadequate to meet metabolic needs, e.g. IHD, heart failure or in the presence of ventricular arrhythmias, valvular problems or cardiomyopathy
6. Blood gas abnormalities		Hypoxaemia or hypercapnia
7. Deconditioning		Lactate accumulates at low levels of exercise causing an increase in ventilation
8. Anaemia		When severe causes dyspnoea on exertion
9. Acute changes in permeability of pulmonary capillaries		Pulmonary oedema
10. Perfusion limitation		The presence of a large $\dot{V}/\dot{Q}$ mismatch or shunt invariably causes dyspnoea, e.g. pulmonary embolus, pulmonary infarction, cyanotic heart disease, pulmonary congestion

$\dot{V}_E$, minute ventilation; ILD, interstitial lung disease; COPD, chronic obstructive pulmonary disease; WOB, work of breathing; $\dot{V}/\dot{Q}$, ventilation/perfusion ratio

6

increase in abdominal effort during expiration, paradoxical breathing and PLB. Characteristically, expiratory time will be prolonged in the presence of airflow limitation (see *Problem – airflow limitation*). The patient may complain of feeling hot and appear sweaty if the WOB is excessive and dyspnoea is associated with fear or panic.

Assessment may reveal signs and symptoms of other problems, most commonly airflow limitation, impaired gas exchange and, in patients with cardiovascular disease, angina may accompany dyspnoea. Exercise tolerance will usually be reduced as a result of dyspnoea on exertion. The chest radiograph will often show signs consistent with the underlying pathology (e.g. lung hyperinflation, effusion, pneumothorax, areas of collapse or consolidation). A laboratory-based incremental exercise test with continuous measurement of ventilatory and cardiovascular variables can be used to differentiate between dyspnoea arising from cardiovascular or respiratory origin. If respiratory muscle weakness is suspected to be a contributing factor this can be confirmed by measuring maximum inspiratory and expiratory mouth pressures (PiMax and PeMax) (Chapter 3 and see *Problem – respiratory muscle dysfunction*).

Special case – problems with bladder and bowel function

The problem of urinary or faecal incontinence may arise in the presence of dyspnoea, decreased exercise tolerance or impaired airway clearance (White et al 2000). Patients who are breathless are often sedentary and have a reduced appetite and fluid intake, and difficulty preparing food. The breathless patient who is also constipated may have difficulty breath holding and assuming an adequate position to enable defecation (Markwell & Sapsford 1995). Reduced fluid intake and frequent or 'just in case' toileting, to prevent stress or urge urinary incontinence, can result in the bladder becoming accustomed to accommodating smaller volumes of urine. This leads to an increased frequency to void. Dyspnoea is likely to intensify when attempting to walk quickly to reach the toilet in time and may also become worse with functional tasks requiring the upper limbs, such as undressing, making urgency worse or resulting in incontinence.

Physiotherapy management

In patients with airflow limitation, bronchodilators may reduce dyspnoea and improve exercise tolerance; therefore, inhaler technique and timing of bronchodilators should be optimized.

Positioning, breathing control and relaxation techniques are used in an attempt to decrease the WOB and eliminate unnecessary muscular activity (Gosselink 2004, O'Neill & McCarthy 1983). Positions such as the forward lean position with the arms supported or high side lying may be useful for patients who are severely distressed, especially when the cause of their breathlessness is COPD. In these patients, the forward lean position increases transdiaphragmatic pressure, improves thoraco-abdominal movements and reduces activity of the scalenes and sternomastoid muscles. In addition, the forward lean position with the arms supported allows the pectoral muscles to significantly contribute to rib cage elevation (Gosselink 2004). Relaxation techniques that do not involve breath holding or the contraction of large muscle groups may be useful for relieving dyspnoea in those who are anxious (Gosselink 2004).

Symptomatic relief may be achieved by increasing the movement of cold air onto the patient's face (e.g. sitting by an open window, use of a fan). This stimulates mechanoreceptors on the face and the decrease in skin temperature may alter afferent feedback to the brain and the perception of dyspnoea (ATS 1999).

Pursed-lip breathing is often spontaneously adopted by patients with COPD and may be very effective in reducing the discomfort associated with dyspnoea. This breathing strategy aims to prevent airway closure and increase expiratory time. This may lead to a decrease in respiratory rate, an increase in tidal volume (V_T) and, in turn, may improve gas exchange at rest. Pursed-lip breathing appears to be most effective when used by patients with COPD who adopt the technique spontaneously (Gosselink 2004). Recovery from dyspnoea following physical activity can be assisted with positioning (e.g. forward lean with the arms supported) together with breathing strategies such as breathing control or PLB. Some patients have a tendency to breath-hold when performing physical tasks and encouraging exhalation during effort is another breathing strategy that may be helpful. For selected patients with severe dyspnoea, education on energy conservation techniques during ADL is important. Conversely, many patients with respiratory or cardiovascular disease adopt a very sedentary lifestyle and, in addition to starting an exercise programme, such patients require encouragement to participate in a greater range of ADL with adequate rests as required to recover from breathlessness. Exercise training is an effective method of relieving dyspnoea in patients with stable chronic lung disease and in those with cardiac failure (ATS /European Respiratory Society (ERS) 2006, Lacasse et al 2006, Rees et al 2004). The underlying mechanisms responsible for the reduction in dyspnoea following exercise training are varied and for the individual may include:

- Physiologic training effect with an increased aerobic capacity of the peripheral muscles associated with decreased lactate production and decreased ventilation at a given submaximal workload

- Decreased oxygen consumption ($\dot{V}O_2$) and ventilation for a given level of physical activity as a result of improved mechanical efficiency (e.g. increased stride length when walking)

- Reduced anxiety as a result of improved self-confidence and desensitization to the intensity of dyspnoea from repeated controlled exposure to a stimulus (e.g. as may occur with regular participation in supervised exercise classes).

Walking aids (e.g. rollator/wheeled walker, gutter frame/pulpit frame) that facilitate the forward lean position and arm support may reduce dyspnoea, increase exercise tolerance and may limit the extent of oxygen desaturation in some patients with COPD (Probst et al 2004, Solway et al 2002). Ambulatory oxygen may be beneficial for patients who are dyspnoeic on exercise and demonstrate oxygen desaturation. Oxygen therapy is only indicated if shown to produce benefit in terms of increased exercise tolerance and reduced breathlessness. The application of non-invasive ventilation (NIV) during exercise may reduce dyspnoea and improve exercise endurance and has been shown to be effective in patients with COPD (van't Hul et al 2002). However, the use of NIV during exercise is cumbersome and often difficult in clinical practice.

For patients with COPD, high-intensity inspiratory muscle training (IMT) has been shown to reduce dyspnoea but the effects of such training on measures of whole body exercise capacity are less convincing (Geddes et al 2005, Hill et al 2006, Lotters et al 2002). Indications for IMT in COPD patients include the presence of severe musculoskeletal problems that prevent participation in a whole body exercise training programme and severe intractable dyspnoea persisting following whole body exercise training.

Outcome measures

The relevant outcome measures include assessment of dyspnoea intensity at rest, during ADL and when exercising. Dyspnoea intensity is most easily quantified using the modified Borg (0–10) Category Ratio Scale (Borg 1982). Changes in exercise tolerance are usually assessed in the clinical setting using a field walking test (Chapter 3). Scales that quantify the functional limitation due to dyspnoea are useful outcome measures of physiotherapy intervention and include the Medical Research Council (MRC) Scale and the New York Heart Association (NYHA) Scale, the University of California San Diego Shortness of Breath Questionnaire, the London Chest Activity of Daily Living Scale and the Pulmonary Functional Status and Dyspnea Questionnaire (Meek 2004). A health-related QoL questionnaire that includes quantification of dyspnoea during ADL is a useful outcome measure for patients who present with dyspnoea and participate in a pulmonary or heart failure rehabilitation programme (Chapters 13 and 14).

PROBLEM – DECREASED EXERCISE TOLERANCE

Exercise tolerance in patients with respiratory or cardiovascular disease is invariably limited by dyspnoea, pain (chest or legs) or fatigue (general or local). This section outlines the pathophysiological basis for exercise limitation occurring in respiratory and cardiovascular diseases. In addition to the pathophysiologic abnormalities that adversely affect exercise tolerance, depression and anxiety often accompany chronic respiratory or cardiovascular disease and may decrease an individual's confidence or motivation to exercise.

Chronic lung disease

Patients with moderate to severe respiratory disease usually terminate exercise due to the development of intolerable symptoms (i.e. dyspnoea or leg fatigue) and fail to reach maximal heart rate (HR) and oxygen consumption. Leg fatigue is more likely to be a limiting factor when cycling is performed as compared with walking. In patients with moderate to severe COPD and chest wall abnormalities (e.g. kyphoscoliosis), respiratory muscle dysfunction may also be present and may contribute to dyspnoea and decreased exercise tolerance (see *Problem – respiratory muscle dysfunction*) (ATS/ERS 2006). Patients with moderate or severe respiratory disease, especially those with COPD, may experience marked dyspnoea when performing ADL that involve the use of the upper limbs, especially when the upper limbs are unsupported (see *Problem – dyspnoea*).

A respiratory impairment to exercise may be due to dysfunction of any or all components of the respiratory system. Normally, the ventilatory demands of exercise are met by an increase in V_T and respiratory rate. Physiological abnormalities present in respiratory disease limit the ability to increase V_T during exercise and thus increases in minute ventilation ($\dot{V}_E$) occur as a result of a disproportionate increase in respiratory rate. This occurs in diseases characterized by airflow limitation such as COPD, ILD, chest wall impairments and respiratory muscle weakness. Thus, for a given level of $\dot{V}_E$ during exercise, V_T tends to be lower and respiratory rate higher than in healthy individuals (Roca & Rabinovich 2005). The excessive increase in respiratory rate is very costly in terms of the oxygen required by the respiratory muscles because of the much larger number of muscle contractions and the increase in dead-space ventilation. In effect, the respiratory muscles may use oxygen at the expense of other skeletal muscles.

In many patients with moderate to severe COPD, functional residual capacity (FRC) is elevated compared with normal even at rest (i.e. the lungs are hyperinflated). Peripheral airway narrowing and loss of lung elastic recoil lead to gas trapping during expiration and are responsible for the increase in FRC. During exercise, the increase in respiratory rate limits the time available for expiration, resulting in a further increase in end-expiratory lung volume. Dynamic hyperinflation is the term used for the increase in gas trapping that occurs in patients with COPD during exercise and acute exacer-

6

bations (see *Problem – airflow limitation*). The associated lung hyperinflation serves to improve ventilation by decreasing airway resistance and increasing expiratory flow rates. However, the main disadvantage of this compensatory mechanism is the altered mechanics of the respiratory muscles that increase WOB. The associated increase in deadspace ventilation and reduction in alveolar ventilation contribute to the impairments in gas exchange observed during exercise.

Healthy subjects maintain normal levels of partial pressure of oxygen in arterial blood (PaO_2) unless extreme levels of exercise are undertaken and partial pressure of carbon dioxide in arterial blood ($PaCO_2$) does not change from resting values until acidosis occurs as a result of high blood lactate levels. When this occurs, ventilation is further increased and $PaCO_2$ falls (ATS/American College of Chest Physicians (ACCP) 2003). In contrast, many patients with chronic lung disease experience oxygen desaturation on exercise especially when the transfer factor of the lung for carbon monoxide (TLCO) is markedly impaired (Hadeli et al 2001, Roca & Rabinovich 2005). A low TLCO is characteristic of ILD and also occurs in some patients with COPD who have predominantly emphysematous changes. In such individuals, hypoxaemia contributes to exercise intolerance both directly through increased chemoreceptor activity and indirectly via stimulation of lactic acid production (ATS/ERS 2006).

In patients with asthma, exercise capacity may be limited by bronchoconstriction and exercise-induced asthma (EIA) may be the only symptom of asthma especially in young patients with mild disease. Usually with exercise there is a mild bronchodilator effect thought to be due to the increase in sympathetic stimulation and withdrawal of vagal control. With EIA, a rapid fall in FEV_1 occurs immediately after the cessation of exercise. The likelihood of developing EIA in susceptible individuals is greater when their asthma control is poor. Exercise performed when an individual has an upper respiratory tract infection or has recently had a cold is more likely to provoke EIA. The types of exercise and environmental conditions most likely to cause EIA are exercise that is continuous and is associated with a high ventilatory demand, for example long distance running or cycling, especially when such exercise takes place in cold and dry conditions or in the presence of high levels of air pollution or known allergens. Following a warm-up, or short bout of exercise, there is a refractory period when protection against EIA occurs (Storms 1999, 2005).

Cardiovascular impairment

Multiple factors contribute to exercise intolerance in patients with cardiovascular disease. These factors include inadequate oxygen delivery, abnormalities in HR response, systolic and diastolic function, abnormal pulmonary vascular responses and peripheral muscle dysfunction (see below) (ATS/ACCP 2003). Compared with healthy subjects, in patients with cardiovascular disease the increase in stroke volume with exercise is often reduced and there is a greater reliance on the HR response to achieve the levels of cardiac output required to meet the metabolic requirements. However, the HR response to exercise may be blunted compared with normal. In more severe disease (e.g. especially chronic heart failure (CHF)), the peak HR achieved declines and during submaximal exercise the HR response is greater for a given level of $\dot{V}O_2$ compared with normal (Pina et al 2003). Ventilatory responses to exercise are often abnormal and are characterized by a greater $\dot{V}_E$ at submaximal $\dot{V}O_2$. In the absence of coexisting lung disease, arterial desaturation during exercise is not observed in patients with stable cardiovascular disease (ATS/ACCP 2003).

Peripheral muscle dysfunction in chronic lung disease and heart failure

Peripheral muscle dysfunction occurs in patients with chronic lung disease and heart failure and contributes to reduced exercise tolerance. Most of the evidence for peripheral muscle dysfunction has been obtained from studies of the quadriceps muscles in patients with COPD and CHF. The documented abnormalities include muscle wasting, decreased strength, a reduction in the proportion of type I fibres (i.e. endurance fibres), a reduction in the number of capillary contacts to muscle fibre cross-sectional area and a decreased concentration of mitochondrial enzymes (ATS/ERS 2006, Gosker et al 2003). Further, in patients with CHF, blood flow to the exercising muscles is reduced as a result of a lower than normal cardiac output and impairment in the endothelium-dependent vasodilatory pathways in these muscles (Pina et al 2003). The changes described above are responsible for the reduced capacity of the peripheral muscles for aerobic metabolism observed in patients with chronic lung disease and CHF. As a consequence, there is a greater increase in lactic acidosis for a given exercise work rate and this contributes to the development of leg fatigue and in turn increases the ventilatory requirements. The aetiology of the peripheral muscle dysfunction is multifactorial and may include inactivity-induced deconditioning, systemic inflammation, oxidative stress, blood gas abnormalities and corticosteroid use (ATS/ERS 2006, Gosker et al 2003).

Peripheral arterial disease

In peripheral arterial disease, the oxygen supply to the exercising muscles is inadequate to meet the metabolic requirements. This oxygen deficiency leads to a build-up of lactic acid and claudication pain occurs during low-intensity weight bearing exercise (i.e. walking).

Marked deconditioning

Marked deconditioning is a common sequela of the prolonged bed rest and decreased mobility that occurs in patients with a protracted recovery following pneumonia, major surgery and time spent in an intensive care unit. Deconditioning is also commonly found in patients with respiratory or cardiovascular disease who avoid exercise because of dyspnoea or fatigue. In a deconditioned individual, the oxygen cost of exercise is higher at any given submaximal exercise intensity than in an individual who is physically fit. This is due to central and peripheral mechanisms that include an increased HR response to exercise, increase in cardiac afterload and a decrease in the aerobic capacity of the peripheral muscles. This leads to the early onset of aerobic metabolism. Further, the avoidance of physical activity and exercise may decrease the skill and efficiency of physical movements.

Other conditions that limit exercise tolerance

Obesity is a common problem in developed countries and is associated with the morbidity and mortality of many conditions including coronary artery disease, type II diabetes and obstructive sleep apnoea. The presence of obesity decreases exercise capacity due to the increase in the metabolic requirements at rest, and the greater respiratory and cardiac work required by an obese individual during exercise.

Many individuals with respiratory or cardiovascular disease are elderly. In addition to the age-related decline in physical work capacity, such individuals may have neurological or musculoskeletal conditions that limit their ability to exercise.

Clinical features

Subjectively the patient with reduced exercise tolerance will report that their performance of ADL or the ability to exercise is limited as a result of breathlessness, fatigue or pain. Patients with EIA will report that respiratory symptoms, i.e. cough, chest tightness or wheeze, occur during or immediately following exercise. If peripheral arterial disease is present, the patient will report pain in the calf and often also in the buttock limiting their ability to walk. The intensity of pain will be increased when walking up inclines, hurrying and walking on uneven ground and barefoot.

On examination, functional exercise capacity, which is most commonly assessed in the clinical setting with a field walking test, will be reduced, abnormal physiolog-ical responses (e.g. oxygen desaturation, blunted or increased HR response) may be present and the patient will report symptoms limiting exercise (i.e. dyspnoea, fatigue or pain). When EIA is present, there will be a reduction in FEV_1 and peak expiratory flow rate (PEFR) measured immediately following exercise. In patients with claudication pain, a marked limp may be noticeable prior to the patient terminating a walking test. In the obese individual, exercise tolerance is usually limited due to breathlessness occurring with low-intensity exercise.

A cardiopulmonary exercise test, including assessment of the physiologic responses, is required to identify the pathophysiological limitation to exercise (Chapters 3, 13 and 14 on assessment, pulmonary rehabilitation and cardiac rehabilitation). The physiologic variables measured usually include $\dot{V}O_2$, carbon dioxide output ($\dot{V}CO_2$), $\dot{V}_E$, V_T, and respiratory rate, oxygenation (measured via oximetry, SpO_2), HR and rhythm (electrocardiogram (ECG)) and systemic blood pressure. In many clinical settings, a full cardiopulmonary exercise test may not be available; however, when a cardiopulmonary exercise test is performed, the data obtained can assist with exercise prescription.

On examination of the patient there may be signs of peripheral muscle wasting and a reduction in muscle strength found on testing. In some patients, respiratory muscle strength may be reduced compared with normal values (Chapter 3).

For the patient with acute cardiopulmonary dysfunction an exercise test is inappropriate. Information regarding the likely responses to interventions aimed at improving oxygen transport (e.g. transferring from bed to chair, standing, ambulating) will be obtained from knowledge of responses to nursing and medical interventions and observation of subjective and objective data over time. Chapter 4 details the therapeutic effects of positioning and mobilization for the patient with acute cardiopulmonary dysfunction.

Physiotherapy management

Identification and optimal medical management of the underlying cause of reduced exercise tolerance (e.g. COPD, IHD, valvular heart disease, CHF) and of comorbid conditions (e.g. osteoarthritis, diabetes, obesity, malnutrition) are essential before starting an exercise programme. Individuals with known or suspected EIA should use an inhaled short-acting β_2-agonist or non-steroidal anti-inflammatory medication before exercise.

There is strong evidence to support the benefits of exercise training for people with respiratory and cardiovascular disease (Lacasse et al 2006, Leng et al 2001, Rees et al 2004, Smart & Marwick 2004). Regular physical

6

6

activity is also effective in preventing cardiovascular disease (Thompson et al 2003). The following section outlines the broad principles of exercise training. The reader is also referred to Chapters 4, 8, 12–14 for further information on the physiotherapy management of specific patient populations.

An exercise programme should be designed to meet the specific requirements of the patient. Supervised exercise training, involving a group of patients with the same or similar condition, can be very helpful. Such training provides peer support that may assist patients to overcome anxiety and improve their motivation to exercise. Further, the supervised setting ensures that the exercise prescription is safe and enables the physiotherapist to adjust the prescription on a regular basis. Concurrent with starting an exercise programme, many patients need encouragement to engage in more physical activity during their everyday life.

The frequency, intensity, duration and modes of exercise should be individually selected for each patient based on assessment findings and established goals. In general, the programme should consist of a warm-up, stretches, an aerobic component, resistive training, when appropriate, and a cool-down. Postural correction is also important (Chapter 5 and see *Problem – musculoskeletal dysfunction: postural abnormalities, decreased compliance or deformity of the chest wall*). Unsupported upper limb exercises are especially important for patients who have respiratory disease and complain of dyspnoea during ADL that involve the upper limbs. Although it is recognized that endurance training is beneficial for most patients, it may be more important for some patients to improve their speed of ambulation over a short distance (e.g. to cross a road or to improve their ability to reach the toilet because of urinary urgency) rather than focusing on improving the distance the patient can walk. Resistance training is an important component of a programme for many patients, as weakness of the peripheral muscles is commonly found in patients with respiratory or cardiovascular disease and may contribute to exercise intolerance (Chapters 13 and 14).

Intermittent exercise and interval training are useful to improve the exercise endurance of patients who are severely deconditioned, extremely dyspnoeic, excessively fatigued or have claudication pain, and are essential when rehabilitating patients in the acute care setting. When marked oxygen desaturation occurs with exercise, the inclusion of frequent rests can assist in maintaining oxygen saturation at an acceptable level.

An adequate warm-up before exercise and including intermittent exercise to provide and make use of the refractory period is very important for those with EIA (Storms 2005).

In the dyspnoeic patient, the use of breathing strategies may assist with improving exercise tolerance and may accelerate the rate of recovery following exercise (see *Problem – dyspnoea*). Walking endurance may be increased with the use of a walking aid that provides arm support and facilitates a forward lean position (see *Problem – dyspnoea*). Ambulatory oxygen therapy during exercise is essential for patients who are receiving long-term oxygen therapy and should be provided in accordance with local guidelines. The flow rate may need to be increased especially during exercise that involves large muscle groups (i.e. walking, step-ups); however, care must be taken to monitor signs of carbon dioxide retention in susceptible patients. In patients who markedly desaturate on exercise but have adequate oxygen saturation levels at rest, formal assessment of the benefits of ambulatory oxygen for exercise is required. A walking test (field test or treadmill test) should be used in preference to a cycle ergometry test to identify exercise-induced hypoxaemia as oxygen desaturation is more marked with walking than cycling (Poulain et al 2003, Turner et al 2004).

In selected patients, the application of non-invasive ventilation (NIV) during exercise may enable exercise to be performed at a greater intensity or duration.

Patients should, whenever possible, exercise in an appropriate environment. Extremes of temperature, very high humidity, very windy conditions and environments with high levels of airborne irritants or pollutants should be avoided. These recommendations are especially important for individuals with EIA.

Other medical conditions

Regular exercise and an overall increase in physical activity are important components of an obesity treatment regimen that also includes dietary control. Regular exercise in the obese individual may improve body image, self-esteem and mood, and assist with more rigorous adherence to a dietary regimen. Even in the absence of weight loss, regular exercise can help blood lipid profiles and reduce the risk of hypertension and mortality from cardiovascular disease (Paffenbarger et al 1983, Sandvik et al 1993). An exercise programme for obese patients should include an aerobic component, and non-weight bearing exercise at a low to moderate intensity to avoid the development of musculoskeletal problems. A component of resistance training is also important. The duration and frequency of exercise should be gradually increased with the overall aim of achieving a high-energy expenditure.

Exercise training in patients with type II diabetes has been shown to improve glycaemic control, decrease body fat and improve plasma lipids even in the absence of weight loss (American Diabetes Association 2004).

Patients with type I and type II diabetes should be able to safely participate in exercise following careful screening and providing they have good control of their blood glucose level. This requires regular blood glucose monitoring before, during and following exercise. Screening of patients with diabetes before starting an exercise programme is required to identify the presence of any complications that may be exacerbated by exercise. These complications comprise cardiovascular abnormalities, including autonomic neuropathy, as these abnormalities may be associated with silent ischaemia and hypotension or hypertension following exercise. Patients with diabetes who are at a high-risk for underlying cardiovascular disease should undergo a graded exercise test with ECG monitoring before starting an exercise programme. Screening for the presence of peripheral arterial disease, retinopathy, ne-phropathy and peripheral neuropathy should also be undertaken in patients with diabetes. The presence of retinopathy requires individuals to avoid exercise that involves straining or Valsava-like manoeuvres. Peripheral neuropathy and peripheral arterial disease are more common in people with diabetes and precautionary measures for the feet, such as special socks and proper footwear, are essential to avoid trauma to the area. Adequate hydration is essential to avoid any adverse effects of exercise on the cardiovascular system or glucose levels; thus, fluid replacement during exercise is important to compensate for fluid loss from sweating (American Diabetes Association 2004).

Outcome measures

Commonly used measures for evaluating the effects of an exercise programme include the assessment of anthropometric variables (e.g. weight, body mass index, waist : hip ratio) in selected patients, resting blood pressure, peripheral muscle strength, functional exercise capacity including assessment of HR response to exercise and symptoms (dyspnoea, fatigue, pain) and QoL using disease-specific questionnaires where available. The ability to perform ADL may be assessed via patient self-report or quantified using validated questionnaires. The economic benefits of an exercise programme for people with CHF or COPD may be evaluated by recording hospital admissions and length of stay before and following rehabilitation.

Chapters 13 and 14 detail specific outcome measures for patients participating in pulmonary or cardiac rehabilitation programmes.

PROBLEM – REDUCED LUNG VOLUME

Reduced lung volume refers to the inability to expand lung tissue and includes a reduction of residual volume (RV), V_T, expiratory reserve volume (ERV) and/or a reduction in inspiratory reserve volume (IRV). There are two main clinical consequences of these reduced lung volumes: a reduction in total lung capacity (TLC) and vital capacity (VC), as a patient may be unable to increase inhaled volume sufficiently to expand lung tissue, and a reduction in FRC, as a patient may be unable to sustain alveolar inflation. A reduction in lung volume occurs in a variety of situations and may be short-lived (e.g. when FRC is reduced following major surgery) or chronic (e.g. when all lung volumes and hence TLC are reduced as a consequence of ILD). On occasions the cause is a disease process affecting the lung parenchyma but in many situations the reduction in lung volume arises from processes affecting other structures, such as the chest wall, respiratory muscles or the pleura. A decrease in FRC is an almost universal finding following upper abdominal surgery or cardio-thoracic surgery.

Many patients with reduced lung volumes and capacities present with the problems of dyspnoea and decreased exercise tolerance, due to the inability to meet the ventilatory demands of physical activity (for example, patients with ILD may present with dyspnoea on ADL). Alternatively, they may present with the problem of impaired airway clearance due to the inability to take a sufficiently deep breath resulting in reduced expiratory flow and an ineffective cough. Impaired gas exchange and orthopnoea may also be present in patients with reduced lung volume.

The pathophysiological basis for a reduction in lung volume and clinical examples are given in Table 6.7.

A reduction in lung volumes is only problematic when it significantly affects gas exchange, the ability to clear the airways or causes dyspnoea. The main consequences of a decrease in lung volume are:

- Impaired oxygenation due to $\dot{V}/\dot{Q}$ mismatching. This occurs because the small airways in the dependent lung regions may close during normal tidal volume breathing. In some cases, wasted perfusion, where blood passes through consolidated, collapsed or damaged lung without being oxygenated (intrapulmonary shunt), may also contribute to impaired oxygenation, especially if hypoxic vasoconstriction is ineffective. Low tidal volume breathing may be associated with a failure to clear the anatomic dead space, resulting in impaired gas exchange.

- Ineffective cough due to the reduction in VC, which reduces the ability to generate an adequate expiratory airflow.

- Increased WOB as airway resistance is increased and lung compliance is reduced.

6

■ Dyspnoea during physical activity due to the inability to meet the ventilatory demands of exercise.

Clinical features

Subjectively the patient may report that breathing requires effort. On examination there will be an adaptive breathing pattern characterized by a small V_T and increased respiratory rate. In the presence of pain, or fear of pain (e.g. in the patient with a surgical incision, fractured ribs or pleuritic pain), there will be an absence of periodic sighs. Chest expansion will be reduced overall such as with ILD or may be a localized finding, for example in the area overlying a collapsed lobe.

On auscultation there will be absent, diminished or bronchial breath sounds. The cough will be weak, due mainly to the inability to achieve an adequate inhaled volume and expiratory airflow (e.g. in spinal cord injury, quadriplegia). Chest radiograph findings may identify the cause of the reduction in lung volumes such as a pleural disorder, ILD, lobar or lung collapse.

Clinical features resulting from acute lobar collapse depend on the extent of the collapse, the abruptness of onset and the underlying respiratory impairment. A slowly developing segmental or lobar collapse may produce few symptoms if the patient has otherwise normal lungs. If a similar magnitude of lung collapse occurs acutely in a patient with chronic lung disease, severe respiratory distress may develop in which case the clinical features of hypoxaemia will be present (see *Problem – impaired gas exchange*). If however, there is a decrease in perfusion to the collapsed lung as a result of hypoxic pulmonary vasoconstriction, hypoxaemia may be minimal or absent.

Lung function test results show a decrease in lung volumes (RV) and capacities (FRC, VC and TLC).

Table 6.7 Pathophysiological basis of a reduction in lung volume and clinical examples

	Pathophysiological basis		Clinical examples
Decrease in compliance	1. Lung		ILD
	2. Chest wall		Kyphoscoliosis, ankylosing spondylitis, spinal cord injury – quadriplegia, disruption to the integrity of the chest wall due to trauma, e.g. flail chest
Atelectasis	1. Postoperative period: normal consequence of UAS and cardiothoracic surgery		Due to the general anaesthetic, surgery and changes occurring in the postoperative period including a lack of periodic deep breaths, absence of sighs, diaphragm dysfunction, supine position
	2. Reduced function of surfactant		ARDS, smoke inhalation, high FiO_2, effect of general anaesthesia and opioids
	3. Airway obstruction		Foreign body, mucus plugging, hilar adenopathy, mediastinal masses
	4. Negative airway pressure		Endobronchial suctioning
Compression of lung tissue	1. Pleural space encroachment		Effusion, empyema
	2. Mediastinal structures		Tension pneumothorax causing mediastinal shift
	3. Cardiomegaly		Decreases ventilation to left lower lobe when supine, e.g. CHF
	4. Abdominal distension		Obesity, ascites, following abdominal surgery, running-in phase of peritoneal dialysis, pregnancy
Pain			Causes shallow breathing, e.g. postoperatively, chest trauma, rib fractures
Decreased ability of respiratory muscles to generate sufficient negative pressure			Respiratory muscle weakness causing an ineffective cough (see *Problem – respiratory muscle dysfunction*)

ILD, interstitial lung disease; UAS, upper abdominal surgery; ARDS, acute respiratory distress syndrome; FiO_2, fraction of inspired oxygen; CHF, chronic heart failure

Hypoxaemia may be present, particularly when there is an inability to expand a large portion of lung tissue, primarily as a result of $\dot{V}/\dot{Q}$ mismatching arising from changes in the FRC/closing volume relationship. Hypercapnia is often absent but will occur if there is associated hypoventilation or chronic lung disease.

Physiotherapy management

When gas exchange is reduced or WOB is increased, physiotherapy management is largely focused on the optimization of lung volumes achieved by upright positioning. As upright positions increase FRC and therefore alveolar inflation, high sitting, sitting out of bed and ambulation are encouraged. The side-lying position is preferred to slumped or supine positions and may be modified by tilting the patient towards prone to further decrease compression on lung tissue. This is especially so in patients with abdominal distension (Jenkins et al 1988). Functional residual capacity may also be increased with the use of continuous positive airway pressure (CPAP).

Short-lived increases in V_T and inspiratory capacity may occur with the use of breathing techniques (e.g. thoracic expansion exercises, sustained maximal inspirations with or without the use of an incentive spirometer, intermittent positive airway pressure (IPPB)) and manual hyperinflation in the intubated patient. These breathing techniques assist in re-expansion of lung tissue and will be more efficient if performed in upright positions. In addition, upright positioning will assist patients to increase inhaled volume sufficiently to generate adequate expiratory airflow and produce an effective cough.

For patients with fixed and irreversible chest wall or lung pathology (e.g. kyphoscoliosis, ILD), physiotherapy is unable to influence lung volume; however, the associated problems of dyspnoea and reduced exercise tolerance can be treated (see *Problem – dyspnoea* and *Problem – decreased exercise tolerance*).

Ambulation increases $\dot{V}_E$ (Chapter 4) and when ambulating, patients should be encouraged to take frequent deep breaths to ensure that the increased $\dot{V}_E$ is not solely due to an increase in respiratory rate (Orfanos et al 1999, Zafiropoulos et al 2004) and to assist in lung re-expansion.

Patients at increased risk of developing clinically significant atelectasis following surgery should be identified and prophylactic physiotherapy started (Chapter 12).

Obese patients may benefit from exercise programmes designed to achieve weight reduction provided that exercise is accompanied by dietary control (see *Problem – decreased exercise tolerance*).

Outcome measures

Following physiotherapy intervention there may be a change in cough effectiveness. Auscultatory findings may reflect changes in lung volume. Chest radiographs may reflect resolution of the underlying problem but are not always good indicators of clinical progress; for example, following coronary artery surgery, small pleural effusions or atelectasis may persist for a considerable time after the patient has recovered clinically. Pulmonary function tests will reflect changes in lung volume if the underlying lung pathology is reversible. Improvements in associated problems such as impaired gas exchange, reduced exercise tolerance and dyspnoea may be evident. In the high-risk surgical patient, the outcome will be prevention of PPCs and reduced length of hospitalization.

PROBLEM – IMPAIRED GAS EXCHANGE

Impaired gas exchange is common in patients with respiratory or cardiovascular disease. In some patients, abnormalities may only become evident when increased demands are imposed on the respiratory and cardiovascular systems such as during physical activity, an infection or when changes in ventilation occur as a normal consequence of sleep (Chapter 11). Gas exchange abnormalities rarely occur in the absence of one or more of the other problems described in this chapter. Impaired gas exchange presents as hypoxaemia, hypercapnia or hypocapnia (West 2005). When the respiratory system is unable to provide adequate gas exchange for metabolic requirements, respiratory failure occurs.

Although changes in ventilation arise in response to hypoxaemia and hypercapnia, dyspnoea is not necessarily present. The physiotherapist does not always have a role in the management of impaired gas exchange; for example, in the patient with acute pulmonary embolus.

Hypoxaemia

Hypoxaemia may be acute or chronic and is seen in a wide range of conditions. Type I respiratory failure is present in a patient who is awake and at rest when PaO_2 is below 8 kPa (60 mmHg); values at sea level. The pathophysiological basis of hypoxaemia and clinical examples are given in Table 6.8.

Hypercapnia

Hypoxaemia always occurs in the presence of hypercapnia in the spontaneously breathing patient unless the patient is receiving oxygen therapy. For the patient who is awake and at rest, a raised $PaCO_2$ is the hallmark of type II respiratory failure, which is present when $PaCO_2$

Table 6.8   Pathophysiological basis of hypoxaemia and clinical examples

	Pathophysiological basis	Clinical examples
$\dot{V}/\dot{Q}$ mismatch	Commonest cause in respiratory disease	
	1. Decrease in FRC	Reduced lung volumes secondary to UAS or cardiothoracic surgery, obesity, ascites, atelectasis, supine position, ILD
	2. Increase in CV	Small airway closure due to airflow limitation (e.g. cigarette smoking, COPD), pulmonary oedema, increased age
	Wasted ventilation (perfusion limitation)	Occurs when a perfusion defect prevents inspired oxygen from reaching arterial blood e.g. pulmonary embolus
	Wasted perfusion (intrapulmonary shunt)	Occurs when blood is shunted through non-ventilated lung tissue (e.g. atelectasis or consolidation), somewhat attenuated by hypoxic pulmonary vasoconstriction
	Cardiac shunt	Atrial septal defect, ventricular septal defect
Hypoventilation	Site of abnormality:	
	1. Respiratory centre	Depression of hypercapnic and hypoxic ventilatory drives by drugs, general anaesthesia, as a normal consequence of sleep
	2. Medulla	Trauma, neoplasm
	3. Spinal cord	Trauma, neoplasm
	4. Anterior horn cell	Trauma, neoplasm, poliomyelitis
	5. Innervation of the respiratory muscles	Phrenic nerve paralysis
	6. Disease of the myoneural junction	Myasthenia gravis
	7. Respiratory muscles	Weakness or fatigue (see *Problem –respiratory muscle dysfunction*)
	8. Upper airway obstruction	Foreign body, obstructive sleep apnoea
	9. Excessive WOB	When an added load on the mechanics of breathing occurs such as in the patient with acute severe asthma who is exhausted, acute exacerbation of COPD
Diffusion limitation	Decrease in alveolar–capillary surface area	Emphysema
	Decrease in diffusion gradient	Low FiO_2 as occurs at high altitude
	Increased thickness of alveolar–capillary membrane	Scarring or fluid in the interstitial space, e.g. pulmonary oedema, ILD
	Decreased transit time of red blood cell in pulmonary capillary	May cause hypoxaemia on exercise in the presence of another cause of diffusion limitation
Decrease in FiO_2	High altitude	
	Malfunctioning of respiratory equipment	Disconnection of gas supply
	Endotracheal suctioning	
Mixed causes	Combination of $\dot{V}/\dot{Q}$ mismatch, diffusion limitation, shunt and hypoventilation	Seen in severe chronic lung disease
Imbalance between $\dot{V}O_2$ and DO_2 (i.e. oxygen consumption and delivery)	This causes a reduction in PvO_2. Low PvO_2 magnifies the effects of $\dot{V}/\dot{Q}$ mismatch and shunt on a patient's level of oxygenation	Low cardiac output states, severe anaemia

WOB, work of breathing; COPD, chronic obstructive pulmonary disease; $\dot{V}/\dot{Q}$, ventilation/perfusion ratio; FRC, functional residual capacity; CV, closing volume; UAS, upper abdominal surgery; ILD, interstitial lung disease; ARDS, acute respiratory distress syndrome; FiO_2, fraction of inspired oxygen; $\dot{V}O_2$, oxygen consumption, PvO_2, mixed venous oxygen tension; DO_2, oxygen delivery

exceeds 6.7 kPa (50 mmHg) and is accompanied by a PaO_2 of less than 8 kPa (60 mmHg); values at sea level. Type II respiratory failure can be acute or chronic. The pathophysiological basis of hypercapnia and clinical examples are given in Table 6.9 (Haslet et al 2002).

Under normal conditions, $PaCO_2$ is an important factor in the chemical control of ventilation and the relationship between $PaCO_2$ and $\dot{V}_E$ is linear (Schwartzstein & Parker 2006). The ventilatory response to $PaCO_2$ is reduced during sleep, in elderly individuals and there is a wide variation in the ventilatory response to $PaCO_2$ among individuals. When the $PaCO_2$ is normal, there is little increase in ventilation until PaO_2 has fallen below 8 kPa (60 mmHg). When hypercapnia is present, the ventilatory response to hypoxaemia is heightened. When $PaCO_2$ is chronically elevated, for example in some patients with COPD, the ventilatory response to $PaCO_2$ is significantly decreased and hypoxaemia becomes the chief stimulus to ventilation (Lumb 2005, West 2005). When high levels of inspired oxygen are administered to such patients to relieve the hypoxaemia (i.e. those with type II respiratory failure), ventilation may become depressed resulting in a decrease in $\dot{V}_E$ and a subsequent worsening of gas exchange.

Hypocapnia

In clinical practice, a low $PaCO_2$ is a far less common occurrence than a raised $PaCO_2$. In an individual who is spontaneously breathing an increase in the rate or depth of breathing may not result in hypocapnia. For example, a large V_T accompanied by a low respiratory rate may not reduce $PaCO_2$ below normal levels. Conversely, a small V_T and high respiratory rate, such as when panting, may not lower $PaCO_2$ or may even raise $PaCO_2$ if the V_T fails to clear the anatomic dead space. The underlying mechanism involved in alveolar hyperventilation and thus hypocapnia is an increased respiratory drive mediated through a behavioural or metabolic respiratory control system (Phillipson 2005).

Special case – the ventilated patient

In the mechanically ventilated patient, hypocapnia or hypercapnia may be a treatment strategy (e.g. permissive hypocapnia or hypercapnia) or may occur due to iatrogenic causes.

Clinical features

Patients may adapt to chronic changes in arterial blood gas tensions whereas acute hypoxaemia and hypercapnia are less well tolerated.

There are few clinical features associated with mild hypoxaemia; however, if associated with severe anaemia or impaired cardiac output, mild hypoxaemia may be poorly tolerated. At moderate degrees of hypoxaemia (PaO_2 between 4.5 and 8 kPa (34 and 60 mmHg)) ventilation may be increased to twice the normal level (Schwartzstein & Parker 2006). The features of moderate or severe hypoxaemia that develop acutely are tachypnoea, restlessness, confusion, sweating, tachycardia, hypertension, skin pallor and cyanosis. With severe hypoxaemia, bradycardia, arrhythmias and hypotension may develop. Worsening neurologic signs associated with acute severe hypoxaemia include blurred vision, tunnel vision, loss of coordination, impaired judgement, convulsions, coma and permanent brain damage. Hypoxaemia exacerbates cardiac arrhythmias and angina in patients with IHD and may predispose to

6

Table 6.9   Pathophysiological basis of hypercapnia and clinical examples

Pathophysiological basis		Clinical examples
Hypoventilation	1. Reduced central drive	Obesity-hypoventilation syndrome, depression of the respiratory centre due to reduced conscious state, general anaesthesia, narcotics, barbiturates
	2. Respiratory muscle dysfunction	See *Problem – respiratory muscle dysfunction*
	3. Added load on the mechanics of breathing	Changes in compliance of the lung or chest wall, e.g. chest wall trauma, pulmonary oedema, large pleural effusion, ILD Increase in airways resistance, e.g. severe COPD
Increased $\dot{V}CO_2$		Increased metabolism, e.g. fever, sepsis, trauma, burns, exercise Metabolic acidosis
Increased dead space as a fraction of V_T		COPD, pulmonary embolus, low lung volume breathing, e.g. with pain, respiratory muscle weakness

ILD, insterstitial lung disease; COPD, chronic obstructive pulmonary disease; $\dot{V}CO_2$, carbon dioxide production; V_T, tidal volume

6

heart failure. The long-term cardiovascular consequences of chronic hypoxaemia are pulmonary hypertension and cor pulmonale.

The clinical features of hypercapnia are determined more by the onset of the raised $PaCO_2$ rather than the severity. Chronic hypercapnia may not be clinically manifest until a more rapid rise is induced by infection, sedation, or oxygen administration. Signs and symptoms associated with hypercapnia include those consistent with vasodilatation, for example warm peripheries, the appearance of flushed skin and a full and bounding pulse. The cardiac system may respond with episodes of extrasystoles. The resulting increase in cerebral blood flow is responsible for headache (this occurs especially on waking and can occur during exercise), a raised cerebrospinal fluid pressure and sometimes papilloedema (oedema of the optic disc). Impaired concentration and drowsiness may also be present. Rapid accumulation of CO_2 and the accompanying acidosis may quickly lead to convulsions and coma. The clinical features of hypercapnia may be less obvious in patients with COPD who have chronic respiratory failure because metabolic adaptations may occur in response to chronically elevated $PaCO_2$.

The signs and symptoms of hypocapnia are many and varied (Gardner 2003). They include paraesthesia in the hands, face and trunk and tetany. A reduction in central nervous system and cerebral blood flow may be responsible for dizziness, loss of consciousness, visual disturbances, headache, tinnitus, ataxia and tremor. With acute hypocapnia, systemic blood pressure falls and HR increases. Peripheral vasoconstriction is thought to be responsible for the complaint of cold hands.

Impaired gas exchange will be reflected in abnormalities in arterial blood gases, pulse oximetry and transcutaneous measures of $PaCO_2$.

Physiotherapy management

Physiotherapy management is determined by the underlying pathophysiological cause(s) and may be limited. Oxygen therapy is indicated whenever tissue oxygenation is impaired and should be prescribed by the medical practitioner in accordance with established guidelines. Physiotherapists should ensure the correct application of oxygen therapy including the delivery device and flow rate/concentration (Chapter 5). For patients with type II respiratory failure susceptible to oxygen-induced respiratory depression, controlled oxygen therapy should be administered via a fixed performance device (Chapter 5). For these patients, careful administration of oxygen therapy is required when a nebulizer is used (Chapter 5).

Gas exchange may by optimized by positioning patients in an upright position to increase FRC. In spontaneously breathing adults with unilateral lung pathology, $\dot{V}/\dot{Q}$ matching may be improved by positioning in side lying with the unaffected lung dependent. However, hypoxaemia due to hypoventilation may be worsened by positioning in supine lying due to the increased load on the respiratory muscles.

Physical activity may improve gas exchange by enhancing oxygen transport or may result in further impairment in gas transfer (i.e. identified by a fall in oxygen saturation) in some patients with severe cardiopulmonary dysfunction. Oxygen therapy during ambulation may be indicated in some patients and this should be assessed using a walking test (Chapter 3) (Poulain et al 2003, Turner et al 2004). In other patients, NIV applied during ambulation may improve gas exchange. Non-invasive ventilation is also a useful treatment for exacerbations of COPD, some causes of acute respiratory failure and nocturnal hypoventilation (Mehta & Hill 2001). Specifically, CPAP may improve oxygenation in patients with acute cardiogenic pulmonary oedema (Cooper 2004).

Special case – positioning the ventilated patient

Prone positioning may improve oxygenation in acutely ill patients who are mechanically ventilated and sedated (e.g. patients with severe acute respiratory failure or acute respiratory distress syndrome) (Stiller 2000, Wong 1999). However, turning critically ill patients who are mechanically ventilated into the side-lying position may acutely increase $\dot{V}O_2$ and cause transient hypoxaemia evoking exercise and stress-like responses (Horiuchi et al 1997).

Outcome measures

Arterial blood gases, oximetry and transcutaneous end-tidal measures of $PaCO_2$ will reflect changes in gas exchange. Short-term changes in cognitive function and symptoms such as headache may be evident when abnormalities in gas exchange are corrected.

In patients with long-term abnormalities in gas exchange, changes in QoL may occur in response to interventions such as NIV or long-term oxygen therapy. In this patient group, a reduction in healthcare utilization and improved survival may also occur.

PROBLEM – AIRFLOW LIMITATION

Airflow limitation can be described as an abnormal resistance or obstruction to airflow. This problem generally occurs together with other physiotherapy problems such as dyspnoea, decreased exercise tolerance or impaired airway clearance. Airflow limitation can be caused by factors inside the airway, changes in the airway wall and factors outside the airway. The pathophysiological basis for airflow limitation is presented in Table 6.10 together with clinical examples (West 2003). Airflow limitation may be reversible (e.g. asthma without fixed airflow obstruction), partially reversible (e.g. chronic bronchitis) or irreversible (e.g. emphysema).

Special case – lung hyperinflation in COPD

Lung hyperinflation is an abnormal increase in the volume of air remaining in the lungs at the end of relaxed expiration. In patients with COPD, static lung hyperinflation, which develops over time, results from an increase in expiratory airflow resistance and a reduction in elastic recoil giving rise to air trapping (Ferguson 2006).

Dynamic hyperinflation is related to the degree of airflow limitation and the time available for exhalation. The increased metabolic demands of exercise, for example, require an increase in $\dot{V}_E$ which is achieved by an increase in V_T and respiratory rate. The increase in respiratory rate reduces the time available to exhale. Exhalation is already prolonged due to the increased resistance to expiratory airflow. The resultant incomplete exhalation causes air trapping and an increase in end-expiratory lung volume, which leads to the development of intrinsic positive end-expiratory pressure (PEEP). As end-expiratory lung volume increases, there is a decrease in inspiratory capacity. With limited inspiratory capacity, increases in $\dot{V}_E$ can only be achieved by an increase in respiratory rate. This further reduces expiratory time and a vicious cycle of air trapping and progressive hyperinflation occurs.

During an acute exacerbation of COPD there is an increase in expiratory airflow resistance due to inflammation and mucus plugging and so dynamic hyperinflation may occur at a lower level of physical activity than usual. Similarly, when a patient becomes emotional or anxious, respiratory rate often increases and the cycle of air trapping and progressive hyperinflation may occur.

Dynamic hyperinflation increases the WOB in order to initiate inspiratory airflow, the inspiratory muscles are required to generate a pleural pressure in excess of the intrinsic PEEP. This imposes an additional threshold load at the start of inspiration because the inspiratory muscles have to overcome this positive pressure. As lung hyperinflation increases there is a decrease in lung compliance leading to a further increase in the WOB on inspiration. As a result of lung hyperinflation, the diaphragm fibres are shortened and the altered length–tension relationship may decrease the ability to generate muscle tension and inspiratory pressure.

Table 6.10 Pathophysiological basis for airflow limitation and clinical examples

Pathophysiological basis		Clinical examples
Causes inside the airway	Partial or total occlusion of the airway lumen	Mucus, e.g. chronic bronchitis, cystic fibrosis, bronchiectasis, asthma
		Inhaled foreign body
		Bronchial tumour
Changes in the airway wall	Smooth muscle contraction	Asthma
	Smooth muscle hypertrophy and hyperplasia	Asthma
	Inflammation of the mucosa	Asthma, infective exacerbation of COPD
	Hypertrophy of mucus glands	Chronic bronchitis
	Thickening of the bronchial wall	Chronic bronchitis, asthma
	Dilation and destruction of airway wall	Cystic fibrosis, bronchiectasis
	Infiltration of the bronchial mucosa with eosinophils and lymphocytes	Asthma
	Changes in the osmolarity of normal airway fluid produced by cooling	Exercise-induced asthma – see *Problem – decreased exercise tolerance*
Causes outside the airway	Loss of radial traction due to a decrease in elastic recoil secondary to increases in lung compliance	Emphysema
	Compression	Enlarged lymph nodes, tumour

COPD, chronic obstructive pulmonary disease

6

Some patients with severe hyperinflation, especially during exercise, may use the abdominal release mechanism to decrease the work of the diaphragm while still maintaining its output. To effect this mechanism, the patient contracts the abdominal muscles at the end of expiration, thus pushing the contents of the abdomen up against the diaphragm and improving its length–tension relationship. The increase in lung volume during the subsequent inspiration occurs by a sudden release of the abdominal pressure that acts to passively pull the diaphragm downwards (McCarren 1992).

Clinical features

The patient with airflow limitation may report chest tightness or wheeze, cough and breathlessness, limiting their ability to undertake ADL and exercise. In asthma, cough and breathlessness may be particularly evident at night or early morning and may lead to sleep disruption. Patients may report that their cough is 'tight' and they have difficulty clearing secretions.

On examination, patients may display signs of an increased WOB to overcome the increase in airway resistance. Respiratory rate may be increased and expiration may be active, with contraction of the abdominal muscles, and prolonged expiration (increased I : E ratio). Recruitment of the accessory respiratory muscles may be evident and indrawing of the intercostal spaces and supraclavicular fossae visible. Pursed-lip breathing is adopted by some patients with severe airflow limitation (e.g. COPD).

With long-standing disease, examination of the chest may reveal signs of hyperinflation such as a barrel-shaped chest with an increase in the anteroposterior diameter and a raised shoulder girdle. Paradoxical movement of the lower chest wall can occur in patients with severe hyperinflation as the diaphragm is unable to descend and contraction of the diaphragm during inspiration leads to indrawing of the lower ribs (Hoover's sign).

Wheezing may be audible. Auscultatory findings often reveal widespread, polyphonic wheezes; however, patients with hyperinflation may have reduced breath sounds.

The chest radiograph may show signs of hyperinflation as well as signs consistent with the underlying condition; for example, the presence of emphysematous bullae or bronchiectatic changes.

Abnormalities in pulmonary function indicative of airflow limitation comprise a reduction in FEV_1, FEV_1/FVC, PEFR and forced expiratory flow at 25–75% of forced expiratory flow (FEF_{25-75}). Characteristic patterns can be seen in the flow–volume loop and may help with identifying the cause and site of the airflow limitation (Chapter 3). Functional residual capacity, RV and TLC are often increased and the ratio of RV to TLC may be elevated.

Physiotherapy management

Where airflow limitation is reversible, optimal medical management with medication is essential. Patient education is an important aspect of the management of airflow limitation, particularly in asthma, and may be undertaken by a physiotherapist in some settings. A simple explanation about the mechanism(s) of airflow limitation, the importance of avoiding trigger factors including cigarette smoke and allergens, and the use and effects of medications are essential. Self-management should be encouraged and, in particular for patients with asthma, the physiotherapist's role includes reinforcing the patient's action plan that has been developed by a medical officer to manage their changing symptoms (Gibson et al 2002).

Education and instruction in the correct method of using inhaled medications to reduce airflow limitation is necessary to ensure maximal deposition of the medication. A large range of devices is available for the delivery of inhaled respiratory medications and the physiotherapist should be familiar with these (Chapter 5). Airway clearance techniques with prior, effective delivery of an inhaled bronchodilator may help to overcome airflow limitation due to retained bronchial secretions and bronchospasm. Where necessary airway clearance techniques should be adapted to ensure that no increase in airflow limitation occurs. Increasing the length of periods of breathing control between huffs in the forced expiration technique (FET) may help to prevent an increase in airflow limitation. For patients with COPD it may be necessary to modify the huff to prevent dynamic airway collapse by decreasing expiratory force or increasing inspiratory volume (van der Schans 1997). Alternatively, positive expiratory pressure (PEP) therapy has been suggested as an appropriate airway clearance technique for patients with COPD as it provides positive mouth pressure to splint open collapsible airways (Holland & Button 2006). Further details on these airway clearance techniques are provided in Chapter 5 on physiotherapy techniques.

Breathing strategies such as PLB may be encouraged in patients who spontaneously adopt the technique (Gosselink 2004). This technique aims to splint the airways open and increase expiratory time, thereby reducing dyspnoea. Other breathing strategies may be directed towards the management of dyspnoea associated with airflow limitation (see physiotherapy management in *Problem – dyspnoea*). For patients with asthma a number of breathing 'retraining' strategies (such as the Buteyko technique; Chapter 17) have been advocated although there is no consistent evidence for improved asthma control (Holloway & Ram 2004).

For the management of EIA, see *Problem – decreased exercise tolerance.*

Where the cause of airflow limitation is a tumour or enlarged lymph nodes, physiotherapy management is not indicated.

Outcome measures

Changes in symptoms related to airflow limitation, particularly in asthma, can be measured with a health-related QoL questionnaire. A number of widely used questionnaires exist, including:

- Asthma Quality of Life Questionnaire (AQLQ) (Juniper et al 1993)
- Mini AQLQ (Juniper et al 1999a)
- Marks Asthma Quality of Life Questionnaire (AQLQ–M) (Marks et al 1993)
- Modified AQLQ–M (Adams et al 2000)
- Asthma Control Questionnaire (Juniper et al 1999b).

For patients with COPD, the SGRQ includes a section that quantifies symptoms of wheeze/chest tightness (Jones et al 1992).

Short-term changes in airflow limitation, as reflected by wheeze, may be evident on auscultation.

Pulmonary function tests may reflect changes in the degree of airflow limitation depending upon the underlying aetiology and whether the condition is reversible.

PROBLEM – RESPIRATORY MUSCLE DYSFUNCTION

Respiratory muscle dysfunction (i.e. reduced strength or endurance) may be present in a range of clinical conditions including neuromuscular disorders (e.g. motor neuron disease, multiple sclerosis, Guillain–Barré syndrome, myasthenia gravis, muscular dystrophy, tetraplegia), connective tissue diseases (e.g. systemic lupus erythematosus), chronic lung disease (e.g. COPD, cystic fibrosis), chest wall disorders (e.g. kyphoscoliosis) and CHF. The problem may also occur in patients treated with oral corticosteroids and in those who are malnourished (Troosters et al 2005). Respiratory muscle dysfunction becomes a physiotherapy problem when the patient presents with problems such as dyspnoea, impaired airway clearance or inability to wean from mechanical ventilation.

Clinical features

Mild respiratory muscle dysfunction is often difficult to detect using simple clinical measures. Weakness of the respiratory muscles is often advanced before clinical symptoms are present because the pressure required to initiate inspiratory flow represents only a small proportion of the maximum force-generating capacity of the inspiratory muscles (Troosters et al 2005). The main clinical features and patient problems associated with respiratory muscle weakness are an unexplained reduction in VC, abnormal breathing pattern, nocturnal hypoxaemia and hypercapnia in the absence of chronic lung disease, dyspnoea, decreased exercise tolerance and impaired airway clearance.

Subjectively, the patient may report breathlessness, especially when supine or standing in water up to their chest, for example when entering the sea or a swimming pool. The weight of water causes pressure on the chest and the abdominal wall and thus the load on the inspiratory muscles, especially the diaphragm, is increased. Marked breathlessness during ADL that involve unsupported upper limb activities may be reported by patients with diaphragm weakness or bilateral phrenic nerve palsy. Daytime somnolence, early morning headaches and impaired mental function may be present if hypoxaemia and hypercapnia occur during sleep. Abnormalities in breathing pattern may be present and include increased respiratory rate, decreased V_T, reduced chest expansion, use of accessory muscles and respiratory alternans (periods of breathing using only chest wall muscles alternating with periods of breathing using the diaphragm). Profound diaphragm weakness or paralysis gives rise to paradoxical movement of the abdomen occurring during inspiration and is most easily seen with the patient supine (Moxham 1999). This occurs when the diaphragm is unable to match the negative intrapleural pressure generated by the other inspiratory muscles, resulting in passive transmission of this pressure during inspiration and causing the abdominal contents to be pulled upwards. When upright, recruitment of the abdominal muscles may occur during expiration in order to elevate the diaphragm so that gravity and chest wall and lung recoil pressure can assist diaphragm descent during inspiration. The patient may have a weak cough due to an inadequate inspired volume or weakness of the expiratory muscles resulting in a reduction in expiratory airflow. The weak cough may in turn lead to the problem of impaired airway clearance.

The plain chest radiograph is a useful diagnostic tool in unilateral diaphragm paralysis as the affected dome is elevated. In addition to respiratory muscle weakness there may also be signs of generalized muscle wasting and assessment may reveal a reduction in peripheral muscle strength. The ability to perform ADL and participate in exercise will be impaired as a result of dyspnoea reflecting the difficulties of the inspiratory muscles to cope with the required increase in ventilation. Depending on the underlying pathological process, peripheral muscle dysfunction may also contribute to exercise intolerance.

Lung function

Lung function may be normal in the absence of marked weakness. The most frequently noted abnormality in lung function is a marked reduction in VC. In the presence of severe bilateral diaphragm weakness, the VC is low when the patient is upright and typically falls by more than 50% when supine, whereas in normal subjects the reduction in VC when supine is less than 10% (ATS/ERS 2002). The fall in VC is due to the weight of the abdominal contents in supine exerting an upward pressure on the diaphragm. Measurement of VC is especially useful in the management of progressive disorders such as Guillain–Barré syndrome. The pattern of abnormality of other lung capacities and volumes is less consistent. Residual volume is normal or may be increased, especially if there is marked expiratory muscle weakness. As a consequence, TLC is reduced to a lesser extent than VC and the RV/TLC and FRC/TLC ratios are often increased (ATS/ERS 2002). In the absence of lung disease, airway resistance to expiratory airflow is normal as indicated by a normal FEV_1/FVC ratio. Gas transfer (i.e. TLCO) is usually normal or only mildly reduced as a result of the inability to fully distend the lungs at TLC and thus enable the entire alveolar surface to be exposed to carbon monoxide (ATS/ERS 2002). Depending on the underlying aetiology, inspiratory and/or expiratory muscle strength (i.e. *PiMax* and *PeMax*) will be reduced compared with normal values (Chapter 3). Assessment of respiratory muscle endurance is more complex and is rarely performed outside of specialized laboratories.

Gas exchange abnormalities

In the awake patient with chronic muscle weakness, even when severe, only a mild reduction in PaO_2 is present and $PaCO_2$ is usually normal. When respiratory muscle weakness occurs acutely, a more marked reduction is PaO_2 is seen. In the absence of lung disease, daytime hypercapnia is unlikely unless VC is reduced to less than 50% predicted normal value and respiratory muscle strength is reduced to less than 40% predicted normal value (ATS/ERS 2002). During sleep, dips in oxygen saturation occur during periods of rapid eye movement (REM) sleep when the work of the diaphragm is increased due to the reduction in the tone of the intercostals and accessory muscles. In the patient with slowly progressive weakness of the respiratory muscles, hypercapnia often develops insidiously at night and over time leads to persistent daytime hypercapnia and thus type II respiratory failure (Chapter 11).

Physiotherapy management

Targeted respiratory muscle training may be an effective means of increasing the strength and endurance of the respiratory muscles (Chapter 5). Most of the evidence for the benefits of respiratory muscle training has been gained from studies of IMT in patients with COPD. In this patient population, IMT performed using a threshold loading device or a target-flow resistive device has been shown to increase inspiratory muscle strength and endurance and reduce dyspnoea (Geddes et al 2005, Lotters et al 2002). The optimal IMT protocol has not been determined; however, high-intensity interval-based protocols, which include regular rest periods, appear to be more efficient at improving respiratory muscle function than protocols that do not permit rest periods (Hill et al 2004, 2006).

Although unsupported upper limb exercise training increases the reliance on the diaphragm to generate inspiratory flow, such training does not appear to improve diaphragm function. Patients may benefit from whole body exercise training as a result of improvements in peripheral muscle function. For patients with excess bronchial secretions, assistance with airway clearance including the use of assisted coughing techniques is often required (Chapters 5 and 16).

Non-invasive ventilation provided during sleep may be required to rest the respiratory muscles and correct blood gas abnormalities. Some patients may also require periods of NIV during the daytime.

In some patients, the underlying cause of respiratory muscle dysfunction is progressive and the main role of physiotherapy is the successful management of associated and potential problems (e.g. impaired airway clearance).

Outcome measures

The following outcome measures should be considered when evaluating the response to physiotherapy intervention. The patient's perception of dyspnoea during ADL and exercise can be assessed using the Borg Category Ratio Scale or a VAS (see *Problem – dyspnoea*). Perception of dyspnoea during ADL can also be quantified using standardized questionnaires, for example, the dyspnoea domain of the Chronic Respiratory Disease Questionnaire (Guyatt et al 1987). Measurement of *PiMax* and *PeMax* will determine whether changes in respiratory muscle strength have occurred. Observation of breathing pattern and evaluation of cough effectiveness are important outcomes to evaluate. Measurement of VC is a useful outcome measure and simple to perform clinically. Changes in exercise tolerance can be assessed using a field walking test (Chapter 3).

In the mechanically ventilated patient who is having problems weaning, changes in respiratory muscle function may be associated with changes in the tolerance to periods of spontaneous breathing (i.e. duration of periods, arterial blood gas tensions).

In situations where the cause of respiratory muscle dysfunction is a progressive condition, the outcome measures for evaluating physiotherapy intervention often relate to the management of associated problems (such as *Problem – impaired airway clearance*) and may include such measures as the frequency of chest infection.

PROBLEM – DYSFUNCTIONAL BREATHING PATTERN

Dysfunctional breathing pattern rarely occurs in isolation in the physiotherapy problem list but is more commonly associated with other patient problems, some of which are amenable to physiotherapy intervention. Examples of these associated problems include dyspnoea and airflow limitation. Resolution of the associated problems may be accompanied by a return to a more normal breathing pattern. Some breathing patterns result from neurological abnormalities (e.g. Cheyne–Stokes respiration occurring in a brainstem cerebrovascular accident) or metabolic dysfunction. These breathing abnormalities are not amenable to physiotherapy intervention.

Observation of breathing pattern and respiratory effort may provide reliable clues about a patient's underlying problem. For example, the characteristic breathing pattern of patients with reduced lung volume is a low V_T and increased respiratory rate. When ventilatory demand is increased, patients with marked airflow limitation recruit their accessory respiratory muscles and signs of abdominal paradox and intercostal recession may be observed. Patients with airflow limitation may also use PLB (see *Problem – airflow limitation*). The changes in respiratory mechanics and breathing pattern give rise to an increased WOB in patients with reduced lung volume and airflow limitation but are necessary adaptations for the maintenance of adequate ventilation and gas exchange and are not dysfunctional.

Dysfunctional breathing mainly occurs when the WOB is exaggerated such that patients overbreathe or have an abnormally high respiratory rate (e.g. hyperventilation syndrome) for their metabolic require-

ments. The pathophysiology of dysfunctional breathing is complex and may arise due to psychological (e.g. anxiety) or physiological stress. The problem may also occur during exercise (Gardner 1996). This syndrome is often referred to as 'hyperventilation syndrome' and is discussed in detail in Chapter 17. Dysfunctional breathing is also commonly found in patients with asthma (Morgan 2006). In the severely breathless patient, a dysfunctional breathing pattern may become evident when the patient is recovering from breathlessness elicited by physical activity. In such instances, the dysfunctional breathing pattern may be due to anxiety.

Dysfunctional breathing may also result from abnormal functioning of the chest wall (e.g. flail chest or from spinal cord injury) where the normal respiratory mechanics are altered.

Clinical features

These include abnormalities in respiratory rate and depth, including excessive sighing or breath holding, and changes in the I : E ratio. Observation and palpation may reveal asymmetrical chest wall movement, paradoxical chest wall movement, asynchronous movements or respiratory alternans. The patient may overuse their accessory respiratory muscles, and may actively elevate their shoulders during inspiration. Associated excessive muscle activity (e.g. facial grimacing, gripping objects) may also occur.

Arterial blood gas analysis may demonstrate abnormalities consistent with an underlying problem (e.g. hypocapnia in hyperventilation syndrome or hypoxaemia and hypercapnia in spinal cord injury). Diagnostic tests may be used to assess hyperventilation including the voluntary hyperventilation provocation test, Nijmegen questionnaire and breath-holding time (Chapter 17).

Physiotherapy management

Breathing pattern retraining is focused on changing dysfunctional breathing patterns when they are not associated with strategies employed by the patient to reduce other problems such as dyspnoea or airflow limitation. Thus, physiotherapy generally aims to eliminate the exaggerated muscle activity associated with increased WOB or associated responses. Retraining may focus on changing V_T, flow rate and strategies such as relaxation and breathing control are encouraged (Chapter 17).

Dysfunctional breathing patterns associated with abnormalities of the chest wall or spinal cord injury may

6

be managed with positive pressure ventilation if these are associated with abnormal gas exchange.

Outcome measures

Physiotherapy intervention can be evaluated using the Nijmegen questionnaire, breath-holding time, diaries recording disability/distress/symptoms and QoL measures (Thomas et al 2003) (Chapter 17).

Arterial blood gas analysis, transcutaneous CO_2 and oximetry may reflect concomitant changes in gas exchange.

PROBLEM – PAIN

This section outlines pain of respiratory and cardiovascular origin as well as other causes of pain located in the chest. Information regarding claudication pain and the physiotherapy management is included in the *Problem – decreased exercise tolerance*.

Chest pain of respiratory origin

The origin and characteristic features of pain due to respiratory causes, together with clinical examples, are given in Table 6.11 (Murray & Gebhart 2000). Pain of respiratory origin arises from the parietal pleura and from stimulation of the mucosa of the trachea and main bronchus. The lung parenchyma and visceral pleura are insensitive to pain. However, inflammatory processes in peripheral regions of the lung that involve the overlying visceral pleura often gives rise to pain as a result of involvement of the adjacent parietal pleura. Chest wall pain is often reported by patients who have chronic cough or dyspnoea as a result of the associated musculoskeletal pathology.

Chest pain of cardiovascular origin

Table 6.12 outlines the main causes and characteristic features of pain due to cardiovascular causes.

Chest pain which may be unrelated to respiratory or cardiovascular disease

Neural, muscular or skeletal pain. Examples of causative factors are disc degeneration, bony metastases, muscle injuries, inflammation of soft tissues and disorders of the costal cartilages. Pain in the chest wall also occurs following insertion of an intercostal catheter and following cardiothoracic surgery, fractured ribs, musculoskeletal disorders and tumours involving the ribs or soft tissues. The pain is usually localized to the affected area and the area is usually tender on palpation. The patient usually reports that the pain is a dull ache or may be described as a sharper pain. The pain is usually increased on respiratory movements including deep inspiration and cough, and is exacerbated by trunk and shoulder movements.

Oesophageal pain. The causes of pain arising from the oesophagus are:

1. Heartburn – this pain is felt in the centre of the chest and the epigastrium. The pain is increased when lying down and relieved by sitting upright and by taking antacids. The commonest causes are GORD and hiatus hernia.
2. Oesophageal spasm – when this occurs the pain may last up to 1 hour and there may not be an obvious provoking factor. The pain closely resembles that of unstable angina and is often relieved by nitroglycerin.

| Table 6.11   Origin and characteristic features of pain due to respiratory causes ||||
Origin	Characteristic features	Stimulus	Clinical examples
Pleura Tends to be limited to the affected region but may be referred to the ipsilateral cervical or shoulder tip or to the upper abdomen or lower back	Sharp stabbing pain due to inflammation or stretching of the parietal pleura Described as sharp, dull, ache, burning or a catching pain	Exacerbated by deep inspiration, coughing and sneezing	Pneumonia, carcinoma, pulmonary tuberculosis, pneumothorax, pleurisy, pulmonary embolus
Tracheobronchial tree	Generally described as a raw, retrosternal discomfort or a dull ache	Deep inspiration, coughing	Usually acute inflammation from infection, inhalation of irritant fumes or radiotherapy for bronchial carcinoma May occur with high-flow oxygen therapy

3. Oesophageal tear – this may occur in association with prolonged vomiting. The pain is felt centrally in the chest.

Peptic ulceration and gallbladder disease. Diseases of the stomach, duodenum or biliary system may give rise to pain felt in the chest although this pain is more commonly confined to the abdomen.

With peptic ulceration the pain is burning in nature, occurs following meals and is relieved by antacids.

Pain of biliary origin is usually colicky in nature and felt on the right side of the abdomen, the front and back of the chest. The pain may be related to the ingestion of certain foods; for example, fatty foods.

'Pseudoangina' due to hyperventilation syndrome. Hyperventilation may cause atypical chest pain, which may mimic angina.

Clinical features

The clinical features associated with pain of respiratory or cardiovascular origin are outlined in Tables 6.11 and 6.12. Subjective assessment will identify the clinical features of the pain and factors that elicit pain or increase the intensity of the pain.

Quantification of the pain intensity can be made using a VAS, a verbal rating of pain severity on a 0–10 or 0–5 scale. On examination of the patient there may be signs of an abnormal breathing pattern and systemic signs such as sweating, pallor and tachycardia. Chest expansion may be reduced over the painful area and there may be an associated reduction in breath sounds on auscultation and pleural rub.

Physiotherapy management

Diagnosis and management of the underlying cause are essential. Anti-inflammatory agents or analgesics

6

Table 6.12   Causes and characteristic features of chest pain due to cardiovascular causes

Cause	Characteristic features	Stimuli
Myocardial ischaemia	Myocardial ischaemia does not always cause pain	
1. Stable angina pectoris	Described as severe pressure, squeezing, ache, tightness or retrosternal burning	Physical exertion – often occurs at the same RPP
	Maximal intensity is felt retrosternally or to the left of the sternum but may radiate to the neck, jaw, shoulder or down the inner aspects of the arms, more commonly the left	Emotional stimuli Heavy meal Inhalation of cigarette smoke With rest, the pain tends to subside within 2–10 minutes
	Often associated with dyspnoea	Relieved by nitroglycerin
	Can be described as epigastric pain	
2. Unstable angina	As for stable angina	Unpredictable pattern and may occur at rest
		Not always relieved by nitroglycerin
3. Acute myocardial infarction	Pain is similar to that of angina but is generally more severe and of longer duration	Usually requires large doses of opiates to control the pain
Pericarditis due to inflammation of parietal pericardium from a variety of causes – bacterial, viral, neoplasm, post-myocardial infarction	Sharp stabbing pain, central or left side of chest and left arm and may radiate to neck, back and upper abdomen May be associated with friction rub in the absence of effusion	Deep inspiration, supine and left side-lying positions Sitting and leaning forwards may decrease pain
Diseases of the aorta		
1. Aortic stenosis	Produces angina-like pain	Exertion
2. Dissection of the aorta	Searing severe pain of sudden onset May present in upper back and may radiate to neck and face	May be associated with exertion

RPP, rate pressure product (systolic blood pressure × heart rate)

are used for musculoskeletal, pleuritic and pericardial pain.

Direct methods of pain management used by physiotherapists include heat modalities, interferential, transcutaneous electrical nerve stimulation, Entonox, acupuncture and manual therapy. Knowledge of pain management, for example medications and their onset and duration of action, route of administration, is required so that physiotherapy interventions can be provided when pain management is optimal.

The physiotherapy management of patients with stable angina is described in Chapter 14.

Outcome measures

These may include assessment of pain and function obtained via subjective questioning and objectively using a VAS or other pain scale. The dose and frequency of analgesics or anti-inflammatory medications required by the patient should be recorded. Outcome measures for evaluating the effects of physiotherapy for the patient with angina are given in Chapter 14.

PROBLEM – MUSCULOSKELETAL DYSFUNCTION

Chest wall stiffness and abnormal posture are commonly seen in patients with neuromuscular disease or chronic lung disease especially when this is associated with lung hyperinflation. Also at risk are patients following sternotomy or thoracotomy and patients who receive prolonged mechanical ventilation. Changes in muscle length, strength and endurance will occur as a result of chest wall and postural abnormalities. Further, in the elderly, there are age-related changes affecting the musculoskeletal system. With increased age, there is a decrease in the range of movement of the costovertebral joints and a decrease in the elasticity of the cartilage in the thoracic spine. These changes increase thoracic kyphosis.

Patients with severe chronic lung disease who adopt the forward-lean position to relieve breathlessness may develop a stiff, kyphotic thoracic spine and abnormal posture of the neck. This in turn will limit the range of movement possible in the cervical and thoracic spine and shoulder girdle.

Neuromuscular disorders lead to progressive muscle weakening, which in turn may cause postural abnormalities, for example, scoliosis or kyphoscolio-

sis, further limiting chest wall muscle strength and mobility.

Clinical features

The patient may present with an abnormal posture, reduced range of movement of the cervical spine, thoracic spine and glenohumeral joint and may report pain or stiffness resulting in decreased function. The assessment of pain, associated functional limitation, posture, muscle length, strength and endurance and joint range of movement are covered elsewhere (Chapter 5).

Physiotherapy management

Physiotherapy management should include, where appropriate, postural correction, stretching techniques (for example, hold-relax), of tight muscles, mobilizations to the cervical spine and thoracic spine, costotransverse, costochondral and sternochondral joints, to the ribs and to the glenohumeral joint (Bray et al 1995, Vibekk 1991) and muscle strengthening exercises. Postural correction and stretches to improve chest wall mobility should be incorporated into other active exercises and ADL. Where possible, especially when chronic lung disease is present, patients should be taught to manage their own condition with clear instructions on appropriate stretches and exercises to carry out daily at home (Chapter 5).

The patient's position during treatment will need to be carefully selected as many patients will not be able to lie prone or supine due to dyspnoea and mobilizations will have to be performed in sitting or forward lean sitting.

Following a sternotomy or thoracotomy, advice should be given on postural correction and upper limb exercises (Chapter 12).

For patients with neuromuscular disorders, physiotherapy management is targeted to the underlying condition.

Clinical outcomes

Range of movement of the cervical spine, thoracic spine and glenohumeral joints can be measured before and following physiotherapy intervention. Muscle length and strength can also be measured where appropriate. Short-term changes in pain can be measured on a VAS. Longer-term changes can be measured with a generic QoL scale such as the Short Form–36 Health Survey (SF–36) (Ware & Gandek 1998).

References

Adams RJ, Ruffin RE, Smith BJ 2000 Validity of a modified version of the Marks Asthma Quality of Life Questionnaire. Journal of Asthma 37(2): 131–143

Ambrosino N, Scano G 2001 Measurement and treatment of dyspnoea. Respiratory Medicine 95: 539–547

American Diabetes Association 2004 Physical activity/exercise and diabetes. Diabetes Care 27: S58–S62

American Thoracic Society 1999 Dyspnea. Mechanisms, Assessment, and Management: A Consensus Statement. American Journal of Respiratory and Critical Care Medicine 159: 321–340 www.thoracic. org/sections/publications/statements/ pages/respiratory-disease-adults/ dyspnea1–20.html (Accessed 9 July 2007)

American Thoracic Society/American College of Chest Physicians 2003 ATS/ACCP statement on cardiopulmonary exercise testing. American Journal of Respiratory and Critical Care Medicine 167: 211–277. www.thoracic.org/sections/publications/ statements/pages/pfet/cardioexercise.html (Accessed 9 July 2007)

American Thoracic Society/European Respiratory Society 2002 ATS/ERS Statement on respiratory muscle testing. American Journal of Respiratory and Critical Care Medicine 166: 516–624 www.thoracic.org/sections/publications/ statements/pages/respiratory-disease- adults/respmuscle.html (Accessed 9 July 2007)

American Thoracic Society/European Respiratory Society Statement on Pulmonary Rehabilitation 2006 American Journal of Respiratory and Critical Care Medicine 173: 1390– 1413. www.thoracic.org/sections/ publications/statements/pages/ respiratory-disease-adults/atserspr0606. html www.thoracic.org/sections/ publications/statements/pages/ respiratory-disease-adults/respmuscle. html

Barker AF 2002 Bronchiectasis. New England Journal of Medicine 346(18): 1383–1393

Borg GAV 1982 Psychophysical basis of perceived exertion. Medicine and Science in Sports and Exercise 14: 377–381

Bray CE, Partridge JE, Banks SK 1995 Thoracic mobilisation in the management of respiratory and cardiac patients. Proceedings of the Australian Physiotherapy Association Cardiothoracic Special Group, 4th National Conference, 22–24 April, Melbourne

Celli BR 1994 Physical reconditioning of patients with respiratory diseases: legs, arms, and breathing retraining. Respiratory Care 39(5): 481–495

Clarke S 1990 Physical defences. In: Brewis RAL, Gibson GJ, Geddes DM (eds) Respiratory medicine. Baillière Tindall, London, pp 176–189

Conway JH, Fleming JS, Perring S et al 1992 Humidification as an adjunct to chest physiotherapy in aiding tracheo-bronchial clearance in patients with bronchiectasis. Respiratory Medicine 86(2): 109–114

Cooper CB 2004 Respiratory failure. Medicine 32(1): 95–98

Elkins M, Robinson M, Rose BR et al 2006. A controlled trial of long-term hypertonic saline in patients with cystic fibrosis. New England Journal of Medicine 354(3): 229–240

Ferguson GT 2006 Why does the lung hyperinflate? Proceedings of the American Thoracic Society 3: 176–179

Gardner WN 1996 The pathophysiology of hyperventilation disorders. Chest 109: 515–534

Gardner WN 2003 Hyperventilation: a practical guide. Medicine 31(11): 7–8

Geddes EL, Reid WD, Crowe J et al 2005 Inspiratory muscle training in adults with chronic obstructive pulmonary disease: a systematic review. Respiratory Medicine 99:1440–1458

Gibson PG, Powell H, Coughlan J et al 2002 Self-management education and regular practitioner review for adults with asthma. Cochrane Database of Systematic Reviews Issue 3. Art. No.: CD001117. DOI: 10.1002/14651858. CD001117. Aug 2006

Gosker HR, Lencer NHM, Franssem FME et al 2003 Striking similarities in systemic factors contributing to decreased exercise capacity in patients with severe chronic heart failure or COPD. Chest 123: 1416–1424

Gosselink R 2004 Breathing techniques in patients with chronic obstructive pulmonary disease. Chronic Respiratory Disease 1: 163–167

Guyatt GH, Berman LB, Townsend M et al 1987 A measure of quality of life for clinical trials. Thorax 42: 773–778

Hadeli KO, Siegel EM, Sherrill DL et al 2001 Predictors of oxygen desaturation during submaximal exercise in 8,000 patients. Chest 120: 88–92

Haslet C, Chilvers ER, Corris PA 2002 Respiratory Disease. In: Haslet C, Chilvers ER, Boon NA et al (eds) Davidson's principles and practice of medicine. Churchill Livingstone, Edinburgh, ch 13

Hill K, Jenkins SC, Hillman DR et al 2004 Dyspnoea in COPD: can

inspiratory muscle training help? Australian Journal of Physiotherapy 50: 169–180

Hill K, Jenkins SC, Philippe D et al 2006 High-intensity inspiratory muscle training in chronic obstructive pulmonary disease. European Respiratory Journal 27: 1119–1128

Holland AE, Button BM 2006 Is there a role for airway clearance techniques in chronic obstructive pulmonary disease? Chronic Respiratory Disease 3: 83–91

Holloway E, Ram FSF 2004 Breathing exercises for asthma. Cochrane Database of Systematic Reviews Issue 1. Art. No.: CD001277. DOI: 10.1002/14651858.CD001277. pub2. Aug 2006

Horiuchi K, Jordan D, Cohen D et al 1997 Insights into the increased oxygen demand during chest physiotherapy. Critical Care Medicine 25(8): 1347–1351

Houtmeyers E, Gosselink R, Gayan-Ramirez G et al 1999a Regulation of mucociliary clearance in health and disease. European Respiratory Journal 13: 1177–1188

Houtmeyers E, Gosselink R, Gayan-Ramirez G et al 1999b Effects of drugs on mucus clearance. European Respiratory Journal 14: 452–467.

Irwin RS, Widdicombe J 2000 Cough. In: Murray J F, Nadel JA (eds) Textbook of respiratory medicine, vol 1, 3rd edn. WB Saunders, Philadelphia, ch 21

Jenkins SC, Soutar SA, Moxham J 1988 The effects of posture on lung volumes in normal subjects and in patients pre- and post-coronary artery surgery. Physiotherapy 74(10): 492–496

Jones AP, Rowe BH 1998 Bronchopulmonary hygiene physical therapy for chronic obstructive pulmonary disease and bronchiectasis. Cochrane Database of Systematic Reviews Issue 4. Art. No.: CD000045. DOI: 10.1002/14651858. CD000045. Jul 2006

Jones AP, Wallis CE, Kearney CE 2003 Recombinant human deoxyribonuclease for cystic fibrosis. Cochrane Database of Systematic Reviews Issue 3. Art. No.: CD001127. DOI: 10.1002/14651858.CD001127. Jul 2006

Jones PW, Quirk FH, Baveystock CM et al 1992 A self-complete measure of health status for chronic airflow limitation. The St. George's Respiratory Questionnaire. American Review of Respiratory Disease 145: 1321–1327

Juniper EF, Guyatt GH, Ferrie PJ et al 1993 Measuring quality of life in

6

6

asthma. American Review of Respiratory Disease 147: 832–838

Juniper EF, Guyatt GH, Cox FM et al 1999a Development and validation of the Mini Asthma Quality of Life Questionnaire. European Respiratory Journal 14: 32–38

Juniper EF, O'Byrne PM, Gyatt GH et al 1999b Development and validation of a questionnaire to measure asthma control. European Respiratory Journal 14: 902–907

Lacasse Y, Brosseau L, Milne S et al 2006 Pulmonary rehabilitation for chronic obstructive pulmonary disease. Cochrane Database of Systematic Reviews Issue 4. Art. No.: CD003793. DOI: 10.1002/14651858.CD003793 pub. 2 15 Sept 2007

Leng GC, Fowler B, Ernst E 2001 Exercise for intermittent claudication. Cochrane Database of Systematic Reviews Issue 2. Art. No.: CD000990. DOI: 10.1002/14651858.CD000990 3 Aug 2006

Lotters F, van Tol B, Kwakkel G et al 2002 Effects of controlled inspiratory muscle training in patients with COPD: a meta-analysis. European Respiratory Journal 20: 570–578

Lumb AB 2005 Nunn's applied respiratory physiology, 6th edn. Elsevier Butterworth-Heinemann, Philadelphia

Marks GB, Dunn SM, Woolcock AJ 1993 An evaluation of an asthma quality of life questionnaire as a measure of change in adults with asthma. Journal of Clinical Epidemiology 46 (10): 1103–1111

Markwell S, Sapsford R 1995 Physiotherapy management of obstructed defaecation. Australian Journal of Physiotherapy 41(4): 279–283

McCarren B 1992 Dynamic pulmonary hyperinflation. Australian Journal of Physiotherapy 38(3): 175–179

Meek PM 2004 Measurement of dyspnea in chronic obstructive pulmonary disease. Chronic Respiratory Disease 1: 29–37

Mehta S, Hill NS 2001 State of the art: noninvasive ventilation. American Journal of Respiratory and Critical Care Medicine 163: 540–577

Morgan MDL 2006 Dysfunctional breathing in asthma: is it common, identifiable and correctable? Thorax 57(Suppl II): ii31–ii35

Moxham J 1999 Respiratory muscles. Medicine 126–129

Murray JF, Gebhart GF 2000 Chest pain. In: Murray JF, Nadel JA (eds) Textbook of respiratory medicine, vol 1, 3rd edn. WB Saunders, Philadelphia, ch 22

O'Neill S, McCarthy DS 1983 Postural relief of dyspnoea in severe chronic airflow limitation: relationship to respiratory muscle strength. Thorax 38: 595–600

Orfanos P, Ellis ER, Johnston C 1999 Effects of deep breathing exercises and ambulation on pattern of ventilation in post-operative patients. Australian Journal of Physiotherapy 45: 173–182

Paffenbarger R, Wing A, Hyde R et al 1983 Physical activity and incidence of hypertension in college alumni. American Journal of Epidemiology 117: 245–247

Phillipson EA 2005 Disorders of ventilation. In: Kasper DL, Braunwald E, Fauci AS et al (eds) Harrisons's principles of internal medicine, 16th edn. McGraw-Hill, New York, ch 246

Pina IL, Apstein CS, Balady GJ et al 2003 Exercise and heart failure. A statement from the American Heart Association Committee on exercise, rehabilitation, and prevention. Circulation 107: 1210–1225

Poulain M, Durand F, Palomba B et al 2003 6-minute walk testing is more sensitive than maximal incremental cycle testing for detecting oxygen desaturation in patients with COPD. Chest 123: 1401–1407

Probst VS, Troosters T, Coosemans I et al 2004 Mechanisms of improvement in exercise capacity using a rollator in patients with COPD. Chest 126: 1102–1107

Rees K, Taylor RS, Singh S et al 2004 Exercise based rehabilitation for heart failure. Cochrane Database of Systematic Reviews Issue 3. Art. No.: CD003331. DOI: 10.1002/14651858. CD00331. pub2 30 Jul 2006

Roca J, Rabinovich R 2005 Clinical exercise testing. European Respiratory Monograph 31: 146–165

Sandvik L, Erikssen J, Thaulow E et al 1993 Physical fitness as a predictor of mortality among healthy middle aged Norweigan men. New England Journal of Medicine 328: 533–537

Scano G, Stendardi L, Grazzini M 2005 Understanding dyspnoea by its language. European Respiratory Journal 25: 380–385

Schwartzstein RM, Parker MJ 2006 Respiratory physiology. A clinical approach. Lippincott Williams & Wilkins, Philadelphia

Smart N, Marwick TH 2004 Exercise training for patients with heart failure: a systematic review of factors that improve mortality and morbidity. American Journal of Medicine 116: 693–706

Solway S, Brooks D, Lau L et al 2002 The short-term effect of a rollator on functional exercise capacity among individuals with severe COPD. Chest 122: 56–65

Stiller K 2000 Physiotherapy in intensive care: towards an evidence-based practice. Chest 118: 1801–1813

Storms WW 1999 Exercise induced asthma: diagnosis and treatment for the recreational or elite athlete. Medicine and Science in Sports and Exercise 31(1)(Suppl): S33–S38

Storms WW 2005 Asthma associated with exercise. Immunology and Allergy Clinics of North America 25: 31–43

Thomas M, McKinley RK, Freeman E et al 2003 Breathing retraining for dysfunctional breathing in asthma: a randomised controlled trial. Thorax 58: 110–115

Thompson PD, Buchner D, Pina IL et al 2003 Exercise and physical activity in the prevention and treatment of atherosclerotic cardiovascular disease. Circulation 107: 3109–3116

Troosters T, Gosselink R, Decramer M 2005 Respiratory muscle assessment. European Respiratory Monograph 31: 51–71

Turner SE, Eastwood PE, Cecins NM et al 2004 Physiologic responses to incremental and self-paced exercise in COPD. A comparison of three tests. Chest 126: 766–773

van der Schans CP 1997 Forced expiratory manoeuvres to increase transport of bronchial mucus: a mechanistic approach. Monaldi Archives of Chest Disease 52(4): 367–370

van der Schans CP, Postma DS, Koeter GH et al 1999 Physiotherapy and bronchial mucus transport. European Respiratory Journal 13: 1477–1486

van der Schans C, Prasad A, Main E 2000 Chest physiotherapy compared to no chest physiotherapy for cystic fibrosis. Cochrane Database of Systematic Reviews Issue 2. Art. No.: CD001401. DOI: 10.1002/14651858. CD001401. Jul 2006

van't Hul A, Kwakkel G, Gosselink R 2002 The acute effects of noninvasive ventilatory support during exercise on exercise endurance and dyspnea in patients with chronic obstructive pulmonary disease. A systematic review. Journal of Cardiopulmonary Rehabilitation 22: 290–297

Vibekk P 1991 Chest mobilization and respiratory function. In: Pryor JA (eds) Respiratory care. Churchill Livingstone, Edinburgh, pp 103–119

Ware JE, Gandek B 1998 Overview of the SF–36 health survey and the international quality of life assessment (IQOL) project. Journal of Clinical Epidemiology 51(11): 903–912

Wark PAB, McDonald V, Jones AP 2005 Nebulised hypertonic saline for cystic fibrosis. Cochrane Database of Systematic Reviews, Issue 3. Art. No.:

CD001506. DOI: 10.1002/14651858. CD001506. pub2. Jul 2006

West JB 2003 Pulmonary pathophysiology – the essentials, 6th edn. Lippincott Williams & Wilkins, Baltimore

West JB 2005 Respiratory physiology: the essentials, 7th edn. Lippincott Williams and Wilkins, Philadelphia

White D, Stiller K, Roney F 2000 The prevalence and severity of symptoms of incontinence in adult cystic fibrosis patients. Physiotherapy Theory and Practice 16: 35–42

Wills P, Greenstone M 2006 Inhaled hyperosmolar agents for bronchiectasis. Cochrane Database of Systematic Reviews Issue 2. Art. No.: CD002996. DOI: 10.1002/14651858. CD002996.pub2. Jul 2006

Wong WP 1999 Use of body positioning in the mechanically ventilated patient with acute respiratory failure: application of Sackett's rules of evidence. Physiotherapy Theory and Practice 15: 25–41

Zafiropoulos B, Alison JA, McCarren B 2004 Physiological responses to the early mobilisation of the intubated, ventilated abdominal surgery patient. Australian Journal of Physiotherapy 50: 95–100

6

Chapter 7

Psychological aspects of care

Mandy Bryon, Elizabeth Steed

INTRODUCTION

In managing any physical health problem it is important to consider not only the biological mechanisms involved in the disease process but also the impact of that condition on the individual person, and the extent that the individual person influences the process of the illness. This broader approach to managing an illness is based on the biopsychosocial model (Engel 1980), which recognizes that an individual's psychological and social worlds are key influences on both the process and management of illness. An illustration of this is the patient with coronary heart disease whose behaviour of smoking, eating a high-fat diet and living a stressful lifestyle may contribute to both development and progression of the disease. This approach to health problems contrasts with the more traditional biomedical model which views illness management purely in terms of the biological mechanisms at work. This chapter therefore aims to discuss some of the key psychological and social issues pertinent to cardiac and respiratory conditions. In doing this an illness trajectory approach i.e. from diagnosis to death, is taken with issues specific to both paediatric and adult populations highlighted throughout.

GIVING A DIAGNOSIS

There is a great deal of anxiety among health care professionals at the prospect of holding a meeting with a patient or parents to give a medical diagnosis. The anxiety stems from anticipation of the reactions produced by the bad news. The prediction is that the recipients will display high levels of distress and the deliverer of the bad news will be the target of their emotions. It is important to remember that the meeting to disclose diagnosis has a very specific purpose and there is no need to ensure that all angles are covered at this first meeting. The patient and/or parents are unlikely to remember much about the content of the meeting and more about the manner in which the information was given (Brewin 1991, Bush 2001, Quine & Pahl 1986). There has been much written on how to deliver 'bad news' but it is important to remember that there are two key aims for the content of the disclosure meeting:

1. To clearly state the confirmed diagnosis.
2. To inform about immediate treatment plans.

Much of the information given will not be taken in initially; it can be given at follow-up meetings when the patient/parents are ready for it and when it is relevant to their own or child's needs.

Impact of diagnosis in childhood

Diagnoses of cardiorespiratory conditions made within the first few months of life have a particular impact as they come at a time when parents are feeling intense emotions towards their newborn infant, and they are asked to assimilate the information that their baby has a potentially life-limiting illness such as cystic fibrosis (CF) or heart problems. Parents who had been prepared for acquiring childrearing skills now must learn nursing and medical skills and incorporate a group of uninvited strangers comprising the medical team. Clearly, this time will be one of stress and sorrow for parents and a frequently asked question is: 'Does a diagnosis of a medical condition given early in the child's life carry with it a risk for damage to the parent–child bond?'

Simmons et al (1995) conducted a study to evaluate whether the mother–child bond was affected when the child has CF. They used Ainsworth et al's (1978) gold standard assessment of mother–child attachment, which examines the infant's behaviour following separation and reunion with mother, to compare a group of children with CF against healthy controls. Their findings revealed that the majority of infants (60.5%) demonstrated a secure attachment with mother, with some showing an insecure–avoidant pattern where the child shows little distress on separation and actively avoids the mother on reunion. A small number show insecure–resistant patterns where the child shows extreme distress on separation and then a mixture of contact and rejection on reunion, generally being very unsettled. There were no significant differences in rates of insecure attachments found from the healthy controls, but the implications are that those children with insecure attachments to a primary caregiver will be vulnerable at times of stress.

This suggests that the parent–child instinctive drives to form a bond are not affected by the diagnosis of CF and the same could be said to be true for other cardiorespiratory conditions. Concerns have been raised that the infant diagnosed with CF via newborn screening techniques may harm the mother–child attachment by disrupting the relationship with the disclosure of a life-threatening illness in an infant that had not displayed any symptoms of disease (Young et al 2001). Studies that have begun to examine that question have found no evidence to support this hypothesis (Boland & Thompson 1990). It has been reported, however, that mothers of children diagnosed by newborn screening have higher frequencies of 'at-risk' scores for parenting stress than mothers of traditionally diagnosed children (Baroni et al 1997) though these authors suggest that the significant variables influencing maternal well-being are the way in which the diagnosis is communicated and subsequent parental support.

Parents of children with a medical condition are at risk for over-protection of their children. A fear of infection can result in parents restricting the physical movements and toys of their young children. Attendance at playschools and nurseries may be denied; possibly even contact with other healthy children may be limited. Studies of the play interactions of parents of preschool children with CF indicate that mothers are much more interfering and less supportive of their children and the child correspondingly shows less persistence and compliance in play activities (Goldberg et al 1995). The child-rearing practices of parents of children with CF may be affected by the overwhelming need to protect the child. All daily interactions from dressing to feeding to bedtimes may be indirectly altered by the diagnosis.

Talking to children about their diagnosis

Originally, developmental theorists sensibly proposed that a child's understanding of illness would follow a stage approach mirroring the stages of intellectual development proposed by Piaget (1952). Bibace & Walsh (1980) proposed a six-stage approach from phenomenism at the first stage where the child believes that illness is spatially remote from the person who has the illness to the most advanced stage – termed psychophysiological – in which children recognize an interaction between physical and psychological health. As such, a child in the preschool years would be considered as capable only of concrete operations; i.e. their thought processes are tied to the immediately observable cause and effect relationships. Their understanding of illness arises from observed links: when unwell, see the doctor, who will give medicine that will make you better. There is no concept that the illness is physically within them. Clearly, within this theoretical framework

7

there is no room for a concept of illness *prevention*, which is the level of understanding required for an illness like CF; you are well but take this medicine to prevent you from being ill.

Anecdotal reports that young children with chronic illnesses have developed a precocious comprehension of their own condition and have a much more competent understanding of illness has led to a re-consideration of the applicability of the stage theory which appears too simplistic (Kalish 1996, Springer 1994, Springer & Ruckel 1992). For sick children a more comprehensive understanding of their medical condition comes about by virtue of their frequent experience with hospital and illness (Eiser 1989). Studies have found that even young children can understand and operate the concept of contagion as originating from invisible sources and they can accept germs causing illness (Eiser 1989, Rosen & Rozin 1993) though they do not fully understand the causal processes (Soloman & Cassimatis 1999).

Children with chronic illness are capable of a more sophisticated understanding of their illness than previously thought. However, there is a barrier to effective communication with children. On interview about their condition, children with CF tend to give consistently similar responses to questions irrespective of age; they know that CF affects the respiratory (85%) and digestive (80%) systems, though don't know why or how and the majority don't know the importance of nutrition (70%) (Angst 1993). This suggests that they are repeating received information without assimilating true understanding. Children tend to hold a glossary of CF terms that is separate from how it affects them personally. Although they are quite capable of a decent knowledge of their own health and engage in patient–clinician discussions about treatment, the tendency is to avoid this. Children with CF define themselves as 'healthy' irrespective of actual health status and this phenomenon is also found in other chronic health conditions: asthma (Frey 1996) and heart disease (Veldtman et al 2001).

This dual comprehension of CF – a knowledge of the physical components of the disease but an unwillingness to apply them to the self – comes about in part from a parental desire to protect the child from the potentially distressing aspects of CF, what Bluebond-Langner (1991) terms a 'conspiracy of silence' and in part from the reluctance of CF health professionals to include the child in consultations. Parents are used by children as envoys and information brokers; they act as buffers from unpleasant information (Young et al 2003).

Impact of diagnosis in adulthood

Diagnosis in adulthood, although also often associated with emotional upset, can be different from a parent receiving diagnosis for their child. This is because the adult will often come to the consultation with thoughts and beliefs about the symptoms that have led to the diagnosis meeting. How the individual's thoughts match the information that is presented, may determine whether the diagnosis is received with acceptance, distress or in some situations relief.

Our knowledge of how patients think about their health has been influenced by a range of theories over the years (Ajzen 1985, Becker 1974, Leventhal et al 1984). Considerable research exploring patients' thoughts about physical health problems suggest that for any condition an individual will have a 'common sense' understanding about the condition, which has been termed an illness representation (Leventhal et al 1984). This is a set of beliefs that revolves around five key themes. These are:

- *Identity* – which describes the symptoms and label that the individual associates with an illness

- *Time-line* – which is related to how long the condition is thought to last for, i.e. whether it is acute, chronic or cyclical

- *Consequences* – which incorporates thoughts about how serious the condition is and the effect that it will have on the lives of both themselves and individuals close to them

- *Control* – including thoughts about the extent that they as an individual can control their illness and thoughts about whether treatment can control the illness

- *Cause* – beliefs relating to what the person attributes the cause of their condition.

These thoughts are a way for individuals to make sense of any symptoms they experience and will influence the behaviours that they conduct; they may be present even before diagnosis. For example, if an individual has chest pain and identifies it as due to indigestion, they may be unlikely to visit a doctor. However, if the pain was interpreted as a heart attack, a very different response might be expected. Such beliefs are important at all stages of illness from diagnosis to the end stages of a condition and are related to outcomes both physical and psychological. For example, the more chronic in nature the condition is perceived to be, the poorer the psychological reaction to the condition. In contrast if the individual perceives that the condition will be controllable or is caused by factors which may be amenable to change, e.g. by changing lifestyle factors such as diet or exercise, their reaction to the condition is generally more positive (Hagger & Orbell 2003, Moss-Morris et al 2002).

The development of such illness beliefs comes from a range of sources, including:

- general lay information about health, such as might be gained through the media or increasingly the internet
- information from the social environment, including authoritative advice such as from medical personnel
- knowledge of other individuals with similar symptoms
- personal experience which relates to the individual's own previous experience of such symptoms (Leventhal 1984).

The range of sources that feed illness beliefs may explain the variability in reaction to diagnosis of physical health problems and differences in management. Such beliefs must therefore be taken into account at all stages of managing physical illness.

One particularly difficult form of diagnosis in adulthood is that which would normally have been made during childhood, such as late diagnosis of CF. Widerman (2002) reports that CF patients diagnosed as adults can be left feeling confused as often there is uncertainty around diagnosis with perhaps multiple tests before diagnosis is confirmed. Emotional reactions that have been reported include anger, depression, fear and relief (Widerman 2002). For the health care professional working with adults diagnosed with CF over the age of 18, it is important to recognize the significant effect of such a diagnosis and to acknowledge that informational needs may be different from that of a patient diagnosed as a child. Providing time for questions and being alert to the meaning of this for both the patient and their plans for the future, e.g. reproductive health, will be important.

Post–diagnosis

Diagnosis of a chronic medical condition is only the beginning of a potentially long-term relationship between the patient, parents, doctor and a range of other health care professionals. Fundamental to the relationship is good communication and the building of a strong doctor–patient relationship. Unlike the outmoded traditional approach of paternalistic practice, nowadays the shift in the doctor–patient relationship is from prescription to collaboration (Bodenheimer et al 2002, Kuther 2003). Such a patient-centred approach sees the health care professional and patient as the meeting of two experts, the patient an expert on the impact of the illness on their individual lives and the doctor an expert on the clinical management of the condition. Evidence of the benefits of a collaborative or patient-centred approach is demonstrated on a range of outcomes including satisfaction, treatment adherence, quality of life and physical health outcomes (Michie et al 2003). Accurate understanding of one's own medical condition correlates with less distress, less confusion, improved relationships with the medical team, better adherence to medication and an improved emotional well-being (Rushforth 1999, Stewart 1995, Veldtman et al 2001).

Collaboration may be more straightforward with the adult patient than the child. How to involve the child in such a collaborative relationship is therefore often something the health care professional may need to guide the parents on. This process can be complex and requires ongoing support. Towle and Godolphin (1999) recommend the following guidelines:

- develop a collaboration with the parents for ongoing information-sharing with the child
- establish the parents' preferences for managing communication
- inform parents of the advantages of including the child as collaborator in their medical treatment
- ensure parents have accurate knowledge
- avoid jargon and technical explanations
- expect that information will be forgotten – ensure repetition at consultations
- when speaking to a child, ask them what they know about a subject first, and expand that knowledge using their own words.

Although targeted at involving children in care, these principles apply equally well when the patient is an adult.

One further aspect of post-diagnosis care is to recognize the social and emotional impact of the diagnosis. In some situations specific support programmes may be implicated. Sawyer and Glazner (2004) have evaluated such a support programme and suggest the essential components of a post-diagnosis support programme should include:

- prompt timing immediately after the diagnosis
- engagement of both parents (if involved)
- clear, comprehensive communication at all stages
- the opportunity for supervised skill development for treatments
- the expertise of the multidisciplinary medical team
- the provision of written material.

LIVING WITH CARDIORESPIRATORY ILLNESS

Following diagnosis with a cardiac or respiratory condition the adult patient, parent or child will be faced with a number of demands in managing their condition. The challenges inherent in living with a physical illness have been described by Holman & Lorig (2004) as:

- having to manage persistent symptoms without cure
- continuous medication use
- adapting to behavioural changes, e.g. diet/exercise
- undergoing changes to social and work circumstances
- managing emotional distress
- participating in decisions about medical treatment.

Given these significant effects, it is perhaps not surprising that individuals with cardiac or respiratory conditions typically experience reduced quality of life compared with individuals without health conditions (Ekici et al 2006, Garrido et al 2006, Simko & McGinnis 2003). A key objective in working with people with respiratory or cardiac conditions should therefore be helping to improve quality of life while managing these demands.

Behavioural demands

Adherence

Compared with 20 or more years ago, both adults and children diagnosed with cardiorespiratory disease are likely to have a far greater life expectancy. Children with conditions such as CF or congenital heart disease now often live into adulthood. However, maintaining relative health in cardiorespiratory illness is not necessarily straightforward and it is increasingly time-consuming. The main reasons for this improved survival are new surgical techniques and in medical respiratory conditions much more aggressive therapy for the chest (including prescription of daily oral and nebulized antibiotics and regular courses of intravenous antibiotics). In addition daily physiotherapy, exercise and adequate nutrition are often essential to maintain good health (Bilton et al 1992, Durie & Pencharz 1989, Valerius et al 1991, Webb & David 1994).

While these treatments offer greater life expectancy, poor adherence to treatment regimen is perhaps the best-documented area of difficulty in managing chronic cardiorespiratory health conditions no matter what age the patient (Geiss et al 1992, Hillyard 2001). Much focus has been placed on how well individuals follow the advice they are given by health professionals which has variously been termed compliance, adherence or concordance. Generally there is good evidence that in adults, like children, adherence is less than optimal. For example adherence to physiotherapy in CF on a daily basis has been reported to be only 29.5% (Myers & Horn 2006). Other studies (Abbott et al 1994, Conway et al 1996, Shepherd et al 1990) have reported adherence to oral antibiotics to be between 68–93% and exercise to be between 69–75%. Similar findings are found for adherence in other cardiac and respiratory conditions (Hersberger et al 2001). The level of poor adherence to CF treatment, especially with physiotherapy and diet, and to a lesser extent with nebulized therapy (Geiss et al 1992), indicates that patients are making decisions about treatment management based on factors other than purely clinician advice. Patients or parents may deliberately alter treatment regimens according to their own beliefs and personal quality of life assessment, which may not match the aims of treatment held by health professionals. Importantly there is little evidence to suggest that adherence is associated with either the seriousness of the condition or sociodemographic variables such as education levels (Abbott et al 1994, Myers & Horn 2006).

The prescribers of treatment must therefore accept that a degree of non-adherence will be normal. A traditional prescriptive approach will fail to uncover any incompatibility between medical criteria and the patients' criteria for treatment success. Recent recommendations have suggested that a more fruitful approach, in line with collaborative care, is to understand the patient's illness behaviours in terms of self-management (Bodenheimer et al 2002). This encompasses the idea that people manage their condition, including its treatments, in a social and emotional world, and good quality of life is achieved by balancing all of these aspects.

Although adult patients are encouraged to become active collaborators in treatment decision-making, adolescents are not often awarded the same status. A medical relationship with a teenager is more complicated than with an adult above the legal age for consent (Kuther 2003). There are cognitive differences between children and adults in their ability to actively consent to or refuse treatment and this underpins the legal directives.

Improving self-management

Given that individuals make decisions about the management of their illness based on their priorities within their broader day to day life, the role of the health care professional is to support the individual to make informed decisions and address the patient's identified priorities. Understanding a patient's or parent's treatment beliefs is key to this. Studies suggest that thoughts about the *necessity* of the medication or treatment and secondly *concerns* about the medication or treatment – e.g. worries about side effects – are particularly important in predicting adherence. In both asthma and cardiac conditions, patients' greater belief in necessity and lower concerns about medication have been shown to be related to greater adherence (Horne & Weinman 1999). Where concerns outweigh beliefs in necessity then adherence will be lower.

In addition, the meaning associated with treatment is important, particularly as an illness progresses and treatments become more demanding. For example, the requirement of an individual to use oxygen is often associated with an adverse reaction by the patient. Frequently this is less to do with the practicalities of oxygen use, but more significantly the representation of this as an indicator that health is deteriorating. At this point understanding what the treatment represents and aiding adjustment to deterioration in health may be an important factor in facilitating use of the treatment.

Another sort of belief that is associated with self-management is self-efficacy. This refers to the confidence an individual has in carrying out a behaviour (Bandura 1986). Self-efficacy can be developed through successful experience, through verbal persuasion such as from health care professionals or through seeing similar others carry out the behaviour. Generally the higher an individual's self-efficacy, the better the self-management behaviours (Zimmerman et al 1996) and the better the physical outcomes such as walking distances and perceptions of dyspnoea (Scherer & Schmieder 1997).

The implications of these findings for practice are that in working with patients or parents to improve self-management their beliefs about the behaviour including worries, concerns and self-efficacy must be elicited. This should supplement traditional approaches of general education and advice giving which, although important, are often insufficient for behaviour change (Kolbe et al 1996). Psychological interventions that target beliefs include cognitive behavioural interventions and recently attention has been given to the value of motivational interviewing as a cognitive behavioural strategy to improve adherence (Miller 1983, Miller & Rollnick 1991). Motivational interviewing is a person-centred intervention which views motivation as a fluctuating state which can be targeted through trained health care professionals facilitating individuals to understand and resolve their ambivalence about behaviour change. It also draws on the concept that individuals may vary in their readiness to change behaviour and has been shown to have use in a range of health care settings (Britt et al 2003).

For children and families, techniques such as a Behavioural Family Systems approach (Robin & Foster 1989) lends itself to this sort of problem as it combines the behavioural techniques of skills training with a systemic focus on structural problems in the family, such as weak parental coalitions and negative belief systems. The approach also allows for the alterations of prescribed treatment. The intervention has been evaluated for families with an adolescent with CF (Quittner et al 2000).

Behavioural challenges in childhood

Although the above issues apply to children and adolescents as well as adults, additional behavioural challenges can be seen in childhood as managing treatment demand is mixed with the normal challenges of raising a child. Levels of parental stress, as measured by the Parenting Stress Index (PSI) (Abidin 1986), have been found to positively correlate with reported child behaviour difficulties, as measured by the Child Behaviour Checklist (CBCL) (Achenbach 1992), but not to correlate with severity of illness, number of hospitalizations or time taken for treatment (Simmons et al 1993). The daily demands of childrearing become a major strain especially around 2 years of age when the child begins to assert autonomy. Oppositional behaviour around treatment can be a major difficulty. As observed at mealtimes, parents inadvertently attend to non-compliant behaviours, so increasing perceived behaviour problems and level of stress. When parents face daily challenges to their authority they lose confidence and become coerced into withdrawing their commands for compliance to any instruction whether or not connected with delivering treatment (Patterson 1984). Behaviour therapy, such as behavioural contracting, parent management training and modelling, has been found to be empirically supported as an effective intervention for use with children and parents (Weisz et al 1995). Parent management training, in particular, is advantageous for the medical team as it can be standardized and implemented from a manual by non-psychologists (Kendall & Chambless 1998, Kendall et al 1998).

Managing well siblings

Although parents are expected to administer their child's medical treatment, this can be time-consuming, disruptive to the family routine and cause parent–child conflict. The parents' reaction to illness can greatly affect all children in the family (Bluebond-Langner 1996). In many cases the administration of medical treatment is incorporated into the daily routine without great difficulty and there is little differentiation between the sick child and other healthy siblings. In some families, however, this is not achieved. It has been documented that mothers differentially respond to their well children and those with CF (Quittner & Opipari 1994). The

7

well child may well feel bereft of maternal attention and young children will be unable to rationalize this difference. Well siblings may discover behaviours that guarantee a response from parents as a means of correcting the perceived deficit. Generally, these behaviours will be negative (Dunn & Munn 1986).

Risk factors for the development of poor sibling relationships have been identified (Foster et al 1998):

- the differential responding of parents between well children and those who are unwell
- the exclusion of the well child from information about the illness
- limitations of family activity without due explanation
- poor communication about the medical condition with all family members.

Parents can be informed of these potential risks and assessment of well sibling behaviours can be incorporated into a clinic review.

Social and work demands

Social and peer relationships

Although for the health care professional helping patients follow treatments may be a key priority, for the child or adult this treatment must occur within their social world. Qualitative research indicates that one of the most pervasive emotional difficulties facing the school age child with a chronic medical condition is a feeling of difference compared with peers (Angst 2001, Christian & D'Auria 1997). Children will go to great lengths to minimize observable differences between themselves and their peers, and this puts them at risk from failing to conduct necessary treatments.

Strong peer relationships (with children without a medical condition) have been found to be a protective factor from social competence problems (Eiser 1993). For all children, peer relationships provide the arena for the development of social skills and a positive self-concept (Hartup 1983). Children with CF tend to avoid discussion of their illness with peers unless forced and this may restrict the opportunity to have their diagnosis accepted by friends (Zeltzer et al 1980). Again this is a question of managing the balance between accepting the imposition of a chronic illness while trying to make life as normal and routine as possible. School age children can be helped to include their friends in knowledge about their condition and this is more likely to sustain and strengthen a relationship than, as is often feared, result in rejection. Friends can help the school age child with CF to incorporate CF into their self-image and learn to live with a chronic illness (Christian & D'Auria 1997). The importance of school attendance is obvious

and the multidisciplinary team needs to enquire about absence rates and ensure that parents are promoting school attendance.

In adults again social relationships are key, and there is now considerable evidence to suggest that an individual's social context and particularly the support the patient or parent receives from their social network can significantly affect adjustment to chronic illness (McNally & Newman 1999). In general the important factor is not necessarily how large the social network is, but how satisfied the individual is with their relationships (DiMatteo 2004). This may reflect the fact that although a social network may be present, if interactions are negative or unhelpful then support will not be received from the network, for example conflict within a relationship has been shown to be associated with poorer health outcomes (Smith & Ruiz 2002).

The illness itself can also put considerable strain on relationships or act as barriers to developing relationships. For example, adult patients with CF may have worries about entering into friendships or sexual relationships because of concern that others may not be able to cope with their illness. The possibility of not being able to have children may also be of concern within a relationship. Evidence suggests however that although rates of marriage may be lower than in individuals without CF it is still common with up to 45% of adults reported to be, or have been, married (Yankaskas & Fernald 1999). Again a difficulty that can arise for adults, as with children, is when patients avoid telling friends and family about their condition. Although this may be manageable at early stages of an illness, as health deteriorates and treatment requirements increase, this can become increasingly difficult. Interventions targeted at communication and relationship issues can be helpful although an individual's autonomy in making such decisions must also be respected. Interventions directed at family members have also been shown to be useful (Martire et al 2004). These may be focused either directly at the needs of the family member or at helping family members provide support to the patient.

Employment

Living with a cardiac or respiratory condition can also have significant implications for employment. As illness progresses the individual may become too physically unwell to work full-time and may need to work fewer hours, change their line of work or ultimately give up work. The implications of this can be both financial and social. From a financial perspective loss of earnings can place significant burden on a family. Although welfare benefits are available, these may not equate with previous earnings. In addition some individuals may associate the receipt of benefits with stigma. Helping individuals overcome the psychological barrier to receiving benefits is important to help individuals maintain as good a quality of life as possible.

Role changes

In understanding the social impact of illness it is important to understand the concept of roles and the changes that can occur when diagnosed with a cardiac or respiratory condition, or when illness deteriorates. Most individuals will fulfil a number of roles at any point in their life, e.g. as parent, child, carer, financial provider. When diagnosed with a physical illness or as an illness progresses, these roles can be challenged due to the physical limitations the illness exerts. For example, adults who worked to provide an income for their family may feel they have lost their role of provider if they have to give up work. Similarly the individual who cared for the family but then – due to illness – requires care, may find this reversal of role difficult. Changes in roles can lead individuals to feel their identity has been challenged and can result in negative emotions if not managed well. It is therefore important to understand the different roles that are challenged by the individual's illness and work with patients to both accept the loss and to help identify new roles that may be undertaken. In addition, helping individuals to see that some roles remain the same regardless of illness, for example friend, partner, etc., can be important in retaining well-being.

Although role changes are often thought of in terms of those undergone by the patient, significant role changes may also be experienced by those close to the patient. For example, the partner or spouse of an ill individual may have to take up employment to support the family or conversely may feel they are unquestioningly forced into a caring role. Although for many people this is done without resentment, in some instances it may cause difficulties and it is important that these individuals are provided with sufficient support.

EMOTIONAL IMPACT OF A MEDICAL ILLNESS

Given the areas of life that can be affected by illness, it is perhaps not surprising that cardiac and respiratory conditions have an impact on psychological well-being in both adults and children. These effects can lead to either general stress and difficulty coping or more formal diagnoses of anxiety or depression.

Stress and coping

The term coping has often been used to refer to how well individuals manage both the physical and emotional impact of their health condition. Theoretical approaches to stress and coping such as that used by Lazarus and Folkman (1984) talk in terms of people making an assessment of the demands a situation presents (primary appraisal) and then the resources they have to meet these demands (secondary appraisal). Where demand outstrips resources, the situation is said to be perceived as stressful and actions are then needed to manage the situation. Coping refers to those actions taken to manage the stress. In cardiorespiratory illness people have many demands placed on them and hence it is not surprising people find the situation stressful. For example, parents of recently diagnosed children and preschoolers report higher levels of parenting stress and depressive symptoms than normal controls (Quittner et al 1992, Simmons et al 1993). Parent stress levels have been found to have a negative effect on the physical health of a child. Problems with family, friends, school and finances correlated with lower pulmonary function and lower height/weight indices over a 15-month prospective study (Finkelstein et al 1992).

In coping with the stress of illness people use a wide range of strategies. Table 7.1 shows a range of different strategies. The table has been split into two columns: active, problem-focused coping strategies versus more passive, avoidant coping strategies. Research in a range of cardiac and respiratory conditions tends to suggest that more problem-focused coping is associated with better psychological adjustment, while avoidant strategies are less helpful. For example, Abbott et al (2001) reported avoidant strategies to be associated with poorer adherence to physiotherapy and enzyme regimens; Barton et al (2003) report emotion-focused coping to be associated with poorer adherence, more hospital admissions and more frequent asthma attacks in patients with asthma; and Hesselink et al (2004) found emotional coping style to be associated with poorer health-related quality of life in both asthma and COPD. These studies must be treated with caution, however, as the

7

Table 7.1 Summary of different coping strategies	
Active/problem–focused coping	Passive/avoidant coping
Seeking information	Withdrawal
Problem solving	Wishful thinking
Cognitive reinterpretation	Avoidance
Seeking emotional support	Denial

usefulness of a coping strategy will very often be dependent on the particular situation.

One particular coping strategy that has variously been described as both helpful and unhelpful is denial. Denial has been described as when an individual does not acknowledge the reality of a situation and acts as if the situation does not exist. Particularly in the field of cancer, denial has been said to help an individual maintain hope and provide time for adjustment to the reality of their situation (Morley 1997). However, others have argued that it can provide barriers to communication (Fallowfield et al 2002), can prevent uptake of beneficial treatments and can act as a barrier to acceptance of the health condition. In working with denial it is important to understand exactly what is behind this and the purpose it holds for the individual. Given the complexity of this it may often be most appropriate to refer to a specialist trained in this area, such as a psychologist. It should be pointed out as well that denial may be less frequent than typically believed by the health care professional and may actually reflect that the patient has simply not 'heard' or understood information that has been told to him about his condition. This may particularly be the case where individuals have been given bad news in a way that has not accounted for the time required to process this information.

If an individual is seen to be having difficulty coping it may be appropriate to refer him to a trained member of the team who can work on positive coping strategies. For example, individuals may be taught problem-solving techniques, can be taught how to manage emotions through exercises such as expressive writing, can be taught social skills and communication which facilitate increasing social support and may be aided in cognitive re-interpretation of symptoms.

Anxiety

Anxiety and panic are common in both respiratory and cardiac conditions, with prevalence typically higher than in individuals without physical health problems (Brenes 2003, Goodwin et al 2004, MacMahon & Lip 2002). The causal relationship between anxiety and particularly respiratory conditions is often not clear: for example, in some instances the experience of breathlessness may precipitate anxiety, whereas in other instances anxiety precipitates breathlessness. In asthma for example there is some evidence that anxiety may precipitate an attack (Lehrer 1998).

Correct diagnosis of anxiety is important for treatment. However, the similarity of the symptoms of anxiety, such as increased breathing and heart rate, sweating, etc., with physiological characteristics of disease can complicate this. In diagnosing anxiety it is

therefore important to also focus on the thoughts and feelings associated with anxiety such as feelings of nervousness or dread.

Although anxiety can be related to a range of factors in respiratory and cardiac conditions it is commonly precipitated by increased exertion and the fear that activity will cause breathlessness. If individuals fear that they cannot manage breathlessness they may then avoid activity, and this can engender a vicious cycle whereby through lack of activity the person becomes physically deconditioned and hence more easily breathless on exertion, which reinforces the sense of panic and anxiety (Fig. 7.1).

In managing anxiety a range of interventions may be useful. Explanation of the cycle of anxiety and reduced functioning can be beneficial as can education to help individuals differentiate symptoms due to anxiety versus those caused by their physical illness. Relaxation and distraction techniques exercises have also been shown to be effective in some respiratory conditions (Stetter & Kupper 2002). Attendance at cardiac or pulmonary rehabilitation programmes where individuals have the opportunity to build confidence in exercising can also be helpful. Further, work with individuals to elicit their worries or concerns are important. Where anxiety is chronic or interfering with daily functioning, it may be necessary to refer the individual for specialist psychological input where techniques such as cognitive behaviour therapy have been shown to be of benefit (NICE Guidance 2004).

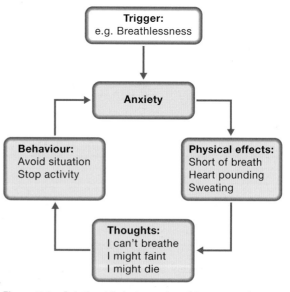

Figure 7.1   Relationship between breathlessness and anxiety.

Procedure–related distress

One area where anxiety commonly occurs is in relation to procedures. This is true for both adults and children. Treatments for procedure-related distress and phobia have developed over recent years. Initially attention was focused on hospital education programmes (Harbeck-Weber & McKee 1995), which typically provided information specifically on the procedures to be encountered using modelling, photographs or video. These programmes were found to be particularly effective for patients who had no previous experience of hospitals (Melamed 1992). Patients undergoing painful procedures, however, require more specific coping strategies to help reduce distress. The predominant treatment involves cognitive behaviour modification and there has been a high degree of consistency in the type of treatments used across medical specialties:

Deep breathing exercises (Jay et al 1985). These are aimed at helping the patient to actively learn mastery over pain and anxiety rather than becoming passive and submissive. Breathing exercises help the patient to divert attention from the procedure and to relax. The procedure is best taught using modelling along with an instruction to pretend to be, for example, a balloon – to slowly breathe in to fill the balloon, then slowly breathe out to make the air leak out again.

Distraction (Blount et al 1994). This is found to work best in the early, anticipatory phase and can be incorporated with the breathing exercise, for example using a party blower. Distraction techniques can be any number of items dependent on the patient's age and interest. Younger children can be distracted by moving objects and toys, older children and adults use counting forwards and backwards as a means of occupying the mind on an alternative activity.

Guided imagery (Lazarus and Abramovitz 1962). Patients are first asked about their favourite superhero, cartoon character, role model or film star. A story is then developed that includes the character using their powerful, special skills to help the child cope with the medical procedure. Older children and adults can produce their own fantasy image that is incompatible with pain, for example, a favourite place. The guided imagery is often used in conjunction with breathing exercises and is worked out before the procedure. The health professional or parent then prompts the patient to use their imagery during the procedure.

Filmed modelling (Jay et al 1985). A film is made of a patient with the same medical condition (or in some cases a model) undergoing a painful procedure. The patient describes his/her thoughts and feelings and how they are using coping strategies to reduce their worries. The film includes the health professional guiding the patient through the procedures.

Reinforcement/incentive (Manne et al 1990). The patient rehearses the events of the procedure beforehand, including the stages of the procedure, each coping strategy and how they might feel; they then undergo the procedure using their techniques of pain management. The patient receives an agreed reward at the end of the procedure, usually a trophy or certificate, though in the case of adults the satisfaction of undergoing the treatment successfully can be reward in itself.

Active coaching and positive self-statements (Powers et al 1993). This is particularly useful with children but can be adapted for adults. The child pretends to be the doctor and to implement the procedure on a doll. The child coaches the doll to use breathing exercise and distraction. At each stage positive coping statements are made as observations of the doll's progress. Parents are involved to describe and promote coping skills used by the doll. This process is conducted for several sessions before the actual procedure and parents are then used to help coach the child at the event.

Packages of cognitive behavioural interventions for pain management with children have been found to be superior to diazepam, watching cartoons prior to the procedure or general anaesthesia (Dalquist et al 1985, Jay et al 1987, Kazak et al 1996). The use of cognitive behavioural strategies is efficacious but time-consuming and impractical in a busy clinic setting. These therapeutic techniques need to be conducted outside the clinic to treat severe cases. Some of the simpler methods of distraction or a combination of distraction with pharmacologic approaches may be equally as good as a series of cognitive behaviour desensitization training sessions for some procedural anxiety (Cohen et al 1997).

Depression

Like anxiety, depression is common in individuals with chronic illness. In heart failure prevalence rates have been estimated to range from 13% to 77%, depending on how depression is assessed (Thomas et al 2003). However, if a major depressive episode is the criterion it is estimated that 20% of individuals hospitalized with heart failure will have depression. High prevalence rates are also common in respiratory conditions (Goodwin et al 2004). In a major study looking at long-term risk for depressive symptoms following diagnosis from a range of medical conditions, individuals diagnosed with respiratory and cardiac disease were at higher risk 2 years after initial diagnosis than those diagnosed with a number of other conditions including diabetes, hypertension, stroke or arthritis (Polsky et al 2005).

Depression has been shown to be associated with significantly poorer physical outcomes than in individuals without depression. For example, in patients with coronary heart disease depression is associated with poorer adherence (Gehi et al 2005), in heart disease with higher mortality (Murberg et al 1999) and reduced prognosis (Rozanski 1999), and in COPD with increased morbidity (Yohannes et al 2003).

Although detection of depression is essential for adequate management it is often underdetected, in part because physical symptoms of depression such as weight loss, loss of energy and disrupted sleep patterns overlap with symptoms caused by the illness. While moods may fluctuate with changes in health, and depression may be prevalent, this does not mean it should simply be considered normal or that it should be ignored (Rosenfeld et al 2005). Diagnosis can be aided by looking at the individual's thoughts. With depression these are typically negative with view to self, the world and the future. There may also be evidence of feelings of guilt, hopelessness and loss of interest in previously enjoyed activities, and withdrawal from social contexts and are all associated with depression. Unfortunately the physical limitations that cardiac and respiratory conditions place on individuals can trigger a vicious cycle of withdrawal from activity, negative evaluations of life, deepening depression and further withdrawal. Where depression is mild, rehabilitation programmes that incorporate mood and adjustment have been shown to reduce emotional distress and subsequent morbidity and mortality. This is true for both cardiac (Denollet & Brutsaert 2001) and pulmonary rehabilitation programmes (Alexopoulos et al 2006). Alternatively, if depression is more severe, referral to a psychologist may be beneficial. Work may then focus on recognizing the association between limitations from the illness and mood state, managing changes in activity levels, scheduling pleasurable events, addressing negative thoughts and focusing on coping strategies to aid adjustment to the current physical state. For individuals where depression is severe and a more cognitive approach is not appropriate, antidepressant medication may be beneficial although interaction with any current medications for the cardiac or respiratory condition should be taken into account.

Cognitive functioning

In managing an individual with cardiac or respiratory illness it is important to also consider cognitive functioning. Cardiac and respiratory conditions can themselves influence cognitive functioning through, for example, hypoxia, which is common in cardiac or respiratory disease (Bennett et al 2005). Cognitive functions that may be affected are attention, concentration, memory, academic progress, communication and decision-making. If concern over an individual's cognitive functioning is apparent, specialized assessment should be sought and with children, liaison with the local educational authority or communication with the school special needs coordinator. This is particularly important if an individual is to undergo procedures where informed consent must be obtained or where complex decisions such as whether to be placed on a transplant waiting list are being considered.

TRANSITIONAL CARE

One specific form of role change is that undergone by the adolescent in transition between being a dependent child and an independent adult. This is a particularly important period and its recognition within cardiorespiratory services is increasing. Well-established transitional care initiatives have come from CF services and these will be used as an example here. The issues identified within CF are directly applicable to a range of services where medical knowledge and expertise originates in the paediatric setting.

Adolescent issues

The adolescent stage of development is perhaps one of the most challenging for children and parents to negotiate; when the teenager also has a life-threatening chronic illness the potential for even greater problems is enormous. The most significant emotional development at this stage is to achieve complete autonomy from their parents as childrearers. There are similarities with the preschool years in that the parents must provide a secure base from which the adolescent can explore the world. Parents of healthy adolescents find this stage particularly challenging (Birch 1996) and those with adolescents with cardiac or respiratory conditions have larger battles to contend with. The cognitive developments that occur at this stage of childhood enable more abstract thought, facilitating analysis and synthesis of ideas and holding mature representations of the world (Piaget 1952). The adolescent is no longer an accepting recipient of the opinions of his elders, but will think for himself. This developmental process necessitates challenging and rejecting previously held beliefs as the adolescent becomes an adult. Of course, that first major target for rejection is the opinions of parents. It is an indication that the parents are providing a safe base if the adolescent can rebel. Many parents see this as a failure of their parenting, but it is quite the opposite (Wolman et al 1994).

Adolescents with chronic illness must undergo the same developmental tasks as their healthy peers: physical and sexual growth, personal individuation, intimate relationships, finding a comfortable social group, educational goals and preparation for an occupation. The medical progress and continued optimism for treatments for CF, in particular, mean that it is a different disease from that of a few years ago; the emotional and behavioural preparation of adolescents and young adults has not kept pace (Mullins et al 1994). There is a paucity of guidance for psychosocial support of adolescents with CF relative to that available for younger age groups (Drotar 1995).

Many adolescents with CF have delayed puberty and are smaller and thinner than their peers. Adequate nutrition becomes a greater problem and there is increasing evidence that adolescents are at greater risk than their healthy peers for developing eating disturbance (Shearer & Bryon 2004), a negative body image and poor self-esteem (Bywater 1981, Shearer & Bryon 2004). Concomitant with a delayed puberty are reported delays in developing a sexual identity and forming intimate relationships, especially in girls (Orr et al 1984, Sawyer et al 1995).

Adolescents with CF may find the process of separation and individuation more challenging than their healthy peers, as the parent–child relationships established following diagnosis tend to be overprotective and enmeshed (Goldberg et al 1995, Matas et al 1978). Parents of adolescents with CF may be more restrictive of their adolescent's social independence than they would be otherwise. Consequently, adolescents with CF may be less well prepared for independent adult life than their healthy peers in terms of moving from home, seeking financial independence and managing their own health. The potential conflict between natural maturation and restriction imposed by parents and CF treatment could well spark a rebellion, the risk-taking behaviour that illustrates this stage of development (Jessor 1991).

A combination of a perceived unreceptive social group, parental overprotection, physical differences, demands of daily treatment and personality factors will affect adjustment during this stage of development. Studies of the prevalence of risk-taking behaviours in adolescents with chronic illness find, however, that they are less likely to engage in such behaviours than their healthy peers (Alderman et al 1995, Frey et al 1997) and more likely to engage in injury-prevention (Britto et al 1997). Adolescents with CF first attempt smoking, alcohol and sexual intercourse later than their age- and race-matched controls and are less likely to have unprotected sex (Britto et al 1997). In summary, adolescents

with cardiorespiratory conditions are not at greater risk for increased teenage rebellion than their healthy peers; perhaps the scrutiny of their parents and the medical teams, which often include a mental health professional, prevent this. It is clear though that they engage in the same sort of risk-taking behaviours as their peers and these behaviours may have great health risks, particularly smoking and unplanned pregnancy. Paediatric and adult medical teams must be equipped to discuss these potential health risks in confidence with their adolescent patients.

Implications for health care teams

Paediatric teams typically communicate via parents about the child patient; the philosophy of care is prescriptive, nurturing and protective. Adult health care systems focus contact on the patient with a philosophy that is collaborative and empowering. Expectations are for shared decision-making for treatment with all the implied independent responsibility (Rosen 1995). Clearly there is a need to bridge the gap between the paediatric system and the adult one. A process of transition needs to begin in the paediatric setting to prepare the adolescent with skills to negotiate the adult system and then to continue in the adult setting to facilitate gradual adaptation.

A simple administrative transfer of care from one doctor to another is an inadequate method for patients with a chronic illness who have received multidisciplinary care in the paediatric setting. A transitional method that emphasizes a guided educational and therapeutic process is required. Acceptance of the need for transition has not resulted in consistent development of services and there are wide variations in practice (Viner 1999).

Most paediatric CF teams will be aware of the developmental challenges that adolescents bring and their need for resources that are frequently unavailable within a paediatric setting (Sawyer et al 1997). Young people with CF have drives to leave home, learn to live with a partner, start an occupation, manage a home, find a congenial social group and assume civic responsibility, plan for a family and/or cope with infertility. It is essential for health care providers to have a working knowledge of the emotional impact that CF will have on the lifestyle and expectations of young people.

Barriers to effective transition

Although there is an acceptance that transitional programmes should be part of the paediatric service resulting in the eventual transfer of care to an adult setting, one of the most frequent barriers to transition comes from the paediatricians themselves, who refuse to hand over their adult patients. This may stem from a long-term attachment to the patient and family, a lack of confidence in the medical skills of the adult physician in adequately caring for the medical condition, or fears that numbers in the paediatric clinic will drastically reduce (Schidlow & Fiel 1990).

Parents and the adolescent patient may also hinder the transition process. Transition is a difficult process that can cause a great deal of stress; to leave trusted health professionals with whom strong relationships have been formed, and face the prospect of the potentially anxiety-provoking task of forming new relationships is quite aversive. Parents may fear that their child will receive inadequate care. Adolescents themselves may fear that the adult services take them one step closer to death. The adult service will undoubtedly have differences in delivery of care that may cause concern, particularly in advocating the withdrawal of parents from the medical consultations (Bryon & Madge 2001). Clearly, there is little incentive to make the change.

Models of transition

Policies of transition are developing, but as yet there is no consistency and most are constrained by local resources with little evidence on programme efficacy (Sawyer et al 1997). The first model is one where little or no transition occurs; either the patient continues to receive their care from the paediatrician or is simply transferred to an adult pulmonary/cardiac clinic rather than a specialist team. Such a model is inadvisable and may result in anxiety and poor medical management. An adult multidisciplinary team is essential to ensure the needs of the adult CF patient are met and the relationship between patient and health professional has a good start (Mahadeva et al 1998).

The second model currently in practice is the adolescent clinic. In this model, patients between 14 and 19 years attend a separate clinic from younger children. The focus is on more adolescent-type issues and the aim is for intermediate preparation before the final move to an adult clinic. Adolescent clinics are usually located at the same hospital as the paediatric clinic and run by the same staff. The clinics are organized differently, however, with facilitation of greater autonomy for the patient and confidentiality to discuss psychosocial issues (Viner 2001).

The third model is the transition clinic where care is provided concurrently by paediatricians and adult physicians for patients within the transition age range; this varies between centres but is generally over the age of 14 years. An example is where the adult team visits the paediatric clinic to see adolescents and families jointly with their corresponding health care professionals. The idea is that the adult team are introduced to patients and families before transfer of care occurs. The patient and family similarly gain knowledge of the adult team and assurance that treatment management will continue along the same lines (Webb et al 2001).

Transition is a 'rite of passage' for people with chronic cardiorespiratory conditions who must have access to developmentally appropriate care. Transition is a process that begins in the paediatric service and continues into the adult clinic. Transition policies must become an expected part of the paediatric and adult services (Blum et al 1993).

DEATH AND DYING

End stage of life

One of the final challenges for any individual with cardiac or respiratory disease is managing the terminal phase of illness and impending death. It has been theorized that when faced with the certain knowledge of one's end of life, the individual goes through a sequence of reactions (Kubler-Ross 1969). It is now known that this is not an exact series of steps, although many patients find the description of the feelings reassuring. These were described as:

- *Denial* – represented by a lack of acknowledgement of the prognosis

- *Anger* – this may be directed at a range of people or situations or may be turned inwards towards oneself and occurs once the reality of the situation begins to be accepted

- *Bargaining* – often with relation to God

- *Depression* – once bargaining is unsuccessful the patient is said to experience a period of sadness, sometimes to the level of depression

- *Acceptance* – this final stage is said to be where the person accepts the reality and can become at peace with the situation.

In working with people at the end stage of their lives it is important that the health care professional gives the patient, whether adult or child, the space to ask questions and also gives permission to discuss this stage of their illness (see von Gunten et al (2000) for discussion of communication techniques at end of life). In discussing dying with patients it is important to elicit specific fears the individual has; for example, these may be related to how they may die, whether they will experience pain or more existential issues. Only by identifying the individual's unique worries will appropriate intervention be possible.

A common challenge when working with people who are dying is when family members request that the patient is not told of what is happening. This request may be particularly common with relatives of child patients but can occur with adults as well. Evidence suggests, however, that individuals want information about their health status and that this can help both the patient and family avoid uncertainty, maximize control, bring order to chaos and make sense of the illness (Fallowfield et al 2002). In working with families who request the patient is not told it is important to help the family member understand the advantages of telling the patient, such as allowing open communication about worries and concerns, and the risks of not discussing information with the patient: for example, not providing an opportunity to say goodbye.

Bereavement

Bereavement is the process which an individual goes through when they experience the loss or death of someone they love; grief is the reaction associated with this and mourning the behavioural and emotional reactions to grief (Payne et al 2000). It is important that although bereavement and grief are common across cultures, the form that mourning takes may vary among cultures and differences in behaviour should be understood in terms of cultural norms.

In understanding bereavement, a number of theories and models have been put forward. Stage models similar to that described above by Kubler-Ross have been described; however, they suffer from the same limitations as previously discussed. Another well-known theory by Parkes (1988) has described bereavement as a psychosocial transition. This suggests that everybody has a set of assumptions of how the world and life should be. This is called an internal model or 'schema'. If something occurs which requires us to make changes to our assumptions about the world and these changes are going to be long term and occur over a relatively short period, then the individual is said to undergo a psychosocial transition. Bereavement is one such psychosocial transition, as individuals have to change a number of their assumptions about the other person being around and the subsequent implications. This

requires a period of adjustment and can be a painful process as is experienced in grief. Payne et al (2000) have described a range of reactions to bereavement such as:

- *Physical* – fatigue, disrupted sleeping, changes in appetite, muscular pains, nausea, increased colds and infections

- *Behavioural* – searching, restlessness, crying, social withdrawal, irritability

- *Cognitive* – poor concentration and memory, repetitive thoughts about the deceased, helplessness, hopelessness

- *Emotional* – depression, anxiety, anger, guilt, loneliness.

It is important to recognize that reactions vary among individuals and that there is no correct way to grieve. Explaining this to individuals may help take away anxiety that they are not responding appropriately. Providing the bereaved person with space to talk about his feelings will be helpful. In some instances where the bereaved person has feelings of anger or guilt these may come out as blame, particularly towards the health care professional. Understanding the basis of such expressions and using this to be able to listen and help the bereaved person work through his feelings can be a more helpful approach than taking any accusations to heart and being defensive.

CONCLUSION

The impact of living with a cardiothoracic illness, whether as a parent or a patient, has been outlined above. Theoretical models and research have expanded the knowledge base such that a thorough understanding of the psychological and emotional correlates of living with disease is obtained. Physical health status can be affected by the individual's emotional well-being, directly via anxiety or depressive reactions and indirectly in terms of coping styles and perceptions of health status. This chapter has aimed to outline the emotional and psychological components of cardiac and respiratory disease, to aid the multidisciplinary health professionals in their relationship with their patients.

References

Abbott J, Baumann U, Conway S et al 2001 Cross-cultural differences in health related quality of life in adolescents with cystic fibrosis. Disability and Rehabilitation 23: 837–844

Abbott J, Dodd M, Bilton D, Webb AK 1994 Treatment compliance in adults with cystic fibrosis. Thorax 49: 115–120

Abidin RR 1986 Parenting Stress Index Manual. Pediatric Psychology Press, Charlottesville, VA

Achenbach TM 1992 Manual for the Child Behaviour Checklist. University of Vermont, Burlington, VT

Ainsworth MDS, Blehar MC, Waters E, Wells S 1978 Patterns of attachment: a psychological study of the strange situation. Lawrence Eribaum, Hilsdael, NJ

Ajzen I 1985 From intentions to action: a theory of planned behavior. In Kuhl J, Beckman J (eds) Action control: from cognitions to behaviors. New York, Springer, pp 11–39

Alderman EM, Lauby JL, Coupey SM 1995 Problem behaviours in inner city adolescents with chronic illness. Journal of Developmental and Behavioral Pediatrics 16: 339–344

Alexopoulos GS, Sirey JA, Raue PJ et al 2006 Outcomes of depressed patients undergoing inpatient pulmonary rehabilitation. American Journal of Geriatric Psychiatry 14: 466

Angst DB 1993 The school age child with cystic fibrosis. Pediatric Pulmonology (Suppl 9): 104–105

Angst DB 2001 School-age children. In: Bluebond-Langner M, Lask B, Angst DB (eds) Psychosocial aspects of cystic fibrosis. Arnold, London, pp 125–138

Bandura A 1986 Social foundations of thought and action: a social cognitive theory. Prentice Hall, Englewood Cliffs, NJ

Baroni MA, Anderson YE, Mischler E 1997 Cystic fibrosis newborn screening: impact of early screening on parental stress. Pediatric Nursing 23: 143–151

Barton C, Clarke D, Sulaiman N, Abramson M 2003 Coping as a mediator of psychosocial impediments to optimal management and control of asthma. Respiratory Medicine 97: 747–761

Becker MH 1974 The health belief model and sick role behavior. Health Education Monographs 2: 409–419

Bennett SJ, Sauve MJ, Shaw RM 2005 A conceptual model of cognitive deficits in chronic heart failure. Journal of Nursing Scholarship 37: 222–228

Bibace R, Walsh ME 1980 Development of children's concept of illness. Pediatrics 66: 912–917

Bilton D, Dodd ME, Abbott J, Webb AK 1992 The benefits of exercise combined with physiotherapy in the treatment of adults with cystic fibrosis. Respiratory Medicine 86: 507–511

Birch DML 1996 Adolescent behaviour and health. Current Paediatrics 6: 80–83

Blount RL, Powers SW, Cotter MW, Swan S, Free K 1994 Making the system work: training pediatric oncology patients to cope and their parents to coach them during BMA/LP procedures. Behaviour Modification 18: 6–31

Bluebond-Langner M 1991 Living with cystic fibrosis: a family affair. In: Morgan J (ed) Young people and death. Charles Press, Philadelphia, pp 46–62

Bluebond-Langner M 1996 In the shadow of illness: parents and siblings of the chronically ill child. Princeton University Press, Princeton, NJ

Blum R, Garell D, Hogman C 1993 Transition from child-centred to adult health-care systems for adolescents with chronic conditions. A position paper for the Society for Adolescent Medicine. Journal of Adolescent Health 14: 570–576

Bodenheimer T, Lorig K, Holman H, Grumbach K 2002 Patient self-management of chronic disease in primary care. Journal of the American Medical Association 288(19): 2469–2475

Boland C, Thompson NL 1990 Effects of newborn screening of cystic fibrosis on reported maternal behaviour. Archives of Disease in Childhood 65: 1240–1244

Brenes GA 2003 Anxiety and chronic obstructive pulmonary disease: prevalence, impact, and treatment. Psychosomatic Medicine 65: 963–970

Brewin TB 1991 Three ways of giving bad news. Lancet 337: 1207–1209

Britt E, Hudson SM, Blampied NM 2003 Motivational interviewing in health settings: a review. Patient Education and Counselling 53: 147–155

Britto MT, Garrett JM, Dugliss MAJ, Daeschner Jr CW 1997 Risky behaviour in teens with cystic fibrosis or sickle cell disease: a multicenter study. Pediatrics 101: 250–256

Bryon M, Madge S 2001 Transition from paediatric to adult care: psychological principles. Journal Royal Society Medicine 94(Suppl): 5–7

Bush A 2001 Giving the diagnosis. In: Bluebond-Langner M, Lask B, Angst DB (eds) Psychosocial aspects of cystic fibrosis. Arnold, London, pp 97–109

Bywater EM 1981 Adolescents with cystic fibrosis: psychological adjustment. Archives of Disease in Childhood 56: 538–543

Christian BJ, D'Auria JP 1997 The child's eye: memories of growing up with cystic fibrosis. Journal of Pediatric Nursing 12: 3–12

Cohen LL, Blount RL, Panopoulos G 1997 Nurse coaching and cartoon distraction: an effective and practical intervention to reduce child, parent and nurse distress during immunizations. Journal of Pediatric Psychology 22: 355–370

Conway S, Pond MN, Hamnett T, Watson A 1996 Compliance with treatment in adult patients with cystic fibrosis. Thorax 51: 29–33

Dalquist LM, Gil KM, Armstrong FD, Ginsberg A, Jones B 1985 Behavioural

management of children's distress during chemotherapy. Journal of Behaviour Therapy and Experimental Psychiatry 16: 325–329

Denollet J, Brutsaert DL 2001 Reducing emotional distress improves prognosis in coronary heart disease: 9-year mortality in a clinical trial of rehabilitation. Circulation 104: 2018–2023

DiMatteo MR 2004 Social support and patient adherence to medical treatment: a meta-analysis. Health Psychology 2: 207–218

Drotar D 1995 Commentary: cystic fibrosis. Journal of Pediatric Psychology 20: 413–416

Dunn J, Munn P 1986 Siblings and the development of prosocial behaviour. International Journal of Behavioral Development 9: 265–284

Durie PR, Pencharz PB 1989 A rational approach to the nutritional care of patients with cystic fibrosis. Journal of the Royal Society of Medicine 82(Suppl): 11–20

Eiser C 1989 Children's understanding of illness: a critique of the 'stage' approach. Psychology and Health 3: 93–101

Eiser C 1993 Growing up with a chronic disease: the impact on children and their families. Jessica Kingsley, London

Ekici A, Ekici M, Kara T, Deles H, Kocyigit P 2006 Negative mood and quality of life in patients with asthma. Quality of Life Research 15(1): 49–56

Engel B 1980 The clinical application of the biopsychosocial model. American Journal of Psychiatry 137: 535–544

Fallowfield L, Jenkins V, Beveridge H 2002 Truth may hurt but deceit hurts more: communication in palliative care. Palliative Medicine 16: 297–303

Finkelstein S, Petzel J, Budd S, Kujawa S, Warwick WA 1992 Comparative study of physical and behavioral status in cystic fibrosis. Pediatric Pulmonology Suppl 8: 221

Foster CL, Bryon M, Eiser C 1998 Correlates of wellbeing in mothers of children and adolescents with cystic fibrosis. Child Care, Health and Development 24: 41–56

Frey M 1996 Behavioural correlates of health and illness in youths with chronic illness. Applied Nursing Research 9: 167–176

Frey M, Guthrie B, Loveland-Cherry C, Park PS, Foster C 1997 Risky behaviour and risk in adolescents with IDDM. Journal of Adolescent Health 20: 38–45

Garrido PC, Diez JM, Gutierrez JR et al 2006 Negative impact of chronic obstructive pulmonary disease on the health-related quality of life of patients: results of the EPIDEPOC study. Health and Quality of Life Outcomes 4: 31

Gehi A, Haas D, Pipkin S, Whooley MA 2005 Depression and medication adherence in outpatients with coronary heart disease: findings from the Heart and Soul study. Archives of Internal Medicine 165: 2508–2513

Geiss SK, Hobbs SA, Hammersley-Maercklein G, Kramer JC, Henley M 1992 Psychosocial factors related to perceived compliance with cystic fibrosis. Journal of Clinical Psychology 48: 99–103

Goldberg S, Gotowiec A, Simmons RJ 1995 Behaviour problems in chronically ill children. Journal of Development and Psychopathology 7: 267–282

Goodwin RD, Fergusson DM, Horwood CJ 2004 Asthma and depressive and anxiety disorders among young people in the community. Psychological Medicine 34: 1465–1474

Hagger MS, Orbell S 2003 A meta-analytic review of the common-sense model of illness representations. Psychology and Health 18(2): 141–184

Harbeck-Weber C, McKee D 1995 Prevention of emotional and behavioural distress in children experiencing hospitalization and chronic illness. In: Roberts MC (ed) Handbook of pediatric psychology, 2nd edn. Guilford Press, New York, pp 167–184

Hartup WW 1983 Peer relations. In: Mussen PH, Hetherington EM (eds) Handbook of child psychology, vol 4: socialization, personality and development: Wiley, New York, pp 103–196

Hersberger RE, Nauman DJ, Burgess D et al 2001 Prospective evaluation of an outpatient heart failure management program. Journal of Cardiac Failure 7: 64–74

Hesselink AE, Penninx BWJH, Schlosser MAG et al 2004 The role of coping resources and coping style in quality of life of patients with asthma and COPD. Quality of Life Research 13: 509–518

Hillyard S 2001 Genetically programmed to self-destruct. Lancet 358: 20

Holman H, Lorig K 2004 Patient self-management: a key to effectiveness and efficiency in care of chronic disease. Public Health Reports 119: 239–243

Horne R, Weinman J 1999 Patients' beliefs about prescribed medicines and their role in adherence to treatment in chronic physical illness.

Journal of Psychosomatic Research 47: 555–567

Jay SM, Elliott CH, Ozolins M, Olson RA, Pruitt SD 1985 Behavioural management of children's distress during painful medical procedures. Behaviour Research and Therapy 23: 513–520

Jay SM, Elliott CH, Katz E, Siegel SE 1987 Cognitive behavioural and pharmacologic interventions for children's distress during painful medical procedures. Journal of Consulting and Clinical Psychology 55: 860–865

Jessor R 1991 Risk behaviour in adolescence: a psychosocial framework for understanding and action. Journal of Adolescent Health 12: 597–605

Kalish C 1996 Causes and symptoms in preschoolers' concepts of illness. Child Development 67: 1646–1670

Kazak AE, Penati B, Boyer BA et al 1996 A randomized controlled prospective outcome study of a psychological and pharmacological intervention protocol for procedural distress in pediatric leukemia. Journal of Pediatric Psychology 21: 615–631

Kendall PC, Chambless DL 1998 Empirically supported psychological therapies. Journal of Consulting and Clinical Psychology 66: 3–167 (special edition)

Kendall PC, Chu B, Gifford A, Hayes C, Nauta M 1998 Breathing life into a manual: flexibility and creativity with manual-based treatments. Cognitive and Behavioral Practice 5: 177–198

Kolbe J, Vamos M, Fergusson W, Elkind G, Garrett J 1996 Differential influences on asthma self-management knowledge and self-management behavior in acute severe asthma. Chest 110: 1463–1468

Kubler-Ross E 1969 On death and dying. Tavistock/Routledge, London

Kuther T 2003 Medical decision-making and minors: issues of consent and assent. Adolescence 38: 343–351

Lazarus AA, Abramovitz A 1962 The use of emotive imagery in the treatment of children's phobias. Journal of Mental Science 108: 191–192

Lazarus RS, Folkman S 1984 Stress appraisal and coping. Springer, New York

Lehrer PM 1998 Emotionally triggered asthma: a review of research literature and some hypotheses for self-regulation. Applied Psychophysiology and Biofeedback. 23: 13–41

Leventhal H, Nerenz DR, Steele DF 1984 Ilness representations and coping with health threats. In: Baum A, Singer J (eds) A handbook of psychology and health. Erlbaum, Hillsdale, NJ, pp 19–252

MacMahon KMA, Lip GYH 2002 Psychological factors in heart failure: a review of the literature. Archives of Internal Medicine 162: 509–516

Mahadeva R, Webb AK, Westerbeek RC 1998 Clinical outcome in relation to care in centres specializing in cystic fibrosis: cross sectional study. British Medical Journal 316: 1771–1785

Manne SL, Redd WH, Jacobsen PB et al 1990 Behavioural intervention to reduce child and parent distress during venipuncture. Journal of Consulting and Clinical Psychology 58: 565–572

Martire LM, Lustig AP, Schulz R, Miller GE, Helgeson VS 2004 Is it beneficial to involve a family member? A meta-analysis of psychosocial interventions for chronic illness. Health Psychology 23: 599–611

Matas L, Arend RA, Sroufe LA 1978 Continuity and adaptation in the second year. The relationship between quality of attachment and later competence. Child Development 49: 549–56

McNally ST, Newman SP 1999 Objective and subjective conceptualizations of social support. Journal of Psychosomatic Research 46: 309–314

Melamed BG 1992 Family factors predicting children's reaction to anaesthesia induction. In: LaGreca MA, Siegel LJ, Wallender JL, Walker CE (eds) Stress and coping in child health. Guilford Press, New York, pp 140–156

Michie S, Miles J, Weinman J 2003 Patient-centredness in chronic illness: What is it and does it matter? Patient Education and Counselling 51: 197–206

Miller WR 1983 Motivational interviewing with problem drinkers. Behaviour and Psychotherapy 11: 147–172

Miller WR, Rollnick SR 1991 Motivational interviewing: preparing people to change behaviour. Guilford Press, New York

Morley C 1997 The use of denial by patients with cancer. Professional Nurse 12: 380–381

Moss-Morris R, Weinman J, Petrie KJ et al 2002 The revised illness perception questionnaire (IPQ-R). Psychology and Health 17(1): 1–16

Mullins LL, Pace TM, Keller J 1994 Cystic fibrosis: psychological issues. In: Olsen RA, Mullins LL, Gillman JB, Chaney JM (eds) The sourcebook

7

of pediatric psychology. Allyn and Bacon, Boston, pp 204–217

Murberg TA, Bru E, Svebak S, Tveteras R, Aarsland T 1999 Depressed mood and subjective symptoms as predictors of mortality in patients with congestive heart failure: a two year follow-up study. International Journal of Psychiatry and Medicine 29: 311–326

Myers LB, Horn SA 2006 Adherence to chest physiotherapy in adults with cystic fibrosis. Journal of Health Psychology 11(6): 915–926

NICE (National Collaborating Centre for Primary Care) 2004 Anxiety: management of anxiety (panic disorder, with or without agoraphobia & generalized anxiety disorder) in adults in primary, secondary & community care. National Institute for Clinical Excellence, London

Orr DP, Weller SC, Satterwaite B, Pless IB 1984 Psychosocial implications of chronic illness in adolescence. Journal of Pediatrics 104: 152–157

Parkes CM 1988 Bereavement as a psychosocial transition: processes of adaptation to change. Journal of Social Issues 44: 53–65

Patterson GR 1984 Siblings: fellow travellers in coercive family process. Advances in the Study of Aggression 1: 173–214

Payne S, Horn S, Relf M 2000 Loss and bereavement. Open University Press, Oxford

Piaget J 1952 The origins of intelligence in children. International Universities Press, New York

Polsky D, Doshi JA, Marcus S et al 2005 Long-term risk for depressive symptoms after a medical diagnosis. Archives of Internal Medicine 165: 1260–1266

Powers SW, Blount RL, Bachanas PJ, Cotter MW, Swan SC 1993 Helping preschool leukemia patients and their parents cope during injections. Journal of Pediatric Psychology 18: 681–695

Quine L, Pahl J 1986 First diagnosis of severe mental handicap: characteristics of unsatisfactory encounters between doctors and parents. Social Science and Medicine 22: 53–62

Quittner AL, DiGirolamo AM, Michel A, Eigen H 1992 Parental response to cystic fibrosis: a contextual analysis of the diagnostic phase. Journal of Pediatric Psychology 17: 683–704

Quittner AL, Drotar D, Iveres-Landis C et al 2000 Adherence to medical treatments in adolescents with cystic fibrosis: the development and evaluation of family-based

interventions. In: Drotar D (ed) Promoting adherence to medical treatment in chronic childhood illness. Earlbaum, Mahwah, NJ, pp 383–407

Quittner AL, Opipari LC 1994 Differential treatment of siblings; interview and diary analysis comparing two family contexts. Child Development 65: 800–814

Robin AL, Foster SL 1989 Negotiating parent adolescent conflict: a behavioural-family systems approach. Guilford, New York

Rosen AB, Rozin P 1993 Now you see it . . . now you don't: the preschool child's conception of invisible particles in the context of dissolving. Developmental Psychology 29: 300–311

Rosen DS 1995 Between two worlds: bridging the cultures of child health and adult medicine. Journal of Adolescent Health 17: 10–16

Rosenfeld B, Abbey J, Pessin H 2005 Depression and hopelessness near the end of life: assessment and treatment. In: Werth JL, Blevins D (eds) Psychosocial issues near the end of life: a resource for professional care providers. APA, Washington

Rozanski A 1999 Impact of psychological factors on the pathogenesis of cardiovascular disease and implications for therapy. Circulation 99: 2192–2217

Rushforth H 1999 Communicating with hospitalized children: review and application of research pertaining to children's understanding of health and illness. Journal of Child Psychology and Psychiatry 40: 683–691

Sawyer S, Blair S, Bowes G 1997 Chronic illness in adolescents: transfer or transition to adult services? Journal of Paediatrics and Child Health 33: 88–90

Sawyer SM, Glazner JA 2004 What follows neonatal screening? An evaluation of a residential education program for parents of infants with newly diagnosed cystic fibrosis. Pediatrics 114: 411–416

Sawyer SM, Rosier MJ, Phelan PD, Bowes G 1995 The self-image of adolescents with cystic fibrosis. Journal of Adolescent Health 16: 204–208

Scherer YK, Schmieder LE 1997 The effect of a pulmonary rehabilitation program on self-efficacy, perception of dyspnea, and physical endurance. Heart and Lung 26: 15–22

Schidlow D, Fiel S 1990 Life beyond pediatrics. Transition of chronically ill adolescents from pediatric to adult health care systems. Medical Clinics of North America 74: 1113–1120

Shearer JE, Bryon M 2004 The nature and prevalence of eating disorders and eating disturbance in adolescents with cystic fibrosis. Journal of the Royal Society of Medicine 97(Suppl): 36–42

Shepherd SL, Hover MF, Harwood IR et al 1990 A comparative study of the psychosocial assets of adults with cystic fibrosis and their healthy peers. Chest 97: 1310–1316

Simko LC, McGinnis KA 2003 Quality of life experienced by adults with congenital heart disease. AACN Clinical Issues 14: 42–53

Simmons RJ, Goldberg S, Washington J 1993 Parenting stress and chronic illness in children. Paper presentation. Society of Behavioural Pediatrics, Providence, Rhode Island

Simmons RJ, Goldberg S, Washington J, Fischer-Fay A, Maclusky I 1995 Nutrition and attachment in children with cystic fibrosis. Journal of Developmental and Behavioral Pediatrics 16: 183–186

Smith TW, Ruiz JM 2002 Psychosocial influences on the development and course of coronary heart disease: current status and implications for research and practice. Journal of Consulting and Clinical Psychology 70: 548–568

Soloman GAE, Cassimatis NL 1999 On facts and conceptual systems: young children's integration of their understanding of germs and contagion. Developmental Psychology 35: 113–126

Springer K 1994 Beliefs about causality among preschoolers with cancer: evidence against immanent justice. Journal of Pediatric Psychology 19: 91–101

Springer K, Ruckel J 1992 Early beliefs about the cause of illness. Cognitive Development 7: 429–443

Stetter F, Kupper S 2002 Autogenic training: a meta-analysis of outcome studies. Applied Psychophysiology and Biofeedback 27: 45–98

Stewart M 1995 Effective physician– patient communication and health outcomes: a review. Canadian Medical Association Journal 152: 1423–1433

Thomas SA, Friedmann E, Khatta M, Cook LK, Lippmann Lann A 2003 Depression in patients with heart failure: physiologic effects, incidence, and relation to mortality. AACN Clinical Issues 14: 3–12

Towle A, Godolphin W 1999 Framework for teaching and learning informed shared decision-making. British Medical Journal 319: 766–771

Valerius NH, Koch C, Hoiby N 1991 Prevention of chronic Pseudomonas aeruginosa colonization in cystic fibrosis by early treatment. Lancet 338: 725–726

Veldtman GR, Matley SL, Kendall L et al 2001 Illness understanding in children and adolescents with heart disease. Western Journal of Medicine 174: 171–174

Viner R 1999 Transition from paediatric to adult care: bridging the gaps or passing the buck? Archives of Disease in Childhood 81: 271–275

Viner R 2001 Barriers to good practice in transition from paediatric to adult care. Journal of the Royal Society of Medicine 94(Suppl): 2–4

von Gunten CF, Ferris FD, Emanuel LL 2000 Ensuring competency in end of life care: communication and relational skills. Journal of the American Medical Association 284: 3051–3057

Webb AK, David TJ 1994 Clinical management of children and adults with cystic fibrosis. British Medical Journal 308: 459–462

Webb AK, Jones AW, Dodd ME 2001 Transition from paediatric to adult care: problems that arise in the adult cystic fibrosis clinic. Journal of the Royal Society of Medicine 94(Suppl): 8–11

Weisz JR, Weiss B, Han SS, Granger DA, Morton T 1995 Effects of psychotherapy with children revisited: a meta-analysis of treatment outcome studies. Psychological Bulletin 117: 450–468

Widerman E 2002 Communicating a diagnosis of cystic fibrosis to an adult: what physicians need to know. Behavioral Medicine 28: 45–52

Wolman C, Resnick MD, Harris LJ, Blum RW 1994 Emotional wellbeing among adolescents with and without chronic conditions. Journal of Adolescent Health 15: 199–204

Yankaskas JR, Fernald GW 1999 Adult social issues. In: Yankaskas JR, Knowles MR (eds) Cystic fibrosis in adults. Lippincott-Raven, Philadelphia

Yohannes AM, Baldwin RC, Connolly MJ 2003 Prevalence of sub-threshold depression in elderly patients with chronic obstructive pulmonary disease. International Journal of Geriatric Psychiatry 18: 412–416

Young B, Dixon-Woods M, Windridge KC, Heney D 2003 Managing communication with young people who have a potentially life-threatening chronic illness: qualitative study of patients and parents. British Medical Journal 326: 305–314

Young SS, Kharrazi M, Pearl M, Cunningham G 2001 Cystic fibrosis screening in newborns: results from existing programs. Current Opinion in Pulmonary Medicine 7: 427–433

Zeltzer L, Kellerman J, Ellenberg L, Dash J, Rigler D 1980 Psychological effects of illness in adolescence, II: impact of illness in adolescents – crucial issues and coping styles. Journal of Pediatrics 97: 132–138

Zimmerman BW, Brown ST, Bowman JM 1996 A self-management program for chronic obstructive pulmonary disease: relationship to dyspnea and self-efficacy. Rehabilitation Nursing 21: 253–257

7

Chapter **8**

Intensive care for the critically ill adult

Alice YM Jones, George Ntoumenopoulos, Jennifer Paratz

INTRODUCTION

There remains a perception by some medical disciplines that physiotherapy patient management in the intensive care unit (ICU) is focused solely on the maintenance and improvement of a patient's cardiopulmonary status. However, the role of the physiotherapist also includes maintenance of musculoskeletal function, optimization of neurological status, and is extending to areas such as extubation/decannulation, ventilator weaning, troubleshooting mechanical ventilation problems and therapeutic fibre optic bronchoscopy (Jones 2001, Norrenberg & Vincent 2000) and involvement in 'patient at risk' and medical emergency teams.

Advances in technology and pharmacology have contributed to the increasing survival of patients from critical illness. Dowdy et al (2005) suggest that ICU survivors have a significantly lower quality of life, both before and after ICU stay, compared with the general population. The impact of post-ICU discharge rehabilitation on a patient's functional capacity and quality of life is as yet unclear.

Physiotherapists may have a role in enhancing functional reserve before patients are admitted to ICU (prehabilitation). This should enable patients to better withstand the stress of ICU procedures and inactivity (Topp et al 2002). It follows that the place of physiotherapy in the management of patients in the ICU comprises a three-segment continuum of care:

- prehabilitation/supportive care
- problem-based physiotherapy management during ICU admission
- post-discharge acute care/rehabilitation.

Irrespective of the evolving direction of the place of physiotherapy in ICU, optimization of the cardiorespiratory status of the patient remains a central objective. It is therefore essential that the physiotherapist has:

- a sound understanding of cardiopulmonary patho-physiology
- an understanding of the optimal means of monitoring and supporting major organ function (cardiac, pulmonary, renal)
- possesses high-quality communication, assessment and clinical reasoning skills
- can accurately identify patient problems
- can formulate a suitable hypothesis and treatment plan.

Physiotherapists should not only acquire competency in techniques necessary for treatment intervention but must also demonstrate the ability to manage complications that might arise as a consequence of their actions.

Furthermore, a greater understanding by the physiotherapist of the relationship between fluid titration, pharmacology and ventilatory management will not only provide the physiotherapist with an opportunity to optimize the quality of patient care but also should entail an extension of the physiotherapist's scope of practice, in liaison with a multidisciplinary team.

This chapter will discuss the optimal means of monitoring and supporting the major organ systems of the body and the implications for physiotherapy intervention. The second section of the chapter adopts a problem-based approach and will focus on the place of physiotherapy in the ICU.

MONITORING AND MECHANICAL SUPPORT

Mechanical ventilation

Mechanical ventilation is essential to maintain life for some patients and is often used for patients with respiratory failure (Box 8.1).

Full ventilatory support should maintain or improve alveolar ventilation (Pilbeam 1992) and reduce the work of breathing. Work of breathing is an important consideration during the provision of mechanical support and can be reduced with various types of inspiratory support. This may be achieved by supporting respiration in various modes such as control, assist-control, synchronized intermittent mandatory ventilation (SIMV) with or without pressure support and bilevel positive airway pressure ventilation (BiPAP). The ventilator pressure waveforms of some common modes of ventilatory support are illustrated in Figure 8.1.

Less conventional methods of ventilation have been introduced with the aim of limiting lung damage and preserving spontaneous breathing. These modes are:

Box 8.1 Types of respiratory failure

Type 1: Hypoxaemia without CO_2 retention
Common in conditions such as lung collapse/consolidation, asthma, pneumonia, pulmonary oedema and pulmonary embolism

Type 2: Hypoxaemia with CO_2 retention
Common in conditions such as chronic bronchitis, chest injuries, drug overdose, postoperative hypoxaemia and neuromuscular disease

Hypoxaemia = PaO_2 <60 mmHg with FiO_2 >0.5

Abbreviations: CO_2, carbon dioxide; PaO_2, partial pressure of oxygen in arterial blood; FiO_2, fractional inspired oxygen concentration

---

- Pressure control–inverse ratio ventilation (PC–IRV)
- Airway pressure release ventilation (APRV)
- Biphasic positive airway pressure (BiPAP) and bilevel ventilation
- High-frequency ventilation (oscillatory or jet or percussive ventilation).

The following descriptions are summarized from the review by Weavind & Wenker 2000.

Pressure control–inverse ratio ventilation (PC–IRV)

This mode of ventilation aims to maintain a constant pressure during ventilation. The physiological basis for adopting this mode of ventilation is that the 'prolonged' inspiration promotes alveolar expansion through alveolar recruitment. The inspiratory:expiratory (I:E) ratio is higher (e.g. 1:1 or 2:1) compared with the traditional 1:2; thus complete exhalation from the alveoli with slower time constants is prevented by the short expiratory time, expansion of the alveoli is maintained by auto-peep (generated by the longer inspiratory time). The combination of decelerating flow and maintenance of airway pressure over time results in the inflation of stiff (non-compliant) lung units with long time constants, for example, in patients with acute respiratory distress syndrome (ARDS). However, there have been no demonstrable benefits in terms of patient outcome using this mode.

Airway pressure release ventilation (APRV)

This mode of ventilation maintains continuous positive pressure in the airway (CPAP) with intermittent release of the pressure (essentially an inverse ratio

8

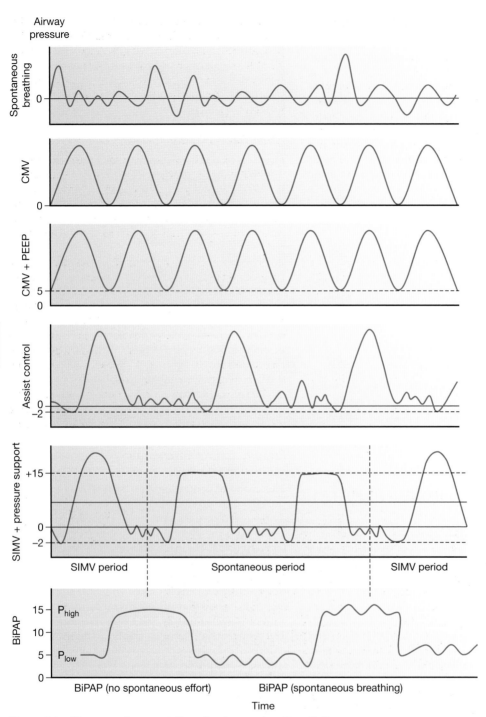

Figure 8.1 Diagrammatic presentation of various modes of ventilation.

form of bilevel ventilation). The duration of release is rather short, and similar to PC–IRV, and results in an inverse I:E ratio mode of ventilation. Patients who are able to breathe spontaneously with a relatively low work of breathing can utilize APRV, thereby minimiz-ing barotrauma and circulatory compromise. This mode of ventilation may not be suitable for patients with asthma or severe COPD because they tend to find difficulty in emptying their lungs during the short release.

Biphasic positive airway pressure (BiPAP) and bilevel ventilation

BiPAP is pressure-controlled ventilation with two levels of continuous positive airway pressure (CPAP) (P_{high} and P_{low}), with a set breathing rate. The I:E ratio can be adjusted. Bilevel ventilation is a combination of APRV and BiPAP. The mandatory breaths are pressure-controlled and the spontaneous breaths can be pressure supported (often only at P_{low}). Thus, bilevel ventilation can be used as pressure-controlled ventilation initially in sedated or paralysed patients, then weaned to CPAP and PS (to allow spontaneous breathing) and then to CPAP. Figure 8.2 shows the biphasic waveform on a monitor screen.

High-frequency ventilation

High-frequency ventilation can be jet ventilation or oscillation. In jet ventilation, a high pressure (30–300 kPa) of air with supplementary oxygen is delivered to the airway via a small-bore catheter at frequencies between 60 and 300 Hz. Expiration is passive. This form of ventilation is mainly used during surgery when the airway is disrupted or placement of a tracheal tube is not possible. High-frequency oscillatory ventilation (HFOV) (Fig. 8.3) is oscillation of a continuous distending pressure at rates of 100–1000/min with active inspiration and expiration. The advantage of high-frequency oscillatory ventilation is a stable continuous positive airway pressure, with control of ventilation at high breath rates and small tidal volumes (50–100 ml). The patient needs to be very heavily sedated and/or paralysed to minimize or prevent spontaneous respiration, often resulting in the cough reflex being abated. Humidification is often inadequate with this form of ventilatory support.

Other forms of ventilation and adjuncts

Liquid ventilation involves filling the lungs with a solution that dissolves oxygen. This form of ventilation is largely experimental at present. *Extracorporeal membrane oxygenation (ECMO)* and *extracorporeal CO_2 removal (ECCO$_2$R)* are other forms of non-conventional ventilation, often used when all other forms of ventilation have failed.

Inhaled *nitric oxide* can be used as a selective pulmonary vasodilator. It has been used for many decades for the management of severe arterial hypoxaemia and pulmonary hypertension in both adults and children. Recent guidelines (Germann et al 2005) recommend inhaled nitric oxide as useful rescue therapy for the management of severe pulmonary arterial hypertension and severe refractory arterial hypoxaemia, but do not confer any survival benefits in adults.

'Protective' and *'open lung'* ventilation are currently used for such conditions as acute lung injury and acute respiratory distress syndrome. This consists of using

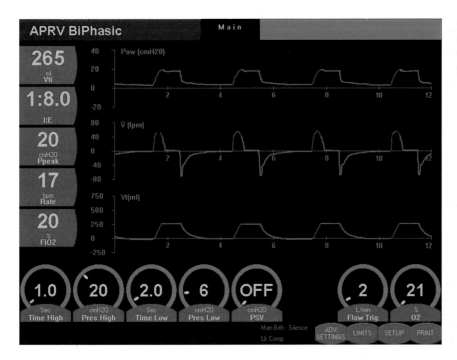

Figure 8.2 A monitor screen displaying the biphasic waveforms (pressure, flow and tidal volume).

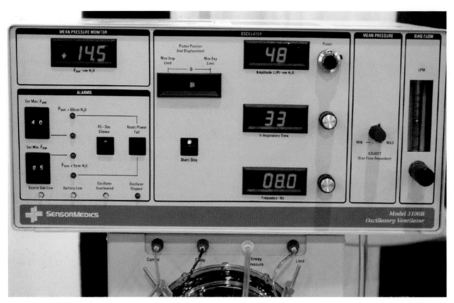

Figure 8.3 Frontal display of a 3100B (Sensor Medics) high-frequency oscillatory ventilator.

8

low tidal volumes (6–8 ml/kg), allowing the partial pressure of carbon dioxide in arterial blood ($PaCO_2$) to rise and ensuring the alveoli remain inflated with optimal positive end-expiratory pressure (PEEP) (Levitt & Matthay 2006). There is Level 1 evidence (Petrie et al 1995) for low tidal volumes causing a decrease in mortality (Petrucci & Iacovelli 2004).

Monitoring of the body systems

Rapid, potentially lethal physiological and pathological changes can occur in an acutely ill patient; hence the performance of the body must be adequately monitored and supported to optimize patient care. While monitors and equipment are essential for primary measurement and support, the interpretation of the data in concert with astute patient observation goes a long way to ensuring that patients will be safely and effectively cared for.

Monitoring of patients on mechanical ventilation

The primary aim of mechanical ventilation is to provide adequate gas exchange. Different forms of mechanical support have been explained above. Careful observation of the patient data and the pressure, flow and volume waveforms will assist the physiotherapist in identifying the level of synchrony between the patient and the mechanical ventilator, including any potential causes of increased work of breathing or changes in lung/thorax compliance or airway resistance in a mechanically ventilated patient.

Monitoring respiratory muscle function. Respiratory muscle weakness is often associated with prolonged mechanical ventilation and the cause of failure or delay in weaning. Diaphragmatic strength can be determined non-invasively in mechanically ventilated patients and can be assessed from the twitch gastric, twitch oesophageal and twitch transdiaphragmatic pressures in response to phrenic nerve stimulation (Mills et al 2001). Maximal static inspiratory and expiratory efforts, electromyography of respiratory muscles, respiratory rate, carbon dioxide (CO_2) level, pressure–time product, vital capacity and maximum voluntary ventilation are all variables which reflect respiratory muscle function. Respiratory rate and tidal volume presently remain the most convenient and frequently used indices of respiratory muscle function (e.g. respiratory rate/tidal volume provides a rapid shallow breathing index) (Spicer et al 1997). These measures may be used to assess the readiness of the patient to breathe spontaneously and to be weaned from ventilatory support.

Lung mechanics. Improvement in lung volume is associated with improvement in the elastic properties of the lung. The relationship between changes in lung volume and transpulmonary pressure is referred to as static lung compliance (l/cmH_2O). Static lung compliance should be measured during 'cessation of air flow', when elastic recoil is independent of airway resistance. Dynamic lung compliance can be measured during 'uninterrupted' respiration.

The change in lung volume and pressure are measured at end-inspiration (compliance) and end-expiration (auto-peep); this is when airflow 'momentarily' ceases during the 'normal' respiratory cycle. Most mechanical ventilators in ICU display/calculate dynamic lung compliance, auto-peep as well as airway resistance.

Assessment of work of breathing. A patient's work of breathing may be described as the amount of muscle activity required to overcome the elastic (lung tissue, chest wall and abdominal compartment) and resistive (airways, flow rate) elements of the respiratory system. It includes any additional loads imposed by the mode of ventilator support, artificial airways and humidification devices (which may contribute additional resistive work, particularly through a heat and moisture exchange filter as compared with a heated humidifier circuit). The work of breathing of the intubated and mechanically ventilated patient depends on factors that are either patient- or ventilator-related. Patient-related factors include the type of pulmonary disease (airway, lung parenchyma, pleural space), cardiovascular dysfunction, altered respiratory drive (fever, pain, anxiety, delirium, acid–base disturbance), level of spontaneous respiratory activity and level of sedation/paralysis. Ventilator-related issues include the mode of mechanical ventilation, settings and, most importantly, the level of synchrony between 'man and machine'.

To optimize mechanical ventilation, the mechanical ventilator must promptly respond to the patient's demand during inspiration and allow an unimpeded expiration. Mechanical ventilation practices vary internationally and hence patient management varies, depending on institutionally driven, airway and ventilator strategies (Esteban et al 2000).

Most modern mechanical ventilators display real-time ventilator waveforms such as pressure, flow and volume across time or as loops (pressure/volume, flow/volume). Waveform/loop monitoring allows the clinician to interpret the interaction between the patient and the mechanical ventilator. Early detection of untoward changes in waveforms may allow the clinician to optimize the ventilator settings (by altering PEEP, trigger sensitivity, pressure support) to minimize any disruption to delivered ventilation (tidal volume, minute volume) and reduce work of breathing during physiotherapy treatment. For adequate synchrony between the patient and the mechanical ventilator, the clinician must ensure that the ventilator responds promptly to the patient inspiratory demand (trigger), provides adequate flow requirements during the inspiratory phase, cycles from inspiration to expiration when the patient starts exhalation and allows full and complete exhalation,

before the next ventilator breath delivery. Detailed bedside waveform analysis of various patient work of breathing scenarios throughout the respiratory phases and suggestions for patient clinical management are illustrated later in this chapter.

Monitoring of the respiratory system

The definitive function of the respiratory system is to ensure adequate gas exchange. Respiratory function is best assessed by analysis of measures of oxygenation and ventilation, such as oxygen saturation and blood gases. An understanding of the mechanics of breathing is essential to determine the work of breathing required to achieve a certain level of gas exchange.

Monitoring oxygenation

Blood gases. Arterial blood gases (partial pressure of oxygen and carbon dioxide, and pH) provide essential information about a patient's metabolic as well as respiratory status. Continuous measurement of arterial blood gases is possible but this technique is not widely practised because of cost, calibration drift and clot formation (Shapiro et al 1993, Zimmerman & Dellinger 1993). Interpretation of arterial blood gases is discussed in Chapter 3.

Transcutaneous gas measurement. This method of measurement is based on the principle that blood flow and oxygen exchange are dependent on skin temperature (Baumburger & Goodfriend 1951). Transcutaneous electrodes include a heating element to maximize local blood flow. When the skin is heated the capillary blood becomes 'arterialized' and the arterialized gases diffuse through the skin to the electrodes (Whitehead et al 1980). More recently, a new sensor (TOSCA monitor) for combined continuous transcutaneous monitoring of arterial oxygen saturation and carbon dioxide tension has been shown to be an accurate and valuable tool for respiratory monitoring (Bernet-Buettiker et al 2005, Senn et al 2005). At present this is used more commonly in neonates.

Oximetry. Non-invasive assessment of oxygen saturation by a pulse oximeter (SpO_2) was introduced clinically in 1975 (Kendrick 2001). Pulse oximetry is now an expected monitoring component for assessment of hypoxaemia. The oxygen saturation of arterial blood [with partial pressure of oxygen (PO_2) of 100 mmHg or 12–13 kPa] is about 97.5% and that of mixed venous blood (with PO_2 of 40 mmHg or 5–5.5 kPa) is about 75% (West 2005). The absorption of light energy by blood varies, depending on the wavelength. Red (660 nm) and infrared (940 nm) light result in the greatest separation between deoxyhaemoglobin and oxyhaemoglobin absorption spectra. Pulse oximetry uses light-emitting diodes set at these wavelengths, and as the emitted light

8

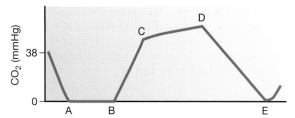

Figure 8.4 A typical capnograph showing normal end-tidal carbon dioxide level. **(A–B)** Dead space (CO_2-free gas); **(B–C)** mixed dead space and alveolar gas; **(C–D)** mostly alveolar gas; **(D)** end-tidal CO_2; **(D–E)** inhaled gas (CO_2-free gas).

Box 8.2   Normal values for blood pressure (BP)
Normal value of systolic/diastolic pressure
95/60–140/90 mmHg
Normal value of mean arterial pressure
Diastolic + [(Systolic − Diastolic)/3] = 70–90 mmHg

---

passes through the finger (or earlobe), the light energy is variably absorbed by the arterial and venous blood. The absorption ratio of the red/infrared light by the blood is proportional to the amount of desaturated haemoglobin, and from these data the pulse oximeter calculates and displays the SpO_2 (Kendrick 2001).

The accuracy of commercial pulse oximeters is about ±2% within the clinical oxygen saturation range of 70–100% (Jensen et al 1998). Pulse oximeter readings may be inaccurate in patients with severe or rapid desaturation, hypotension, hypothermia and low perfusion states. A further limitation of oximetry is that it provides information only on oxygen status, and not on ventilation ($PaCO_2$).

Monitoring carbon dioxide (capnography). The concentration of carbon dioxide expired during different phases of the respiratory cycle provides information on the effectiveness of alveolar ventilation (Fig. 8.4), not only the end-tidal carbon dioxide value but also tube position and breathing circuit integrity.

Detailed 'indications' for capnography can be found in the American Association for Respiratory Care (AARC) Clinical Practice Guidelines on Capnography/Capnometry during Mechanical Ventilation (AARC 1995).

Monitoring of the cardiovascular system

Non-invasive monitoring

Blood pressure. The use of automated non-invasive blood pressure (NIBP) devices is common. The mean arterial pressure (MAP) most closely approximates capillary perfusion pressure and is thus a useful measurement. NIBP devices can give inaccurate results in patients with arrhythmias, cardiac valvular lesions, where there is improper cuff application and when the blood pressure is low (Box 8.2).

Electrocardiogram. The electrocardiogram provides information on the rate and rhythm of the heart; it also assists in the diagnosis, and identification of the possible site of myocardial infarction. The pathological feature of myocardial infarction is necrosis of myocardial muscle. Absolute evidence of myocardial necrosis is the pathological Q wave. Q waves, ST elevation and T wave inversion are all associated with transmural infarction (involvement of whole thickness of the myocardium). For sub-endocardial infarction (involvement of the inner layer of the myocardium, adjacent to the endocardium), Q waves do not appear and changes are confined to ST segments and T waves. Thus subendocardial infarction may be difficult to differentiate from ischaemia of the myocardium. Interpretation of the electrocardiogram is discussed in Chapter 3.

Thoracic electrical bioimpedance and impedance cardiography. Thoracic electrical bioimpedance (TEB) relies on measurement of bidirectional blood flow within the aorta by a laser Doppler velocimeter and an impedance measurement unit which determines the cross-sectional area of the vessel. TEB allows the clinician to view beat-to-beat cardiac output. (Newman and Callister 1999, Tjin et al 2001) and provides information on haemodynamic indices such as systolic time interval, left cardiac work index and end diastolic index (Belott 1999, Weiss et al 1997).

Non-invasive measurement of stroke volume and cardiac output by impedance cardiography (ICG) has been shown to be accurate and significantly correlated to conventional thermodilution method (see Thermodilution cardiac output, below) (Scherhag et al 2005). ICG measures synchronized pulse changes in TEB via simple surface electrodes together with a conventional electrocardiogram.

Partial CO_2 rebreathing cardiac output and NICO. Rather than applying the oxygen Fick method for cardiac output monitoring, the non-invasive CO_2 Fick methods for estimation of cardiac output are receiving increased clinical interest. Adopting the CO_2 version of the Fick equation has the advantage that CO_2 elimination is easier to measure accurately compared with oxygen uptake (Jaffe 1999). The differential Fick partial rebreathing method computes a cardiac output value based on the changes in carbon dioxide elimination and end tidal CO_2 in response to a change in ventilation. The non-invasive cardiac output (NICO system) is the first commercially available cardiac output system making use of the principle of partial rebreathing of CO_2 (Jaffe 1999).

Echocardiography and Doppler. This uses ultrasound to examine the performance of the heart and great vessels. Information from echocardiography can be presented one- (M-mode), two- or three-dimensionally. M-mode is often used in conjunction with a two-dimensional echo to provide a clear illustration of the structures being investigated (Young & Sanderson 1997).

Doppler echocardiography uses ultrasound to measure blood flow velocity and is able to determine pressure gradients, stenotic valve areas, cardiac output, left ventricular contractility, and diastolic function.

Transoesophageal echocardiography can be considered an invasive technique as it involves the introduction of an ultrasound probe (attached to the end of a flexible endoscope) into the oesophagus. This technique avoids image obstructions caused by the lungs and ribs and allows better views of the valves, septa and thoracic aorta.

Urine output. Urine output is an index of renal perfusion and is a guide to adequacy of cardiac output. With normal renal perfusion, the urine output should be at least 0.5 ml/kg/hour.

Invasive monitoring

Arterial pressure. Intra-arterial measurement should normally be considered accurate, but the systolic pressure may be overestimated due to systolic 'overshoot' (a property of the fluid-pressure transducer monitoring system). The 'area' under the arterial tracing can provide a rough estimate of the cardiac output (Gomersall & Oh 1997).

Central venous pressure. Central venous pressure (CVP) reflects right ventricular filling and is usually monitored by a catheter inserted via the internal jugular or subclavian vein, and less frequently via the femoral vein. A quick way to confirm correct placement of the catheter is observed pressure change with respiration (Gomersall & Oh 1997). As the right ventricular preload is determined by the volume and not the pressure, the absolute value of CVP is less meaningful. A high CVP value, however, may be associated with conditions that cause a rise in the right atrial pressure (for example right heart failure, reduced right ventricular diastolic compliance, hypervolaemia and pulmonary hypertension) (Gray et al 2002), whereas a low CVP value may suggest hypovolaemia. Changes in CVP may provide useful guidance for fluid management in patients: for example, a minimal rise of CVP despite fluid loading may suggest the loading volume is insufficient; but a rise of CVP of more than 9.5 cmH$_2$O (7 mmHg) may indicate maximal

Box 8.3   Normal values for central venous pressure (CVP)
Normal CVP 3–15 cmH$_2$O (2.2–11 mmHg)

loading. A raised CVP in response to fluid loading is expected to return to its original value within 10 minutes – an indication that the risk of pulmonary oedema is only moderate (Gomersall & Oh 1997) (Box 8.3).

Pulmonary artery catheter (Swan–Ganz). Pulmonary artery catheters are often used in patients with impaired right or left ventricular function, pulmonary hypertension, septic shock and when measurements of cardiac output or mixed venous saturation are indicated. It can also be used to assist in the diagnosis of an intracardiac shunt, such as a ventricular septal defect. Apart from cardiac output, cardiac index and systemic vascular resistance, a pulmonary artery catheter can provide a measure of mean right atrial pressure, systolic and diastolic right ventricular pressure, systolic, diastolic and mean pulmonary artery pressure, and pulmonary artery occlusion pressure.

Pulmonary artery occlusion pressure (PAOP) (previously referred to as pulmonary capillary wedge pressure (PCWP)) provides an estimation of the left atrial pressure (LAP). PAOP is obtained with the balloon at the catheter tip wedged in a pulmonary capillary. PAOP increases in poor left ventricular function, fluid overload and mitral valve disease (and is low in hypovolaemia). A high pulmonary artery pressure (PAP) may indicate high pulmonary vascular resistance.

 Clinical implication

The physiotherapist should check the pulmonary artery waveform before and after positioning a patient for physiotherapy treatment. The catheter, even though not inflated, may be 'pushed' further into the pulmonary capillary and assume a wedged position.

Thermodilution cardiac output. Non-invasive monitoring of cardiac output has been discussed above. Traditional measurement of cardiac output by the thermodilution method requires the use of a pulmonary artery catheter. Cardiac output can be computed from the decrease in blood temperature in the pulmonary artery after injection of a known volume of cold saline into the right atrium. Computation of cardiac output is based on the principle that the decrease in blood

8

8

temperature is inversely proportional to the extent of dilution of the cold saline (i.e. the higher the cardiac output the less the change in temperature between injection and measurement points).

Continuous thermodilution is possible by monitors that use infusion of heat from a filament in the right atrium rather than injection of cold saline. The monitor displays cardiac output averaged over the previous 3 to 6 minutes (Boldt et al 1994, Yelderman et al 1992).

The most commonly used method of continuous cardiac output monitoring is by PiCCO® technology. This technology is less invasive. It requires the insertion of a thermodilution catheter in the femoral or axillary artery and a central venous catheter. (The use of a right heart catheter is not necessary.) This technology is based on the transpulmonary thermodilution technique and arterial pulse contour analysis and provides specific and quantitative parameters including arterial blood pressure, heart rate, cardiac output, global end-diastolic volume [an indicator of cardiac volume, the normal range of global end-diastolic volume index (GEDVI) is 680–800 ml/m^2], intrathoracic blood volume [an indicator of thoracic blood volume, the intrathoracic blood volume index (ITBVI) is 850–1000 ml/m^2], extravascular lung water [an indicator of pulmonary oedema, extravascular lung water index (EVLWI) is 3.0–7.0 ml/kg], cardiac function index, global ejection fraction, stroke volume, stroke volume variation SVV (an indicator of the potential for a response to intravascular filling, SVV should be less than 10%), pulse pressure variation (also an indicator of the potential for a positive response to intravascular filling) and systemic vascular resistance (an indicator of left ventricular afterload). (Pulsion Medical Systems) (Fig 8.5).

Mixed venous oxygen saturation. Normal oxygen saturation in the venous blood is 75% and mixed venous oxygen saturation (SvO$_2$) reflects the adequacy of tissue perfusion. SvO$_2$ falls when oxygen demand increases (such as stressful procedures, shivering, nursing care) and/or when oxygen delivery is inadequate (poor cardiac output as a result of heart failure). Increased SvO$_2$, however, suggests failure of tissue cells to take up or utilize oxygen from the blood. An SvO$_2$ of 30% or less suggests that oxygen delivery is insufficient to meet tissue oxygen demands and anaerobic metabolism and lactic acidosis will be likely accompaniments in such circumstances.

Monitoring of the neurological system

Level of consciousness The Glasgow Coma Scale (Chapter 1) is the most common way to objectively index the level of consciousness. Pupil size and level of reactivity to light provides an index of neurological integrity (pupils equal and reactive to light (PERL)). A fixed dilated unilateral pupil indicates pressure on the oculomotor nerve and urgent investigation is necessary. Physiotherapy intervention should be delayed. Fixed dilated pupils indicate severe neurological impairment, which may be made worse by hypoxia or biochemical abnormalities and are often a sign of brainstem death.

Cranial computed tomography scan. Computed tomography (CT) of the head provides information about the brain and skull. A plain skull radiograph may identify fractures of the skull and CT with contrast is used for investigation of intracranial space-occupying lesions (haemorrhage, tumour or abscess). Cranial CT permits visualization of the following (Kumar 1997):

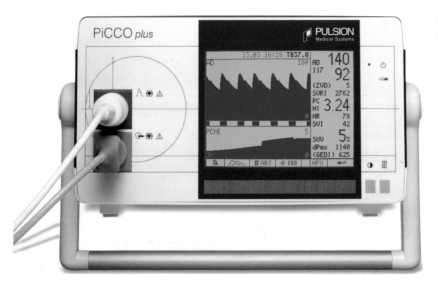

Figure 8.5 PiCCO. (© Pulsion Medical Systems AG)

- cerebral oedema
- hemispheric shift
- hydrocephalus
- subdural haematoma
- extradural haematoma
- intracerebral haematoma
- subarachnoid haemorrhage.

Magnetic resonance imaging (MRI) is now more commonly used when scanning neurological patients.

Intracranial pressure. Intracranial pressure (ICP) is measured by insertion of a catheter through the skull into the lateral ventricle or by means of an extradural or subarachnoid bolt (Turner 2002). ICP is often monitored in patients with head injuries, post-brain surgery and for patients with intracranial and subarachnoid haemorrhage or cerebral oedema. The intraventricular catheter has the advantage of allowing drainage of cerebrospinal fluid when the intracranial pressure is high but because it penetrates the dura, there is a greater accompanying risk of intracranial infection. Any change in the intracranial pressure is dependent upon the relative amounts of blood, brain and CSF within the adult skull. ICP allows determination of global cerebral perfusion pressure (CPP), which relates closely to cerebral blood flow (CBF) (Box 8.4).

Raised PCO_2 results in an increase in cerebral blood flow, which will cause a rise in ICP and a lowering of CPP. Hyperventilation may lower the PCO_2, thus reducing cerebral vasodilatation and CBF, thereby lowering the ICP. Normal ICP is 10–15 mmHg, but baseline levels are often higher in neurosurgical patients. In order to provide adequate perfusion to the brain, it is generally recommended that CPP should be maintained at a level greater than 60 mmHg (Huang et al 2006).

Jugular bulb oxygen saturation. Jugular bulb oxygen saturation (SjO_2) reflects the adequacy of global cerebral oxygen delivery, although monitoring of SjO_2 is now rarely used in neurosurgical ICU. Monitoring of SjO_2 is based on the principle that cerebral arterial and mixed venous oxygen difference (A–VDO_2) is directly proportional to cerebral metabolic rate ($CMRO_2$) but inversely proportional to cerebral blood flow (CBF). The normal values of SjO_2 are between 55–71%. Less than 55% indi-

cates an increase in cerebral oxygen extraction, often due to hypotension or systemic hypoxia. Over 70% indicates hyperaemia. The results have to be interpreted along with other information such as ICP (White & Baker 2002).

Measurement and monitoring of cerebral blood flow

Transcranial Doppler. Transcranial Doppler (TCD) is a non-invasive diagnostic tool that uses sound waves to measure the velocity of blood flow in the basal cranial arteries (Miller 2005). Blood flow velocity, however, is variable and dependent on the diameter of the cerebral arteries. Thus a dimensionless variable, the pulsatility index (PI) is used which is derived from the difference between systolic and diastolic flow velocities divided by the mean velocity. PI is a reflection of the cerebrovascular resistance and a high PI is associated with a low cerebral perfusion pressure (CPP) (Lindegaard 1992). A high correlation between PI and ICP (Voulgaris et al 2005) and CPP (Bellner et al 2004) has been reported. PI has a high predictive value for detecting a CPP of less than 70 mmHg (Voulgaris et al 2005).

Bispectral index (electroencephalographic analysis). The bispectral index (BIS) is a parameter that was developed to measure a patient's level of awareness during sedation (Haug et al 2004) and to determine the probability of recovery of consciousness in patients in coma (Fabregas et al 2004). BIS is derived from an electroencephalogramic parameter, which includes time and frequency domains and higher-order spectral information. With electrode sensors placed on the forehead of the healthiest brain hemisphere, identified by computed tomography scan, a BIS recording can be quantified on a scale from 0 to 10. BIS correlates with clinical signs of hypnosis (Billard et al 1997, Rosow and Manberg 2001) and is reported to be predictive of traumatic brain injury and neurological outcome at discharge (Haug et al 2004).

PROBLEM IDENTIFICATION AND PHYSIOTHERAPEUTIC INTERVENTIONS IN ICU

Quality of patient care depends on appropriate patient assessment and identification of problems associated with presenting symptoms. Appropriate intervention involves complex decision-making processes. This section discusses broad problems encountered by patients in the ICU and the rationale for interventions to be undertaken. Case studies or common patient scenarios are presented to illustrate the principles of intervention.

Broad problems

Chapter 6 has comprehensively detailed potential problems that may occur in the respiratory patient,

---

Box 8.4   Calculation of cerebral perfusion pressure (CPP)

CPP = MAP − ICP

CPP = cerebral perfusion pressure; MAP = mean arterial pressure; ICP = intracranial pressure

Ulatowski 1997

8

mechanisms, medical and physiotherapy management. Apart from the presenting problem, for example, severe pneumonia or multiple trauma, patient's previous comorbidities, immobility, problems associated with intubation, ventilation and impaired nutrition should be considered. Problems particularly relevant to critically ill patients include:

- decreased lung volumes/compliance
- decreased gas exchange
- decreased mucociliary clearance
- weakness of peripheral and respiratory muscles
- increased work of breathing.

Decreased lung volumes, compliance and gas exchange

Intubation, mechanical ventilation and the accompanying sedation can result in a number of adverse effects on the respiratory and cardiovascular system. Ventilation/perfusion mismatching may occur due to preferential ventilation of the non-dependent areas (increased dead space) of the lung while the poorly ventilated dependent areas still receive preferential perfusion (increased shunt) especially in the supine position. The monotonous pattern of positive pressure ventilation without spontaneous respiration may impair gas exchange (Hedenstierna et al 1985) and the absence of sighs during mechanical ventilation will lead to decreased surfactant release, decreased lung compliance and progressive pulmonary atelectasis (Antonaglia et al 2006). Decreased functional residual capacity (FRC) also occurs because of cephalad displacement of the diaphragm and loss of lung volumes, both of which occur predominantly in the dependent zones. Alveoli may develop different levels of resistance, those with high resistance taking a longer time to inflate. The different mechanical properties of alveoli may be interpreted as having varying *time constants* (the product of alveolar *compliance × resistance*). A long time constant indicates an alveolus that opens slowly during tidal inflation.

In the immobilized ventilated patient, progressive atelectasis will result in a further decrease in lung compliance and gas exchange. The patient may also have a diffusion defect due to factors such as pneumonia, alveolar thickening or acute respiratory distress syndrome (ARDS).

Decreased mucociliary/secretion clearance

Normal mucociliary clearance depends on a complex interaction between ciliated columnar cells in the tracheobronchial tree and special viscoelastic properties of the bronchial secretions. As well as the presence of an invasive airway, immobility and decreased conscious level, the intensive care patient may have a number of factors that specifically impair mucociliary clearance, which include:

- ciliary denudation by the endo- or nasotracheal tube
- pharmacological agents, including barbiturates
- activation of the inflammatory mediator system
- high levels of inspired oxygen
- high inspiratory pressures/PEEP
- low tidal volume
- trauma from suctioning
- volatile anaesthetic agents.

Premorbid factors such as a history of smoking, chronic respiratory disease and/or severe neuromuscular disorders other than impaired respiratory muscle strength may also further impair mucociliary/secretion clearance.

Intubation and mechanical ventilation can inhibit the normal mucociliary clearance and be associated with secretion retention and pneumonia (Konrad et al 1994). A patient intubated and ventilated for longer than 48 hours has been shown to be heavily colonized with anaerobic bacteria (Agvald-Ohman et al 2003). The colonization of bacteria may be partly due to suction-induced lesions of mucous membranes. These bacteria are then capable of synthesizing and releasing factors capable of further impairing ciliary mobility and causing a loss in epithelial integrity. It is important that the physiotherapist understands the mechanisms of impaired mucociliary clearance in the intubated ventilated patient and appreciates which methods of intervention are effective.

Mucociliary clearance in the healthy, non-intubated patients includes the cough mechanism. In the intubated patient, mucociliary clearance may be facilitated by the mechanism of annular two-phase gas liquid transport. This is a non-ciliary dependent phasic flow with energy transmitted from moving air to static liquid, resulting in shearing of the secretions.

Weakness of respiratory and peripheral muscles

Mechanical ventilation for as little as 48 hours has been demonstrated to decrease diaphragm strength (Sassoon et al 2002) and endurance of respiratory muscles (Chang et al 2005).

A combination of the catabolic effects of the major illness, stress response, hospital-acquired infections and certain pharmacological agents can result in the loss of large amounts of muscle mass attributed to a proteolytic or protein degradation process or specific critical care weakness syndromes (Latronico et al 2005). General immobility also results in clinically significant bone demineralization and general impairment of orthostatic reflexes. This can result in increased time on mechanical

Table 8.1 Measures of work of breathing, lung thorax/mechanics and metabolic consumption

- $P_{0.1}$ (amount of negative pressure generated (effort) in first 100 msec of inspiration). Most modern ventilators can measure this value automatically, with normal values of 2–5 cmH$_2$O. Increased $P_{0.1}$ indicates excessive work of breathing to trigger inspiration and hence may require increased inspiratory support and/or reduced ventilator trigger sensitivity or increased sedation

- NIF/MIP (maximal inspiratory force generated – effort dependent, normal values 70–100 cmH$_2$O)

- Intrinsic PEEP/gas trapping (amount of PEEP generated at the end of a normal passive expiration estimating the amount of gas trapped in the lung); normal = 0 cmH$_2$O

- Oesophageal balloon monitoring (oesophageal balloon catheter placed to measure negative oesophageal pressures as an estimation of pleural pressure)

- Direct/indirect calorimetry (expired ventilator gas measure of oxygen consumption and carbon dioxide production as a measure of metabolic consumption of the patient)

- Weaning indices – f/Vt (breath frequency in bpm divided by tidal volume as fraction of 1 litre with value of <105 being potentially predictive of weaning success). For example, for a patient with respiratory rate 50 bpm and tidal volume 400 ml, the weaning index will be 50/0.4 = 125, and thus not suitable for weaning

$P_{0.1}$ = effort in first 100 msec in inspiration, NIF = negative inspiratory force, MIP = maximal inspiratory pressure, PEEP = positive end-expiratory pressure, f/Vt = rapid shallow breathing index, bpm = breaths per minute

8

ventilation, longer hospital stay and decreased quality of life on discharge.

Increased work of breathing

The primary reasons for mechanical ventilation are to decrease the work of breathing and optimize gas exchange. Mechanical ventilation can be applied to patients who are or are not making spontaneous respiratory efforts (Georgopoulos et al 2006). The patient's respiratory system may either be passively ventilated (mandatory modes) or the patient may interact with the ventilator and trigger machine-supported breaths (in synchronized modes with set tidal volume or set pressure), or the patient may spontaneously breathe throughout the respiratory cycle interspersed with positive pressure breaths (bilevel ventilation).

There are many means of assessing the lung/thorax mechanics, work of breathing and metabolic cost of breathing in an intubated and mechanically ventilated patient (Table 8.1).

Work of breathing in the mechanically ventilated patient will increase if there is asynchrony between the patient and the ventilator: that is, the ability of the mechanical ventilator to respond promptly to patient demand for flow during inspiration, to cycle from inspiration to expiration and to allow an unimpeded expiration.

An understanding of the basic waveform of ventilatory pattern allows the physiotherapists to obtain much information associated with the patient's work of breathing during mechanical ventilation. This is covered later in this chapter.

Interventions

This section aims to describe interventions that have been specifically developed for critically ill and/or ventilated patients, including the rationale, indications, modifications and precautions of current respiratory techniques in these patients.

Positive pressure

Hyperinflation techniques. The ventilated, critically ill patient often has an underlying problem associated with progressive atelectasis and loss of compliance combined with impaired mucociliary clearance. Hyperinflation techniques, manual hyperinflation (MHI) and ventilator hyperinflation (VHI) have been introduced in an effort to improve ventilation and secretion mobilization in a patient whose normal defensive mechanism is lost.

The aims of hyperinflation techniques are to:

- improve lung thoracic compliance (by increased tidal volume/inspiratory pressure, altered inspiratory:expiratory ratio or by increased positive end-expiratory pressure)

- enhance mobilization of secretions (by increased expiratory flow rate)

- reinflate atelectatic areas (increased tidal volume and inspiratory time)

- improve gas exchange (increased tidal volume and inspiratory time).

Manual hyperinflation (MHI) is a technique whereby the patient is disconnected from the ventilator and given an altered breathing pattern via a valve circuit and reservoir bag (Fig. 8.6). To reduce the risk of barotrauma, it is recommended that a pressure manometer be incorporated into the circuit so that the peak airway pressure can be monitored during the MHI procedure.

The ideal pattern includes a slow inspiration, an inspiratory hold and a fast release. This pattern hypothetically has beneficial effects on volume restoration, compliance and removal of secretions. Evidence and rationale for these mechanisms will be discussed below.

Various types of circuits are utilized. Expiratory flow rate and volume produced by the more pliable Mapleson and Magill circuits and the less pliable Air Viva and Laerdal circuits have been compared, both in laboratory and clinical studies (Jones et al 1991, 1992a, 1992b, Maxwell & Ellis 2003, McCarren & Chow 1998, Rusterholz & Ellis 1998). The Mapleson and Magill circuits provide greater tidal volume and faster expiratory flow. When a pressure manometer is not in use, the latter circuits may be safer.

Ventilator hyperinflation (VHI) has been used as an alternative to manual hyperinflation in ventilated patients. The method consists of leaving the patient attached to the ventilator and altering either the volume, pressure or flow/time characteristics of the breath delivered. This method of ventilation has been shown to result in similar levels of secretions removed and improvements in compliance as manual hyperinflation (Berney & Denehy 2002, Savian et al 2005).

Evidence for hyperinflation techniques

Effect on decreased volumes, compliance and oxygenation. As discussed, the critically ill patient may have low lung volumes and decreased lung compliance due to a number of factors. In order to reverse the process of decreased lung compliance, the inspiratory pressure must exceed a critical opening level to expand collapsed alveoli. A pressure of 40 cmH$_2$O has been stated to be a minimum (Rothen et al 1999); however, other studies have resolved atelectasis using lower pressures (Maa et al 2005).

A slow inspiration procedure used in both MHI and VHI results in laminar flows, which encourage alveoli with prolonged time constants to reinflate. A larger tidal volume and inspiratory plateau promotes release of surfactant, which will reduce the surface tension of alveoli and assist re-expansion. The inspiratory hold also facilitates alveolar expansion via collateral ventilation.

MHI has been demonstrated to result in reversal of atelectasis (Stiller et al 1990), improvement in tidal volumes, improvement in chest radiograph scores (Maa et al 2005), improvements in static and dynamic

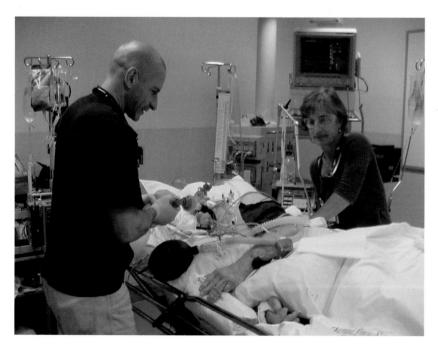

Figure 8.6 An intubated adult receiving manual hyperinflation and chest wall shaking/vibration (note blue pressure manometer, Laerdal MHI circuit with orange spring-loaded PEEP valve).

compliance (Hodgson et al 2000, Jones et al 1992b, Paratz et al 2002, Patman et al 2000) and increased yield of secretions (Choi & Jones 2005, Hodgson et al 2000, Jones 2002).

Effect on mucociliary clearance. The fast release technique during the expiration phase of MHI encourages movement of the secretions in a cephalad direction. Patients on mechanical ventilation are normally sedated, with a consequence of reduced ability to cough. The movement of airway secretions in these patients is impaired and may be improved by an increased expiratory to inspiratory flow ratio (the 'two-phase gas liquid transport'), which is proposed to occur during MHI or VHI (Savian et al 2005).

Laboratory and clinical studies have demonstrated that manual hyperinflation compared with a control manoeuvre results in higher peak expiratory flows, improved lung/thorax compliance and increased removal of secretions (Jones 2002). It appears that a critical expiratory flow must be reached during manual hyperinflation in order for sputum movement to occur and this is linked to the method of delivery of manual hyperinflation, including the type of circuit employed (Maxwell & Ellis 2003, Savian et al 2005); tidal volume; and rapid release of the valve and bag. Research on MHI to date has not established a link between the flow rates generated and the volume of secretions removed.

Inclusion of a positive end-expiratory pressure (PEEP) valve in the manual hyperinflation circuit has been shown to decrease expiratory flow. When the PEEP exceeds 10 cmH$_2$O, MHI may be ineffective as a secretion clearance technique (Savian et al 2005).

Laboratory evidence has suggested that MHI may not be effective in mobilization of thin (low viscosity) secretions and an alternative technique such as gravity-assisted drainage may be more effective (Jones 2002).

A further method of hyperinflation that intensivists and some physiotherapists utilize are 'recruitment manoeuvres' (Mols et al 2006). Lung-protective strategies using low tidal volume ventilation are beneficial and improve survival in patients with acute respiratory distress syndrome. However, the low tidal volumes can cause tidal alveolar de-recruitment and atelectasis. A recruitment manoeuvre is a sustained increase in airway pressure with the goal to recruit atelectatic lung tissue. A number of methods are used, including increases in positive end-expiratory pressure (PEEP), sustained increased inspiratory pressure (e.g. 40 cmH$_2$O PEEP for 40 seconds duration), or sigh breaths. Using these techniques, short-term increases in oxygenation and reversal of atelectasis have been reported (Barbas et al 2005).

Precautions for hyperinflation techniques

Haemodynamic instability. Haemodynamic instability is a vague term and can cover a multitude of events. Each intervention will have a different effect depending on the pathophysiology of the patient. The relationship between hyperinflation techniques and the haemodynamic status highlights the need to consider the following factors:

- an intervention such as manual hyperinflation or ventilator hyperinflation (which causes an increase in intrathoracic pressure) may lead to a decrease in preload and subsequently cardiac output and blood pressure. *This is more likely in a patient who is hypovolaemic, i.e. has a decrease in overall circulating blood volume either absolutely (haemorrhage) or relatively (sepsis, opiates)*

- if the systemic blood pressure is below normal values and supported by inotropes or vasopressors – hyperinflation techniques could further decrease the blood pressure

- a significant drift in the baseline of the arterial blood pressure waveforms before hyperinflation techniques may indicate that the patient may require increased filling (fluids) and may not tolerate hyperinflation techniques.

Undrained pneumothorax. This is usually an absolute contraindication. If an underwater drain is in situ and a large air leak is present, hyperinflation methods may be ineffective and may worsen the air leak. The presence of bullae on a plain chest radiograph may not be an absolute contraindication, but limiting peak inspiratory pressure with the aid of a manometer may ensure safety.

Severe bronchospasm and asthma. If the patient has acute asthma, an increase in positive pressure and tidal volume or the delivery of dry unhumidified gas may further increase intrinsic PEEP and aggravate hyperinflation and bronchospasm, thereby increasing the potential risk of barotrauma.

As a general rule, the manual hyperinflation technique must always be preceded, and followed, by auscultation. Clinicians should always be mindful of pneumothorax as a potential risk of the MHI technique.

High PEEP, nitric oxide, heat and moisture exchanger (HME) and hypoxic pulmonary vasoconstriction (HPV). If the patient is receiving high PEEP (>10 cmH$_2$O) and/or nitric oxide as a ventilatory adjunct, it is advisable not to disconnect the ventilator circuit for manual hyperinflation techniques. Interruption to high levels of PEEP can cause de-recruitment and atelectrauma, especially in conditions such as ARDS (Mols

8

et al 2006). Interruption of nitric oxide can cause sudden increases in pulmonary artery pressure and severe strain on the right side of the heart as well as potential severe hypoxaemia. Ventilator hyperinflation may be an alternative in these situations, but may dilute the amount of nitric oxide the patient is receiving, unless the patient is on an automated nitric oxide delivery device.

The use of a heat and moisture exchanger (passive humidifier) in the MHI circuit may optimize humidification and reduce airway irritation. Inhaled bronchodilators before, during or after MHI may be useful if severe bronchospasm is present.

Resolution of severe atelectasis as a consequence of MHI may, however, induce sudden hypoxemia. This is because the blood flow diverted from an atelectatic area due to hypoxic pulmonary vasoconstriction (HPV) may not respond efficiently to re-perfuse the newly re-inflated alveoli. Mismatch of ventilation and perfusion thus occur, leading to sudden hypoxaemia. The patient may need to be ventilated at a higher FiO_2 until the pulmonary circulation to the recently re-inflated lung improves.

Non-invasive ventilation (NIV)

Biphasic positive airway pressure (BiPAP), continuous positive airway pressure (CPAP) and intermittent positive pressure breathing (IPPB) have been covered earlier and in Chapters 5 & 10. These modes of ventilation are of particular use in the critically ill patient in attempting to prevent intubation in respiratory failure or in weaning and extubation. Patients with chronic obstructive airways disease, chronic heart failure, obesity and renal failure are often at risk of needing reintubation and ventilation following extubation. These patients may benefit from some form of NIV post-extubation.

Manual techniques

Percussion and vibration. Although manual techniques such as percussion of the chest wall and vibration during the expiratory phase are commonly used in intensive care patients, often in conjunction with hyperinflation techniques and positioning, individual studies of their effectiveness in this setting are currently lacking. Vibration has been shown to increase expiratory flow rate (MacLean et al 1989), but there are no clinical studies that demonstrate whether this increases removal of secretions. A series of animal and human studies by Unoki et al (2004) demonstrated that chest wall compression moved secretions in a cephalad direction.

Precautions. Precautions applied to manual techniques have been discussed in Chapter 5. In intensive care patients, precautions also include decreased platelet levels, skin wounds and chest trauma.

Secretion removal techniques

Suction – open/closed. As critically ill patients are usually intubated, regular pulmonary toilet must be applied. Formerly this was always via the open suction technique: that is disconnection of the endotracheal tube, instillation of a sterile catheter and application of a negative pressure. As the patient did not receive ventilation during this period, an efficient technique in less than 15 seconds was necessary. Most intensive care units now utilize the 'in-line' suction technique (closed-suctioning), whereby a sealed catheter is connected to the endotracheal tube and suction is possible without disconnection from the ventilator. This technique has been associated with less risk of desaturation and reduction in lung volume (Cereda et al 2001), fewer arrhythmias, less cardiovascular changes (Lee et al 2001) and less reduction of PEEP (Maggiore et al 2003). However, in pressure-controlled modes of mechanical ventilation, the negative pressure from the suction catheter may trigger ventilator breaths, and the inspiratory flow from the ventilator may force the secretions away from the catheter tip, resulting in fewer secretions being aspirated (Lasocki et al 2006). After suctioning, a lung recruitment technique such as MHI or VHI may be required to minimize the risk of atelectasis induced by the negative pressure suctioning generated by either the open or closed system.

Nasopharyngeal/oropharyngeal suction and mini-tracheotomy. Nasopharyngeal and oropharyngeal suction have been discussed in detail in Chapter 5. These techniques are often necessary before and during extubation, as well as in attempt to prevent intubation in patients with inefficient coughing efforts or increased secretions.

Minitracheotomy is often utilized in intensive care and is invaluable for patients with secretion retention, weak cough and contraindications to or intolerance of oral/nasopharyngeal airways. However, as only size 10 French gauge suction catheters can be used, this may limit suction effectiveness in some patients. Also a mini-tracheostomy is an uncuffed tube, and hence will not prevent the patient from aspirating oropharyngeal secretions.

Increased moisture to airways

Humidification. Humidification has been discussed in Chapter 5. Humidification is mandatory for patients on mechanical ventilation to reverse some of the adverse effects of intubation such as reduced tracheal mucus velocity and cilial impairment.

A critically ill patient on high concentration of inspired oxygen will also benefit from heated humidification. A heat and moisture exchanger (HME) can be used as an alternative but has been associated with increased circuit dead space and resistance to airflow. It may also be associated with an increased work of breathing in spontaneously breathing patients who are on low levels of respiratory support (Boots et al 2006). The use of HMEs may increase $PaCO_2$ in patients with acute lung injury/acute respiratory distress syndromes (Moran et al 2006). Nebulization with normal saline via the ventilator circuit has been reported to increase the yield of airway secretions (O'Riordan et al 2006).

Saline instillation. Direct instillation of normal saline to the endotracheal tube during or prior to suction in an attempt to decrease viscosity of secretions is a frequently used (and yet sometimes controversial) technique. A number of studies have found that this practice results in decreased SaO_2 and/or mixed venous saturation (Ackerman & Mick 1998), no increase in secretion yield (Lerga et al 1997) and possible dislodgement/dispersion of microorganisms into the lower respiratory tract (Hagler & Traver 1994). Schreuder & Jones (2004), however, demonstrated increased sputum wet weight and stable arterial oxygen saturation following use of saline when it was combined with chest physiotherapy. It is recommended that instillation of saline should be reserved for patients with excessively tenacious secretions. In addition, the clinician should anticipate a short-term drop in arterial saturation that may require a temporary increase in FiO_2.

Positioning

The physiological effects and rationale of positioning have been covered in detail in Chapter 4. Altering the position of a critically ill patient is a powerful tool and may result in both beneficial and adverse effects. Cardiovascular changes associated with positional changes, especially in critically ill patients, should be closely monitored during physiotherapy. An adequate understanding of the pathophysiology of positioning and its predicted effects is essential.

Gravity-assisted positioning. Traditional gravity-assisted positions (Chapter 5) are often not utilized in intensive care patients as full positioning is often hindered by cardiovascular instability, equipment and lack of patient cooperation. However, evidence suggests that specifically positioning the patient for the affected lobe results in increased expiratory flow rate, better oxygenation, increased sputum clearance and faster resolution without adverse effects on haemodynamic stability (Berney et al 2004, Krause et al 2000).

Prone positioning. Specific prone positioning for extended periods of time has been advocated as a method to improve oxygenation and lung mechanics in patients with acute lung injury and acute respiratory distress syndrome. There is strong evidence that this method results in improved lung mechanics and oxygenation due to expansion of the collapsed dorsal regions of the lung (Messerole et al 2002). This technique is most useful if used early in the disease process and may also result in increased secretion clearance due to drainage of the collapsed dorsal regions of the lung. Reduction in carbon dioxide with prone positioning is indicative of improved alveolar ventilation and is predictive of better survival (Gattinoni et al 2003).

Lateral positioning. The effects of lateral positioning will depend on pathology of the lung, whether unilateral or bilateral and type of ventilation. To maximize alveolar expansion, lung segments to be expanded are often placed in the upper most (non-dependent) lateral position for facilitation of aeration, especially with positive pressure ventilation. However, blood flow will preferentially move to the dependent lung (even more so during positive pressure ventilation); hence, there may be potent effects on gas exchange dependent upon the extent of pulmonary disease (unilateral or bilateral).

In patients with unilateral lung disease, gas exchange may improve by laying the patient on the non-diseased lung (Ibanez et al 1981, Stiller 2000). This may also facilitate secretion drainage. In adopting lateral positioning to optimize gas exchange, the physiotherapist should be aware of the mode of ventilation, monitored variables (tidal volume, airway pressures), inotropic and vasoactive requirements and cardiovascular status (blood pressure, heart rate). For example re-positioning a heavily sedated intubated patient who is receiving a pressure-controlled mode of ventilation (such as pressure support) and who has copious secretions and a poor cough, may lead to severe reductions in tidal volume (and hence minute ventilation) due to the movement of secretions in the major airways which may alter airway resistance.

Continuous lateral rotation therapy or kinetic therapy. Continuous lateral rotation therapy or kinetic therapy is a relatively new innovation in intensive care and consists of continually changing the position of the patient (to extreme lateral position) in specially designed hydraulic beds. The beds are costly but have been proposed to increase the clearance of airway secretions (Davis et al 2001), reduce the rate of development of ventilator-associated pneumonia (VAP) (Dodek et al 2004, Kirschenbaum et al 2002) and resolve atelectasis if combined with percussion (Raoof et al 1999). However, these beds have not been shown to result in improved patient outcomes such as time on mechanical ventilation or time in the intensive care unit and there are reports of high rates of patient intolerance of the beds.

Precautions in positioning. Precautions in positioning are similar to those of postural drainage (Chapter 5). Each patient should be assessed individually, especially for the presence of severe cardiac disease, as indiscriminate head-down tilt for extended periods in ventilated patients with cardiac failure has been shown to result in major arrhythmias (Artucio & Pereira 1990) and right side lying has been shown to reduce blood pressure in critically ill patients with cardiac decompensation (Bein et al 1996).

Mobilization

Passive/active exercises. While passive movement is commonly employed by physiotherapists in maintenance of joint range and muscle length for unconscious and semi-conscious patients in the ICU, there is minimal evidence to support its use. There is emerging evidence that continuous passive movement or electrical stimulation may prevent protein degradation and/or induce induction of messenger ribonucleic acid and c-fos in immobilized subjects (Griffiths et al 1995, Zador et al 1999). When a patient can actively move his limbs, passive limb mobilization exercise is usually no longer indicated.

Sit out of bed. Sitting up in bed, sitting over the edge of the bed, and sitting the patient out of bed, allows the diaphragm to descend, thus increasing functional residual capacity and facilitating efficient gas exchange. A sitting position also has the advantage of increasing wakefulness and alertness and therapist–patient communication is promoted.

Tilt table. If a patient is unable to stand due to either decreased power in the hip and knee extensors, placing the patient on a tilt table is an option. Tilt tables have been shown to be in common use in the majority of intensive care units in Europe and Australia (Chang et al 2004a, Norrenberg & Vincent 2000). Increased minute ventilation without adverse haemodynamic changes has been demonstrated when patients are placed on a tilt table (Chang et al 2004b). However, at present there is no evidence for long-term benefit from use of this equipment although weight bearing stimuli have been proven to result in prevention and reversal of osteopenia in medical patients (Jorgensen et al 2000).

Stand, walking. As soon as a patient is deemed capable (Box 8.5), standing or mobilizing is ideal for the intensive care patient. This is often initially supported by equipment such as a walking frame, oxygen or portable ventilation. Orthostatic reflexes may be impaired by immobilization and therefore monitoring of haemodynamic changes is essential. Short-term improvements in

---

Box 8.5   Indications for standing /mobilization

- Haemodynamically stable
- Stable airway (tracheostomy)
- Grade 3 muscle power in antigravity muscles
- Alert
- Willing to try
- Stable airway

---

tidal volume, inspiratory flow rate and minute volume with mobilization to standing were demonstrated in intubated, ventilated, abdominal surgical patients (Zafiropoulos et al 2004).

Absence of active mobilization (tilt table, walking or sit out of bed) in intensive care has been shown to be associated with an increased risk of readmission to ICU (Paratz et al 2005). Chiang et al (2006) have demonstrated that daily rehabilitation assisted in reduced time on mechanical ventilation and improved functional status in long-term mechanical ventilator-dependent patients.

Precautions in mobilization. All intensive care patients are potentially unstable and an important aspect of exercise or mobilization is to achieve a fine balance between progressing the patient and not causing any deterioration in cardiovascular status. While these techniques are relatively simple, the ability to judge when critically ill patients are sufficiently stable to begin such rehabilitation requires considerable expertise. The safety aspects of mobilizing intensive care patients have been extensively reviewed by Stiller et al (2004).

Combined management

For optimal patient management, the above methods of intervention are often combined (e.g. positioning, manual hyperinflation, expiratory vibrations and suction of the endotracheal tube). A combination of techniques has been shown to be effective in increasing secretion yield and reducing airway resistance (Choi & Jones 2005). A controversial point in physiotherapy management of the patient in ICU is whether mechanically ventilated patients should be treated prophylactically, i.e. before problems actually arise. Ntoumenopoulos et al (2002) demonstrated that prophylactic physiotherapy treatment could result in a decrease in ventilator-associated pneumonia by as much as 31%, demonstrating that preventative treatment is of value.

Conditions in ICU

This section describes the management of some conditions commonly encountered in the ICU. Common problems associated with the conditions are illustrated as case studies.

Acute lung injury (ALI)/acute respiratory distress syndrome (ARDS)

Acute respiratory distress syndrome refers to 'a clinical syndrome caused by a wide variety of events and characterized by acute onset, refractory hypoxemia, decreased compliance and bilateral diffuse infiltrates on chest radiograph' (Wilson et al 2001). The term acute lung injury (ALI) was often used and confused with acute respiratory distress syndrome (ARDS). The American-European Consensus Conference (AECC) in 1992 recommended that the term ALI should be used in a 'broader' sense and ARDS used for the more severe illness with poor oxygen status. Thus all patients with ARDS suffer ALI but not all patients with ALI will have ARDS. The criteria for diagnosis of ALI and ARDS as set by the AECC are:

- acute onset of lung injury
- diffuse bilateral infiltrates seen on chest radiographs
- PaO_2/FiO_2 <200 mmHg (26 kPa) for ARDS and <300 mmHg (40 kPa) for ALI (Matthay et al 2003)
- pulmonary artery occlusion pressure <19 mmHg
- no clinical evidence of congestive heart failure (Bernard et al 1994).

Thoracic imaging (both plain radiographs and computed tomography) is one of the essential components in diagnosis and assessment of ARDS.

Pathogenesis of acute respiratory distress syndrome. Acute respiratory distress syndrome (ARDS) carries a mortality rate of 50–80% (Metnitz et al 1999) and is often associated with sepsis, further increasing the likelihood of mortality. The exact mechanisms involved in the pathogenesis of ARDS are unknown, although infiltrating leukocytes and widespread endothelial injury are typical. Alveolar and pulmonary microcirculatory endothelial injury leads to normal inflammatory responses characterized by the release of cytokines and recruitment of neutrophils to the area of inflammation (Zimmerman et al 1999). This initiates a number of reactions in the lungs, which lead to hypoxaemia.

Patients with ARDS are often administered high concentrations of oxygen, which may further exacerbate the primary lung injury. The release of reactive oxygen species (ROS) causes damage to the alveolar surfactant system and decreases the ability of cells to transport sodium actively across epithelial membranes – an important process in the removal of alveolar fluid. These detrimental effects on lung function, as a consequence

of prolonged mechanical ventilation and oxygen therapy, are further aggravated by other risk factors such as old age and sepsis (Wilson et al 2001).

These conditions cause a general inflammatory response with damage to the alveolar–capillary interface, leading to leakage of fluid into the interstitial space/alveoli and resulting in reduced compliance and shunting. Patients are often dyspnoeic, tachypnoeic and severely hypoxaemic. Management revolves around 'protective ventilation'; that is low tidal volumes and the maintenance of optimal PEEP (MacIntyre 2005). If high tidal volumes are given and the ventilator is frequently disconnected, barotrauma, volutrauma and and/or atelectrauma may result. These syndromes are basically results of damage from high pressure, high volume and repeated deflation and inflation of alveoli. Biotrauma may also result, where high pressure, volume or shearing of alveoli may result in leaking of inflammatory substances from the lung causing a multi-organ system failure.

ARDS can act as one of two distinct pathological types of disease according to the initial type of insult (Gattinoni et al 1998). Those associated with intrapulmonary causes, for example respiratory burns and aspiration pneumonia, tend to have a non-compliant lung with pathology typical of consolidation. If patients have had an extrapulmonary insult, for example pancreatitis or head injury, the patient will have a stiff thoracoabdominal cage and compliant lung with pathology similar to atelectasis. Studies have shown that the latter type (extrapulmonary) is more amenable to hyperinflation manoeuvres such as manual or ventilator hyperinflation (Paratz et al 2002, Pelosi et al 2003). Prone positioning may be beneficial. In the past physiotherapists were advised that any intervention should occur when the patient was in the subacute stage of ARDS. However it has been found that certain interventions such as recruitment of the lung and prone positioning are more successful when introduced early in the disease (Pelosi et al 2002).

How would you manage the two patients in Case studies 8.1 and 8.2?

Ventilator-associated pneumonia (VAP)

Ventilator-associated pneumonia (VAP) is an infection that can occur more than 48 hours after starting ventilation and has been quoted as occurring in 30–50% of intensive care patients, with a mortality between 20–70%. The condition extends length of ventilation and length of stay in ICU.

Diagnosis of VAP. Clinical criteria for the diagnosis of VAP are new or progressive pulmonary infiltrates and at least two of the following (Chytra 2002):

CASE STUDY 8.1

A 35-year-old male with multiple fractures requires replacement of 5 litres of blood following a motor vehicle accident (MVA). On Day 2 after admission, he develops tachypnoea and bilateral pulmonary infiltrates. His PaO_2/FiO_2 decreases to 220 and his pulmonary arterial occlusion pressure (PAOP) is 14 cmH$_2$O. He is ventilated on SIMV (16 breaths/minute × 500 ml tidal volume, PEEP 7.5 cmH$_2$O, pressure support 10 cmH$_2$O, FiO$_2$ 0.4). His peak pressures on a breath of 500 ml are 27 cmH$_2$O.

CASE STUDY 8.2

A 40-year-old male develops community-acquired pneumonia (right lower lobe) and is admitted to a medical ward with an FiO$_2$ of 0.3 and a PaO_2 of 95 mmHg. He is expectorating sputum and receives secretion mobilization techniques for 3 days. By Day 4 he is non-productive, increasingly tachypnoeic and hypoxaemic (FiO$_2$ 0.4, PaO_2 75) with bilateral infiltrates on chest radiograph. He is ventilated in intensive care and deteriorates further. On examination, he is on pressure-controlled ventilation (inspiratory pressure 32 cmH$_2$O), respiratory rate 15 breaths /minute, FiO$_2$ 0.6, PEEP 10 cmH$_2$O. His tidal volumes on this inspiratory pressure are only 300 ml.

What is your clinical reasoning for the difference in management between these two patients?

Discussion of Case studies 8.1 and 8.2

These two patients differ with respect to the aetiology of their ARDS as well as lung compliance and ventilation method. The patient in Case study 8.2 has lower lung compliance, the ventilation method is aiming to control the pressure and only small volumes are produced by this pressure. As his cause of ARDS was 'intrapulmonary', the pathology of his condition is similar to that of 'consolidation'. If hyperinflation methods are used, very little increase in tidal volume will occur without exceeding a safe pressure. He is also on a high PEEP and, if disconnected, will lose the recruitment gained and be predisposed to atelectrauma. If there was evidence of retained secretions, interventions to mobilize secretions such as percussion or vibrations, while maintaining ventilation and closed suction, could assist.

In contrast, the patient in Case study 8.1 has a less severe form of the disease (ALI P/F ratio, i.e. PaO_2/FiO$_2$ is >200) and has reasonable lung compliance with reserve to provide hyperinflation without exceeding recommended peak inspiratory pressures. His type of lung injury is 'extrapulmonary' and more

amenable to further recruitment. He is not on high PEEP, but a PEEP valve should still be included in the manual hyperinflation circuit. This patient may also benefit from prone positioning, especially as his injury is extrapulmonary and he is in the early stage of the syndrome.

(continued from p 287)

- fever of >38°C or <36°C
- leukocytosis >10 000 cells/mm^3 or leukopenia of <4 000 cells/mm^3
- purulent tracheobronchial secretions
- decrease in PaO_2.

Blood cultures are considered low in both specificity and sensitivity, as critically ill patients in ICU often have multiple potential sources of infection. Cultures of the lower respiratory tract and histological examination of lung tissue are considered a more reliable process for diagnosing VAP. Proximal airway sampling (tracheal tube aspirates) and distal airway sampling (aspiration, brushing and bronchoalveolar lavage) can be achieved using both bronchoscopic and non-bronchoscopic techniques. Both techniques, however, may be subject to error owing to contamination during passage through the upper airway, which is invariably colonized by organisms. Thus 'quantitative cultures' and bronchoscopic 'protected catheter brushing' are often used. Quantitative culture can differentiate 'contaminants' from 'pathogens'. Often a growth threshold of 10^3 cfu/ml is used to define organism growth. This 'quantity' is equivalent to 10^5–10^6 organisms/ml in the secretions.

Treatment of VAP. The mortality attributable to VAP is significant and therefore prompt administration of appropriate empiric antibiotic therapy directed at the most prevalent and virulent pathogens is essential. As the most common pathogens are *Pseudomonas, Enterobacter, Acinetobacter*, as well as gram-positive organisms, multi-drug therapy is often required (Bowton 1999), although the use of monotherapy versus combination therapy remains controversial (Chytra 2002). Chastre (2006) has undertaken a review on antimicrobial management in VAP.

There is strong evidence (Minei et al 2006) that measures such as semi-recumbent positioning, continuous turning, handwashing, aspiration of subglottic secretions, selective digestive contamination and early tracheotomy all result in a decreased incidence of VAP. Physiotherapists have a definite role in the prevention of VAP. Ntoumenopoulos and colleagues (2002) found a decreased incidence of VAP (39% vs 8%) as a consequence of physiotherapy intervention.

Burns

Patients with thermal injury are frequently admitted to intensive care. Even if there is no direct respiratory burn, these patients often require mechanical ventilation, due to haemodynamic problems, decreased immune response, severe infections and secondary respiratory compromise (Monafo 1996). Respiratory burns are indicated by a history of burns in an enclosed space, facial burns, loss of consciousness before evacuation from the fire, stridor or wheezing, carbonaceous sputum, oedema and erythema on bronchoscopy. Damage to the mucosal barrier and release of inflammatory mediators are the major pathophysiological events (Bargues et al 2005). Mucosal sloughing often occurs and along with carbon must be cleared from the lungs. There is therefore a strong indication for respiratory physiotherapy (Sheridan 2000).

Patients with respiratory burns require expert respiratory care in addition to musculoskeletal rehabilitation. A number of considerations apply to the respiratory management:

■ The patient may be haemodynamically unstable – in the first 2 days fluid resuscitation is an issue and measurements such as urine output, blood pressure and CVP will indicate the overall fluid status. Myocardial 'stunning' often occurs in the first 3 days leading to decreased contractility. This is followed by an ongoing hypermetabolic and catabolic state. The patient has a markedly depressed immunological state and is at increased risk of sepsis, especially from a pulmonary source.

■ Chest wall burns and/or grafting may be a precaution for manual techniques such as percussion or vibration. Consideration should be given to the depth of burn, adequacy of pain relief, and type, timing and viability of the graft. Good communication should occur with the burn surgeons regarding the graft. Vibrations have a larger shearing force than percussion and should be used as an intervention at a later stage of graft healing.

■ On extubation patients with burns often exhibit marked tachypnoea, shallow breathing and increased white secretions. Positive pressure (IPPB, BiPAP, CPAP) for a few hours post-extubation may facilitate lung expansion and reduce the risk of reintubation.

Sepsis and systemic inflammatory response syndrome (SIRS)

Patients admitted with, or acquiring an infection in ICU often develop *sepsis*, that is a systemic response to infection. Measurements such as respiratory rate, heart rate

and temperature will change to defined levels. If this condition worsens, *sepsis syndrome*, that is sepsis with evidence of organ dysfunction, for example hypoxaemia or renal failure, may develop.

Septic shock is the most extreme manifestation of this condition and refers to sepsis syndrome with hypotension despite adequate fluid resuscitation. There is widespread fluid leakage, peripheral vasodilatation and often an inadequate circulating volume. Patients require inotropic support to maintain an adequate blood pressure and are often monitored with a pulmonary artery catheter.

An inflammatory reaction may also develop to a non-infectious insult such as pancreatitis, burns or post organ transplantation. This is termed *systemic inflammatory response syndrome (SIRS)*. Criteria for the diagnosis of SIRS include two or more of the following: altered temperature >38.0°C or <36.0°C; heart rate >90 beats / minute; respiratory rate >20/min; $PaCO_2$ <32 mmHg; white cell count >12 × 10^9/l (Worthley 2000). This syndrome can overlap with syndromes of sepsis, but the important difference is that patients with SIRS are more haemodynamically stable than those patients with sepsis and can tolerate most physiotherapy interventions.

In 2002, at the European Society of Intensive Care Annual Congress, the 'Surviving Sepsis Campaign' was launched, leading to publication of a document for critical care providers and health agencies to reduce the sepsis mortality rate by 25% in 5 years. The recommendations include a 'sepsis care bundle' to optimize patient care. Some of the measures in the 'bundle' are the early provision of oxygen therapy, intravenous access, blood cultures, serum lactates, immediate intravenous fluids, blood glucose control, nursed 30-degrees head-up and protective lung ventilatory strategy (to minimize airway pressures/tidal volumes). It has been demonstrated that lack of adherence to 'sepsis care bundles' in the first 24 hours of sepsis, results in worse patient outcome (Gao et al 2005).

The scenarios in Case studies 8.3 and 8.4 are common in patients with SIRS and/or sepsis.

Chest trauma

Chest trauma can range from a single rib fracture to multiple rib fractures with a 'flail' segment and underlying contusions. Accompanying injuries may also include haemothoraces, pneumothoraces and solid organ injury (for example to the liver). Patients are admitted to intensive care based on whether they can effectively maintain ventilation, but other criteria depend on whether there are other injuries such as head trauma or laceration to organs such as the liver or spleen. Further risk factors for deterioration following chest trauma include age

8

8

CASE STUDY 8.3

A 24-year-old male received second- and third-degree burns to 40% of his arms and legs and respiratory burns, in an industrial accident 2 weeks ago. He remains intubated on spontaneous ventilation PEEP 5 cmH$_2$O and pressure support (PS) 10 cmH$_2$O, FiO$_2$ 0.3. He has had grafting to the burns and these have healed. However his vital signs are: temperature 39.5°C, heart rate 135 beats/min (regular) and BP 120/80 mmHg (unsupported). The high heart rate and temperature have persisted for 1 week with no evidence of an infective site despite multiple testing.

These vital signs above and time period described are typical of SIRS. Note the stable blood pressure. This patient could be mobilized, tilted, sat out of bed or given MHI if required. It would be advisable to monitor the heart rate and blood pressure, but his circulation should remain stable during these procedures.

CASE STUDY 8.4

A 46-year-old female is admitted in respiratory failure following diagnosis of severe community-acquired pneumonia and ventilated on synchronized intermittent mandatory ventilation (SIMV) 12 breaths × 600 ml, PEEP 7.5 cmH$_2$O, FiO$_2$ 0.4 and pressure support 10 cmH$_2$O. On Day 6 in ICU, her blood pressure decreases to 85/60 mmHg and heart rate increases to 110/minute. A pulmonary artery catheter is inserted and the following values are noted: cardiac index (CI) = 4.3 l/min/m^2 (normal: 2.5–4.2 l/min/m^2), systemic vascular resistance index (SVRI) = 1800 dyn · sec/cm^{-5} · m^2 (normal: 1970–2390 dyne · sec/cm^{-5} · m^2) and pulmonary artery occlusion pressure (PAOP) = 6 mmHg (normal: 4–12 mmHg). She is given a large volume of fluid resuscitation and the blood pressure increases to 95/60mmHg. Noradrenaline 5 µg/min increasing to 9 µg/min over 2 hours is administered.

This patient obviously has developed septic shock and she is in a 'hyperdynamic state.' The low SVRI indicates that the peripheral circulation is widely vasodilated and the patient does not have adequate circulating fluid. If an intervention of either increased positive pressure (MHI or VHI) or mobility against gravity was given at this stage, there would be inadequate compensatory reflexes and the circulation would fail. The physiotherapist needs **to delay these procedures until fluid resuscitation is complete; inotrope/vasopressors levels are decreasing;** *and blood pressure and SVRI values are in the normal range* (Paratz & Lipman 2006, Paratz et al 2002).

greater than 65 years old and pre-existing respiratory disease. Elderly patients with three or more rib fractures have been shown to have a 5 times greater increase in mortality and a 4 times greater increase in the incidence of pneumonia (Stawicki et al 2004).

The current management of chest trauma is directed towards effective pain relief, avoidance of fluid overloading, early mobilization and avoidance of invasive ventilation if possible. If a flail segment is present, an adequate end-expiratory pressure is required to 'splint' the flail segment in order for the patient to ventilate effectively.

Figures 8.7A and 8.7B describe the pathophysiological changes present in a severe chest trauma with a lung contusion and the physiological consequences.

These consequences often do not occur until Day 2 or 3, leading to a late deterioration. Management of the chest trauma patient must therefore be proactive and aimed at restoring effective ventilation, reversing atelectasis and mobilizing secretions, using a combination of management techniques. Transcutaneous electrical stimulation (TENS) can be an effective adjunct for pain relief even with an epidural in situ.

Critical illness weakness syndromes

Critical illness weakness syndromes often occur following multisystem organ failure and result in the patient surviving the initial acute problem, but having a major peripheral weakness (including cranial nerves) which often prevents weaning and mobilization. Both critical illness polyneuropathy and myopathy may occur (Latronico et al 2005). The syndrome appears to be related to use of neuromuscular blocking agents, steroids and sedation especially following ventilation for severe asthma. These patients usually require admission to a rehabilitation unit; however, there is no evidence as to whether this accelerates recovery or to the optimal method of rehabilitation. The syndrome can affect function and quality of life for 12 months post-ICU discharge. There is some preliminary evidence that proactive treatment during the paralysis stage, for example continuous passive movement, may prevent this problem (Griffiths et al 1995). With the use of spontaneous modes of mechanical ventilation, and decreased use of steroids or neuromuscular blocking agents, this syndrome may prove less of a problem in intensive care.

Haematological problems

Patients with haematological conditions (e.g. leukaemia) often develop secondary respiratory problems following bone marrow transplants and require admission to intensive care as well as mechanical ventilation. This is more likely in patients with decreased lung volumes due to pulmonary fibrosis caused by pre-transplant irra-

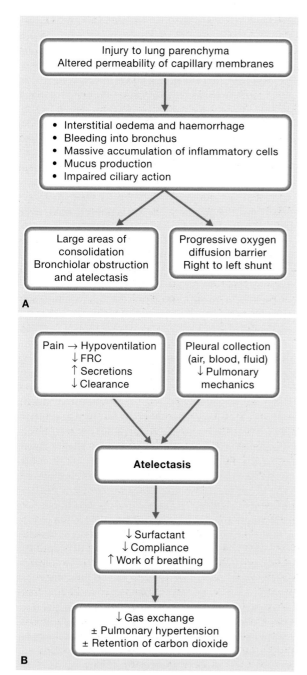

management of patients with haematological conditions warrant further investigation.

It is essential for the platelet count of these patients to be checked before interventions. Patients with a low platelet count ($<20 \times 10^9/l$) may bleed spontaneously and manual techniques such as percussion, vibration and resisted exercise should be avoided. Soft-tipped catheters should be used for suction in patients with low platelet counts. Alternative methods of secretion removal such as the active cycle of breathing techniques, positive expiratory pressure (PEP), oscillatory PEP and autogenic drainage should be considered if the patient is able to cooperate.

Brain injury

Injury to the brain may occur due to trauma (local haematoma or diffuse brain injury) or post subarachnoid haemorrhage. It is important to remember that while primary damage is irreversible, the outcome can also be affected by indirect or secondary brain damage to the brain due to such events as hypoxaemia, hypercarbia, cerebral oedema or hypotension. The brain injury patient therefore needs to be expertly managed. Normal management of the head-injured patient involves the following principles (Dutton & McCunn 2003):

- control of intracranial volume
- ensuring adequate oxygenation and perfusion of brain
- minimizing metabolism of the brain.

This is achieved by the following management strategies which may address either one or all three of the above aims:

- nursing 30 degrees head up

- monitoring of intracranial pressure

- drainage of cerebrospinal fluid via the external ventricular drain, if indicated

- maintaining the patient in a hypernatraemic state (less water content in brain cells)

- sedation and paralysis in the early stage (days 1–3) in order to limit increases in ICP from coughing and struggling and also to decrease brain metabolism

- prevention of seizures

- hypothermia

- ensuring optimal arterial blood gases

- hyperventilation to maintain $PaCO_2$ 30–35 mmHg

- ensuring cerebral perfusion pressure >60 mmHg using noradrenaline

Figure 8.7 (A) Pathophysiological changes following chest trauma with lung contusion. (B) Physiological consequences of severe chest trauma.

diation (Shankar & Cohen 2001). It has been demonstrated that non-invasive ventilation applied proactively to haematological patients with lung infiltrates and hypoxaemia results in decreased mortality (Hilbert et al 2001). The benefits of non-invasive ventilation in the

■ barbiturates*

■ decompression craniotomy (removal of frontal lobe)*

These last two methods of management are only used in cases of uncontrollable ICP.

Factors such as ICP, CPP, brain CT scan, changes on chest radiograph and arterial blood gases need to be noted in order to balance the significance of injury of one system over the other. For example a patient with chest X-ray changes, borderline arterial blood gases and low to medium ICP may be given active intervention but a patient with a clear chest radiograph, normal arterial blood gases and high ICP may be treated with position changes only.

When planning intervention in the acute severe head injury patient, consideration should be given to the following:

■ Patient should be treated in a maximally sedated state.

■ Treat when ICP is low, <20 mmHg if possible.

■ Keep neck strictly in midline – rotation will block CSF and venous blood and increase ICP. Nurse with head-up 30 degrees.

■ Suction will increase ICP; severe increases in ICP following suction may be prevented by intravenous or topical lidocaine (lignocaine) (Brucia et al 1992).

■ ICP is likely to increase during a combined physiotherapy intervention (MHI, suction, manual techniques) as a rate of time. Short treatment sessions (<8 minutes) are preferable to a long session (Paratz & Burns 1993, Rudy et al 1991).

■ Percussion or vibration as sole techniques do not increase ICP (Paratz & Burns 1993).

■ Coordinate management – do not allow patient to receive too many interventions e.g. chest X-ray, turning, physiotherapy in quick succession. This is more likely to cause increased ICP.

■ During manual hyperinflation an end tidal CO_2 monitor should be used in order to control the $PaCO_2$ between 30–35 mmHg or baseline value.

■ Head-down postural drainage or prone positions are likely to increase ICP. Research has shown that prone positioning may be well tolerated (in terms of ICP) in head-injured patients (Nekludov et al 2006, Thel-andersson et al 2006).

Severe neuromuscular disease

Acute chest infection with an increase in respiratory secretions may precipitate an acute or chronic episode of respiratory failure in patients with chest wall and or neuromuscular disease (i.e. motor neuron disease, Duchenne muscular dystrophy, amyotrophic lateral sclerosis). Mechanical ventilation further impairs secretion clearance and increases the risk of ventilator-associated pneumonia (Konrad et al 1994) and patients with neuromuscular disease often require prolonged weaning from mechanical ventilation (Bach 1993). Improved secretion clearance may be important in the recovery process, but has yet to be proven. Boitano (2006) provides a comprehensive review of the factors necessary for, and optimal means of, enhancing secretion clearance in the neuromuscular diseased patient.

Manual or ventilator hyperinflation, combined with patient positioning and airway suctioning, have been demonstrated to produce significant improvements in static lung/thorax compliance and wet weight of sputum (Berney et al 2004, Hodgson et al 2000) compared with patient positioning and airway suctioning alone, in general medical surgical intubated and ventilated patients. These techniques alone may not be sufficient in the patient with severe neuromuscular weakness.

Patients with severe neuromuscular dysfunction often have a combination of problems, including reduced inspiratory and expiratory muscle strength, increased volume and tenacity of airway secretions, bulbar dysfunction (non-intubated), increased airway resistance and reduced lung/thorax compliance (Boitano 2006). For these patients, conventional chest physiotherapy techniques may be less effective. Hence, newer mechanical devices such as the mechanical in/exsufflator (JH Emerson Co, Mass, USA) have been introduced. This technique combines two approaches: a positive pressure (usually 40 cmH₂O) is first applied to produce a maximum inspiration capacity; then, once the patient is 'fully inflated,' a sudden negative pressure (usually −40 cmH₂O) is employed to assist the patient cough. The in/exsufflation device has been reported to improve peak cough expiratory flow rates in non-intubated patients with severe respiratory muscle weakness due to various neuromuscular disorders (Bach & Saporito 1996, Chatwin et al 2003) but the technique has been poorly investigated to date in intubated patients (Pillastrini et al 2006, Sancho et al 2003). However, one retrospective study (Garstang et al 2000) investigated tracheostomized spinal cord injury (C1-T3) patients' preference for in/exsufflation for secretion management. In a direct comparison, the results indicated that 89% of patients preferred in/exsufflation to suctioning. In addition, 89% of patients found in/exsufflation faster, 78% found in/exsufflation more convenient and 72% found in/exsufflation more effective than suctioning. Manual-assisted cough (abdominal compression during the expiration phase following a maximal inspiration)

(Chapter 15) is another effective means of enhancing expiratory flow and hence secretion clearance (Boitano 2006).

PHYSIOTHERAPY MANAGEMENT OF WORK OF BREATHING AND CONCEPTS OF WEANING FROM MECHANICAL VENTILATION

The primary reasons for mechanical ventilation are to decrease the work of breathing and optimize gas exchange. Synchronized intermittent mandatory ventilation (SIMV) and assist control were the traditional ventilatory modes (Esteban et al 2000). Dual modes (combination of pressure and volume-controlled) of ventilation are becoming more commonly used and it appears that evolution of mechanical ventilation is in the direction of computer-driven protocolized weaning (Lellouche et al 2006).

While increased sedative and narcotic use can achieve greater patient–ventilator synchrony, in the short term (Richman et al 2006) these agents, as well as neuromuscular blocking agents, have been shown to be associated with an increased duration of mechanical ventilation, weaning time and time in the ICU (Arroliga et al 2005). During activities when the patient's demand of ventilation may increase (e.g. physiotherapy or situations such as anxiety and sepsis) a simple manoeuvre such as increasing the inspiratory flow rate or a change over to a pressure-controlled mode may ensure patient comfort and assist in the reduction of sedative requirement. A better understanding of the interaction between the ventilator and the patient will thus facilitate the role of the physiotherapist in the management of patients under mechanical ventilation. This section will discuss the concepts of work of breathing in patients under mechanical ventilation and issues that facilitate the weaning of patients from mechanical ventilation.

Work of breathing

Work of breathing may include the work undertaken by the patient as well as the work by the ventilator. The active contraction of the respiratory muscles causes the thoracic compartment to expand, inducing a negative pleural pressure. This negative pressure, generated by the respiratory muscles, produces lung expansion through a decrease in alveolar pressure, causing air to flow into the lungs (Cabello & Mancebo 2006). This driving pressure can be generated in three ways:

1. entirely by the ventilator (positive pressure during controlled mechanical ventilation)
2. entirely by the patient's respiratory muscles during spontaneous unassisted breathing
3. a combination of 1 and 2 (Cabello & Mancebo 2006).

While minimizing the patient's work of breathing is the main interest for most clinicians, the optimal balance between the level of work from the patient and the level of support from the ventilator is still unknown. The patient's work of breathing is dependent on the type of pulmonary disease, respiratory muscle strength, airway (and/or tracheal tube) diameter, airway secretions, anxiety, sedatives, narcotics, neuromuscular blocking agents, the mode of mechanical ventilation/settings and the level of synchrony between the patient and the mechanical ventilator.

A patient's work of breathing may be described as the amount of muscle activity required to overcome the elastic (lung tissue, chest wall and abdominal compartments) and resistive (airways, flow rate) elements of the respiratory system.

The waveform of the patient's ventilatory pattern can provide much information about the lung/thoracic compliance and airway resistance. Figure 8.8 illustrates a typical volume-delivered breath with an inspiratory pause (generated by closure of the ventilator valves at the end of inspiration).

The main cause of high peak airway pressure (in volume-controlled mode) or low tidal volume (in pressure-controlled mode) in an intubated patient is often related to problems with airways resistance: for example, a small endotracheal tube (ETT), high flow rates, secretions, bronchospasm. In patients with volume-

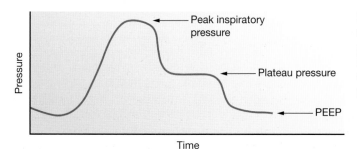

Figure 8.8 The waveform of a typical volume-controlled breath, illustrating a reliable plateau pressure that allows measurement of dynamic lung/thorax compliance (= TV / [PIP − PEEP]) and static lung/thorax compliance (= TV / [Plateau pressure − PEEP]).

controlled or dual mode ventilation, if both the peak and plateau pressures are high relative to the tidal volume delivered (5–6 ml/kg), this may indicate diffuse parenchymal disease such as ALI/ARDS or pneumonia.

A more accurate measure of static lung/thorax compliance requires the delivery of a volume-controlled breath with a known plateau/pause pressure using the formula:

Tidal volume/(Plateau pressure – PEEP)

An accurate plateau pressure exists only if a long enough inspiratory pause (zero flow) of 1–3 seconds is incorporated in the ventilatory pattern (Barberis et al 2003). Patient respiratory effort should be minimal during this measurement, and the patient usually needs to be heavily sedated.

Abdominal distension can severely impair diaphragmatic excursion and reduce FRC and may also lead to reduced lung/thorax compliance, which would increase the work of breathing.

In order to optimize mechanical ventilation, it is important to ensure patient–ventilator synchrony (ability of the mechanical ventilator to promptly respond to patient demand for flow during inspiration and to allow an unimpeded expiration), which may reduce the requirements for sedation.

Waveform analysis – assessment of patient–ventilator synchrony

Considering that most mechanical ventilators now display real-time ventilator waveforms such as pressure, flow and volume across time or as loops (pressure/volume, flow/volume), it is imperative that physiotherapists familiarize themselves with basic waveform analysis and the expected changes with therapy or alterations to mechanical ventilatory support.

Specific patient interventions, such as patient re-positioning and secretion movement, may adversely affect ventilation (reduced tidal volume, minute volume), particularly in pressure-controlled modes such as PCV or BiPAP. The early detection of untoward changes in waveforms allows the clinician to optimize the ventilator settings (by altering the PEEP or pressure support settings), modify treatment (increase the head-up tilt) and provide intervention (airway suctioning) to minimize any disruptions to the ventilation delivered.

Bedside waveform analysis (Tables 8.2 and 8.3) can be used to determine the presence of specific clinical problems such as excessive patient trigger, inadequate inspiratory flow, asynchrony with cycling from inspiration to expiration, bronchospasm/gas trapping and airway secretions.

The following section will discuss the commonly encountered clinical problems in the intubated and mechanically ventilated patient, and how these problems can be detected through bedside waveform analysis. For this section it will be assumed that the patient is able to breathe in an assisted mode of ventilation (e.g. SIMV with pressure support). The normal pressure waveform is shown in Figure 8.1.

The three variables that determine how effectively a mechanical ventilator delivers a breath are:

- initiation of inspiratory flow (flow or pressure trigger) – the 'trigger' variable
- the volume or pressure to be delivered – the 'set inspiratory' variable, and
- the transition from inspiration to expiration phase – the 'cycling off' variable (Georgopoulos et al 2006).

Troubleshooting for ventilator triggering. The clinician should suspect a problem with triggering in the patient who displays excessive accessory muscle use, especially at the start of inspiration. Analysis of the start of the breath delivery on the pressure/time waveforms will detect the amount of negative pressure deflection (Table 8.2 Curve A). If the trigger effort required from the patient is excessive, then 'missed breath' attempts may be the result (Table 8.2 Curve B), Case study 8.5.

Troubleshooting – cycling from inspiration to expiration. The factors that determine the ventilator cycling from inspiration to expiration normally depend on the mode of ventilation (pressure, volume or dual mode). The cycling parameters are either:

- inspiratory time (in pressure control mode of ventilation)
- tidal volume/flow rate (in volume control mode of ventilation)
- percentage reduction of peak inspiratory flow rate (e.g. when inspiratory flow is reduced to 25% of peak value) in pressure support mode of ventilation.

If a patient attempts to exhale while the ventilator is still delivering inspiratory flow, the contraction of the muscles of expiration will lead to an increase in the work of breathing. Bedside detection of the pressure/time waveforms may demonstrate a positive pressure deflection (pressure/time waveform) at the end of the inspiratory cycle (Table 8.2 Curve D). Reduction of the set inspiratory time, tidal volume or inspiratory pressure should facilitate transition to expiration. However, care should be taken as a reduction in set inspiratory time or inspiratory pressure may lead to significant reductions in tidal volume, which must be monitored.

Troubleshooting – gas trapping/intrinsic–PEEP. The full relaxed respiratory cycle must include enough time for

Table 8.2 Pressure waveforms of common clinical problems, causes and clinical signs (volume-controlled)

Abnormal ventilator waveform appearance	Description and potential causes
A Pressure curve (triggering) *Excessive trigger* 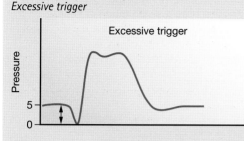	**Pressure curve** At the start of pressure curve there is a negative deflection greater than 1–2 cmH$_2$O, followed by positive pressure breath delivery Potential causes: • excessive trigger settings (e.g. pressure trigger set at −4 cmH$_2$O) • patient distress/agitation/ETT intolerance • inadequate inspiratory support • respiratory muscle weakness Clinical signs: • accessory muscle use at start of breath • increased work of breathing/patient distress
B Pressure curve (breath attempts) *Missed breath attempts* 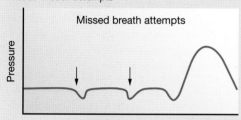	**Pressure curve** Negative deflection(s) in the pressure curve (arrows), below PEEP level without inspiratory flow or positive pressure being delivered Potential causes: • excessive trigger setting (pressure or flow setting) • intrinsic PEEP • ineffective patient effort Clinical signs: • respiratory distress/accessory muscle use • paradoxical respiratory attempts • mismatch between respiratory rate on ventilator and actual patient respiratory rate/attempts at breathing (e.g. total ventilator respiratory rate 12, but calculated rate on basis of observation 22 bpm).
C Pressure curve (flow rate) *Inadequate flow rate* 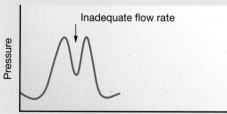	**Pressure curve** Negative inflection in the pressure curve during inspiratory phase (arrow), due to patient inspiratory effort exceeding set ventilator flow rate, often coined 'bunny ears' in appearance with no change in inspiratory flow rate Potential causes: • volume controlled mode with inadequate fixed inspiratory flow rate Clinical signs: • patient appears to be triggering an additional breath during ventilator breath • paradoxical respiratory attempts during ventilator
D Pressure curve (inspiratory time) *Prolonged inspiration* 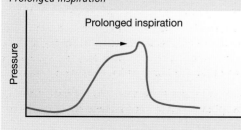	**Pressure curve** A positive inflection at the end of inspiration on the pressure/time curve (arrow), indicating the patient is attempting to exhale while the ventilator is still delivering inspiratory flow. Potential causes: • prolonged inspiratory time or excessive inspiratory pressure/tidal volume Clinical signs • expiratory muscle activation at end of inspiratory phase of respiration of ventilator

8

Table 8.3 Flow waveforms of common clinical problems, causes and clinical signs (volume–controlled)

Abnormal ventilator waveform appearance	Description and potential causes
E Flow curve (expiratory flow) *Gas trapping* 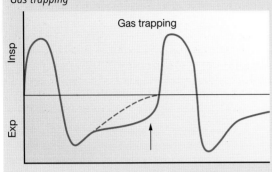	**Expiratory flow curve (end curve)** Expiratory gas trapping (arrow indicates that expiratory flow is still occurring before next positive pressure breath is delivered). Normal exhalation Potential causes: • bronchospasm • COPD • ARDS/ALI • high set respiratory rate, long inspiratory time, with insufficient expiratory time • insufficient PEEP Clinical signs: • expiratory muscle use during expiration • hyperinflated appearance. May result in reduced blood pressure due to raised intrathoracic pressure *(Note: some intensivists disconnect the patient from mechanical ventilator at end of expiration to assess a rebound increase in blood pressure)*
F Flow curve (expiratory flow) *Missed breath attempts* 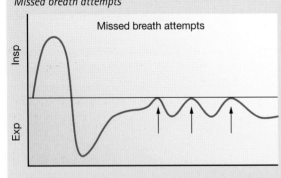	**Expiratory flow curve** Missed breath attempts (arrows) – patient attempts to trigger inspiratory flow Potential causes: • bronchospasm • COPD • ALI/ARDS • insufficient PEEP Clinical signs: • respiratory distress/accessory muscle use • paradoxical respiratory attempts • mismatch between respiratory rate on ventilator and actual patient respiratory rate/attempts at breathing (e.g. total ventilator respiratory rate 12 mismatches patients' actual breath attempts of 22 bpm)
G Flow curve (expiratory flow) Saw-tooth pattern 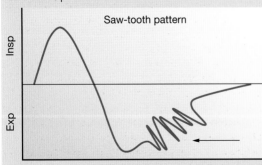	**Expiratory flow curve** Saw-tooth pattern (arrow) on expiration Potential causes: • indicative of secretions in major airways • condensate in ventilator tubing. Clinical signs • palpable fremitus (chest wall or ventilator tubing) • auscultatory signs of airway secretions (crackles, wheezes)

8

CASE STUDY 8.5

Troubleshooting for ventilator triggering (Curve A)

A 60-year-old male patient following upper abdominal surgery, orally intubated and mechanically ventilated in SIMV volume-controlled ventilation, set respiratory rate 10 bpm, flow rate 50 lpm, TV 500 ml, PEEP 5 and FiO_2 0.4. The nursing staff reported that the patient was restless and agitated overnight, and appeared to be intolerant of the endotracheal tube; regular boluses of intravenous sedation were required throughout the evening. The physiotherapist examined the patient and noticed increased accessory muscle use at the start of inspiration (Table 8.2 Curve A). The pressure trigger sensitivity was noted to be at -4 cmH$_2$O and on inspection, the pressure/time waveform was as illustrated in Curve A. The large negative deflection suggested that a relatively high level of work of breathing was required to initiate inspiratory flow. The physiotherapist then reduced the trigger 'sensitivity' from -4 to -1 cmH$_2$O, which resulted in reduced accessory muscle use during inspiration and a reduced negative deflection on the pressure/time curve.

Analysis

This case illustrates that the trigger sensitivity was set too high. Reducing the trigger sensitivity reduced the demand on the work of breathing from the patient and resulted in a lower negative pressure deflection (as shown under Curve A). If these adjustments had not improved the situation, other clinical causes of the increased work of breathing such as intrinsic/auto PEEP should be investigated. Other means of achieving this could be through the use of increased sedation (after discussion with the medical team and dependent on local intensive care unit policy).

Troubleshooting inadequate inspiratory flow delivery (Curve C)

The patient is now being treated by the physiotherapist and has been positioned with the head of the bed flat, in preparation for re-positioning into right sidelying for treatment of his left lower lobe collapse. The physiotherapist notices the patient becoming agitated during repositioning, with increased accessory muscle use and paradoxical chest wall movements. There are also further changes in the pressure/time waveforms (Table 8.2 Curve C). Following a bolus of sedation, the pressure/time curve improved with reduced negative deflection during the inspiratory breath.

Analysis

In patients receiving set volume-controlled modes (SIMV, assist control) with fixed flow rate delivery and with spontaneous breathing effort, the work of breathing will increase if the demand for flow exceeds the set ventilator flow. This may occur during nursing care, exercise or physiotherapy treatments. To reduce the patient inspiratory effort/drive and allow the patient to remain in the same mode of ventilation, the set inspiratory flow rate and sedation could be increased. An alternative way to reduce the demand on the patient's inspiratory effort would be to change to a pressure-controlled mode (variable flow delivery) or dual mode of ventilation (set tidal volume but with variable flow delivery). These decisions, however, should be multidisciplinary, and dependent on the local intensive care unit policy.

(continued from p 294)

complete exhalation to occur, with zero flow at the end of expiration before the next inspiration is delivered. However, in the mechanically ventilated patient, there is often inadequate time for complete exhalation (Blanch et al 2005); hence 'gas trapping' tends to occur (Table 8.3 Curve E).

Gas trapping results in retained gas in the thorax above FRC (causing intrinsic PEEP) which may lead to several cardiac and pulmonary effects:

■ The increase in intrathoracic pressure may lead to reduced cardiac filling pressures and compromise blood pressure and cardiac output.

■ An increase in intrinsic PEEP may increase spontaneous work of breathing, with increased use of expiratory muscles in an attempt to facilitate expiration, and increased use of inspiratory muscles at the start of inspiration due to the generation of increased intrinsic PEEP.

Examination of the expiratory flow waveforms will allow the clinician to determine whether there is near full exhalation before the next inspiration (zero flow, at baseline). A sound understanding of the patient's disease pathology, for example asthma or COPD, will assist the clinician in determining the optimal way of managing gas trapping. For example, if gas trapping is occurring due to inadequate expiratory time, then dependent on the patient status (e.g. normal arterial pH) the set respiratory rate or set tidal volume may be reduced to allow adequate time for full exhalation. On the other hand, gas trapping due to airway narrowing during expiration in patients with asthma, COPD or ARDS may be reduced or avoided by ensuring adequate bronchodilator therapy (again, these decisions should be multidisciplinary and dependent on the local intensive care unit policy).

8

Gas trapping due to intrinsic PEEP may lead to ventilator asynchrony (Dhand 2005). Patients with intrinsic PEEP who are triggering breaths have to generate a large negative intrapleural pressure that is at least equal to the level of intrinsic PEEP plus the trigger sensitivity level of the ventilator, before a breath can be triggered and delivered. Thus if the PEEP is set at 5 cmH_2O, and intrinsic PEEP is 5 cmH_2O, the total PEEP is in fact 10 cmH_2O; i.e. although the set inspiratory trigger is –1 cmH_2O (below PEEP), the patient has to generate a negative intrapleural pressure of at least 6 cmH_2O to trigger a breath. This may result in ineffective or wasted patient effort to trigger a ventilator breath, resulting in patient–ventilator asynchrony.

The expiratory flow waveforms should also be checked to ensure complete exhalation before the next breath delivery (Table 8.3 Curve E). Adequate exhalation before the next inspiration should occur, not only during mandatory breath delivery but also during spontaneous ventilation modes such as CPAP and pressure support. Incomplete exhalation (to zero flow or baseline) puts the patient at risk of attempting to trigger inspiratory gas flow before expiration is complete (Table 8.3 Curves E and F). This may also potentially lead to ineffective triggering efforts and patient–ventilator asynchrony (Table 8.3 Curve F), with missed breath attempts.

Measurement of intrinsic PEEP

The measurement of intrinsic PEEP determines the effect of passive elastic recoil on expiratory flow and hence the patient should be under a mandatory ventilator mode and adequately sedated to minimize any respiratory muscle effort. Most modern mechanical ventilators have the facility to measure intrinsic PEEP either through a manual 'expiratory-hold' or an intrinsic-PEEP diagnostic function. Ventilator waveforms (pressure and flow) must be monitored during the expiratory hold manoeuvre (Fig. 8.9) to ensure the patient is not actively breathing during the pause (normally 2–5 seconds).

Airway secretions. Airway secretions in the mechanically ventilated patient may be difficult to detect through conventional means (auscultation, chest palpation), for the following reasons:

- inability to position the patient properly for examination

- inadequate inspiratory and expiratory flow rates to create turbulent flow (e.g. due to low levels of CPAP and pressure support).

Ventilator flow waveform analysis can assist in the detection of airway secretions. The presence of airway secretions or condensate in the ventilator tubing could induce a 'saw-tooth' pattern or jagged waveform during the expiratory flow (Table 8.3 Curve G and Fig. 8.10). The 'saw-tooth' pattern should disappear with airway suctioning and clearance of secretions or removal of the condensate from the ventilator circuit.

Patient positioning and work of breathing

Supine patient positioning in intensive care is often required when patients are cardiovascularly unstable, have a suspected spinal injury and/or when supported by devices such as an intra-aortic balloon pump. The supine patient position combined with intubation and mechanical ventilation may lead to increased $\dot{V}/\dot{Q}$ mismatch resulting in hypoxaemia. Upright positioning can be used to improve gas exchange and end-expiratory lung volumes even in patients with severe hypoxaemia due to ALI/ARDS (Richard et al 2006), reducing the risk of development of VAP (Drakulovic et al 1999). Head-down positioning, however, is often utilized by physiotherapists for secretion clearance or by medical staff for procedures such as insertion of central venous catheters. Head-down posture may cause reductions in tidal volume and FRC and may be associated with increases in total respiratory resistance and reductions in lung/thorax compliance (Fahy et al 1996). Hence, with the patients on low levels of ventilator support (e.g. 5 cmH_2O CPAP and 5 cmH_2O pressure support), the recumbent position (supine or head down) may result in increased patient work of breathing. The increase in work of breathing may also depend on factors such as

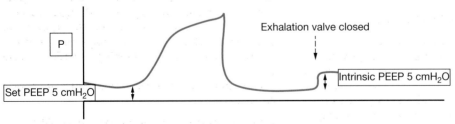

Figure 8.9 Auto-PEEP manoeuvre. The procedure entails closure of the exhalation valve at end exhalation (for up to 3 seconds) to measure the level of intrinsic PEEP (often an automated function in most modern ventilators). The patient should be in a mandatory mode of mechanical ventilation, heavily sedated and/or paralysed to prevent any active respiratory effort. P, pressure; PEEP, positive end-expiratory pressure.

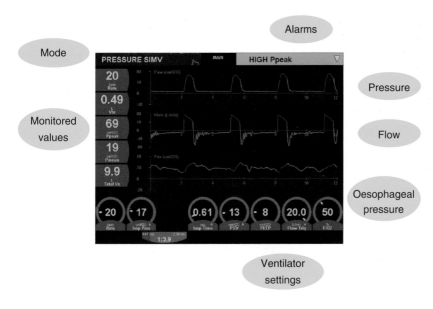

Figure 8.10 Ventilator screen displaying a 'saw-tooth' expiratory flow pattern suggesting the presence of secretions.

8

the level of sedation, diameter of endotracheal tube, muscle strength, lung/thorax compliance (abdominal distension, pulmonary oedema) and airway resistance (airway secretions, bronchospasm).

Appropriately performed physiotherapy is well tolerated from a haemodynamic and metabolic perspective (Berney & Denehy 2003). However, any adverse changes in haemodynamics (blood pressure, heart and pulmonary artery pressure) can be attenuated through increased sedation (Harding et al 1993) or increased pressure support (Harding et al 1995). The increases in metabolic consumption may only be attenuated with neuromuscular blocking agents (Horiuchi et al 1997). But clinicians should be aware that sedation boluses in a pressure-controlled mode of ventilation (e.g. PCV or CPAP and pressure support) may significantly reduce the patient's spontaneous respiratory effort (work of breathing), which may lead to a reduction in tidal volume/minute volume, and additional inspiratory support may be required.

Lung/thoracoabdominal compliance and airway resistance

Reduced lung/thoracoabdominal compliance or increased airway resistance are common causes of increased work of breathing. The physiotherapist's assessment of the patient should identify the problem in this clinical scenario. During repositioning to head down or flat for secretion clearance, the functional residual capacity may be reduced, secretions mobilized and lung/thorax compliance (dynamic) further reduced. This may lead either to reductions

in tidal volume delivered (pressure-controlled modes) or increased peak airway pressures (volume- or dual-controlled modes) and may increase the patient's work of breathing. The mode of ventilation (volume-controlled vs pressure-controlled) may impact on the physiological effects of physiotherapy treatment.

Case study 8.6 examines some issues on ventilation and positioning.

Respiratory muscle strength and weaning

The critically ill patient is predisposed to develop muscle dysfunction/wasting due mainly to inactivity and sepsis, with the consequence of poor activity tolerance, reduced strength and prolonged time on mechanical ventilation in intensive care (Winkelman 2004). The evidence supporting inspiratory muscle training to date has focused on the long-term, difficult to wean patient (Aldrich et al 1989, Martin et al 2002). However, inspiratory muscle training (through reduced trigger sensitivity) in acute critically ill patients from the beginning of mechanical ventilation may not improve respiratory muscle strength or shorten weaning time (Caruso et al 2005).

Interventions aimed at enhancing respiratory muscle strength include:

- respiratory muscle training (Martin et al 2002)
- partially resting the patient overnight (Vassilakopoulos et al 2006) with increased respiratory support (pressure support)

CASE STUDY 8.6

A 70-year-old female patient following abdominal surgery, complicated by sepsis and ALI due to an infected peritoneum. This patient was ventilated in BiPAP mode, set rate 20 bpm, P_{high} 30 cmH$_2$O, P_{low} 10 cmH$_2$O, FiO$_2$ 0.8, with exhaled tidal volume of 400 ml. The morning chest radiograph demonstrated bilateral diffuse pulmonary infiltrates (alveolar shadowing). The physiotherapist examined the patient and reported bilateral crackles on auscultation with palpable fremitus throughout the left hemithorax. The physiotherapist repositioned the patient into right sidelying with the head of the bed flat. The tidal volume reduced from 400 ml to 250 ml, with the respiratory rate unchanged.

What are the implications of the treatment decisions of this physiotherapist?

Analysis

This scenario may commonly occur during physiotherapy treatment and may often be undetected. The reductions in tidal volume may relate to the reduced FRC as a result of altered head-down posturing (from head up to head flat) in combination with a pressure-controlled mode of ventilation. In addition, as the patient had palpable fremitus unilaterally, this is indicative of airway secretions, and repositioning into sidelying may have caused the movement of secretions to the more central airways or caused direct aspiration of secretions into the dependent lung. The set inspiratory pressure in a pressure-controlled mode (such as bilevel ventilation) does not ensure constant tidal volume with changing airways resistance and lung/thorax compliance. The clinician at the bedside must pre-empt and monitor these changes by understanding the disease process, the mode of mechanical ventilation and potential impact of therapy interventions. Inspection of the flow waveforms (reduced inspiratory flow rate and reduced area under the curve) and exhaled tidal volumes (reduced exhaled tidal volume) should alert the clinician to the changing patient status and early recognition/intervention should prevent any untoward changes in gas exchange. Before repositioning the patient head-down, the therapist should have suctioned the airway to clear secretions from central airways and assess cough response. Reassessment of exhaled lung volumes may have demonstrated an increase in tidal volumes with this intervention alone and determined whether there really was a need for repositioning.

The assessment of flow waveforms (saw-tooth) pattern on expiratory flow waveforms, Table 8.3 Curve G) may also have indicated the presence of upper airway secretions, which may have resolved with suctioning alone.

Reduced lung/thorax compliance may be improved with the upright sitting position (Behrakis et al 1983). This, however, does not mean that patients cannot and should not be turned for pressure area care or physiotherapy for secretion clearance. The therapist should, however, be aware of the potent effects of patient repositioning and that changes in mechanical ventilation may be required to minimize any adverse effects (e.g. increased PEEP, FiO$_2$, increased tidal volume or increased inspiratory pressure dependent on the mode of ventilation).

(continued from p 299)

- general exercise training including activities of daily living such as sitting over the edge of the bed, standing and ambulation (Chiang et al 2006, Zafiropoulos et al 2004).

The rehabilitation of the critically ill patient is attracting more and more interest in the literature as a means of minimizing or preventing muscle dysfunction. Activity for the critically ill may be considered along a spectrum of care from passive repositioning into upright or sidelying, to passive range of motion exercises, active assisted exercises, self-care, sitting over the edge of the bed, standing, sitting out of bed and ambulation. The metabolic cost of the activity may therefore be expected to increase as the level of muscle use and participation in activity increases (Weissman & Kemper 1991). However, little is known about the typical level of activity among intensive care unit patients (Winkelman 2004) and there is limited information about the place of activity in preventing complications or improving outcome in ICU (Stiller 2000). The only consistent activity performed by nursing staff may be patient turning for pressure care (Winkelman 2004) with minimal other activities undertaken. Mobilization of an intubated and ventilated patient out of bed (Zafiropoulos et al 2004) can be a useful means of effecting short-term improvements in tidal volume and minute ventilation. Daily rehabilitation/mobilization can significantly improve peripheral and respiratory muscle strength, activities of daily living and reduce time on mechanical ventilation (Chiang et al 2006). Increased pressure support during exercise/physiotherapy may be useful to minimize haemodynamic stress responses.

Evaluation of respiratory muscle strength

The evaluation of respiratory muscle strength in the intubated and mechanically ventilated patient is often complicated by factors such as sedation and lack of cooperation (Man et al 2004).

A basic respiratory strength assessment can be undertaken by the use of a pressure manometer in the circuit or by a diagnostic function on most modern mechanical ventilators. The assessment of maximal inspiratory pressure (MIP), negative pressure generated in the first 100 milliseconds of inspiration ($P_{0.1}$) and forced vital capacity (FVC) manoeuvres are some of the most commonly reported procedures. However, patient cooperation and understanding of the assessment procedures (MIP and FVC) are required and this is not always feasible due to sedation required for the tolerance of the tracheal tube. With the development of magnetic stimulation, it has become possible to non-volitionally assess respiratory muscles in a clinical setting (Man et al 2004). There have not been any reported links between measures of respiratory muscle strength and extubation or weaning outcomes.

Weaning from mechanical ventilation

Although mechanical ventilation may be lifesaving, it is associated with numerous complications such as ventilator-associated pneumonia, cardiovascular compromise, barotrauma and ventilator-induced lung injury (Epstein 2002). Mechanical ventilation may be associated with diaphragmatic dysfunction (Jubran 2006) and reduced inspiratory muscle endurance (Chang et al 2005). Once clinical improvement has occurred, emphasis is placed on weaning or liberating the patient from mechanical ventilation (Epstein 2002). However, the value of weaning the patient from the ventilator as soon as possible must be balanced against the risks of premature withdrawal, which may be associated with re-intubation, in turn associated with increased mortality (MacIntyre 2004). The McMaster Evidence Based Practice Centre (Cook et al 2000) provides a more detailed overview of weaning from mechanical ventilation. The imbalance between increased respiratory workload, decreased respiratory muscle strength and endurance may be important factors associated with ventilator dependence (Caruso et al 2005). Shock on admission, increased APACHE II score

[= (acute physiology score) + (age points) + (chronic health points)]

ARDS and multiple organ dysfunction are variables significantly associated with prolonged time (>21 days) on mechanical ventilation. These patients also suffer from a high rate of failed extubations, unsuccessful weaning, malnutrition and infection (Estenssoro et al 2006).

Key issues in the management of the ventilated patient are outlined in Box 8.6. Suggested guidelines for extubation are given in Box 8.7.

Box 8.6 Key issues that must be addressed in the overall management of the mechanically ventilated patient

When it has been determined that the disease process or processes have begun to stabilize or reverse, clinicians should:

1. Understand the reasons why the patient may still require mechanical ventilation (e.g. respiratory system mechanics, resistance, gas exchange, neuromuscular dysfunction, cardiac failure) and their treatment (e.g. secretions, bronchospasm, pleural effusion, cardiac function).
2. Use assessment techniques to identify whether the patient can tolerate withdrawal of ventilation (e.g. spontaneous breathing trials, wean off pressure support, rapid shallow breathing index).
3. Determine whether the patient requires continued ventilation, and develop an appropriate ventilator management strategy (daily spontaneous breathing trials, mobilization, weaning sedation).
4. Provide for the patient who is likely to remain ventilator-dependent an extended management plan.

(MacIntyre 2004)

Box 8.7 Suggested guidelines for extubation

Ready for extubation?
A simple screening procedure at the bedside to identify a patient's readiness for weaning:

- FiO_2 <0.50
- PEEP ≤5 cmH_2O
- no vasopressor agents
- able to follow simple commands.

The patient may then undergo a short spontaneous breathing trial of CPAP alone or breathing via a T-piece for 30–90 minutes, with the aim to then extubate the patient if he tolerates this trial (Tonnelier et al 2005).
  If the patient fails this trial:

- SaO_2 <90%
- respiratory rate >35 bpm
- variation in heart rate or blood pressure >20%
- agitation

mechanical ventilation is often then reinstituted.

8

Weaning strategies

When the patient's medical condition has been stabilized, weaning off mechanical ventilation is often started. Various approaches to weaning have been adopted by centres around the world (Esteban et al 2000). Bedside measurements of respiratory function (Chapter 3) are often used to assess the suitability of the patient for weaning from mechanical ventilation to extubation, but the predictive success of these measures for the general intensive care population is poor (Conti et al 2004). Recent work by Kuo et al (2006) demonstrated improved predictive accuracy of the measurement of the rapid shallow breathing index at the end of a 2-hour period of spontaneous breathing compared with the traditional method when the measurement is taken at the beginning of the trial. The optimal means to assess appropriateness for weaning and extubation is still evolving.

The requirements for continuing ventilatory support are determined by the balance between the ventilatory capability of the patient and his ventilatory demands (e.g. atelectasis, disease, surgery, sepsis). As the imbalance between ventilatory capability and ventilatory demand begin to resolve (Fig. 8.11), the focus of patient care then concentrates on removing the patient from the ventilator as quickly as possible (MacIntyre 2004). Rehabilitation may play a key role in facilitating weaning from ventilation in long-term patients (Chiang et al 2006).

Controversy exists regarding the most appropriate weaning strategy, the indicators used to assess readiness for weaning/extubation and the use of weaning protocols. Early work (Kollef et al 1997) demonstrated a significantly lower weaning time, when weaning was protocol-led by nurse and therapist compared with physician-led. Weaning protocols may have minimal impact in an intensive care environment where there is a high number of qualified nurses, high physician input, good collaboration between the team members and autonomous nursing decision-making in relation to weaning practices (Rose & Nelson 2006). Other weaning strategies include daily T-piece trials, pressure support and extubation to non-invasive ventilation to facilitate the process (Girault et al 1999).

Tracheostomy

A tracheostomy is often performed in an intensive care patient when long-term ventilation (>7–10 days) is anticipated. Tracheostomy is also performed if there is

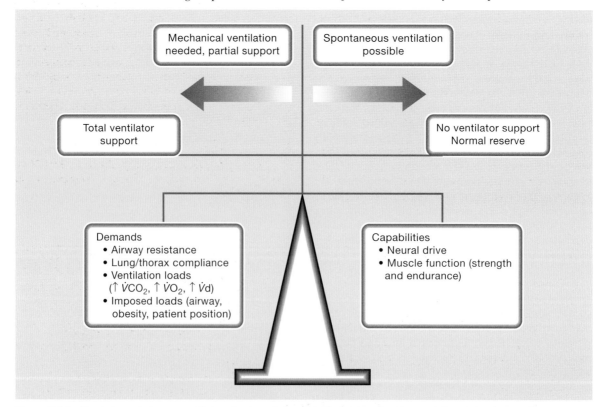

Figure 8.11 The balance between ventilatory loads and demands that determine the need for mechanical ventilator support. Adapted from MacIntyre 2004.

concurrent upper airway obstruction, e.g. tumour, trauma, or if equipment dead space poses an unacceptable hindrance to weaning. A tracheostomy may be instituted either percutaneously or surgically, depending on the urgency and physical features of the patient, such as body mass index, condition and head/neck anatomy. Percutaneous tracheostomy is performed at the bedside and uses a Seldinger dilation technique, which usually leaves only a small residual scar. Surgical tracheostomy requires patient transfer to the operating room, a surgical incision and dissection through to the trachea. In some cases, removal of the cricoid cartilage is necessary but the cosmetic result is less acceptable (Friedman 2006). Tracheostomy assists weaning from mechanical ventilation by reducing dead space, decreasing airway resistance, improving secretion clearance and decreasing the need for sedation (Pierson 2005).

Physiotherapists are usually required to optimize lung function in tracheostomized patients and therefore it is important that they understand the functional characteristics of the tracheostomy tube design and the implications for patient care. Tracheostomy tubes are available in different sizes and styles (Hess 2005). They can be of different diameters and lengths, angled or curved, cuffed or uncuffed, with single or dual tubes (dual-cannula tracheostomy tubes). Fenestrated tracheostomy tubes and tubes which allow subglottic suction are also available (Portex Blue Line Ultra Suctionaid). These latter have a suction port situated above the cuff.

Dimensions of a tracheostomy tube refer to the internal and external diameter, length and curvature of the tube. A patient with a large neck may require a tracheostomy tube with extra proximal length. Too small an internal diameter will increase the resistance to airflow through the tube.

With the cuff deflated, a standard tracheostomy tube allows use of the upper airway and speech (but protection from aspiration is sacrificed). Efficiency of upper airway engagement will be decreased if the outer diameter of the tube is too large.

Dual-cannula tracheostomy tubes have an inner cannula that is disposable or reusable. The use of an inner cannula facilitates regular changing or cleaning and is believed to reduce biofilm formation and the incidence of ventilator-associated pneumonia (Burns et al 1998).

A fenestrated tracheostomy tube is similar to a standard tracheostomy tube except that there is an opening (window) in the posterior portion of the tube above the cuff and the tube is provided with an inner cannula and a plastic plug (decannulation cap). With the cuff deflated, removal of the inner cannula allows the use of the upper airway and permits air to pass through the vocal cords, which facilitates phonation, as does digital occlusion of the tube. A speaking valve can also be placed in the tube for speech training. The decannulation cap allows the patient to breathe through the fenestrations and around the tube and is used to facilitate weaning of the patient from the tracheostomy tube (decannulation). The inner cannula may or may not have a window in situ. Insertion of a non-fenestrated inner cannula allows the tubes to function as an ordinary tracheostomy tube and to be used for suctioning. It should be noted that suction should never be performed with a fenestrated inner cannula in situ, as this will cause damage to the trachea. Fenestrated tracheostomy tubes have also been shown to reduce the work of breathing (Hussey & Bishop 1996). Fenestrated tracheostomy tubes are often used during extended weaning of patients from long-term mechanical ventilation.

Suggested guidelines for decannulation

Pre-weaning criteria have been specified (Heffner 2005, Ladyshewsky & Gousseau 1996) and are summarized in Table 8.4.

Table 8.4   Guidelines for weaning from a tracheostomy

Indications for weaning	Contraindications to weaning
• Original indication for tracheostomy resolving • Spontaneously breathing with regular respiratory pattern and RR <30 breaths/minute • Inspired oxygen <35% with adequate saturation • Strong cough – able to clear to top of tracheostomy tube • Clear chest • Adequate nutrition • Patient swallowing assessed by speech and language therapist and able to cope with own saliva	• Tumour • Upper airway oedema • Absent or inadequate cough or gag reflex • Persistent dysphagia and compromised airway protection • Reduced ability to clear secretions • High respiratory rate >30 breaths/minute

While the management of each patient should be individualized, it has been shown that a multidisciplinary approach with a standardized decisional protocol can result in increased success in weaning (Ceriana et al 2003, Ladyshewsky & Gousseau 1996). The usual progression (although this can vary from centre to centre) of weaning a tracheostomy is:

- cuff deflation/swallow assessment
- fenestrated tube
- downsizing of tube
- capping off
- decannulation.

During each stage, there should be close monitoring of respiratory rate, respiratory muscle work, oxygen saturation and cardiovascular parameters. Presence of wheeze, stridor, drooling and respiratory distress indicate that the patient should not progress to the next stage. A mini-tracheostomy (cuffless tracheal tube) may be appropriate following decannulation, if the patient requires assistance with secretion clearance.

Criteria employed to assess each aspect and stage of weaning are controversial. The 'blue dye' test used to assess swallowing is cited in the major international guidelines (Heffner & Hess 2001) but has been shown to have low sensitivity and may give a false-negative result, especially when compared with video-fluoroscopy (Ceriana et al 2003). Actual cough strength and ability to clear secretions can be subjective; therefore maximal expiratory pressure (MEP) and/or peak flow measurements have been used to predict the likelihood of being weaned from tracheotomy. During mechanical ventilation, in a stable patient, cuff deflation can be used to facilitate verbal communication (termed 'leak speech' without the use of a speaking valve).

The physiotherapist's role in weaning from mechanical ventilation

Non-physician and nurse-led weaning may significantly improve weaning outcomes, but the impact may depend on the medical staffing levels (Krishnan et al 2004). The physiotherapist's role in weaning could be directed towards:

- early assessment of patient rehabilitation potential (strength, endurance, bed mobility, transfer training)
- assistance with secretion clearance
- respiratory muscle training

- ambulatory ventilation where appropriate
- identify readiness for extubation (e.g. minimal secretions, effective cough, airway reflexes present, neurological status)
- facilitate early appropriate endotracheal extubation to institute NIV where appropriate
- assisting with tracheostomy weaning (e.g. periods of spontaneous breathing interspersed with periods of respiratory muscle rest on mechanical ventilation)
- recognizing patients at risk of difficulties in weaning: e.g. COPD, heart failure, obesity, chronic renal failure, flail chest and being proactive in applying NIV
- appropriate respiratory management including titration of PEEP and pressure support settings to facilitate 'leak speech' or the use of speaking valves.

CONCLUSION

The extended role of the physiotherapist in intensive care is currently topical (McPherson et al 2006). While the role and responsibilities of the physiotherapist vary from country to country and even hospital to hospital in the same city, over recent years physiotherapists have successfully gained greater autonomy and their role within the ICU in weaning, extubation, ventilator and tracheostomy management, fibre optic bronchoscopy, ICU outreach, post ICU clinics, and bedside thoracic ultrasound have all received varying amounts of endorsement at different centres.

This chapter has described various means of monitoring and supporting the major organ systems of the body and the implications for physiotherapy intervention, and adopted a problem-based discussion of various physiotherapeutic interventions in the intensive care unit. The inclusion of waveform analysis associated with mechanical ventilation, concepts of weaning from the ventilator and the role of the physiotherapist in optimization of work of breathing, all aim to encourage a greater awareness of the extended scope of their role in intensive care. Tables 8.5 and 8.6 provide a quick reference table for ventilator troubleshooting and management.

In addition to clinical research, it is essential that documentary evidence of the cost-effectiveness of physiotherapy in intensive care is collected, to provide outcomes and to direct clinical practice in the future. Opportunities include engagement in collaborative approaches and large observational databases.

Table 8.5   Troubleshooting – management of patients under mechanical ventilation

Events	Possible causes	Possible action
High-pressure alarm signals (volume- or dual-controlled modes)	Patient is restless and/with asynchronous breathing	• Calm the patient • Auscultate breath sounds – right and left side equal? • Check tidal volume • Check with nurse/doctor for sedation • If the patient has adequate respiratory drive, check with doctor to consider pressure controlled/CPAP/pressure support modes which might be more comfortable for the patient
	Increased airway resistance • Position of ETT • Secretions • Bronchospasm	• Check ETT • Auscultate – coarse crackles/wheezes? • Suction airway • Discuss with medical team – bronchodilators
	Obstruction in airway • Secretions • Patient biting the tube	• Suction airway • Insert Guedel airway or bite block to stop biting of endotracheal tube • MHI and saline lavage
	Poor compliance (stiff lung) • Pulmonary oedema • Pleural effusion • Pneumothorax	• Auscultate breath sounds – right and left side equal? • Check chest radiograph and appropriate management of condition • Consider reducing set inspiratory flow rate in volume-controlled or change over to pressure or dual-controlled ventilation
Low-pressure alarm signals	• Disconnection of circuit • Cuff leak • Large negative pressure patient effort	• Check tidal volume/expired minute volume • Manually ventilate the patient while checking and reconnecting the circuit • Check cuff pressure
	Malfunction of the ventilator	• Check function of ventilator
Slight drop (1 to 2 cmH$_2$O) in airway pressure in volume-controlled mode is normal after physiotherapy (no alarm signal)	The patient's lung compliance and/or airway resistance has improved (e.g. after secretion clearance)	• No action required
Hypoxaemia	Incorrect settings	• Increase FiO$_2$ • Check settings (tidal volume, rate, PEEP) and alter settings if necessary
	Circuit/airway disconnection	• Check tidal volume/expired minute volume • Auscultate breath sounds • Manually ventilate the patient while checking and reconnecting the circuit
	Secretions	• Auscultate breath sounds • Suction airway (if secretions are tenacious and/or poor cough, saline and/or manual hyperinflation may be required)
	Malposition of the tracheal tube (e.g. down right main bronchus)	• Auscultate breath sounds • Check position of ETT at lip level, check ETT ties • Check chest radiograph
	Pneumothorax/pleural effusion	• Auscultate breath sounds – right and left side equal • Check chest radiograph
	Onset of new medical problem (e.g. sputum plugging, atelectasis, pulmonary oedema)	• Check chest radiograph • Auscultate/palpate chest • Bronchoscopy
	Medications (vasodilators)	• Increase FiO$_2$

8

CPAP, continuous positive airway pressure; ETT, endotracheal tube; FiO$_2$, fractional inspired oxygen concentration; PEEP, positive end-expiratory pressure

If the following happens, alert help, and the recommended actions for consideration are:

Table 8.6

If	Action
Cardiopulmonary arrest	Stop intervention and follow basic life support or advanced life support protocols
Sudden drop in blood pressure (possibly associated with manual hyperinflation or patient repositioning)	• Check arterial line • Stop manual hyperinflation but maintain tidal breaths • Return patient to supine • Monitor vital signs (blood pressure and SpO_2)
Accidental removal of chest drain	• Notify nursing staff immediately • Apply immediate constant pressure to drain site • Stop manual inflation • Put patient to supine and back onto ventilator • Monitor vital signs • If patient has spontaneous effort, ask patient to exhale before applying pressure to drain site
Accidental removal or dislodging of central venous line or pulmonary artery catheter	• Notify nursing staff immediately • If line is removed, apply constant pressure to site • If dislodged, prevent further traction on line

Sudden onset of cardiac arrhythmias	• Check chest leads
	• Monitor vital signs
	• Alert help if:
	  — The arrhythmias progress from 2nd degree to 3rd degree/complete block
	  — Arrhythmias are frequent ectopic beats of multiple and/or ventricular origin and impair blood pressure
	• Check electrolytes (K^+, Mg^{2+})

Sudden desaturation	• Check oximeter probe, pulse waveform • Stop intervention and hyperoxygenate • May need to disconnect the patient from ventilator and apply manual lung inflation – to assess respiratory status and determine airway resistance (e.g. blocked tube, biting tube, bronchospasm, secretions) and or lung/thorax compliance problem (pneumothorax) • Check with medical team for consideration of increased FiO_2 or PEEP
Sudden rise in intracranial pressure	• Check ICP tracing • Search for causes (e.g. raised CO_2, agitation, reduced sedation, paralysis ceased, secretions) • Check head and neck alignment and position • Nurse patient with head of bed up 30 degrees • Monitor vital signs – especially arterial saturations • If manual lung ventilation was being delivered, terminate treatment and resume mechanical ventilation • Liaise with medical team
Blocked tracheal tube	• Alert nursing/medical staff • Check positioning of tube • Attempt suction with saline/manual ventilation • Deflate cuff • Assist ventilation with a resuscitation bag with face mask • Monitor vital signs

table continues

If	Action
Dislodged tracheal tube (signs of loss of tidal volume or airway pressure, with evident cuff leak)	• Inform medical team • Hyperoxygenate • Assess if patient can be ventilated by bag/ mask • Do not attempt to advance tracheal tube! – You may advance it into the oesophagus or right main bronchus, thus ventilating only one lung (in which case there will be no breath sound over the left lung)
Sudden onset of 'absent breath sound' over one lung	• Alert nursing/medical staff • Assess cause (collapse, sputum plug, pneumothorax, misplaced tube, effusion) • If effective, continue manual lung inflation • Check chest radiograph (or request for one if required) • Monitor vital signs
Self-extubation	• Alert nursing/medical staff • Terminate treatment and hyperoxygenate via mask • Apply manual lung ventilation via a resuscitation bag with a face mask • Assess vital signs • Assess suitability for non-invasive ventilation (presence of good cough and gag reflex; absence of copious secretions)
Sudden reduction in level of consciousness	• Alert nursing/medical staff • Check vital signs, especially saturations and blood pressure • Terminate treatment and resume mechanical ventilation • If patient has spontaneous breathing with good saturations, administer high level of oxygen via a face mask • Attempt to rouse patient, score Glasgow Coma Scale • Monitor vital signs

CPAP, continuous positive airway pressure; FiO_2, fractional inspired oxygen concentration; PEEP, positive end-expiratory pressure; ETT, endotracheal tube; SpO_2, oxygen saturation; K^+, potassium; Mg^{2+}, magnesium; CO_2, carbon dioxide; ICP, intracranial pressure

References

Ackerman MH, Mick DJ 1998 Instillation of normal saline before suctioning in patients with pulmonary infections: a prospective randomized controlled trial. American Journal of Critical Care 7(4): 261–266

Agvald-Ohman C, Wernerman J, Nord CE, Edlund C 2003 Anaerobic bacteria commonly colonize the lower airways of intubated ICU patients. Clinical Microbiology and Infection 9(5): 397–405

Aldrich TK, Karpel JP, Uhrlass RM et al 1989 Weaning from mechanical ventilation: adjunctive use of inspiratory muscle resistive training. Critical Care Medicine 17(2): 143–147

American Association for Respiratory Care (AARC) 1995 Clinical practice guidelines. Capnography/ capnometry during mechanical ventilation. Respiratory Care 40(12): 1321–1324

Antonaglia V, Pascotto S, Simoni LD, Zin WA 2006 Effects of a sigh on the respiratory mechanical properties in ALI patients. J Clin Monit Comput 20(4): 243–249

Arroliga A, Frutos-Vivar F, Hall J et al 2005 Use of sedatives and neuromuscular blockers in a cohort of patients receiving mechanical ventilation. Chest 128(2): 496–506

Artucio H, Pereira M 1990 Cardiac arrhythmias in critically ill patients: epidemiologic study. Critical Care Medicine 18(12): 1383–1388

Bach JR 1993 Mechanical insufflation-exsufflation. Comparison of peak expiratory flows with manually assisted and unassisted coughing techniques. Chest 104(5): 1553–1562

Bach JR, Saporito LR 1996 Criteria for extubation and tracheostomy tube removal for patients with ventilatory failure. A different approach to weaning. Chest 110(6): 1566–1571

Barbas CS, de Matos GF, Pincelli MP et al 2005 Mechanical ventilation in acute respiratory failure: recruitment and high positive end-expiratory pressure are necessary. Current Opinion in Critical Care 11(1): 18–28

Barberis L, Manno E, Guerin C 2003 Effect of end-inspiratory pause duration on plateau pressure in mechanically ventilated patients. Intensive Care Medicine 29(1): 130–134

Bargues L, Vaylet F, Le Bever H, L'Her P, Carsin H 2005 Respiratory dysfunction in burned patients. Revue des Maladies Respiratoires. 22(3): 449–460

Baumburger JP, Goodfriend RB 1951 Determination of arterial oxygen tension in man by equilibration through intact skin. Federation Proceedings 10: 10–21

Behrakis PK, Baydur A, Jaeger MJ, Milic-Emili J 1983 Lung mechanics in sitting and horizontal body positions. Chest 83(4): 643–646

Bein T, Metz C, Keyl C, Pfeifer M, Taeger K 1996 Effects of extreme lateral posture on hemodynamics and plasma atrial natriuretic peptide levels in critically ill patients. Intensive Care Medicine 22(7): 651–655

Bellner J, Romner B, Reinstrup P et al 2004 Transcranial Doppler sonography pulsatility index (PI) reflects intracranial pressure (ICP). Surgical Neurology 62(1): 45–51

Belott P 1999 Bioimpedance in the pacemaker clinic. AACN Clinical Issues 10(3): 414–418

Bernard GR, Artigas A, Brigham KL et al 1994 The American-European Consensus Conference on ARDS. Definitions, mechanisms, relevant outcomes, and clinical trial coordination. American Journal of Respiratory and Critical Care Medicine 149(3 Pt 1): 818–824

Bernet-Buettiker V, Ugarte MJ, Frey B et al 2005 Evaluation of a new combined transcutaneous measurement of PCO_2/pulse oximetry oxygen saturation ear sensor in newborn patients. Pediatrics 115(1): e64–68

Berney S, Denehy L 2002 A comparison of the effects of manual and ventilator hyperinflation on static lung compliance and sputum production in intubated and ventilated intensive care patients. Physiotherapy Research International 7(2): 100–108

Berney S, Denehy L 2003 The effect of physiotherapy treatment on oxygen consumption and haemodynamics in patients who are critically ill. Australian Journal of Physiotherapy 49(2): 99–105

Berney S, Denehy L, Pretto J 2004 Head-down tilt and manual hyperinflation enhance sputum clearance in patients who are intubated and ventilated. Australian Journal of Physiotherapy 50(1): 9–14

Billard V, Gambus PL, Chamoun N, Stanski DR, Shafer SL 1997 A comparison of spectral edge, delta power, and bispectral index as EEG measures of alfentanil, propofol, and midazolam drug effect. Clinical Pharmacology and Therapeutics 61(1): 45–58

Blanch L, Bernabe F, Lucangelo U 2005 Measurement of air trapping, intrinsic positive end-expiratory pressure, and dynamic hyperinflation in mechanically ventilated patients. Respiratory Care 50(1): 110–23; discussion 23–4

Boitano LJ 2006 Management of airway clearance in neuromuscular disease. Respiratory Care 51(8): 913–22

Boldt J, Menges T, Wollbruck M, Hammermann H, Hempelmann G 1994 Is continuous cardiac output measurement using thermodilution reliable in the critically ill patient? Critical Care Medicine 22(12): 1913–1918

Boots RJ, George N, Faoagali JL et al 2006 Double-heater-wire circuits and heat-and-moisture exchangers and the risk of ventilator-associated pneumonia. Critical Care Medicine 34(3): 687–693

Bowton DL 1999 Nosocomial pneumonia in the ICU – year 2000 and beyond. Chest 115(3 Suppl): 28S–33S

Brucia JJ, Owen DC, Rudy EB 1992 The effects of lidocaine on intracranial hypertension. Journal of Neuroscience Nursing 24(4): 205–214

Burns SM, Spilman S, Wilmoth D et al 1998 Are frequent inner cannula changes necessary? A pilot study. Heart and Lung 27: 58–62

Cabello B, Mancebo J 2006 Work of breathing. Intensive Care Medicine 32(9): 1311–1314

Caruso P, Denari SD, Ruiz SA et al 2005 Inspiratory muscle training is ineffective in mechanically ventilated critically ill patients. Clinics 60 (6): 479–484

Cereda M, Villa F, Colombo E et al 2001 Closed system endotracheal suctioning maintains lung volume during volume-controlled mechanical ventilation. Intensive Care Medicine 27(4): 648–454

Ceriana P, Carlucci A, Navalesi P et al 2003 Weaning from tracheotomy in long-term mechanically ventilated patients: feasibility of a decisional flow chart and clinical outcome. Intensive Care Medicine 29: 845–848

Chang A, Hodges P, Boots R, Paratz J 2004a Standing with assistance of a tilt table in intensive care: a survey of Australian physiotherapy practice. Australian Journal of Physiotherapy 50(1): 51–54

Chang A, Hodges P, Paratz J, Boots R 2004b Using a tilt table improves minute ventilation in critically ill patients. Archives of Rehabilitation Medicine 85(12): 1972–1976

Chang AT, Boots RJ, Brown MG, Paratz J, Hodges PW 2004 Reduced inspiratory muscle endurance following successful weaning from prolonged mechanical ventilation. Chest 128(2): 553–559

Chastre J 2006 Ventilator-associated pneumonia: what is new? Surgical Infection 7(Suppl 2): S81–85

Chatwin M, Ross E, Hart N et al 2003 Cough augmentation with mechanical insufflation/exsufflation in patients with neuromuscular weakness. European Respiratory Journal 21(3): 502–508

Chiang L-L, Wang L-Y, Wu C-P, Wu H-D, Wu Y-T 2006 Effects of physical training on functional status in patients with prolonged mechanical ventilation. Physical Therapy 86: 1271–1281

Choi JS, Jones AY 2005 Effects of manual hyperinflation and suctioning in respiratory mechanics in mechanically ventilated patients with ventilator-associated pneumonia. Australian Journal of Physiotherapy 51(1): 25–30

Chytra I 2002 Ventilator-associated pneumonia. RT International Fall: 30–42

Conti G, Montini L, Pennisi MA et al 2004 A prospective, blinded evaluation of indexes proposed to predict weaning from mechanical ventilation. Intensive Care Medicine 30(5): 830–836

Cook D, Meade M, Guyatt G, Griffith L, Booker L 2000 Criteria for weaning from mechanical ventilation. Evidence Report/Technology Assessment No. 23 (Prepared by McMaster University under Contract No. 290–97–0017). AHRQ Publication No. 01–E010. Rockville MD: Agency for Healthcare Research and Quality

Davis K, Johannigman JA, Campbell RS et al 2001 The acute effects of body position strategies and respiratory therapy in paralyzed patients with acute lung injury. Critical Care 5 (2): 81–87

Dhand R 2005 Ventilator graphics and respiratory mechanics in the patient with obstructive lung disease. Respiratory Care 50(2): 246–261; discussion 59–61

Dodek P, Keenan S, Cook D et al 2004 Evidence-based clinical practice guideline for the prevention of ventilator-associated pneumonia. Annals of Internal Medicine 141(4): 305–313

Dowdy DW, Eid MP, Sedrakyan A et al 2005 Quality of life in adult survivors of critical illness: a systematic review of the literature. Intensive Care Medicine 31(5): 611–620

Drakulovic MB, Torres A, Bauer TT et al 1999 Supine body position as a risk factor for nosocomial pneumonia in mechanically ventilated patients: a randomised trial. Lancet 354(9193): 1851–1858

Dutton RP, McCunn M 2003 Traumatic brain injury. Current Opinion in Critical Care 9(6): 503–509

Epstein SK 2002 Weaning from mechanical ventilation. Respiratory Care 47(4): 454–466

Esteban A, Anzueto A, Alia I et al 2000 How is mechanical ventilation employed in the intensive care unit? An international utilization review. American Journal of Respiratory and

8

Critical Care Medicine 161(5): 1450–1458

Estenssoro E, Reina R, Canales HS et al 2006 The distinct clinical profile of chronically critically ill patients: a cohort study. Critical Care 10(3): R89

Fabregas N, Gambus PL, Valero R et al 2004 Can bispectral index monitoring predict recovery of consciousness in patients with severe brain injury? Anesthesiology 101(1): 43–51

Fahy BG, Barnas GM, Nagle SE et al 1996 Effects of Trendelenburg and reverse Trendelenburg postures on lung and chest wall mechanics. Journal of Clinical Anesthesia 8(3): 236–244

Friedman Y 2006 Percutaneous versus surgical tracheostomy: the continuing saga. Critical Care Medicine 34(8): 2250–225

Gao F, Melody T, Daniels DF, Giles S, Fox S 2005 The impact of compliance with 6-hour and 24-hour sepsis bundles on hospital mortality in patients with severe sepsis: a prospective observational study. Critical Care 9(6): R764–770

Garstang SV, Kirshblum SC, Wood KE 2000 Patient preference for in-exsufflation for secretion management with spinal cord injury. Journal of Spinal Cord Medicine 23(2): 80–85

Gattinoni L, Pelosi P, Suter PM et al 1998 Acute respiratory distress syndrome caused by pulmonary and extrapulmonary disease. Different syndromes? American Journal of Respiratory and Critical Care Medicine 158(1): 3–11

Gattinoni L, Vagginelli F, Carlesso E, Taccone P, Conte V, Chiumello D, Valenza F, Caironi P, Pesenti A: Prone-Supine Study Group 2003 Decrease in $PaCO_2$ with prone position is predictive of improved outcome in acute respiratory distress syndrome. Critical Care Medicine 31(12): 2727–2733

Georgopoulos D, Prinianakis G, Kondili E 2006 Bedside waveforms interpretation as a tool to identify patient-ventilator asynchronies. Intensive Care Medicine 32(1): 34–47

Germann P, Braschi A, Della Rocca G et al 2005 Inhaled nitric oxide therapy in adults: European expert recommendations. Intensive Care Medicine 31(8): 1029–1041

Girault C, Daudenthun I, Chevron V et al 1999 Non-invasive ventilation as a systematic extubation and weaning technique in acute-on-chronic respiratory failure: a prospective, randomized controlled study. American Journal of Respiratory and Critical Care Medicine 160(1): 86–92

Gomersall CD, Oh TE 1997 Haemodynamic monitoring. In: Oh TE (ed) Intensive care manual, 4th edn. Butterworth-Heinemann, Oxford, pp 831–838

Gray HH, Dawkins KD, Morgan JM, Simpson IA 2002 Examination of the cardiovascular system. In: Lecture notes on cardiology, 4th edn. Blackwell Publishing, Denmark, p 12

Griffiths RD, Palmer TE, Helliwell T, MacLennan P, MacMillan RR 1995 Effect of passive stretching on the wasting of muscle in the critically ill. Nutrition 11(5): 428–432

Hagler DA, Traver GA 1994 Endotracheal saline and suction catheters: sources of lower airway contamination. American Journal of Critical Care 3(6): 444–447

Harding J, Kemper M, Weissman C 1993 Alfentanil attenuates the cardiopulmonary response of critically ill patients to an acute increase in oxygen demand induced by chest physiotherapy. Anesthesia and Analgesia 77(6): 1122–1129

Harding J, Kemper M, Weissman C 1995 Pressure support ventilation attenuates the cardiopulmonary response to an acute increase in oxygen demand. Chest 107(6): 1665–1672

Haug E, Miner J, Dannehy M, Seigel T, Biros M 2004 Bispectral electroencephalographic analysis of head-injured patients in the emergency department. Academic Emergency Medicine 11(4): 349–352

Hedenstierna G, Brismar B, Strandberg A, Lundquist H, Tokics L 1985 New aspects on atelectasis during anaesthesia. Clinical Physiology 5 (Suppl 3): 127–131

Heffner JE 2005 Management of the chronically ventilated patient with a tracheostomy. Chronic Respiratory Disease 2(3):151–161

Heffner JE, Hess D 2001 Tracheostomy management in the critically ill patient. Clinical Chest Medicine 22: 55–69

Hess DE 2005 Tracheostomy tubes and related appliances. Respiratory Care 50: 497–510

Hilbert G, Gruson D, Vargas F et al 2001 Noninvasive ventilation in immunosuppressed patients with pulmonary infiltrates, fever, and acute respiratory failure. New England Journal of Medicine 344(7): 481–487

Hodgson C, Denehy L, Ntoumenopoulos G, Santamaria J, Carroll S 2000 An investigation of the early effects of manual lung hyperinflation in critically ill patients. Anaesthesia and Intensive Care 28(3): 255–261

Horiuchi K, Jordan D, Cohen D, Kemper MC, Weissman C 1997 Insights into

the increased oxygen demand during chest physiotherapy. Critical Care Medicine 25(8): 1347–1351

Huang SJ, Hong WC, Han YY et al 2006 Clinical outcome of severe head injury using three different ICP and CPP protocol-driven therapies. Journal of Clinical Neuroscience 13(8): 818–822

Hussey JD, Bishop MJ 1996 Pressures required to move gas through the native airway in the presence of a fenestrated vs a nonfenestrated tracheostomy tube. Chest 110: 494–497

Ibanez J, Raurich JM, Abizanda R et al 1981 The effect of lateral positions on gas exchange in patients with unilateral lung disease during mechanical ventilation. Intensive Care Medicine 7(5): 231–234

Jaffe MB 1999 Partial CO_2 rebreathing cardiac output – operating principles of the NICO system. Journal of Clinical Monitoring and Computing 15(6): 387–401

Jensen LA, Onyskiw JE, Prasad NG 1998 Meta-analysis of arterial oxygen saturation monitoring by pulse oximetry in adults. Heart and Lung 27(6): 387–408

Jones AYM 2001 Intensive care physiotherapy – medical staff perceptions. Hong Kong Physiotherapy Journal 19: 9–16

Jones AYM 2002 Secretion movement during manual lung inflation and mechanical ventilation. Respiratory Physiology and Neurobiology 132(3): 321–327

Jones AYM, Hutchinson RC, Oh TE 1992a A comparison of the peak expiratory flow rates produced by two different circuits in intubated patients. Australian Journal of Physiotherapy 38: 211–215

Jones AYM, Hutchinson RC, Oh TE 1992b Effects of bagging and percussion on total static compliance of the respiratory system. Physiotherapy 78: 661–666

Jones AYM, Jones RDM, Bacon-Shone J 1991 A comparison of the expiratory flow rates in two breathing circuits used for manual inflation of the lungs. Physiotherapy 77(9): 593–597

Jorgensen L, Jacobsen BK, Wilsgaard T, Magnus JH 2000 Walking after stroke: does it matter? Changes in bone mineral density within the first 12 months after stroke. A longitudinal study. Osteoporosis International 11(5): 381–387

Jubran A 2006 Critical illness and mechanical ventilation: effects on the diaphragm. Respiratory Care 51(9): 1054–1061; discussion 1062–1064

Kendrick AH 2001 Non-invasive blood gas measurement. 1. Pulse Oximetry.

In. The buyer's guide. European Respiratory Society, pp 15–23

Kirschenbaum L, Azzi E, Sfeir T, Tietjen P, Astiz M 2002 Effect of continuous lateral rotational therapy on the prevalence of ventilator-associated pneumonia in patients requiring long-term ventilatory care. Critical Care Medicine 30(9): 1983–1986

Kollef MH, Shapiro SD, Silver P et al 1997 A randomized, controlled trial of protocol–directed versus physician–directed weaning from mechanical ventilation. Critical Care Medicine 25(4): 567–574

Konrad F, Schreiber T, Brecht-Kraus D, Georgieff M 1994 Mucociliary transport in ICU patients. Chest 105(1): 237–241

Krause MW, van Aswegen H, de Wet EH 2000 Postural drainage in intubated patients with acute lobar atelectasis: a pilot study. South African Journal of Physiotherapy 56(3): 29–32

Krishnan JA, Moore D, Robeson C, Rand CS, Fessler HE 2004 A prospective, controlled trial of a protocol-based strategy to discontinue mechanical ventilation. American Journal of Respiratory and Critical Care Medicine 169(6): 673–678

Kumar AB 1997 Imaging techniques in intensive care. In: Oh TE (ed) Intensive care manual, 4th edn. Butterworth-Heinemann, Oxford, pp 855–859.

Kuo PH, Wu HD, Lu BY et al 2006 Predictive value of rapid shallow breathing index measured at initiation and termination of a 2-hour spontaneous breathing trial for weaning outcome in ICU patients. Journal of the Formosan Medical Association 105(5): 390–398

Ladyshewsky A, Gousseau A 1996 Successful tracheal weaning. Canadian Nurse 92(2): 35–38

Lasocki S, Lu Q, Sartorius A et al 2006 Open and closed-circuit endotracheal suctioning in acute lung injury: efficiency and effects on gas exchange. Anesthesiology 104(1): 39–47

Latronico N, Shehu I, Seghelini E 2005 Neuromuscular sequelae of critical illness. Current Opinion in Critical Care 11(4): 381–390

Lee CK, Ng KS, Tan SG, Ang R 2001 Effect of different endotracheal suctioning systems on cardiorespiratory parameters of ventilated patients. Annals of the Academy of Medicine, Singapore 30(3): 239–244

Lellouche F, Mancebo J, Jolliet P et al 2006 A multicenter randomized trial of computer-driven protocolized weaning from mechanical ventilation. American Journal of Respiratory and

Critical Care Medicine 174(8): 894–900

Lerga C, Zapata MA, Herce A et al 1997 [Endotracheal suctioning of secretions: effects of instillation of normal serum]. Enfermería Intensiva 8(3): 129–137

Levitt JE, Matthay MA 2006 Treatment of acute lung injury: historical perspective and potential future therapies. Semin Respiratory Critical Care Medicine 27(4): 426–437

Lindegaard K-F 1992 Indices of pulsatility. In: Newell DW, Aaslid R (eds) Transcranial Doppler. Raven Press, New York, pp 67–82

Maa SH, Hung TJ, Hsu KH et al 2005 Manual hyperinflation improves alveolar recruitment in difficult-to-wean patients. Chest 128(4): 2714–2721

MacIntyre NR 2004 Evidence-based ventilator weaning and discontinuation. Respiratory Care 49(7): 830–836

MacIntyre NR 2005 Current issues in mechanical ventilation for respiratory failure. Chest 128(5 Suppl 2): 561S–7S

MacLean D, Drummond G, Macpherson C, McLaren G, Prescott R 1989 Maximum expiratory airflow during chest physiotherapy on ventilated patients before and after the application of an abdominal binder. Intensive Care Medicine 15(6): 396–399

Maggiore SM, Lellouche F, Pigeot J et al 2003 Prevention of endotracheal suctioning-induced alveolar derecruitment in acute lung injury. American Journal of Respiratory and Critical Care Medicine 167(9): 1215–1224

Man WD, Moxham J, Polkey MI 2004 Magnetic stimulation for the measurement of respiratory and skeletal muscle function. European Respiratory Journal 24(5): 846–860

Martin AD, Davenport PD, Franceschi AC, Harman E 2002 Use of inspiratory muscle strength training to facilitate ventilator weaning: a series of 10 consecutive patients. Chest 122(1): 192–196

Matthay MA, Zimmerman GA, Esmon C et al 2003 Future research directions in acute lung injury: summary of a National Heart, Lung, and Blood Institute working group. American Journal of Respiratory and Critical Care Medicine 167(7): 1027–1035

Maxwell LJ, Ellis ER 2003 The effect of circuit type, volume delivered and 'rapid release' on flow rates during manual hyperinflation. Australian Journal of Physiotherapy 49(1): 31–38

McCarren B, Chow CM 1998 Description of manual hyperinflation in intubated patients with atelectasis.

Physiotherapy Theory and Practice 14: 199–210

McPherson K, Kersten P, George S et al 2006 A systematic review of evidence about extended roles for allied health professionals. Journal of Health Services Research and Policy 11(4): 240–247

Messerole E, Peine P, Wittkopp S, Marini JJ, Albert RK 2002 The pragmatics of prone positioning. American Journal of Respiratory and Critical Care Medicine 165(10): 1359–1363

Metnitz PG, Bartens C, Fischer M et al 1999 Antioxidant status in patients with acute respiratory distress syndrome. Intensive Care Medicine 25(2): 180–185

Miller RD 2005 Monitors of cerebral blood flow. In: Miller's anesthesia, 6th edn. Elsevier Churchill Livingstone, Philadelphia, PA [Edinburgh], pp 1540–1542

Mills GH, Ponte J, Hamnegard CH et al 2001 Tracheal tube pressure change during magnetic stimulation of the phrenic nerves as an indicator of diaphragm strength on the intensive care unit. British Journal of Anaesthesia 87(6): 876–884

Minei JP, Nathens AB, West M et al 2006 Inflammation and the host response to injury, a large-scale collaborative project: patient-oriented research core-standard operating procedures for clinical care. II. Guidelines for prevention, diagnosis and treatment of ventilator-associated pneumonia (VAP) in the trauma patient. Journal of Trauma 60(5): 1106–1113

Mols G, Priebe HJ, Guttmann J 2006 Alveolar recruitment in acute lung injury. British Journal of Anaesthesia 96(2): 156–166

Monafo WW 1996 Initial management of burns. New England Journal of Medicine 335(21): 1581–1586

Moran T, Bellapart J, Vari A, Mancebo J 2006 Heat and moisture exchangers and heated humidifiers in acute lung injury/acute respiratory distress syndrome patients. Effects on respiratory mechanics and gas exchange. Intensive Care Medicine 32(4): 524–531

Neklaudov M, Bellander B, Mure M 2006 Oxygenation and cerebral perfusion pressure improved in prone position. Acta Anaesthesiologica Scandinavica 50(8): 932–936

Newman DG, Callister R 1999 The non-invasive assessment of stroke volume and cardiac output by impedance cardiography: a review. Aviation, Space and Environmental Medicine 70(8): 780–789

Norrenberg M, Vincent JL 2000 A profile of European intensive care unit physiotherapists. European Society of

Intensive Care Medicine. Intensive Care Medicine 26(7): 988–994

Ntoumenopoulos G, Presneill JJ, McElholum M, Cade JF 2002 Chest physiotherapy for the prevention of ventilator-associated pneumonia. Intensive Care Medicine 28(7): 850–856

O'Riordan TG, Mao W, Palmer LB, Chen JJ 2006 Assessing the effects of racemic and single-enantiomer albuterol on airway secretions in long-term intubated patients. Chest 129(1): 124–132

Paratz J, Burns Y 1993 The effect of respiratory physiotherapy on intracranial pressure, mean arterial pressure, cerebral perfusion pressure, and end tidal carbon dioxide in ventilated neurosurgical patients. Physiotherapy Theory and Practice 9: 3–11

Paratz J, Lipman J 2006 Manual hyperinflation causes norepinephrine release. Heart and Lung 35(4): 262–268

Paratz J, Lipman J, McAuliffe M 2002 Effect of manual hyperinflation on hemodynamics, gas exchange, and respiratory mechanics in ventilated patients. Journal of Intensive Care Medicine 17(6): 317–324

Paratz J, Zeppos L, Patman S et al 2005 Adverse physiological events in intensive care – is it an issue? Australian and New Zealand Society Intensive Care Medicine, Adelaide

Patman S, Jenkins S, Stiller K 2000 Manual hyperinflation – effects on respiratory parameters. Physiotherapy Research International 5(3): 157–171

Pelosi P, Brazzi L, Gattinoni L 2002 Prone position in acute respiratory distress syndrome. European Respiratory Journal 20(4): 1017–1028

Pelosi P, D'Onofrio D, Chiumello D et al 2003 Pulmonary and extrapulmonary acute respiratory distress syndrome are different. European Respiratory Journal Suppl 42: 48s–56s

Petrie GJ, Barnwell E, Grimshaw J, on behalf of the Scottish Intercolegiate Guidelines Network 1995 Clinical guidelines: criteria for appraisal for national use. Royal College of Physicians, Edinburgh

Petrucci N, Iacovelli W 2004 Ventilation with lower tidal volumes versus traditional tidal volumes in adults for acute lung injury and acute respiratory distress syndrome. Cochrane Database of Systematic Reviews (2): CD003844

Pierson DJ 2005 Tracheostomy and weaning. Respiratory Care 50(4): 526–533

Pilbeam SP 1992 Mechanical ventilation: physiological and clinical applications, 2nd edn. Mosby Year Book, St. Louis, pp 169–170

Pillastrini P, Bordini S, Bazzocchi G, Belloni G, Menarini M 2006 Study of the effectiveness of bronchial clearance in subjects with upper spinal cord injuries: examination of a rehabilitation programme involving mechanical insufflation and exsufflation. Spinal Cord 44(10): 614–616

PULSION Medical Systems AG: PiCCO technology www.pulsion.com/index.php?id=39 (accessed 13 July 2007)

Raoof S, Chowdhrey N, Raoof S et al 1999 Effect of combined kinetic therapy and percussion therapy on the resolution of atelectasis in critically ill patients. Chest 115(6): 1658–1666

Richard JC, Maggiore SM, Mancebo J et al 2006 Effects of vertical positioning on gas exchange and lung volumes in acute respiratory distress syndrome. Intensive Care Medicine 32(10): 1623–1626

Richman PS, Baram D, Varela M, Glass PS 2006 Sedation during mechanical ventilation: a trial of benzodiazepine and opiate in combination. Critical Care Medicine 34(5): 1395–1401

Rose L, Nelson S 2006 Issues in weaning from mechanical ventilation: literature review. Journal of Advanced Nursing 54(1): 73–85

Rosow C, Manberg PJ 2001 Bispectral index monitoring. Anesthesiology Clinics of North America 19(4): 947–966, xi

Rothen HU, Neumann P, Berglund JE et al 1999 Dynamics of re-expansion of atelectasis during general anaesthesia. British Journal of Anaesthesia 82(4): 551–556

Rudy EB, Turner BS, Baun M, Stone KS, Brucia J 1991 Endotracheal suctioning in adults with head injury. Heart and Lung 20(6): 667–674

Rusterholz B, Ellis E 1998 The effect of lung compliance and experience on manual hyperinflation. Australian Journal of Physiotherapy 44(1): 23–28

Sancho J, Servera E, Vergara P, Marin J 2003 Mechanical insufflation-exsufflation vs. tracheal suctioning via tracheostomy tubes for patients with amyotrophic lateral sclerosis: a pilot study. America Journal of Physical Medicine and Rehabilitation 82(10): 750–753

Sassoon CS, Caiozzo VJ, Manka A, Sieck GC 2002 Altered diaphragm contractile properties with controlled mechanical ventilation. Journal of Applied Physiology 92(6): 2585–2595

Savian C, Chan P, Paratz J 2005 The effect of positive end-expiratory pressure level on peak expiratory flow during manual hyperinflation.

Anesthesia and Analgesia 100(4): 1112–1116

Scherhag A, Kaden JJ, Kentschke E, Sueselbeck T, Borggrefe M 2005 Comparison of impedance cardiography and thermodilution-derived measurements of stroke volume and cardiac output at rest and during exercise testing. Cardiovascular Drugs and Therapy 19(2): 141–147

Schreuder FM, Jones UF 2004 The effect of saline installation on sputum yield and oxygen saturation measurement in adult intubated patients. Abstract, Thoracic Society Australia and New Zealand, Sydney, Australia

Senn O, Clarenbach CF, Kaplan V, Maggiorini M, Bloch KE 2005 Monitoring carbon dioxide tension and arterial oxygen saturation by a single earlobe sensor in patients with critical illness or sleep apnea. Chest 128(3): 1291–1296

Shankar G, Cohen DA 2001 Ideopathic pneumonia syndrome after bone marrow transplantation: the role of pre-transplant radiation conditioning and local cytokine dysregulation in promoting inflammation and fibrosis. International Journal of Experimental Pathology 82(2): 101–113

Shapiro BA, Mahutte CK, Cane RD, Gilmour IJ 1993 Clinical performance of a blood gas monitor: a prospective, multicenter trial. Critical Care Medicine 21(4): 487–494

Sheridan RL 2000 Airway management and respiratory care of the burn patient. Internatonal Anesthesiology Clinics 38(3): 129–145

Spicer M, Hughes P, Green M 1997 A non-invasive system to evaluate diaphragmatic strength in ventilated patients. Physiological Measurement 18(4): 355–361

Stawicki SP, Grossman MD, Hoey BA, Miller DL, Reed JF 3rd 2004 Rib fractures in the elderly: a marker of injury severity. Journal of the American Geriatrics Society 52(5): 805–808

Stiller K 2000 Physiotherapy in intensive care: towards an evidence-based practice. Chest 118(6): 1801–1813

Stiller K, Geake T, Taylor J, Grant R, Hall B 1990 Acute lobar atelectasis: a comparison of two chest physiotherapy regimens. Chest 98(6): 1336–1340

Stiller K, Phillips A, Lambert P 2004 The safety of mobilization and its effects on haemodynamic and respiratory status of intensive care patients. Physiotherapy Theory and Practice 20: 175–185

Thelandersson A, Cider A, Nellgard B 2006 Prone position in mechanically ventilated patients with reduced intracranial compliance. Acta

8

Anaesthesiologica Scandinavica 50(8): 937–941

Tjin SC, Ho YC, Lam YZ, Hao J, Ng BK 2001 Continuous cardiac output monitoring system. Medical and Biological Engineering and Computing 39(1): 101–104

Tonnelier JM, Prat G, Le Gal G et al 2005 Impact of a nurses' protocol-directed weaning procedure on outcomes in patients undergoing mechanical ventilation for longer than 48 hours: a prospective cohort study with a matched historical control group. Critical Care 9(2): R83–89

Topp R, Ditmyer M, King K, Doherty K, Hornyak J 2002 The effect of bed rest and potential of prehabilitation on patients in the intensive care unit. AACN Clinical Issues 13(2): 263–276

Turner JS 2002 Monitoring and interpreting medical investigations. In: Pryor JA, Prasad SA (eds) Physiotherapy for respiratory and cardiac problems: adults and paediatrics, 3rd edn. Churchill Livingstone, Edinburgh, pp 132–134

Ulatowski J 1997 Cerebral protection. In: Oh TE (ed). Intensive care manual, 4th edn. Butterworth-Heinemann, Oxford, pp 403–411

Unoki T, Mizutani T, Toyooka H 2004 Effects of expiratory rib cage compression combined with endotracheal suctioning on gas exchange in mechanically ventilated rabbits with induced atelectasis. Respiratory Care 49(8): 896–901

Vassilakopoulos T, Zakynthinos S, Roussos C 2006 Bench-to-bedside review: Weaning failure – should we rest the respiratory muscles with controlled mechanical ventilation? Critical Care 2006 10(1): 204

Voulgaris SG, Partheni M, Kaliora H et al 2005 Early cerebral monitoring using the transcranial Doppler pulsatility index in patients with severe brain trauma. Medical Science Monitor 11(2): CR49–52

Weavind L, Wenker OC 2000 Newer modes of ventilation: an overview. The Internet Journal of Anesthesiology 4: 4

Weiss SJ, Kulik JP, Calloway E 1997 Bioimpedance cardiac output measurements in patients with presumed congestive heart failure. Academic Emergency Medicine 4(6): 568–573

Weissman C, Kemper M 1991 The oxygen uptake–oxygen delivery relationship during ICU interventions. Chest 99(2): 430–435

West JB 2005 Gas transport by the blood – how gases are moved to the peripheral tissues. In: Respiratory physiology: the essentials, 7th edn. Lippincott Williams & Wilkins, Philadelphia, PA, p 77

White H, Baker A 2002 Continuous jugular venous oximetry in the neurointensive care unit – a brief review. Canadian Journal of Anaesthesia 49(6): 623–629

Whitehead MD, Halsall D, Pollitzer MJ et al 1980 Transcutaneous estimation of arterial PO_2 and PCO_2 in newborn infants with a single electrochemical sensor. Lancet 1(8178): 111–114

Wilson JN, Pierce JD, Clancy RL 2001 Reactive oxygen species in acute respiratory distress syndrome. Heart and Lung 30(5): 370–375

Winkelman C 2004 Inactivity and inflammation: selected cytokines as biologic mediators in muscle dysfunction during critical illness. AACN Clinical Issues 15(1): 74–82

Worthley LI 2000 Shock: a review of pathophysiology and management. Part II. Critical Care and Resuscitation 2(1): 66–84

Yelderman ML, Ramsay MA, Quinn MD et al 1992 Continuous thermodilution cardiac output measurement in intensive care unit patients. Journal of Cardiothoracic and Vascular Anesthesia 6(3): 270–274

Young RJ, Sanderson JE 1997 Echocardiography in intensive care. In: Oh TE (ed) Intensive care manual, 4th edn. Butterworth-Heinemann, Oxford, pp 197–205

Zador E, Dux L, Wuytack F 1999 Prolonged passive stretch of rat soleus muscle provokes an increase in the mRNA levels of the muscle regulatory factors distributed along the entire length of the fibers. Journal of Muscle Research and Cell Motility 20(4): 395–402

Zafiropoulos B, Alison JA, McCarren B 2004 Physiological responses to the early mobilisation of the intubated, ventilated abdominal surgery patient. Australian Journal of Physiotherapy 50(2): 95–100

Zimmerman GA, Albertine KH, Carveth HJ et al 1999 Endothelial activation in ARDS. Chest 116(1 Suppl): 18S–24S

Zimmerman JL, Dellinger RP 1993 Initial evaluation of a new intra-arterial blood gas system in humans. Critical Care Medicine 21(4): 495–500

8

Chapter 9

Paediatric mechanical support

Tomás Iolster, Robert C Tasker

INTRODUCTION

The technique of respiratory support in children needs to be informed by an understanding of age-specific pathophysiology. In contrast to adults, the most common causes of respiratory failure in children vary with age. In the newborn infant, prematurity, hyaline membrane disease, asphyxia and aspiration pneumonia are the most common causes of breathing difficulty. Under 2 years of age, bronchopneumonia, bronchiolitis, croup, status asthmaticus, foreign body inhalation and congenital heart and airway anomalies are important; compared with asthma, accidental poisoning and central nervous system infection, trauma and cerebral hypoxia/ischaemia in the over 2 year olds. Although the principles of when and how mechanical support should be undertaken in such patients are, broadly speaking, similar to those applied in adults, there are differences in epidemiology, pathophysiology and management that warrant consideration. The emphasis, therefore, of this chapter will be a paediatric perspective of respiratory supportive therapy.

EPIDEMIOLOGY OF ACUTE RESPIRATORY FAILURE IN CHILDREN

Respiratory failure develops when the rate of gas exchange between the air and the blood fails to match the body's metabolic demands. The patient therefore loses the ability to provide sufficient oxygen to the blood and develops hypoxaemia, or the patient is unable to ventilate adequately and develops hypercarbia. Epidemiologically, there is little information in children about the incidence of acute respiratory failure. Adult definitions using blood gas parameters may be appropriate for certain age groups but in others they may not be useful. For example, in infants with acute bronchiolitis, acute respiratory failure is usually defined as:

$PaCO_2 = 8$ kPa (60 mmHg) with $PaO_2 = 8$ kPa (60 mmHg) when using $F_iO_2 = 0.6$

(where $PaCO_2$ = partial pressure of carbon dioxide in arterial blood, PaO_2 = partial pressure of oxygen in arterial blood, FiO_2 = fractional inspired oxygen concentration) or, in the case of patients with respiratory arrest, a preceding history of severe respiratory distress accompanied by cyanosis.

However, when trying to look at large populations, in the absence of blood gases, a more pragmatic definition for acute respiratory failure is needed. For example, when using the definition of 'acute airway management necessitating endotracheal tube intubation' (Tasker 2000) it is possible to explore issues such as the pattern and time course of paediatric disease that have some bearing on how mechanical support should be undertaken.

Pattern of and time course of disease

Table 9.1 summarizes a retrospective analysis of 1000 infants and children (aged older than 28 days and younger than 17 years) who required endotracheal intubation for acute respiratory failure complicating acutely acquired medical, rather than surgical, disease (Tasker 2000). The three major categories relate to the system or problem underlying respiratory failure (respiratory tract disorder, central nervous system disorder or systemic disorder) and the subcategories relate to the clinical diagnostic entities commonly encountered in intensive care. Respiratory tract problems due to infection are, not surprisingly, the most common problems seen. The time course of recovery in survivors is influenced by the site within the airways that infection has reached. This is reflected by an increase in the length of stay in the intensive care unit (ICU) with more distally affected tissues (i.e upper airway compared with lower airway). In relating such information to clinical practice one can use the expected time course to decide on an agenda for treatment or 'care pathway'. For example, given that the expected time course for intensive care recovery in pneumonia necessitating intubation is around 8 days (interquartile range 5–12 days) one can then predict when certain targets should be met. The same applies to the other 11 distinct diagnosis-related

Table 9.1 Diagnostic distribution of 1000 children requiring endotracheal tube intubation during acute medical illness ordered by number (n), age and length of stay on the intensive care unit in survivors

System disorder	n	Age in months median (IQR)	Length of stay in survivors median (IQR) days m : f
Respiratory tract	521	13 (4–40)	
Upper airway infection	80	21 (12–35)	4 (3–5) : 3 (3–5)
Bronchiolitis	89	3 (2–6)	5 (4–9) : 6 (3–9)
Asthma	25	37 (21–86)	4 (3–5) : 4 (3–5)
Pneumonia	90	10 (4–40)	8 (5–12) : 9 (4–14)
Pneumonia and immunodeficiency	120	16 (5–51)	9 (5–16) : 9 (7–14)
Neuromuscular disease	66	22 (7–88)	10 (5–19) : 8 (5–20)
Non-infective LRTD	51	16 (7–69)	5 (3–8) : 6 (4–10)
Central nervous	342	18 (6–62)	
Infection	117	22 (8–65)	4 (2–6) : 4 (3–7)
Hypoxia-ischaemia	78	14 (4–34)	5 (2–10) : 3 (1–8)
Other encephalopathy	147	17 (6–70)	5 (3–8) : 5 (2–8)
Systemic	137	19 (6–52)	
Septicaemia	90	19 (4–69)	6 (4–10) : 6 (4–12)
Inflammatory syndromes	47	19 (6–32)	4 (3–9) : 5 (3–8)

IQR, interquartile range; LRTD, lower respiratory tract disease

entities. This idea will be revisited later in this section where three clinical examples are discussed.

Acute hypoxaemic respiratory failure

Acute hypoxaemic respiratory failure (AHRF) signifies respiratory failure at the more severe end of the patho-physiological spectrum, irrespective of underlying aetiology. For paediatric practice we identify this state by using diagnostic criteria that have been modified from the American-European Consensus Conference diagnostic criteria for acute respiratory distress syndrome (ARDS) (Bernard et al 1994). These criteria include:

- acute onset of respiratory failure over less than 48 hours
- evidence of a severe defect in oxygenation (PaO_2/ F_iO_2 of less than 26.7 kPa, 200 mmHg) for at least 6 consecutive hours on the day of admission
- no evidence of left atrial hypertension
- four-quadrant interstitial shadowing on chest radiograph.

Children meeting all the above criteria except the characteristic chest radiographic appearances of ARDS (last criterion) are described as cases of AHRF. The significance of AHRF is that it implies a certain severity of illness and risk of mortality, factors which are important when it comes to deciding which ventilatory strategy should be adopted and the use of adjunctive therapies (see section on 'ventilation strategies for specific disease'). For example, in a prospective, epidemiological study, Peters and colleagues (1998) found that out of 850 mechanically ventilated infants and children, AHRF occurred in 118 patients (14%, 95% confidence interval (CI) 12–16%). Of these 118 patients, 52 met the criteria for ARDS (44%, 35–53%). In all 850 patients, mortality was four times higher than the mortality seen in those patients without AHRF. In the AHRF patients, mortality was three times higher for those with ARDS (Peters et al 1998). In a study from North America, the PALISI network (Pediatric Acute Lung Injury and Sepsis Investigators) reported a mortality from ARDS of 4.3% (Randolph et al 2003). This coincides with the adoption of protective modes of ventilation for this condition. Therefore, identifying these entities (i.e. AHRF and ARDS) at an early stage is important so as to institute the most appropriate method or mode of ventilation.

INDICATIONS FOR SUPPORTIVE RESPIRATORY THERAPY

For practical purposes we can consider the treatment of respiratory dysfunction in terms of treating hypoxia and hypercarbia. Appropriate management is aimed first at prevention, second at early diagnosis and third at a clear understanding of the pathophysiology and way in which the proposed treatment works to maintain or restore good lung function.

Hypoxia

Hypoxia must be treated first; give oxygen. At the same time attempts should be made to correct the underlying problem. Local processes in the lung, such as atelectasis and bronchopneumonia, can result in a portion of the pulmonary blood flow perfusing unventilated alveoli (i.e. intrapulmonary shunt), which in some cases may be effectively treated by pulmonary toilet and postural change. With a large shunt fraction – greater than 25% of pulmonary blood flow – PaO_2 is not significantly improved by solely increasing the FiO_2. In these cases a diffuse pulmonary process is usually present and a form of assisted positive airway pressure is required. Such assistance may also be required for severe impairment of chest wall mechanics (e.g. rib fractures, pain, weakness, etc.) even in the absence of pulmonary parenchymal disease.

In infants and children, there are several methods of administering oxygen (Table 9.2). Young patients do not usually tolerate nasal catheters and cannulae. Face-masks with a reservoir and a non-rebreathing valve can be used to increase the FiO_2. Alternatively, high-flow oxygen via the appropriate Venturi-valve mask can be used. Oxygen delivered via the oxygen inlet of an incubator rarely exceeds an FiO_2 of 0.4. When supplemental oxygen is delivered into an tent the concentration varies depending on any leaks in the system. Regardless of the technique, it is essential that the administered oxygen is

9

Table 9.2 Methods of oxygen administration	
Method	Maximum achievable FiO$_2$ at 6–10 l/min of oxygen (%)
Nasopharyngeal catheter	50
Nasal prongs	50
Mask without reservoir bag	50
Mask with reservoir bag (partial rebreathing)	70
Mask with reservoir bag (non-rebreathing)	95
Venturi	24, 28, 35, 40
Incubator	40
Canopy tent	50
Head box	95

FiO$_2$, fractional inspired oxygen concentration

warmed and humidified. To avoid damage to the lungs, oxygen administration should be discontinued as soon as possible (as indicated by blood gas measurements). An FiO_2 below 0.6 is preferred, to minimize the risk of oxygen toxicity. Reduction in the FiO_2 should be carried out cautiously in a stepwise manner. To facilitate this process both the concentration and duration of oxygen therapy must be recorded accurately. A well-calibrated oxygen analyser is used to check the inspired concentration every 2 hours when using a tent, head box or when adding oxygen into an incubator. The need for monitoring PaO_2 in preterm newborn infants is related to the potential for pulmonary oxygen toxicity and the danger of retrolental fibroplasia. So, in any patient, oxygen should be administered at the lowest concentration sufficient to maintain the PaO_2 between 6.7 and 13.3 kPa (50–100 mmHg). Continuous measurement or monitoring of transcutaneous oxygen or pulse oximetry arterial oxygen saturation (SpO_2) are essential additions to the direct, and intermittent, measurement of arterial blood gases. In some instances, supplemental oxygen may cause respiratory depression if there has been chronic respiratory failure and the patient has a hypoxic-drive to ventilation (as opposed to the normal situation where the $PaCO_2$ is the most important factor in the control of ventilation). This phenomenon is generally uncommon in paediatric practice, but has been encountered in children with cystic fibrosis, cerebral palsy and bronchopulmonary dysplasia.

In addition to oxygen, some type of positive pressure may be useful in the management of hypoxia. Mask and nasal continuous positive airway pressure (CPAP) or bilevel positive airway pressure (BiPAP) increase lung compliance by recruiting additional areas of the lung for ventilation. Also, lung recruitment improves oxygenation by decreasing intrapulmonary shunt. These modes of non-invasive ventilation (NIV) are being used more frequently as the step before invasive mechanical ventilation. When invasive mechanical ventilation is used, the addition of some positive end-expiratory pressure (PEEP) is a common practice in maintaining adequate functional residual capacity. However, PEEP may adversely affect the patient lung mechanics if hyperinflation occurs. This problem results in impaired pulmonary perfusion and further accentuates any ventilation–perfusion $(\dot{V}/\dot{Q})$ mismatch. Therefore PEEP above 4 cmH_2O should be used judiciously if there is already regional hyperinflation, such as occurs in bronchopulmonary dysplasia (Box 9.1). In this context a strategy for treating hypoxia is outlined in Box 9.2.

Hypercarbia

When shallow (or ineffectual) breathing is present, the dead space (i.e. ventilated but non-perfused regions)

> **Box 9.1   Positive end-expiratory pressure**
>
> *Advantages*
> Increased functional residual capacity
> Recruits additional lung units, improving compliance
> Reduces pulmonary shunt fraction
> Allows for a decrease in FiO_2
>
> *Disadvantages*
> Increases mean airway pressure, leading to reduced venous return
> Can increase 'dead space' by impairing perfusion to hyperinflated regions
> Can increase pulmonary vascular resistance and right heart dysfunction
> Altered renal blood flow with increase in antidiuretic hormone release
> Barotrauma caused by increased airway pressure

> **Box 9.2   Initial treatment of hypoxia**
>
> 1. Increase FiO_2 to maintain SaO_2 >90% (Table 9.2)
> 2. Consider positive pressure and PEEP, if large shunt. Indications:
>   hypoxaemia with FiO_2 >0.5
>   diffuse lung disease
>   maintain lung volume
> 3. Initiate aggressive pulmonary toilet
> 4. Eliminate the underlying cause:
>   pain
>   fluid overload
>   atelectasis
>   bronchopneumonia
> 5. Correct systemic abnormalities:
>   hypovolaemia
>   sepsis
>   carbon monoxide poisoning
>
> SaO_2, arterial oxygen saturation; FiO_2, fractional inspired oxygen concentration

becomes a larger fraction of each breath. This change results in a decrease in alveolar ventilation, even if the lung parenchyma is normal. When hypercarbia has been found and its cause considered, NIV can be tried a step before invasive mechanical ventilation. This may be useful when hypercarbia is secondary to neuromuscular weakness. If the patient needs invasive mechanical ventilation, then increasing tidal volume or respiratory rate can bring about increased alveolar ventilation. However, these changes may increase mean airway pressure that may generate detrimental effects on pulmonary vascular resistance and $\dot{V}/\dot{Q}$ matching.

If the patient is treated with full mechanical ventilation, the first step is to make sure that the patient is receiving an appropriate tidal volume and minute ventilation. Ventilatory system leaks and loss of a portion of the tidal volume through compressive loss in the tubing, as well as abnormalities in endotracheal tube function, are common problems that need rectifying. Having excluded mechanical factors, the other causes of hypercarbia may be related to an increase in CO_2 production or an increase in dead-space ventilation. An increase in dead space may be due to excessive PEEP (particularly when there is already hyperinflation or hypovolaemia) and it may be corrected by intravenous volume to increase preload to the heart.

Endotracheal intubation

There are four absolute indications for controlling the airway by endotracheal intubation:

- maintaining the patency of the airway where problems are present or anticipated (e.g. direct airway trauma, oedema or infection)

- to protect the airway from aspiration in states of altered consciousness, where airway-protective mechanisms may be lost or impaired

- to facilitate pulmonary toilet and avoid airway obstruction when there is marked atelectasis and pulmonary infection – an inadequate cough might necessitate more direct access to the airways for suctioning

- when positive pressure breathing is indicated because of inadequate spontaneous ventilation.

In practice, experienced staff should carry out establishing airway and respiratory support for the acutely ill child, because such patients can deteriorate rapidly, particularly at the time of inducing anaesthesia. Following preoxygenation with 100% inspired oxygen, a variety of agents are used to facilitate endotracheal intubation, including intravenous induction with drugs such as fentanyl, midazolam and suxamethonium, or inhalational induction with gases such as halothane or isoflurane. Table 9.3 provides a guide to the appropriate endotracheal tube size, length and suction catheter used in the paediatric age range and Figure 9.1 illustrates a commonly used method of endotracheal tube fixation.

MECHANICAL VENTILATION

Many of the ventilatory techniques are similar for children and adults. However, there are some differ-

9

Table 9.3 Endotracheal tube size and suction catheters

Age	Weight (kg)	Endotracheal tube (mm)	Length at lip (cm)	Length at nose (cm)	Suction catheter (French gauge)
Newborn	<0.7	2.0	5.0	6.0	5.0
	<1	2.5	5.5	7.0	5.0
	1	3.0	6.0	7.5	6.0
	2	3.0	7.0	9.0	6.0
	3	3.0	8.5	10.5	6.0
	3.5	3.5	9.0	11	7.0
3 months	6.0	3.5	10	12	7.0
1 year	10	4.0	11	14	8.0
2 years	12	4.5	12	15	8.0
3 years	14	4.5	13	16	8.0
4 years	16	5.0	14	17	10
6 years	20	5.5	15	19	10
8 years	24	6.0	16	20	12
10 years	30	6.5	17	21	12
12 years	38	7.0	18	22	12–14
14 years	50	7.5	19	23	14

9

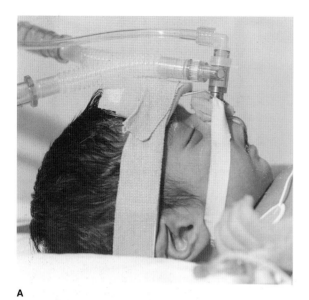

A

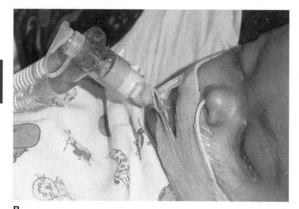

B

Figure 9.1 Endotracheal tube fixation for (**A**) nasal and (**B**) oral tubes.

ences between these two groups that are highlighted below.

General ventilatory care

A variety of ventilators can be used in paediatric mechanical ventilation (Fig. 9.2). There are specific ventilators designed for neonates and small infants that are used mainly in neonatal units to ventilate premature babies. Fortunately most modern ventilators can be used across the whole age spectrum and they can deliver different modes of pressure control ventilation (PCV) and volume control ventilation (VCV).

One of the main goals during mechanical ventilation is to minimize and optimize patient–ventilator interaction. Adequate patient comfort will potentially decrease the need for pharmacological sedation and may help to

minimize the duration of mechanical ventilation. The addition of PEEP at 3–5 cmH$_2$O above atmospheric pressure is routinely used unless there is a contraindication. This helps to avoid alveolar collapse during mechanical ventilation. The amount of PEEP may need to be increased in conditions associated with low lung volume, such as hyaline membrane disease, atelectasis, severe pneumonia (e.g. viral, *Pneumocystis carinii*) or ARDS.

Complications of ventilator therapy occur frequently and all intensive care staff should be continually aware of the potential hazards (Box 9.3). Aseptic technique is important for tracheal airway care because nosocomial infection constitutes a large and preventable problem. The application of PEEP, increased tidal volumes and increased airway pressure can also produce complications. Potential disruption of normal $\dot{V}/\dot{Q}$ matching seen with spontaneous breathing can occur with lung overexpansion and leads to regional hypoperfusion. A decrease in venous return, an increase in pulmonary vascular resistance and a decrease in left ventricular output can impair cardiac output and oxygen delivery. The more compliant the lung or the less compliant the chest wall, the greater the transmission of positive airway pressure to the mediastinum and the greater the negative effect on cardiac function. Volume loading or inotropic support can overcome the concomitant decrease in cardiac output, in large part.

The significance of ventilator-induced lung injury (VILI) has been appreciated more during the last few years. It now seems clear that the pathogenesis of respiratory failure is greatly influenced by the way the lungs are ventilated. Barotrauma and volutrauma have been used to describe VILI. However, there is some controversy as to which of these is the more damaging. Both can produce overdistension and it is this problem that appears to cause the injury. To complicate matters, another factor appears to be 'atelectrauma,' i.e. where the repeated collapse and re-expansion of areas of the lung produce shearing injury that contributes to inflammation and lung damage. The best ventilator strategy should therefore aim to keep tidal volume to a minimum with optimum PEEP and, sometimes, neuromuscular blockade. Theoretically, these manoeuvres should reduce atelectasis and patient–ventilator interactions.

In regard to other problems, pulmonary interstitial emphysema, pneumomediastinum, pneumoperitoneum and subcutaneous emphysema do not require specific treatment unless there is significant haemodynamic impairment. Poor renal function, as exhibited by decreased glomerular filtration rate, urine production and sodium excretion, can be a consequence of hypoxia and hypercarbia. This may be further compounded by the effects of mechanical ventilation with PEEP on pro-

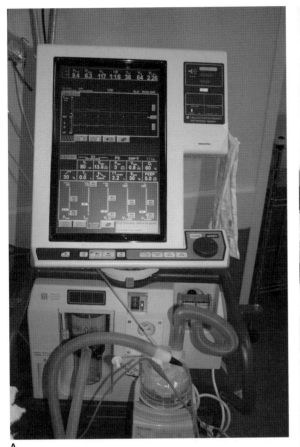 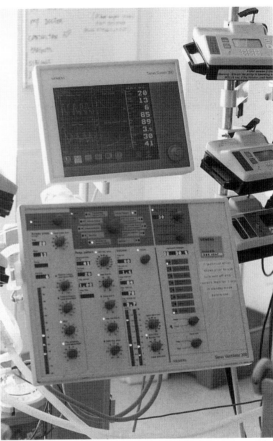

A   B

Figure 9.2   (A) Puritan Bennett 840 ventilator and (B) the Servo 300 ventilator.

9

ducing an antidiuretic hormone-mediated salt and water-retaining effect (probably secondary to decreased cardiac output), an increased renal vein pressure and a neural reflex from the pressure-distorted atrial wall.

Acute deterioration and 'troubleshooting'

In mechanically ventilated patients, the adequacy of gas exchange and ventilation should be assessed frequently. Changes in therapy should then be titrated against expected parameters or targets (Table 9.5). When there is an acute deterioration during mechanical ventilation, problem solving or 'troubleshooting' should begin with making the patient safe. In the first instance this means disconnecting the patient from the ventilator and support breathing with bag-ventilation using FiO_2 of 1.0. Easy ventilation and patient stabilization with the bag suggests a ventilator problem that should be systematically addressed (e.g. check the circuit for leaks, check ventilator function, check gas flow). However, it

should be remembered that 'hand-bagging' might result in increased tidal volume, which can also be responsible for the patient's improvement. Patients with stiff lungs are frequently dyspnoeic, despite adequate gas exchange. Increasing the tidal volume will correct this subjective feeling and may also account for patient improvement. Difficult bagging at the time of disconnecting the ventilator strongly suggests a problem with the endotracheal tube or the lung to chest-wall complex. A suction catheter (Table 9.3) should be passed down the endotracheal tube to check for narrowing or blockage. Chest examination, blood gases and chest radiography should be ordered. A blocked endotracheal tube should be replaced. A pneumothorax requires chest tube placement. If neither of these is the cause for deterioration, then the possibilities may include new problems such as an increased oxygen demand due to sepsis, impaired oxygen delivery due to heart failure or acute pulmonary injury due to gastric aspiration. These and other causes need to be sought and treated appropriately.

9

Box 9.3 Complications associated with mechanical ventilation

Respiratory
Tracheal lesions, e.g. erosions, oedema, stenosis, granuloma, obstruction
Accidental endotracheal tube displacement into bronchus, oesophagus or hypopharynx
Infection
Air leaks, e.g. pneumothorax, pneumomediastinum, interstitial emphysema
Air trapping causing hyperinflation
Excessive secretions resulting in atelectasis
Oxygen hazards, e.g. depression of ventilation, bronchopulmonary dysplasia
Pulmonary haemorrhage

Circulatory
Impaired venous return resulting in decreased cardiac output and systemic hypotension
Oxygen hazards, e.g. retrolental fibroplasia, cerebral vasoconstriction
Septicaemia
Intracranial haemorrhage, e.g. intraventricular, subarachnoid
Hyperventilation leading to decreased cerebral blood flow

Metabolic
Increased work of breathing because of 'fighting' the ventilator
Alkalosis due to potassium depletion or excessive bicarbonate therapy

Renal and fluid balance
Antidiuresis
Excess water in the inspired gas

Equipment malfunction (mechanical)
Ventilator leaks or valve dysfunction
Overheating of inspired gases
Kinked or disconnected tubes

Commonly used modes of mechanical ventilation in children

Pressure versus volume control

In VCV a set tidal volume is delivered and the peak inspiratory pressure (PIP) will depend on lung compliance, inspiratory flow and airway resistance. The plateau pressure is a more accurate measurement of actual alveolar pressure and it will be mainly influenced by lung compliance. The ventilator rate and inspiratory time are set by the clinician. This mode has the advantage of guaranteeing minute ventilation, especially in conditions when optimum minute ventilation is required (e.g. head injury). However, a decrease in compliance can lead to excessively high pressures with risk of lung injury (Table 9.4).

In PCV the delivered breath is limited by pressure. The tidal volume is determined by preset pressure limit, inspiratory time and lung compliance; it may also vary with the condition of the lung. The flow is decelerating, meaning that it slows down progressively after reaching the set inspiratory pressure. As in VCV, the ventilator rate and inspiratory time are set by the clinician. PCV has the advantage of decelerating flow and it has been considered to be less injurious because lower pressures are usually achieved, compared with volume control. However, a decrease in lung compliance, such as that caused by accumulation of secretions, may be associated with a decrease in tidal volume. This situation may go unrecognized because the ventilator will continue to cycle at the preset pressure (Table 9.4).

There are few controlled studies in children comparing these various modes of ventilation. Usually the final choice of ventilator mode depends on personal experience, the availability of technology and the underlying disease. Whatever mode is chosen it is essential to ensure that the expected tidal volume, minute ventilation and pressures are achieved.

Low tidal volume ventilation

In patients with AHRF or ARDS, ventilation using low tidal volumes has been widely accepted. In 2000, the ARDS network reported a decreased mortality in adults

Table 9.4	Advantages and disadvantages of pressure–limited and volume–limited ventilation	
	Pressure–limited	**Volume–limited**
Advantages	Avoids excessive inflating pressures	Constant volume delivered
	Decreased risk of barotrauma	High inflating pressures reflect changes in mechanics
Disadvantages	Variable volume delivered	Capable of generating very high inflating pressures
	No signs of altered mechanics	Increased risk of barotrauma

Table 9.5 Normal values

	Newborn	Up to 3 years	3–6 years	>6 years
Respiratory rate (breaths/minute)	40–60	20–30	20–30	15–20
Arterial blood pH	7.30–7.40	7.30–7.40	7.35–7.45	7.35–7.45
$PaCO_2$ (mmHg)	30–35	30–35	35–45	35–45
(kPa)	4.0–4.7	4.0–4.7	4.7–6.0	4.7–6.0
PaO_2 (mmHg)	60–90	80–100	80–100	80–100
(kPa)	8.0–12.0	10.7–13.3	10.7–13.3	10.7–13.3
Heart rate (beats/minute)	100–200	100–180	70–150	70–150
Systolic blood pressure (mmHg)	60–90	75–130	90–140	90–140
Diastolic blood pressure (mmHg)	30–60	45–90	50–80	50–80

$PaCO_2$, partial pressure of carbon dioxide in arterial blood; PaO_2, partial pressure of oxygen in arterial blood

when using tidal volumes of 6 ml/kg as compared to 12 ml/kg (Acute Respiratory Distress Syndrome Network 2000). These results are probably applicable to children. The risk of using smaller tidal volumes for mechanical ventilation is that it can lead to insufficient gas exchange and hypercarbia. Therefore, the strategy commonly adopted when using low tidal volume ventilation is to accept a higher $PaCO_2$ provided the arterial pH is 7.25. In practice, the ventilator is set so that peak inspiratory pressures are limited below 30 cmH$_2$O (30 cmH$_2$O of plateau pressure when using volume control) while employing high mean airway pressures to ensure maximum lung volume recruitment via the use of PEEP.

Pressure–regulated volume control (PRVC) ventilation

This mode of ventilation is now available in some newer ventilators. This mode delivers a preset tidal volume in a pressure-limited manner using the lowest possible pressure with a decelerating flow. To guarantee the set tidal volume, the gas flow and pressure change constantly in each delivered breath, depending on lung compliance and airway resistance. This method has the advantage of guaranteeing tidal volume and using decelerating flow. As lung compliance improves during the course of pulmonary disease, the ventilator will automatically wean inspiratory pressures. Even though PRVC seems to have advantages over other modes, clinical controlled trials to evaluate its benefits are still lacking in children.

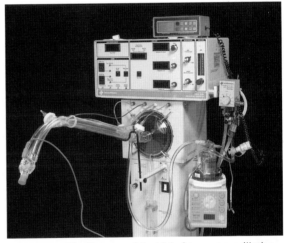

Figure 9.3 Ventilator used for high-frequency oscillation.

NEWER VENTILATORY SUPPORT TECHNIQUES

High-frequency oscillatory ventilation

High-frequency ventilation techniques, including high-frequency positive pressure ventilation, high-frequency jet ventilation and high-frequency oscillatory ventilation (HFOV), achieve adequate ventilation by employing tidal volumes that are often less than actual dead space and respiratory rates of 60–3000 cycles/minute (Fig. 9.3). The most widely used of these modes in children is the HFOV. The theoretical advantage of HFOV is that it keeps the lungs open by using a relatively high mean airway pressure and it delivers very low tidal volumes, thereby minimizing lung damage caused by high volumes and high inspiratory pressures. The high mean airway pressure allows lung-volume recruitment and improves oxygenation.

The most common indication for this form of ventilation is refractory hypoxaemia. However, HFOV has been used in bronchopleural fistula and some types of obstructive disease and bronchiolitis (Kneyber et al 2005, Slee-Wijffels et al 2005). Unfortunately there is a paucity of published clinical trials on the use of HFOV in the paediatric population and its benefits have not been clearly established as compared with conventional mechanical ventilation. Despite this lack of evidence, HFOV is frequently used in the treatment of hypoxemic respiratory disease. When used, early institution of this therapy seems to be more beneficial in this group of patients (Arnold et al 1994). The experience reported by Watkins and colleagues (2000) in 100 courses of such ventilation would suggest that, in the presence of AHRF or ARDS, a threshold mean airway pressure of 16 cmH$_2$O is an appropriate indication.

Extracorporeal membrane oxygenation

Extracorporeal membrane oxygenation (ECMO) is designed to provide a variable degree of cardiopulmonary support for a predetermined period of time over which the underlying pulmonary disorder is expected to recover. Potentially, ECMO allows recovery without subjecting the lungs to the risks of VILI or oxygen toxicity. Venoarterial systems may be used to completely take over the child's own heart and lung function (Fig. 9.4), although in practice extracorporeal flows may be limited by venous drainage (usually from the right internal jugular vein). Venovenous systems have been used for CO$_2$ removal, although a retrospective study concluded that venovenous ECMO could effectively provide adequate oxygenation for children with severe acute respiratory failure (Pettignano et al 2003). In the complete absence of pulmonary function, venovenous ECMO will provide SpO$_2$ of 80%. Using extracorporeal support, success has been achieved in some children with acute lung injury (Pearson et al 1993). However, appropriate patient selection is a critical and contentious issue. One method, proposed by Bartlett (1982, 1990), is to identify

9

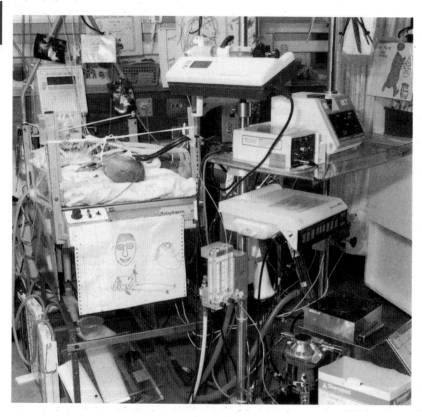

Figure 9.4 Extracorporeal membrane oxygenation.

neonates at high risk for failing to respond to conventional therapy by applying an index of oxygenation, which is related to the mean airway pressure and the FiO_2 during mechanical ventilation, and the achieved PaO_2:

Oxygenation index (OI) = (mean airway pressure × FiO_2 × 100)/PaO_2 (mmHg)

In Bartlett's proposal (1990), OI greater than 25 predicted 50% mortality and OI greater than 40 predicted 80% mortality. Anecdotally, in children, Goldman and colleagues (1997) have found in meningococcal sepsis that ARDS that fails to respond to HFOV may be reasonably treated with ECMO.

VENTILATION STRATEGIES FOR SPECIFIC DISEASE

In paediatric practice there are some specific diseases or problems that do require a specific ventilatory strategy. These issues are illustrated by the examples that follow.

Acute bronchiolitis

The typical features of bronchiolitis are:

- acute generalized peripheral airway obstruction ('air trapping') with tachypnoea, decreased breath sounds and low hemidiaphragms on chest radiography

- infant less than 2 years of age

- little or no evidence of past similar episodes.

Respiratory syncytial virus (RSV) is the most frequent cause of bronchiolitis. Other viral causes include adenovirus, influenza and parainfluenza viruses and rhinovirus. Cytomegalovirus can produce a bronchiolitis or pneumonitis-like illness in immunocompromised children. Rare non-viral causes of the bronchiolitis syndrome include *Mycoplasma pneumoniae* and *Bordetella pertussis* infection.

Sixteen per cent of infants hospitalized for RSV have apnoea and its course is usually short-lived. Clinically these episodes are diaphragmatic or non-obstructive with complete absence of respiratory effort. In these cases, endotracheal intubation with minimal support is required until the problem resolves. In patients with worsening respiratory distress due to pulmonary parenchymal changes, mechanical support does not necessarily require endotracheal intubation. In some instances, nasopharyngeal prong CPAP, which maintains positive transpulmonary pressure during spontaneous breathing, can be used to avoid mechanical ventilation. When infants with RSV infection require mechanical ventilation, there are many similarities with mechanical ventilation of adults with status asthmaticus (Box 9.4). Clinical observation of inspiratory and expiratory chest excursion as well as regular auscultation is important if overventilation, with associated hyperinflation and barotrauma, is to be avoided. The aim is to maintain or achieve adequate arterial oxygenation and control of respiratory acidosis. This may even necessitate ventilating at slow rates with prolonged expiratory times to permit adequate CO_2 clearance. Low levels of PEEP are used to decrease airway resistance and improve gas exchange, although in studies of lung mechanics this has not been verified. The presence of inadvertent or auto-PEEP requires that extrinsic PEEP be applied to the same level in order to maintain expiratory flow.

In patients with hyperinflation the ventilatory strategy should aim to limit ventilator-associated dynamic hyperinflation and impaired minute ventilation. The ventilator should be set at a slow rate (10–15 breaths/minute) and with a prolonged expiratory time. Time-cycled, PCV is used in this instance while aiming for an arterial pH >7.25 and a SpO_2 88–92%. When indicated, neuromuscular blockade and antibiotics will need to be prescribed. All patients should receive adequate analgesia and sedation during mechanical ventilation. Bronchodilators can be administered if patients demonstrate a therapeutic response to an initial trial dose. In the acute phase of illness, fluids, electrolytes and hydration must be closely monitored while generally restricting fluid to 67–75% of maintenance requirements. In the weaning phase, patients can be removed from ventilatory support when safe to do so. In regard to blood gas parameters this means, in general, adequate oxygenation in an FiO_2 <0.4 and normal pH, with good respiratory drive, in the absence of hypercarbia. Discharge from the intensive care unit can then be considered once the patient has managed at least 12–24 hours without any respiratory assistance. Overall these patients will, on average, spend about 7 days (interquartile range 4–8 days) on the intensive care unit (Tasker et al 2000).

In about one-fifth of mechanically ventilated patients with RSV more severe disease is seen (Tasker et al 2000). In this instance, more extensive pulmonary pathology results in a picture of pneumonitis with diffuse alveolar consolidation rather than bronchiolitis with lung hyperinflation. These infants have the clinical features of ARDS as they exhibit four-quadrant consolidation on chest radiograph. The aim of mechanical support should be to recruit lung volume with the addition of PEEP. Sometimes HFOV or ECMO is required if lung injury becomes more extensive with likely development of interstitial emphysema and pneumothorax. The time course of this problem is very different to the usual

9

9

course of bronchiolitis and, on average, patients spend at least 2 weeks on the intensive care unit (Tasker et al 2000).

Acute hypoxaemic respiratory failure

In patients with AHRF or ARDS the low tidal volume strategy in addition to PEEP helps to minimize VILI. The level of PEEP should be adjusted so as ensure maximum lung volume recruitment. Adequate recruitment improves oxygenation and avoids repeated alveolar collapse and reopening that lead to shear injuries. If oxygenation continues being inadequate with a mean airway pressure of 16 cmH_2O or greater, then HFOV should be considered, particularly if the problem is one of diffuse parenchymal changes or consolidation. A

series of adjunctive therapies have been proposed for this condition.

Prone positioning

Prone positioning has been shown to improve oxygenation during hypoxaemic respiratory disease in a number of adult and paediatric studies (Curley et al 2005, Pelosi et al 2002). These observations together with the simplicity of the procedure have justified the inclusion of this technique as standard practice. The incidence of serious adverse effects has not been reported to increase during prone position and only mild complications (e.g. facial oedema and pressure ulcers) have been described. During ventilation in the supine position the dorsal areas of the lung become preferentially consolidated or collapsed. The change to prone position allows recruitment of the dorsal areas of the lung and generates a more even distribution of ventilation and improved $\dot{V}/\dot{Q}$ matching. Unfortunately, even though the change in position seems to improve oxygenation during acute lung injury (ALI), it does not appear to have an impact on outcome. A recent study failed to show a reduction in ventilator-free days or mortality in children with ALI ventilated in prone position as compared with supine position (Curley et al 2005).

Recruitment manoeuvres

Recruitment manoeuvres are aimed at recovering collapsed areas of the lung during ALI, especially after specific manipulations such a suctioning and disconnection of the ventilator. A variety of manoeuvres have been described including increases in the level of PEEP while maintaining constant inspiratory pressures, prolonged increases in pressure (i.e. 40 mmHg for 40 seconds) as a single manoeuvre or using stepwise increases, and the use of high tidal volumes. There are no controlled studies and there is no consensus regarding these manoeuvres and their safety in children.

Nitric oxide

Nitric oxide (NO) is an endogenous, endothelium-derived vasodilator. Inhaled NO has the theoretical advantage of producing selective reduction in pulmonary vascular resistance. The fact that inhaled NO acts on the vessels of the aerated areas of the lung during ARDS suggests that it should improve $\dot{V}/\dot{Q}$ mismatch and therefore should be helpful during the management of this condition. Unfortunately, even though NO has shown to transiently improve oxygenation in ARDS, it does not seem to improve outcome (Sokol et al 2003).

Surfactant

The use of exogenous surfactant in adults with ARDS has been shown to be feasible and safe; however, it has not proven to be effective in adult ALI. A recent multi-centre, randomized, blinded trial of calfactant (extract of natural surfactant from calf lungs) compared with placebo in 153 infants with ALI showed improvement in oxygenation and a decrease in mortality in the patients that had received surfactant (Willson et al 2005).

Other considerations during mechanical ventilation

Position during mechanical ventilation

Changes in position during mechanical ventilation can be used to improve lung volumes, $\dot{V}/\dot{Q}$ matching, the clearance of airway secretions or to improve comfort and work of breathing. Changes in position can also be used to avoid or treat pressure lesions. Elevation of the bed head may also help to reduce gastro-oesophageal reflux and pulmonary aspiration (Torres et al 1992).

Humidification

During mechanical ventilation most of the upper airway is bypassed by the endotracheal tube or tracheostomy tube, and the rest of the airway may not be able to supply enough heat and moisture to the delivered gases that are dry and colder than body temperature. Humidification and heating is therefore essential to avoid complications such as hypothermia, inspissation of airway secretions, destruction of airway epithelium and atelectasis. In adults humidifying filters (which operate passively by storing heat and moisture from the patient's exhaled gas) are frequently used for this purpose; however, in children, active heating of humidified air is necessary. In order to achieve this, a humidifier that operates to increase the heat and water vapour content of the gases is interposed in the inspiratory limb of the ventilator circuit and the temperature is usually set to deliver approximately 37°C to the distal area of the circuit.

Suctioning

Suctioning of the airway to remove secretions is part of the routine care of patients receiving artificial ventilation. However, suctioning can lead to side effects including hypoxaemia, haemodynamic instability, mucosal damage, increase in intracranial pressure and patient discomfort. The use of adequate sedation, reassurance, preoxygenation and a good technique may help to minimize these complications.

Physiotherapy

Physiotherapy is frequently used as an integral part of the management of children receiving mechanical ventilation. However, the place, frequency and techniques of physiotherapy vary widely among units. Frequent techniques used in mechanically ventilated patients are manual hyperinflation, percussion, vibration and positioning, all of which are believed to increase the clearance of secretions (Chapter 10).

Monitoring during mechanical ventilation

Adequate monitoring of the parameters affected by mechanical ventilation is essential. The information helps to characterize the pathophysiology of the underlying condition, to improve ventilation, to enhance patient comfort, and to guide weaning. Blood gas measurement is the gold standard for assessing pulmonary gas exchange, but this technique is limited by the fact that measurements are not continuous, because they require invasive techniques. The use of pulse oximeters and end-tidal carbon dioxide concentration helps to minimize the number of blood gas samples. Transcutaneous carbon dioxide measurement is another way of continuously monitoring the CO_2 status.

Monitoring of the respiratory mechanics and analysis of the patient–ventilator interaction should be part of the routine care during mechanical ventilation. Most modern mechanical ventilators provide a graphical display of gas flow, airway pressures and tidal and minute volumes. In small infants and neonates, the information obtained with a pneumotachometer positioned at the end of the endotracheal tube instead of inside the mechanical ventilator can be more reliable. These data, together with measurements of pulmonary gas exchange, help to assess the adequacy of ventilation.

A new technique, electroimpedance tomography, analyses the distribution of ventilation and can be used at the bedside. This technique used 16 electrodes placed around the chest. Injection of an alternating electrical current between sequential pairs of adjacent electrodes and the repeated measurement of the differences in voltage through the array of electrodes permits the detection of changes in impedance. Since air is a poor conductor of electricity compared with other tissues, computer-assisted use of a mathematical algorithm then allows the reconstruction of a spatial image of a section of the chest. This method has the advantage of being non-invasive, radiation free, portable and dynamic. Different studies have shown its usefulness to assess regional lung ventilation (Victorino et al 2004).

Weaning from mechanical ventilation

Stopping mechanical ventilation as soon as the child is ready to be weaned from support is essential to avoid complications. Prolonged mechanical ventilation has been associated with higher risk of nosocomial pneumonia, progressive ventilator-associated lung

9

injury, airway injury, physiological dependence on sedative and narcotic drugs, and even higher mortality. In children who need mechanical ventilation for respiratory failure, the usual approach is to wean the ventilator settings gradually, until the patient is considered to be ready for extubation. However, this gradual weaning process is now being questioned.

A randomized controlled trial comparing weaning protocols versus standard physician-guided weaning in children did not show any impact on the duration of mechanical ventilation. This study also showed that gradual weaning may not be indicated for the majority of children receiving mechanical ventilation due to respiratory failure, and that a large group of children were ready to be extubated when the physicians determined that they were ready to begin a weaning process (Randolph et al 2002). Readiness for extubation can be evaluated using a daily test as soon as the patient meets the criteria for testing (Box 9.5). Different tests for extubation readiness have been proposed. In one paediatric study, patients were extubated if they passed a trial of spontaneous breathing with either pressure support of 10 cmH$_2$O, or T-piece for up to 2 hours. Mechanical ventilation was reinstituted if any of the following signs appeared:

1. respiratory rate higher than the 90th centile for the age
2. signs of increased respiratory work
3. diaphoresis and anxiety
4. heart rate higher than the 90th centile for the age
5. change in mental status
6. blood pressure lower than the 3rd centile
7. oxygen saturation lower than 90%
8. $PaCO_2$ more than 50 mmHg or an increase of more than 10 mmHg
9. arterial pH lower than 7.30 (Farias et al 2002).

Box 9.5 Eligibility criteria for readiness for extubation testing

1. Spontaneous respiratory effort
2. Gag or cough reflexes with suctioning
3. Presence of air leak around the ET tube
4. pH of 7.32–7.47 on blood gas
5. PEEP of 7 or lower
6. FiO$_2$ of 0.6 or less
7. Acceptable level of consciousness
8. Improvement of the underlying process that led to intubation
9. No need of increased ventilation during the last 24 hours
10. No planned administration of heavy sedation during the next 12 hours

---

Use of sedation has an impact on the duration of mechanical ventilation. Improved management of sedatives, including the use of objective sedation scores, should be part of the standard care for children receiving mechanical ventilation.

Non-invasive support

Non-invasive ventilation is the delivery of supportive ventilation without the use of an endotracheal airway. NIV is usually delivered as positive pressure ventilation using CPAP or BiPAP; however, negative pressure ventilation by mean of a cuirass is still useful for some conditions. Initially the use of NIV was mostly used in children with neuromuscular disease. Now, it is used in most types of respiratory failure.

In neonates and small infants the most frequent way of delivering non-invasive positive pressure ventilation (NPPV) is by means of nasal CPAP, although modern technology also incorporates the possibility of delivering BiPAP. The most frequent indication is bronchiolitis and other infections with apnoea. In bigger children NPPV is frequently delivered as BiPAP (Fig 9.5),

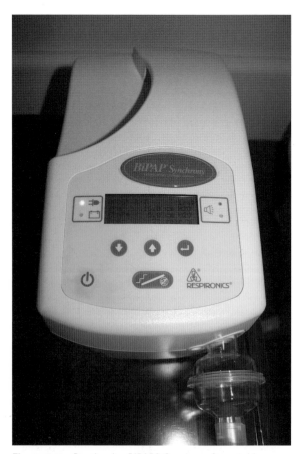

Figure 9.5 Respironics BiPAP® Synchrony®, portable.

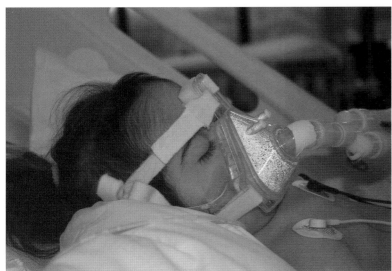

Figure 9.6 Facemask for non-invasive ventilation.

although CPAP can also be used. In this age it is used for different forms of acute hypoxaemic or hypercarbic respiratory failure including asthma, neuromuscular disease, or after extubation in children that have received long periods of mechanical ventilation. The usual way of applying this form of support is via a nasal mask or a facemask. Nasal masks are better tolerated, but many patients with respiratory distress are mouth breathers and therefore a facemask might be necessary (Fig. 9.6). In order to tolerate NPPV some sedation is needed in the young infant. In older children, explanation, reassurance and familiarity with the therapy should suffice. To increase the tolerance, NPPV can be started at low-pressure settings that are then increased progressively until the target pressures are obtained. Nasogastric tubes can be used when the accumulation of air in the stomach is a concern, especially in children with facemasks. However, many clinicians prefer not to use nasogastric tubes as their placement with tapes can reduce the tightness of the seal between the mask and the face.

A review of clinical studies using NPPV has shown that improvement usually occurs after the first 3 hours of therapy (Akingbola & Hopkins 2001). NPPV is not recommended in ARDS (Essouri et al 2006). The contraindications for NPPV include respiratory arrest, inability to use the mask because of trauma or surgery, difficult secretion management, haemodynamic instability, altered mental state, risk of aspiration, intolerance to the therapy and life-threatening refractory hypoxaemia or hypercarbia.

Finally, one technique that has historically been used effectively in children with neuromuscular disease since the poliomyelitis epidemics in the 1950s is extrathoracic negative pressure ventilation with a cuirass (Lassen 1953). In the past decade there has been renewed interest in this form of ventilation (Meessen et al 1994). There are many physiological reasons why negative pressure support should be beneficial, such as its ability to increase tonic activity in the diaphragm and intercostal muscles. In children with neuromuscular disease, who are on positive pressure mechanical support, it has been found that, when it comes to weaning, extubation and the introduction of negative pressure support means that analgesia and sedation can be discontinued quite quickly (Chisakuta & Tasker 1998). This approach should limit the unavoidable iatrogenic worsening of respiratory drive that results from the co-administration of analgesia and sedation (which is invariably necessary for children in order that they may tolerate the endotracheal tube). In myasthenic patients the time course of mechanical ventilatory support can be more than halved using this technique. Regarding bronchiolitis-related apnoeas, a retrospective analysis comparing two centres, one using negative pressure ventilation and the other using conventional therapies, concluded that the use of NPV was associated with a reduced rate of endotracheal intubation, and shorter paediatric intensive care unit (PICU) stay (Al-balkhi et al 2005). As more portable and easier-to-use ventilators become available, this form of respiratory support may be used more frequently.

9

References

Acute Respiratory Distress Syndrome Network 2000 Ventilation with lower tidal volumes as compared with traditional tidal volumes for acute lung injury and the acute respiratory distress syndrome. New England Journal of Medicine 342(18): 1301–1308

Akingbola OA, Hopkins RL 2001 Pediatric noninvasive positive pressure ventilation. Pediatric Critical Care Medicine 2(2): 164–169

9

Al-balkhi A, Klonin H, Marinaki K et al 2005 Review of treatment of bronchiolitis related apnoea in two centres. Archives of Disease in Childhood 90(3): 288–291

Arnold JH, Hanson JH, Toro-Figuero LO et al 1994 Prospective, randomized comparison of high-frequency oscillatory ventilation and conventional mechanical ventilation in pediatric respiratory failure. Critical Care Medicine 22(10): 1530–1539

Bartlett RH 1990 Extracorporeal life support for cardiopulmonary failure. Current Problems in Surgery 27(10): 621–705

Bartlett RH, Andrews AF, Toomasian JM et al 1982 Extracorporeal membrane oxygenation for newborn respiratory failure: forty-five cases. Surgery 92(2): 425–433

Bernard GR, Artigas A, Brigham KL et al 1994 The American-European consensus conference on ARDS: definitions, mechanisms, relevant outcomes and clinical trial coordination. American Journal of Respiratory and Critical Care Medicine 149(3 Pt 1): 818–824

Chisakuta A, Tasker RC 1998 Respiratory failure in myasthenia gravis and negative pressure support. Pediatric Neurology 19(3): 225–226

Curley MA, Hibberd PL, Fineman LD et al 2005 Effect of prone positioning on clinical outcomes in children with acute lung injury: a randomized controlled trial. Journal of the American Medical Association 294(2): 229–237

Essouri S, Chevret L, Durand P et al 2006 Non-invasive positive pressure ventilation: five years of experience in a pediatric intensive care unit. Pediatric Critical Care Medicine 7(4): 329–334

Farias JA, Alias I, Retta A et al 2002 An evaluation of extubation failure predictors in mechanically ventilated infants and children. Intensive Care Medicine 28(6): 752–757

Goldman AP, Kerr SJ, Butt W et al 1997 Extracorporeal support for intractable cardiorespiratory failure due to meningococcal disease. Lancet 349(9050): 466–469

Kneyber MC, Plötz FB, Sibarani-Ponsen RD, Markhorst DG 2005 High-frequency oscillatory ventilation (HFOV) facilitates CO_2 elimination in small airway disease: the open airway concept. Respiratory Medicine 99(11): 1459–1461

Lassen HC 1953 A preliminary report on the 1952 epidemic of poliomyelitis in Copenhagen with special reference to the treatment of acute respiratory insufficiency. Lancet 1(1): 37–41

Meessen NE, van der Grinten CP, Luijendijk SC et al 1994 Continuous negative airway pressure increases tonic activity in diaphragm and intercostal muscles in humans. Journal of Applied Physiology 77(3): 1256–1262

Pearson GA, Grant, J, Field, D et al 1993 Extracorporeal life support in paediatrics. Archives of Disease in Childhood 68(1): 94–96

Pelosi P, Brazzi L, Gattinoni L 2002 Prone position in acute respiratory distress syndrome. European Respiratory Journal 20(4): 1017–1028

Peters MJ, Tasker RC, Kiff KM, Yates R, Hatch DJ 1998 Acute hypoxemic respiratory failure in children: case mix and the utility of respiratory severity indices. Intensive Care Medicine 24(7): 699–705

Pettignano R, Fortenberry JD, Heard ML et al 2003 Primary use of the venovenous approach for extracorporeal membrane oxygenation in pediatric acute respiratory failure. Pediatric Critical Care Medicine 4(3): 291–298

Randolph AG, Meert KL, O'Neil ME et al 2003 (Pediatric Acute Injury and Sepsis Investigators Network). The feasibility of conducting clinical trials in infants and children with acute respiratory failure. American Journal of Respiratory and Critical Care Medicine 167(10): 1334–1340

Randolph AG, Wypij D, Venkataraman ST et al 2002 (Pediatric Acute Lung Injury and Sepsis Investigators (PALISI) Network). Effect of mechanical ventilator weaning protocols on respiratory outcomes in infants and children: a randomized controlled trial. Journal of the American Medical Association 288(20): 2561–2568

Slee-Wijffels FYAM, van der Vaart KRM, Twisk JWR et al 2005 High-frequency ventilation in children: a single-center experience of 53 cases. Critical Care 9(3): R274–279

Sokol J, Jacobs SE, Bohn D 2003 Inhaled nitric oxide for acute hypoxemic respiratory failure in children and adults. Cochrane Database of Systematic Reviews Issue 1. Art. No.: CD002787. DOI: 10.1002/14651858. CD002787

Tasker RC 2000 Gender differences and critical medical illness Acta Paediatrica 89(5): 621–623

Tasker RC, Gordon I, Kiff K 2000 Time course of severe respiratory syncytial virus infection in mechanically ventilated infants. Acta Paediatrica 89(8): 938–941

Torres A, Serra-Batlles J, Ros E et al 1992 Pulmonary aspiration of gastric contents in patients receiving mechanical ventilation: the effect of body position. Annals of Internal Medicine 116(7): 540–543

Victorino JA, Borges JB, Okamoto VN et al 2004 Imbalances in regional lung ventilation: a validation study on electrical impedance tomography. American Journal of Respiratory and Critical Care Medicine 169(7): 777–778

Watkins SJ, Peters MJ, Tasker RC 2000 One hundred courses of high frequency oscillatory ventilation: what have we learned? European Journal of Pediatrics 159(1–2): 134

Willson DF, Thomas NJ, Markovitz BP et al (Pediatric Acute Lung Injury and Sepsis Investigators) 2005 Effect of exogenous surfactant (calfactant) in pediatric acute lung injury: a randomized controlled trial. Journal of the American Medical Association 293(4): 470–476

Chapter 10

Paediatrics

S Ammani Prasad, Eleanor Main

INTRODUCTION

The respiratory system in children differs significantly from adults, both anatomically and physiologically. These differences have important consequences for the physiotherapy care of children in terms of respiratory assessment, treatment and choice of techniques.

The principal reason for hospital admissions in children aged 0–4 years is respiratory illness and the management of children with acute or chronic respiratory disorders has become a specialized area of respiratory physiotherapy. The inexperienced physiotherapist working with children will require the support and mentorship of an experienced paediatric physiotherapist in order to develop the necessary skills.

Assessment and treatment of children requires skillful age-appropriate communication with the child, the family and within the multidisciplinary team. It is essential to include parents, relatives and carers as part of the care team and children and their parents should have a full explanation of why treatment is required and what it involves. Treating children can be difficult and challenging and these sessions are easier when children are cooperative and compliant. Cooperation can often be obtained by persuasion, distraction with games, television, cassette tapes or reading books suited to the child's age and interest. It may be helpful in some situations to reward good behaviour or bravery, but occasionally children do refuse treatment. In these cases, if the benefits of treatment are considered to outweigh the risks, treatment must be given after thorough and careful explanation to the child and their carers.

Parents are able to refuse physiotherapy treatment for their child but this rarely occurs in practice. Parents of sick children often feel extremely vulnerable and anxious. Therapists should ensure their communication is always professional, empathetic and understanding. Parental stress may manifest in different ways, including apparent lack of concern or anger. Some parents may need special help to cope with their feelings of fear and anxiety and the regular contact between the physiotherapist and family is often an important source of support.

Children's awareness of the implications of chronic illness and treatment develop as they grow older and they should be encouraged to take on more responsibility for their treatment. Teenagers, particularly, have a more sophisticated understanding and may be beginning to think about the future and the impact of illness on school, social life and body image.

DEVELOPMENT OF THE LUNGS

The development of the lung can be divided into four stages (Inselman & Mellins 1981):

- Embryonic period (weeks 3–5)
- Pseudoglandular period (weeks 6–16)
- Canalicular period (weeks 17–24)
- Alveolar sac period (week 24–term).

Embryonic period (weeks 3–5). The lung bud starts as an endodermal outgrowth of fetal foregut. The single tube thus formed soon branches into two, forming the major bronchi. By cell division, the process of growth continues until, at the end of this period, the major lung branches are formed.

Pseudoglandular period (weeks 6–16). During this period the airways grow by dichotomous branching so that by week 16 all generations of the airway from trachea to terminal bronchioles (i.e. the preacinus) are formed. During this period the pulmonary circulation also develops, cartilage and lymphatic formation occur and cilia appear (week 10 onwards) (Langman 1977).

Canalicular period (weeks 17–24). The respiratory bronchioles, alveolar ducts and alveoli (i.e. the acinus) start to develop during this time, simultaneously with the lung capillaries, thus preparing the lungs for their future role in gas exchange (Hislop & Reid 1974). The air–blood barrier first appears at week 19 and towards the end of this period surfactant synthesis begins.

Terminal sac period (week 24–term). Development of the pulmonary circulation continues and the respiratory bronchioles subdivide to form air spaces. Two different cell types (types I and II pneumocytes) line the air spaces. Type I pneumocytes flatten and elongate to cover the majority of the surface area of the saccular air spaces. Type II cells only occupy approximately 2% of the surface and are responsible for surfactant synthesis and storage (Greenough 1996). Surfactant is a phospholipid, which stabilizes surface tension in the alveolus and prevents alveolar collapse on expiration. Small quantities of surfactant are present at weeks 23–24 of gestation and the amount present gradually increases until a surge at about week 30. Birth itself and the onset of respiration stimulate surfactant production.

Towards the end of the terminal sac period, the air spaces have developed into primitive multilocular alveoli. After birth, alveoli increase in size and number. The average number of alveoli in the newborn is 150 million. By the age of 3–4 years, the adult number of 300–400 million alveoli has been reached, but alveolar growth continues for the first 7 years (Hislop et al 1986). More recent estimations of mean alveolar number in adulthood have been 480 million (range 274–790 million), with alveolar number closely related to lung volume (Ochs 2004).

RESPIRATORY SYSTEM: ANATOMICAL AND PHYSIOLOGICAL DIFFERENCES BETWEEN CHILDREN AND ADULTS

The respiratory anatomy and physiology of infants and children is very different from that of adults. The principles of adult cardiorespiratory physiotherapy management cannot be transposed directly to an infant with pulmonary pathology.

Anatomical differences

Rib cage and chest shape

The cross-sectional shape of the infant thorax is cylindrical and not elliptical as in adolescents or adults. The ribs of the newborn infant are relatively soft and cartilaginous compared with the more rigid chest wall of older children and adults. They are also placed horizontally in relation to the sternum and vertebral column compared with the more oblique rib angle of adults (Fig. 10.1). The bucket handle rib movement seen in older children and adults is therefore not possible. As the infant grows, and begins to develop an upright posture, the ribs develop a more oblique angle and the transverse diameter of the rib cage increases. The adult chest shape is achieved by 3 years of age (Openshaw et al 1984).

The intercostal muscles are poorly developed in infancy and contraction of the intercostal muscles is inefficient at improving thoracic volumes either by increasing the anteroposterior or transverse diameters of the chest. Increased ventilatory requirements have to be met by increasing the respiratory rate rather than depth (Konno & Mead 1967).

Diaphragm

The angle of insertion of the infant diaphragm is horizontal compared with older children or adults, placing it at a mechanical disadvantage. The infant diaphragm has a lower relative muscle mass and a lower content of high-endurance muscle fibres, and thus is much more vulnerable to fatigue.

Maximal diaphragmatic activity during severe respiratory distress or respiratory obstruction leads to an inward movement of the lower rib cage instead of a downward movement of the diaphragm, as well as intercostal and sternal recession (Muller & Bryan 1979). Despite these disadvantages, the diaphragm is the main muscle of inspiration in the infant, since the intercostals are poorly developed. Ventilation in the infant is also more affected by impaired diaphragmatic function, for example by abdominal distension, hepatomegaly or phrenic nerve damage.

Preferential nasal breathing

The shape and orientation of head and neck in babies (large head, prominent occiput, short neck, large tongue, smaller retracted lower jaw, high larynx) mean that the airway is prone to obstruction in young infants. Young infants up to about 6 months of age are preferential nasal breathers and studies suggest that up to half of all neonates are unable to breathe through their mouths, except when crying, for the first few weeks of life (King & Booker 2004) The small nasal passages account for between 30% and 50% of the total airway resistance in neonates. The narrowest portion of the nasal airway has a cross-sectional area of about 20 mm². Therefore, even a small amount of swelling or obstruction of the nasal passages of infants compromises breathing considerably and causes a disproportionate and detrimental effect on the work of breathing. Some young infants with upper respiratory tract infections and partial

10

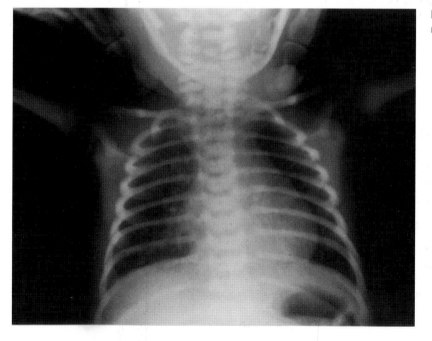

Figure 10.1 Normal chest radiograph.

obstruction of their nasal passages can develop respiratory distress.

Position of larynx

In the newborn infant, the larynx and hyoid cartilage are higher in the neck and closer to the base of the epiglottis, being at the level of C3 in a premature infant and C4 in a child compared with C5–6 in the adult. The larynx descends with age, but its high position enables the infant to feed and breathe simultaneously for approximately the first 4 months of age.

This high position also provides some protection of the airway in infants younger than 4–6 months because it acts as a valve, which helps keep food in the mouth until the pharyngeal swallow is initiated. The airway has less anatomical protection as the larynx assumes its lower position in the neck and is not as directly protected by the epiglottis. Then, poor closure of the airway or partial paralysis of the vocal folds may become more evident and coughing, choking or aspiration may occur.

Airway diameter

The neonatal trachea is short (4–9 cm) and directed downward and posteriorly. The diameter of the trachea in the newborn is 4–5 mm and the diameter of an infant trachea is only about one-third that of an adult. This makes respiratory resistance higher and the work of breathing greater. Since the resistance to airflow through a tube is directly related to the tube length and inversely related to the fourth power of the radius of the tube, halving the radius of the trachea will increase its resistance (reduce flow) 16 times. Tracheal swelling as a result of endotracheal intubation or suction can therefore dramatically increase resistance to breathing. These factors give the lungs less reserve, so that a well-oxygenated infant with upper airway obstruction can become cyanotic in a matter of seconds.

In contrast to adolescents and adults, the narrowest part of the infant's airway is not the vocal cords, but the cricoid ring. Thus an uncuffed endotracheal tube provides a larger internal diameter compared with a cuffed tube and in children will successfully seal against in the circular subglottic ring. However, the inflexible cricoid ring also leaves children more vulnerable to mucosal oedema and post-extubation stridor. The right main bronchus is less angled than the left, making right mainstem intubation more likely.

At birth there is no further increase in the number of airways formed but there is growth and development in their size. In the first few years of life there is a significant increase in the diameter of the larger, more proximal airways (Hislop & Reid 1974). The smaller, more distal airways do not increase in diameter until nearer 5 years of age. This higher peripheral airways resistance is exacerbated by respiratory infections, which cause inflammation of the airways, for example in bronchiolitis, or in the presence of secretions.

Bronchial walls

The bronchial walls are supported by cartilage, which begins to develop from 12 weeks' gestation and continues throughout childhood. The cartilaginous support of an infant's airways is much less than that of an adult, and predisposes the airways to collapse. The bronchial walls contain proportionally more cartilage, connective tissue and mucous glands than do those of adults, but less smooth muscle; this makes the lung tissue less compliant. The lack of bronchial smooth muscle, particularly in the smaller bronchioles, may be one reason for the lack of response to bronchodilators under the age of 12 months. The β-receptors in infants are also immature, which further reduces any response to β-adrenergic bronchodilator therapy (Reid 1984). The high proportion of mucous glands in the major bronchi of infants makes the airways more susceptible to mucus obstruction.

Cilia

At birth the cilia are poorly developed, which increases the risk of secretion retention, especially in the premature infant. The airway obstruction caused by secretions in a neonate is much greater than in an adult whose airways are relatively large.

Alveoli and surfactant

The respiratory system is not fully developed at birth, even in the term neonate, and postnatal maturation continues for a significant time. Although by 20–27 weeks' gestation lung acinar have formed, several types of epithelial cells can be differentiated, and the air–blood barrier is thin enough to support gas exchange; true alveoli develop only after about 36 weeks' gestation. A term newborn has an average of 150 million alveoli. The remainder of the eventual average of 400 million alveoli develop after birth, the vast majority within the first 2 years of life. Both the number and size of alveoli continue to increase postnatally until the chest wall stops growing. By 4 years of age, the adult number of 300 million may exist, although growth can continue until 7 years of age. The smaller alveolar size of an infant makes the infant more susceptible to alveolar collapse, and the smaller number of alveoli reduces the area available for gaseous exchange (Reid 1984).

Pulmonary surfactant is a mixture of phospholipids (90%) and apoproteins (10%), which act to reduce surface tension at the air–liquid interface in the alveolus, thereby preventing collapse of lung parenchyma at the end of expiration. Type II alveolar cells synthesize and secrete surfactant from 23 to 24 weeks' gestation. In preterm newborns, a deficiency of surfactant is a major factor in the development of neonatal respiratory distress syndrome (RDS). Male gender is a risk factor for neonatal RDS, bronchopulmonary dysplasia (BPD) and mortality. Boys with neonatal RDS seem to have more health problems than girls during the neonatal period.

Collateral ventilation

Collateral ventilation is the means by which a distal lung unit can be ventilated, despite blockage of its main airway. Collateral ventilatory pathways are achieved by a network of interconnecting pathways linking different structures. Respiratory bronchioles are linked by channels of Martin. Canals of Lambert connect respiratory and terminal bronchioles with alveoli and their ducts; and adjacent alveoli are joined by openings in the alveolar wall, called pores of Kohn (Menkes & Traystman 1977). However, none of these pathways exists at birth. The pores of Kohn develop between years 1 and 2, and the canals of Lambert do not appear until about 6 years of age. The collateral ventilatory channels between alveoli, respiratory bronchioles and terminal bronchioles are poorly developed until 2 and 3 years of age, predisposing towards alveolar collapse.

Internal organs and lymphatic tissue

The lymphatic tissue (adenoids and tonsils) may be enlarged in the infant and the tongue is also relatively large. These factors may contribute to upper airway obstruction. The heart and other organs are also relatively large in infants, leaving less space for lung expansion. The heart can occupy up to half the transverse diameter of the chest in chest radiographs.

Height and exposure to air pollution

Because children breathe more rapidly compared with adults and because they spend more time outdoors being physically active, they tend to be more exposed to outdoor air pollution and allergens than do adults and have greater deposition of particulate matter. Their reduced height means they are also more exposed to vehicle exhausts and heavier pollutants that concentrate at lower levels in the air. There is substantial evidence linking air pollution with respiratory health problems and children are more vulnerable (Brauer et al 2007, Pénard-Morand et al 2005).

Physiological differences

Respiratory compliance

Respiratory compliance is a measure of the pressure required to increase the volume of air in the lungs and reflects a combination of lung and chest wall compliance. The lung compliance of a child is comparable to that of an adult, being directly proportional to the child's size. However, compliance is reduced in the infant

because of the high proportion of cartilage in the airways. The premature infant, who lacks surfactant, demonstrates a further significant decrease in compliance. The chest wall of an infant is cartilaginous and therefore very soft and compliant in comparison with the more calcified and rigid adult structure. The intercostal muscles are also less well equipped to stabilize the rib cage during diaphragmatic contraction. Neonates therefore have an imbalance between a relatively low outward recoil of their chest wall and normal inward elastic recoil, which means that they are prone to airway collapse. An awake, spontaneously breathing neonate will maintain its functional residual capacity (FRC) by active measures including laryngeal braking, the initiation of inspiration before the end of passive expiration (intrinsic PEEP) and persistent inspiratory muscle activity throughout the respiratory cycle. These active mechanisms are lost during anaesthesia and result in a fall in FRC, airway closure, atelectasis and ventilation/perfusion mismatch.

Closing volume

The closing volume is the lung volume at which closure of the small airways occurs. This volume plus the residual volume (the volume of gas left in the lungs following maximum expiration) is known as the closing capacity (CC). In the adult, CC is less than FRC, i.e. the volume of gas left in the lungs following tidal expiration, whereas in the infant it is greater than FRC. The higher closing volumes apparent in infants are due to greater chest wall compliance and reduced elastic recoil of the lungs than in the adult. Therefore, airway closure may occur before the end of expiration, e.g. during expiratory chest vibrations, putting the infant at a much greater risk of developing widespread atelectasis, especially in the presence of lung disease, where lung volume is further reduced. In the event of respiratory distress, the infant grunts on expiration, adducting the vocal cords in an attempt to reduce the amount of gas expired, thus maintaining a higher FRC and minimizing alveolar collapse (Pang & Mellins 1975). Re-inflation of alveoli, once collapsed, is more difficult in the infant, who has to work considerably harder to overcome the effects of the compliant chest wall.

Ventilation and perfusion

In the adult, both ventilation and perfusion are preferentially distributed to the dependent lung. The best gas exchange and ventilation/perfusion match will therefore be in the dependent region of the lung (Zack et al 1974). In the infant, however, ventilation is preferentially distributed to the uppermost lung (Davies et al 1985), whereas the perfusion remains best in the dependent regions. This leads to greater gas exchange in the uppermost lung (Heaf et al 1983) but an imbalance

10

between ventilation and perfusion (Bhuyan et al 1989). In acutely ill children with unilateral lung disease, oxygenation may be optimized by placing the 'good' lung uppermost. However, this is contrary to the goal of improving ventilation to the diseased lung and facilitating secretion clearance, in which positioning and postural drainage would require the diseased lung to be uppermost. The therapist would have to balance their decision based on the stability, tolerance and current therapeutic priorities.

The difference in ventilation distribution between infants and adults is most likely due to the more compliant rib cage of the infant, which compresses the dependent areas of lung. In addition, while in the adult the weight of the abdominal contents provides a preferential load on the dependent diaphragm and therefore improves its contractility, in the infant this does not happen. The effect on both hemidiaphragms is similar, due to the abdomen being so much smaller and narrower (Davies et al 1985). It has been shown in adults that, when the diaphragm is inactivated, e.g. when ventilated under anaesthetic, the ventilation distribution changes to that of an infant (Rehder et al 1972). It is not yet known exactly when the ventilation distribution in the infant changes to that of an adult, but it may be as late as 10 years of age.

Oxygen consumption, cardiac output and response to hypoxia

Infants have a higher resting metabolic rate than adults and consequently have a higher oxygen requirement. Children have a higher cardiac output and oxygen consumption per kilogram than adults; in infants this may exceed 6 ml/kg/min, twice that of adults. They support this higher output with a higher baseline heart rate but lower blood pressure than adults.

Neonatal myocardium has a large supply of mitochondria, nuclei and endoplasmic reticulum to support cell growth and protein synthesis, but these are non-contractile tissues, which render the myocardium stiff and non-compliant. This may impair filling of the left ventricle and limit the ability to increase the cardiac output by increasing stroke volume (Frank Starling mechanism). Stroke volume in infants is therefore relatively fixed and the only way of increasing cardiac output is by increasing heart rate.

The sympathetic nervous system is not well developed predisposing the neonatal heart to bradycardia. An infant responds to hypoxia with bradycardia and pulmonary vasoconstriction, whereas the adult becomes tachycardic with systemic vasodilation. The bradycardic response in infants is probably due to myocardial hypoxia and acidosis, but leads to an immediate reduction in cardiac output and the development of further hypoxia.

Although anatomical closure of the foramen ovale can occur as early as 3 months of age, the channel remains 'probe patent' in 50% of children up to 5 years of age, and persists in about 30% of adults. Similarly, anatomical closure of the ductus arteriosus usually occurs between 4 and 8 weeks of age. Any stimulus, such as hypoxia or acidosis, that causes an increase in pulmonary vascular resistance during the neonatal period may allow these two potential channels to reopen, resulting in right-to-left shunting and increasing hypoxia (King & Booker 2004).

Muscle fatigue

The respiratory muscles of infants tire more quickly than those of adults due to a much smaller proportion of fatigue-resistant muscle fibre (Keens & Ianuzzo 1979). There are two main muscle fibre types, type I and type II. Type I muscle fibres are slow twitch, high oxidative and slow to fatigue. Type II fibres are fast twitch, slow oxidative and tire quickly. Of the muscle fibres in the adult diaphragm, 55% are type I compared with only 30% in the infant. Premature infants tire even more easily as, at 24 weeks' gestation, only 10% of their muscle fibres are fatigue resistant (Muller & Bryan 1979). Excessive muscle fatigue results in apnoea. By 12 months of age the number of type I fibres equals that of an adult.

Breathing pattern and rapid eye movement sleep

Irregular breathing patterns and episodes of apnoea are relatively common in neonates, especially if premature, and are related to immature cardiorespiratory control. Short spells of apnoea can be considered normal in these circumstances, but need careful monitoring as they may reflect hypoxic conditions.

During rapid eye movement (REM) sleep there is a reduction in postural tone and tonic inhibition of the infant's intercostal muscles such that the rib cage is even less well equipped to counteract the contraction of the diaphragm during inspiration (Muller & Bryan 1979). This reduces the efficiency of respiration, causes a drop in functional residual capacity and increases the work of breathing, predisposing the infant to apnoeic episodes (Muller & Bryan 1979). The premature infant is most at risk, spending up to 20 hours a day asleep, 80% of which may be in active REM sleep compared with 20% in adult sleep.

Response to cold

Paediatric patients have an increased surface area per kilogram and lose heat to the environment more readily than adults. This is compounded by cold intravenous fluids, dry anaesthetic gases and exposure. Non-shivering thermogenesis in brown adipose tissue is the major mechanism of heat production during the first few months of life. Brown fat is specialized tissue located in the posterior of the neck, along the interscapular and vertebral areas, and surrounding the kidneys and adrenal glands. Metabolic heat production can increase up to two and a half times during cold stress. Shivering is a less economical form of heat production but does occur in severely hypothermic neonates. Hypothermia is a serious problem that can result in increased oxygen consumption, cardiac irritability and respiratory depression (King & Booker 2004).

RESPIRATORY ASSESSMENT OF THE INFANT AND CHILD

Careful assessment is essential to identify problems requiring physiotherapy intervention. Many aspects of assessment will be the same as in adults (Chapter 1), but specific differences are listed below.

Medical notes

Information can be extracted from the medical notes relating to present and past medical history. When assessing a neonate, history of pregnancy, labour and delivery are relevant as well as gestational age and weight. In addition, the Apgar score at birth should be noted. This score relates to heart rate, respiratory effort, muscle tone, reflex irritability and colour and gives an indication of the degree of asphyxiation suffered by the infant at birth.

Discussion with the relevant carers

Discussion with medical staff, nursing staff and the parent/carer is essential to obtain correct information about recent changes. In chronically ill children who require home physiotherapy, liaison with the primary healthcare team is essential.

When assessing the hospitalized child, information should be obtained about:

- the stability of the child's condition over the last few hours
- how well the infant tolerates handling. Does the infant become rapidly hypoxic or bradycardic?
- how long does the child take to recover from the handling episode?
- whether the child is fed via the oral, nasogastric or intravenous route and the timing of the last feed
- whether the child is sufficiently rested to tolerate a physiotherapy treatment.

Observation charts and investigations

Pyrexia may indicate a possible respiratory infection. The core-to-peripheral temperature gradient should be noted, particularly in the critically ill patient as it is a reflection of peripheral vasoconstriction which can occur as a response to cold, hypovolaemia, sepsis or low cardiac output.

Tachycardia may be due to sepsis or shock. It may also be caused by inadequate levels of sedation or analgesia. In preterm infants, bradycardias may be due to many causes, including retention of secretions.

Apnoeic spells in the infant may indicate respiratory distress, sepsis or presence of secretions in the upper or lower respiratory tract.

The trend of arterial gases and their relationship to oxygen saturation and transcutaneous oxygen should be noted, together with the degree and type of respiratory support.

Results of investigations and other relevant observations should be referred to as appropriate.

Examination

Examination of the older child is similar to that of the adult (Chapter 1). The following specific factors should be considered in younger children.

Clinical signs

Clinical signs of respiratory distress are listed in Box 10.1.

10

Box 10.1   Clinical signs of respiratory distress

Respiratory
- Recession
  - intercostal
  - subcostal
  - sternal
- Nasal flaring
- Tachypnoea
- Expiratory grunting
- Stridor
- Cyanosis
- Abnormal breath sounds

Cardiac
- Tachycardia/bradycardia
- Hypertension/hypotension

Other/general
- Neck extension
- Head bobbing
- Pallor
- Reluctance to feed
- Irritability/restlessness
- Altered conscious level
- Headache

Recession occurs when high negative intrathoracic pressure during inspiration pulls the soft, compliant chest wall inward. It may be sternal, subcostal or intercostal. Mild recession may be normal in preterm infants but in older infants is a sign of increased respiratory effort.

Nasal flaring is a dilatation of the nostrils by the dilatores naris muscles and is a sign of respiratory distress in the infant. It may be a primitive response attempting to decrease airway resistance.

Tachypnoea (respiratory rate greater than 60 breaths/min) may indicate respiratory distress in infants. Normal values are listed in Table 10.1.

Grunting occurs when an infant expires against a partially closed glottis. This is an automatic response which increases functional residual capacity in an attempt to improve ventilation.

Stridor is heard in the presence of a narrowing of the upper trachea and/or larynx. This may be due to collapse of the floppy tracheal wall, inflammation or an inhaled foreign body. It is most commonly heard during inspiration, but in cases of severe narrowing it may be heard during both inspiration and expiration.

Cyanosis refers to the bluish colour of the skin and mucous membranes caused by hypoxaemia. In infants and young children it is an unreliable sign of respiratory distress as it depends on the relative amount and type of haemoglobin in the blood and the adequacy of the peripheral circulation. For the first 3–4 weeks of life, the newborn infant has an increased amount of fetal haemoglobin, which has a higher affinity for oxygen than adult haemoglobin. The result is a shift of the oxygen saturation curve to the left in infants.

Auscultation of the infant and young child is sometimes complicated by the easy transmission of sounds. In the infant who is ventilated, referred sounds such as water in the ventilator tubing may be transmitted to the chest. In the older child, secretions in the nose or throat may lead to referred sounds in both lung fields. Wheezing in the younger child or infant may be due to bronchospasm, but could also be due to retained secretions partially occluding smaller airways. It is sometimes very difficult to hear breath sounds in the spontaneously breathing preterm infant.

Cardiac manifestations of respiratory distress include an initial tachycardia and possible increase in systemic blood pressure. This changes with worsening hypoxia to bradycardia and hypotension.

Neck extension in an infant with respiratory distress may represent an attempt to reduce airway resistance.

Head bobbing occurs when infants attempt to use the sternocleidomastoid and the scalene muscles as accessory muscles of respiration. It is seen because the relatively weak neck extensors of infants are unable to stabilize the head.

Pallor is commonly seen in infants with respiratory distress and may be a sign of hypoxaemia or other problems, including anaemia.

Reluctance to feed is often associated with respiratory distress and infants may need to take frequent pauses from sucking when tachypnoeic.

Alterations in levels of consciousness should be noted. A reduction in activity may be due to neurological deficit or as a result of opiate analgesia but may also be due to hypoxia. It may be accompanied by an inability to feed or cry. Irritability and restlessness may also be indicative of a hypoxic state.

Other relevant observations

The behaviour of a child can often give important clues about their respiratory status. Agitation or irritability may be a sign of hypoxia, while the child in severe respiratory distress may be withdrawn and lie completely still.

It is important to note muscle tone in the infant or child with respiratory distress. A hypotonic child may have increased difficulty with breathing, coughing and

Table 10.1	Normal values		
Age group	Heart rate mean (range) (beats/min)	Respiratory rate – range (breaths/min)	Blood pressure systolic/diastolic (mmHg)
Preterm	150 (100–200)	40–60	39–59 / 16–36
Newborn	140 (80–200)	30–50	50–70 / 25–45
<2 years	130 (100–190)	20–40	87–105 / 53–66
>2 years	80 (60–140)	20–40	95–105 / 53–66
>6 years	75 (60–90)	15–30	97–112 / 57–71

expectorating, while hypertonia may also be associated with difficulty in clearing secretions.

Abdominal distension can cause or exacerbate respiratory distress, because the diaphragm is placed at a mechanical disadvantage. In infants this is of greater concern as the diaghragm is the primary muscle of respiration.

PHYSIOTHERAPY TECHNIQUES IN INFANTS AND CHILDREN

Most physiotherapy techniques used in adults can be applied in children and the same contraindications apply (Chapters 5 & 6). Treatment should never be performed routinely as it may have potentially detrimental effects (Horiuchi et al 1997, Krause & Hoehn 2000, Stiller 2000). Ideally treatment should occur before feeds or adequate time allowed following a feed to avoid problems associated with vomiting and aspiration.

Chest percussion

Chest percussion (sometimes referred to as chest clapping) using the hand, fingers or a facemask is generally well tolerated and widely used in children. Percussion with one hand is used in small children and babies (Fig. 10.2A). In neonates and preterm infants 'tenting' (using the first three or four fingers of one hand with slight elevation of the middle finger) or the use of a soft plastic cup-shaped object such as a facemask may be more appropriate (Fig. 10.2B) (Tudehope & Bagley 1980).

Vibrations and shaking

Chest wall vibrations involve the application of a rapid extrathoracic compressive force at the beginning of expiration, followed by oscillatory compressions until expiration is complete. The compressions and oscillations applied during chest wall vibrations are believed to aid secretion clearance via a number of physiological mechanisms, including increasing peak expiratory flow to move secretions towards the large airways for removal by suction or cough (Kim et al 1987, King 1998, McCarren et al 2006, Ntoumenopoulos 2005, van der Schans et al 1999, Wanner 1984).

Chest wall vibrations remain objectively undefined and may vary considerably between practitioners and units. The terms chest vibrations, compressions, shaking and expiratory flow increase techniques have been used variously in the literature (Almeida et al 2005, Sutton et al 1985, Wong et al 2003).

Chest wall vibrations appear to be used more frequently in ventilated children than percussion, probably because the glottis is held open by the endotracheal tube, facilitating rapid expiratory flow during vibra-

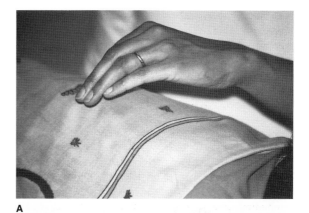

A

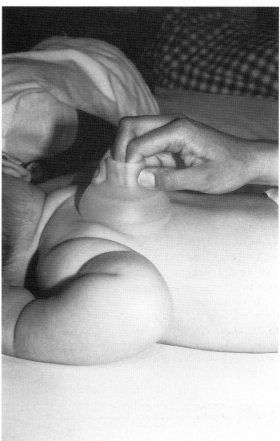

B

Figure 10.2 (A) Single-handed percussion. (B) Percussion with facemask.

tions that improve mucus clearance. There is a strong linear relationship between the maximum force applied during chest wall vibrations and the age of the child, most likely reflecting modification of techniques to accommodate changes in chest wall compliance (Gregson et al 2007a). Maximum force applied during

10

10

physiotherapy can vary substantially between physiotherapists. Similarly there is marked variability in the pattern of force–time profiles between physiotherapists with respect to the duration of vibration, and amplitude, number and frequency of oscillations. Figure 10.3 illustrates the style of force profiles delivered to four infants, all aged between 5 and 14 months by four different physiotherapists. However, there is remarkable consistency within and between each physiotherapist's treatment sessions (Gregson et al 2007b). The clinical consequences for such variation in treatment profiles remain unclear.

In children who are not intubated, vibrations can be applied effectively when reflex glottic closure does not occur and when the respiratory rate is normal or near normal (30–40 breaths/min). If infants are breathing very rapidly, the expiratory phase is so short that vibrations are more difficult to perform.

Precautions for chest percussion and vibratory techniques

In children with dietary deficiencies, liver disease, bone mineral deficiency (e.g. rickets) or coagulopathies,

manual techniques should be applied with caution. Manual techniques may not be appropriate in extremely premature infants and specific issues related to this group of patients are discussed later.

Chest percussion has been reported to cause an increase in bronchospasm in adults with chronic lung disease (Campbell et al 1975, Wollmer et al 1985). Premedication with bronchodilator therapy may reduce this effect but in severe cases percussion should be avoided.

Postural drainage (gravity-assisted positioning)

The use of gravity-assisted positioning, including a head-down tip, has traditionally been a component of airway clearance in babies and children. However, the use of the head-down tipped position has been the focus of considerable debate in recent years. Very few studies have examined specifically the efficacy of gravity-assisted positioning in infants and children. An Australian study of 20 babies with cystic fibrosis reported an increase in gastro-oesophageal reflux in

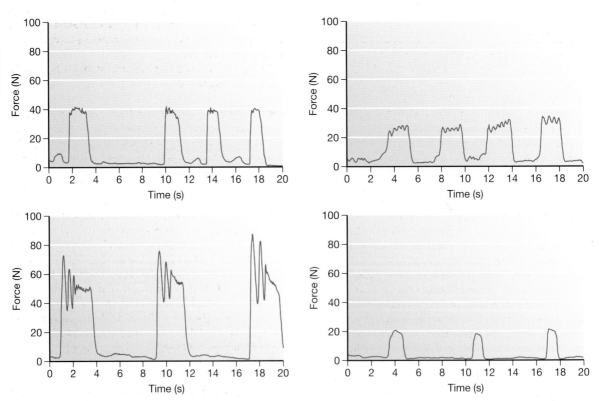

Figure 10.3 Force–time profiles of chest wall vibrations delivered by four different physiotherapists to four infants (5–14 months). The patterns are repeatable within each treatment but vary considerably between therapists with respect to magnitude and duration of vibration, and amplitude, number and frequency of oscillations.

those receiving postural drainage (PD) using a head-down tipped position compared with modified PD without a head-down tilt (Button et al 1997). Another study also undertaken in babies with cystic fibrosis (CF) (Phillips 1996) reported no adverse effect of the head-down tipped position on gastroesophageal reflux. This discrepancy could be attributed to the differences between the two study populations. Despite the inconsistency between these two studies, the concerns raised have led to a significant change in practice in many CF centres. This has to some extent been extrapolated to other paediatric respiratory disorders with the result that the head-down tipped position is now used much less in paediatric practice. A head-down tip should never be used in children with raised intracranial pressure or in preterm infants because of the risk of periventricular haemorrhage. Abdominal distension places the diaphragm at a mechanical disadvantage and a head-down tilt is likely to exacerbate this further.

Where appropriate, modified gravity-assisted positions can be used in children to assist clearance of bronchial secretions. The upper lobes, particularly the right side, are more frequently affected by respiratory problems and appropriate positioning may be helpful.

Positioning

Positioning may be used to optimize respiratory function. The supine position has been shown to be the least beneficial, while prone positioning has been shown to improve respiratory function (Chapter 4), decrease gastro-oesophageal reflux (Blumenthal & Lealman 1982) and reduce energy expenditure (Brackbill et al 1973). It is often used in closely monitored infants with respiratory problems in a hospital setting, but parents should be advised against using this position when babies are sleeping unattended because of its association with sudden infant death (Southall & Samuels 1992).

Patterns of regional ventilation in infants differ significantly from adults (Davies et al 1985), with ventilation in infants and small children being preferentially distributed to the uppermost regions of the lungs. In acutely ill children with unilateral lung disease, care should be taken if positioning the child with the affected lung uppermost as this may cause rapid deterioration of respiratory status. Spontaneously breathing newborn infants are better oxygenated when tilted slightly head up (Thoresen et al 1988) and show a drop in PaO_2 if placed flat or tilted head down.

It is suggested that the redistribution of ventilation, which occurs with a change in body position, results in optimized ventilation to specific lung regions and localized improvement in airway patency. This may result in enhanced secretion clearance from these regions,

which are not necessarily those positioned in such a way to allow gravitational drainage (Lannefors & Wollmer 1992).

Manual ventilation

Manual lung inflation involves disconnection of the patient from mechanical ventilation to provide temporary manual ventilation. The same contraindications apply for children and adults (Chapters 5 & 8). However, special consideration should be applied in preterm infants whose lung tissue is easily damaged by high inflation pressures and in children with hyperinflated lungs (e.g. asthma and bronchiolitis) in whom there is a greater risk of pneumothorax. For infants, 500 ml bags should be used and 1 litre bags for older children. They may be valved or open-ended, so that expulsion of excess pressure is controlled by the operator's fingers. A manometer should be placed in the circuit whenever possible to monitor the inflation pressures (Fig. 10.4). As a general guideline, manual ventilation pressures during physiotherapy should not exceed 10 cmH$_2$O above the ventilator pressure. In order to prevent airway collapse, some positive end-expiratory pressure (PEEP) should be maintained in the bag. Self-inflating bags are used in some units. The flow rate of gas is adjusted according to the size of the child: 4 l/min for infants increasing to 8 l/min for children.

In paediatric patients manual ventilation is used to achieve the following:

Hyperinflation – a long inspiration with an inspiratory pause followed by rapid release of the bag. The aim of this technique is to recruit lung units by improving collateral ventilation and increasing lung volume. However in acute respiratory distress, the proportion of recruitable lung may be extremely variable (Gattinoni et al 2006). Following hyperinflation, a high expiratory flow may assist in mobilizing secretions towards central airways. Some studies support the use of hyperinflation for improving respiratory mechanics (Choi & Jones 2005, Marcus et al 2002). However there remains some controversy over the safety and effectiveness of manual lung hyperinflation as the volumes, pressures and FiO$_2$ are not always controlled and there are inherent dangers of barotrauma (Berney & Denehy 2002, Gattinoni et al 1993, Savian et al 2006). In children with compromised cardiac output, the long inspiratory phase with pause may be contraindicated.

Hyperoxygenation – may be used before suction in order to reduce suction-induced hypoxia or pulmonary hypertension. A review of the efficacy of ventilator versus manual hyperinflation in delivering hyperoxygenation

10

10

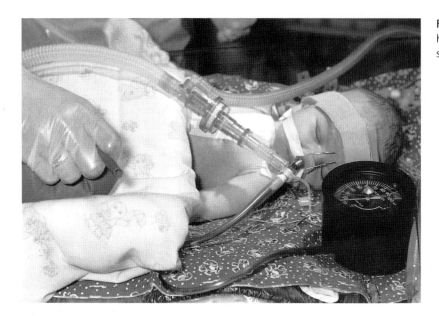

Figure 10.4 Manual hyperinflation in a small child showing pressure gauge in circuit.

or hyperinflation breaths before, during and/or after endotracheal suctioning found that hyperoxygenation or hyperinflation breaths at 100% oxygen delivered via the ventilator were either superior or equivalent to manually delivered breaths in preventing suction-induced hypoxaemia. However, delivery of manual hyperinflation breaths resulted in increased airway pressure and increased haemodynamic consequences (Stone 1990, Stone & Turner 1989). In the presence of pulmonary hypertension, it is generally not advisable to use an FiO_2 of 1.0 during manual hyperinflation as this may further increase blood flow to the lungs.

Hyperventilation – in order to reduce the carbon dioxide in patients with head injury, so that physiotherapy can be safely undertaken, the carbon dioxide should not be allowed to drop too low as this may lead to excessive reduction in cerebral blood flow. In those patients with a large cardiac shunt, hyperventilation may be contraindicated.

Independently performed airway clearance techniques

Over the past two decades, several modalities of airway clearance have been developed. The aim of all of these techniques is to effectively enhance clearance of bronchial secretions and at the same time to facilitate independence with treatment. The majority of techniques were developed for chronic lung disease, in particular cystic fibrosis, but their use has become widespread in both acute and chronic disorders and they are commonly used in paediatric practice (Fig. 10.5). The various

techniques are described in detail in Chapter 5 and include:

- active cycle of breathing techniques
- autogenic drainage
- high-frequency chest wall oscillation
- oscillatory positive expiratory pressure
  — flutter
  — acapella
  — cornet
- positive expiratory pressure.

Airway clearance for children with neurological and neuromuscular impairment

Impaired cough, as a consequence of weakness from neuromuscular disease such as Duchenne muscular dystrophy and spinal muscular atrophy or neurological impairment, can cause serious respiratory complications including atelectasis, pneumonia, airway obstruction and acidosis (Miske et al 2004). Chronic respiratory insufficiency and respiratory failure will ultimately result from chronic weakness of respiratory muscles, shallow breathing and ineffective cough. For these children, independently performed airway clearance techniques are not usually feasible, but options such as the 'cough assist' (mechanical insufflation/exsufflation device) and other non-invasive forms of positive pressure ventilation are safe and well tolerated in this client group, with growing evidence to support their efficacy (Chatwin et al 2003, Panitch 2006, Vianello et al 2005). They are discussed more comprehensively in Chapters 5 & 11. Not all patients with neuromuscular disease are

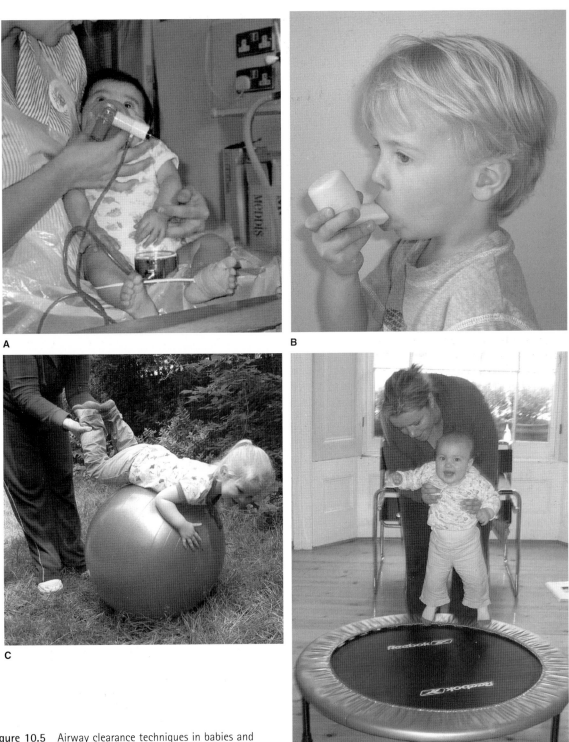

Figure 10.5 Airway clearance techniques in babies and children. **(A)** PEP in an infant. **(B)** Flutter. **(C)** and **(D)** Physical activity.

A

B

C

D

10

good candidates for the use of non-invasive respiratory aids. Potential contraindications include an inability to manage oropharyngeal secretions, mental status changes or cognitive impairment, and cardiovascular instability. For some patients, including those with the most severe spinal muscular atrophy, sole reliance on non-invasive methods of assisted cough and ventilation is inadequate, and they may require repeated episodes of intubation and mechanical ventilation in the intensive care unit to prolong survival (Birnkrant 2002).

Breathing exercises

It is possible to encourage children to deep breathe from about 2 years of age by using games such as bubbles, paper windmills or incentive spirometers, although the efficacy of these treatments is unproven. Laughing is a very effective means of lung expansion in infants. As children get older, they are able to play a more active role in their treatment and appropriate airway clearance techniques can be introduced (Chapter 5).

Coughing

Younger children are not able to cough to command and although children from about 18 months of age often mimic coughing if asked to do so, the cough is often ineffective. Tracheal compression is occasionally used to try and stimulate a cough in babies. Gentle pressure applied briefly to the trachea, below the thyroid cartilage, causes apposition of the soft and pliant tracheal walls and may stimulate the cough reflex. This technique must be used with care in small infants as this can potentially trigger a vagal response and bradycardia. If a cough cannot be stimulated or if it is ineffective, airway suction may be necessary to remove thick or copious secretions. Changing position or physical activity can be very effective in mobilizing secretions and stimulating a cough reflex in toddlers and older children. Children under the age of 4 or 5 do not usually have the ability to expectorate voluntarily and usually swallow secretions. Even older children can find it difficult to mobilize secretions far enough in to the mouth to expectorate.

Airway suction

Airway suction is discussed in Chapters 5 and 8. Suction techniques may be either naso- or oropharyngeal or endotracheal, depending on whether there is an artificial airway in situ. Adverse effects have frequently been reported and include hypoxaemia, mechanical trauma, apnoea, bronchospasm, pneumothorax, atelectasis, cardiac arrhythmias and even death on rare occasions (Clark et al 1990, Clarke et al 1999, Czarnik et al 1991, Kerem et al 1990, Shah et al 1992, Singer et al 1994, Stone & Turner 1989, Wood 1998). Practice varies widely among centres and where available local guidelines should be taken in to consideration (Sole et al 2003).

Complications associated with suction may be reduced by:

- Preoxygenation before suction using ventilator or manually delivered breaths with a higher FiO_2 (Chulay & Graeber 1988, Goodnough 1985). Preoxygenation with ventilator breaths has been recommended in preference to disconnection and manual hyperinflation because of the reduced risk of barotrauma, loss of PEEP and FiO_2 (Glass et al 1993, McCabe & Smeltzer 1993, Stone et al 1991). Particular care should be taken in preterm infants to avoid hyperoxia, as this is associated with retinopathy of prematurity (Roberton 1996).

- Suctioning via a port adapter or closed suction systems in patients who require maintenance of PEEP and/or positive pressure ventilation during suction (Harshbarger et al 1992).

- Avoiding cross-infection, particularly in vulnerable infants, by meticulous hand washing and adherence to local infection control policies.

- Keeping suction pressures as low as possible, without compromising the efficacy of secretion clearance. High vacuum pressures have been associated with mechanical trauma of the tracheal mucous membranes (Kleiber et al 1988).

- Selecting a suction catheter with an external diameter which does not exceed 50% of the internal diameter of the airway (Imle & Klemic 1989). Most commonly used catheters are 6 and 8 French gauge (FG). Size 5 FG and below are usually ineffective in removing thick secretions. Size 10 FG and above should be reserved for use with older children.

- Using graduated catheters with centimetre markings to gauge how far the catheter has been passed. Pneumothorax due to direct perforation of a segmental bronchus by a suction catheter has been reported in intubated preterm infants (Vaughan et al 1978).

- Positioning in side lying and restraining the non-intubated child who requires nasopharyngeal suction, to avoid potential aspiration of gastric contents (Fig. 10.6). Constant reassurance should be given throughout the procedure. Supplemental oxygenation and resuscitation equipment should be available. Nasopharyngeal suction of neonates may cause reflex bradycardia and apnoea.

- Avoiding nasopharyngeal suction if the child has stridor or has recently been extubated, as this may precipitate laryngospasm.

Saline instillation

Saline instillation into the tracheal tube of ventilated patients aims to loosen thick or sticky secretions to facilitate easy removal with suction (Schreuder & Jones 2004). Evidence for the practice is variable and therefore saline should be used only where there is a clear indication. Some suggest that saline instillation at best is not effective and at worst is harmful (Blackwood 1999, Hagler & Traver 1994, Kinloch 1999, McKelvie 1998, Ridling et al 2003), while others suggest it is well tolerated even in infants and may be helpful in removing secretions adherent to the chest wall (Shorten et al 1991). Other mucolytics (*N*-acetylcysteine) in aliquots of 0.5–5 ml may be used to enhance secretion clearance. Larger quantities of irrigants are sometimes used as part of bronchoalveolar lavage procedures.

Passive movements

Passive movements and two-joint muscle stretches should be considered in older children in intensive care, although they are at less risk of developing joint stiffness than adults. Care should be taken when handling children and infants who are hypotonic in order to avoid soft tissue damage. Preterm infants are hypotonic and require minimal handling, so passive movements are not usually indicated.

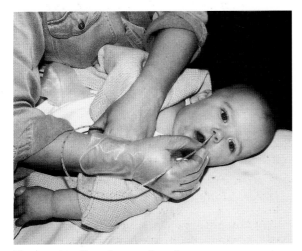

Figure 10.6 Nasopharyngeal suction.

RESPIRATORY DISEASE IN CHILDHOOD

Respiratory disease in childhood is very common and is one of the major causes of morbidity and mortality in children worldwide. Outside of the developing countries, most illnesses are mild; only a small proportion are more serious, involving the lower respiratory tract. The overall mortality rate per 100 000 children aged between 1–16 years due to respiratory illness in England and Wales has declined from 8.6 in 1968 to 1.3 in 2000. Asthma, pneumonia and cystic fibrosis (CF) together accounted for 73% of respiratory deaths in this age group (Panickar et al 2005). Respiratory disease is more common in children: from a poor socioeconomic background; with a family history of respiratory disease; from an urban rather than country environment; with a school-age sibling; or with a mother who smokes during pregnancy. The highest morbidity and mortality from lower respiratory tract disease occur in the first year of life. Respiratory disease is more severe in infants with congenital heart or lung abnormalities, immunodeficiency, cystic fibrosis or chronic lung disease.

Asthma

There is considerable global variation in the prevalence rates of asthma, with the highest rates reported in America, Australasia and the United Kingdom. Much lower rates are reported in prevalence studies from Africa and Asia. Prevalence also varies considerably within countries regionally. In the 1980s to early 1990s, several cross-sectional studies from widely varying regions of the world reported an increase in the prevalence of asthma. Although many of these studies relied on self-reported symptoms, there were also reports of a parallel increase in hospitalizations and mortality rates. However, repeat cross-sectional studies over the past decade have suggested a leveling off or even a decrease in prevalance (Toelle & Marks 2005). Atopic (allergic) disease in general has increased over the past few decades and possible explanations for this rise include outdoor pollution, social deprivation/socioeconomic status, dietary factors and passive smoking (particularly maternal smoking during pregnancy). In addition, modern Westernized homes, which tend to be highly insulated (e.g. double glazing) and have increased humidity, have been recognized to be 'dust mite-friendly' environments. Thick pile carpets, heavily padded furniture and conventional bedding are all potential sites for dust mite activity, a known trigger for allergic reaction.

The main pathophysiological mechanism of asthma in children is inflammation within the airway, resulting in recurrent episodes of wheezing, breathlessness and cough. There is an increased responsiveness of the smooth muscle in the bronchial wall to various stimuli. Hypertrophy of the mucous glands may lead to mucus plugging. These changes cause variable airway obstruction, which may become chronic and severe.

Aetiology

Children are more likely to develop asthma if parents or close relatives are asthmatic or atopic. There is an important link between atopy and bronchial hyperreactivity, and children with asthma often have other atopic features such as eczema, food allergy, hay fever or urticaria. Exposure to specific allergens such as house dust mite, pollen and animal dander can precipitate bronchospasm and wheeze. Exercise, particularly running, can precipitate an acute attack (exercise-induced asthma, EIA), as can emotional upset or upper respiratory tract infections.

Management

The mainstay of asthma treatment is drug therapy. There are agreed guidelines on the management of asthma (British Thoracic Society & Scottish Intercollegiate Guidelines Network (SIGN) 2003, National Asthma Education and Prevention Programme (NAEPP) 2002). The aims of therapy are to obtain optimal asthma control with few or no symptoms, undisturbed sleep, normal lung function with no limitation to daily activity and no severe, acute exacerbations. Poor asthma control has been attributed to suboptimal adherence to treatment guidelines both by physicians and families (Rabe et al 2004).

Short-acting inhaled β_2-agonists may be all that is required in children who have mild intermittent asthma, but inhaled corticosteroids are the mainstay of asthma therapy in those with persistent symptoms and are given in addition to short-acting β_2-agonists. Administration of corticosteroids by the inhaled route is safer and results in fewer systemic effects. It is important when using inhaled corticosteroids in children that growth is carefully monitored. In more severe asthma, long-acting β_2-agonists should be added to the treatment regimen. Leukotriene receptor antagonists may also be useful in a proportion of cases. Higher doses of inhaled corticosteroids may be needed. The use of continuous (preferably alternate day) oral steroids for prophylaxis is rarely needed nowadays. More severely affected children may require them intermittently on a continuous daily basis, for short periods, during acute exacerbations.

Inhalation of asthma medications provides effective topical therapy, which usually requires smaller doses and has fewer systemic effects. However, the method of drug delivery is very important and has been extensively reviewed (O'Callaghan 2000).

The choice of device depends both on the drug to be delivered and the patient, particularly in relation to age. In children the preferred method for delivery of both inhaled corticosteroids and β_2-agonists is by metered dose inhaler (MDI) along with a spacer device. Metered dose inhalers can be manually or breath-actuated and contain a mixture of propellant and drug which is emitted at a high velocity. Breath-actuated devices require an adequate inspiratory flow to trigger the device and the manual devices require coordination of the actuation of the device with inspiration. This makes them inherently difficult to use in children and therefore a valved spacer device should be incorporated into the system. The spacer allows the infant or child to inhale from a reservoir of drug within a chamber.

In babies, a facemask is required and should be held gently over the nose and mouth with the device held upright, at an angle greater than 45°, to ensure the valve is open. The drug can then pass effectively through the open valve to be inhaled (Fig. 10.7A & B). Once the child is older (usually from the age of 2 or 3), the spacer device can be used conventionally with a mouthpiece (Fig. 10.7C). The click of the valve opening will be heard with each breath. It should be noted that different spacer devices have been shown to deliver varying drug doses (Barry & O'Callaghan 1996).

Nebulized drug delivery systems for asthma are now rarely used in the home setting. They may be used in circumstances where medication cannot be delivered effectively using an MDI and spacer and in severe cases or during an acute exacerbation. It is preferable to use a mouthpiece (if the child is able) so as to avoid drug deposition on the face.

Children with a severe asthma attack usually display signs of acute respiratory distress; they may not be able to complete a sentence in one breath or may not be able to talk, and infants show difficulty in feeding due to breathlessness. The respiratory rate is usually high (>30/minute age 5 years and above, >50/minute – age 2–5 years) and the child is tachycardic. Obvious wheezing may not necessarily be present. In life-threatening attacks, when airway obstruction in the presence of hyperinflation is severe, the airflow may be so low that wheezing is not heard, the respiratory rate is lower than expected and the chest is 'silent'. The child may be cyanotic and is often exhausted. Children with either severe or life-threatening asthma require immediate admission to hospital. It is important to note that if nebulized bronchodilator therapy is given during an acute attack it should be oxygen driven to avoid hypoxaemia (Inwald et al 2001).

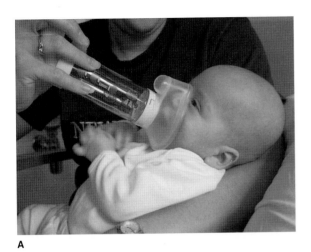

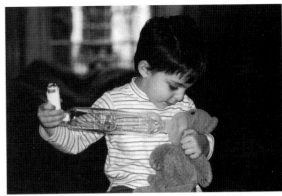

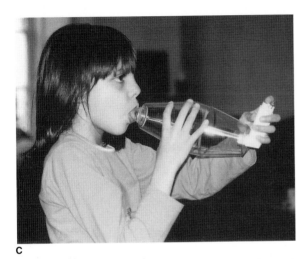

10

Figure 10.7 Administration of bronchodilator by spacer device to (**A**) an infant; (**B**) a teddy bear, to familiarize a young child with the device; (**C**) a young child.

Exercise-induced asthma

Exercise-induced asthma (EIA) is a common symptom associated with childhood asthma. However there is considerable controversy around the subject of EIA. Seear et al (2005) in a study of 52 asthmatic children concluded that the clinical diagnosis of EIA was often inaccurate mainly due to the unreliability of children's initial reporting of symptoms.

Physiotherapy

A crucial part of the management of asthma is education of the child and parents about the condition and its treatment. Often much of this is undertaken by the primary care team. The role of specialist nurses has also increased greatly in this field, although physiotherapists are sometimes still involved in teaching children how to take their medication.

Physiotherapists should also be able to advise on exercise, which is important in the asthmatic child to maintain general fitness. Improvements in aerobic capacity following exercise programmes have been documented in asthmatic patients (Bingol Karakoc et al 2000, Matsumoto et al 1999, Neder et al 1999), but there is no clear evidence to suggest that exercise training can influence the dose of medication required or improve asthma control in some other way (Carrol & Sly 1999). A systematic review of physical training in asthma concluded that physical training improved cardiopulmonary fitness, although it had no effect on lung function. No adverse effects of exercise were found and the authors stated that there are no reasons why those with asthma should not participate in regular physical activity (Ram et al 2005). A 'warm-up' should be recommended before starting vigorous activity (such as football, hockey, running), particularly in children with

EIA. The use of a pre-exercise inhaled β-agonist may also be helpful.

A systematic review of the use of breathing exercises was also not conclusive as to the efficacy of this form of intervention in asthma, primarily because the studies included used a wide variety of treatment interventions and outcome measures (Holloway & Ram 2004).

The child with acute asthma may need to be admitted to hospital and in severe cases may require mechanical ventilation (Chapter 9). Often the situation will resolve with careful medical management and appropriate respiratory support. Physiotherapy intervention is not always necessary. However, if problems arise, due to mucus plugging or retained secretions, chest physiotherapy may be of benefit. It is essential that bronchospasm is adequately controlled before physiotherapy techniques are started. Treatment should proceed cautiously and if bronchospasm increases, treatment should be discontinued until bronchospasm can be controlled. Although there is no routine indication for chest physiotherapy in asthma (Hondras et al 2000), children with persistent areas of lung collapse following an acute attack may respond well to an appropriate airway clearance technique. Parents may need to continue physiotherapy at home if bronchial hypersecretion persists.

Bronchiolitis

10

Bronchiolitis caused by human respiratory syncytial virus (RSV) is the most common severe lower respiratory tract disease in infancy. It is a seasonal disorder, occurring most frequently in the winter months and mainly affects infants under 2 years of age. The cause is viral, with RSV being the main agent in more than 70% of cases. As many as 1–2% of infants require hospital admission for management of RSV infection (Hodge & Chetcuti 2000) and of these 90% are under 12 months. Bronchiolar inflammation occurs with necrosis and destruction of cilia and epithelial cells, leading to obstruction of the small airways. Ventilation/perfusion mismatch may cause hypoxia and hypercapnia. Guidelines for the diagnosis and management of bronchiolitis have been published by the Scottish Intercollegiate Guidelines Network (2006).

Clinical features

The initial presenting symptoms are coryzal, such as the common cold. The infant develops a dry irritating cough and has difficulty in feeding. As the disease progresses, the infant becomes tachypnoeic and wheezy with signs of respiratory distress. The chest radiograph shows hyperinflation and patchy areas of collapse or pneumonic consolidation. Widespread inspiratory cre-pitations and expiratory wheezes can be heard on auscultation.

Management

Management of this condition is mainly supportive. The infant is given humidified oxygen via a head box as required. In those with severe respiratory distress, blood gas monitoring and even ventilatory support may be necessary. Intensive care management of the infant with acute bronchiolitis is discussed in Chapter 9.

Most infants have difficulty with feeding due to respiratory distress. Milder cases may tolerate small, frequent nasogastric feeds, although the nasogastric tube causes obstruction of one nostril and may itself significantly increase the work of breathing. For this reason some centres prefer to use orogastric tubes. Small-volume feeds lessen the risk of vomiting and aspiration. More severely affected infants may require intravenous nutrition.

Antibiotics are not required as the cause of the illness is viral, although they are often used if there is suspicion of secondary bacterial infection. The risk of this is increased if the infant is ventilated and many centres would use intravenous antibiotics for those requiring mechanical ventilation. Bronchodilators or inhaled corticosteroids have not been proven to be of any value in the treatment of acute bronchiolitis (Scottish Intercollegiate Guidelines Network 2006).

Ribavirin is an antiviral agent, which may be effective in reducing severity and duration of the disease. It is delivered as an aerosol by a small particle aerosol generator for long periods (>3–5 days). The drug is expensive and its efficacy has not been proven and it is therefore not currently recommended for use in acute bronchiolitis in infants (Scottish Intercollegiate Guidelines Network 2006).

Physiotherapy

Physiotherapy is not indicated in the acute stage of bronchiolitis when the infant has signs of respiratory distress. Studies that have examined the efficacy of physiotherapy intervention compared to no treatment in these patients have not shown any benefit in terms of the course of the disease (Nicholas et al 1999, Webb et al 1985). A systematic review based on the results of three randomized controlled trials concluded that chest physiotherapy using vibration and percussion techniques does not reduce length of hospital stay, oxygen requirements, or improve the clinical severity score in infants with acute bronchiolitis who are not under mechanical ventilation and who do not have any other comorbidity (Perrotta et al 2005). The ventilated infant with bronchiolitis needs careful assessment, and physiotherapy techniques should be applied only when sputum retention or mucus plugging is a problem.

Pertussis

Pertussis, commonly called 'whooping cough', is caused by the organism *Bordetella pertussis*. It occurs in epidemics every 3–4 years and is largely preventable by immunization, although immunity may not be lifelong (Raguckas et al 2007), with the highest incidence of pertussis since 1959 being reported in 2004. Pertussis is particularly dangerous in infants less than 6 months of age and in children with underlying cardiopulmonary problems, for example congenital heart disease, asthma, chronic lung disease and cystic fibrosis.

Clinical features

The disease starts with coryza lasting 7–10 days during which the child is most infectious. The cough then becomes paroxysmal and can be provoked by crying, feeding or any other disturbance. It is particularly bad at night. The spasms of coughing may cause hypoxia and apnoea, especially in infants, and may lead to further problems such as convulsions, intracranial bleeding and encephalopathy.

At the end of the coughing spasm, the inspiratory whoop may occur followed by vomiting, when thick, tenacious sputum can be expectorated. This phase of paroxysmal coughing may last for 6–8 weeks and is exhausting for the child and parents. The Chinese call pertussis the '100-day cough'.

Bronchopneumonia is the most common complication, particularly in infants, and is due to the primary disease itself or to secondary bacterial infection with other organisms such as *Staphylococcus, Haemophilus* or *Pneumococcus*. The chest radiograph in severe cases shows hyperinflation and patchy areas of collapse and consolidation.

Management

Most children with pertussis will be managed at home. Infants and children with pneumonia may need admission to hospital. Treatment is supportive. Minimal handling in a quiet environment is essential for the infant with pertussis in order to reduce disturbance, which may precipitate coughing spasms. Nutritional and fluid support should be given throughout the stage of paroxysmal coughing. Antibiotics do not affect the course of the disease, but erythromycin may reduce infectivity and it can also be given prophylactically to close contacts. A small number of cases, particularly infants who have had frequent apnoeic attacks or hypoxic convulsions, will need intensive care and mechanical ventilation.

Physiotherapy

Any physiotherapy manoeuvre, during the acute phase, can precipitate the paroxysmal cough with its complications. Treatment is therefore contraindicated in children during this stage.

If the child or infant requires ventilation, physiotherapy is very important to remove the extremely tenacious secretions, which easily block large and small airways and endotracheal tubes. The paroxysmal cough is not a problem when the child is paralysed in order to be ventilated.

When the stage of paroxysmal coughing is over, there may occasionally be persistent lobar collapse. This lung pathology often responds to an appropriate airway clearance technique. Parents can be taught how to treat the child at home.

Pneumonia

The most common cause of pneumonia in the neonate is *Staphylococcus aureus;* in the infant, RSV or *Mycoplasma pneumoniae* and in the child *Mycoplasma, Streptococcus pneumoniae* or *Haemophilus influenzae*. However, in a significant number of cases no pathogen is identified (British Thoracic Society 2002).

Clinical features

Presenting signs are pyrexia, dry cough, tachypnoea and not infrequently recession of the ribs and sternum. The chest radiograph shows areas of consolidation. Chest signs are often minimal compared with the degree of illness. Children with underlying pulmonary disease are particularly at risk from pneumonia.

Management

Treatment is supportive with adequate fluid intake and humidified oxygen, if required. In younger children it is impossible to distinguish between viral and bacterial pneumonia and broad-spectrum antibiotics are usually given.

Physiotherapy

In many cases of pneumonia there is consolidation of lung tissue with no excess secretions and there is no evidence that physiotherapy is of benefit (Stiller 2000). Where sputum retention is a problem, an appropriate airway clearance technique may be used. Copious amounts of sputum may be cleared in one treatment, following which the pyrexia may settle and the child will feel better. Reassessment of the child is often necessary, as retention of secretions may become a recurrent problem as the pneumonia resolves.

10

Pleural infection

Pleural infections, although relatively uncommon, have become more prevalent in the United Kingdom and the United States of America in recent years. Empyemas are a significant cause of morbidity in children, but differ from pleural infections in adults in that the final outcome is usually very good (Balfour-Lynn et al 2005). A pleural effusion in a relatively well child is usually a secondary occurrence to an acute bacterial pneumonia. The effusion is usually unilateral. Very occasionally pleural effusions in children represent an underlying malignancy; otherwise, most effusions are associated with an underlying infection. Once the presence of an effusion has been confirmed by chest radiograph or chest ultrasound and other causes ruled out, most children are started on intravenous antibiotics. A loculated effusion is treated either locally, with chest drain insertion and intrapleural fibrinolytics, or surgically with video-assisted thoracic surgery (VATS) or mini-thoracotomy.

Physiotherapy

Although these children do not always have a primary problem with bronchial secretions, immobility and the presence of a chest drain can result in retained secretions and a weak cough. Airway clearance may be necessary, using an appropriate technique. Breathing exercises and advice on coughing are also important parts of treatment. As soon as the clinical condition allows, the child should be encouraged to mobilize as much as possible.

Acute laryngotracheobronchitis (croup)

Croup is a common problem occurring between the ages of 6 months and 4 years. The illness is usually viral and produces acute inflammation and oedema of the upper airways.

Clinical features

The presenting symptoms are coryzal and later include fever, a harsh barking cough and a hoarse voice. Stridor, initially inspiratory only, is much worse at night and may become inspiratory and expiratory. Signs of respiratory obstruction are seen and the severely affected child may develop respiratory failure. The acute stage of respiratory obstruction may only last 1–2 days but the stridor and cough may continue for 7–10 days. Some children have recurrent bouts of croup.

Management

Mild cases can be managed at home. Extra humidity is often given, for example by sitting with the child in a warm steamy bathroom, although there is no objective evidence of benefit from inhaled moist air in emergency settings (Moore & Little 2006). More severely affected infants will be admitted to hospital and given humidified oxygen if hypoxic or distressed. Treatment is supportive, but with minimal handling as any disturbance that upsets the child will increase the laryngeal obstruction.

Glucocorticoids (dexamethasone and budesonide) have rapid beneficial effects on symptoms (Russell et al 2004). Nebulized adrenaline may be given with careful observation, in case of rebound and an acute collapse, and has been shown to provide short-term relief, but is probably not useful in the long term. Antibiotics are not usually required unless there is more specific evidence of a bacterial cause, for example purulent secretions.

Very few children with croup who are admitted to hospital go on to require intubation to maintain the airway due to severe respiratory obstruction. A few of these, particularly infants, may also require some additional form of respiratory support, e.g. intermittent positive pressure ventilation or continuous positive airway pressure.

Physiotherapy

Physiotherapy is contraindicated in the non-intubated child with croup. Treatment may be required when the child is intubated, if secretions cannot be cleared by suction alone.

Acute epiglottitis

Epiglottitis is caused by *Haemophilus influenzae* but is now rarely seen due to the introduction of the Hib *(Haemophilus influenzae)* vaccine. It is, however, a very dangerous condition, which occurs between the ages of 1 and 7 years.

Clinical features

The onset is sudden, with a severe sore throat and high temperature. Stridor and dysphagia develop rapidly, the child is unable to swallow saliva and drools. The neck is held extended in an attempt to open the airway. Acute and possibly fatal obstruction of the airway can develop.

Management

The child with suspected epiglottitis should not be disturbed in any way. No attempt should be made to examine the throat, as this may precipitate acute life-threatening obstruction. Usual management is intubation with a nasotracheal tube. In extreme circumstances tracheostomy may be necessary, but should only be required for 3–4 days, following which there is usually complete recovery.

10

Physiotherapy

Physiotherapy techniques may be required in the intubated child, if secretions cannot be removed by suction alone.

Bronchopulmonary dysplasia

Infants who remain oxygen-dependent and have abnormal findings on chest radiograph are described as having bronchopulmonary dysplasia (BPD). BPD covers a broad range of disease and a variety of terminology have been used to describe this disorder, including chronic lung disease (CLD). Although both CLD and BPD are both still commonly used, it is felt that BPD distinguishes this disorder as a neonatal lung process rather than other chronic respiratory diseases (Jobe & Bancalari 2001, Ryan 2006). The classification of BPD into mild, moderate and severe, depending on oxygen and positive pressure requirement, may offer a better description of underlying pulmonary disease and has been reported to correlate with the infant's maturity, growth and overall severity of illness (Ehrenkranz et al 2005). BPD is seen in extremely low birthweight infants and is inversely related to gestational age (Johnson et al 2002). Reported incidence of BPD varies from 15–50%, although this is likely to be related to the difference in populations (i.e number of very premature infants) among the studies.

The pathology of BPD has changed considerably over the past few decades, since the use of newer modalities of mechanical ventilation, introduction of new treatments (such as surfactant) and also due to improved survival of extremely premature infants. The pathology of BPD used to be associated with fibrosis and airway obstruction but in the present population of BPD babies, the problem is one of abnormal lung growth (in particular a marked reduction in alveolar numbers) (Kotecha 2000). This pathological picture is often termed 'new' BPD (Greenough et al 2006).

In addition to prematurity and low birthweight there are several other risk factors for BPD, in particular the requirement of mechanical ventilation and oxygen therapy. High peak pressures in positive pressure ventilation cause barotrauma and high inspired oxygen concentrations cause an acute inflammatory response leading to local tissue damage. Other factors that also influence the pathogenesis of BPD include the presence of a persistent arterial duct – patent ductus arteriosus (PDA) and infection.

Despite several studies, the optimum ventilation mode whereby BPD can be prevented has not been identified. Preventative strategies aim to mimimize lung injury. These include using less mechanical ventilatory support, refining the methods of mechanical ventilation and using alternative techniques: permissive hypercapnia, minimal peak pressures, rapid ventilatory rates, early use of continuous positive airway pressure (CPAP) and rapid weaning and extubation (Ambalavanan & Carlo 2006). High-frequency ventilation, in particular high-frequency oscillation, may have a place in preventing BPD but this is as yet unclear (Greenough et al 2006). The infant with BPD shows an increased oxygen requirement and carbon dioxide retention and has decreased lung compliance with increased airway resistance. Tachypnoea and persistent sternal and costal recession are often present. The condition may be progressive, requiring more ventilatory support and eventually leading to respiratory and cardiac failure. Radiographic appearance can vary but in classic BPD shows interstitial fibrosis and cystic abnormalities. The radiographic appearance in 'new' BPD is often of small volume and hazy lung fields.

Supplementary oxygen is the mainstay of the baby with BPD. The most appropriate target for the oxygen saturation level requires further study (Greenough et al 2006). Good nutrition is essential and the infant may require fluid restriction and diuretics. Some infants respond to bronchodilators and steroids, although the effect of long-term steroids on lung and brain growth is an issue of concern. Antibiotics may be required as these infants are prone to recurrent chest infections. Babies with a chronic oxygen requirement but who have a reasonable growth rate and do not have frequent episodes of desaturation can be discharged with home oxygen. These families require appropriate community support.

The long-term prognosis for those who survive the first 2 years is good, although infants with BPD have significant pulmonary sequelae during childhood and adolescence (Bhandari & Panitch 2006).

Physiotherapy

Infants with CLD are particularly prone to chest infections and have an increased rate of hospital admission in the first 2 years of life. Physiotherapy may be indicated if secretion retention is a problem. However these infants often wheeze and may have airway collapse. Detailed assessment is important before any intervention. If wheezing is not too severe, careful treatment may be possible. Inhaled β_2-agonists may temporarily improve lung function in these babies (Ng et al 2001) and may be useful as a premedication before physiotherapy. Modified gravity-assisted positions with chest percussion may be useful in infants, but nasopharyngeal suction may be required if retained secretions are a cause for concern. In older children an appropriate airway clearance technique should be used, either during episodes of infection or if retained secretions are a persistent problem. Children, particularly infants in

10

whom supplemental oxygen is delivered via nasal cannulae, often have a problem with thick, dry nasal secretions and may need humidification (Chapter 5).

Inhaled foreign body

Aspiration of a foreign body into the respiratory tract can occur at all ages, but is most common between the ages of 1 and 3 years. All types of foodstuffs may be aspirated, for example peanuts, pieces of fruit and vegetables, as well as small plastic or metal toys. Objects are most commonly aspirated into the right main bronchus. The left main bronchus and trachea are the next most common, and smaller objects may be inhaled into right middle and lower lobe bronchi or occasionally into the left lower lobe bronchus.

When aspiration has been witnessed by parents or carers, the child should be taken immediately to hospital. On examination there may be wheeze and some signs of respiratory distress. Breath sounds may be reduced over the affected lung. The chest radiograph, taken on expiration, may show gas trapping in the area distal to the blockage.

In some cases, the aspiration is not witnessed and the acute changes just described may be assumed to be the onset of a respiratory infection. The bronchial wall becomes oedematous, especially if the inhaled object is vegetable matter. Total obstruction of the bronchus gradually occurs and secondary pneumonic changes develop in the area distal to the obstruction. After a few days the child may become unwell with a persistent cough. The longer the obstruction remains, the more permanent the lung damage, eventually leading to bronchiectasis (Dinwiddie 1997). An inhaled foreign body should be suspected in any child with a pneumonia that does not respond to conventional treatment.

Management

All children who have aspirated a foreign body into the airway should have an urgent rigid bronchoscopy for removal of the foreign body. If symptoms persist, a repeat bronchoscopy may be necessary to ensure complete removal. Rarely bronchoscopic removal may fail and thoracotomy may be required.

Physiotherapy

Physiotherapy is not indicated to attempt to remove the object before bronchoscopy. Usually physiotherapy is ineffective as the object is firmly wedged in the bronchus. However, if the object is dislodged by physiotherapy manoeuvres, it may travel up the bronchial tree and obstruct the trachea, leading to respiratory arrest.

Following bronchoscopy, gravity-assisted positioning and chest clapping may be necessary to clear excess secretions, particularly if the object has been aspirated for some time and secondary bacterial infection has occurred.

Primary ciliary dyskinesia

Primary ciliary dyskinesia (PCD) is a rare, genetic disorder in which cilial motility is severely reduced because of structural defects within the cilia (Chapter 18), leading to disease of the upper and lower respiratory tract. Disorders of ciliary structure or function result in recurrent sinusitis and bronchiectasis due to decreased clearance of secretions (Cowan et al 2001). Males may be infertile because of reduced cilial motility of the sperm tails. Visceral mirror image arrangement occurs in approximately 50% of patients. Cilia can be examined for motility using nasal epithelial brushings.

Infants with this condition may present in the neonatal period with persistent rhinitis or pneumonia, but many children present later with chronic upper and lower respiratory tract infection. This condition is not curable, so treatment is directed towards preventing infection and chronic lung damage (Ferkol et al 2006). Appropriate antibiotic therapy is required during periods of infection. Children often require daily physiotherapy to clear bronchial secretions. An individualized programme of airway clearance should be formulated using an appropriate airway clearance technique (Chapter 5). There has been very little work published on chest physiotherapy in this condition, but it has been suggested that airway clearance techniques may be useful (Gremmo & Guenza 1999) (Chapter 18).

Cystic fibrosis

Cystic fibrosis (CF) is the most common inherited recessive condition in Caucasians, occurring in about 1 in 2500 births. The disorder results from a defective gene on chromosome 7, which encodes for the CF transmembrane conductance regulator (CFTR) protein. One of the functions of this protein (as a chloride channel) is to regulate ion transport. The absence or dysfunction of CFTR leads to defective ion transport and may result in either low volume or abnormal salt concentration of the airway surface fluid (Boucher 2004) (Chapter 18). This results in increased mucus viscosity and impaired mucociliary clearance, contributing to recurrent bacterial infection with gradual lung destruction. The survival of patients with CF has increased dramatically over the past five decades and this improvement has been attributed largely to improved nutrition and early aggressive treatment of the chest (Jaffe & Bush 2001). The primary areas affected are the respiratory and digestive tracts, but CF is a multisystem disorder with complications such as liver disease, diabetes and low bone mineral density.

10

CF may be identified in some babies before birth when echogenic bowel is seen on routine antenatal ultrasound scan or where there is a family history of CF and parents choose to have antenatal diagnosis. Others are identified as having CF through regional or national neonatal screening programmes. Twelve to fifteen per cent of children present at birth with meconium ileus, where thickened inspissated meconium causes blockage of the colon and ileum. The infant may present in the first day or two of life with abdominal distension, vomiting and failure to pass meconium. The obstruction can often be managed conservatively by the use of Gastrografin enema but occasionally laparotomy may be required. Other modes of presentation include recurrent chest infections and/or failure to thrive. Diagnosis of CF is confirmed with blood sampling for identification of two CF mutations and/or a sweat test.

Much focus has been placed on the early detection of lung disease in babies with CF. Traditionally the assessment of clinical status involved relying on symptoms, physical signs and investigations such as chest radiography, until the child was old enough to undertake respiratory function testing (approximately age 5–6 years). However, it is now possible to measure infant lung function and these studies along with early bronchoscopy and high-resolution computed tomography show clearly that infants with CF, who have no overtly detectable signs of respiratory disease, do have abnormalities in airway function and structure, and evidence of inflammation and even infection, within the early months of life (Armstrong et al 1995, Lum et al 2007, Martinez et al 2005, Ranganathan et al 2001). It is therefore important that these changes are detected and appropriate treatment instigated early. This may also be important in the future, when novel therapies such as gene therapy, manipulation of CFTR function and perhaps stem cell therapy are likely to work best at an early stage of the disease process, before irreversible lung damage has occurred.

Physiotherapy

Improvements in survival in CF have been attributed to regular monitoring, attention to nutrition and early, aggressive multidisciplinary treatment of CF lung disease. Most babies and young children attending cystic fibrosis centres now have good nutritional status, with body mass index (BMI) within normal limits, and do not display any recognizable signs of respiratory disease. Traditionally, airway clearance (usually in the form of postural drainage (PD) and percussion) was instigated on diagnosis. This approach is still taken by many physiotherapists, although many centres no longer use the head-down tipped position in these

babies, as a consequence of a small study which suggested that a head-down tip may exacerbate gastro-oesophageal reflux and may have both short- and long-term consequences to the child's respiratory status (Button et al 2003, 2004). In addition, these babies often have very little in the way of secretions and justification for postural drainage with a head-down tip is questionable.

Although there is considerable evidence that inflammation and infection are present from an early stage in CF and that changes in lung function and structure occur long before the onset of obvious clinical signs, the early pathophysiological picture is not associated with copious secretions or other symptoms which respond to airway clearance therapy. This has led many to question the appropriateness of a routine daily airway clearance regimen in these babies and it remains unclear whether airway clearance treatments are effective in asymptomatic babies with CF or whether a routine regimen of chest physiotherapy should be instigated regardless of clinical status (Prasad & Main 2006). An alternative approach is that these babies are very carefully monitored and active treatment applied only when symptoms warrant it. Parents and carers should always be taught an appropriate airway clearance technique soon after diagnosis and this should be practised and expertise maintained. They should also be taught how to check the child's chest and when to instigate treatment (Chapter 18). The importance of physical activity should be emphasized from the time of diagnosis. Even if the child is not receiving a daily regimen of airway clearance, parents should be encouraged to engage in some sort of physical activity on a daily basis, even in infancy. In addition to modified postural drainage and percussion (Fig. 10.8), the use of other airway clearance techniques such as positive expiratory pressure, assisted autogenic drainage and the use of physical activity (e.g. bouncing on a gym ball) are becoming more widely used in these babies (Chapter 5).

As children grow older, they can begin to play a more active role in their treatment. Many different airway clearance modalities are now available and the treatment regimen should be individualized depending on clinical status, age and social circumstances. The overall physiotherapy treatment and the various airway clearance techniques are discussed in detail in Chapters 5 and 18.

MANAGEMENT OF THE ACUTELY ILL INFANT OR CHILD

Babies and children with a wide variety of medical and surgical problems are admitted to neonatal, general paediatric or cardiac intensive care units. Respiratory failure

10

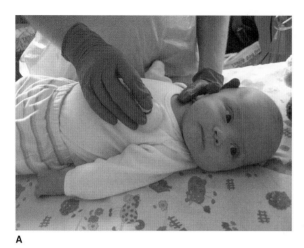
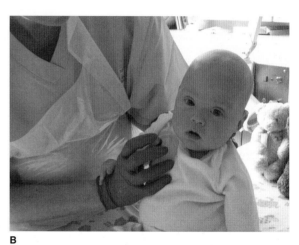

A

B

Figure 10.8   Modified postural drainage in an infant, using a facemask for percussion (**A**) in supine and (**B**) in sitting for the upper lobes.

10

in acutely ill infants and children may have various aetiologies. In the neonate the most common causes are prematurity, respiratory distress syndrome, asphyxia and aspiration pneumonia. Under 2 years of age bronchopneumonia, bronchiolitis, asthma, croup, foreign body inhalation and congenital heart or pulmonary anomalies are more common aetiologies. In children over 2 years' asthma, central nervous system infection (e.g. meningitis) and trauma are more frequent.

The effects of surgery, anaesthesia and immobility are the same in infants and children as in adults (Chapter 12). However, anatomical and physiological differences between these populations make children more vulnerable to respiratory complications. Infants and children undergoing major surgery should therefore be regularly assessed by a physiotherapist.

Physiotherapy treatments for ventilated children involving manual techniques have been shown to have an advantage over routine suction in reducing respiratory resistance, which may be of substantial benefit in patients with evidence of acute atelectasis (Main et al 2004). Within individuals, physiotherapy treatments are also more likely to produce improvements in tidal volume, respiratory compliance and resistance than suction alone, but both physiotherapy and suction procedures can produce short-term deterioration in almost one-third of children. Sensitive tools still need to be identified for selection of patients most likely to benefit from physiotherapy (Main et al 2004).

Physiotherapists working in an intensive care unit should be familiar with the equipment used on that unit (Fig. 10.9). They should be able to respond when a problem is indicated by the monitors and be able to

ascertain whether the problem is patient or equipment related. Details of oxygen delivery and paediatric mechanical support are described in Chapter 9. Standard monitoring equipment is often similar to those used on adult intensive care units (Chapter 8), although normal values vary according to age (see Table 10.1).

Children can have either nasal or oral endotracheal tubes (Fig. 10.10). The narrowest part of the upper airways in babies and small children is the circular cricoid ring. Thus, perfectly sized uncuffed tubes can be passed nasally and form a good seal in the cricoid and reduce the risk of damage to the tracheal mucosa from larger cuffed tubes (Deakers et al 1994, Khine et al 1997). Another advantage to nasal intubation is that the mouth is free to suck a sponge or pacifier during ventilation, so that normal feeding can be started as soon after extubation as possible. An important disadvantage to ill-fitting uncuffed tubes is the potential risk of endotracheal tube leak, in terms of both inconsistent delivery of ventilation and inaccurate monitoring of respiratory function (Kuo et al 1996, Main et al 2001).

Neonatal intensive care

The reasons for admission to a neonatal intensive care unit (NICU) include the following:

Preterm delivery: defined as less than 37 completed weeks of gestation (full term is defined as 38–42 weeks). Preterm infants who require admission to a NICU are usually less than 32 weeks of gestation with a birthweight less than 2500 g. Some infants are born as early as 23 weeks' gestation and are considered at the edge of viability. Causes of preterm birth include antepartum

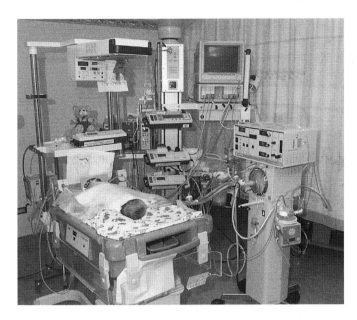

Figure 10.9 Equipment used in a paediatric intensive care unit. Figure shows an infant undergoing high-frequency oscillatory ventilation.

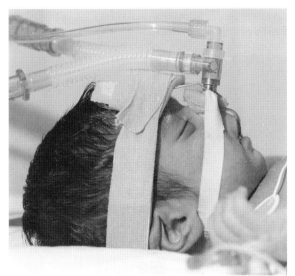

A

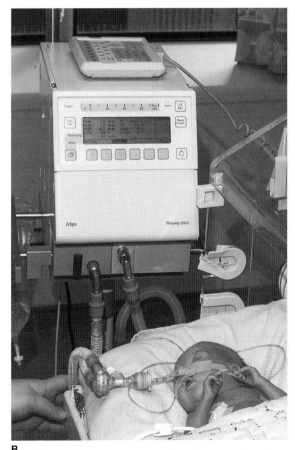

B

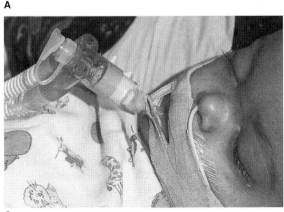

C

Figure 10.10 (A) and (B) Nasal intubation. (C) Oral intubation.

10

haemorrhage, cervical incompetence, multiple pregnancies or infection. There is also an association with deprived socioeconomic circumstances and in some cases the cause of preterm delivery is unknown.

Low birth weight is often due to prematurity but more mature infants may also be of low birth weight due to intrauterine growth retardation. Causes include placental dysfunction, smoking and intrauterine infection, e.g. rubella.

Perinatal problems such as birth asphyxia or meconium aspiration.

Congenital abnormalities include congenital heart disease and diaphragmatic hernia.

General problems of infants in the NICU

Infection

The preterm infant is particularly vulnerable to infection. Early-onset sepsis can occur during the first days of life. Infection can occur at any time during a NICU stay and may occur as a complication of invasive therapies in immature immune systems. The most important means of preventing and reducing cross-infection is by meticulous attention to hygiene by both staff and visitors.

Physiological jaundice

Physiological jaundice is common in the normal full-term infant owing to the breakdown of fetal haemoglobin causing a raised level of unconjugated bilirubin in the blood. It usually begins 2 days after birth and disappears after 1 week to 10 days. High levels of unconjugated bilirubin may diffuse into the basal ganglia and lead to a condition called kernicterus, characterized by athetoid cerebral palsy, deafness and mental retardation. Preterm infants are particularly prone to developing jaundice and run an increased risk of subsequent kernicterus, though this condition is now extremely rare. Serum bilirubin levels are closely monitored and phototherapy may be required. Phototherapy units consist of white or blue lamps, which emit light of wavelength 400–500 nm. Light of these wavelengths oxidizes unconjugated bilirubin into harmless derivatives. Infants receiving phototherapy have to be nursed naked, which can cause problems of temperature control. There is also increased insensible fluid loss and a theoretical risk of eye damage, so eye shields are placed on the infant. Advances in technology have led to a new phototherapy system that enables effective treatment to be given without the inconveniences of conventional phototherapy. The BiliBlanket® system uses fibre optics to provide therapeutic light for the treatment of physiological jaundice, filtering out the more harmful ultraviolet

and infrared light. The fibre optics are covered with a pad of woven fibres and the pad is placed directly against the baby. In severe cases of jaundice an exchange transfusion (where small amounts of blood are replaced by donor blood until twice the infant's blood volume has been exchanged) may be required.

Nutrition

Adequate calorie intake and weight gain are important in preterm and low birthweight infants to avoid hypoglycaemia, persistent jaundice and delayed recovery from respiratory distress syndrome. Feeding should be started as soon as possible, either enterally in those who can tolerate it, or intravenously. Preterm infants have poor sucking, gag and cough reflexes so will be fed nasogastrically until these develop. Continuous infusion of milk may be preferable to bolus feeds, which can increase respiratory distress, regurgitation and aspiration because of abdominal distension. Feeds are often better tolerated when the infant is lying in the prone position. Orogastric tubes may be used rather than nasogastric ones in order to avoid blockage of the nostril in spontaneously breathing infants with respiratory distress.

Temperature control

Preterm and low birthweight infants have difficulty in maintaining their body temperature because they have a large surface area relative to their body mass and easily lose heat through the skin by evaporation and radiation. They also have a smaller proportion of brown fat in comparison with full-term infants. Hypothermia may cause acidosis, hypoglycaemia, increased oxygen consumption and decreased surfactant production. Infants should therefore be kept in a thermoneutral environment (incubators or under radiant warmers) to maintain body temperature. Heat shields may be used to reduce radiant heat loss and the ambient room temperature is kept high at 27–28°C. A core temperature of less than 36.5°C in preterm infants indicates that non-essential handling should be delayed until the infant's temperature has risen. Infants, especially preterm babies, may have difficulty maintaining their temperature and are therefore nursed in incubators or under radiant warmers.

Pulmonary haemorrhage

Pulmonary haemorrhage is defined as acute intrapulmonary bleeding. It is relatively uncommon but may be a life-threatening event. Physiotherapy is contraindicated, although regular suctioning may be required to keep the airway clear. When fresh blood is no longer being aspirated, physiotherapy techniques may assist removal of residual blood. Prognosis is often poor.

Patent ductus arteriosus

Patent ductus arteriosus (PDA) occurs in up to a third of all preterm infants of less than 1500 g at birth (Zahka & Patel 2002). In the full-term infant the duct, which is a fetal circulatory vessel, closes within the first 24 hours of life. A persistent patent duct in the preterm infant may lead to increased pulmonary blood flow. If symptomatic, a PDA can be treated medically (using indomethacin) or surgically (with ligation), depending on the infant's clinical status.

Periventricular haemorrhage and periventricular leucomalacia

The incidence of intraventricular bleeding in preterm infants is inversely proportional to birth weight, occurring most frequently and severely in the smallest and least mature infant. Haemorrhage in the capillaries in the floor of the lateral ventricles is common in very low birthweight infants. The bleeding may extend into the ventricles and subarachnoid space. Several factors contribute to the risk of bleeding. These include hypoxia, fluctuation in blood pressure and cerebral blood flow and venous congestion. Cerebral ultrasound scanning is used to diagnose periventricular bleeds and is often the only way that small bleeds are detected. Periventricular haemorrhage is graded according to the extent of the bleeding seen on the ultrasound scan:

- Grade I   bleeding into the floor of the ventricle
- Grade II   bleeding into the ventricle (intraventricular haemorrhage (IVH))
- Grade III–IVH with dilatation of the ventricle
- Grade IV–IVH   and bleeding into the cerebral cortex causing areas of ischaemia.

The smaller bleeds (grades I and II) have a good prognosis. They usually require no treatment and have no long-term sequaelae. Neurological development following a grade I or II bleed seems to be similar to that of an infant with a comparable gestation. Larger bleeds may need treatment with shunting and the outcome is dependent on the grade of the bleed. More severe bleeds are associated with ischaemic brain damage and therefore have a high mortality and morbidity.

Periventricular leucomalacia (PVL) may occur on its own or associated with PVH. Ischaemia of cerebral tissue adjacent to the ventricles causes formation of cystic lesions. There is an association with neurological problems, particularly diplegia.

Respiratory distress

Respiratory distress syndrome (RDS) is a common complication of preterm infants, primarily caused by structural and biochemical immaturity of the lung, in particular a lack of surfactant. The incidence of RDS increases with decreasing gestational age. Symptoms can develop within 4 hours of delivery with sternal and costal recession, nasal flaring, grunting and tachypnoea. Steroids are usually administered to women in preterm labour in an attempt to enhance lung maturation (Roberts & Dalziel 2006).

Pulmonary surfactant production usually begins 36–48 hours after birth, regardless of gestational age. The more mature infant will start to recover at this time. Very preterm infants who have other problems compounding their respiratory distress or infants who have developed complications of treatment may require ventilatory support for much longer. Surfactant therapy has significantly altered the treatment of RDS. Both prophylactic and early surfactant replacement therapy have been shown to reduce mortality and pulmonary complications in ventilated infants with RDS. A systematic review has reported advantages of early surfactant replacement therapy with extubation to nasal continuous positive airway pressure (CPAP) (Stevens et al 2004).

As lung collapse in RDS is primarily caused by lack of surfactant, physiotherapy is not required for this condition. Secretions may become a problem after the infant has been intubated for more than 48 hours, owing to irritation of the tracheal mucosa by the endotracheal tube. These secretions may be cleared easily by suction alone. Physiotherapy may be indicated if suction is not adequately clearing secretions.

Respiratory distress in the preterm infant can also be caused by pneumonia. Organisms causing pneumonia may be bacterial, viral or fungal and may be acquired before, during or after birth. The most serious bacterial cause is group B streptococcus. The presenting features of this pneumonia are similar to RDS with an indistinguishable chest radiograph. Group B streptococcal pneumonia can be rapidly fatal unless antibiotic therapy is started early. For this reason all infants presenting with respiratory distress are given antibiotics.

Parent–infant bonding

Infants who have been resuscitated and require immediate admission to a NICU shortly after birth will not have had the chance for physical contact with their parents. Incubators and other equipment may be a further barrier to contact. Parents will need to be supported by the NICU team through this difficult period

10

and should be encouraged to have as close contact as possible with their baby and help with routine care.

Neonatal mechanical ventilation

Prophylactic ventilation is often started from birth in infants <1000 g, although wherever possible CPAP delivered via nasal prongs would be the intervention of choice. Other indications for ventilation are: deteriorating blood gases (hypoxaemia or hypercapnia) despite a high FiO$_2$, recurrent or major apnoea, major surgery pre- or postoperatively for congenital anomalies.

The goals of mechanical ventilation in the NICU are to achieve and maintain adequate gas exchange, to reduce the work of breathing and to minimize the risk of secondary lung injury. Achieving synchrony between the baby's breathing pattern and the ventilator is important, as asynchrony is associated with alterations in arterial and cerebral blood flow and an increased incidence of pneumothorax. Attempts to achieve synchrony include fast ventilatory rates and paralysing agents to suppress the infant's respiratory drive. Time-cycled, pressure-limited devices have largely been replaced by newer ventilators which offer pressure control or volume limitation and patient triggering (Donn & Sinha 2003). Volume-limited ventilation enables the measurement of very small tidal volumes and the provision of very low flows.

The use of high-frequency ventilation has also increased over the past decade. Whether high-frequency oscillation (Chapter 9) can reduce the incidence of bronchopulmonary dysplasia remains unclear, but it is regarded as a useful rescue technique.

Complications of mechanical support in neonates

Pneumothorax may be caused by many factors including high peak inspiratory pressures, high positive end-expiratory pressure and long inflation times or ventilator asynchrony. Predisposing factors include hyperinflation of alveoli occurring in conditions such as meconium aspiration and respiratory distress syndrome (RDS). A tension pneumothorax is likely to cause a sudden deterioration and usually requires immediate insertion of an intercostal drain. Very small pneumothoraces may not require drainage.

Pulmonary interstitial emphysema used to be common in preterm infants, with the incidence being inversely proportional to gestational age. It has been seen less frequently since the introduction of treatment of preterm infants with exogenous surfactant, which improves lung compliance. Pulmonary interstitial emphysema is still seen occasionally in infants who require long-term ventilation and who have uneven aeration and gas trapping.

Retinopathy of prematurity is a condition of preterm infants seen when the capillaries in the retina proliferate, leading to haemorrhage, fibrosis and scarring. In the most severe form, this may result in permanent visual impairment. The cause is unknown, but periods of hyperoxia (exact length of time unknown) with a PaO$_2$ of above 12 kPa are thought to be a major predisposing factor (Roberton 1996). Careful oxygen monitoring is essential to attempt to prevent this condition.

Prolonged ventilatory support and oxygen dependency may result in bronchopulmonary dysplasia (BPD), discussed earlier in this chapter.

Perinatal problems and congenital anomalies

Meconium aspiration

Meconium aspiration usually occurs in full-term infants who become hypoxic due to a prolonged and difficult labour. Hypoxia causes the infant to pass meconium into the amniotic fluid and to make gasping movements, thereby drawing meconium into the pharynx. The irritant properties of meconium can cause a chemical pneumonitis and meconium aspiration can also lead to significant gas trapping and thoracic air leak. In severe cases it can result in secondary persistent pulmonary hypertension of the newborn (PPHN). A severely affected infant is likely to require mechanical ventilation and may require extracorporeal membrane oxygenation.

Physiotherapy is very important when meconium aspiration has occurred in order to remove the extremely thick and tenacious green secretions. In milder cases treatment consists of gravity-assisted positioning, as tolerated, with chest percussion. Treatment is usually well tolerated soon after aspiration. In more severe cases where pneumonitis develops, these babies are often very sick, require significant respiratory support, do not tolerate handling and should only be treated with caution.

Congenital diaphragmatic hernia

Diaphragmatic herniation occurs when abnormal fetal development of the diaphragm weakens the muscular barrier. The abdominal contents (usually stomach or small bowel) are displaced into the thoracic cavity, posteriorly and most commonly on the left side. The incidence is approximately 1 in 3000 births with mortality rates up to 50% (Schultz et al 2007). The abnormality may be diagnosed antenatally by ultrasound or postnatally in significant defects when the infant presents with neonatal respiratory distress. A chest radiograph will show abdominal viscera in the thoracic cavity. Unless the herniation has occurred late in pregnancy, which is very unusual, there will be associated pulmonary hypoplasia on the affected side as the abdominal viscera occupy the space normally available for the growing lung. Pulmonary hypoplasia is the main determinant of survival. The contralateral lung is also smaller than expected because of compression due to mediastinal shift during fetal development. There are also commonly other associated anomalies such as persistent fetal circulation and abnormalities of the pulmonary vasculature.

The infant with diaphragmatic hernia is often very unwell, particularly as the bowel in the chest distends with air and further compresses the lungs, and requires immediate gastric decompression with simultaneous intubation and ventilation. Surgery is not usually carried out until the infant's condition is stabilized and extracorporeal membrane oxygenation may be required to support the infant until surgery is possible. A systematic review has reported a reduction in early mortality with extracorporeal membrane oxygenation but no overall long-term benefit (Morini et al 2006). Surgical correction is via a laparotomy. The abdominal viscera are carefully returned to the abdominal cavity and the defect in the diaphragm is closed. High-frequency oscillation has been reported as a beneficial elective ventilation strategy but as yet there have been no large randomized controlled trials (Smith et al 2005).

Postoperatively, the infant may require ventilation for some time, depending on the amount of pulmonary hypoplasia. Prognosis is variable and mortality for isolated hernias is about 45% (Wenstrom et al 1991). Physiotherapy may be indicated if retention of secretions is a problem. Manual hyperinflation techniques should avoid generating excess pressures within the hypoplastic lungs.

Congenital anomalies of the lung

Congenital conditions of the lung such as lobar emphysema, lung cysts and adenomata are relatively rare. They may be diagnosed by ultrasound antenatally or by chest radiography postnatally. Treatment may involve surgical resection (lobectomy) if the condition is severe, but in some cases the lesions appear to resolve spontaneously in infancy.

Acquired lobar emphysema and lung cysts are more common as complications of respiratory distress syndrome and its treatment. Many cases resolve with medical management, although some do require resection. Physiotherapy may be indicated postoperatively if there is sputum retention, but manual hyperinflation is contraindicated if cysts are present.

Oesophageal atresia and tracheo–oesophageal fistula

There are five recognized types of this anomaly. In the most common variety the oesophagus ends in a blind proximal pouch (atresia) and there is a fistula between the trachea and the lower section of the oesophagus. About 10% of affected infants have oesophageal atresia with a tracheal fistula. The incidence is approximately 1 in 3000 births (Depaepe et al 1993).

The infant presents postnatally with episodes of choking, coughing and respiratory distress due to an inability to swallow saliva or feeds and consequent aspiration into the larynx or trachea. It is often difficult to pass a nasogastric tube, which on chest radiograph appears curled in the upper oesophagus.

Surgical correction is usually attempted as soon as possible and involves division of the fistula and anastomosis of the ends of the oesophagus. Some anastomoses may have to be performed under tension and the infant has to be electively ventilated and paralysed with the neck kept in flexion postoperatively. In a few cases, where the gap between the two ends of the oesophagus is too large, primary anastomosis is not possible and a feeding gastrostomy is performed. Oesophageal anastomosis or replacement by colonic, jejunal or gastric interposition is delayed.

If recurrent or continuous aspiration occurs before corrective surgery, physiotherapy (in the head-up position) may be indicated to clear excess secretions or treat lung collapse due to reflux of gastric contents. Preoperatively the airway is often kept clear by continuous suction of the upper pouch and the infant should be nursed head-up to prevent reflux of gastric contents through the fistula.

Postoperatively, head-down postural drainage is contraindicated and patients are often nursed in the head-up position for the first few days, to reduce the risk of reflux. Care must be taken not to extend the neck, especially in patients with a tight oesophageal anastomosis. Naso- or oropharyngeal suction should not in general exceed the external distance between the nasal cavity and the ear. This distance is effective at producing cough and inadvertent damage to the oesophageal anastomosis is avoided.

Gastroschisis and exomphalos (omphalocele)

These conditions are relatively rare abdominal wall defects, occurring in approximately 1 : 5000 births (Baird & MacDonald 1982). Gastroschisis refers to a full thickness abdominal wall defect next to the umbilical opening, through which the small and large bowel herniate, not usually covered by a membrane. Exomphalos

10

occurs when the anterior abdominal wall fails to close at the base of the umbilical cord, allowing the abdominal contents and sometimes the liver to herniate through the umbilical ring and develop externally in utero. A translucent membranous sac encloses the hernial contents. The defect is usually diagnosed antenatally by ultrasound and is classified as major or minor depending on whether the defect is bigger or smaller than 5 cm. Affected infants often have other major associated anomalies.

Immediately after birth, the abdominal contents are covered to prevent heat and fluid loss until corrective surgery can be undertaken. In most cases primary repair is possible but where the defect is large a staged procedure is required, with gradual reduction of the bowels into the abdominal cavity.

Postoperatively the infant may require ventilation as the tightly packed, rigid abdomen causes respiratory embarrassment and compromises venous return. Where a staged procedure is necessary, prolonged ventilation may be required. Some infants have impaired antenatal lung growth and a proportion continue to have abnormal lung function during infancy.

These infants are particularly at risk from retention of secretions and lobar collapse due to the distended abdomen and predominantly supine nursing position (with the abdominal contents suspended above the abdomen). If treatment is required, techniques that increase intrathoracic pressure and consequently intra-abdominal pressure, such as vibrations or manual hyperinflation, should be used very cautiously. Postoperative respiratory compromise, if related to increased abdominal pressure, is unlikely to respond to physiotherapy. A slightly head-up position may relieve the thorax of some of the weight of the abdominal contents and reduce the work of breathing.

Cardiac intensive care

Congenital heart problems in infants and children

Congenital heart disease is the most common congenital anomaly with the incidence of moderate and severe forms about 6 in 1000 live births, and of all forms about 75 in 1000 live births (Hoffman & Kaplan 2002). Roughly one-third of these will require surgical intervention, with the rest either resolving spontaneously or being haemodynamically insignificant. Major congenital cardiac defects can often be detected antenatally by ultrasound examination, while more minor defects may not be detected until the postnatal period. Diagnosis is usually confirmed by echocardiography. Postnatally most cardiac defects are amenable to surgery and overall

mortality has fallen to less than 5% in the best units (Elliott & Hussey 1995, Stark et al 2000). Early complete repair is attempted whenever possible, with the majority of operations being performed in the first year of life.

Management of congenital heart defects must involve agreement between cardiologist, surgeon, family and the child, if he is old enough. Each aspect of the child's care is an integrated process requiring the skills of a multidisciplinary team before, during and after surgery.

Common paediatric cardiac surgery procedures

The normal anatomy of the heart is shown in Figure 10.11.

Palliative procedures

When a primary repair is not possible, palliative or staging procedures will provide temporary or extended relief of symptoms. They are usually indicated to deal with excessive pulmonary blood flow, inadequate pulmonary blood flow or inadequate mixing between oxygenated and deoxygenated blood in the heart.

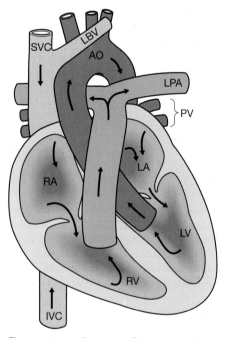

Figure 10.11 Anatomy of the normal heart: AO, aorta; PA, pulmonary artery; SVC, superior vena cava; IVC, inferior vena cava; RA, right atrium; LA, left atrium; RV, right ventricle; LV, left ventricle; LPA, left pulmonary artery; PV, pulmonary veins; LBV, left brachiocephalic vein.

Pulmonary artery band. The pulmonary artery band is designed to restrict excessive blood flow to the lungs by reducing the diameter of the pulmonary artery with a constricting tape. A child with excessive pulmonary blood flow (ventricular and atrioventricular septal defects or truncus arteriosus) may present with poor feeding, heart failure, tachypnoea and, if uncorrected, pulmonary hypertension. If a corrective procedure is not possible, pulmonary artery banding may be performed via a left thoracotomy, to protect the lungs from the progression of pulmonary vascular disease. The pulmonary artery pressure is reduced to approximately one-third of the systemic pressure.

The modified Blalock–Taussig shunt. The modified Blalock–Taussig shunt (MBTS) is the most common palliative procedure used to improve pulmonary blood flow by placing a conduit between the subclavian artery and the pulmonary artery via sternotomy or thoracotomy. Inadequate pulmonary blood flow will result in poorly oxygenated blood and central cyanosis (e.g. tetralogy of Fallot, pulmonary or tricuspid atresia). If primary repair is not possible, the MBTS temporarily improves pulmonary perfusion, thereby significantly improving oxygen saturation (80–85%). The shunt is usually ligated at the time of definitive repair.

Septostomy. In defects such as transposition of the great arteries, where there is inadequate mixing of oxygenated and deoxygenated blood within the heart, the foramen ovale may be enlarged using either a balloon atrial septostomy in neonates or surgically in older children via a Blalock–Hanlon septectomy.

Corrective surgery: closed procedures

Patent ductus arteriosus. The ductus arteriosus is the fetal vascular connection between the main pulmonary trunk and the aorta (usually distal to the origin of the left subclavian artery), which normally closes soon after birth. If it remains open, excessive blood shunts from the aorta to the lungs causing pulmonary oedema and, in the long term, pulmonary vascular disease. Symptoms may be mild or severe, depending on the magnitude of the left-to-right shunt. This defect occurs very commonly in premature infants and may cause difficulty weaning from ventilation or congestive cardiac failure.

In some circumstances (for instance, neonates with transposition of the great arteries) it is desirable to delay closure of the ductus arteriosus and this may be achieved by the administration of prostaglandin.

It may also be possible to induce closure of the duct in preterm infants with indomethacin. Surgical correction involves a left thoracotomy and ligation. In older

infants closure may be achieved via cardiac catheterization using a double umbrella device.

Coarctation of the aorta. This is a congenital narrowing of the aorta. It usually occurs proximal to the junction of the ductus arteriosus and distal to the left subclavian artery origin. Neonatal presentation with symptoms of congestive heart failure requires early surgical repair. This is usually performed by resection of the stenosis and end-to-end anastomosis. If the aortic arch is extensively hypoplastic, aortic arch angioplasty may be necessary. Repair of simple coarctation carries almost zero mortality. For severe forms of coarctation such as interrupted aortic arch (where upper and lower aortic arches are separated) mortality is higher. Paraplegia is an extremely rare complication specific to correction of this defect (Brewer et al 1972) and may be associated with longer cross-clamping times.

Vascular ring. This defect is caused when malformations of the aorta or pulmonary artery compresses the trachea, oesophagus or both (examples include double aortic arch, abnormally positioned innominate artery or abnormal course of the left pulmonary artery crossing behind the trachea). Symptoms include stridor, respiratory difficulties, repeated chest infections or feeding problems. Surgical decompression of the vascular ring will often improve symptoms, but tracheal stenosis or malacia are frequently associated with vascular rings and further surgery may be required to repair tracheal or bronchial obstruction.

Corrective surgery: open procedures

Open procedures require cardiopulmonary bypass, modified for children in terms of size, flow rate, perfusion, temperature and drugs (Elliott & Hussey 1995).

Atrial septal defect (ASD). Atrial septal defect is one of the most common congenital cardiac anomalies, characterized by a hole in the septum that separates the left and right atria. Types of ASD include ostium primum defects, also referred to as partial atrioventricular septal defects (AVSDs), discussed below, and ostium secundum defects due to failure of fusion of the two atrial septa and patency of the foramen ovale. Ostium secundum ASD may be associated with one or more of the superior pulmonary veins draining into the superior vena cava.

Children with ASD are generally asymptomatic and diagnosis is usually made after a murmur is detected at routine examination. If undiagnosed, slow development of symptoms may occur with rising pulmonary artery pressure and pulmonary vascular disease. If pulmonary vascular disease becomes severe and pulmonary hypertension is irreversible, then corrective surgery is not possible and heart-lung transplantation is the only pal-

10

liative option. Because of the severe late consequences of pulmonary hypertension, repair is usually undertaken before the age of 5 years via median sternotomy or right anterior thoracotomy. Late diagnosis and surgical intervention are rare in developed countries. The septal defect is usually closed by direct suture, pericardial or synthetic patch. Umbrella or balloon devices have also been used successfully to close small, round defects via cardiac catheterization.

Ventricular septal defect (VSD). Ventricular septal defects are the most common congenital cardiac lesions, defined by a hole in the septum that separates left and right ventricles. VSDs are often found in conjunction with other cardiac defects and the clinical presentation will depend on the size of the VSD and the presence or absence of other cardiac anomalies. Infants may present with congestive cardiac failure, recurrent chest infections and failure to thrive. More than half of all VSDs close spontaneously and do not require surgery (Elliott & Hussey 1995). However, as with ASDs, undiagnosed larger defects can lead ultimately to severe irreversible pulmonary hypertension.

VSDs (Fig. 10.12) are defined according to their position in either the perimembranous inlet, the trabecular portion or the muscular outlet of the ventricular septum. Primary repair is usually performed using synthetic or bovine pericardial patches via median sternotomy, with the cardiac approach varying according to the position of the defect. Conduction disturbances are common following surgery.

Although operative mortality approaches zero for isolated septal defects, multiple VSDs or 'Swiss cheese' defects carry a higher risk (De Leval 1994a).

Atrioventicular septal defect (AVSD). Incomplete development of the inferior atrial septum, superior ventricular septum and atrioventricular valves results in a spectrum of anomalies termed atrioventricular septal defects. Symptoms vary in severity according to the magnitude and direction of the shunt and the extent of the ASD, VSD, valve incompetence or combination of these. They may be associated with other cardiac defects (transposition of the great arteries, tetralogy of Fallot) and are also strongly associated with chromosomal abnormalities such as Down's syndrome. Some patients may be asymptomatic despite high pulmonary vascular resistance, but a high left-to-right shunt causes dyspnoea, recurrent chest infection and congestive cardiac failure.

Partial AVSD refers to an ostium primum type of ASD above the mitral and tricuspid valves that are displaced into the ventricles and may be incompetent. The development of pulmonary vascular disease is uncommon.

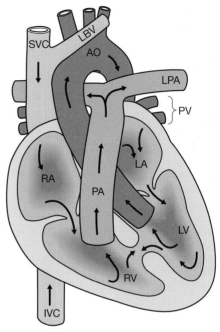

Figure 10.12 Ventricular septal defect, showing mixing of blood between the left and right ventricle: AO, aorta; PA, pulmonary artery; SVC, superior vena cava; IVC, inferior vena cava; RA, right atrium; LA, left atrium; RV, right ventricle; LV, left ventricle; LPA, left pulmonary artery; PV, pulmonary veins; LBV, left brachiocephalic vein.

Complete AVSD is distinguished by a single six-leafed atrioventricular valve between the right and left atrioventricular chambers and continuous with the ASD above and VSD below. Over 50% of infants with this defect will die within the first year of life because of pulmonary vascular disease if left untreated. The remaining children will almost all have died within 5 years.

Both types of AVSD are repaired with patches on cardiopulmonary bypass via a median sternotomy. Hospital mortality is usually less than 10% but may be greater in patients with major associated anomalies. Early complete repair is preferred so that irreversible development of pulmonary vascular disease may be avoided but conduction problems and valve incompetence are relatively common postoperatively.

Tetralogy of Fallot. The four components of Fallot's tetralogy are classically described as a large VSD, right ventricular (infundibular) outflow or valve obstruction, overriding aorta and right ventricular hypertrophy (Fig. 10.13).

Inadequate blood flow to the pulmonary circulation and preferential flow of deoxygenated blood to the

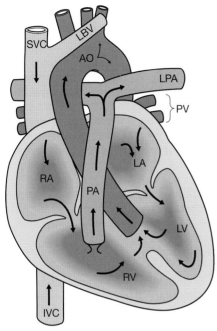

Figure 10.13   Tetralogy of Fallot, showing VSD, right ventricular hypertrophy, aorta overriding both ventricles and stenosis of the pulmonary artery: AO, aorta; PA, pulmonary artery; SVC, superior vena cava; IVC, inferior vena cava; RA, right atrium; LA, left atrium; RV, right ventricle; LV, left ventricle; LPA, left pulmonary artery; PV, pulmonary veins; LBV, left brachiocephalic vein.

aorta may cause cyanosis, but severity of symptoms will depend on the degree of obstructed pulmonary blood flow. The majority of infants are pink at birth but become progressively cyanosed as they grow. Periodic spasm of the infundibulum prevents blood flow to the lungs and may cause 'spelling' episodes in which infants become irritable. Continued crying leads to increasing cyanosis and eventual loss of consciousness. The spasm then relaxes and the child gradually recovers. These episodes are dangerous and may lead to death or cerebral anoxia. Older undiagnosed children may intuitively squat following exercise, which reduces blood flow to and from the lower extremities in an effort to compensate for the large oxygen debt accrued during physical activity. In the presence of cyanosis, this behaviour may suggest diagnosis of this defect.

Some controversy exists about whether it is better to do primary repair or palliative shunt with repair when the child is older. Corrective surgery will involve closure of the VSD, resection of the hypertrophied infundibulum and reconstruction of the pulmonary arteries. Long-

term results are good with actuarial survival of 93% at 15 years and good quality of life (Castenda 1994).

Pulmonary atresia.   The infant with pulmonary atresia may be cyanosed at birth and this may become rapidly worse as the ductus arteriosus closes. Palliation in the form of a modified Blalock–Taussig shunt is the immediate treatment of choice so that adequate blood supply to the lungs can be established. Prostaglandins may be used to delay closure of the ductus arteriosus until surgery. In the absence of right ventricular hypoplasia and coronary artery abnormalities, mortality is very low. However, this defect can occur with a VSD, in which case the right ventricle may be hypertrophied or hypoplastic and the pulmonary valve atretic. Sometimes the coronary arteries are supplied with desaturated blood from the right ventricle and major aortopulmonary collateral arteries (MAPCAs) can augment pulmonary blood flow. The technique used for definitive surgical repair is variable depending on the size of the right ventricle.

Transposition of the great arteries (TGA).   This defect is characterized by the aorta originating from the right ventricle and the pulmonary artery from the left (Fig. 10.14). Oxygenated pulmonary blood recirculates through the lungs without reaching the body and deoxygenated blood recirculates through the body without reaching the lungs. The two closed circulations would quickly lead to death but there is usually a degree of mixing through the PDA and, if present, associated anomalies such as ASD or VSD. Babies therefore present soon after birth with cyanosis and immediate treatment aims include keeping the ductus arteriosus open with prostaglandins until surgery. Before corrective surgery, cardiac catheterization and balloon atrial septostomy may also be necessary.

The arterial switch operation has been performed with good results since 1985 and is the preferred option for simple TGA or for TGA with VSD. It is generally performed in the first 2–3 weeks of life, while the pulmonary vascular resistance is high and the left ventricle is 'trained' to receive the systemic workload. The aorta and pulmonary arteries (above the level of the coronary vessels) are transected and transferred to their correct anatomical positions. The coronary arteries are also transferred to their appropriate positions. Operative mortality is low (<2%) and long-term results appear to be far superior to the earlier Mustard or Senning operations, which redirected blood flow via intra-atrial tunnels (Freed et al 2006).

Interrupted aortic arch.   This rare condition is characterized by a discontinuous aortic arch and will result in death within the first month if left untreated. The most

10

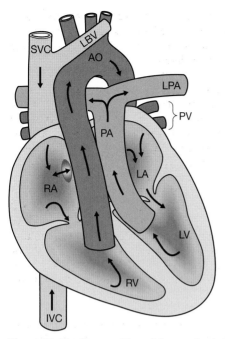

Figure 10.14 Transposition of the great arteries. Shaded area shows either position of a patent foramen ovale or site of balloon septostomy allowing some mixing of oxygenated and deoxygenated blood between the systemic and pulmonary circulations: AO, aorta; PA, pulmonary artery; SVC, superior vena cava; IVC, inferior vena cava; RA, right atrium; LA, left atrium; RV, right ventricle; LV, left ventricle; LPA, left pulmonary artery; PV, pulmonary veins; LBV, left brachiocephalic vein.

common site for interruption is distal to the left carotid artery. A VSD is almost always present, as is a PDA through which blood flows to the distal aorta. Soon after birth, when the ductus arteriosus begins to close, the pulmonary vascular resistance increases and severe congestive cardiac failure develops. Early surgical repair is the treatment of choice, but is technically difficult and the postoperative course is often prolonged.

Partial or total anomalous pulmonary venous connection (PAPVC or TAPVC). These anomalies are rare and involve some or all four pulmonary veins connecting to the systemic venous circulation. Supracardiac connections (50%) involve blood draining to the innominate vein or the superior vena cava. Cardiac connections (20%) involve blood draining into the coronary sinus or directly into right atrium. Infradiaphragmatic connections (20%) drain into the portal or hepatic veins. The final 10% are mixed connections. The reduced left atrial pressure keeps the foramen ovale open postnatally and mixed arterial and venous blood is transported systemically. Thus symptoms in the first few days of life will

include congestive cardiac failure and cyanosis. There are often associated cardiac anomalies and surgical repair will depend on the nature of these, if present.

Truncus arteriosus. Truncus arteriosus is characterized by a single arterial trunk arising from both ventricles and from which the aorta and pulmonary arteries originate via a single semilunar valve. A VSD permits flow up the common trunk. Congestive cardiac failure and irreversible pulmonary vascular disease rapidly develop in early infancy and untreated infants rarely survive beyond their first year. Surgical treatment involves the closure of the ventricular septal defect with a patch to divert the left ventricular flow up the aorta. The pulmonary arteries are then detached from the common artery (truncus arteriosus) and connected to the right ventricle using a conduit.

Cardiac valve abnormalities

Aortic stenosis. Obstruction to left ventricular outflow may occur in isolation or in combination with other cardiac defects. They may be found at valvular, subvalvular, supravalvular or combined levels. Critical stenoses present neonatally with congestive cardiac failure and reduced peripheral pulses and require immediate intervention. Relief of aortic stenosis may be obtained with aortic valvotomy, aortic valve replacement, homograft insertion or balloon dilatation. However, mortality is high (10%) and reoperation common (Elliott & Hussey 1995). Aortic stenosis may not cause problems until adulthood, although, by then, a degree of left ventricular hypertrophy may have developed.

Pulmonary stenosis. The neonate with pulmonary stenosis may become progressively more cyanosed as the PDA closes and this may be reversed or delayed by the use of prostaglandins to keep the PDA patent. Management is similar to that of pulmonary atresia, with surgery dependent on the nature and extent, if any, of associated cardiac anomalies. Homograft valve replacement may be required at a later stage. Less critical pulmonary stenosis may present later in life with breathlessness on exertion and fatigue.

Tricuspid valve. Tricuspid valve disease is rare in childhood but is seen in Ebstein's anomaly. Patients present with severe cardiac failure, cyanosis and dysrhythmia. Neonatal surgery carries a high mortality and a palliative approach with a later Fontan procedure may be preferred (De Leval 1994b). In the older child it is possible to perform a more complex repair of the anomaly.

Mitral valve. Mitral valve problems present either as stenosis or incompetence, usually associated with other cardiac anomalies. Repair is the preferred option though replacement may be the only option. Early replacement is associated with a high mortality (20%) (Carpenter 1994).

Hypoplastic left heart syndrome.   This defect is defined by aortic valve stenosis or atresia associated with severe left ventricular hypoplasia. Early mortality in untreated patients is high. The systemic blood flow derives almost entirely from the right ventricle through the ductus arteriosus and, depending on the size of it, peripheral pulses may be normal, reduced or absent. Immediate management involves keeping the ductus arteriosus open with prostaglandins. Surgical management options include early heart-lung transplantation or a three-staged surgical procedure that makes the child's circulation function with only two of the heart's four chambers. The first step (Norwood procedure) makes the right ventricle pump blood to the whole body and to the lungs. The second stage (Glenn procedure) allows greater blood flow to the upper body and reduces some of the workload from the right ventricle. The final procedure (Fontan procedure or total cavopulmonary connection) allows blood to return passively to the lungs (rather than being pumped there) and allows the right ventricle to only pump blood out to the body (Norwood & Jacobs 1994). The Norwood procedure is generally performed within a week of birth, the second stage at 3–6 months of age, and the Fontan at 18 months to 4 years of age. Success of these types of surgery depends on the lungs being free of pulmonary vascular disease and a good balance between pulmonary and systemic circulations.

Transplantation surgery in children

The problems of cardiac, lung and heart-lung transplant surgery in children are similar to those in adults, and are discussed in detail in Chapter 15.

General paediatric intensive care

Trauma & head injury

Accidents are the most common cause of child death after the first year of life and 50% are road traffic accidents. Children who have been severely injured may require intensive care and mechanical ventilation, particularly after head injury.

In the acutely head-injured child the primary injury refers to the damage sustained during trauma caused by bleeding, contusion or neuronal shearing. Secondary injury is due to the resultant complicating events. These may be intracranial factors such as bleeding, swelling, seizures and raised intracranial pressure (ICP) or systemic factors such as hypoxia, hypercarbia, hyper- or hypotension, hyper- or hypoglycaemia and fever. In the United Kingdom, 90–95% of injuries are managed

without the need for neurosurgical intervention (Tasker et al 2006). When required, for example in the presence of an acute subdural bleed, surgical evaluation should be facilitated immediately.

The most common presentation of acute, severe head injury in children is coma. Clinical scores, such as the paediatric modifications of the Glasgow Coma Scale (GCS) (Tasker 2000, Teasdale & Jennett 1974), allow bedside assessment of neurological function and the degree of impairment of consciousness in children. Such scores are designed to allow early identification of pathology when it is still potentially reversible by medical or surgical intervention.

Coma in children may present after a longer interval than in adults. Continued extradural bleeding following a relatively minor injury may lead to a deteriorating level of consciousness. Cerebral oedema may be focal or generalized; the latter may result in an increase in intracranial pressure and cause a more rapid deterioration.

Raised intracranial pressure

Raised intracranial pressure (ICP) represents an increase in the volume of the intracranial contents. In addition to trauma, it can be caused by space-occupying lesions or encephalopathy. Normal values for ICP fall below 15 mmHg. The cerebral perfusion pressure (CPP) is the driving pressure for cerebral blood flow and is defined as the difference between mean arterial blood pressure and ICP. It is a crucial parameter, which lies within the range of 50–70 mmHg. A variety of methods to monitor ICP can be used including intraventricular catheters, subdural or subarachnoid monitors and cerebral intraparenchymal catheters.

Once the child is stabilized, medical management aims to avoid or minimize secondary brain injury. Factors that may precipitate a rise in ICP, resulting in a potential fall in CPP, should be avoided. Intubation and mechanical hyperventilation have been sometimes been used to reduce ICP. This has been controversial as hyperventilation (and hypocapnia) may induce cerebral ischaemia. In general, this is still sometimes used for short periods during acute deterioration or when intracranial hypertension is unresponsive to other therapy.

The management of children with acute head injury has been reviewed extensively (Tasker 2001). Many of the strategies for management are similar to adults and discussed in Chapter 8.

Pulmonary problems following liver transplantation

Liver transplantation is used for chronic end-stage liver disease and fulminant hepatic failure. Shortage of paediatric donors means that more and more grafts are reductions of adult livers. In some situations one donor

10

liver can be used for two patients. Postoperative complications include bleeding and splinting of the right side of the diaphragm. Patients invariably develop a pleural effusion which is usually right-sided but may be bilateral. Acute rejection is common 5–7 days post-transplant. Some patients develop chronic rejection and require retransplantation (Salt et al 1992).

Physiotherapists may have the opportunity to assess these patients preoperatively, but often patients with fulminant hepatic failure are operated on as an emergency or are too ill to be seen preoperatively.

Postoperatively, the risk of bleeding in some patients means that handling is kept to a minimum. Patients are assessed regularly and treated as appropriate. Following extubation, ambulation is encouraged as soon as possible. Large pleural effusions coupled with ascites mean patients are often very breathless and unable to mobilize.

KEY ISSUES FOR PHYSIOTHERAPISTS TREATING ACUTELY ILL CHILDREN

Paediatric intensive care units are often stressful and demanding environments. When children are critically ill, intubated and ventilated, therapists often have to use complex clinical reasoning to make difficult decisions. Classic contraindications to certain treatment techniques may sometimes be superceded by more compelling clinical needs, for example a small or moderate pneumothorax may be considered less important than acute lobar atelectasis.

Thorough assessment before to any physiotherapy intervention in ventilated children is essential. A report from the nurse in charge of the baby will provide important information about the current haemodynamic status and stability of the child. A recent chest radiograph will be helpful in identifying any focal areas of respiratory compromise and should be used in conjunction with thorough auscultation in order to decide on the appropriateness of intervention. Evaluation of fluid status, urine output, heart rate and rhythm, blood pressure, platelets, bleeding, inotropic support, level of sedation, will all contribute to a decision on how any treatment should be performed.

Successful treatments depend on accurate assessment and then thorough and continuous evaluation of clinical data during treatment from a multitude of different sources, including haemodynamic and respiratory information, observation and auscultation. Experience and competence are essential in the management of the most critically ill babies, as is a complete knowledge of underlying anatomical and physiological processes likely to influence the outcome of treatment. For example, treating a child with a univentricular pulmonary and systemic circulation with high bagging pressures or high oxygen concentration would dramatically influence the flow of blood to the lungs with potentially life-threatening consequences. Similarly, treating a child with head injury without appreciating the relationship between intracranial pressure, mean arterial pressure and cerebral perfusion pressure could have serious immediate and long-term consequences for their recovery.

Technological advances in recent years have meant that modern ventilators often incorporate pressure and flow sensors which allow continuous monitoring and calculation of tidal breathing parameters or respiratory mechanics from which an assessment of respiratory function can be made (MacNaughton & Evans 1999). It is imperative that physiotherapists familiarize themselves with these devices, the interpretation of data generated from them and their limitations in the clinical environment (Castle et al 2002). There is great potential for such equipment to provide objective feedback about efficacy and tolerance of treatments in individual patients and to provide excellent tools for systematic evaluation of physiotherapy treatment in mechanically ventilated infants.

Physiotherapy management of surgical patients

Preoperative management

In some hospitals preoperative visits and handbooks are available which help to reduce some of the fear of being in hospital. Except in emergency admissions, it is desirable for children and their parents to be seen by a physiotherapist before their surgery. Appropriate explanation of postoperative procedures should be given at the level of the child's age and understanding, but overloading the child with information they do not understand may increase stress and anxiety. It is important that parents understand the need for postoperative physiotherapy intervention as they can play an important role in encouraging postoperative mobility.

Physiotherapy assessment should include cardiorespiratory status and physical and motor development. The assessment of respiratory status provides an opportunity to evaluate postoperative risks and the need for preoperative treatment. If indicated, older children may be taught an airway clearance technique. Incentive spirometry can be useful in reducing atelectasis in children after cardiac surgery, especially those techniques specifically designed for children (Krastins et al 1982).

When a child has pre-existing pulmonary disease, for example cystic fibrosis, they may need to be admitted some time before surgery for prophylactic antibiotics and for effective airway clearance. Such children may require physiotherapy and suction in the anaesthetic room following intubation and before surgery (Tannenbaum et al 2007).

Several congenital cardiac anomalies are associated with a broader spectrum of embryological malformations, some of which result in developmental delay. These children may require long-term developmental follow-up. Any preoperative neurological problems or developmental delay should be documented and appropriate management plans formulated.

Postoperative management

In addition to the altered pulmonary dynamics and respiratory insufficiency seen after general anaesthesia, open heart surgery with cardiopulmonary bypass leads to further changes in respiratory function. The lungs may be compressed during surgery, contributing to atelectasis, loss of perfusion and diminished surfactant production, all of which contribute to poor respiratory compliance postoperatively. Children and infants should be regularly reviewed and treated as required.

As sedation is reduced and children are able to take a more active role in their treatment, effective pain relief is essential. Pain due to the incision and presence of intercostal drains may cause splinting of the chest wall and reduced excursion. Adequate pain relief can be provided through continuous infusion or patient-controlled systems in older children. It may be difficult to assess the severity of pain in children, although the development of specific paediatric pain scales has made it easier in recent years (Razmus & Wilson 2006). Children in pain can be withdrawn and immobile and infants in pain may be tachycardic and tachypnoeic. Some children who have a fear of needles will deny pain in order to avoid injections.

Treatment is directed towards early extubation and mobilization. When in bed, children should be comfortably positioned in alternate side lying or sitting upright and the 'slumped posture' should be avoided. As soon as possible, children should be sat out of bed and walking encouraged when appropriate. Drips, drains and catheters can all be carried to allow early ambulation. Attention to posture is important, particularly following thoracotomy when arm and shoulder exercises to the affected side are also essential.

If sputum retention is a problem postoperatively, airway clearance techniques may be required. A child may prefer not to have his wound supported or to support his own wound when coughing.

Prematurity

Preterm and critically ill neonates tolerate handling poorly and should therefore be handled as little as possible. The skin of a preterm baby is very thin and easily damaged. Manual techniques should be applied with

care. Physiotherapy and suction should only be carried out when indicated and careful assessment is essential before any intervention.

The positioning of infants receiving mechanical ventilation in NICU may have an impact on clinical outcome. The lateral decubitus positions, prone and supine are all used, although there is a tendency to nurse ventilated infants in the prone position. A systematic review of 11 trials involving 206 infants reported that prone positioning did have some advantage in terms of improved oxygenation but that there was no evidence to suggest that any one position during mechanical ventilation was more effective in producing a clinically relevant and sustained improvement (Balaguer et al 2006).

An active programme of pre- and post-extubation chest physiotherapy may result in a lower incidence of lobar collapse and reintubation within 24 hours (Flenady & Gray 2002). However a large randomized controlled trial testing the effects of a neonatal post-extubation programme on the incidence of post-extubation collapse found no differences between the physiotherapy and control group in terms of the rate of post-extubation collapse, adverse events (apnoea or bradycardia), duration of requirement of supplemental oxygen or the need for re-intubation within 24 hours (Bagley et al 2005).

An association between chest physiotherapy and encephaloclastic porencephaly in extremely preterm infants was reported by Harding et al in 1998. This study involved a retrospective analysis of 454 infants with birth weights less than 1500 g delivered between 24 and 27 weeks' gestation. Affected subjects received two to three times as many chest physiotherapy treatments as did the control group, but the group also had more prolonged and severe episodes of hypotension in the first week than controls and were less likely to have had a cephalic presentation at delivery. The lesions were considered to be caused by impact of the brain with the skull during shaking movements, which could occur during chest physiotherapy with percussion (Harding et al 1998). Since this publication, however, several authors have disputed the association between encephaloclastic porencephaly and chest physiotherapy (Beby et al 1998, Gray et al 1999, Vincon 1999). The significant methodological errors in this work have been highlighted and it is possible that these lesions occurred only in the sickest infants and the fact that they had more chest physiotherapy may be a reflection of their degree of illness (Gray et al 1999). No cases of encephaloclastic porencephaly were reported over the same 3-year period in two separate studies, despite similar criteria for initiation of chest physiotherapy (Beby et al 1998, Gray et al 1999). Follow-up data from the centre in New Zealand which first reported this problem later suggested that identification of encephaloclastic porencephaly emerged at a time when the use of chest physiotherapy had

10

already decreased and that the cluster of cases seen between 1992 and 1994, although associated with the number of chest physiotherapy treatments given, may have been due to some other factor (Knight et al 2001). Although an association between chest physiotherapy and encephaloclastic porencephaly seems unlikely, it highlights the need for very careful assessment of preterm infants and a judicious approach to treatment. If chest physiotherapy is indicated and chest percussion thought appropriate, the baby should be kept in a stable position, with the head and shoulders well supported, and vital signs carefully monitored throughout treatment.

Head injury

Immobility, impaired cough, depression of the respiratory centre and pulmonary dysfunction due to anaesthetic and paralysing agents predispose patients to pulmonary complications. The frequency of pneumonia in severely head-injured patients requiring prolonged mechanical ventilation has been reported to be as high as 70% (Demling & Riessen 1993).

Safe and effective treatment should be based on careful assessment and judicious use of appropriate physiotherapy techniques (Prasad & Tasker 1990). The use of bolus doses of analgesics and sedatives or, in more unstable cases, thiopental before an intervention can help reduce acute swings in ICP. Length of treatment time is an important factor, with longer treatment more likely to produce larger elevations of ICP. Sustained increases in ICP during cumulative interventions should be avoided by allowing a return to baseline values between procedures. Careful monitoring of CPP during treatment is essential and treatment should be withheld or abandoned if levels fall below 50 mmHg.

A head-down position is generally contraindicated and any change in position should maintain the head midline in relation to body position. A 30° head-up tilt has been shown to significantly reduce ICP in the majority of patients (Feldman et al 1992). The presence of a bone flap from decompressive craniotomy may limit options for positioning. Chest clapping may be better tolerated than vibrations and manual hyperinflation may be used with careful monitoring (Prasad & Tasker 1995). Endotracheal suctioning may have severe prolonged effects on ICP (Gemma et al 2002) and great care must be taken to avoid hypoxia. A protocol for physiotherapy management is shown in Figure 10.15.

Passive movements to maintain joint mobility may be felt necessary and it has been shown that these can be undertaken without detrimental effect on ICP in adults, provided that Valsalva-like manoeuvres are avoided (Brimioulle et al 1997).

Extracorporeal membrane oxygenation

Extracorporeal membrane oxygenation (ECMO) provides complete or partial cardiopulmonary bypass support for the heart and lungs or lungs alone when extremely ill children have severe but potentially reversible cardiac or respiratory failure (Huang et al 2007) (Chapter 9). It has been reported to be beneficial in both neonates and children with acute lung injury and respiratory failure (Pearson et al 1993, Swaniker et al 2000, UK Collaborative ECMO Trial Group 1996).

In some respects, physiotherapy treatments for children on ECMO may seem relatively less stressful for the physiotherapist. Children on full cardiopulmonary ECMO support are not reliant on mechanical ventilation for adequate oxygenation and it may not be as important to connect ventilation circuits quickly or complete suction cycles quickly. However, children on ECMO are heparinized and thus very vulnerable to bleeding, with potentially devastating consequences for survival or long-term outcome. Too much movement or coughing during physiotherapy may raise intracranial pressure and cause brain or pulmonary bleeding. If the nursing report suggests active haemorrhage, therapists should consider whether it is appropriate to apply manual techniques or treat at all. Adequate blood flow through the ECMO circuit is often dependent upon body position and the therapist should ensure that turning during treatments does not compromise flow through the cannulae.

Frequently children on ECMO for respiratory failure demonstrate a complete 'whiteout' of the lung fields on chest radiograph within the first day of ECMO support. During this time respiratory compliance is extremely low and little chest movement is seen or achieved during treatments. Children are often on 'resting' ventilation with low respiratory pressures and rates. During this time physiotherapy treatments may only consist of a quick assessment during the day, until it becomes apparent that the chest wall is beginning to move and air bronchograms are beginning to appear on chest radiograph. At this time it is appropriate to start more regular treatments in order to recruit functional airways and to facilitate early weaning from ECMO.

High-frequency oscillatory ventilation

High-frequency oscillatory ventilation (HFOV) theoretically provides gentle ventilatory support by employing very small tidal volumes and high respiratory rates (1–15 Hz) with high mean airway pressures to achieve adequate ventilation. It has been shown to be safe and effective in the treatment of respiratory failure in paediatric practice (Arnold 1996).

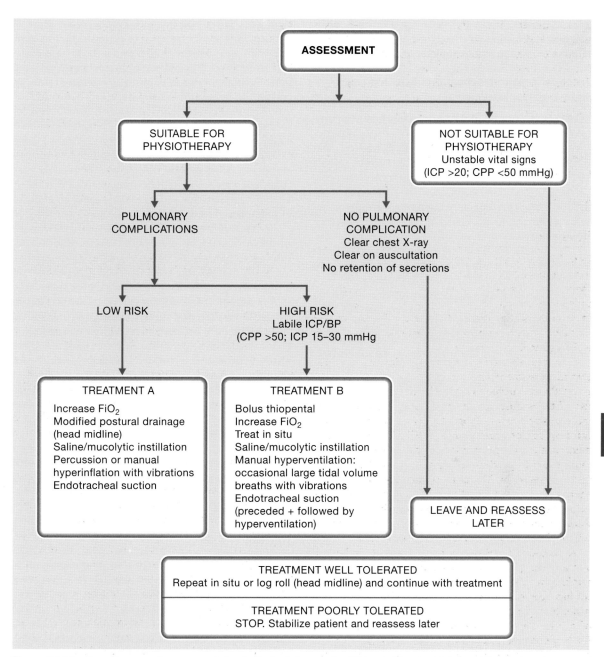

Figure 10.15 Flow diagram of an approach to chest physiotherapy in children with raised intracranial pressure. (Reproduced with permission from Prasad and Tasker 1990)

In theory, disconnecting infants from such ventilation for physiotherapy treatments, including manual inflation techniques, would contradict the principles of reducing volume loss, bulk flow of air and the shearing forces associated with such ventilation (Lindgren et al 2007). However many experienced physiotherapists find that unless children are disconnected for brief and effective treatments, these children are vulnerable to airway obstruction and atelectasis. The loss of volume after disconnection and suction is significant but transient (Tingay et al 2007). The key to successful physiotherapy treatments of children on HFOV lies in adequate

10

preoxygenation, proper assessment and quick, competent and effective treatments, which do not permit derecruitment within any treatment cycle.

Tracheal repair: tracheal stenosis and slide tracheoplasty

Subglottic stenosis occurs in some infants following prolonged intubation and leads to upper airway obstruction. It could be avoided by attention to tracheal tube placement and fixation and care with suction (Albert 1995). Acquired neonatal tracheobronchial stenosis (particularly in preterm infants) has a poor outcome. Stridor is often present and may respond to adrenaline via a nebulizer. In more severe cases a tracheostomy may be necessary until the airway has increased sufficiently in size to allow adequate ventilation. Some patients will also require surgical laryngotracheoplasty before successful decannulation of the tracheostomy can be achieved. More recently, primary repair of subglottic stenosis with laryngotracheal reconstruction has been successfully developed.

Children born with tracheal stenosis have had a high mortality. Now the development of various surgical tracheal reconstructions, replacements and slide tracheoplasty procedures has provided a new hope for such patients (Beierlein & Elliott 2006). ECMO may be required pre- or postoperatively to provide ventilatory support for patients undergoing critical tracheobronchial reconstruction. Manual hyperinflation following tracheal repair may be associated with greater risk of pneumothorax, because of the tracheal anastomosis. In addition, the tracheal anastomosis may extend distally to the tracheal tube and suction procedures should avoid traumatizing the site.

Some degree of tracheomalacia is often present and the fact that children are either paralysed or very well sedated in the early postoperative period means there is often air trapping and impaired airway clearance. It is thus essential that treatments are quick, competent and effective and include decompression, if necessary, of any trapped air. In the long term, such children may need follow-up in the community and may continue to have noisy breathing and problems with airway clearance.

Pulmonary hypertensive crisis

Pulmonary hypertensive crisis is described as an acute elevation of the pulmonary artery (PA) pressure (owing to contraction of the pulmonary arteriolar musculature), which restricts blood flow through the lungs. It is associated with a fall in left atrial pressure and a dramatic fall in cardiac output. PA pressure may approach or even exceed systemic pressure. It is seen in the presence of hypertrophic reactive arteriolar muscle in the lungs and is therefore common in those patients who have had

significant left-to-right shunts (VSD, AVSD, truncus arteriosus). This phenomenon is a critical, life-threatening event and prevention of such an incident is desirable. Airway suction and chest physiotherapy have the potential both for precipitating a hypertensive crisis (by creating an imbalance in the pulmonary/systemic flow ratio) and for correcting an imbalance (caused by excess secretions). The partial pressures of blood oxygen and carbon dioxide relative to each other will determine the ratio of systemic–pulmonary blood flow. Low oxygen and high carbon dioxide will increase pulmonary vascular resistance and reduce pulmonary blood flow. High oxygen and low carbon dioxide cause an increase in pulmonary blood flow.

In children prone to pulmonary hypertensive crisis, treatment should be undertaken with great caution. Inspired oxygen should be increased during chest physiotherapy (but not too much if a child is dependent on a univentricular circulation) and treatment times kept to a minimum. Particular attention should be paid to oxygen saturation and the PA pressure in relation to systemic blood pressure. Often children will require a bolus of sedation before treatment and if there is already nitric oxide entrained in the ventilator circuit, care should be taken to ensure this supply is maintained during manual ventilation with a bag. Nitric oxide gas (NO) has a potent pulmonary vasodilatory effect and can be delivered directly to the lungs via the ventilator circuit, for the effective relief of pulmonary hypertension in infants and children. Very small doses are used to reduce pulmonary arterial pressures, while systemic blood pressure is not affected (doses larger than 80 parts per million can be toxic) (Cheifetz 2000, Haddad et al 2000, Kinsella & Abman 2000).

Delayed sternal closure

Occasionally postoperative closure of the sternum is impeded by pulmonary, myocardial or chest wall oedema (due either to prolonged bypass times or particularly complicated intracardiac repairs). If sternal closure is likely to constrict cardiopulmonary function, closure may be delayed for days or even weeks. During this period children are paralysed or very well sedated and are preferentially nursed in supine. They are therefore at much greater risk of pulmonary complications. However, if stable and if the sternum is stented (to keep its edges separate), the child can with care be quarter turned from supine. Manual hyperinflation is usually well tolerated and gentle posterior and posterolateral vibrations may be applied. When the sternum is finally closed, there is often short-term deterioration in respiratory function and it may be useful to suggest an increase in ventilatory support if treatments are to be undertaken soon after sternal closure or to delay physiotherapy treatments until respiratory function has stabilized again (Main et al 2001).

Phrenic nerve damage

Damage to the phrenic nerve is a well-documented complication of paediatric cardiac surgery (Mok et al 1991). It occurs most commonly where dissection is required close to the mediastinal vessels and pericardium with which its course is closely associated. The result may be difficulty weaning from mechanical ventilation or severe respiratory compromise once extubated. Paradoxical movement during inspiration may compress the ipsilateral lung and cause mediastinal shift to the contralateral side, causing a further loss in lung volume. Physiotherapy intervention will depend on clinical symptoms, but it is important that the patient is positioned head up to relieve the pressure from the abdominal viscera and reduce the work of breathing. It is sometimes necessary to surgically plicate the affected diaphragm.

Acknowledgements

We would like to thank Dr Robert Dinwiddie and Catherine Dunne for their invaluable assistance with the preparation of this chapter.

References

Albert D 1995 Management of suspected tracheobronchial stenosis in ventilated neonates. Archives of Disease in Childhood 72: 1–2

Almeida CC, Ribeiro J D, Almeida-Junior AA, Zeferino AM 2005 Effect of expiratory flow increase technique on pulmonary function of infants on mechanical ventilation. Physiotherapy Research International 10(4): 213–221

Ambalavanan N, Carlo WA 2006 Ventilatory strategies in the prevention and management of bronchopulmonary dysplasia. Seminars in Perinatology 30(4): 192–199

Armstrong DS, Grimwood K, Carzino R et al 1995 Lower respiratory tract infection and inflammation in infants with newly diagnosed cystic fibrosis. British Medical Journal 310: 1571–1572

Arnold JH 1996 High frequency oscillatory ventilation: theory and practice in paediatric patients. Paediatric Anaesthesia 6: 437–441

Bagley, CE, Gray PH, Tudehope DI et al 2005 Routine neonatal post-extubation chest physiotherapy: a randomized controlled trial. Journal of Paediatric and Child Health 41(11): 592–597

Baird PA, MacDonald EC 1982 An epidemiologic study of congenital malformations of the anterior abdominal wall in more than half a million consecutive live births. American Journal of Human Genetics 34: 517–521

Balaguer A, Escribano J, Roque M 2006 Infant position in neonates receiving mechanical ventilation. Cochrane Database of Systematic Reviews Issue 4 Art No: CD003668 DOI: 10.1002/14651858 CD003668.pub2

Balfour-Lynn IM, Abrahamson E, Cohen G et al 2005 BTS Guidelines for the management of pleural infection in children (on behalf of the Paediatric Pleural Diseases Subcommittee of the BTS Standards of Care Committee). Thorax 60: 1–21

Barry P, O'Callaghan C 1996 Inhalational drug delivery from seven different spacer devices. Thorax 51: 835–840

Bauer M, Hoek G, Smit HA et al 2007 Air pollution and development of asthma, allergy and infections in a birth cohort. European Respiratory Journal 29: 879–888

Beby PJ, Henderson-Smart DJ, Lacey JL, Rieger I 1998 Short and long term neurological outcomes following neonatal chest physiotherapy. Journal of Paediatric and Child Health 34: 60–62

Beierlein W, Elliott MJ 2006 Variations in the technique of slide tracheoplasty to repair complex forms of long-segment congenital tracheal stenoses. Annals of Thoracic Surgery 82: 1540–1542

Berney S, Denehy L 2002 A comparison of the effects of manual and ventilator hyperinflation on static lung compliance and sputum production in intubated and ventilated intensive care patients. Physiotherapy Research International 7(2): 100–108

Bhandari A, Panitch HB 2006 Pulmonary outcomes in bronchopulmonary dysplasia. Seminars in Perinatology 30(4): 219–226

Bhuyan U, Peters AM, Gordon I, Helms P 1989 Effect of posture on the distribution of pulmonary ventilation and perfusion in children and adults. Thorax 44: 480–484

Bingol Karakoc G, Yilmaz M, Sur S et al 2000 The effects of daily pulmonary rehabilitation program at home on childhood asthma. Allergology Immunopathology (Madr) 28: 12–14

Birnkrant DJ 2002 The assessment and management of the respiratory complications of pediatric neuromuscular diseases. Clinical Pediatrics (Philadelphia) 41(5): 301–308

Blackwood B 1999 Normal saline instillation with endotracheal suctioning: primum non nocere (first do no harm). Journal of Advanced Nursing 29: 928–934

Blumenthal I, Lealman GT 1982 Effects of posture on gastro-oesophageal reflux in the newborn. Archives of Disease in Childhood 57: 555–556

Boucher RC. 2004 New concepts of the pathogenesis of cystic fibrosis lung disease. European Respiratory Journal 23: 146–158

Brackbill Y, Douthitt TC, West H 1973 Psychophysiological effects in the neonate of prone versus supine placement. Journal of Pediatrics 82: 82–83

Brewer LA, Fosburg RG, Mulder GA, Verska JJ 1972 Spinal cord complications following surgery for coarctation of the aorta – a study of 66 cases. Journal of Thoracic and Cardiovascular Surgery 64: 368

Brimioulle S, Moraine JJ, Norrenberg K, Kahn RJ 1997 Effect of positioning and exercise on intracranial pressure in a neurosurgical intensive care unit. Physical Therapy 77: 1682–1689

British Thoracic Society Standards of Care Committee 2002 Guidelines for the management of community acquired pneumonia in childhood. Thorax 57: 1–24

British Thoracic Society (BTS), Scottish Intercollegiate Guidelines Network (SIGN) 2003 British guideline on the management of asthma. Thorax 58 (Suppl I): i1–i94

Button BM, Heine RG, Catto-Smith AG Phelan PD, Olinsky A 1997 Postural drainage and gastro-oesophageal reflux in infants with cystic fibrosis. Archives of Disease in Childhood 76: 148–150

Button BM, Heine RG, Catto-Smith AG et al 2003 Chest physiotherapy in infants with cystic fibrosis: to tip or not? A five-year study. Pediatric Pulmonology 35(3): 208–213

10

Button BM, Heine RG, Catto-Smith AG et al 2004 Chest physiotherapy, gastro-oesophageal reflux, and arousal in infants with cystic fibrosis. Archives of Disease in Childhood 89(5): 435–439

Campbell AH, O'Connell JM, Wilson F 1975 The effect of chest physiotherapy upon the FEV_1 in chronic bronchitis. Medical Journal of Australia 1: 33–35

Carpenter A 1994 Congenital malformation of the mitral valve. In: Stark J, De Leval M (eds) Surgery for congenital heart defects, 2nd edn. WB Saunders, Philadelphia, pp 599–614

Carrol N, Sly P 1999 Exercise training as an adjunct to asthma management? Thorax 54: 190–191

Castenda AR 1994 Tetralogy of Fallot. In: Stark J, De Leval M (eds) Surgery for congenital heart defects, 2nd edn. WB Saunders, Philadelphia, pp 405–416

Castle RA, Dunne CJ, Mok Q et al 2002 Accuracy of displayed values of tidal volume in the pediatric intensive care unit. Critical Care Medicine 30(11): 2566–2574

Chatwin M, Ross E, Hart N et al 2003 Cough augmentation with mechanical insufflation/exsufflation in patients with neuromuscular weakness. European Respiratory Journal 21(3): 502–508

Cheifetz IM 2000 Inhaled nitric oxide: plenty of data, no consensus. Critical Care Medicine 28: 902–903

Choi JS, Jones AY 2005 Effects of manual hyperinflation and suctioning in respiratory mechanics in mechanically ventilated patients with ventilator-associated pneumonia. Australian Journal of Physiotherapy 51: 25–30

Chulay M, Graeber GM 1988 Efficacy of a hyperinflation and hyperoxygenation suctioning intervention. Heart and Lung 17: 15–22

Clark AP, Winslow EH, Tyler DO, White KM 1990 Effects of endotracheal suctioning on mixed venous oxygen saturation and heart rate in critically ill adults. Heart and Lung 19: 552–557

Clarke RC, Kelly BE, Convery PN, Fee JP 1999 Ventilatory characteristics in mechanically ventilated patients during manual hyperventilation for chest physiotherapy. Anaesthesia 54: 936–940

Cowan MJ, Gladwin MT, Shelhamer JH 2001 Disorders of ciliary motility. American Journal of Medical Science 321: 3–10

Czarnik RE, Stone KS, Everhart CJ, Preusser BA 1991 Differential effects of continuous versus intermittent suction on tracheal tissue. Heart and Lung 20: 144–151

Davies H, Kitchman R, Gordon G, Helms P 1985 Regional ventilation in infancy. Reversal of the adult pattern. New England Journal of Medicine 313: 1627–1628

De Leval M 1994a Ventricular septal defects. In: Stark J, De Leval M (eds) Surgery for congenital heart defects, 2nd edn. WB Saunders, Philadelphia, pp 55–371

De Leval M 1994b Tricuspid valve. In: Stark J, De Leval M (eds) Surgery for congenital heart defects, 2nd edn. WB Saunders, Philadelphia, Ch 23, pp 453–466

Deakers TW, Reynolds G, Stretton M, Newth CJ 1994 Cuffed endotracheal tubes in pediatric intensive care. Journal of Pediatrics 125: 57–62

Demling RH, Riessen R 1993 Respiratory failure after cerebral injury. Critical Care Medicine 1: 440–446

Depaepe A, Dolk A, Lechat MF 1993 The epidemiology of tracheo-oesophageal fistula and oesophageal atresia in Europe. Archives of Disease in Childhood 68: 743–748

Dinwiddie R 1997 Aspiration syndromes. In: The diagnosis and management of paediatric respiratory disease, 2nd edn. Churchill Livingstone, New York, pp 247–260

Donn SM, Sinha SK 2003 Invasive and non-invasive neonatal mechanical ventilation. Respiratory Care 48(4): 426–441

Ehrenkranz RA, Walsh MC, Vohr BR et al 2005 National Institutes of Child Health and Human Development Neonatal Research Network. Validation of the National Institutes of Health consensus definition of bronchopulmonary dysplasia. Pediatrics 116(6): 1353–1360

Elliott M, Hussey J 1995 Paediatric cardiac surgery. In: Prasad SA, Hussey J (eds) Paediatric respiratory care. Chapman & Hall, London, pp 122–141

Feldman Z, Kanter MJ, Robertson CS et al 1992 Effect of head elevation on intracranial pressure and cerebral blood flow in head injured patients. Journal of Neurosurgery 59: 206–211

Ferkol T, Mitchison HM, O'Callaghan C et al 2006 Current issues in the basic mechanisms, pathophysiology, diagnosis and management of primary ciliary dyskinesia. European Respiratory Monograph 37 11: 291–313

Flenady VJ, Gray PH 2002 Chest physiotherapy for preventing morbidity in babies being extubated from mechanical ventilation. Cochrane Database of Systematic Reviews, No. 2, article CD000283

Freed DH, Robertson CM, Sauve RS et al 2006 Intermediate-term outcomes of the arterial switch operation for transposition of great arteries in neonates: alive but well? Journal of Thoracic and Cardiovascular Surgery 132(4): 845–852

Gattinoni L, Caironi P, Cressoni M et al 2006 Lung recruitment in patients with the acute respiratory distress syndrome. New England Journal of Medicine 354(17): 1775–1786

Gattinoni L, Pesenti A, Bombino M, Pelosi P, Brazzi L 1993 Role of extracorporeal circulation in adult respiratory distress syndrome management. New Horizons 1: 603–612

Gemma M, Tommasino C, Cerri M et al 2002 Intracranial effects of endotracheal suctioning in the acute phase of head injury. Journal of Neurological Anesthesiology 14: 50–54

Glass C, Grap MJ, Corley MC, Wallace D 1993 Nurses' ability to achieve hyperinflation and hyperoxygenation with a manual resuscitation bag during endotracheal suctioning. Heart and Lung 22: 158–165

Goodnough SK 1985 The effects of oxygen and hyperinflation on arterial oxygen tension after endotracheal suctioning. Heart and Lung 14: 11–17

Gray PH, Flenady VJ, Blackwell L 1999 Potential risks of chest physiotherapy in preterm infants. Journal of Pediatrics 135: 131

Greenough A 1996 Lung maturation. In: Greenough A, Roberton NRC, Milner A (eds) Neonatal respiratory disorders. Arnold, London, pp 13–26

Greenough A, Kotecha S, Vrijlandt E 2006 Bronchopulmonary dysplasia: current models and concepts. In: Frey U, Gerritsen J (eds) Respiratory diseases in infants and children. European Respiratory Monograph 11: 217–229

Gregson R, Shannon H, Main E et al 2007a The relationship between age and forces applied during chest physiotherapy in mechanically ventilated children. Physiotherapy 93: S517

Gregson RK, Stocks J, Petley GW et al 2007b Simultaneous measurement of force and respiratory profiles during chest physiotherapy in ventilated children. Physiological Measurement 28: 1017–1028

Gremmo ML, Guenza MC 1999 Positive expiratory pressure in the physiotherapeutic management of primary ciliary dyskinesia in the paediatric age. Monaldi Archives of Chest Disease 54: 255–257

Haddad E, Lowson SM, Johns RA, Rich GF 2000 Use of inhaled nitric oxide perioperatively and in intensive care patients. Anesthesiology 92: 1821–1825

Hagler DA, Traver GA 1994 Endotracheal saline and suction

10

catheters: sources of lower airway contamination. American Journal of Critical Care 3: 444–447

Harding JE, Miles FK, Becroft DM, Allen BC, Knight DB 1998 Chest physiotherapy may be associated with brain damage in extremely premature infants. Journal of Pediatrics 132: 440–444

Harshbarger SA, Hoffman LA, Zullo TG, Pinsky MR 1992 Effects of a closed tracheal suction system on ventilatory and cardiovascular parameters. American Journal of Critical Care 1: 57–61

Heaf DP, Helms P, Gordon I, Turner HM 1983 Postural effects on gas exchange in infants. New England Journal of Medicine 308(25): 1505–1508

Hislop A, Reid L 1974 Development of the acinus in the human lung. Thorax 29: 90–94

Hislop A, Wigglesworth JS, Desai R 1986 Alveolar development in the human fetus and infant. Early Human Development 13: 1–11

Hodge D, Chetcuti PAJ 2000 RSV: management of the acute episode. Paediatric Respiratory Reviews 1: 215–220

Hoffman JIE, Kaplan S. 2002 The incidence of congenital heart disease. Journal of the American College of Cardiology 39(12): 1890–1900

Holloway E, Ram FSF 2004 Breathing exercises for asthma. Cochrane Database of Systematic Reviews, Issue 1: CD001277, pub2

Hondras MA, Linde K, Jones AP 2000 Manual therapy for asthma (Cochrane Review). In: The Cochrane Library, 4. Update Software, Oxford

Horiuchi K, Jordan D, Cohen D, Kemper MC, Weissman C 1997 Insights into the increased oxygen demand during chest physiotherapy. Critical Care Medicine 25: 1347–1351

Huang SC, Wu ET, Chi NH et al 2007 Perioperative extracorporeal membrane oxygenation support for critical pediatric airway surgery. European Journal of Pediatrics E-pub DOI 10.1007/500431-006-0390-y

Imle PC, Klemic N 1989 Methods of airway clearance: coughing and suctioning. In: Mackenzie CF, Imle PC, Ciesla N (eds) Chest physiotherapy in the intensive care unit. Williams and Wilkins, Baltimore, pp 153–187

Inselman LS, Mellins RB 1981 Growth and development of the lung. Journal of Pediatrics 98: 1–15

Inwald D, Roland M, Kuitert L, McKenzie S, Petros A 2001 Oxygen for all in acute severe asthma. British Medical Journal 27: 722–729

Jaffe A, Bush A 2001 Cystic fibrosis: review of the decade. Monaldi

Archives of Chest Disease 56: 240–247

Jobe AH, Bancalari E 2001 Bronchopulmonary dysplasia. American Journal of Respiratory and Critical Care Medicine 163: 1723–1729

Johnson AH, Peacock JL, Greenough A et al 2002 United Kingdom Oscillation Study Group. High frequency oscillatory ventilation for the prevention of chronic lung disease of prematurity. New England Journal of Medicine 347: 633–642

Keens TG, Ianuzzo CD 1979 Development of fatigue-resistant muscle fibers in human ventilatory muscles. American Review of Respiratory Disease 119(2): 139–141

Kerem E, Yatsiv I, Goitein KJ 1990 Effect of endotracheal suctioning on arterial blood gases in children. Intensive Care Medicine 16: 95–99

Khine HH, Corddry DH, Kettrick RG et al 1997 Comparison of cuffed and uncuffed endotracheal tubes in young children during general anesthesia. Anesthesiology 86: 627–631

Kim CS, Iglesias AJ, Sackner MA 1987 Mucus clearance by 2-phase gas–liquid flow mechanism – asymmetric periodic-flow model. Journal of Applied Physiology 62(3): 959–971

King H, Booker PD 2004 General principles of neonatal anaesthesia. Current Anaesthesia and Critical Care 15: 302–308

King M 1998 Experimental models for studying mucociliary clearance. European Respiratory Journal 11(1): 222–228

Kinloch D 1999 Instillation of normal saline during endotracheal suctioning: effects on mixed venous oxygen saturation. American Journal of Critical Care 8: 231–240

Kinsella JP, Abman SH 2000 Clinical approach to inhaled nitric oxide therapy in the newborn with hypoxemia. Journal of Pediatrics 136: 717–726

Kleiber C, Krutzfield N, Rose EF 1988 Acute histologic changes in the tracheobronchial tree associated with different suction catheter insertion techniques. Heart and Lung 17: 10–14

Knight DB, Bevan CJ, Harding JE et al 2001 Chest physiotherapy and porencephalic brain lesions in very preterm infants. Journal of Paediatric and Child Health 37(6): 554–558

Konno K, Mead J 1967 Measurement of the separate volume changes of rib cage and abdomen during breathing. Journal of Applied Physiology 22: 407–422

Kotecha S 2000 Lung growth: implications for the newborn infant. Archives of Disease in Childhood Fetal & Neonatal Edition 82: F69–F74

Krastins I, Corey ML, McLeod A et al 1982 An evaluation of incentive spirometry in the management of pulmonary complications after cardiac surgery in a pediatric population. Critical Care Medicine 10: 525–528

Krause MF, Hoehn T 2000 Chest physiotherapy in mechanically ventilated children: a review. Critical Care Medicine 28: 1648–1651

Kuo CY, Gerhardt T, Bolivar J, Claure N, Bancalari E 1996 Effect of leak around the endotracheal tube on measurements of pulmonary compliance and resistance during mechanical ventilation: a lung model study. Pediatric Pulmonology 22: 35–43

Langman J 1977 Medical embryology. Williams and Wilkins, Baltimore

Lannefors l, Wollmer P 1992 Mucus clearance with three chest physiotherapy regimes in cystic fibrosis: a comparison between postural drainage, PEP, and physical exercise. European Respiratory Journal 5: 748–753

Lindgren S, Odenstedt H, Olegard C et al 2007 Regional lung derecruitment after endotracheal suction during volume- or pressure-controlled ventilation: a study using electric impedance tomography. Intensive Care Medicine 33(1): 172–180

Lum S, Gustafsson P, Ljungberg H et al 2007 Early detection of cystic fibrosis lung disease: multiple-breath washout versus raised volume tests. Thorax 62(4): 341–347

MacNaughton PD, Evans TW 1999 Pulmonary function in the intensive care unit. In: Hughes JMB, Pride NB (eds) Lung function tests: physiological principles and clinical applications. London, WB Saunders, pp 185–199

Main E, Castle R, Newham D, Stocks J 2004 Respiratory physiotherapy vs. suction: the effects on respiratory function in ventilated infants and children. Intensive Care Medicine 30(6): 1144–1151

Main E, Castle R, Stocks J et al 2001 The influence of endotracheal tube leak on the assessment of respiratory function in ventilated children. Intensive Care Medicine 27(11): 1788–1797

Main E, Elliott MJ, Schindler M, Stocks J 2001 Effect of delayed sternal closure after cardiac surgery on respiratory function in ventilated infants. Critical Care Medicine 29(9): 1798–1802

Marcus RJ, van der Walt JH, Pettifer RJ 2002 Pulmonary volume recruitment restores pulmonary compliance and resistance in anaesthetized young children. Paediatric Anaesthesia 12: 579–584

10

Martinez TM, Llapur CJ, Williams TH et al 2005 High-resolution computed tomography imaging of airway disease in infants with cystic fibrosis. American Journal of Respiratory and Critical Care Medicine 172: 1133–1138

Matsumoto I, Araki H, Tsuda K et al 1999 Effects of swimming training on aerobic capacity and exercise induced bronchoconstriction in children with bronchial asthma. Thorax 54: 196–201

McCabe SM, Smeltzer SC 1993 Comparison of tidal volumes obtained by one-handed and two-handed ventilation techniques. American Journal of Critical Care 2: 467–473

McCarren B, Alison JA, Herbert RD 2006 Vibration and its effect on the respiratory system. Australian Journal of Physiotherapy 52(1): 39–43

McKelvie S 1998 Endotracheal suctioning. Nursing in Critical Care 3: 244–248

Menkes HA, Traystman RJ 1977 Collateral ventilation. American Review of Respiratory Disease 116: 287–309

Miske LJ, Hickey EM, Kolb SM et al 2004 Use of the mechanical in-exsufflator in pediatric patients with neuromuscular disease and impaired cough. Chest 105(3): 741–747

Mok Q, Ross-Russell R, Mulvey D et al 1991 Phrenic nerve injury in infants and children undergoing cardiac surgery. British Heart Journal 65(5): 287–292

Moore M, Little P 2006 Humidified air inhalation for treating croup. Cochrane Database of Systematic Reviews, Issue 3. Art. No: CD002870. DOI: 10.1002/14651858.CD002870. pub2.

Morini F, Goldman A, Pierro A 2006 Extracorporeal membrane oxygenation in infants with congenital diaghragmatic hernia. European Journal of Pediatric Surgery 16: 385–391

Muller NL, Bryan AC 1979 Chest wall mechanics and respiratory muscles in infants. Pediatric Clinics of North America 26(3): 503–516

National Asthma Education and Prevention Programme (NAEPP) Expert Panel 2002 Guidelines for the diagnosis and management of asthma – update on selected topics. NIH publication 02–5075, National Institutes of Health, Bethesda, MD

Neder JA, Nery LE, Silva AC, Cabral ALB, Fernandes ALG 1999 Short-term effects of aerobic training in the clinical management of moderate to severe asthma in children. Thorax 54: 202–206

Ng GYT, da Silva O, Ohlsson A 2001 Bronchodilation for the prevention

and treatment of chronic lung disease in preterm infants. Cochrane Database of Systematic Reviews 23: CD003214

Nicholas KJ, Dhouibe MO, Marchall TG, Edmunds AT, Grant MB 1999 Physiotherapy in patients with bronchiolitis. Physiotherapy 85(12): 669–674

Norwood WI, Jacobs ML 1994 Hypoplastic left heart syndrome. In: Stark J, De Leval M (eds) Surgery for congenital heart defects, 2nd edn. WB Saunders, Philadelphia, pp 587–598

Ntoumenopoulos G 2005 Indications for manual lung hyperinflation (MHI) in the mechanically ventilated patient with chronic obstructive pulmonary disease. Chronic Respiratory Disease 2(4): 199–207

O'Callaghan C 2000 How to choose delivery devices for asthma. Archives of Disease in Childhood 82: 185–191

Ochs M, Nyengaard J, Jung A et al 2004 Number of alveoli in the human lung. American Journal of Respiratory and Critical Care Medicine 169: 120–124

Openshaw P, Edwards S, Helms P 1984 Changes in rib cage geometry during childhood. Thorax 39: 624–627

Pang LM, Mellins RB 1975 Neonatal cardiorespiratory physiology. Anesthesiology 43(2): 171–196

Panickar JR, Dodd SR, Smyth RL, Couriel JM 2005 Trends in deaths from respiratory illness in children in England and Wales from 1968–2000. Thorax 60: 1035–1038

Panitch HB 2006 Airway clearance in children with neuromuscular weakness. Current Opinion in Pediatrics 18(3): 277–281

Pearson GA, Grant J, Field D, Sosnowski A, Firmin RK 1993 Extracorporeal life support in paediatrics. Archives of Disease in Childhood 68: 94

Pénard-Morand C, Charpin D, Raherison C et al 2005 Long-term exposure to background air pollution related to respiratory and allergic health in schoolchildren. Clinical and Experimental Allergy 35(10): 1279–1287

Perrotta C, Ortiz Z, Roque M 2005 Chest physiotherapy for acute bronchiolitis in paediatric patients between 0 and 24 months old. Cochrane Database of systematic Reviews, Issue 2. Art. No: CD004873. pub2

Phillips G 1996 To tip or not to tip? Physiotherapy Research International 1(1): 1–6

Prasad SA, Main E 2006 Routine airway clearance in asymptomatic infants and babies with cystic fibrosis: obligatory or obsolete? Physical Therapy Reviews 11: 11–20

Prasad SA, Tasker RC 1990 Guidelines for physiotherapy management of critically ill children with acutely raised intracranial pressure. Physiotherapy 76(4): 248–250

Prasad SA, Tasker RC 1995 Neurological intensive care. In: Prasad SA, Hussey J (eds) Paediatric respiratory care. Chapman & Hall, London, pp 142–149

Rabe KF, Adachi M, Lai CK et al 2004 Worldwide severity and control of asthma in children and adults: the global asthma insights and reality surveys. Journal of Allergy and Clinical Immunology 114: 40–47

Raguckas SE, Vandenbussche HL, Jacobs C, Klepser ME 2007 Pertussis resurgence: diagnosis, treatment, prevention, and beyond. Pharmacotherapy 27(1): 41–52

Ram FSF, Robinson SM, Black PN, Picot J 2005 Physical training for asthma. Cochrane Database of Systematic Reviews, Issue 4. Art. No.: CD001116. DOI: 10.1002/14651858.CD001116. pub2

Ranganathan SC, Dezateux C, Bush A et al 2001 Airway function in infants newly diagnosed with cystic fibrosis (London Collaborative Cystic Fibrosis Group). Lancet 358(9297): 1964–1965

Razmus I, Wilson D 2006 Current trends in the development of sedation/analgesia scales for the pediatric critical care patient. Pediatric Nursing 32: 435–441

Rehder K, Hatch DJ, Sessler AD, Fowler WS 1972 The function of each lung of anesthetized and paralyzed man during mechanical ventilation. Anesthesiology 37(1): 16–26

Reid L 1984, Lung growth in health and disease. British Journal of Diseases of the Chest 78: 113–132

Ridling DA, Martin LD, Bratton SL 2003 Endotracheal suctioning with or without instillation of isotonic sodium chloride solution in critically ill children. American Journal of Critical Care 12(3): 212–219

Roberton NRC 1996 Intensive care. In: Greenough A, Roberton NRC, Milner A (eds) Neonatal respiratory disorders. Arnold, London, pp 174–195

Roberts D, Dalziel S 2006 Antenatal corticosteroids for accelerating fetal lung maturation for women at risk of preterm birth. Cochrane Database of Systematic Reviews 2006, Issue 3. Art. No: CD004454. DOI: 10.1002/14651858.CD004454.pub2

Russell K, Wiebe N, Saenz A et al 2004 Glucocorticoids for croup. Cochrane Database of Systematic Reviews Issue 1. Art. No: CD001955. DOI: 10.1002/14651858.CD001955.pub2

Ryan RM 2006 A new look at bronchopulmonary dysplasia

classification. Journal of Perinatology 26: 207–209

Salt A, Noble-Jameson G, Barnes ND et al 1992 Liver transplantation in 100 children: Cambridge and King's College Hospital series. British Medical Journal 304: 416–421

Savian C, Paratz J, Davies A 2006 Comparison of the effectiveness of manual and ventilator hyperinflation at different levels of positive end-expiratory pressure in artificially ventilated and intubated intensive care patients. Heart Lung 35(5): 334–341

Schreuder FM, Jones UF 2004 The effect of saline instillation on sputum yield and oxygen saturation measurement in adult intubated patients: single subject design. Physiotherapy 90: 109

Schultz CM, Digeronimo RJ, Yoder BA Congenital Diaphragmatic Hernia Study Group 2007 Congenital diaphragmatic hernia: a simplified postnatal predictor of outcome. Journal of Pediatric Surgery 42: 510–516

Scottish Intercollegiate Guidelines Network 2006 Bronchiolitis in children: a national clinical guideline. Scottish Intercollegiate Guidelines Network, Edinburgh

Seear M, Wensley D, West N 2005 How accurate is the diagnosis of exercise induced asthma among Vancouver schoolchildren? Archives of Disease in Childhood 90: 898–902

Shah AR, Kurth CD, Gwiazdowski SG, Chance B, Delivoria-Papadopoulos M 1992 Fluctuations in cerebral oxygenation and blood volume during endotracheal suctioning in premature infants. Journal of Pediatrics 120: 769–774

Shorten DR, Byrne PJ, Jones RL 1991 Infant responses to saline instillations and endotracheal suctioning. Journal of Obstetric, Gynecological and Neonatal Nursing 20: 464–469

Singer M, Vermaat J, Hall G, Latter G, Patel M 1994 Hemodynamic effects of manual hyperinflation in critically ill mechanically ventilated patients. Chest 106: 1182–1187

Smith NP, Jesudason EC, Featherstone NC et al 2005 Recent advances in congenital diaghragmatic hernia. Archives of Disease in Childhood 90: 426–428

Sole ML, Byers JF, Ludy JE et al 2003 A multisite survey of suctioning techniques and airway management practices. American Journal of Critical Care 12(3): 220–230

Southall DP, Samuels MP 1992 Reducing risks in the sudden infant death syndrome. British Medical Journal 304: 260–265

Stark J, Gallivan S, Lovegrove J et al 2000 Mortality rates after surgery for congenital heart defects in children

and surgeons' performance. Lancet 355(9208): 1004–1007

Stevens TP, Blennow M, Soll RF 2004 Early surfactant administration with brief ventilation vs selective surfactant and continued mechanical ventilation for preterm infants with or at risk for respiratory distress syndrome. Cochrane Database of Systematic Reviews, Issue 3. Art. No.: CD003063. DOI: 10.1002/14651858. CD003063.pub2

Stiller K 2000 Physiotherapy in intensive care: towards an evidence-based practice. Chest 118: 1801–1813

Stone KS 1990 Ventilator versus manual resuscitation bag as the method for delivering hyperoxygenation before endotracheal suctioning. AACN: Clinical Issues in Critical Care Nursing 1: 289–299

Stone KS, Talaganis SA, Preusser B, Gonyon DS 1991 Effect of lung hyperinflation and endotracheal suctioning on heart rate and rhythm in patients after coronary artery bypass graft surgery. Heart and Lung 20: 443–450

Stone KS, Turner B 1989 Endotracheal suctioning. Annual Review of Nursing Research 7: 27–49

Sutton PP, Lopezvidriero MT, Pavia D et al 1985 Assessment of percussion, vibratory-shaking and breathing exercises in chest physiotherapy. European Journal of Respiratory Diseases 66: 147–152

Swaniker F, Kolla S, Moler F et al 2000 Extracorporeal life support outcome for 128 pediatric patients with respiratory failure. Journal of Pediatric Surgery 35: 197–202

Tannenbaum E, Prasad SA, Dinwiddie R, Main E 2007 Chest physiotherapy during anaesthesia for children with cystic fibrosis: effects on respiratory function. Pediatric Pulmonology 42(12): 1152–1158

Tasker RC 2000 Neurological critical care. Current Opinion in Pediatrics 12(3): 222–226

Tasker RC 2001 Neurocritical care and traumatic brain injury. Indian Journal of Paediatrics 68: 257–266

Tasker RC, Morris KP, Forsyth RJ et al 2006 Severe head injury in children: emergency access to neurosurgery in the United Kingdom. Emergency Medicine Journal 23(7): 519–522

Teasdale G, Jennett B 1974 Assessment of coma and impaired consciousness: a practical scale. Lancet 2: 81–84

Thoresen M, Cavan F, Whitelaw A 1988 Effect of tilting on oxygenation in newborn infants. Archives of Disease in Childhood 63: 315–317

Tingay DG, Copnell B, Mills JF et al 2007 Effects of open endotracheal suction on lung volume in infants receiving HFOV. Intensive Care Medicine 33(4): 689–693

Toelle BG, Marks GB 2005 The ebb and flow of asthma. Thorax 60(2): 87–88

Tudehope DI, Bagley C 1980 Techniques of physiotherapy in intubated babies with RDS. Australian Paediatric Journal 16: 226–228

UK Collaborative ECMO Trial Group 1996 UK collaborative randomised trial of neonatal extracorporeal membrane oxygenation. Lancet 348: 75–81

van der Schans CP, Postma DS, Koeter GH, Rubin BK 1999 Physiotherapy and bronchial mucus transport. European Respiratory Journal 13(6): 1477–1486

Vaughan RS, Menke JA, Giacoia GP 1978 Pneumothorax: a complication of endotracheal suctioning. Journal of Pediatrics 92: 633–634

Vianello A, Corrado A, Arcaro G et al 2005 Mechanical insufflation-exsufflation improves outcomes for neuromuscular disease patients with respiratory tract infections. American Journal of Physical Medicine and Rehabilitation 84(2): 83–88

Vincon C 1999 Potential risks of chest physiotherapy in preterm infants. Journal of Pediatrics 135: 131–132

Wanner A 1984 Does chest physical therapy move airway secretions? American Review of Respiratory Disease 130: 701–702

Webb MSC, Martin JA, Cartlidge PHT, Ng YK, Wright NA 1985 Chest physiotherapy in acute bronchiolitis. Archives of Disease in Childhood 6: 1078–1079

Wenstrom KD, Weiner CP, Hanson JW 1991 A five-year statewide experience with congenital diaphragmatic hernia. American Journal of Obstetrics and Gynecology 165: 838–842

Wollmer P, Ursing K, Midgren B, Eriksson L 1985 Inefficiency of chest percussion in the physical therapy of chronic bronchitis. European Journal of Respiratory Disease 66: 233–239

Wong WP, Paratz JD, Wilson K, Burns YR 2003 Hemodynamic and ventilatory effects of manual respiratory physiotherapy techniques of chest clapping, vibration, and shaking in an animal model. Journal of Applied Physiology 95(3): 991–998

Wood CJ 1998 Endotracheal suctioning: a literature review. Intensive Critical Care Nursing 14: 124–136

Zack MB, Pontoppidan H, Kazemi H 1974 The effect of lateral positions on gas exchange in pulmonary disease: a prospective evaluation. American Review of Respiratory Disease 110: 49–55

Zahka KG, Patel CR 2002 Congenital defects. In: Fanaroff A, Martin RJ (eds) Neonatal–perinatal medicine: diseases of the fetus and infant, 7th edn. Mosby, St Louis

10

Chapter **11**

Non-invasive ventilation

Amanda Piper, Elizabeth Ellis

INTRODUCTION

The application of non-invasive ventilatory support to improve ventilation is not a new idea. The tank ventilator or 'iron lung', which provides negative pressure to the chest wall, was first developed in the 19th century (Woollam 1976). Further developments and modifications occurred, but it was not until the poliomyelitis outbreaks of the 1940s and 1950s that such devices became widely used. Continuous positive airway pressure (CPAP) through a facemask for patients with pulmonary oedema and other forms of acute respiratory failure was extensively described in the 1930s (Barach et al 1938). However, with the development of positive pressure ventilators and the introduction of the endotracheal tube in the 1960s, use of non-invasive forms of ventilatory support for acute respiratory failure declined. Negative pressure devices continued to be used in patients with severe respiratory muscle impairment following poliomyelitis and in other patient groups presenting with chronic respiratory failure where long-term ventilatory support in the home was required (Garay et al 1981, Weirs et al 1977).

Since the mid-1980s, interest in non-invasive ventilatory support has again flourished, specifically the use of positive airway pressure devices and facemask interfaces. Although this interest had its genesis in the area of sleep-disordered breathing and chronic respiratory failure, clinicians have rapidly recognized the value of this therapy in acute medical and surgical conditions where respiratory failure develops, in weaning from conventional ventilatory support and as an adjunct to established respiratory care programmes. In this chapter we will outline the mechanisms by which abnormal sleep-breathing contributes to the development of awake respiratory failure and the place nocturnal ventilatory support plays in reversing this. We will also look at the potential application of this technique in a broadening range of clinical conditions.

BREATHING, SLEEP AND RESPIRATORY FAILURE

It has been recognized for many years that significant changes in breathing and ventilation can occur during sleep (Gastaut et al 1966). The contribution abnormal breathing, during sleep, can play in the development of awake hypercapnia is now more fully appreciated. Our understanding of what happens to breathing during sleep has been greatly enhanced by three major developments in technology:

- The routine use of accurate oximeters (Trask & Cree 1962), which have allowed the continuous monitoring of arterial oxygenation over prolonged periods of time.

- The development of a comfortable and acceptable nasal mask interface (Sullivan et al 1981) has provided a simple yet effective means by which abnormalities of breathing can be reversed.

- The development of portable ventilatory support systems suitable for home use.

These developments made it possible to continuously monitor changes in breathing associated with sleep state and to provide patients with a treatment intervention that is both effective and acceptable on a long-term basis.

Changes in breathing during sleep

Sleep is associated with a number of normal physiological events that have little effect on individuals with normal respiratory drive and mechanics. However, in patients with a range of respiratory abnormalities, sleep can lead to worsening respiratory function and gas exchange.

The awake state itself is associated with an additional stimulus to breathe, over and above that determined by the metabolic control system. This is known as the wakefulness drive to breathe and is lost with the onset of sleep. General postural muscle tone is also reduced at sleep onset, resulting in increases in upper airway resistance and reductions in ventilatory drive. At the same time, ventilatory responses to both hypoxia and hypercapnia are reduced so that there is an attenuated response to changes in gas exchange compared with wakefulness. As a result, a small fall in ventilation occurs with sleep in the range of 10–15% (Douglas et al 1982).

Although reduced, ventilation during non-rapid eye movement (NREM) sleep is steady, particularly during periods of slow-wave sleep. However, even in normal subjects there is substantial variation in breathing during rapid eye movement (REM) sleep, most pronounced during periods of phasic eye movements. During these episodes, alveolar ventilation may fall by as much as 40% (Douglas et al 1982). REM sleep is also associated with alterations in respiratory control, caused by descending inhibition of alpha and gamma motor neurons. This produces hypotonia of postural muscles, including the intercostal and accessory respiratory muscles and a reduction in the rib cage contribution to ventilation. As a result, ventilation during REM sleep becomes heavily reliant on diaphragmatic activity.

In patients with severely compromised lung function or significant inspiratory muscle weakness, recruitment of other inspiratory and accessory muscles, including the abdominals, may occur to augment breathing. By this compensatory mechanism, individuals are usually able to maintain adequate ventilation during wakefulness and NREM sleep for prolonged periods. In those with significant lung disease, recruitment of the intercostal muscles occurs not only to augment ventilation but to maintain end-expiratory lung volume, thereby preventing small airway closure. With the transition into REM sleep, this postural muscle activity will be lost, resulting in a reduction in minute ventilation, worsening ventilation–perfusion relationships and a deterioration in gas exchange. Falls in saturation will be more severe in those patients with awake saturation values already near the steep portion of the oxyhaemoglobin dissociation curve. The degree of abnormal breathing which then occurs will depend upon the patient's arousal response. Arousal causes a change in state from sleep to transient wakefulness, permitting the re-emergence of accessory muscle activity and restoration of ventilation, albeit briefly. In this way, arousal acts as a defensive mechanism, limiting the degree of gas exchange abnormality that is permitted to occur. However, this response also leads to sleep fragmentation, which in itself can alter respiratory drive and arousal thresholds, so that eventually more extreme blood gas derangement must occur before the arousal response is activated.

The role of sleep in the development of awake hypercapnic respiratory failure

It is now well recognized that disturbed breathing first becomes apparent in REM sleep (Bye et al 1990). However, as REM sleep takes up only a relatively small proportion of total sleep time, patients with REM

11

hypoventilation, even if severe, may remain clinically stable for months or even years before significant daytime hypercapnia becomes apparent. Initially, ventilation and sleep between periods of REM hypoventilation are usually normal, often through the recruitment of accessory respiratory muscles. In addition, the arousal mechanism operates to defend ventilation by limiting the amount of time spent in REM sleep and therefore the degree of abnormal gas exchange that occurs. Characteristically, awake blood gases remain normal during this initial stage.

Progression of abnormal breathing into NREM sleep heralds the second stage in the evolution of sleep-induced respiratory failure (Piper & Sullivan 1994a). Mechanisms responsible for this progression include not only a deterioration of the underlying disease itself but also the appearance of other factors that may load breathing such as ageing, weight gain, upper airway dysfunction or the development of an intercurrent illness such as a chest infection. Sleep fragmentation from abnormal breathing events has the capacity to further alter respiratory control and depress arousal. These factors allow more severe sleep-disordered breathing to occur, with less arousal between events. This begins a vicious cycle whereby resetting the sensitivity of the ventilatory control system occurs so that higher levels of carbon dioxide and lower levels of oxygen are tolerated without stimulating a change in respiration, not only asleep but during wakefulness as well. During this stage, daytime CO_2 retention becomes apparent (Fig. 11.1).

The final stage in the development of sleep-induced hypercapnia is characterized by unstable respiratory failure both awake and asleep. During this stage, changes in blood gases during sleep are extreme and sleep architecture may be profoundly disturbed. By this stage, the clinical condition of the patient may deteriorate considerably, which can be mistaken for a progression of the underlying disease process. It is crucial that clinicians recognize patients with nocturnal hypoventilation early and treat appropriately, in order to prevent the complications associated with an acute respiratory crisis (Box 11.1).

NON-INVASIVE VENTILATION

Rationale and methods

Non-invasive ventilation (NIV) is a technique whereby positive pressure is applied to the airways and lungs without the need for an endotracheal or tracheostomy tube. Whether used for the management of acute or chronic conditions, during awake or sleep states, the aim of this therapy is the same: to improve gas exchange

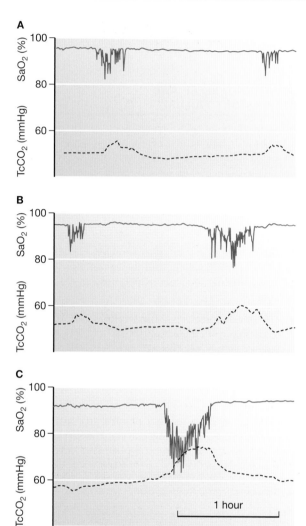

Figure 11.1   Serial recordings of oxygen saturation (SaO_2) (solid green line) and transcutaneous carbon dioxide ($TcCO_2$) (dotted line) from a patient with Duchenne muscular dystrophy showing progressive nocturnal respiratory failure. **(A)** Mild sleep-disordered breathing, with modest falls in SaO_2. **(B)** Eight months later more substantial oxygen desaturation was apparent during REM sleep, with rises in carbon dioxide. **(C)** Severe REM desaturation occurs, with failure of SaO_2 to return to baseline values between periods of abnormal breathing. This was accompanied by large rises in CO_2. Over the same period, awake CO_2 had risen from 40 to 45 mmHg (5.3 to 6.0 kPa), with no change in inspiratory muscle pressures.

by assisting inspiratory efforts and reducing the work of breathing.

In patients presenting with acute respiratory failure there is a deterioration in gas exchange accompanied by changes in pulmonary mechanics with increased

Box 11.1 Common conditions where nocturnal hypercapnic respiratory failure is likely to occur

Neuromuscular	Myopathies ■ Duchenne muscular dystrophy ■ Acid maltase deficiency Neuropathies ■ Poliomyelitis ■ Motor neurone disease ■ Bilateral phrenic nerve palsy
Chest wall	Kyphoscoliosis Thoracoplasty Obesity hypoventilation syndrome
Impaired ventilatory control	Brainstem injury Primary alveolar hypoventilation
Airway obstruction	Severe obstructive sleep apnoea
Lung disease	Chronic obstructive pulmonary disease Cystic fibrosis Bronchiectasis

respiratory loads. As a consequence a shallow, rapid breathing pattern develops with shortening of inspiratory time and reductions in tidal volume. Non-invasive ventilatory support in this setting aims to augment the patient's tidal volume while reducing the amount of effort or work performed. In addition, maintaining a low level of positive pressure during expiration can subsequently reduce inspiratory effort by counterbalancing intrinsic PEEP (the end-expiratory recoil pressure of the respiratory system due to incomplete expiration). The improved breathing pattern with NIV should improve alveolar ventilation while preventing respiratory muscle fatigue. Ventilators that provide a range of settings and features can be desirable in the acute situation in order to ensure the machine has the capability of addressing the individual's breathing needs.

The mechanism by which NIV improves awake spontaneous breathing in patients with chronic respiratory failure is a little less clear. Three possible hypotheses have been put forward (Hill 1993). The first relates to chronic muscle fatigue and proposes that the use of NIV permits intermittent rest of fatigued muscles, restoring function. The second hypothesis proposes that NIV increases lung volumes and compliance. Finally, the respiratory centre sensitivity to CO_2 may be blunted during the development of chronic respiratory failure. Non-invasive ventilation, by preventing hypoventilation during sleep, may work by restoring ventilatory

sensitivity to carbon dioxide and hence improve awake breathing. In a study designed to determine the relative importance of each of these mechanisms, Nickol et al (2005) found there was no change in measures of inspiratory muscle strength, lung function or respiratory system compliance with the commencement of NIV in patients with restrictive thoracic disease despite significant improvements in awake blood gases. However, they did find an increase in ventilatory sensitivity to CO_2 supporting this as a principle mechanism for the improvements in breathing seen in patients with chronic respiratory failure who had been started on NIV.

Ventilator systems

Primarily two types of ventilator systems are available for mask ventilation: volume-preset and pressure-preset devices. Each type of support has its own advantages and limitations. A successful outcome using mask ventilation will depend upon the clinician's understanding of the underlying pathological processes that have contributed to the patient's respiratory deterioration, and choosing a machine and mode of ventilatory support which best meet the respiratory needs of the patient.

Volume-preset machines such as the PLV®-102 (Respironics, Inc, Murrysville, PA, USA), the PV501 (Breas™, Molnycke, Sweden) or the BromptonPAC (PneuPAC Ltd, Luton, Beds, UK) operate as time-cycled flow generators and deliver a fixed tidal volume irrespective of the airway pressure generated, provided that leaks from the system are minimized. Pressure-preset systems include bilevel positive pressure devices, the most widely recognized being the BiPAP® machines (Respironics, Inc, Murrysville, PA, USA). Other pressure-preset devices include the Vivo30® (Breas™, Molnycke, Sweden), VS Integra™ (ResMed, Bella Vista, NSW, Australia), and the VPAP™ III device (ResMed, Bella Vista, NSW, Australia) (Fig 11.2A). With these devices, tidal volume will vary according to the preset inspiratory pressure, the inspiratory–expiratory pressure difference and the chest wall and lung compliance of the patient. Bilevel devices are reported to compensate better for mild to moderate leaks than volume-preset devices (Mehta et al 2001). However, leaks are common during mask ventilation, particularly during sleep, and this may adversely affect the quality of ventilation and sleep architecture even with bilevel positive pressure devices (Piper & Willson 1996, Teschler et al 1999).

In studies comparing the efficacy of these two systems, little difference has been found either in acute (Girault et al 1997) or chronic respiratory failure (Tuggey & Elliott 2005), although many patients find pressure preset devices easier to tolerate. Poor tolerance to

11

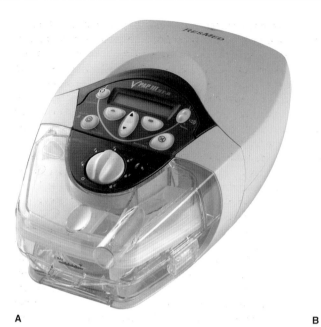

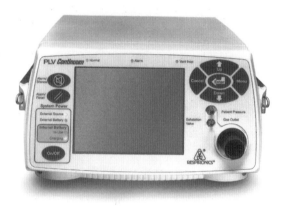

A **B**

Figure 11.2 Examples of two types of ventilatory support systems: **(A)** VPAP™ III ST-A (ResMed), a bilevel positive pressure device; **(B)** PLV® Continuum™ ventilator able to deliver both volume and pressure ventilation. (Image **A** used with the permission of ResMed Limited, North Ryde, Australia; image **B** used with permission of Respironics, Inc, Murrysville, PA, USA)

volume-preset devices may be related to an increase in airway resistance causing an elevation of inspiratory pressure in the mask, which may be uncomfortable or may cause leaks, thus limiting the effectiveness of ventilation. On the other hand, in patients with low chest wall compliance, higher airway pressures may be needed to maintain optimal ventilation. In these patients, volume-preset ventilators can prove more reliable and effective in delivering a stable tidal volume despite changing chest wall mechanics or airway resistance. A change to a volume-preset device should always be considered if hypoventilation persists on bilevel ventilatory support (Schonhofer et al 1997).

Criteria for choosing mode of ventilatory support

A number of criteria need to be considered when choosing a machine and mode of ventilatory support. These include:

- the clinical condition of the patient on presentation
- the primary diagnosis
- the patient's respiratory drive
- the compliance of the lungs and chest wall
- the degree of synchronization that can be achieved between the patient and the device
- the familiarity of the staff with the equipment.

Sleep study data are useful in patients requiring long-term ventilation in identifying any degree of upper airway dysfunction that may be present as well as determining the patient's respiratory drive during sleep. Understanding the features and limitations of the various machines available and the modes of ventilatory support in which they can operate will assist in selecting the appropriate system to meet the patient's needs. A recent development is the availability of portable ventilators that are able to deliver both pressure and volume ventilation, allowing flexibility with regard to changing the mode of ventilatory support with changes in the patient's condition (e.g. PLV® Continuum™ (Fig. 11.2B), Respironics, Inc, Murrysville, PA, USA; PV403, Breas™, Molnycke, Sweden; VS Ultra™, ResMed, Bella Vista, NSW, Australia).

Settings

The mode of support needs to be set so that the breaths delivered will be either machine-triggered or patient-triggered. With bilevel devices, a spontaneous mode of support is available, where the machine cycles into inspiration in response to the patient's spontaneous inspiratory effort. The volume-preset and a number of the bilevel devices can also be set to deliver a preset respiratory rate should the patient fail to trigger the device. Titration of the inspiratory positive airway pressure (IPAP) for a patient on a bilevel device or the tidal volume for a patient using a volume-preset device is made on the basis of patient tolerance and the effect such a setting has on ventilation and gas exchange. However, when setting pressures or volumes it should be borne in mind that excessively high inspiratory pressures will promote leakage of air from the mouth, reducing the effectiveness of ventilatory support. Excessive hyperventilation can also occur, which may induce upper airway obstruction and the appearance of central apnoea. The use of expiratory positive airway pressure (EPAP) may be advantageous in a number of clinical conditions, including controlling upper airway closure, recruiting collapsed alveoli or to overcome intrinsic end-expiratory pressure. Where inspiratory time or flow can be set, this will be based on the patient's own respiratory pattern, taking into account the effect short inspiratory times can have on gas exchange.

In patients where the compliance of the alveoli is heterogeneous, delivered tidal volume may be directed towards those alveoli with short filling times, producing overdistension of already inflated units and therefore not contributing to improved gas exchange. Prolonging the inspiratory time allows the recruitment of alveoli with slower filling times, so that increased ventilation can contribute to improved gas exchange.

Timing of intervention

There is extensive evidence to support the use of NIV as first-line therapy in patients with acute exacerbations of COPD (Lightowler et al 2003). However, the technique is not universally successful, with a proportion of patients continuing to deteriorate despite appropriate support. The likelihood of failure increases as acidosis worsens (Ambrosino et al 1995, Plant et al 2001). Instituting NIV in mild exacerbations has not been shown to be beneficial and may be poorly tolerated (Keenan et al 2003). Therefore, identifying and intervening during this window of therapeutic opportunity is important to achieve the best clinical outcomes with NIV. Generally speaking, patients with a pH in the range of 7.25–7.35 are the best candidates for the procedure.

Determining when to start NIV in patients with chronic respiratory failure is less clear cut. Most would agree that the presence of daytime hypercapnia ($PaCO_2$ >6 kPa (45 mmHg)) or daytime symptoms of nocturnal hypoventilation such as daytime sleepiness, early

morning headaches, severe orthopnoea or alterations in cognitive function would be clear indications for assessment and appropriate intervention. However, for many patients the onset of nocturnal respiratory failure occurs over an extended period of time, in some cases even years. With such an insidious onset, the signs and symptoms of chronic hypoventilation may be overlooked or incorrectly attributed to the ongoing progression of the primary disease process.

One study looked at the 'preventative' use of NIV in patients with Duchenne muscular dystrophy (DMD), free of daytime respiratory failure (Raphael et al 1994). No benefit was found from early intervention with this technique, with the treated group showing a similar rate of deterioration in blood gases and pulmonary function as the control group. However, nocturnal monitoring was not performed either at baseline or during therapy in these patients. A more recent study looking at patients with neuromuscular disease, including patients with DMD, found that those with nocturnal hypoventilation despite daytime normocapnia were likely to deteriorate and develop daytime respiratory failure and/or progressive symptoms within 2 years if NIV was not introduced (Ward et al 2005). This suggests that the timing of NIV intervention is important, with identification of those patients at risk of developing nocturnal hypoventilation, monitoring of nocturnal gas exchange in these individuals and intervention with NIV before the development of awake respiratory failure ensues. In this way, the chances of the patient presenting with an acute respiratory crisis may be minimized.

11

INDICATIONS FOR NON-INVASIVE VENTILATION IN CHRONIC RESPIRATORY FAILURE

Assessment of chronic hypoventilation

Although a number of investigators have tried to use daytime pulmonary function tests as a predictor of the degree of abnormal breathing occurring during sleep, no strong correlation has been found (Bye et al 1990). However, it has been shown that a low vital capacity, a significant fall in vital capacity from erect to supine or a maximum inspiratory pressure of less than 30 cmH$_2$O are all indicators that sleep-disordered breathing and hypoventilation may be present (Bye et al 1990, Ragette et al 2002). Each of these tests can be easily carried out at the bedside as part of the overall assessment of a patient presenting in respiratory failure. Strong use of the accessory respiratory muscles at rest, including the sternomastoid and the abdominal muscles, should raise the possibility that respiratory function may worsen during sleep.

In general, if there is awake hypercapnia then there will be substantial sleep-linked worsening of respiratory failure (Piper & Sullivan 1994a), although the converse does not necessarily hold true. Many subjects with awake CO_2 within the normal range will have significant sleep-linked respiratory failure. The failure of clinicians to recognize this and intervene appropriately puts a patient at risk of developing daytime respiratory failure within the following 12–24 months (Ward et al 2005).

The limitations of daytime indices as predictors of nocturnal hypoventilation mean that more detailed sleep investigations may be required in order to accurately assess the severity and nature of the breathing disorder. While hypoventilation and desaturation are likely to occur predominantly in REM sleep, upper airway obstruction may also be present and needs to be identified and appropriately managed in order for NIV to be maximally effective. In patients with suspected nocturnal hypoventilation, monitoring of carbon dioxide is important looking at evening to morning changes in arterial values or continuous monitoring with transcutaneous measures (Ward et al 2005). Regardless of the investigations used, a high index of suspicion in patients with diagnoses known to be associated with nocturnal hypoventilation is warranted. In these individuals, baseline and serial testing of respiratory function should be performed with the view to identifying any deterioration early so that more specific investigation can be undertaken.

Conditions

Kyphoscoliosis

The final stages of severe kyphoscoliosis have been characterized by progressive respiratory failure associated with severe nocturnal hypoventilation (Ellis et al 1988). REM hypoventilation is probably caused by a combination of a very high work of breathing due to low chest wall compliance for a diaphragm that is at a significant mechanical disadvantage. In some patients sleep-disordered breathing is also complicated by upper airway obstruction. Mask ventilation is particularly suitable for these patients as other methods of assisted ventilation are very difficult. Tracheostomy can be problematic because of the loss of the extrathoracic trachea and the fitting of a cuirass is made exceptionally difficult by the chest wall deformity. Non-invasive ventilation can be readily achieved with a mask in this group despite the stiffness of the chest wall (Ellis et al 1988).

Cystic fibrosis

Although low-flow oxygen therapy has been the mainstay of treatment for patients with cystic fibrosis (CF) who develop respiratory failure, several reports have shown that, at least acutely during sleep, oxygen therapy can promote CO_2 retention (Gozal 1997, Milross et al 2001). The beneficial effects of nocturnal non-invasive ventilation for patients with end-stage CF are recognized. Non-invasive ventilation has been shown to be of value during periods of acute deterioration, where marked pulmonary deterioration occurs despite maximum conventional therapy (Piper et al 1992). Use of mask ventilatory support in this setting can correct hypoxaemia without inducing additional CO_2 retention. In addition, this technique may also be used to stabilize the patient in the short term while donor organs become available (Hodson et al 1991) or on a longer-term basis, allowing the patient to return home (Piper et al 1992). Although in initial reports volume preset machines were used, bilevel pressure devices are now being increasingly used with similar outcomes (Gozal 1997, Milross et al 2001).

Some patients report improved sputum clearance after initiation of nasal ventilatory support, possibly related to better tolerance of longer chest physiotherapy sessions (Piper et al 1992). Improved lung expansion and chest wall excursion while on the machine may also play a part. Studies have shown that use of nasal ventilatory support during chest physiotherapy was able to ameliorate adverse effects such as reduced respiratory muscle performance and oxygen desaturation (Fauroux et al 1999, Holland et al 2003).

Duchenne muscular dystrophy

Ventilatory support is often reluctantly prescribed for patients with progressive neuromuscular disease, owing to a perceived lack of quality of life for these patients. However, health professionals often underestimate quality of life in such patients. The use of long-term non-invasive ventilation has been shown to stabilize pulmonary function and prolong life expectancy while improving quality of life in patients with Duchenne muscular dystrophy (DMD) and awake hypercapnia (Simonds et al 1998). Non-invasive ventilation has also been initiated early in this disorder in an attempt to prevent the decline in lung function that occurs with increasing respiratory muscle weakness. However, no benefits from such a strategy could be identified (Raphael et al 1994). Therefore, NIV is an effective long-term therapy in this group of patients once nocturnal hypoventilation occurs, but may not have a prophylactic role.

Chronic obstructive pulmonary disease

Nocturnal nasal ventilation has been used effectively in selected patients with stable chronic obstructive pulmonary disease (COPD). However, this form of therapy is not tolerated as well as in other diagnostic groups and longer-term outcomes are not as favourable as in patients with neuromuscular and chest wall disorders (Simonds & Elliott 1995). Those patients most likely to benefit from nocturnal ventilatory support appear to be those with significant daytime hypercapnia, who have symptomatic sleep problems and in whom nocturnal hypercapnia can be successfully reduced by overnight ventilation. Meecham Jones et al (1995) reported a randomized crossover study of nasal pressure support ventilation plus oxygen therapy compared with domiciliary oxygen therapy alone in 18 hypercapnic patients with COPD. Improvements in daytime arterial blood gas tensions, overnight transcutaneous carbon dioxide ($TcCO_2$), total sleep time and sleep efficiency were seen during non-invasive ventilation and oxygen therapy compared with oxygen therapy alone, suggesting that control of hypoventilation with non-invasive ventilation can be achieved. Importantly, these authors found that those who showed the greatest reduction in nocturnal hypercapnia with ventilation were likely to gain the greatest benefit from the treatment. However, a number of other randomized trials in this population have failed to find a clinically significant benefit of NIV (Casanova et al 2000, Clini et al 2002). These discrepant results may be due to patient selection or the way in which NIV was delivered and monitored. It would seem that patients with high daytime CO_2, with a higher likelihood of nocturnal hypoventilation, are more likely to respond to this therapy than patients with near normal awake CO_2 levels. In addition, data from Meecham Jones et al (1995) as well as uncontrolled trials (Windisch et al 2005) highlight the importance of using sufficiently high inspiratory pressures to control CO_2 during sleep in order to achieve improvements in daytime ventilation and symptoms.

Motor neuron disease

Respiratory insufficiency usually occurs as a late manifestation of this disorder, when global peripheral and respiratory muscle weakness has occurred. However, in a small number of patients, presentation with hypercapnia, severe orthopnoea and sleep fragmentation may be seen. Although nasal ventilatory support has been shown to be effective in relieving these symptoms in this group, its use also raises some ethical and clinical concerns that need to be discussed with the patient and their caregiver (Polkey et al 1999). There has been reluc-

tance to initiate such therapy for a condition that is known to be relatively rapidly progressive and where many will experience involvement of the bulbar muscles and swallowing difficulties (Meyer & Hill 1994). However, a recent randomized controlled trial has shown that NIV improves survival while maintaining and even improving quality of life in these patients (Bourke et al 2006). In those with severe bulbar impairment there was no survival benefit with NIV, but quality of life related to symptoms did improve.

Non-invasive ventilation appears to have a place as a management alternative in motivated patients with appropriate home supports, where established respiratory failure is present or where quality of life is impaired by sleep disruption or severe orthopnoea (Polkey et al 1999). However, before undertaking such therapy in this group, frank discussion with the patient and caregiver needs to occur. Potential benefits of NIV in palliating symptoms should be discussed as well as its limitations in the face of progressively worsening respiratory and general muscle strength and disability.

Obesity hypoventilation syndrome

Another group that responds rapidly and positively to non-invasive ventilation are those patients with obesity hypoventilation syndrome (Perez de Llano et al 2005, Piper & Sullivan 1994b). This syndrome is characterized by extreme obesity, excessive daytime sleepiness and severe derangement of awake blood gases. Patients frequently present grossly decompensated with right heart failure, lower limb oedema and hypercapnia. Use of non-invasive ventilatory support in these patients may result in improved awake blood gases and clinical condition within days of starting therapy, improving quality of life and daily function. The aim of therapy in these patients is to maintain upper airway stability while improving alveolar ventilation. Bilevel ventilatory support is usually required initially, particularly in those with severely deranged nocturnal and awake blood gases. However, after a short period of nocturnal ventilatory support, a proportion of patients can be transferred to the more simple CPAP therapy for longer-term domiciliary use (Perez de Llano et al 2005, Piper & Sullivan 1994b).

INDICATIONS FOR NON-INVASIVE VENTILATION IN ACUTE RESPIRATORY FAILURE

In order to reduce the problems associated with endotracheal intubation and ventilation, an increasing number of centres are now using non-invasive ventila-

11

tion as a treatment alternative for patients with acute respiratory failure. It avoids the complications of endotracheal intubation, is more comfortable for the patient, allowing speech and swallowing, and avoids the need for sedation and immobilization. Treatment does not have to be instituted in the intensive care or emergency department environment and is increasingly started on general medical or surgical wards (Bott et al 1993, Lightowler et al 2003, Piper & Willson 1996, Plant et al 2000).

Assessment of acute respiratory failure

Appropriate patient selection is essential for a successful treatment outcome. Non-invasive ventilation should be seen as a therapy to prevent the need for intubation rather than an alternative to it. Therefore, when undertaking this therapy it is important to be able to identify those patients who are unlikely to respond well, in order that a delay in mandatory intubation does not occur (Box 11.2). The ideal patient should be cooperative enough to tolerate a mask and to follow simple instructions. A successful outcome depends to a large degree on the ability to rapidly correct acidosis, decrease CO_2 and reduce respiratory rate (Lightowler et al 2003). This in turn will be influenced by the ability of the patient and the therapist to minimize mouth/mask leaks and to coordinate breathing with the ventilator. A common reason for failure of this therapy is the inability of the patient to effectively remove secretions. Identification of those patients with secretion retention and prompt intervention by the physiotherapist to aid in clearing the airways can be pivotal in increasing the likelihood of therapy being successful. However, if hypercapnia and acidosis fail to improve within the first few hours of treatment, longer-term success is unlikely (Ambrosino et al 1995, Anton et al 2000, Lightowler et al 2003).

In patients who are hypoxaemic but retain carbon dioxide, the use of non-invasive ventilation permits higher levels of inspired oxygen to be introduced without unduly worsening hypercapnia. Under these circumstances, the use of non-invasive ventilation supports patients until their acute deterioration can be reversed (Conway et al 1993).

Conditions

Chronic obstructive pulmonary disease

The majority of studies reported to date have involved patients with chronic obstructive pulmonary disease (COPD) during an acute exacerbation. Evidence from a number of randomized trials have shown that NIV is

---

> **Box 11.2   Characteristics of patients with acute respiratory failure unlikely to do well on non-invasive ventilation**
>
> - Agitation, encephalopathic, uncooperative
> - Severe illness, including extreme acidosis (pH <7.2)
> - Presence of excessive secretions or pneumonia
> - Multiple organ failure
> - Haemodynamic instability
> - Inability to maintain a lip seal
> - Inability to protect the airway
> - Overt respiratory failure requiring immediate intubation
>
> (Ambrosino et al 1995, Brochard et al 1995, Kramer et al 1995)

clearly beneficial, with significant reductions in mortality, endotracheal intubation, complication rates and shorter length of hospital stay compared with standard medical therapy (Lightowler et al 2003). It appears that the type of ventilator (volume preset or bilevel pressure support) or the type of interface chosen (nose or full face mask) is not pivotal in determining the success of treatment. However, results will be influenced by the patient's tolerance and adaptation to the machine and some patients may find the bilevel pressure support devices easier to adapt to. Very dyspnoeic patients tend to be mouth breathers and where it is not possible for the patient to maintain lip closure, a full facemask needs to be used to ensure machine–patient synchronization and delivery of an effective tidal volume. The technique has been used with equal success both in high dependency (Brochard et al 1995) and general ward situations (Bott et al 1993, Plant et al 2000). However, when considering location of care, the degree of acidosis, the therapeutic goals of NIV for the individual and the experience and level of staffing must be taken into account. While NIV may be a highly effective technique in patients with COPD, failure of therapy still occurs and arrangements for escalation of management or institution of a more palliative treatment approach need to made at the time NIV is first initiated (British Thoracic Society 2002).

Pulmonary oedema

Cardiogenic pulmonary oedema has also been shown to respond well to mask positive pressure therapy, either in the form of continuous positive airway pressure

(CPAP) or bilevel ventilatory support (Masip et al 2005, Nava et al 2003, Peter et al 2006). Both therapies have been shown to reduce the need for intubation and reduce mortality compared to standard medical care, including oxygen supplementation, although the evidence for CPAP is stronger (Masip et al 2005, Peter et al 2006). A recent meta-analysis suggested a trend towards a higher occurrence of new cases of myocardial infarction with NIV compared with CPAP (Peter et al 2006). Therefore, current guidelines suggest CPAP should be used as first-line therapy in patients presenting with acute pulmonary oedema (British Thoracic Society 2002). Bilevel ventilatory support should be reserved for those in whom CPAP is unsuccessful (British Thoracic Society 2002, Peter et al 2006), or for the subgroup of patients who are hypercapnic (Nava et al 2003).

Hypoxaemic respiratory failure

Although the majority of initial work with NIV has been carried out in patients with hypercapnic respiratory failure, a number of recent randomized controlled trials have provided evidence that NIV can provide similar benefits in selected patients presenting with hypoxaemic respiratory failure (Antonelli et al 2000, Ferrer et al 2003), including those with community-acquired pneumonia (Confalonieri et al 1999). However, given the variability in pathophysiology leading to hypoxaemia, it is not surprising that the benefits of using NIV in patients with hypoxaemic respiratory failure have been mixed. Despite some promising preliminary results, the role of NIV in acute asthma remains controversial (Ram et al 2005) and requires further investigation. The current evidence suggests that NIV is most likely to be effective in patients with an underlying diagnosis of COPD (Confalonieri et al 1999) or in those who are immunosuppressed (Hilbert et al 2001). In patients developing acute respiratory failure following solid organ transplantation (Antonelli et al 2000) or after lung resection (Auriant et al 2001), use of NIV has been found to reduce the need for intubation and improve survival. However, as therapy failure is higher in patients with hypoxaemic respiratory failure treated with NIV compared to patients with hypercapnia (Delclaux et al 2000), treatment is best carried out and monitored in a high-dependency area rather than on a general ward.

Obesity hypoventilation syndrome

Although some patients with obesity hypoventilation syndrome (OHS) will present with stable chronic respiratory failure, the diagnosis is frequently overlooked until the patient presents with acute respiratory failure. Despite significant reductions in chest wall compliance

and, in most cases, increased upper airway loading secondary to the presence of upper airway obstruction, these patients can be effectively managed with NIV in the acute setting, avoiding the need for intubation and its subsequent complications (Perez de Llano et al 2005). Even patients with simple obesity are at risk of developing postoperative respiratory failure following major surgery. Many of these patients probably have pre-existing sleep-disordered breathing. The affects of anaesthesia and analgesia may worsen an already compromised upper airway, producing apnoea and its sequelae such as hypoxaemia and blood pressure fluctuations. In addition, diaphragm inhibition after upper abdominal surgery can exacerbate REM hypoventilation. These patients generally respond well and rapidly to positive pressure, improving gas exchange and pulmonary function.

'Do-not-intubate' patients

While NIV is generally applied with the aim of avoiding the need for intubation rather than a substitution for it, for patients in whom intubation and ICU is considered inappropriate or futile, NIV may be used as a ceiling therapy (British Thoracic Society 2002). However, when applied in this way, higher failure rates have to be expected, with data suggesting a hospital mortality of 37% in COPD patients, 39% in acute cardiogenic pulmonary oedema, 68% in non-COPD hypercapnic respiratory failure and 86% in hypoxaemic failure (Schettino et al 2005). If applying NIV in this situation, it is important to bear in mind that the therapy and monitoring take time to set up and treatment is not without some possible discomfort to the patient. These factors need to be considered carefully if thinking about using NIV in patients with a likely terminal condition.

PRACTICAL ISSUES IN THE APPLICATION OF NON-INVASIVE VENTILATION

Interfaces

Both nasal and full facemasks may be used to deliver ventilatory support (Figs 11.3A & B , 11.4) and advances in design of both types have meant a greater degree of comfort and choice for the patient. Evidence from the literature suggests that successful outcomes in acute respiratory failure can be achieved with either type of interface (Kwok et al 2003), although the full facemask is often preferred in the acute setting to better control mouth leaks and ensure the effective delivery of ventilatory support (Kwok et al 2003, Navalesi et al 2000). In a study looking at various interfaces in patients with

11

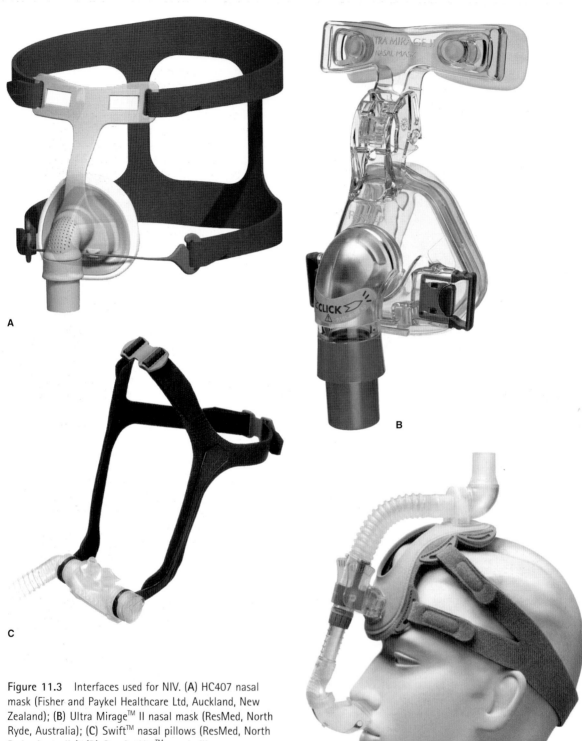

Figure 11.3 Interfaces used for NIV. (**A**) HC407 nasal mask (Fisher and Paykel Healthcare Ltd, Auckland, New Zealand); (**B**) Ultra Mirage™ II nasal mask (ResMed, North Ryde, Australia); (**C**) Swift™ nasal pillows (ResMed, North Ryde, Australia); (**D**) ComfortLite™ nasal pillows (Respironics, Inc, Murrysville, PA, USA). (Use of the Ultra Mirage™ II and Swift™ nasal pillow images made with the permission of ResMed Limited. Use of the ComfortLite™ image made with the permission of Respironics, Inc, Murrysville, PA, USA).

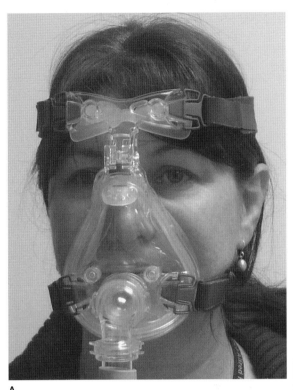
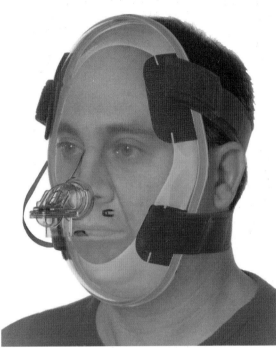

A   **B**

Figure 11.4   Examples of facemasks. (**A**) Ultra Mirage™ II full facemask (ResMed, North Ryde, Australia); (**B**) Total face-mask™. (Image used with the permission of Respironics, Inc, Murrysville, PA, USA.)

chronic hypercapnic respiratory failure, the nasal mask was the best tolerated although the oronasal and nasal plug interfaces were associated with significantly lower $PaCO_2$ levels (Navalesi et al 2000). Chinstraps may be useful in those cases where the patient prefers a nasal mask but where mouth leaks remain problematic (Fig. 11.5).

Often overlooked is the impact that mask design can have on the effectiveness of ventilatory support. Ventilators designed specifically for non-invasive applications generally operate using a single circuit with an expiratory port placed either within the mask itself or close to the mask at the end of the ventilator circuit. In a lung model, Schettino and colleagues (2003) demonstrated that the use of an oronasal mask with the exhalation port within the mask generated less CO_2 rebreathing than when the exhalation was placed in the ventilator circuit itself. In a later study, also using a modified lung model, Saatci and co-workers (2004) found that the use of facemasks with expiratory ports over the nasal bridge produced beneficial flow characteristics within the facemask and nasal cavity, resulting in a decrease in dead space. Expiratory ports placed at other sites such as at the cheeks or at the mask–circuit connection were not as effective. In addition, having some level of constant pressure throughout the expiratory phase was benefi-

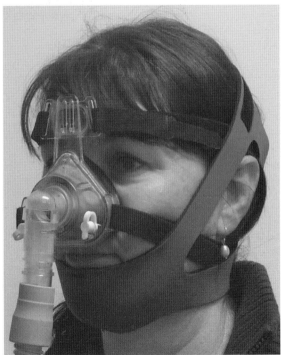

Figure 11.5   Nasal mask (ProfileLite™, Respironics, Inc, Murrysville, PA, USA) with chinstrap (Seatec Aquasuits, Australia).

cial in reducing the total dynamic dead space close to or even below physiological dead space. While these factors may not be of great clinical significance for most patients using NIV, in those with a borderline response to NIV, a change in mask to one with lower dynamic dead space or more favourable positioning of the expiratory ports may be the difference between success and failure of the technique.

Humidification, nebulization and oxygen therapy

In some patients, the high flows of cold dry air across the nasal passages can cause distressing nasal symptoms that may affect compliance with therapy, or increase nasal resistance (Richards et al 1996). Patients may report sneezing, nasal stuffiness or rhinorrhoea and erroneously believe they are developing a head cold. The use of an in-line humidifier such as an HC–150 (Fisher & Paykel Healthcare Ltd, Auckland, New Zealand), that can both warm and moisten the air, will largely improve these symptoms. Nasal symptoms frequently point to the presence of significant mouth leaks and this should be rectified, as leaks may reduce the effectiveness of ventilation. In patients with bronchial hypersecretion, such as cystic fibrosis or bronchiectasis, the addition of in-line humidification while using nasal ventilatory support may be useful in ensuring secretions are well hydrated. Patients with acute respiratory failure may become dehydrated and can also benefit from additional humidification of the airways to improve secretion clearance (Wood et al 2000). Heated humidifiers are preferable to heat moisture exchangers as the latter have been shown to increase dead space, resulting in a higher $PaCO_2$ despite significant increases in minute ventilation (Jaber et al 2002).

In patients who require ventilatory support on a continuous basis, nebulized bronchodilators and normal saline can be given during mask ventilatory support by adding the nebulizer chamber in-line close to the mask interface. Bilevel ventilatory support devices have been used to deliver β_2-agonists in the emergency department for patients with bronchospasm with a greater increase in peak expiratory flow rates compared with aerosols delivered by small-volume nebulizers alone (Pollack et al 1995). Fauroux and colleagues (2000) have shown that delivery of a nebulized aerosol by NIV enhances total lung aerosol deposition without increasing particle impaction in the proximal airways in patients with cystic fibrosis.

Generally, supplemental oxygen is not required in those patients with chronic respiratory failure from neuromuscular or chest wall disorders. However, in patients with parenchymal disease or those with acute respiratory failure, additional oxygen is likely to be needed and can be added either into the ventilator tubing or into a port on the mask itself. In some portable ventilator systems, it may be possible to dial up an exact FiO_2. However, most simple bilevel devices do not have this feature and the concentration of oxygen being delivered can only be estimated. Factors such as where along the circuit the oxygen is injected, the ventilator settings, the type of leak port and the oxygen flow will all influence the delivered oxygen concentration. In practice, the flow rate of oxygen used is determined by the oxygen saturation achieved in the patient.

Monitoring and initiating therapy

When commencing mask ventilation in the acute situation, careful monitoring is mandatory in order to gauge the effectiveness of ventilatory support. Continuous monitoring of oxygen saturation should be carried out for at least the first 24 hours, with transcutaneous carbon dioxide monitoring if available (British Thoracic Society 2002) (Fig. 11.6). Direct measurements of arterial blood gases should be taken before starting ventilation, then again at 1 hour, 6 hours, 24 hours and as needed thereafter depending on the patient's clinical condition. In addition, heart rate, respiratory rate and FiO_2 should be recorded hourly for the first few hours until the patient is stable. Blood pressure measurements may also be necessary, particularly if there is any question of the patient's haemodynamic stability. Monitoring in the acute situation is crucial to identify early any deterioration in the patient's clinical situation or to uncover any technical problems with NIV so that prompt and appropriate action can be taken.

Initial reports found that NIV in the acute care setting was a time-consuming procedure (Chevrolet et al 1991). While more recent experience suggests that this is not necessarily the case (Kramer et al 1995, Nava et al 1997), it does need to be appreciated that a time commitment from a member of the NIV team is necessary to initially coach the patient, check the efficacy of the technique and make adjustments to the machine settings. Nevertheless, it has been shown that the use of this technique can be transferred to the general ward environment without a reduction in efficacy (Plant et al 2000), while achieving significant cost savings (Plant et al 2003). This, however, requires adequate training and the opportunity for staff to develop sufficient skills and knowledge to perform the technique effectively and safely (British Thoracic Society 2002). Non-invasive ventilation in the acute setting is usually continued until blood gases have stabilized for several hours, then trial periods off the mask

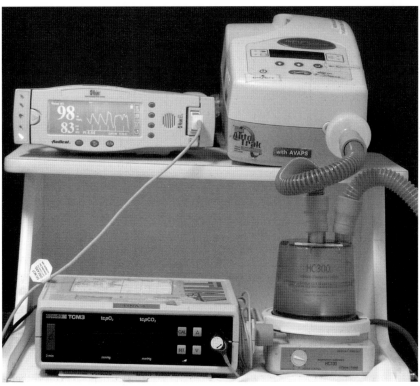

Figure 11.6 Monitoring set up for NIV trials. Oximeter and transcutaneous carbon dioxide monitor (lower left of picture) used to measure the physiological response to nasal ventilatory support. An active humidifier has been placed in the circuit between the bilevel ventilator and the patient (bottom right-hand corner).

11

are started. The patient's response to spontaneous ventilation is monitored and mask ventilatory support re-instituted if breathing deteriorates. In some cases, almost continuous use of the mask during the first day or two may be necessary. There is then a gradual withdrawal of awake ventilatory support to nocturnal use only. Prior to hospital discharge, investigation into the need for domiciliary therapy should be undertaken.

In patients with chronic respiratory failure, acclimatization to the mask and machine can be carried out during the day, with monitoring of oxygen saturation and preferably CO_2, either end-tidal or transcutaneous. Low pressures, commonly IPAP 9–10 cmH$_2$O and EPAP 4 cmH$_2$O, are trialled initially, with increases in the inspiratory pressure based on patient tolerance and the impact on saturation (Box 11.3). Once the patient has a broad understanding of the sensations to expect when using mask ventilation, adjustments to other settings, such as pressurization times or inspiratory trigger levels, can be undertaken to improve comfort and synchronization.

Frequently the patient will fall asleep during these initial trials and problems such as mouth leaks or the development of upper airway obstruction may be identified at this time, and alterations to machine settings made. Once the patient is able to sleep for a number of hours on the machine, a sleep study or nocturnal respiratory monitoring should be performed. Although some centres base machine settings on ventilation achieved during wakefulness, such settings may not be adequate during sleep for patients with chronic respiratory failure. This may relate to changes in the behaviour of the glottis, mouth leaks, alteration in respiratory drive or compliance of the respiratory system associated with changes in sleep state. Depending on the monitoring system used, a number of respiratory variables can be recorded, including mask pressure, leak, oxygen saturation, chest wall motion, diaphragmatic and other respiratory muscle electromyograms or inspiratory/expiratory tidal volumes. This information is useful in determining the efficacy of ventilatory support and in troubleshooting. If ventilation is not being adequately supported,

---

Box 11.3 Steps in initiating NIV therapy for home ventilatory support

- Introduce the patient slowly to the equipment and all its parts
- Ensure the mask fits comfortably and that the patient can experience the mask on their face without the ventilator connected
- Allow the patient the opportunity to feel the operation of the machine through the mask on their hand or cheek before applying it over their nose or mouth
- Allow the patient the opportunity to practise breathing with the ventilator, either holding the mask in place or allowing them to hold it in place before applying the straps
- Adjust settings initially for comfort and establish whether the patient can relax comfortably in a sleeping posture
- Provide opportunities for the patient to feed back any discomfort or uncertainty with regard to the use of the equipment
- Assess and adjust the performance of the ventilator during an afternoon nap to optimize gas exchange and patient comfort
- Progress to an overnight study, continuing to monitor and optimize gas exchange and sleep quality

---

a change in the mode or type of ventilator can be made.

Studies have shown that NIV will be effective in improving arterial blood gases and offloading the inspiratory muscles irrespective of whether settings are determined on the basis of the patient's comfort and tolerance or by invasive monitoring of respiratory mechanics (Fanfulla et al 2005, Vitacca et al 2000).

Adverse effects

A number of complications and adverse effects can arise during attempts to establish patients on non-invasive ventilation. Mouth leaks during the inspiratory phase of the ventilator cycle are probably the most common problem. This leak can reduce effective ventilation and may only be obvious during certain sleep stages. Leaks may be seen in the presence of upper airway obstruction, if asynchrony between the patient and the ventilator develops or if the lips and palate fail to provide a seal. If the leak is significant it can usually be remedied by the use of a chinstrap which should cradle the chin

and hold the lower jaw up (Fig. 11.5). The chinstrap is designed to have elastic sections on the sides so that patients can still move their jaw comfortably and call out and breathe should their nose become blocked or the ventilator fail. Other solutions for this problem include repositioning of the neck, taping the lips, mouth guards and full facemasks. Full facemasks are usually preferred once the patient's confidence has been established. The presence of leaks will not only reduce the degree of effective ventilation reaching the lungs but also may cause sleep fragmentation (Teschler et al 1999). Upper airway obstruction can occur particularly if the cycling pressure is allowed to drop below the closing pressure of the upper airway. It is very difficult to establish effective ventilation when this occurs, although it can, in some very mild cases, be reduced by positioning the patient's head so that the neck is slightly more extended. Sometimes a chinstrap alone is effective in lifting the jaw and thereby opening the upper airway. An increase in end-expiratory pressure usually ensures adequate ventilation.

Mask leaks commonly occur on either side of the bridge of the nose and can cause significant irritation to the eyes. If the leak is small it can be compensated for by the machine and this is preferable to pulling the mask too tightly onto the face. Patients usually learn to eliminate the leaks by repositioning the mask or by adjusting the strap alignment. Elastic straps of the head harnesses usually need regular replacement to ensure effective mask pressures. Other solutions include custom-built masks and a change in sleeping posture.

Mask pressure can cause pressure sores or pressure marks on the bridge of the nose or across the top lip in particular. These are best prevented by careful selection of mask for size and skin sensitivity. The areas respond well to standard pressure care including gentle massage, being left clean, dry and open and getting a regular amount of sunshine. The bridge of the nose often becomes thick and tough with time, although some people have recurring problems. For these patients the bridge of the nose can be protected with special pressure-absorbing materials that are commonly used with prostheses. Alternatively the patient may need to use a mouthpiece or nasal pillows (e.g. Swift™, ResMed, North Ryde, Australia; ComfortLite™, Respironics, Inc, Murrysville, PA, USA) (Fig. 11.3C & D) which fit securely into the nares without pressure on the nasal bridge, permitting pressure areas to heal. Head harness or strap pressure can cause abrasions over the back of the neck or over the ears. This can be simply relieved by re-designing the head harness to realign the straps or to include cotton wadding or a pad over the tender parts. If patients require NIV for extended periods of time, alternating between two types of interface such as a nasal mask and mouthpiece can help avoid sustained pressure on the skin.

Abdominal distension can be caused by air in the stomach, particularly when high cycling pressures are required for effective ventilation. This problem is less frequent now but would be more likely with volume-cycled ventilators. It appears that air can track through the stomach to the bowel and cause considerable discomfort. Every effort should be made to lower the cycling pressure without compromising effective ventilation. Some patients find relief from lying on their left side at night, some from having an empty stomach and others resort to medications including charcoal and acidophilus tablets. Pulmonary barotrauma is another potential but rarely encountered complication of positive pressure therapy. In some disorders managed by NIV, such as cystic fibrosis and COPD, subpleural cysts may be present, increasing the possibility of rupture due to or coincident with the use of positive pressure therapy. Patients with Duchenne muscular dystrophy have also been reported to have an increased risk of spontaneous pneumothorax. Although the risk is small it is potentially life threatening for a patient with limited respiratory reserve. Clinicians and patients should be aware of the potential for this occurring, with prompt investigation of any sudden shortness of breath and chest pain the patient experiences (Simonds 2004).

Home management

Once the patient is tolerating the machine during sleep and ventilator settings are finalized, patients should be encouraged to manage the equipment themselves and solve any problems that may arise prior to home discharge. Alternatively, if individuals remain dependent on some assistance the home carers should be brought in for at least part of the night to develop skills in setting up and troubleshooting.

Most people adapt well to ongoing ventilatory support in the home. However, acceptance of therapy may differ depending on the underlying pathology, the patient's response to therapy and relief of symptoms. Initial experience with mask ventilation may also influence outcome. A number of hospitals start ventilation on an inpatient basis to provide the patient with maximum support while minimizing problems (Meecham Jones et al 1995, Piper & Willson 1996).

It is important to provide full information to patients and families at the time of considering ongoing ventilation to ensure that an informed choice is made, especially in patients with progressive disorders. Some patients may need time to adapt to the idea of assisted ventilation, and will initially reject ongoing therapy.

Others may find it beyond their resources and capabilities to acquire and manage the technology or may fear it will weaken their muscles further, causing them to become ventilator-dependent. Each of these beliefs needs to be explored and discussed without judgement. They can be resolved in a number of ways. Patients need to be allowed to make their own choice and when the symptoms of respiratory failure or sleep deprivation become severe enough they may then seek relief and ask to try therapy again. Alternatively patients can be counselled, often with the help of other patients, that the benefits outweigh any real or perceived detriments. For most patients, compliance is usually dependent on relief of symptoms, and once they are sleeping on the ventilator overnight with control of blood gases, the improvement in daytime function often sustains continuing use of ventilation.

Ongoing review of the patient once discharged home on ventilatory support is essential to ensure therapy remains effective and appropriate. This is especially important for patients with progressive disorders and for children, as their circumstances and needs will change with time. Monitoring of basic lung function such as spirometry and arterial blood gases can identify any deterioration in the patient's condition and signal the need for more extensive investigation. In many of the newer home ventilators, objective compliance with therapy can be monitored using data stored within the device itself. This is important when trying to determine whether return of symptoms or deterioration in awake blood gases are a consequence of inadequate nocturnal use or progression of the underlying disorder. Other issues such as weight control, enrolment in a rehabilitation programme or referral to other services may also need to be discussed during these reviews. For patients with progressive neuromuscular disorders, review of swallowing and nutritional status is also necessary, and these patients will require extensive input from a number of specialties as their muscle weakness increases. Equipment needs to be inspected and reviewed regularly, and worn masks, filters and accessories replaced.

While patients are not ventilator-dependent, many express considerable anxiety about the risk of being without the ventilator even for one night. They may be anxious about the symptoms of sleep deprivation and hypercapnia. Those who are geographically isolated or live alone are particularly vulnerable if there is equipment failure. Back-up systems and emergency plans are valuable and need to be worked out with each individual. Patients should be encouraged to enter into a regular maintenance agreement with the companies or hospitals supplying the equipment. All relevant instructions for cleaning and maintenance should be provided in writing and in their preferred language. In a recent

11

study looking at the performance of ventilation equipment in the patient's home, considerable differences between the settings prescribed, the values set on the control panel of the machines and the actual ventilation settings delivered were found (Farre et al 2006). This highlights the importance of both the patient and the prescribing centre developing regular equipment review procedures to ensure therapy is both safe and effective.

SPECIAL APPLICATIONS OF NON-INVASIVE VENTILATION

Children and infants

Although non-invasive ventilatory support is now seen as a first-line therapy for adults with hypercapnic respiratory failure, this technique has, to date, been less commonly used by paediatric centres. To some extent this is due to a lack of randomized controlled trials of NIV in children, although an increasing number of published reports would suggest use of the technique in children is increasing (Teague 2005). In addition, some reports have suggested that infants and young children may not be tolerant of mask therapy (Heckmatt et al 1990), limiting the application of this technique. However, one of the earliest reports of mask ventilation use involved a 6-year-old-child with congenital central hypoventilation syndrome (Ellis et al 1987a). Since that time, a number of studies have appeared in the literature describing the successful use of nasal masks for both CPAP and NIV in more than 300 children. Many of those described were under 6 years of age, yet tolerated therapy well both in the short and long term (Fortenberry et al 1995, Simonds et al 2000, Waters et al 1995).

Reports of nasal ventilation use in paediatric patients have included children with upper airway obstruction, cystic fibrosis, congenital central hypoventilation syndrome and neuromuscular disorders (Ellis et al 1987b, Fauroux et al 2005, Simonds et al 2000). Prior to the introduction of mask ventilation, children with chronic respiratory failure from these disorders were managed with tracheostomy in order to deliver positive pressure to the lungs. Although effective, the tracheostomy tube can also interfere with speech development and may predispose the child to chest infections. While mask ventilation can also be associated with side effects, most commonly skin breakdown and leak, these problems are generally minor or manageable. In the largest study of its kind to date, Simonds and colleagues (2000) reported the use of domiciliary mask ventilation in 40 children with respiratory failure secondary to congenital neuromuscular and skeletal disorders. The youngest

child commenced on therapy was 9 months of age. Thirty-eight tolerated mask ventilatory support in the long term, resulting in reversal of nocturnal hypoventilation and significant improvements with daytime spontaneous CO_2 and O_2 levels.

Mask ventilation has also been used in children presenting with acute hypoxaemic or hypercapnic respiratory failure (Fortenberry et al 1995, Padman et al 1998). As with adults, therapy has been instituted to improve gas exchange, reduce the work of breathing and avoid intubation. It has also been used successfully to wean patients who failed attempted extubation or to facilitate extubation in those likely to have difficulty resuming spontaneous ventilation (Brinkrant et al 1997). In circumstances where there are ethical or medical concerns about the use of invasive ventilation techniques in children with severe neurological dysfunction or terminal diseases, mask ventilation offers a realistic active treatment alternative (Teague 2005). Although randomized trials are lacking, mounting clinical evidence suggests mask ventilation in children with acute respiratory failure is both feasible and safe.

Increasingly, bilevel devices rather than volume preset are used in this population due to simplicity, portability and cost. These devices are flow-initiated and therefore can be easier to trigger and more comfortable than volume-preset devices. In addition, the availability of setting EPAP with bilevel devices can be valuable in patients requiring stabilization of the upper airway as well as ventilatory support. The principles of adjusting settings for NIV in children are no different from those used with adults. Initial IPAP and EPAP pressures are set to achieve both patient comfort and the goals of ventilatory support, and are altered later depending on clinical response and patient acceptance. Many of the modern bilevel devices now have internal alarms and these should be set to alert carers to the loss of airway pressure associated with mask removal or machine malfunction. External alarm systems may need to be added to those devices without internal alarms.

Generally, children tolerate masks well, although initially extra time and effort may be needed to encourage the child to keep the mask in place. Imagination and patience, from both the clinician and the child, help. Compared with adult masks, there is a limited range for children and even fewer for neonatal use. Most 'children's' masks are simply scaled-down versions of the adult model. Although this is not much of a problem for the older, larger child, it can make fitting a mask for the younger patient (<2 years) a little more challenging. Medium-sized adult nasal masks can be used as full facemasks for the smaller child (Simonds et al 2000). Care needs to be taken when choosing a mask to ensure dead space is minimized and sufficient carbon dioxide washout is occurring. However, as the technique becomes more widely accepted for this population, a larger choice of mask should become available.

A specific problem that can arise in children using long-term mask therapy is that of altered facial skeletal development resulting from the application of tightly fitting headgear and nasal mask. Although only mild effects have been reported (Fauroux et al 2005, Simonds et al 2000), the impact of mask therapy on craniofacial development should be taken into consideration when choosing and fitting mask equipment. Simonds and colleagues (2000) reported four cases of mild mid-facial hypoplasia in their series of 40 children treated long-term with mask ventilation. Fauroux and colleagues (2005) found that global facial flattening was present in 68% of children using home mask ventilation. Strategies to minimize these side effects include using different masks rotated on a weekly basis to reduce and vary the pressure over the maxillary region and reducing the amount of time NIV is used daily (Fauroux et al 2005, Simonds et al 2000). Regular maxillofacial evaluation and follow-up is essential in this population (Fauroux et al 2005). In those patients requiring long-term therapy, frequent review is necessary to ensure the ventilator settings and the mask size remain adequate as the child grows and develops. In addition, the child's parents/carers need to be trained to supervise therapy and solve problems as they arise.

There is no doubt that as clinicians become more experienced and confident with the technique, more paediatric centres will come to accept mask ventilation as a suitable modality for children. As a consequence, increasingly more children will be offered mask ventilation as first-line therapy for the management of respiratory failure, in hospital as well as in the home. The success of this therapy relies heavily on initiation of treatment by skilled therapists and training both the child and family in its use.

Weaning and early extubation

Most patients can be weaned from mechanical ventilation without incident. However, a small number will require a prolonged weaning period, particularly when there is a history of underlying lung, chest wall or neuromuscular disease. Although various weaning strategies have been developed to facilitate the resumption of spontaneous breathing, some patients will not tolerate removal of ventilatory support without developing unacceptably high levels of carbon dioxide retention. Non-invasive ventilatory support can be a useful tool in the weaning of such patients from conventional mechanical ventilation, permitting the earlier removal of the endotracheal tube than with conventional invasive

pressure support techniques (Girault et al 1999, Nava et al 1998). Data from three randomized controlled trials have shown that early extubation and application of NIV results in shorter length of stay, reduces the incidence of complications and improves survival, especially in patients with underlying COPD (Ferrer et al 2003, Girault et al 1999, Nava et al 1998). However, the application of NIV to unselected patients in the post-extubation period either prophylactically (Jiang et al 1999) or after respiratory failure develops within 48 hours of extubation (Esteban et al 2004, Keenan et al 2002) and does not appear to be of benefit. In contrast, in patients with a high risk of post-extubation failure, the use of NIV applied immediately following extubation has been shown to reduce the need for reintubation (Ferrer et al 2006, Nava et al 2005) and to improve survival in those with hypercapnia at extubation (Nava et al 2005). Therefore, based on current evidence, there does not appear to be a place for the routine use of NIV in all patients following extubation (Jiang et al 1999). However, NIV should be considered in any patient considered at risk of developing post-extubation respiratory difficulties, with therapy initiated immediately post-extubation rather than waiting for signs of respiratory distress to develop (Ferrer et al 2006, Nava et al 2005).

In patients already tracheostomized and on partial ventilatory support, nasal mask ventilation may be substituted for tracheal support (Restrick et al 1993). This is usually started on a continuous basis, with the patient removing the mask for short periods for eating, speaking and coughing. Periods of spontaneous breathing are then interspersed with periods on the nasal mask, the balance being determined by patient tolerance and clinical response. Once nasal ventilatory support has been shown to be acceptable and to effectively support ventilation, the tracheostomy tube is removed. Non-invasive ventilation is then used nocturnally and for any rest/sleep period during the day as required. Although many patients may be weaned entirely from the mask, some will have an underlying process which features sleep-disordered breathing. Therefore, investigation into the presence of nocturnal breathing abnormalities and discharge home on nocturnal ventilatory support should be considered.

Physiotherapy intervention during non-invasive ventilation

Physiotherapists have long been involved in the application of positive pressure therapy to patients with respiratory problems with the aim of improving gas exchange, mobilizing secretions or reducing dyspnoea. Through until the mid-1970s physiotherapists routinely

11

administered respiratory medications by intermittent positive pressure breathing (IPPB) through a mask or mouthpiece (Bennett et al 1976), or used IPPB to increase ventilation in patients with severe pain or with poor ventilatory control. The mid-1980s saw the introduction of nocturnal mask ventilation as a feasible and effective method of supporting breathing during sleep, resulting in improved awake gas exchange, daytime function and quality of life. Physiotherapists were central in introducing and applying this technique in a wide range of respiratory disorders (Ellis et al 1987a, 1987b, 1988, Holland et al 2003, Keilty et al 1994, Milross et al 2001, Piper & Sullivan 1994b, Piper & Willson 1996, Piper et al 1992). When the potential for this technique in the management of acute respiratory failure was realized, physiotherapists were again amongst the forerunners in applying and evaluating therapy (Bott et al 1993, Conway et al 1993).

In daily practice, physiotherapists may become involved with the application of this technique in a number of different ways (Box 11.4). Data from a survey looking at physiotherapy practice in European intensive care units found that almost half the respondents reported physiotherapy involvement in implementing and supervising NIV (Norrenberg & Vincent 2000). In a survey of physiotherapy involvement in non-invasive ventilation hospital services in the British Isles, more than 90% of respondents reported physiotherapy involvement in some aspect of the management of patients using NIV, with around half contributing to implementation of the technique (Moran et al 2005). The skills and knowledge base of physiotherapists regarding respiratory disease and its management place them in a good position to be key members contributing to any non-invasive ventilation service.

Even where therapists are not directly involved in implementing NIV, the widespread use of this technique both in high dependency and ward areas means that at some point most will be involved in the care of patients using this therapy (Moran et al 2005). In the acute setting one of the most common causes of NIV failure is the inability to manage secretion clearance effectively (Carlucci et al 2000). While there is currently limited published data confirming the efficacy of various airway clearance techniques during acute NIV use, the practice is widespread (Moran et al 2005). In a small randomized trial in patients with acute hypercapnic respiratory failure, Inal-Ince and colleagues (2004) found that the addition of the active cycle of breathing techniques (ACBT) to NIV resulted in a small reduction in the length of time NIV was required (5 vs 6.7 days, $p = 0.03$). However, this did not impact on any other outcome measure such as length of ICU stay. In patients with acute exacerbations of COPD and large amounts

---

Box 11.4 Role of the physiotherapist in home ventilation services

Assessment of the patient
- Identification of symptoms of sleep-disordered breathing
- Bedside pulmonary function testing including respiratory muscle strength
- Exercise tolerance (e.g. 6-minute walking test, shuttle test)
- Level of dyspnoea during daily activities

Initiating therapy
- Choice of device and setting
- Acclimatizing patient to mask and machine
- Education of patient and family regarding therapy
- Monitoring response to therapy

Planning a concurrent rehabilitation programme
- Need for oxygen or ventilatory support required during activities
- Upper limb and whole body training
- Lifestyle modification
- Use of ventilatory support as part of secretion clearance

Discharge planning
- Training patient and/or caregivers in the care and operation of the equipment
- Home exercise programme
- Ongoing appointments and emergency plans

Follow-up
- Assessment of daytime symptoms and pulmonary function including arterial blood gases, spirometry, etc.
- Exercise tolerance
- Troubleshooting problems: technical problems versus changes in clinical condition

---

of sputum, the addition of positive expiratory pressure (PEP) and assisted coughing to routine NIV management resulted in greater amounts of sputum removed and a shorter period of NIV use (Bellone et al 2002). These interesting, preliminary results illustrate the potential benefits of traditional airway clearance techniques in conjunction with NIV in the management of patients with acute respiratory failure and require further exploration.

It has also been shown that NIV may have a place in selected patients as a stand-alone method to aid in secretion removal (Fauroux et al 1999, Holland et al 2003). For the breathless patient who is unable to lie flat, use of NIV may permit the use of postural drainage positions that would otherwise not be tolerated (Piper et al 1992). Anecdotally, patients report being able to tolerate longer physiotherapy sessions when using ventilatory support, which is important in patients who tire easily but who have retained or copious secretions. In patients with severe muscle weakness and poor cough, mask ventilation may be used to assist deep breathing and mobilization of secretions. In these circumstances techniques such as overpressures, breath stacking and mechanical in-exsufflation may be used. The tidal volume or inspiratory pressure of the device may be increased during physiotherapy sessions to aid chest wall expansion and assist the mobilization of secretions (Piper & Moran 2006).

Exercise

By the time patients with chronic respiratory failure present for nocturnal ventilatory support they are usually severely debilitated. Their presentation is usually characterized by severe shortness of breath on exertion, excessive daytime sleepiness, fatigue, prolonged illness and regular hospitalization. Consequently significant peripheral deconditioning has likely occurred which will limit their tolerance to daily activities and exercise performance. After a period of nocturnal ventilatory support, patients are able to perform a great deal more work without fatigue (Fuschillo et al 2003, Schonhofer et al 2001). Survey data has shown that exercise is commonly used as part of the physiotherapy management for patients using NIV (Moran et al 2005). However, fewer centres use the technique routinely during exercise training. The beneficial effects of posi-

tive pressure during exercise in patients with severe lung disease have been reported (Keilty et al 1994, van't Hul et al 2002). Acute benefits include reduced breathlessness, increased exercise time and improved oxygen saturation. However, the long-term benefits of routine application of this technique during exercise training remain unclear and await further investigation.

CONCLUSION

Non-invasive ventilation is a technique which can improve gas exchange and reduce the work of breathing and is becoming increasingly used to manage both chronic and acute respiratory failure. Evidence for the effectiveness of this technique in a wide range of clinical situations has seen it become an integral part of the respiratory management for patients with respiratory failure. Physiotherapists working in respiratory care require knowledge of and skills with the equipment and its applications in order to continue to provide holistic and effective treatment programmes to manage these patients.

Acknowledgements

We would like to thank the following companies for their kind permission to use images of their products: Fisher and Paykel Healthcare Ltd, Auckland, New Zealand; ResMed Limited, North Ryde, Australia and Respironics, Inc, Murrysville, PA. ResMed Limited owns the copyright of the ResMed images and ResMed Limited reserves all rights.

11

References

Ambrosino N, Foglio K, Rubini F et al 1995 Noninvasive mechanical ventilation in acute respiratory failure due to chronic obstructive pulmonary disease: correlates for success. Thorax 50: 755–757

Anton A, Guell R, Gomez J et al 2000 Predicting the result of noninvasive ventilation in severe acute exacerbations of patients with chronic airflow limitation. Chest 117: 828–833

Antonelli M, Conti G, Bufi M et al 2000 Noninvasive ventilation for treatment of acute respiratory failure in patients undergoing solid organ transplantation. Journal of the American Medical Association 283: 235–241

Auriant I, Jallot A, Herve P et al 2001 Noninvasive ventilation reduces mortality in acute respiratory failure following lung resection. American

Journal of Respiratory and Critical Care Medicine 164: 1231–1235

Barach AL, Martin J, Eckman M 1938 Positive-pressure respiration and its application to the treatment of acute pulmonary edema. Annals of Internal Medicine 12: 754–795

Bellone A, Spagnolatti L, Massobrio M et al 2002 Short-term effects of expiration under positive pressure in patients with acute exacerbations of chronic obstructive pulmonary disease and mild acidosis requiring non-invasive positive pressure ventilation. Intensive Care Medicine 28: 581–585

Bennett L, Heath J, Mitchell R 1976 An inpatient observation and comparison of the Bennett's IPPB and aerosol methods of administering salbutamol. Australian Journal of Physiotherapy 23: 111–113

Bott J, Carroll MP, Conway JH et al 1993 Randomized controlled trial of nasal ventilation in acute ventilatory failure due to chronic obstructive airways disease. Lancet 341: 1555–1557

Bourke SC, Tomlinson M, Williams TL et al 2006 Effects of non-invasive ventilation on survival and quality of life in patients with amyotrophic lateral sclerosis: a randomized controlled trial. Lancet Neurology 5: 140–47

Brinkrant DJ, Pope JF, Eiban RM 1997 Pediatric noninvasive nasal ventilation. Journal of Child Neurology 12: 231–236

British Thoracic Society Standards of Care Committee 2002 Non-invasive ventilation in acute respiratory failure. Thorax 57: 192–211

Brochard L, Mancebo J, Wysocki M et al 1995 Noninvasive ventilation for acute exacerbations of chronic obstructive pulmonary disease. New England Journal of Medicine 333: 817–822

Bye PTP, Ellis ER, Issa FG, Donnelly PD, Sullivan CE 1990 The role of sleep in the development of respiratory failure in patients with neuromuscular disease. Thorax 45: 241–247

Carlucci A, Richard JC, Wysocki M, Lepage E, Brochard L 2000 Noninvasive versus conventional mechanical ventilation. An epidemiologic survey. American Journal of Respiratory and Critical Care Medicine 163: 874–880

Casanova C, Celli BR, Tost L et al 2000 Long-term controlled trial of nocturnal nasal positive pressure ventilation in patients with severe COPD. Chest 118: 1582–1590

Chevrolet JC, Jolliet P, Abajo B, Toussi A, Louis M 1991 Nasal positive pressure ventilation in patients with acute respiratory failure. Difficult and time-consuming procedure for nurses. Chest 100: 775–782

Clini E, Sturani C, Rossi A et al 2002 The Italian multicentre study noninvasive ventilation in chronic obstructive pulmonary disease patients. European Respiratory Journal 20: 529–538

Confalonieri M, Potena A, Carbone G et al 1999 Acute respiratory failure in patients with severe community acquired pneumonia: a prospective randomized evaluation of non-invasive ventilation. American Journal of Respiratory and Critical Care Medicine 160: 1585–1591

Conway JH, Hitchcock RA, Godfrey RC, Carroll MP 1993 Nasal intermittent positive pressure ventilation in acute exacerbations of chronic obstructive pulmonary disease – a preliminary study. Respiratory Medicine 87: 387–394

Delclaux C, L'Her E, Alberti C et al 2000 Treatment of acute hypoxemic nonhypercapnic respiratory insufficiency with continuous positive airway pressure delivered by a face mask. A randomized controlled trial. Journal of the American Medical Association 284: 2352–2360

Douglas NJ, White DP, Pickett CK, Weil JV, Zwillich CW 1982 Respiration during sleep in normal man. Thorax 37: 840–844

Ellis ER, McCauley VB, Mellis C, Sullivan CE 1987a Treatment of alveolar hypoventilation in a six-year-old girl with intermittent positive pressure ventilation through a nose mask. American Review of Respiratory Disease 136: 188–191

Ellis ER, Bye PTP, Bruderer JW, Sullivan CE 1987b Treatment of respiratory failure in patients with neuromuscular disease. American Review of Respiratory Disease 135: 148–152

Ellis ER, Grunstein RR, Chan CS, Bye PTP, Sullivan CE 1988 Treatment of nocturnal respiratory failure in kyphoscoliosis. Chest 94: 811–815

Esteban A, Frutos-Vivar F, Ferguson ND et al 2004 Noninvasive positive-pressure ventilation for respiratory failure after extubation. New England Journal of Medicine 350: 2452–2460

Fanfulla F, Delmastro M, Berardinelli A, Lupo ND, Nava S 2005 Effects of different ventilator settings on sleep and inspiratory effort in patients with neuromuscular disease. American Journal of Respiratory and Critical Care Medicine 172: 619–624

Farre R, Navajas D, Prats E et al 2006 Performance of mechanical ventilators at the patient's home: a multicenter quality control study. Thorax 61: 400–404

Fauroux B, Boule M, Lofaso F et al 1999 Chest physiotherapy in cystic fibrosis: improved tolerance with nasal pressure support ventilation. Pediatrics 103: E32

Fauroux B, Itti E, Pigeot J, Isabey D et al 2000 Optimization of aerosol deposition by pressure support in children with cystic fibrosis: an experimental and clinical study. American Journal of Respiratory and Critical Care Medicine 162: 2265–2271

Fauroux B, Lavis J-F, Nicot F, Picard A, Boelle P-Y, Clement A, Vazquez M-P 2005 Facial side effects during noninvasive positive pressure ventilation in children. Intensive Care Medicine 31: 965–969

Ferrer M, Esquinas A, Leon M et al 2003 Non-invasive ventilation in severe hypoxemic respiratory failure. A randomized clinical trial. American Journal of Respiratory and Critical Care Medicine 168: 1438–1444

Ferrer M, Valencia M, Nicolas JM et al 2006 Early noninvasive ventilation averts extubation failure in patients at risk. American Journal of Respiratory and Critical Care Medicine 173: 164–170

Fortenberry JD, Del Toro J, Jefferson LS, Evey L, Haase D 1995 Management of pediatric acute hypoxemic respiratory failure with bilevel positive pressure (BiPAP) nasal mask ventilation. Chest 108: 1059–1064

Fuschillo S, De Felice A, Gaudiosi C, Balzano G 2003 Nocturnal mechanical ventilation improves exercise capacity in kyphoscoliotic patients with respiratory impairment.

Monaldi Archives for Chest Disease 59: 281–286

Garay SM, Turino GM, Goldring RM 1981 Sustained reversal of chronic hypercapnia in patients with alveolar hypoventilation syndromes: long-term maintenance with noninvasive mechanical ventilation. American Journal of Medicine 70: 269–274

Gastaut H, Tassinari CA, Duron B 1966 Polygraphic study of the episodic diurnal and nocturnal manifestations of the Pickwick syndrome. Brain Research 1: 167–186

Girault C, Daudenthun I, Chevron V et al 1999 Noninvasive ventilation as a systematic extubation and weaning technique in acute-on-chronic respiratory failure. American Journal of Respiratory and Critical Care Medicine 160: 88–92

Girault C, Richard JC, Chevron V et al 1997 Comparative physiologic effects of noninvasive assist-control and pressure support ventilation in acute hypercapnic respiratory failure. Chest 111: 1639–1648

Gozal D 1997 Nocturnal ventilatory support in patients with cystic fibrosis: comparison with supplemental oxygen. European Respiratory Journal 10: 1999–2003

Heckmatt JZ, Loh L, Dubowitz V 1990 Night-time nasal ventilation in neuromuscular disease. Lancet 335: 579–582

Hilbert G, Gruson D, Vargas F et al 2001 Noninvasive ventilation in immunosuppressed patients with pulmonary infiltrates, fever, and acute respiratory failure. New England Journal of Medicine 344: 481–487

Hill N 1993 Noninvasive ventilation. Does it work, for whom, and how? American Review of Respiratory Disease 147: 1050–1055

Hodson ME, Madden BP, Steven MH, Tsang VT, Yacoub MH 1991 Non-invasive mechanical ventilation for cystic fibrosis patients – a potential bridge to transplantation. European Respiratory Journal 4: 524–527

Holland AE, Denehy L, Ntoumenopoulos G, Naughton MT, Wilson JW 2003 Non-invasive ventilation assists chest physiotherapy in adults with acute exacerbations of cystic fibrosis. Thorax 58: 880–884

Inal-Ince D, Savci S, Topeli A, Arikan H 2004 Active cycle of breathing techniques in non-invasive ventilation for acute hypercapnic respiratory failure. Australian Journal of Physiotherapy 50: 67–73

Jaber S, Chanques G, Matecki S et al 2002 Comparison of the effects of heat and moisture exchangers and heated humidifiers on ventilation

11

and gas exchange during non-invasive ventilation. Intensive Care Medicine 28: 1590–1594

Jiang JS, Kao SJ, Wang SN 1999 Effect of early application of biphasic positive airway pressure on the outcome of extubation in ventilator weaning. Respirology 4: 161–165

Keenan SP, Powers C, McCormack DG, Block G 2002 Noninvasive positive-pressure ventilation for postextubation respiratory distress. A randomized controlled trial. Journal of the American Medical Association 287: 3238–3244

Keenan SP, Sinuff T, Cook DJ, Hill NS 2003 Which patients with acute exacerbation of chronic obstructive pulmonary disease benefit from noninvasive positive-pressure ventilation? A systematic review of the literature. Annals of Internal Medicine 138: 861–870

Keilty SEJ, Ponte J, Fleming TA, Moxham J 1994 Effect of inspiratory pressure support on exercise tolerance and breathlessness in patients with severe stable chronic obstructive pulmonary disease. Thorax 49: 990–994

Kramer N, Meyer TJ, Mehang J, Cece RD, Hill NS 1995 Randomized, prospective trial of noninvasive positive pressure ventilation in acute respiratory failure. American Journal of Respiratory and Critical Care Medicine 151: 1799–1806

Kwok H, McCormack J, Cece R, Houtchens J, Hill NS 2003 Controlled trial of oronasal versus nasal mask ventilation in the treatment of acute respiratory failure. Critical Care Medicine 31: 468–473

Lightowler JV, Wedzicha JA, Elliott MW, Ram FSF 2003 Non-invasive positive pressure ventilation to treat respiratory failure resulting from exacerbations of chronic obstructive pulmonary disease: Cochrane systematic review and meta-analysis. British Medical Journal 326: 185–189

Masip J, Roque M, Sanchez B et al 2005 Noninvasive ventilation in acute cardiogenic pulmonary edema. Systematic review and meta-analysis. Journal of the American Medical Association 294: 3124–3130

Meecham Jones DJ, Paul EA, Jones PW, Wedzicha JA 1995 Nasal pressure support ventilation plus oxygen compared with oxygen therapy alone in hypercapnic COPD. American Journal of Respiratory and Critical Care Medicine 152: 538–544

Mehta S, McCool FD, Hill NS 2001 Leak compensation in positive pressure ventilators: a lung model. European Respiratory Journal 17: 259–267

Meyer TJ, Hill NS 1994 Noninvasive positive pressure ventilation to treat respiratory failure. Annals of Internal Medicine 120: 760–770

Milross MA, Piper AJ, Norman M et al 2001 Low-flow oxygen and bilevel ventilatory support. Effects on ventilation during sleep in cystic fibrosis. American Journal of Respiratory and Critical Care Medicine 163: 129–134

Moran FM, Bradley JM, Elborn JS, Piper AJ 2005 Physiotherapy involvement in non-invasive ventilation hospital services: a British Isles survey. Int J Clin Pract 59: 453–456

Nava S, Ambrosino N, Clini E et al 1998 Noninvasive mechanical ventilation in the weaning of patients with respiratory failure due to chronic obstructive pulmonary disease. Annals of Internal Medicine 128: 721–728

Nava S, Carbone G, DiBattista N et al 2003 Noninvasive ventilation in cardiogenic pulmonary edema. A multicenter randomized trial. American Journal of Respiratory and Critical Care Medicine 168: 1432–1437

Nava S, Evangelisti I, Rampulla C et al 1997 Human and financial costs of noninvasive mechanical ventilation in patients affected by COPD and acute respiratory failure. Chest 111: 1631–1638

Nava S, Gregoretti C, Fanfulla F et al 2005 Noninvasive ventilation to prevent respiratory failure after extubation in high-risk patients. Critical Care Medicine 33: 2465–2470

Navalesi P, Fanfulla F, Frigerio P, Gregoretti C, Nava S 2000 Physiologic evaluation of noninvasive mechanical ventilation delivered with three types of masks in patients with chronic hypercapnic respiratory failure. Critical Care Medicine 28: 1785–1790

Nickol AH, Hart N, Hopkinson NS et al 2005 Mechanisms of improvement of respiratory failure in patients with restrictive thoracic disease treated with non-invasive ventilation. Thorax 60: 754–760

Norrenberg M, Vincent JL 2000 A profile of European intensive care unit physiotherapists. Intensive Care Medicine 26: 988–994

Padman R, Lawless ST, Kettrick RG 1998 Noninvasive ventilation via bilevel positive airway pressure support in pediatric practice. Critical Care Medicine 26: 169–173

Perez de Llano LA, Golpe R, Ortiz Piquer M et al 2005 Short-term and long-term effects of nasal intermittent positive pressure ventilation in patients with obesity-hypoventilation syndrome. Chest 128: 587–594

Peter JV, Moran JL, Phillips-Hughes J, Graham P, Bersten AD 2006 Effect of non-invasive positive pressure ventilation (NIPPV) on mortality inpatients with acute cardiogenic pulmonary oedema: a meta-analysis. Lancet 367: 1155–1163

Piper AJ, Moran FM 2006 Non-invasive ventilation and the physiotherapist: current state and future trends. Phys Ther Rev 11:37–43

Piper AJ, Sullivan CE 1994a Sleep breathing in neuromuscular disease. In: Saunders N, Sullivan CE (eds) Sleep and breathing, 2nd edn. Marcel Dekker, New York, pp 761–821

Piper AJ, Sullivan CE 1994b Effects of short-term NIPPV in the treatment of patients with severe obstructive sleep apnea and hypercapnia. Chest 105: 434–440

Piper AJ, Parker S, Torzillo PJ, Sullivan CE, Bye PTP 1992 Nocturnal nasal IPPV stabilizes patients with cystic fibrosis and hypercapnic respiratory failure. Chest 102: 846–850

Piper AJ, Willson G 1996 Nocturnal nasal ventilatory support in the management of daytime hypercapnic respiratory failure. Australian Journal of Physiotherapy 42(1): 17–29

Plant PK, Owen JL, Elliott MW 2000 Early use of non-invasive ventilation for acute exacerbations of chronic obstructive pulmonary disease on general respiratory wards: a multicentre randomized controlled trial. Lancet 355: 1931–1935

Plant PK, Owen JL, Elliott MW 2001 Non-invasive ventilation in acute exacerbations of chronic obstructive pulmonary disease: long term survival and predictors of in–hospital outcome. Thorax 56: 708–712

Plant PK, Owen JL, Parrott S, Elliott MW 2003 Cost effectiveness of ward based non-invasive ventilation for acute exacerbations of chronic obstructive pulmonary disease: economic analysis of randomized controlled trial. British Medical Journal 326: 956–960

Polkey MI, Lyall RA, Davidson AC, Leigh PN, Moxham J 1999 Ethical and clinical issues in the use of home non-invasive mechanical ventilation for the palliation of breathlessness in motor neurone disease. Thorax 54: 367–371

Pollack CV, Fleisch KB, Dowsey K 1995 Treatment of acute bronchospasm with beta-adrenergic agonist aerosols delivered by a nasal bilevel positive airway pressure circuit. Annals of Emergency Medicine 26: 552–557

Raphael JC, Chevret S, Chastang C, Bouvet F 1994 Randomized trial of preventive nasal ventilation in Duchenne muscular dystrophy. Lancet 343: 1600–1603

Ragette R, Mellies U, Schwake C, Teschler H 2002 Patterns and

11

predictors of sleep disordered breathing in primary myopathies. Thorax 57: 724–728

Ram FS, Wellington S, Towe B, Wedzicha JA 2005 Non-invasive positive pressure ventilation for treatment of respiratory failure due to severe acute exacerbations of asthma. Cochrane Database of Systematic Reviews 3: CD004360

Restrick LJ, Scott AD, Ward EM et al 1993 Nasal intermittent positive-pressure ventilation in weaning intubated patients with chronic respiratory failure from assisted intermittent, positive-pressure ventilation. Respiratory Medicine 87: 199–204

Richards GN, Cistulli PA, Ungar G, Berthon-Jones M, Sullivan CE 1996 Mouth leak with nasal continuous positive airway pressure increases nasal airway resistance. American Journal of Respiratory and Critical Care Medicine 154: 182–186

Saatci E, Miller D, Stell IM, Lee KC, Moxham J 2004 Dynamic dead space in face masks used with noninvasive ventilators: a lung model study. European Respiratory Journal 23: 129–135

Schettino G, Altobelli N, Kacmarek RM 2005 Noninvasive positive pressure ventilation reverses acute respiratory failure in select 'do-not-intubate' patients. Critical Care Medicine 33: 1976–1982

Schettino GPP, Chatmongkolchart S, Hess DR, Kacmarek RM 2003 Position of exhalation port and mask design affect CO_2 rebreathing during noninvasive positive pressure ventilation. Critical Care Medicine 31: 2178–2182

Schonhofer B, Sonneborn M, Haidl P, Bohrer H, Kohler D 1997 Comparison of two different modes for noninvasive mechanical ventilation: volume vs pressure controlled device. European Respiratory Journal 10: 184–191

Schonhofer B, Wallstein S, Wiese C, Kohler D 2001 Non-invasive mechanical ventilation improves

endurance performance in patients with chronic respiratory failure due to thoracic restriction. Chest 119: 1371–1378

Simonds AK 2004 Pneumothorax: an important complication of non-invasive ventilation in neuromuscular disease. Neuromuscular Disorders 14: 351–352

Simonds AK, Elliott MW 1995 Outcome of domiciliary nasal intermittent positive pressure ventilation in restrictive and obstructive disorders. Thorax 50: 604–609

Simonds AK, Muntoni F, Heather S, Fielding S 1998 Impact of nasal ventilation on survival in hypercapnic Duchenne muscular dystrophy. Thorax 53: 949–952

Simonds AK, Ward S, Heather S, Bush A, Muntoni F 2000 Outcome of paediatric domiciliary mask ventilation in neuromuscular and skeletal disease. European Respiratory Journal 16: 476–481

Sullivan CE, Berthon-Jones M, Issa FG, Eves L 1981 Reversal of obstructive sleep apnea by continuous positive airway pressure applied through the nose. Lancet 1: 862–865

Teague WG 2005 Non-invasive positive pressure ventilation: current status in paediatric patients. Paediatric Respiratory Review 6: 52–60

Teschler H, Stampa J, Ragette R, Konietzko N, Berthon-Jones M 1999 Effect of mouth leak on effectiveness of nasal bilevel ventilatory assistance and sleep architecture. European Respiratory Journal 14: 1251–1257

Trask CH, Cree EM 1962 Oximeter studies on patients with chronic obstructive emphysema, awake and during sleep. New England Journal of Medicine 266: 639–642

Tuggey JM, MW Elliott 2005 Randomised crossover study of pressure and volume non-invasive ventilation in chest wall deformity. Thorax 60: 859–864

van't Hul A, Kwakkel G, Gosselink R 2002 The acute effect of non-invasive ventilatory support during exercise

on exercise endurance and dyspnea in patients with chronic obstructive pulmonary disease. A systematic review. J Cardiopulm Rehab 23: 307–313

Vitacca M, Nava S, Confalonieri M et al 2000 The appropriate setting of noninvasive pressure support ventilation in stable COPD patients. Chest 118: 1286–1293

Ward S, Chatwin M, Heather S, Simonds AK 2005 Randomised controlled trial of non-invasive ventilation (NIV) for nocturnal hypoventilation in neuromuscular and chest wall disease patients with daytime normocapnia. Thorax 60: 1019–1024

Waters KA, Everett FM, Bruderer JW et al 1995 Obstructive sleep apnea: the use of nasal CPAP in 80 children. American Journal of Respiratory and Critical Care Medicine 152: 780–785

Weirs PWJ, LeCoultre R, Dallinga OT et al 1977 Cuirass respirator treatment of chronic respiratory failure in scoliotic patients. Thorax 32: 221–228

Windisch W, Kostic S, Dreher M, Virchow JC, Sorichter S 2005 Outcome of patients with stable COPD receiving controlled noninvasive positive pressure ventilation aimed at a maximal reduction of $PaCO_2$. Chest 128: 657–662

Wood KE, Flaten AL, Backes WJ 2000 Inspissated secretions: a life-threatening complication of prolonged non-invasive ventilation. Respiratory Care 45: 491–493

Woollam CHM 1976 The development of apparatus for intermittent negative pressure respiration Anaesthesia 31: 537–547

Further reading

Mehta S, Hill NS 2001 Noninvasive ventilation. American Journal of Respiratory and Critical Care Medicine 163: 540–577

Turkington PM, Elliott MW 2000 Rationale for the use of non-invasive ventilation in chronic ventilatory failure. Thorax 55: 417–423

11

Chapter **12**

Surgery for adults

Linda Denehy

INTRODUCTION

Perioperative physiotherapy aims to prevent or mini-mize the adverse physiological changes associated with major surgical procedures. In these patients, physio-therapy has played a significant part in minimizing the adverse effects of anaesthesia and surgery on the respi-ratory system for more than 50 years. This role of the physiotherapist has been supported by evidence from clinical trials reported since 1947. The evidence advo-cated pre- and postoperative physiotherapy for all patients having major surgery, to reduce the incidence of postoperative pulmonary complications (PPC) and thereby reduce patient morbidity and prolonged hospi-tal admission.

Recent advances in both surgical and pain manage-ment, the evolution of new forms of postoperative phys-iotherapy support and a reduction in the incidence of clinically significant PPC have provided the stimulus for a re-evaluation of the place of physiotherapy in surgery. The incidence of PPC has shown a gradual reduction over time in these patient populations. In part this is due to a change in the method for the measurement of PPC, and also because anaesthetic and surgical techniques have improved. The use of epidural and patient-con-trolled analgesic techniques on the ward has also had a profound impact on the incidence of PPC. The incidence of PPC is stated to be 5–10% (Brooks-Brunn 1995), whereas earlier it was reported to be 20–30% (King 1933, Wightman 1968). The introduction of 'fast track' postop-erative management and minimally invasive abdominal, thoracic and cardiac surgery has also impacted on the physiotherapy management in these patient popula-tions, although more research is needed in these areas.

This chapter outlines the effects of the surgical process, pain and pain management on the respiratory system, the development of PPC, evidence for the physiotherapy treatment of different surgical populations, use of a variety of physiotherapy treatment techniques, management of surgical drips and drains, including underwater seal drainage and brief notes on different types of surgical procedures and lung cancer. The chapter has been written to aid both undergraduate physiotherapy students and cardiorespiratory clinicians in better understanding the area of physiotherapy and surgery. The evidence base underpinning the place of physiotherapy in surgery has been reviewed by Denehy & Browning (2007).

THE SURGICAL PROCESS

General anaesthesia

General anaesthesia (GA) provides the patient with sleep, amnesia and analgesia. Constant monitoring of the patient's vital signs allow these to be kept within physiological limits. General anaesthesia can be divided into three different stages: induction, maintenance and reversal or emergence. Before induction an intravenous (IV) administration of a combination of an anxiolytic drug with amnesic power such as midazolam, together with a narcotic such as fentanyl, is often given. The narcotic given preoperatively helps to prevent nerve impulses, arising from intraoperative events, from sensitizing central neuronal structures and is called pre-emptive analgesia (Katz 1993). There is some evidence that analgesia given before the painful stimulus reduces subsequent pain, but this remains controversial.

Induction of anaesthesia: Anaesthesia is usually achieved by IV administration of a short-acting, coma-inducing drug such as propofol or thiopental. Intubation may be performed if the surgery requires administration of muscle relaxants to cause paralysis (as is the case in major surgical procedures such as abdominal surgery). Maintenance of anaesthesia is achieved using inhalational agents such as sevoflurane with nitrous oxide or air with a suitably high inspired oxygen concentration (FiO_2). Total intravenous anaesthesia using propofol may be used for maintenance and instead of an inhalation agent. During maintenance, muscle relaxants are often used to aid the surgical procedure and narcotics given for both intraoperative and postoperative analgesia. The process of reversal begins well before the surgeon has finished. Inspired anaesthetic concentrations are scaled back and drugs to reverse paralysis such as neostigmine are given. Analgesia is provided using narcotics or regional analgesia and extubation occurs once the patient can

protect their airway (gag reflex) (Euliano & Gravenstein 2004).

Induction of anaesthesia causes unavoidable changes in lung mechanics, lung defences and gas exchange. The most profound effect on the lung of a GA is the reduction in lung volumes, particularly functional residual capacity (FRC). These are discussed in a later section.

Management of acute postoperative pain

It has been suggested that pain in the early postoperative period may be the most important factor responsible for ineffective ventilation, poor cough, impaired ability to breath deeply and sigh, atelectasis, hypoxaemia and respiratory distress postoperatively (Sabanathan et al 1999). It is clear that pain is an important factor that can be modified postoperatively to attenuate some of the above physiological changes associated with surgery. For this reason it is critically important that postoperative pain management is optimum. Inadequate analgesia may delay discharge from hospital, cause sleep disturbances and limit early mobilization.

Reduction in acute postoperative pain facilitates improved patient comfort and satisfaction, reduced length of hospital stay and rehabilitation. Acute postoperative pain is the result of local tissue damage with release of algesic substances (prostaglandins, histamine, serotonin, bradykinin) and generation of noxious stimuli, which are transduced by nociceptors and transmitted by A-delta and C nerve fibres to the neuraxis. Complex modulating influences occur in the spinal cord, producing segmental responses including increased sympathetic stimulation, muscle spasm and increased gastrointestinal tone. Other impulses are transmitted to higher centres via the spinothalamic and spinoreticular tracts producing cortical and suprasegmental responses. These result in further increased sympathetic tone increasing metabolism and oxygen consumption (Ready 1985). The major anatomical targets for relief of postoperative pain are the peripheral tissues, nerve axons in peripheral nerves and dorsal nerve roots, the dorsal horn of the spinal cord and the brain. Many different methods of pain relief, directed to these different anatomical sites are available to patients. Several other factors may modify postoperative pain: these include the site and duration of surgery and the extent of the incision and surgical trauma. However, the physiological and psychological makeup of the patient and past pain experience also play a part. Postoperative pain is often accompanied by changes in autonomic activity, which are sympathetically mediated and include hypertension, tachycardia, sweating and decreased gut motility (National Health and Medical Research Council 2005).

12

Drug management of postoperative pain

Many different methods of pain relief are available, using several different routes of administration. Opiates and derivatives (such as morphine, pethidine, fentanyl) make up a large proportion of these drugs and morphine arguably remains the benchmark drug (Barrat 1997). Table 12.1 gives a summary of common routes of administration of drugs. In Table 12.2 a list of the common drugs used for postoperative pain is shown, together with their potential side effects.

Opioids are drugs that bind with specific opioid receptors. They mimic endogenous peptide transmitters involved in pain modulation and act principally within the central nervous system. Non-steroidal anti-inflammatory drugs (NSAIDs), such as indomethacin, are also used in management of acute postoperative pain and can act as opioid sparing agents. They decrease production of prostaglandins that sensitize nociceptor nerve endings to inflammatory mediators and also have an antipyretic effect (reduce fever). Local anaesthetic

Table 12.1   Common routes of drug administration for postoperative analgesia

Route	Description	Drug examples
Oral	Slow acting, drug is absorbed from the small intestine and therefore need a working gut for absorption (often not the case immediately after major surgery)	Paracetamol NSAIDs Codeine
IM	Maximum blood concentrations in 15–60 minutes. Absorption variable. Given 3–4 hourly. May only provide adequate analgesia for 35% of the 4 hours	Morphine Pethidine
IV (infusion)	The IV route provides a more rapid onset of action. Lower dose continuous infusion eliminates the peaks and troughs of IM administration. Need a loading bolus to reach analgesic blood concentration. Respiratory depression is high with continuous IV opioids	Morphine Pethidine Fentanyl Ketamine
PCA	The self-administration of small doses of analgesics by patients when they feel pain. Microprocessor pumps triggered by depressing a button. Pump is programmed to deliver a preset bolus dose but has a minimum period between doses called lock-out interval. Patients receive no drug if button is depressed during lock-out **Advantages:** Patient autonomy, elimination of delay of delivery of pain relief, less total narcotic dose, better pain relief than conventional parenteral regimens **Disadvantages:** Some patients cannot use, improper programming	Morphine Pethidine Fentanyl Ketamine
Epidural	A fine-bore catheter is inserted into the thoracic or lumbar epidural space (Fig. 12.2) by the anaesthetist at time of operation. Insertion site is sealed with OpSite dressing, and catheter is taped along its length up the patients back and over one shoulder. A pump is used to continuously infuse drugs via a bacterial filter. Nerve roots are blocked as they course from the spinal cord to IV foramina. Epidural can also be administered using a patient-controlled system (PCEA). The PCEA results in lower cumulative doses compared with continuous epidural infusions **Side effects:** hypotension, respiratory depression, total spinal block, causes motor and sensory block – patient unable to lift or feel legs. Block may be positional, nausea/vomiting, urinary retention, headache and neck stiffness	Fentanyl Bupivacaine Morphine Ropivacaine
Peripheral blocks	Have the advantage of less central side effects such as drowsiness. **Intercostal nerve blocks:** injection of local anaesthetic into main nerve supplying operative area or incision. Used for patients whose incisions are limited to thoracic dermatomes and are effective for incisional but not visceral pain **Intrapleural analgesia:** a catheter is placed in the interpleural space and local anaesthetic is administered to produce unilateral pain relief as it spreads through parietal pleura. Best for surgery with intact pleura. Not commonly used	Bupivacaine Ropivacaine

NSAIDs, non-steroidal anti-inflammatory drugs; IV, intravenous; IM, intramuscular; PCA, patient-controlled analgesia; PCEA, patient-controlled epidural analgesia

12

Table 12.2 Information about commonly used analgesic drugs

Drug	Dosage	Route of administration	Analgesic effect	Complications/side effects
Morphine Natural agonist opioid	5–20 mg, weight dependent: also adjusted for age and tolerance	IM: 10 mg (may vary) IV: 2–10 mg bolus, 1–3 mg/hour Infusion delivers more constant pain relief	Peak effect 3–40 min Lasts 4–6 hours	Respiratory depression, nausea, vomiting, sedation, hypotension, pinpoint pupils, decreased cough reflex, decreased sensitivity to hypercapnia or hypoxaemia
Pethidine Synthetic agonist opioid	Mean range 25–100 mg	IM: 25, 50 or 100 mg IV: 25–50 mg bolus, 10–40 mg/hour infusion	Onset 10 min post, lasts 2–4 hours, peak 20–30 min	As for all opioids
Fentanyl Synthetic agonist opioid	50–100 mcg	Often used in epidurals. Rarely given IM May be administered transdermally (e.g. cancer pain)	2–3 min onset, lasts 30–60 min Half-life 20 min	Reported decreased nausea and hypotension compared with morphine/pethidine
Codeine Low-efficacy opioid	10% converted to morphine	500 mg paracetamol + 8 mg codeine phosphate. Adults 1–2 tabs 3–4 hourly PRN, maximum 8/day or 500 mg paracetamol + 30 mg codeine. Adults 2 tabs 4/24, maximum 8/day	Most actions 1/6th those of morphine	Constipation. Large doses have an excitatory effect compared with morphine
Oxycodone Semi-synthetic narcotic	analgesic oral 5–10 mg, 4–6 hourly suppository dose = 30 mg, 6–8 hourly	Suppository (Prolodone) Oral (OxyContin or Endone)		As for morphine
Tramadol Synthetic opioid	50–100 mg 4–6 hourly (maximum 600 mg/day)	Oral – immediate release or slow release (for chronic or persistent pain) and IV	1 hour (approx) with peak effect 1–3 hours. Half-life: 4–6 hours	No respiratory depression but nausea and dizziness. CI – history of epilepsy or predisposition to seizures. Precautions: renal and hepatic impairment, raised ICP. Drug interactions – codeine

Table continues

Drug	Dosage	Route of administration	Analgesic effect	Complications/side effects
NSAIDs Non-steroidal anti-inflammatory drugs	e.g. Indometacin (Indocid) 50–200 mg daily	Suppository (100 mg) Oral (25 mg)	2–4 hours for full absorption (faster PR) Half-life 4.5 hours	GI ulcers/bleeding, tinnitus, oedema, dizziness, headache, rash, blurred vision, oedema. Can have adverse renal effects esp. if pre-existing renal dysfunction. *Contraindicated if active GI bleed or ulcer*
Bupivacaine Local anaesthetic	Bupivacaine hydrochloride maximum 2 mg/kg	Epidural infusion Local blocks, e.g. intercostal block	Anaesthetic agent	CNS, cardiovascular, respiratory and GI disturbances. Used with caution in hypotensive/bradycardic patients or those with cardiac problems, the elderly and children
Ketamine General anaesthetic and analgesic	Ketamine hydrochloride	IV or IM	Anaesthetic agent in larger doses Analgesic in low doses Useful for short procedures	Hypertension, arrhythmias, respiratory depression with rapid doses
Paracetamol	1 g in 4–6 hours maximum of 4 g in 24 hours	Oral or suppository	Analgesic	Liver toxicity in very high doses

(With permission from the School of Physiotherapy, University of Melbourne, Cardiorespiratory manual, School of Physiotherapy, 2006a)

mg, milligram; IV, intravenous; IM, intramuscular; CI, contraindication; ICP, intracranial pressure; GI, gastrointestinal; PRN, as necessary: min, minute; mcg, microgram; g, gram; CNS, central nervous system; PR, per rectal

12

agents such as bupivacaine, block the initiation and propagation of action potentials by blocking sodium channels. They are used to produce nerve root blocks and to depress action potentials in sensory neurons, thereby reducing pain (NHMRC 2005).

The use of multimodality analgesia rather than single analgesic administration is more common in the new millennium as is the existence of hospital pain management teams led by anaesthetists and nurses.

Opiates have significant respiratory depression effects (Sabanathan et al 1999) and they are only partially effective in relieving pain. Richardson and Sabanathan (1997) report that since opioids may only relieve pain transmitted by C fibres, where opioid receptors exist, the sharp pain transmitted by A fibres still exists. More recently, use of local anaesthetics (bupivacaine, ropivacaine) by the epidural route has gained more favour in postoperative pain management, often used

in combination with opioids. The introduction of these multimodal methods has also seen an increase in the use of NSAIDs such as indometacin. These are used as opioid sparing agents, but have also been shown to improve analgesia by a reduction in inflammation and stress inhibition (Richardson & Sabanathan 1997). There is level 1 evidence that oral administration of NSAIDs is as effective as intravenous (National Health and Medical Research Council 2005). Oral paracetamol or narcotic drugs may also be added to these regimens. Multimodal or balanced analgesia has been developed in response to the commonly associated side effects of monotherapy – nausea, vomiting, paralytic ileus and respiratory depression in the case of opioids and urinary retention, motor block and hypotension in the case of local anaesthetic agents. Balanced analgesia was also developed to allow early postoperative ambulation and enteral feeding, which minimize the respiratory and gut complications associated with use of opioids, leading to earlier patient discharge from hospital. The drugs are used in smaller doses than if used separately and provide effective pain relief as a result of their synergistic actions (Peeters-Asdourian & Gupta 1999).

The most common methods for pain control following abdominal surgery are patient-controlled analgesia (PCA) with intravenous opioids (Fig. 12.1) and continuous epidural analgesia delivering a combination of local anaesthetic and opioids (Fig. 12.2). In a recent systematic review it was concluded that continuous epidural analgesia is superior to PCA in relieving postoperative pain for up to 72 hours in patients undergoing intra-abdominal surgery. Similarly a large review of analgesia reports that all techniques of epidural analgesia provide better postoperative pain relief compared with parenteral opioid administration (NHMRC 2005). However, PCA remains a common method of analgesic delivery,

as patients often prefer it (Werawatganon & Charuluxanun 2005). Continuous infusion may be associated with increased risk of respiratory depression compared with bolus IV administration and evidence for improved pain relief with continuous administration is lacking (NHMRC 2005).

Non-pharmacological methods for managing postoperative pain are generally perceived to be adjuncts to pharmacological methods, but there is growing evidence for the value of their contribution (National Health and Medical Research Council 2005). Education including providing procedural information about treatment (such as provided by physiotherapists preoperatively), combined with sensory information describing the sensory experiences a patient may expect and information regarding coping strategies, may be effective in reducing negative affect, pain medication use and improving clinical recovery after surgery (National Health and Medical Research Council 2005). Preoperative education may encourage a more positive attitude toward pain relief, although there is no evidence that preoperative education about pain has any effect on postoperative pain after cardiac surgery (National Health and Medical Research Council 2005). Implementation of an acute pain management service may also improve pain relief.

Measurement of pain

Pain is difficult to measure as it is a purely individual and sensory experience (Dodson 1985). Postoperative pain is acute and initiated by tissue injury during surgery, but reduces with time and the natural healing process. The measurement of pain is often necessary to assess the results of an intervention or to measure intensity of pain, such as postoperative pain. Regular measurement of pain leads to improved acute pain management. Most measures of pain are based upon self-report but can provide sensitive and consistent results if performed properly (National Health and Medical Research Council 2005).

Several different instruments may be used to measure pain, these include:

- numerical rating scales
- verbal descriptor scales (VDS)
- pain questionnaires, such as the McGill
- the visual analogue scale (VAS).

Except for the McGill pain questionnaire, these methods are unidimensional; that is, they only measure intensity of pain in absolute terms or changes in pain intensity. Verbal scales may use words that have different meanings for different people, such as mild, moderate or severe pain. These categorical scales are quick and simple but less sensitive than numerical rating scales

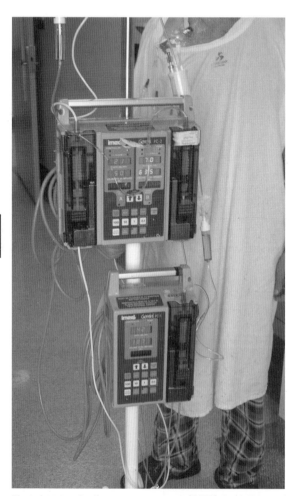

Figure 12.1 A microprocessor pump (IMED) for delivery of patient-controlled analgesia.

12

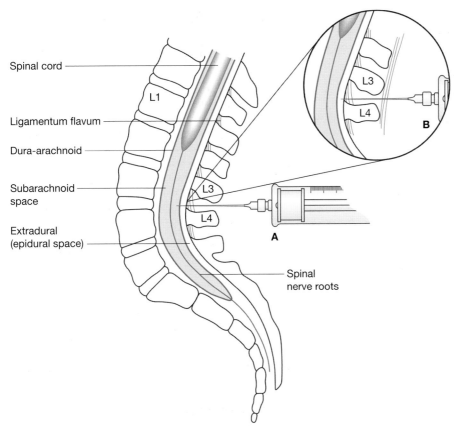

Spinal cord

L1

Ligamentum flavum

Dura-arachnoid

Subarachnoid space

Extradural (epidural space)

L3

L4

A

Spinal nerve roots

L3

L4

B

Figure 12.2 Spinal and epidural anaesthesia. (A) Position of needle in subarachnoid space for spinal anaesthesia. (B) Position of needle in epidural space for epidural anaesthesia/analgesia.

such as the visual analogue scale (VAS) (National Health and Medical Research Council 2005). The McGill questionnaire uses 20 groups of two to six words and the patient is asked which word in each group best describes their pain. While this offers more valid information than VDS, it is very time consuming and it not used extensively for the measurement of acute postoperative pain. Verbal rating scales are commonly used in clinical practice and use of the VAS is the most commonly used method. Visual analogue scales usually consist of a straight line, 10 cm long, the extremes of which are taken to represent the limits of the subjective experience being measured. In the case of pain measurement, one end of the line may be defined as 'no pain' and the other as 'severe pain' or 'worst possible pain'. The subject is asked to place a mark on the line corresponding to the severity of their pain. The distance from the mark to the end of the scale is taken to represent pain severity. The most common way to use a VAS in the study of postoperative pain is to ask the patient to score the pain they are experiencing at the time of completion of the VAS. Visual analogue scales may also be used to obtain a pain score that reflects pain or pain relief over the preceding 24 hours. Commonly, physiotherapists ask patients to rate their pain on activity in the postopera-

tive period to provide more meaningful information. The VAS has been shown to be a linear scale for patients with postoperative pain of mild to moderate intensity. Therefore results are equally distributed across the scale so that the difference between each number on the scale is equal. It is reported that values greater than 70 mm are indicative of severe pain while values between 45 and 74 mm represent moderate pain and those between 5 and 44 mm mild pain (National Health and Medical Research Council 2005).

Box 12.1 shows the physiotherapy key points with regard to analgesia.

Effects of the surgical process on respiratory function

The intra- and postoperative periods are frequently associated with alterations in pulmonary function (Craig 1981). Furthermore, altered physiological function of the respiratory system is an expected finding, especially after upper abdominal and thoracic surgery (Ford et al 1993). The combined effects of the GA, postoperative pain, recumbency, immobility and administration of drugs after surgery lead to several respiratory abnormalities.

12

Lung volumes

The characteristic abnormality of respiratory mechanics following major surgery is a restrictive ventilatory defect manifest by changes in vital capacity (VC) and functional residual capacity (FRC) (Wahba 1991). The

VC can reduce to 40% of preoperative values, while the FRC may gradually reduce to be 70% of preoperative value at 24 hours postoperatively. These changes may persist for 5–10 days following surgery (Craig 1981). The timing of greatest reduction in FRC, while varying between studies, is generally on the first or second postoperative day. In morbidly and even mildly obese patients there is a significant reduction in FRC compared with patients within the ideal weight range (Jenkins & Moxham 1991). Although most other lung volumes also reduce following major surgery, it is thought that the reductions in FRC represent the most clinically important changes because of the functional consequences. The alteration in lung volumes after lower abdominal and laparoscopic surgery is less pronounced.

Functional residual capacity and closing capacity

FRC may be affected by a number of factors. It is linearly related to height and is 10% less in females for the same body height (Nunn 1993). The FRC is affected by gravity and therefore body position. In supine the abdominal contents push the diaphragm cephalad, reducing intrathoracic volume and FRC. In normal subjects FRC is reduced by approximately 500–1000 ml upon adopting the supine position (Macnaughton 1994). It is highest in standing and reduces with recumbency (Fig. 12.3). A change in body position from bed to sitting in a chair increased the FRC by 17% in 10 patients following upper abdominal surgery.

The relationship of FRC with the closing capacity of the lungs explains the functional significance of periop-

12

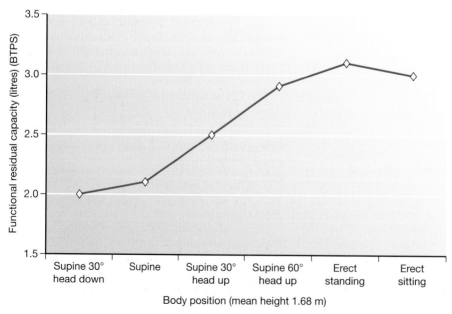

Figure 12.3 Functional residual capacity in different body positions. (Adapted from Nunn 1993 p 55 with permission from Butterworth-Heinemann, Oxford)

erative reductions in FRC. Closing capacity (CC) is defined as the lung volume at which dependent airways begin to close, or cease to ventilate (Macnaughton 1994). The small airways (less than 1.0 mm diameter) in the periphery of the lung are not supported by cartilage and are therefore influenced by transmitted pleural pressures. Normally the transpulmonary pressure or distending pressure is less than atmospheric, producing a positive pressure, which distends the lungs. Breathing at lower lung volumes produces a higher pressure in gravity-dependent lung regions. This produces a negative distending pressure and causes small, unsupported airways to narrow or close, resulting in reduced ventilation. The relationship between FRC and CC is an important determinant of dependent airway closure. If the CC exceeds the FRC, as it does during tidal breathing in the upright position in people over 70 years of age, then dependent lung regions underventilate, resulting in $\dot{V}/\dot{Q}$ mismatch and hypoxaemia. The relationship between CC and FRC is responsible for the reduction in arterial oxygen tension (PaO_2) with increasing age. Closing capacity increases with age due to loss of elastic lung tissue. It also increases in chronic lung disease and with cigarette smoking, due also to changes in lung elasticity. In combination with these increases in CC, any factor which at the same time reduces FRC will significantly affect the relationship between the two volumes, such that dependent airway closure occurs during normal tidal breathing (Macnaughton 1994) (Fig. 12.4).

Anaesthesia, surgery and recumbency reduce FRC. The reduction in FRC together with possible increases in CC in some subjects may account for the regional changes in ventilation that occur perioperatively and lead to reduced compliance, altered ventilation and perfusion ($\dot{V}/\dot{Q}$), arterial hypoxaemia and atelectasis from absorption of trapped gas behind closed airways. Postoperative hypoxaemia is inevitable, but usually subclinical, and like FRC, is usually lowest on the first and second days after surgery. Therefore supplemental oxygen is routinely given postoperatively (Craig 1981, Fairshter & Williams 1987).

The mechanisms for the perioperative reductions in FRC and VC in upper abdominal surgery (UAS) are thought to be: mechanical disruption of the thorax and abdomen, absence of spontaneous sighs, shallow breathing, pain and inhibition of diaphragmatic function (Wahba 1991). Abdominal distension, presence of a nasogastric tube and the use of analgesics to control postoperative pain may impact on ventilatory function.

Mucociliary clearance

Mucociliary clearance is a major function of the airway epithelium. This important function depends both on the physicochemical properties of the airway mucus and on the activity of the cilia (Kim 1997). Anaesthesia, intubation, mechanical ventilation reduced lung volumes and reduced cough effectiveness perioperatively present a significant insult to the mucociliary escalator. A summary of the perioperative contributions to altered mucociliary clearance is given in Box 12.2.

Respiratory muscle function

Diaphragmatic excursion has been shown in research literature to be reduced following abdominal and thoracic surgery and postoperative pain may contribute to diaphragm dysfunction. This is associated with reduced VC, changed pattern of ventilation to predominately rib cage movement rather than abdominal movement and postoperative hypoxaemia. The reduced function may last up to 1 week following surgery. Reflex inhibition of

12

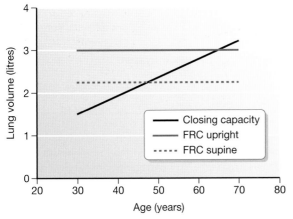

Figure 12.4 The relationship between functional residual capacity (FRC) and closing capacity. (Adapted from Nunn 1993 p 56 with permission from Butterworth-Heinemann, Oxford)

Box 12.2   Factors promoting postoperative mucociliary dysfunction

- Anaesthetic agents
- Endotracheal intubation
- Pain medication
- Higher inspired oxygen concentrations and airway humidification
- Atelectasis
- Reduced lung volumes
- Reduced cough efficiency
- Increased viscosity of secretions

(Adapted from Denehy and van de Leur 2004)

the phrenic nerve may occur after UAS, but research findings are inconsistent. The breathing pattern observed after abdominal surgery may act as a protective mechanism by splinting the abdomen, allowing faster healing of abdominal incisions and reducing the risk of peritoneal infection (Ford et al 1993).

Postoperative pulmonary complications

One of the aims of physiotherapy in the perioperative period is to counteract the adverse pulmonary changes produced as a result of the surgical process (Stiller et al 1994). The factors described above; dependent atelectasis, hypoxaemia and altered $\dot{V}/\dot{Q}$, although occurring in most patients, can lead to clinically significant PPC in some patients after surgery. Two basic theories have been proposed to explain the pathogenesis of PPC following major surgery. Firstly, regional hypoventilation and blockage of airways by mucus and, secondly, absorption of alveolar air distal to a mucus plug in the proximal airways, may lead to eventual collapse unless fresh air enters through collateral channels (Marini 1984). Regional hypoventilation results from reductions in FRC and the altered relationship between FRC and CC together with diaphragmatic dysfunction postoperatively as discussed above. The precise sequence and relative contributions of each of the two mechanisms for developing PPC is unclear. It is possible that they vary among patients and that both alveolar hypoventilation and secretion plugging coexist to contribute to postoperative lung changes (Denehy & Browning 2007). Other risk factors that may predispose to increased risk of mucus plugging may be a history of cigarette smoking, weak cough, prolonged intubation, presence of a nasogastric tube and prolonged postoperative atelectasis (Smith & Ellis 2000).

The definition of PPC can include atelectasis or pneumonia (atelectasis and collapse are terms that are often used interchangeably). Significant PPCs have been defined as complications that alter the patient's clinical course (O'Donohue 1992). PPC may be defined by using radiological and bacteriological criteria, clinical signs and symptoms, or a combination of these (Pasquina et al 2006). The definition of PPC impacts on the incidence obtained. Using only radiological evidence of atelectasis for example, gives a higher incidence of complications than using a combination definition. To date, no valid definition has been established and as a result the definitions used are variable.

The clinical signs and symptoms of PPC may include the following:

- arterial desaturation (measured using a pulse oximeter), often defined as <90% on two consecutive days

- radiological evidence of atelectasis or pneumonia (routine chest X-rays are not common after surgery)

- raised oral temperature (febrile is >37.5°C), often defined as >38°C on more than one consecutive day as a raised temperature on the first day after surgery is a common finding resulting from the surgical insult

- production of yellow or green sputum (where different to preoperative)

- abnormal lung auscultation (given that the majority of patients have some dependent atelectasis, reduced breath sounds are commonly found in the first 2 days after surgery)

- bacterial growth on sputum microbiology

- otherwise unexplained raised white cell count (>11 × 10^9/l)

- prescription of an antibiotic specific for lung infection (many patients are given routine antibiotics immediately postoperatively depending on type of surgery).

Many of these signs and symptoms occur in patients after major surgery and a combination of three or four, occurring together, could be considered as clinically significant PPC.

The incidence of postoperative atelectasis is reported to be 70% following UAS but the incidence of clinically significant complications is reported to range from 5% to 20% (Denehy et al 2001). There is a lower reported incidence following cardiac surgery of around 5%–7% (Brasher et al 2003, Pasquina et al 2003). The incidence following thoracic surgery varies but is reported to be 8–32% (Gosselink et al 2000). A higher incidence of 16% (Law & Wong 2006) to 30% (Gosselink et al 2000) is reported in patients following oesophageal surgery.

Risk factors for postoperative pulmonary complications

Advances in operative technique and postoperative patient management have led to surgery of increasing complexity being performed routinely in patient populations with more severe comorbidities. Estimation of surgical risk is therefore important for all health professionals involved in the management of surgical patients. Surgical risk is the probability of morbidity and mortality secondary to the presence of pre-, intra- and postoperative risk factors. This discussion will be limited to the development of PPC that most affects physiotherapists. Assessment of risk of developing PPC is important for the physiotherapist as it allows prioritized respiratory care for high-risk subjects and more appropriate use of often scarce resources in physiotherapy staffing. Surgical complications such as wound breakdown, bleeding, renal failure and other respiratory problems such as development of pulmonary embolus (PE) will not be discussed in detail. However, it is important to consider a PE in differential diagnosis of a respiratory complication such as pneumonia. The symptoms of both may be quite similar and include pleuritic chest pain, moderate to severe hypoxaemia, breathlessness and fever. Anticoagulation with heparin and then warfarin is indicated for PE. The identification of any pain in the calf on assessment is also important as it may indicate a deep vein thrombosis (DVT), although clinical diagnosis of DVT is unreliable with 50% of patients with DVT on venography showing symptoms.

Several patient characteristics are associated with an increased risk of developing complications. There is a large volume of literature published on this topic. In a systematic review (Fisher et al 2002), 40 variables were reported as possible risk factors for patients having non-thoracic surgery. There have been attempts to find a group of risk factors (model) that predict most complications in a particular patient population; several different models currently exist and none provide perfect prediction. The most common patient, operation and postoperative factors considered to increase risks of developing a PPC are described below. In physiotherapy research, a weighted model was developed to predict the risk of patients having abdominal surgery developing PPC (Scholes et al 2006). Five main risk factors (all these risk factors occurring together in one patient) were identified in this model, which predicted 82% of patients who developed a PPC in a population of 268 patients having upper abdominal surgery. Patients predicted as high risk were eight times more likely than those predicted to be at low risk of developing a PPC. The risk factors identified were:

- duration of anaesthesia >180 minutes
- type of surgery performed (upper abdominal)
- presence of preoperative respiratory problems, e.g. COPD
- current smoking (within last 8 weeks)
- reduced level of preoperative activity (measured using a questionnaire).

In addition to the risk factor model above, a systematic review of non-cardiopulmonary surgery (Smetana et al 2006) reports *good* evidence for the following risk factors to increase incidence of PPC:

- advanced age
- American Society of Anestheologists (ASA) classification of comorbidity of class 3–5
- functional dependence

- respiratory and cardiac disease
- serum albumin <3 g/dl.

Procedure-related risk factors that were supported by *good* evidence were thoracic, abdominal, emergency and prolonged surgery. There is *fair* evidence for significant intraoperative blood loss, oesophageal surgery and abnormal chest radiograph. However, in this systematic review, which presents the highest level of evidence, there was *good* evidence that the following were **not** important risk factors: obesity, asthma, hip and gynaecological surgery (lower abdominal surgery). These results challenge some traditional views, especially that of obesity being considered a risk factor. The results from this systematic review support the risk factors identified in the model by Scholes et al (2006). In patients having oesophageal surgery, age, operation duration and location of tumour in the proximal oesophagus were identified in one study as risk factors for PPC in 421 patients (Law et al 2004).

The ASA score (1–5) divides patients into five groups and collectively rates patient risk from anaesthesia. It was developed as a standardized way for anaesthetists to convey information about the patients' overall health status and to allow outcomes to be stratified by a global assessment of their severity of illness. In practice, the ASA score may be the only overall documentation of preoperative condition that is used widely. Generally, the attending anaesthetist ascribes a score to each patient upon preoperative assessment.

The classification of physical status recommended by the House of Delegates of the American Society of Anesthesiologists (1963) is:

1. a normal healthy patient
2. a patient with mild to moderate systemic disease
3. a patient with a severe systemic disease that limits activity, but is not incapacitating
4. a patient with an incapacitating systemic disease that is a constant threat to life
5. a moribund patient not expected to survive 24 hours with or without operation.

Box 12.3 shows key points in the surgical process.

TYPES OF SURGERY

Generally, surgical incisions are placed to optimize access to the target organ (Fig. 12.5). Understanding surgery involves an appreciation of the anatomy of the abdominal and thoracic organs and the muscles and bony structures surrounding them. An appreciation of nomenclature also aids understanding descriptions of operations. The prefix of words can help to locate the surgery: for example, *enter-* relates to small intestine,

12

gaster- to stomach, *pneum-* to lung. Surgical procedures may also be named for the person who first performed or reported them: for example, *Nissen* fundoplication, a wrap of fundus of the stomach around the intra-abdominal oesophagus; a *Whipple's* procedure, a pancreatico-duodenectomy; and *Hartmann's* procedure, a sigmoid colectomy with a colostomy.

Box 12.3　Key points in the surgical process

- Functional residual capacity (FRC) is reduced perioperatively as a result of anaesthesia, surgery and recumbency.
- FRC is increased in sitting and standing positions.
- The altered relationship between FRC and closing capacity is an important determinant of dependent airway collapse.
- Ventilation/perfusion ($\dot{V}/\dot{Q}$) mismatch and arterial hypoxaemia commonly occur after major surgery, although increases in CO_2 are rare unless patients are narcotized.
- Mucociliary clearance and cough effectiveness are reduced after surgery.
- Changes in pulmonary function after surgery generally resolve spontaneously with time from surgery.
- Clinically relevant postoperative pulmonary complication (PPC) may develop in a subset of patients having major surgery.
- A combination of clinical signs and symptoms is used to diagnose a PPC.
- Assessment of risk factors for developing PPC is important for the physiotherapist as it allows prioritized respiratory care for high-risk patients.

Understanding 'endings' of words also helps to work out the type of surgery (Table 12.3).

Abdominal surgery

Understanding abdominal surgery requires an appreciation of the anatomy of abdominal organs. The abdomen is a cavity lined by peritoneum and surrounded by muscle and skin. Abdominal organs may be intraperitoneal, and thus nourished via a mesentery (e.g. stomach), or extraperitoneal (e.g. pancreas). Some organs are both (e.g. liver).

Access to abdominal organs may be via their lumen, when there is one. This is called endoscopy (Greek *skopein* = to look at) where a fibre-optic telescope containing a light source and instruments are inserted. Examples are gastroscopy, colonoscopy and endoscopic retrograde choliangiopancreatography (ERCP). This may be used for diagnosis or therapy.

Laparoscopy involves insufflation of the peritoneal cavity with CO_2 gas (pneumoperitoneum), insertion of a camera through a 5–10 mm subumbilical incision and inspection of the abdominal contents using the transmitted picture and a monitor. Commonly three ports are used to introduce the instruments and perform the procedure. The technique is performed under general anaesthesia and the most common laparoscopic technique is for the removal of the gall bladder (cholecystectomy), but many other procedures are now performed this way including hernia repair, appendicectomy, splenectomy and oophorectomy (Harris 2006). The term minimal access surgery has been used to reflect the fact that the operations themselves are the same, but the surgical approach is less invasive, which impacts on the postoperative recovery of the patient. It has been well established in the literature that laparoscopic cholecys-

12

Table 12.3　Surgical terminology		
Ending	Meaning	Example
-tomy	Cut, cut out	Thoracotomy
-ect	Outside or extra	Gastrectomy (removal of stomach)
-stom	Mouth	Colostomy (an opening between the colon and skin)
-rraphy	Sew or suture	Herniorraphy (hernia repair)
-plasty	Mould or shape	Thoracoplasty (removal of ribs to collapse underlying diseased lung which reshapes the thorax)
-plico	To fold	Fundoplication (a wrap or fold of fundus of stomach)
-scop	To look at	Mediastinoscopy (look at mediastinum)

tectomy is associated with a low incidence of PPC (Sharma et al 1996).

Until the publication of a large randomized controlled trial (RCT) in 2004, there was a moratorium placed on laparoscopic cancer surgery owing to concerns regarding the oncological outcomes. This large (1200 cases) RCT reported that that there were no differences found in tumour recurrence using laparoscopic compared with open surgery. The benefits of this minimal access surgery have been reported, in a systematic review, to lead to lower morbidity, reduced postoperative pain, faster recovery of respiratory function, earlier recovery of bowel function and shorter length of hospital stay (laparoscopic patients were discharged a mean of 1.7 days earlier). Laparoscopic surgery, however, took 30% longer to perform (Tjandra & Chan 2006). There is an expanding interest in laparoscopic colorectal surgery but more research on the longer-term outcomes and standardizing surgical expertise are needed. Indeed, the more recent trend toward early postoperative rehabilitation also reduces length of hospital stay with improved patient quality of life after surgery. Therefore the integration of early 'fast tracking' rehabilitation with laparoscopic colorectal surgery may be required to fully evaluate the justification of the application of this surgery on a larger scale (Kehlet & Kennedy 2006).

A narrative literature review conducted by Olsen (2000) concluded that routine prophylactic chest physiotherapy is not necessary after laparoscopic upper gastrointestinal surgery such as fundoplication and vertical banded gastroplasty. The efficacy of physiotherapy in other forms of laparoscopic surgery such as colorectal surgery has not been investigated. A survey found that 58% of physiotherapists in Australian hospitals where laparoscopic colorectal surgery is performed routinely assess and treat these patients postoperatively (Browning, personal communication, 2006). However, future research examining the need for physiotherapy in this patient group is recommended.

Where minimally invasive procedures are not appropriate or possible, the abdominal cavity may be opened (laparotomy) through a variety of incisions placed to maximize access to the target organ. A midline incision is the most often used, as it allows access to most areas and may be easily extended to allow access to the whole of the abdominal cavity. The length and site of the incision has important implications for the amount of pain the patient may experience postoperatively and for the methods of controlling pain. Closing the surgical wound using different types of sutures may be achieved using continuous methods as in abdominal wounds or interrupted methods as in sternal wires. Staples are also used – they are faster but more expensive and produce a scar with a poorer cosmetic result than sutures. Many of the surgical complications that may occur are related to the incision, such as wound infection or dehiscence.

Abdominal surgery includes all operations involving the abdominal viscera. Colorectal and hepatobiliary surgery are most commonly encountered by physiotherapists, since they generally involve an incision above the umbilicus and are considered UAS (Celli et al 1984). Risk of PPC is greater in UAS than in lower abdominal operations such as hysterectomy. Many colorectal procedures are performed to remove cancer, colorectal cancer being the most common cause of cancer death (in non-smokers) in many Western countries. Conditions such as diverticulitis and ulcerative colitis are also common reasons for surgical intervention. Hepatobiliary procedures are performed for both malignant and benign diseases of the biliary tree. These include operations involving the liver, pancreas, spleen, duodenum, bile duct and gall bladder. Box 12.4 describes several commonly encountered abdominal operations.

Thoracic surgery

Thoracic surgery encompasses topics related to disorders of the chest wall, pleural space, lungs, oesophagus, mediastinum and chest trauma (Smith 2006). It has developed extensively in the past 50 years and now also includes lung transplantation (Chapter 15), video-assisted thoracoscopic surgery (VATS) and lung volume reduction surgery.

Most commonly, removal of part or all of the lung is performed to remove a carcinoma. Of over 3000 lung resections performed in 27 European centres, two-thirds of these were for lung cancer (Berrisford et al 2005). In Australia, the total number of new cases of lung, tracheal and bronchial cancers in 2005 was 9000 and this is predicted to increase (particularly in females) by 30% in 2011 with an ageing population. Lung cancer was the fourth most common cancer in both men and women in Australia in 2003 and presents a significant disease burden (AIHW & AACR 2007). It is reported to be the leading cause of cancer-related death in men and women worldwide (Hassan 2006).

Carcinoma of the lung

Cigarette smoking is the single most common predisposing factor for lung carcinoma, but other factors such as environmental or occupational exposure to hydrocarbons or asbestos are also implicated. There are several different pathological types of lung carcinoma; these are divided into non-small cell and small cell carcinoma. The non-small cell types are squamous cell, adenocarcinoma, large cell and adenosquamous carcinoma. Of these, squamous cell and adenocarcinoma are most

12

Box 12.4 Some commonly performed abdominal surgical procedures

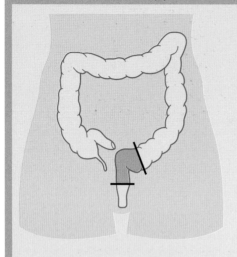

Anterior resection
Indication: Ca upper portion of rectum
Sigmoid colon to lower part of rectum

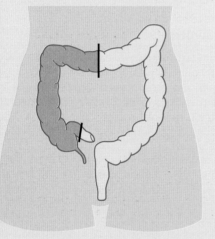

Right hemicolectomy
Indications: Ca right colon, terminal ileum
Incision: Right paramedian, midline, right oblique
Continuation restored by: Anastomosis of ileum to transverse colon

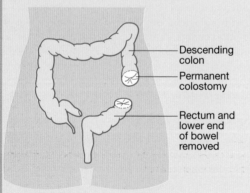

Descending colon

Permanent colostomy

Rectum and lower end of bowel removed

Abdomino-perineal (AP) resection/sigmoid colostomy
Indication: Ca lower portion large bowel and rectum, ulcerative colitis
Incisions: Laparotomy and perineal

12

box continues

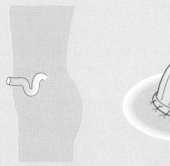

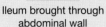

Ileum brought through
    abdominal wall

Valve with sutures

Ileostomy
Most are permanent (small bowel)

Indications: Ulcerative colitis, Crohn's disease, Ca of bowel

    Incision: Left paramedian or midline

    Operation: Continent pouch ileostomy

Reservoir constructed out of distal ileum: removal of
large colon and rectum

Outlet from reservoir is arranged as a valve so that
fluid cannot escape on to the abdominal wall

Colostomy
May be temporary

Indications: Ca, trauma, Crohn's disease, to rest bowel

Incision: Depends on site of colostomy

Operation: Stoma formed from colon. Names according to section of colon it is situated in, e.g. ascending
Types of sigmoid colostomy permanent (performed for abdomino-perineal resection – Ca rectum)

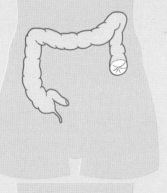

Single-barrelled colostomy
Permanent if bowel distal to colostomy is resected

Double-barrelled colostomy
Both loop distal and proximal are opened, may be
permanent or temporary depending on disease

12

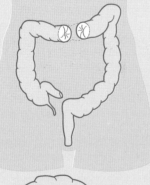

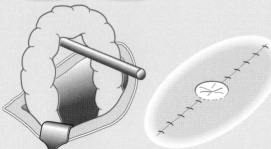

Loop colostomy
Usually formed in transverse colon. Loop of bowel brought
out through incision, plastic

box continues

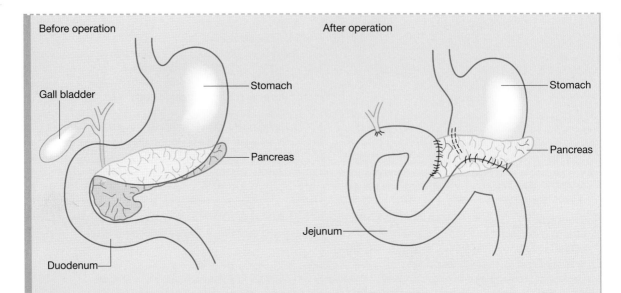

Before operation

Gall bladder

Stomach

Pancreas

Duodenum

After operation

Stomach

Pancreas

Jejunum

Whipple's procedure (pancreaticoduodenectomy)
May be required when severe pancreatitis is confined to the head of the gland or in Ca
Resection of the distal stomach, common bile duct, duodenum, gall bladder and the pancreas to the mid-body

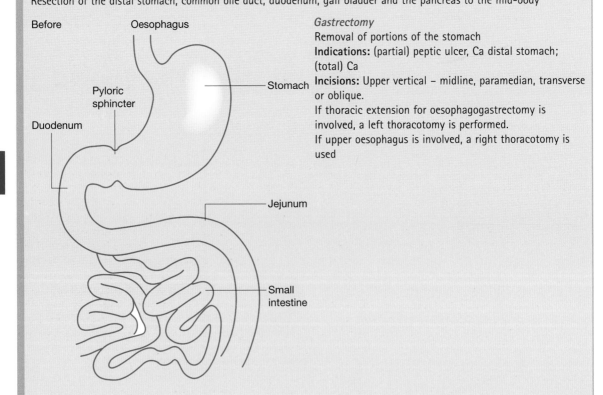

Before

Oesophagus

Pyloric
sphincter

Duodenum

Stomach

Jejunum

Small
intestine

Gastrectomy
Removal of portions of the stomach
Indications: (partial) peptic ulcer, Ca distal stomach; (total) Ca
Incisions: Upper vertical – midline, paramedian, transverse or oblique.
If thoracic extension for oesophagogastrectomy is involved, a left thoracotomy is performed.
If upper oesophagus is involved, a right thoracotomy is used

12

box continues

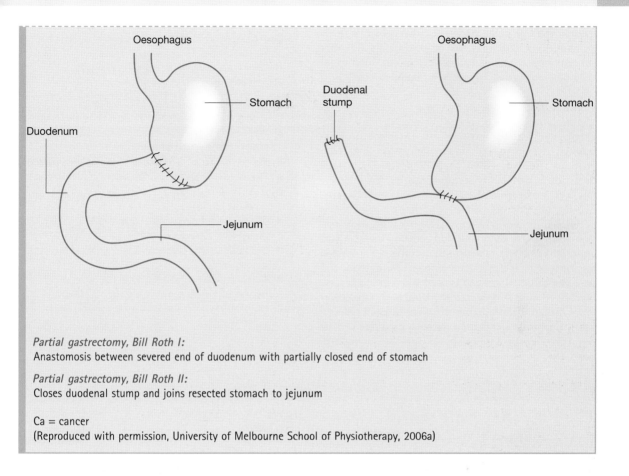

Partial gastrectomy, Bill Roth I:
Anastomosis between severed end of duodenum with partially closed end of stomach

Partial gastrectomy, Bill Roth II:
Closes duodenal stump and joins resected stomach to jejunum

Ca = cancer
(Reproduced with permission, University of Melbourne School of Physiotherapy, 2006a)

common, making up approximately 80% of all lung cancers (Smith 2006). Small cell carcinomas are the most malignant and make up about 10% of presentations of lung cancers. Extrathoracic spread is common at the time of presentation.

Thoracic clinical signs and symptoms of lung cancer include: cough, haemoptysis, chest pain, hoarse voice (if recurrent laryngeal nerve involved), shortness of breath, arm pain and weakness. There may be other symptoms depending on the extent and site of metastases at presentation, such as bone, liver or central nervous system involvement. Physical findings may include loss of weight, fatigue, finger clubbing, pleural effusion or lung collapse. Several investigations may be undertaken to determine the cell type, extent and location of the carcinoma; these include chest radiograph, pulmonary function tests, computed tomography (CT) scan, needle biopsy of tumour under CT control, bronchoscopy, mediastinoscopy, positron emission tomography (PET) scan, ventilation/perfusion scan, and sputum cytology.

Lung cancer is staged depending on the size and location of the tumour (T), the amount of spread to lymph nodes in the thorax (N), and the presence or absence of metastases (M). Each of these is further divided and scored from 0 to 4 (for example $T_1N_0M_0$). The TNM classification is used internationally for all non-small cell lung cancers to give information about prognosis and to guide therapy (Hassan 2006). The most prognostic indicator in lung cancer is the extent of the disease. Early-stage cancer lung cancer ($T_1N_0M_0$ and $T_2N_0M_0$) have a potentially high curability with surgery (Hassan 2006). The common sites for distant spread are to mediastinal lymph nodes, brain, liver, bones, kidneys and pancreas.

For those presenting with localized tumours and an adequate respiratory reserve, surgical resection offers the only curative treatment. However, only about one-third of presentations are considered for surgery. The 5-year survival (number of patients still surviving at 5 years) from curative surgery is about 30%, but the overall 5-year survival is only 15% (Smith 2006). Radio-

12

therapy may be given and is usually palliative, as is chemotherapy. Both may also be used before and after surgical resection. For small cell carcinoma, multiagent chemotherapy is the only current treatment.

Surgical resection

Thoracotomy allows access to the lung. A full posterolateral thoracotomy involves an extensive incision through the 5th or 6th intercostal space (Fig. 12.5) including muscular division of trapezius, latissimus dorsi, lower rhomboids, serratus anterior, the intercostals and erector spinae. A rib retractor is used to separate the ribs and sometimes a partial rib resection is performed to improve exposure of the lung. This incision is used less commonly but remains the standard approach. A lateral (axillary) thoracotomy is a limited muscle sparing incision made between the anterior and posterior axillary lines and is used when limited access is required as in surgery of the pleura such as pleurectomy. Anterior thoracotomy involves a small incision below the breast and is used for open lung biopsy. The common thoracic surgical procedures are defined in Box 12.5.

Box 12.5   Common thoracic surgical procedures

The types of thoracic operations that may be performed are:

- Pneumonectomy (removal of whole lung)
- Lobectomy (removal of an entire lobe of the lung)
- Wedge and segmental resections (removal of a segment or a wedge of lung tissue)
- Pleurectomy (partial stripping of the parietal pleura)
- Pleurodesis (application of an irritant to the pleura)
- Decortication (removal of thickened pleura ± drainage of pus)
- Video-assisted thorascopic surgery (VATS) (minimally invasive surgery)
- Oesophagectomy (removal of part or all of the oesophagus)
- Oesophagogastrectomy (removal of the lower portion of the oesophagus and the stomach)

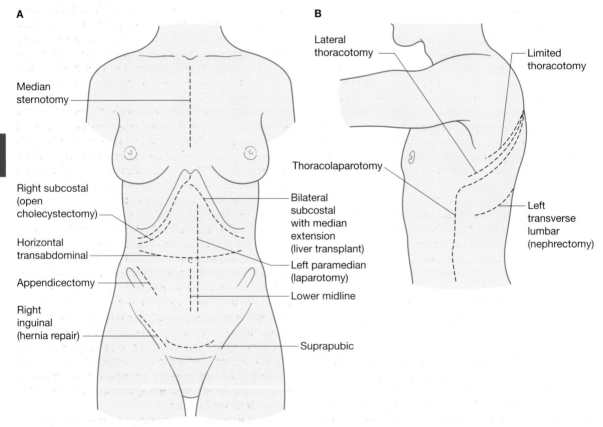

Figure 12.5   Common surgical incisions.

Minimally invasive surgery using thoracoscopy is now used where possible. This technique offers less surgical trauma and reduced recovery time and is the thoracic equivalent of laparoscopy. Video-assisted thorascopic surgery (VATS) simultaneously uses a light source, camera and telescope through several ports of access made by 2 cm incisions in the chest wall. Commonly three ports are used: one for the telescope, light and camera and two for surgical instruments. This technique is used commonly for pleural surgery such as pleurectomy performed for recurrent pneumothorax, as well as increasingly for smaller lung resection procedures.

Oesophageal surgery

Oesophageal surgery is generally performed for carcinoma and has a high mortality usually due to late disease presentation. Surgery may be performed after combined treatment of chemotherapy and radiotherapy or may be palliative to provide symptom relief. Patients generally present with symptoms of dysphagia (problems with swallowing); other common symptoms include loss of weight, regurgitation and substernal pain. The sites of metastases are similar to the lung and include cervical lymph nodes, lungs, liver, bones and other viscera.

The surgical approach for carcinoma of the middle and lower thirds of the oesophagus is by laparotomy (to mobilize and prepare the stomach) and right thoracotomy (to resect the oesophagus); this is commonly known as an Ivor Lewis oesophagectomy. The stomach is delivered up into the thorax to anastomose with the remaining proximal oesophagus through the diaphragmatic hiatus. In carcinoma of the upper oesophagus, a neck incision is used in conjunction with the laparotomy and thoracotomy to allow anastomosis (Law & Wong 2006).

Placement of a prosthetic tube or now more commonly a stent to restore luminal patency provides symptom relief of dysphagia for carcinoma that is not otherwise suitable for other treatments. Laser therapy to vaporize the tumour is also used.

Surgery of the pleura

Pleural surgery is commonly performed for recurrent pneumothorax, pleural effusion and empyema.

Pneumothorax

Pneumothorax is defined as the presence of air in the pleural space. The common types of pneumothorax are primary spontaneous, secondary spontaneous, tension and traumatic (Smith 2006). *Primary spontaneous pneumothorax* is the most common and usually results from the rupture of a tiny bleb at the apex of the lung. Clinical

signs may include acute chest pain and shortness of breath or shortness of breath on exertion. It commonly occurs in tall thin individuals of either sex. The size of the pneumothorax will usually dictate the management approach. This may include observation and repeat chest radiographs, needle aspiration of air directly from the pleural space or insertion of intercostal drainage. Spontaneous pneumothorax may be recurrent, with figures suggesting that about 30% recur. After a second episode this figure increases to 70%. Surgical management is usually indicated after two pneumothoraces on the same side and this most commonly involves pleurectomy or pleurodesis to allow the visceral pleura to adhere to the parietal, which thereby obliterates the 'potential' pleural space.

Secondary pneumothorax occurs as a result of underlying lung disease such as COPD or lung abscess. *Traumatic pneumothorax* occurs after penetrating trauma such as by a rib fracture, knife or gunshot wound. Traumatic pneumothoraces are usually accompanied by *haemothorax*, which is defined as an accumulation of blood in the pleural space. Bleeding may be from the chest wall, heart, major vessels or lungs. When it occurs in conjunction with a pneumothorax it is called a haemopneumothorax. *Lung contusion* is also common in traumatic lung injury and involves injury to lung parenchyma, oedema and blood collecting in the alveoli and an inflammatory reaction to blood components in the lung. Gas exchange may be significantly affected by contusion, which may lead to acute respiratory distress syndrome (Trauma.org 2004).

Tension pneumothorax results when the site of air leak acts as a one-way valve so that air enters the pleural space during inspiration but cannot escape during expiration. The volume of air and pressure in the hemithorax increase, resulting in compression of the ipsilateral lung, mediastinal shift away from the side of pneumothorax including shift of the trachea, and possible kinking of the great vessels if the mediastinal shift is large. Clinical signs include deviation of the trachea, absent breath sounds, acute respiratory distress, raised jugular venous pressure and hypotension, Tension pneumothorax can be life threatening and should be relieved as soon as possible by insertion of a large-bore needle to let the air escape under pressure followed by insertion of an intercostal drain (Smith 2006). Figure 12.6 shows different types of pneumothorax and flail chest.

Following open thoracic surgical procedures (including VATS), intercostal drainage tube(s) are positioned in the pleural space before surgical closure and connected to a closed drainage system called underwater sealed drainage (UWSD).

Key points for physiotherapy in thoracic surgery are shown in Box 12.6.

12

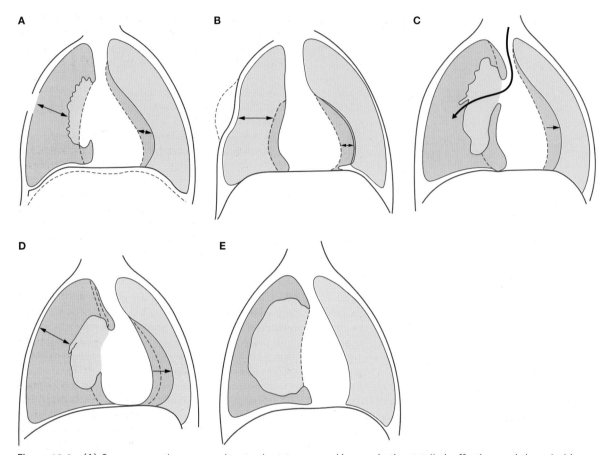

Figure 12.6 (A) Open pneumothorax secondary to chest trauma making respiration totally ineffective as air is sucked in and out of the open wound. (B) Flail chest secondary to multiple anterior and posterior rib fractures, resulting in chest wall instability. (C) Tension pneumothorax allowing air to enter the pleural space with each inspiratory breath. (D) Tension pneumothorax on expiration. The hole in the lung closes on expiration, resulting in a build-up of pressure in the pleural space with mediastinal shift. (E) Partial pneumothorax. Partial collapse of the lung away from the chest wall but not under tension.

12

Underwater seal drainage units are a system used specifically to drain air and/or fluid from the thoracic cavity in order to regain and/or maintain re-expansion of the lung by re-establishing normal negative pressure in the pleural space. Effective gas exchange will only occur if the lungs are able to expand sufficiently to allow adequate ventilation. The pleural membranes assist with this vital function. Each lung sits in its own pleural cavity and is attached to the mediastinum. The exterior surface of the lung is covered by a thin, serous membrane called the visceral pleura. At the root of the lung, the visceral pleura become continuous with the parietal pleura, which line the wall of the pleural cavity. Separating the two membranes is approximately 10 ml of serous pleural fluid, produced by the pleural membranes. This fluid acts to lubricate the pleural surfaces and reduces friction between the parietal and visceral pleura during respiration.

A negative pressure exists between the visceral and parietal pleura. It acts to provide a suction between the two membranes, counteracting the tendency of the lungs to recoil. Intrapleural pressure varies slightly throughout the different phases of the ventilatory cycle. Before inspiration, the intrapleural pressure is approximately -5 cmH$_2$O. During inspiration the chest wall expands, decreasing the negative pressure to approximately -8 cmH$_2$O, which allows the lung to expand and air to flow inward. During expiration, the intrapleural pressure decreases to approximately -4 cmH$_2$O, allowing the air to flow from the lung to the atmosphere.

While the intrapleural space remains intact and free of all but a small amount of pleural fluid, the negative

Box 12.6   Key points for physiotherapy in thoracic surgery

- Attention to pain management is essential for effective treatment outcomes.
- Pulmonary reserve is reduced in patients having pneumonectomy.
- Care must be taken with positioning patients after pneumonectomy. In general, patients may be positioned on to their operation side (so that the remaining lung is uppermost). However, the protocol in some units requires patients to remain sitting for the first 3–6 days until the fluid in the hemithorax which replaces the removed lung has become more organized (fibrous). Once this has occurred there is much less risk of fluid entering the anastomosis of the bronchial stump and potentially spilling into the remaining lung. Physiotherapists must check with individual surgeons/units regarding local protocol.
- A serious complication of pneumonectomy is pulmonary oedema. Postoperative fluid balance is important since the entire cardiac output is directed through only one lung. A positive fluid balance together with signs of tachypnoea, tachycardia and hypoxaemia should be reported immediately.
- After pneumonectomy, the fluid in the hemithorax is controlled by clamping and releasing the intercostal catheter (ICC). This management is different to that after other thoracic surgery where the ICCs are on gravity drainage ± suction.
- Patients having oesophageal surgery are often undernourished preoperatively and this may affect anastomotic healing and general progress after surgery.
- The head-down position is usually avoided after oesophageal surgery to prevent gastric reflux which may lead to aspiration or affect the integrity of the anastomosis. Head-up positions (for example on two pillows) are preferred.
- Neck extension should be avoided in patients after oesophageal surgery that involve neck incisions.
- Nasopharyngeal suction should be avoided if possible.
- Positive pressure should be applied with caution and not at all unless a functioning nasogastric tube is in situ and on free drainage.
- The nasogastric tube is placed intraoperatively to provide drainage. If removed accidentally it cannot be replaced, so care must be taken when moving the patient.
- There is no absolute contraindication to positioning a patient in side lying or head down after lobectomy or pleurectomy.

pressure required to hold the membranes together will be maintained. However, if air or fluid of any kind is allowed to enter the pleural space, the negative pressure will be lost and the affected lung will partially or fully collapse. In such cases, an underwater seal drain may be indicated to remove the fluid or air from the pleural space, thus restoring the negative pressure necessary to allow lung expansion.

Underwater sealed drainage is indicated in the presence of any surgery or trauma where there has been a significant disruption to the integrity of the pleural space. The most common substances to enter the intrapleural space are air, blood, pus or an excess of pleural fluid. These may appear alone or in combination, and cause an increase in intrapleural pressure from negative to positive, thus terminating the suctioning effect and resulting in collapse of the lung.

Intercostal catheters (chest tubes)

A chest tube is generally made of clear pliable plastic into which a radio-opaque strip may be incorporated. The diameter of the tube will vary depending on the size of the patient and on what is being drained. A smaller drain is usually employed to evacuate air while a larger drain is used for fluids (Miller & Sahn 1987).

The location of the substance to be drained usually determines the placement of the tube. When the patient is upright, fluids in the pleural space will generally gravitate to the lower zones of the thorax, while air will usually rise to the apex. Therefore, for drainage of a pneumothorax the tube is usually inserted anteriorly in the mid clavicular line into the 2nd or 3rd intercostal space or in the mid axillary line in the 3rd to 5th space and is directed towards the apex of the thorax. When fluids are to be drained, the tube is usually inserted slightly lower, in the mid axillary line and the 6th space, and directed basally. Following surgery such as lobectomy or pleurectomy, two intercostal catheters are inserted: one is usually directed apically and one basally.

Principles of underwater seal drainage

The underwater seal

The underwater seal prevents air re-entering the pleural space. Usually, the distal end of the drain tube is submerged 2 cm under the surface level of water in the drainage (or collection) chamber. This creates a hydrostatic resistance of $+2 \, cmH_2O$ in the drainage chamber.

Creation of a pressure gradient

Normal intrapleural pressure is negative. However, if air or fluid enters the pleural space, intrapleural pressure becomes positive. Air is eliminated from the pleural

12

space into the drainage chamber when intrapleural pressure is greater than +2 cmH$_2$O. Thus, air moves from a higher (intrapleural) to lower pressure (within the drainage chamber) along a pressure gradient. The drainage chamber has a vent to allow air to escape the chamber, and not build up within the chamber.

Gravity

Fluids will drain by gravity into the drainage chamber, and will not spill back into the pleural space if the bottle is always kept below the level of the patient's chest. If the bottle needs to be lifted above the chest (e.g. during a patient transfer), the tubing should be briefly double clamped as close to the patient as possible. The movement and unclamping should take place as quickly as possible to minimize clamping time.

Types of underwater seal drainage systems

One-bottle system

The simplest form of UWSD is a one-bottle system. This system can drain both air and fluid. The distal end of the drainage tube must remain under the water surface level. There is always an outlet (vent) to the atmosphere to allow air to escape. A problem with this system is that when fluid starts to fill the chamber it creates a more positive (hydrostatic) pressure due to a rise in the fluid level (Fig. 12.7). Thus it is more difficult for air to escape from the pleural space into the drainage chamber due to a reduced pressure gradient (in this situation, a two-bottle system is preferable). A single-bottle system is suitable for use with a simple pneumothorax, when the vent is left open to the atmosphere, or following a pneumonectomy when the tubing is clamped and released hourly.

Two-bottle system

This system is suitable for drainage of air and fluid (Fig. 12.7). The first chamber is for collection of fluid and the second is for the collection of air. As the two are separate, fluid drainage does not adversely affect the pressure gradient for evacuation of air from the pleural space. A separate chamber for fluid collection enables monitoring of volume and expelled matter (e.g. pus, blood clots).

Three-bottle system

When air or fluid needs a greater pressure gradient to move from the pleural space to the collection system (e.g. excess volume of fluid or a large air leak), suction is required. Suction may be applied via a third bottle or suction chamber. (The first two bottles are as described above.) With this system, suction is regulated by the depth of the tube under the water in the suction chamber (rather than the pressure setting at the wall). As the wall suction is applied, air is pulled into the suction chamber from the atmosphere and bubbling occurs. Note: it is the depth of water that regulates the amount of negative pressure (suction) not the wall suction pressure. The difficulties with the systems described are that they are complex and have many connections, all of which must be intact. With these systems there is a danger that the glass bottles will break or tubing becomes disconnected.

Disposable (all-in-one) three-bottle systems

This refers to the combination of the three-bottle system into one device for easier connection and management. There are many different systems used in clinical practice and when examining these systems it is useful to remember that they are simply a three-bottle system: one chamber collects fluid, one chamber collects air and has the underwater seal and the other is the suction control chamber. These systems are easier to move around and carry during patient ambulation as they have carrying handles and hooks.

Waterless 'dry' suction systems

There are some systems in use that operate on a waterless suction system. The level of suction is set on a dial; then the wall suction is turned on slowly to the point where an indicator denotes that suction is set at the required level. The column of water is replaced with a calibrated spring mechanism accurate to ±1 cmH$_2$O. If suction from the wall exceeds the level set on the suction dial, a chamber opens allowing excessive sucking to be applied to the atmosphere and not the patient. It has some advantages over water-sealed drains: it is silent, has no water levels to evaporate, a high level of suction is available and it is easy to set up.

Patient assessment and underwater seal drainage systems

As part of a physiotherapy objective assessment, specific examination of a UWSD system should be performed. There are four important aspects of examination – swing, bubbling, drainage, and suction.

Swing. The intrapleural pressure changes that occur during inspiration and expiration are transmitted to the drainage system. During inspiration, when a more negative pressure is generated, fluid moves up the tube of the drainage collection chamber and during expiration the movement is in the opposite direction. This movement of fluid along the tube during normal breathing is termed 'swing'. It may be a small movement during quiet breathing or a large movement when the patient is coughing or during an increased inspiratory effort. If

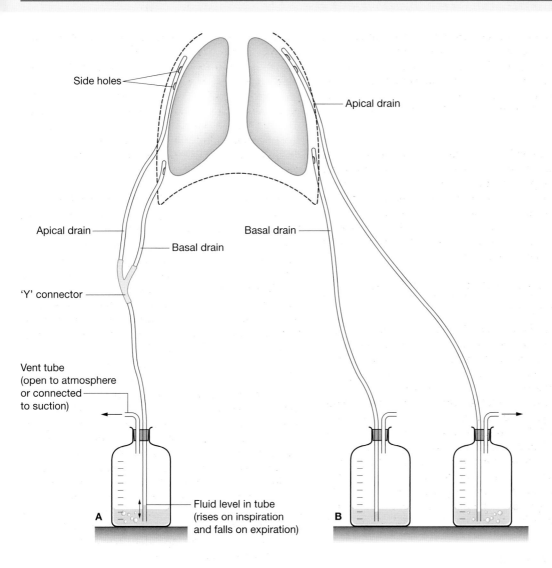

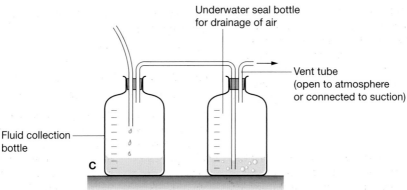

Figure 12.7   Underwater seal chest drainage. (**A**) Single-bottle system allowing use of one bottle via a 'Y' connector to drain fluid and air. (**B**) Two separate bottles enabling drainage of air from the apical drain and fluid from the basal drain. (**C**) Two-compartment drainage system where two bottles are connected in series, the first collecting fluid and the second acting as the underwater seal drainage for air.

12

the patient is attached to suction, pressure is more regulated and swing is reduced.

If no swing is seen:

- the tubing may be kinked
- the patient may be lying on the tube
- there may be a dependent fluid-filled loop of tubing
- the lung may be re-expanded (lung tissue blocks off the eyelets).

Bubbling. The presence or absence of bubbling in the underwater seal chamber of the system should be determined. Bubbling in the underwater seal chamber indicates an air leak (from the pleural space). It is important not to confuse the bubbling in the underwater seal chamber with the bubbling in the suction chamber. The bubbling in the suction chamber indicates suction is applied to the system at the correct level. The following points should be considered:

- no bubbling indicates absence of an air leak
- bubbling on coughing indicates a small air leak
- bubbling on expiration indicates a moderate air leak
- bubbling throughout inspiration and expiration indicates a large air leak.

When examining the underwater sealed drainage system, ask the patient to take a deep breath and observe for swinging and bubbling. If there is no bubbling at this time, ask the patient to cough and observe for bubbling. Assessment for air leak (from the pleural space) must include observation of the underwater seal chamber during coughing.

Drainage. It is important to note the pattern of drainage of fluid from the chest drain for two reasons:

- when drainage is reduced to 100 ml over 24 hours the tube may (usually) be removed
- large amounts of blood draining over a short period of time may indicate haemorrhage.

Large amounts of haemoserous drainage may also be associated with hypovolaemia, hypotension and low haemoglobin. It is not uncommon for some drainage to occur during patient movement: e.g. transfers and exercise. Generally, drainage of more than 100 ml per hour or a sudden increase in drainage is cause for concern and medical staff should be informed if this occurs.

Suction. As previously mentioned, it is the level of water in the suction chamber that regulates the amount of suction. When the wall suction is applied, this should result in gentle bubbling only (in the suction chamber). Vigorous bubbling will not increase the amount of suction applied and will cause evaporation of the water in the suction tube. No bubbling in the suction chamber indicates that the wall suction is not sufficiently high and needs to be increased. (It is very important to check that all tubing connections are intact before increasing the suction.) In some cases of persistent air leak, suction may be switched off to facilitate healing. The more common systems used now are integrated all-in-one disposable systems. General criteria for removal of intercostal catheters and underwater sealed drains are outlined in Box 12.7, while Box 12.8 gives key points for underwater sealed drainage.

Cardiac surgery

Cardiac surgery has been performed since the 1960s following the introduction of cardiopulmonary bypass. It is performed for both congenital (Chapter 10) and acquired heart diseases and can be closed surgery (without the need for cardiopulmonary bypass) or open-heart surgery (OHS). The most common adult cardiac surgery is performed for ischaemic heart disease. Table 12.4 lists common types of congenital abnormalities that require cardiac surgery. This chapter will focus on the management of coronary artery disease and valve pathology.

Coronary artery disease

Coronary atherosclerosis is a significant disease, particularly of Western countries. Atherosclerosis is the hardening and narrowing of arteries due to atheroma (from the Greek word meaning 'porridge'). It develops in larger vessels (>2 mm internal diameter) mainly as a result of longer-term injury to the endothelium. An initial 'fatty streak' lesion is caused by increased permeability of the endothelial cells. Following this, accumulation of oxidized low-density lipoprotein by macrophages and infiltration of T lymphocytes leads to the development of a white fibrolipid plaque. This plaque may ulcerate and a thrombus can form and may embolize. The risk of rupture and haemorrhage of the plaque (fissuring) is high. Coronary vessels commonly develop lesions proximally at the origins of the main coronary

---

Box 12.7   General criteria for removal of intercostal catheters and underwater sealed drains

- Less than 100 ml of drainage in 24 hours
- Minimal swing
- Chest X-ray establishing full lung expansion
- Breath sounds present over the whole thorax on auscultation
- No air leak

Box 12.8   Key points for underwater sealed drainage

- The water seal must remain intact at all times. Therefore, the water seal chamber must always be in an upright position. If the water seal chamber is tipped over such that the tip of the tube is above the water surface level, air can re-enter the pleural cavity.
- The drainage system must always be kept below the patient's chest or clamped briefly if it must be raised above this level.
- If a patient with an air leak needs to lie on the drain tubing, it is important to ensure that air may continue to drain from the pleural space into the UWSD system, and that the weight of the patient does not result in occlusion of the tubing. If the latter were to occur, a tension pneumothorax could result.
- If the tubing becomes disconnected, it should be clamped by hand as close to the patient as possible. The drain may be immediately reconnected only if the ends of the tubing have avoided contact and contamination. A nurse should be called to help with reconnection. The risk of this occurring can be minimized by checking all connections of the chest drain before moving the patient. When a patient is getting out of bed or moving around in the bed, care should be taken that the patient does not lean on the chest tubing.
- If the chest drain falls out, the wound should be covered immediately with a gloved hand and urgent assistance called for.
- If positive pressure is being used (continuous positive airway pressure, bilevel positive airway pressure,

intermittent positive pressure breathing and manual hyperinflation) in the presence of an air leak, the air leak needs to be constantly monitored as it may be exacerbated by these techniques. For example, during application, the air leak may be present on expiration when previously it was observed only on coughing.
- The pain from a chest drain can be quite severe and may limit the patient's ability to cooperate with physiotherapy treatment.
- Patients should be able to move around with their chest drain in situ. They should be encouraged to keep the shoulder of the affected side moving, and generally discouraged from adopting protective postures.
- Patients may be disconnected from suction and taken for a walk, but communication with the medical and nursing team is essential regarding unit policy. It is important to ensure that the underwater sealed drainage system is kept below the level of the chest at all times.
- If the patient cannot be disconnected from suction, walking within the confines of the suction tubing or marching on the spot may be attempted.
- If a patient is being disconnected from suction, it is essential that the tubing from the collection chamber to the suction is disconnected rather than just switching the wall suction off. (If the patient is left connected to the wall suction with the suction switched off, there is no vent to the atmosphere through which air may escape from the pleural space and a tension pneumothorax may occur).

12

Table 12.4   Common congenital abnormalities of the heart

Abnormality	Description
Patent ductus arteriosus (PDA)	Persistent large PDAs at birth allow shunting of blood from the aorta back into the pulmonary circulation. The ductus is closed using endovascular techniques or thoracotomy
Coarctation of the aorta	A narrowing of the aorta, most commonly distal to the left subclavian artery. Treated by angioplasty or resection with grafting
Atrial septal defects (ASDs) and ventricular septal defects (VSDs)	Incomplete or failure of development of the interatrial (ASD) or interventricular (VSD) septa. The defects are closed with a prosthetic patch during open heart surgery

branches or at major branch points. A narrowing (>50%) of coronary arteries causes reduced blood flow to the area supplied by that vessel. Common sites of obstruction are the left anterior descending artery, the right coronary artery and the circumflex artery.

Angina occurs when the heart muscle is underperfused and lacks the required oxygen supply as a result of obstruction of a coronary vessel. Angina pectoris is acute pain described as 'crushing, vice-like, tight, or squeezing pain'; it may be retrosternal or radiate to the jaw, left arm or neck. The reason for this distribution of pain is that during embryonic development the heart originates in the neck, as do the arms. Therefore, these structures receive pain nerve fibres from the same spinal cord segments. Angina commonly occurs on exertion/exercise and is relieved by rest and medication such as sublingual glycerol trinitrate. The myocardial perfusion is reversible and does not cause permanent damage.

Myocardial infarction (MI) occurs with prolonged or permanent occlusion, causing severe chest pain at rest (which may be 'silent'), which lasts several hours and is accompanied by autonomic responses such as sweating, nausea and vomiting. Myocardial infarction involves necrosis of cardiac muscle followed by inflammatory cell infiltration and eventual fibrous repair. The classical cause of infarction is atheromatous plaque with thrombosis and vasospasm leading to complete occlusion of the vessel lumen. Myocardial infarction can vary from mild to fatal and may lead to arrhythmias. Typical diagnostic changes associated with MI are ST segment elevation on electrocardiograph (Chapter 3) and raised levels of serum proteins released from disrupted myocardial cells, particularly the isoenzyme of creatine kinase (CK) more specific to cardiac muscle (CK-MB). This is raised from about 4 hours to 72 hours following infarction. More specific markers, troponin T and I, are found only in myocardial cells and are the gold standard diagnostic test for MI; the blood levels peak at 14–20 hours following MI (Noble et al 2005).

Frequent or unstable angina (angina at rest) commonly requires the coronary artery occlusion to be either dilated or bypassed. There are several approaches to coronary revascularization: these are by immediate fibrinolysis using pharmacological agents such as streptokinase or alteplase (within 6–12 hours of the event), using percutaneous transluminal coronary angioplasty (PTCA) with or without stenting the vessel(s) or by bypassing the occlusion during OHS. The use of thrombolytic therapy positively promotes activation of the fibrinolytic system, helping to break down clots. Greatest benefits are reported if the drugs are administered (intravenously) within 70 minutes of the onset of pain. PTCA is used for discreet lesions in one or two vessels. A balloon-tipped catheter is placed at the blockage guided by a fine wire and the balloon is inflated. This pushes the plaque against the artery wall, enlarging the lumen. This procedure has a high rate of restenosis. A stent (expandable wire cage) may be placed during PTCA to keep the lumen patent and this has been more successful in reducing the rate of restenosis (Noble et al 2005). Investigations used include chest X-ray, 12-lead ECG, stress test, thallium scans, positive emission tomography (PET) scan with coronary angio-

graphy being the definitive diagnostic investigation (Chapter 3).

Coronary artery bypass surgery

Several severe coronary stenoses associated with unstable or uncontrolled angina may be treated with OHS and bypass grafting. This operation involves access via a median sternotomy, requires cardiopulmonary bypass (although 'off-pump' operations are now performed) and uses conduits, commonly the left and right internal thoracic arteries, the radial artery and saphenous vein, to bypass the coronary occlusion. The operative mortality is 1%, with perioperative stroke, myocardial ischaemia, arrhythmias, cardiovascular instability, sternal infection and haemorrhage being the most common complications. Respiratory complications include low lung volumes, basal atelectasis and pleural effusion. Long-term survival is excellent with 90–95% alive at 5 years and 80–85% at 10 years but is significantly influenced by age at surgery, diabetes, left ventricular function and risk factor modification after surgery (Tatoulis & Smith 2006).

Cardiopulmonary bypass

Cardiopulmonary bypass ('heart–lung machine') was developed to allow operations on a still and empty heart. Cardiopulmonary bypass (CPB) involves the use of a mechanical pump and an oxygenating device to supply oxygenated blood to the body while the heart is empty. Blood is removed from the right atrium (using gravitational flow), oxygenated across a membrane and returned to the ascending aorta. A heat exchanger cools and rewarms blood and a centripetal pump or roller propels the blood (at 4–6 l/min) back into the aorta. A vent may be placed in the left ventricle to remove blood collecting from the coronary sinus and operative field. Complete arrest of the heart requires cross clamping of the aorta, during which the myocardium is protected with hypothermia to reduce oxygen requirements. This is achieved by infusion of cold (4°C) cardioplegic solution (usually potassium with oxygenated blood and other products) into the coronary arteries, topical cold solution and using the heat exchanger on the CPB machine. The cardioplegic solution arrests the heart in diastole. The duration of CPB is usually between 1 and 2 hours, although up to 3 hours is possible. After 2 hours, problems such as blood cell destruction by the roller pump, coagulation problems, neurological, hepatic and renal dysfunction may occur.

The preferred conduits for grafting are arteries, since they have a higher patency. The right internal thoracic artery is commonly anastomosed to the important, left anterior descending artery. The patency of the right

12

internal thoracic artery at 5 years is 96% and at 10 years is still 95% compared with the saphenous vein (75%, reducing to 50% at 10 years) (Tatoulis & Smith 2006). Once surgery is completed, the patient is rewarmed and sinus rhythm restored. The sternum is wired together, and drains are placed behind the sternum and into the pleural cavities (with UWSD) if necessary. A typical operation usually takes 3–4 hours and the average number of vessels bypassed is three or four. The postoperative length of hospital stay is approximately 5–7 days for uncomplicated surgery and many patients are referred to outpatient (Phase III) cardiac rehabilitation after discharge following hospital (Chapter 14).

Acquired valvular heart disease

Acquired valvular heart disease is limited to the aortic, mitral and occasionally tricuspid valves. The most common form of valvular disease in Western countries is stenosis (narrowing), which is generally calcific and incompetence/regurgitation as a result of degeneration and ageing. The two forms may occur together. The incidence of rheumatic heart disease (caused by rheumatic fever) has declined in Western countries but is still high in developing regions such as China, India and South America. The two most common presentations of valvular dysfunction are aortic stenoses and mitral regurgitation (Tatoulis & Smith 2006). The main symptom of valve disease is dyspnoea, but it may manifest late in the disease process because of adequate ventricular reserve. Angina and syncope may occur in aortic stenosis and cerebral emboli or endocarditis may also complicate valve lesions. Echocardiography is the investigation and transoesophageal echocardiography provides anatomical detail of pathology and may be used intraoperatively. It is common for patients to also have investigations for coronary artery disease since both valve and coronary artery bypass surgery occur together in about 30% of patients (Tatoulis & Smith 2006).

Aortic valve surgery involves OHS via a median sternotomy and CPB. A prosthetic valve replaces the diseased one and the operation takes approximately 3 hours with 80 minutes of CPB.

Mitral valve surgery. Mitral stenosis may be treated by valvuloplasty, where a balloon is passed via catheterization of the femoral vein into the left atrium and mitral valve and then inflated. However, OHS is required for severe disease and may involve debridement of calcification, resection of portions of the thickened chordae or may require replacement with a prosthetic valve. Mitral regurgitation is usually due to elongated and ruptured chordea, leading to a prolapsed and flail valve. In severe disease, valve replacement is necessary.

Cardiac valve prostheses. Both tissue and mechanical valves are used for valve replacement surgery. Mechanical valves (such as St Jude) are durable but the patient needs to continue, for life, on anticoagulation therapy. Tissue valves (bioprostheses) may be human allografts or xenografts from specially treated porcine or bovine valves. With these valves no anticoagulation is necessary and they have long durability.

Operative mortality is 1–3% in valve surgery and 3–5% for combined valve and coronary artery surgery, and long-term results are excellent. Morbidity of valve surgery is relatively high, with problems of anticoagulant-related haemorrhage, thromboembolism, endocarditis and perivalvular leaks occurring in 1% of patients annually.

Monitoring following cardiac surgery

Pacing wires may be inserted at the time of the operation and the patient is returned to the cardiothoracic intensive care with ECG, blood pressure, right atrial pressure, pulmonary artery pressure and cardiac and urine output monitoring. The patient is initially mechanically ventilated (4–12 hours), then weaned and supported with oxygen therapy. Some patients require inotropic circulatory support including dopamine and afterload reducing agents such as nitroprusside. In cases where the function of the left ventricle is very poor postoperatively, an intra-aortic balloon pump (IABP) may be used to support the heart.

The IABP is a circulatory device providing support for the left ventricle. It consists of a single or multichamber balloon attached to an external pump console via a large lumen catheter. The balloon is inflated during diastole and deflated during systole. Inflation and deflation of the balloon is synchronized to the patient's cardiac rhythm via the ECG trace. The physiological aims of the IABP are to improve myocardial perfusion and reduce afterload, resulting in a reduction in myocardial oxygen demand, improved cardiac contractility and decreased risk of ongoing myocardial ischaemia. These aims are achieved by increasing the blood flow through the coronary arteries from the counterpressure exerted by the inflated balloon. This in turn reduces the volume of blood in the aortic arch, thus decreasing the work of the left ventricle to eject the cardiac output. The large lumen catheter is inserted into the femoral artery with the balloon positioned in the aorta between the subclavian and renal arteries. Patients usually begin on a cycle of 1:1 (i.e. inflation/deflation every heart contraction) and are weaned off to 1:2, and then 1:3, usually over a period of several days before the pump is removed. Patients with the IABP in situ should be treated by physiotherapists as indicated following discussion with the ICU consultant. Their myocardial

12

dysfunction may result in an inability of oxygen supply to meet demand, a condition known as circulatory shock. Situations that put these patients under greater physiological stress should therefore be avoided (i.e. activities that increase the work of their myocardium). If the patient is repositioned, great care should be taken not to kink the IABP catheter. Aggressive anticoagulation is required while the IABP is in situ and therefore patients should remain resting in bed for 24 hours following removal of the pump. The ICU physiotherapist must alert ward physiotherapists as to when mobilization is allowed, as often the pump will be removed and the patient transferred to the ward during this 24-hour bed rest period (School of Physiotherapy 2006b). Ventricular assist devices (VADs), which perform the work of the left ventricle, are used when inotropes and balloon pump are insufficient to maintain adequate circulation.

Newer concepts in coronary artery surgery

Performance of surgery on a beating heart without the use of cardiopulmonary bypass (CPB) is called 'off pump' surgery and its use is becoming more common in many cardiac units worldwide. Minimally invasive techniques using an endoscope and robotics (avoiding a median sternotomy) are being utilized in some centres, and endoscopic harvesting of the saphenous vein to minimize incisions and pain is being performed. The use of these newer techniques will impact on the physiotherapy management of this patient population, as it is probable that these patients will require less physiotherapy intervention after surgery. However, this means that those patients who ultimately undergo open-heart surgery with CPB in the future may represent a much sicker population who will need increased physiotherapy resources. Research into physiotherapy management and outcomes for patients having heart surgery needs to continue as the populations being treated change with the introduction of new surgical techniques.

Box 12.9 shows key points in cardiac surgery

Common surgical intravenous access and drains

Postoperatively, surgical patients have several different intravenous lines and drains. These are:

Surgical wound or cavity drains to remove blood or serous fluid from around the operative site. These drains may be open and drain into gauze or dressing, such as a drain placed in an abscess cavity, or closed and drain into a collection bag with or without added suction to enhance drainage. The drains are removed when minimal fluid is being drained, by cutting the suture

---

> **Box 12.9 Key points in cardiac surgery**
>
> - There is no evidence to support the effectiveness of physiotherapy treatment while the patient is intubated and ventilated in the intensive care unit after return from open-heart surgery (OHS).
> - Level 1 evidence from systematic reviews does not support the use of prophylactic respiratory physiotherapy treatment to reduce the incidence of postoperative pulmonary complications after OHS.
> - There is insufficient evidence to support or refute the role of thoracic mobilizing exercises in improving function or range of movement after open-heart surgery; therefore these exercises are still recommended.
> - Patients with the intra-aortic balloon pump (IABP) in situ should be treated by physiotherapists as indicated only following discussion with the intensive care consultant.
> - If the patient with an IABP is repositioned, great care should be taken not to kink the IABP catheter.
> - Due to aggressive anticoagulation while the IABP is in situ, patients should remain resting in bed for 24 hours following removal of the pump.

---

that anchors them and withdrawing the tube from the patient (Tjandra 2006).

Intravenous (IV) cannulation is used for administration of fluids and drugs such as analgesics, usually into the forearm or hand. Thrombophlebitis develops at the insertion site after about 3 days and IV cannulas should be resited if infusions are required for longer periods.

Central venous catheterization is used for longer-term venous access or for administration of total parenteral nutrition or chemotherapy and also for short-term monitoring of central venous pressure (CVP). The cannula may be inserted into the subclavian or jugular veins. The catheter tip sits in the superior vena cava.

Infusion pumps are used to deliver drugs with mechanical assistance. Three types are commonly seen:

> patient-controlled analgesia (PCA)
> syringe pumps
> 'IMED' (see Fig. 12.1).

Catheterization of the bladder involves introducing a tube through the urethra and into the bladder. An indwelling catheter is most commonly seen in the hospital setting. These catheters are equipped with a balloon, which is inflated following induction to anchor the catheter. It remains in situ until a patient is able to void completely and voluntarily. A suprapubic catheter is placed directly into the bladder through an incision in the abdominal wall. It is indicated for long-term management of urinary tract dysfunction.

Nasogastric tubes may be used either to deliver enteral feeds, medications or fluid or to drain/aspirate gastric contents. Fine-bore or wide-bore tubing is passed nasally down the oesophagus into the stomach. If a nasogastric tube is being used for the purpose of feeding, it will be attached to feed or will be spigotted. If it is being used as a drain, a drain bag will be connected to the end of the tubing.

Enteral feeding is feeding directly into the digestive system. It requires a functioning gastrointestinal system and is preferred over parenteral nutrition as it maintains gut mucosal barrier integrity, mucosal structure and function and gut hormones. Feeding tubes may be inserted into several structures. In the stomach (nasogastric tube), the duodenum (gastrostomy) or the small intestine (jejunostomy).

Total parenteral nutrition (TPN) is delivered via a central line and nutrients are given intravenously. IV feeding can be supplementary or complete.

Stoma.   A stoma is an artificial orifice or opening surgically created between a hollow organ, e.g. bowel, and the abdominal wall. A bag is attached to the external opening. Its purpose is to replace the function of a non-functioning or excised natural orifice. Two types of stoma are commonly seen:

- A *colostomy* is the formation of a stoma by fixing a portion of the colon to the abdominal wall. Its purpose is to act as an artificial anus, evacuating the bowel of its contents.

- An *ileostomy* is the formation of a stoma by fixing a part of the ileum to the abdominal wall. This is usually performed when the entire colon is resected. Its purpose is to evacuate the contents of the small bowel.

A stoma can be temporary or permanent depending on the pathology. *Temporary stomas* are created to relieve acute bowel obstruction, rest an inflamed distal bowel or to prevent bowel contents escaping into the peritoneal cavity following cases of bowel perforation. When the underlying problem has been corrected, the stoma is usually surgically closed and normal bowel evacuation is resumed. *Permanent stomas* are indicated when the bowel distal to the stomas has been removed. A stomal therapist or specialist nurse usually performs

stomal care and extensive education of the patient (School of Physiotherapy 2006b).

Box 12.10 shows key points for the physiotherapist in managing drips and drains.

Box 12.10   Key points for the physiotherapist in managing drips and drains

- Ensure there is adequate tubing to roll, sit up and ambulate the patient without pulling lines.
- Take care when positioning patients to ensure you do not dislodge or kink the lines.
- Note dosage/rate of drugs being delivered especially by infusion pumps. For patient controlled analgesia (PCA) note if the system is in patient 'lock-out mode'. Patients will be unable to use delivery button until the lockout signal is cleared.
- For pumps note the alarm silence button. If the alarm sounds, contact the nursing staff.
- All pumps can run on battery but ensure cords are plugged into wall supply when patients are non ambulant.
- All pumps can be transferred to mobile intravenous poles. Nursing staff may need to assist with some types of PCA pump transfer, as they need to be unlocked with keys.
- Care and consultation is required if you plan to use the head down position with a patient who is being enterally fed.
- For patients with a colostomy or ileostomy observe for leakages before moving the patient. If full of air or fluid, the bag will require emptying before mobilizing or rolling the patient.
- Ensure a nasogastric tube is always supported after positioning a patient so there is no traction on the patients nose to reduce the risk of disconnecting the tubing. Dislodging a nasogastric tube may lead to aspiration and may not be possible to replace the tube for example following oesophageal surgery.
- In relation to drips and drains, the following points are not in your responsibility but should be noted:
  - Check patency of drip: Is it running?
  - Is there blood tracking in the tubing? This is a sign that the drip may be too slow, hence not causing enough pressure to resist arterial flow. Notify nursing staff.
  - Has the IV tissued? The entrance point is allowing fluid to enter subcutaneously rather than intravenously. The skin around the insertion site become swollen and tender. Notify nursing staff.

12

PHYSIOTHERAPY FOR PATIENTS HAVING SURGERY

Evidence

In many countries physiotherapists see patients awaiting major surgical procedures (upper abdominal, thoracic, cardiac, oesophageal) prophylactically with a 'blanket' referral system from medical staff. The physiotherapist may assess and educate the patient preoperatively and then treat postoperatively, using a variety of techniques. However, in the past 15 years research evidence has challenged components of this traditional prophylactic approach. Advances in surgery and pain management, together with a reduction in the incidence of clinically significant postoperative pulmonary complications, have also impacted on physiotherapy management. In this section, the evidence for physiotherapy intervention will be outlined with reference specifically to abdominal and cardiothoracic surgery. In reviewing the evidence for physiotherapy there are three strands of knowledge necessary to consider:

- basic science
- published evidence from high-quality clinical trials
- knowledge generated from professional practice (Herbert et al 2005).

Sackett et al (2000) and Herbert et al (2005) describe in depth the steps of evidence-based practice.

From the previous discussion of the surgical process it is clear that the physiological changes occurring in the lungs following major surgery and the proposed theories of pathogenesis of PPC provide empirical support for the place of physiotherapy intervention to counteract these changes (Denehy & Browning 2007).

To review evidence from clinical trials an extensive database search is needed. A review of literature can be undertaken using electronic searches including MEDLINE, CINAHL, ISI Web of Science, PEDro and evidence-based medicine reviews (Cochrane, DARE). The search terms that could be entered include pulmonary complications, atelectasis, pneumonia and surgery, respiratory therapy, chest physiotherapy, chest physical therapy, deep breathing exercises (DBE), early mobilization, early ambulation, continuous positive airway pressure (CPAP), incentive spirometry (IS) and positive expiratory pressure (PEP), together with the type of surgery of interest.

Evidence in abdominal surgery

Using the above search terms, six randomized controlled trials (with a no-treatment control group) can be accessed from 1980 to 2006 in upper abdominal surgery (UAS). These provide Levels 1b and 2b evidence (Sackett et al 2000) for the place of physiotherapy management and are summarized in Table 12.5. Older data were not included because it was thought that these would no longer reflect current practice either in physiotherapy or pain and surgical management. Five of these six research papers are of moderate methodological quality but only three represent convincing evidence in support of the use of physiotherapy treatment to reduce the incidence of PPC following abdominal surgery (these are presented in italics in Table 12.5). Based on these trials, the provision of physiotherapy treatment to reduce the incidence of PPC in patients having UAS will on average prevent one respiratory complication in every four or five patients treated.

The evidence from these trials is further supported by three systematic reviews (Lawrence et al 2006, Overend et al 2001, Thomas & McIntosh 1994). Systematic reviews provide combined evidence from several trials using systematic and explicit methodology and therefore offer the highest level of evidence while narrative reviews may introduce bias in interpretation. One systematic review (Pasquina et al 2006) examines the evidence for the place of respiratory physiotherapy to prevent PPC. Of the 35 papers available between 1952 and 2005, only 13 included a no-treatment control group and of these, six included both upper and lower abdominal surgery populations. The authors concluded that routine physiotherapy following abdominal surgery was not justified. However several major shortcomings of this review were evident: the inclusion of papers from the 1950s, inclusion of lower abdominal surgery (routine physiotherapy is not performed for patients after lower abdominal surgery) and the omission of a large randomized controlled trial by Olsen et al (1997). The 368 subjects in the Olsen study represent more than half of the number of patients reported in the six RCTs with an endpoint of pneumonia. Inclusion of this study may have altered the conclusions of this review, which are in contrast to the findings of another review by Lawrence and co-workers (2006). In summary, on the basis of the above evidence the place of physiotherapy treatment in reducing PPC after upper abdominal surgery is supported.

Evidence in cardiac surgery

Following cardiac surgery, the evidence obtained from a large body of research clearly challenges the continued traditional approach of prophylactic physiotherapy intervention. A search of the physiotherapy evidence database (PEDro) using 'cardiac surgery' reveals four systematic reviews regarding the place of respiratory physiotherapy for patients having cardiac surgery (Brooks et al 2001, Jonasson & Timmermans 2001, Moore 1997, Pasquina et al 2003) in addition to numerous

12

Table 12.5   Randomized controlled trials of physiotherapy in upper abdominal surgery since 1980

(reports in italics present convincing evidence from methodologically sound research)

Author/date	Sample size	Intervention	PPC incidence	Conclusion
Olsen et al (1997)	*368 UAS*	*Treatment:* preoperative physiotherapy, breathing exercises with pursed lips, huffing and coughing hourly and information about the importance of early mobilization. PEP for high-risk patients *Control:* no intervention	*Treatment: 6%* *Control: 27%*	*Preoperative chest physiotherapy reduced the incidence of PPC and improved mobilization and oxygen saturation after major abdominal surgery*
Condie et al (1993)	130 (310 total, only 130 major UAS)	**Treatment:** preoperative, daily physiotherapy for 3 days postoperatively **Control:** preoperative, no postoperative supervision , just followed information sheet	Treatment: 8.2% Control: 17.4%	The value of the routine provision of supervised postoperative chest physiotherapy in non-smoking patients undergoing elective abdominal surgery is questionable
Chumillas et al (1998)	81 UAS	**Treatment:** respiratory rehabilitation including FET, DBE, SMI and early mobilization **Control:** no intervention	Treatment: 7.5% Control: 19.5%	Respiratory rehabilitation protects against PPC and is more effective in moderate and high-risk patients, but does not affect surgery-induced functional alterations
Celli et al (1984)	*81 (172 total, 81 UAS)*	*Treatment:* preoperative, 4 times daily for 4 postoperative days *IPPB:* 15 min IPPB *IS:* 10 breaths up to 70% VC *DBE:* 6 × 10 DBE with SMI and cough *Control:* no intervention	*IPPB: 30.4%* *IS: 33.3%* *DBE: 33.3%* *Control: 89.5%*	*IPPB, IS and DBE, when compared with an untreated control group, were equally effective in significantly decreasing the incidence of PPC after abdominal surgery*
Roukema et al (1988)	153 UAS	**Treatment:** preoperative, postoperative DBE, FET and coughing and dead space rebreathing. **Control:** no intervention	All grades combined Treatment: 19% Control: 60% Only grades 2 and 3: Treatment: 4% Control: 35%	Pre- and postoperative breathing exercises as a prophylactic treatment in all patients scheduled for UAS are recommended
Morran et al (1983)	*102 UAS*	*Treatment:* 15 min DBE, assisted coughing and vibration *Control:* no intervention	***Chest infection*** *Treatment: 14%* *Control: 37%* ***Pulmonary atelectasis*** *Treatment: 22%* *Control: 35%* ***Combined*** *Control: 59%* *Treatment: 49%*	*Routine prophylactic postoperative chest physiotherapy decreased significantly the frequency of chest infection*

UAS, upper abdominal surgery; DBE, deep breathing exercises; FET, forced expiration technique; IPPB, intermittent positive pressure breathing; IS, incentive spirometry; PEP, positive expiratory pressure; PPC, postoperative pulmonary complication; SMI, sustained maximal inspiration; Temp, temperature; VC, vital capacity

12

clinical trials. The most recent systematic review concluded that there is no clear evidence that prophylactic respiratory physiotherapy reduces the incidence of PPC following cardiac surgery (Pasquina et al 2003). In a randomized clinical trial, Stiller and colleagues (1994) found no difference in the incidence of PPC between a group of cardiac surgery patients receiving physiotherapy and a group receiving no physiotherapy intervention. Based on this evidence, it is recommended that postoperative treatment that aims to reduce PPC, such as breathing exercises, is not routinely included in physiotherapy management of this patient population. A Swedish paper (Westerdahl et al 2005) presented evidence that deep breathing exercises may reduce the degree of atelectasis following cardiac surgery. However, the authors commented that the value of this short-term improvement in influencing the patient's clinical recovery and length of stay was not the aim of the study. Based on the current evidence, in many centres the assessment and monitoring of mobility is the only intervention. Provision of rehabilitation for these patients is supported by a large body of evidence and is discussed in detail in Chapter 14. The place and effectiveness of shoulder and thoracic mobilizing exercises has not been studied extensively in this population and presents opportunity for research. Stiller et al (1997) reported that active range of movement exercises of the trunk and upper limb in the early postoperative period did not affect the incidence of musculoskeletal problems up to 10 weeks after surgery. The incidence of musculoskeletal complications in this study was 30%. Others report a relatively high incidence of musculoskeletal problems after cardiac surgery, particularly after internal mammary artery grafts (El-Ansary et al 2000, LaPier & Schenk 2002).

Evidence in thoracic and oesophageal surgery

Literature pertaining to the place of physiotherapy for patients having thoracic and oesophageal surgery is scant and inconclusive. A randomized clinical trial examining physiotherapy intervention is much needed in these patient populations. Currently, given the lack of definite evidence either way, it is recommended that patients undergoing these operations are treated both pre- and postoperatively. In general the site (both a thoracotomy and abdominal incision for oesophageal surgery) and extent of these operations, the positioning of the stomach within the thorax after oesophageal resection, together with patient factors such as cachexia, particularly in patients presenting for oesophageal surgery, mean that they represent a high-risk group for developing PPC. The incidence of PPC in these patients has been reported to be between 8 to 30% (Gosselink et al 2000).

> **Box 12.11 Key points in evidence for physiotherapy for the surgical patient**
>
> - There is a large body of evidence that supports the place of physiotherapy treatment to reduce the incidence of postoperative pulmonary complication (PPC) after upper abdominal surgery.
> - There is no clear evidence that prophylactic respiratory physiotherapy reduces the incidence of PPC following cardiac surgery.
> - There is insufficient evidence to draw conclusions about the place of physiotherapy in reducing the incidence of PPC after thoracic and oesophageal surgery: pre- and postoperative physiotherapy treatment should still be provided.

Box 12.11 shows key points in evidence for physiotherapy for the surgical patient.

Physiotherapy treatment techniques

The main presenting problems found on assessment of patients who have had a major surgical procedure are reduced lung volumes, which may lead to impaired gas exchange, and less commonly impaired airway clearance. The research described above presents a variety of different treatment techniques that are aimed at improving these problems in patients undergoing surgery. The definition and uses of these different techniques are described in Chapters 4, 5 and 6. In the management of surgical patients the physiotherapy techniques commonly used include preoperative education, deep breathing exercises (DBE), incentive spirometry (IS), positive expiratory pressure (PEP), continuous positive airway pressure (CPAP), early positioning and mobilization and less commonly intermittent positive pressure breathing (IPPB). The current research into the comparative efficacy of these techniques in preventing PPC after major surgery provides Level 3 evidence (Sackett et al 2000) that no one particular physiotherapy technique appears to be most effective. This is supported by a meta-analysis and systematic review (Thomas & McIntosh 1994), which concluded that there were no significant differences in the incidence of PPC using either IS, DBE or IPPB after upper abdominal surgery. Furthermore both IS and DBE were found to be more effective than no treatment. A second systematic review (Overend et al 2001) examined the effect of IS in preventing PPC and reported that the balance of evidence from the best available studies (10 out of 46 studies) failed to support the use of IS for reducing the incidence of PPC following UAS.

In this section the use of these techniques specifically for surgical patients will be presented. In the research discussed in this section it is difficult to isolate the effects of individual techniques, since most results are confounded by the effects of body positioning and mobilization. It is only recently that attention has been paid to mobilization as a treatment technique in its own right, despite the early work of Dean & Ross (1992). The inclusion of early mobilization is important since it is also beneficial in treating deconditioning following surgery.

Preoperative assessment and education

With the advent of same-day surgery and preadmission clinics it has become more difficult for the physiotherapist to see patients before surgery. However, patients undergoing higher-risk operations such as those having liver transplantation, upper abdominal, ear, nose and throat, aortic aneurysm repairs, thoracic or oesophageal surgery should be treated preoperatively.

The aims of preoperative physiotherapy treatment are to:

- gain the patient's confidence and reduce anxiety
- educate the patient regarding postoperative routine
- assess the patient's risks of developing PPC
- assist in the prevention of respiratory complications
- assist in the prevention of deep vein thrombosis.

Following a thorough assessment of the patient (Chapter 1), including documentation of patient risk factors:

Explain:
- the role of the physiotherapist within the team
- the probable site of the incision
- presence of drips/drains/oxygen therapy/catheter/ intercostal catheter (if uncertain, be non-specific or ask if the surgeon or anaesthetist has explained these)
- type of analgesia administered
- effects of general anaesthesia, surgery and pain on the cardiorespiratory system, e.g. atelectasis, pneumonia, deep vein thrombosis
- the importance of optimal postoperative positioning, e.g. high-sitting, sitting out of bed and the importance of regular deep inspirations and early mobilization for making an uncomplicated recovery.

Demonstrate/practise:
- deep breathing exercises to increase lung volumes
- forced expiration technique (FET) and cough with support using a pillow or towel

- foot and ankle circulatory exercises
- recommend the frequency and number of times for the deep breathing exercises, FET, supported cough and foot and ankle exercises
- provide the patient with a written practice routine or information booklet, taking into consideration the language skills of the patient
- for surgery such as cardiothoracic, upper limb and trunk exercises should be included in addition to education regarding underwater sealed drainage and discussion of rehabilitation on discharge
- for patients having ear, nose and throat surgery, information about tracheostomy care, particularly oxygen therapy and suction, should be provided.

Note: If the patient exhibits respiratory symptoms that require physiotherapy for airway clearance, for example patients with bronchiectasis, full treatment is imperative preoperatively. Patients with acute exacerbations of respiratory disease rarely undergo general anaesthesia until they are in a stable condition.

Postoperative management

Assessment.   All patients should be assessed thoroughly following surgery by the attending physiotherapist (Chapter 1), and a prioritized problem list and treatment plan developed. A brief overview of possible treatment techniques that can be used follows. More information on these techniques can be found in Chapters 4, 5 and 6.

Deep breathing exercises to improve lung volumes.   Application of breathing exercises after upper abdominal and thoracic surgery is an integral part of most physiotherapy treatments. The use of inconsistent terminology is a feature of the literature describing breathing exercises. Traditionally, deep breathing exercises may include bilateral basal expansion, thoracic expansion exercises, diaphragmatic breathing and sustained maximal inspiration. The aim of a deep breath is to produce a large and sustained increase in transpulmonary pressure, which distends the lungs and reinflates collapsed lung units (Duggan & Kavanagh 2005), and deep breathing exercises have been the mainstay of physiotherapy treatment for these patient groups for over 50 years.

Most deep breathing exercises that aim to improve lung volume are performed from functional residual capacity (FRC) to total lung capacity (TLC). As a result of the effect of body position on lung volume they are most often performed in erect sitting, but may also be used in combination with gravity-assisted drainage and forced expiratory manoeuvres. If airway clearance is the

12

main aim of treatment then an appropriate airway clearance technique, such as the active cycle of breathing techniques (ACBT), should be used. It is important to note that when using ACBT in surgical populations, the emphasis would be focused more on the deep breathing component to improve ventilation and less on the forced expiratory manoeuvres such as FET when compared with patients with excess secretion production. For example, in surgical patients it may be more effective to perform three sets of DBE before the FET. Variations in inspiratory flow rates are thought to alter the distribution of ventilation; so, to improve ventilation to the dependent lung regions that are most affected following major surgery, a slow inspiratory flow rate is recommended (Tucker & Jenkins 1996).

The importance of periodic deep breaths in people with normal lungs has been evaluated and has shown that regular large breaths to TLC are essential to maintain inflation. Furthermore, it was reported that five consecutive breaths to TLC were needed for effective inflation of alveoli (Ferris & Pollard 1960). In addition, a sustained maximal inspiration (SMI) mimics a sigh or yawn and also aims to increase transpulmonary pressure (Bakow 1977). Sustained maximal inspirations have been reported to redistribute gas into areas of low lung compliance, thus enhancing lung expansion through lung interdependence and by using collateral ventilation pathways (Menkes & Traystman 1977). It may also allow time for alveoli with slow time constants to fill and the addition of a 3-second SMI at TLC is therefore recommended (Denehy & Browning 2007). Based on this research, the common treatment regimen used for deep breathing exercises is five deep breaths, with a 3-second inspiratory hold to maintain increased transpulmonary pressure, once every waking hour (Platell & Hall 1997).

Physiotherapists may choose to perform deep breathing exercises by using tactile stimulation over the patient's lower ribs, or anteriorly on the costal margin. The addition of resistance through the hands and application of a quick stretch is thought to encourage a maximal inspiration (Levenson 1982). Studying diaphragmatic motion using ultrasonography showed a significant increase in diaphragmatic excursion following surgery when tactile or 'hands-on' breathing techniques were used (Blaney & Sawyer 1997).

The regimen of breathing exercises used was found to be reasonably uniform across studies included in a meta-analysis of the effectiveness of physiotherapy techniques in the prevention of PPC (Thomas & McIntosh 1994) indicating that the treatment regimen, based upon physiological principles and developed in the 1960s, is still common in clinical practice today. The lack of current research evidence to support the method of

implementation of breathing exercises means that this technique may be used suboptimally by physiotherapists, and this in turn may affect treatment efficacy. It is not clear whether the depth of inspiration achieved during deep breathing exercises is more important than dose and frequency of breaths. Additionally, while there is good evidence that lung expansion techniques are important as part of the postoperative treatment (Fig. 12.8), it is not yet clear whether lung expansion can be achieved just as well by mobilizing the patient.

Incentive spirometry (IS) was developed to stimulate the patient to perform deep breathing exercises under supervision or independently. The additional effects of IS compared with deep breathing exercises have been widely discussed in the literature. The use of IS has been evaluated in different patient diagnostic groups such as adult cardiothoracic surgery, UAS and paediatrics (Overend et al 2001). The additional value of IS over other forms of postoperative prophylaxis has not been supported in these patient groups. It was reported that the addition of IS to physiotherapy, including deep breathing exercises and early mobilization, did not significantly alter the incidence of PPC following thoracic and oesophageal surgery (Gosselink et al 2000). Based on the current available evidence, use of IS is therefore not supported when deep breathing exercises and mobilization are possible.

Positive pressure techniques for postoperative patients

PEP and IR-PEP. Research evidence reporting the clinical efficacy of positive expiratory pressure (PEP) mask physiotherapy is conflicting and most of the research has been undertaken in patients with chronic sputum production rather than in surgical patients. Conclusions from these data are hampered by use of different treatment regimens, and the lack of equivalence in frequency of the other physiotherapy techniques with which PEP was compared. The physiological effects of PEP are thought to be that application improves gas mixing in the lungs leading to improved lung function and oxygenation, together with improved forced expiratory flow (Darbee et al 2004). In the treatment of patients undergoing UAS, PEP has been compared with conventional pre- and postoperative physiotherapy. The effect of adding PEP to conventional physiotherapy was measured in 71 patients following elective abdominal surgery and the incidence of PPC was found to be 31% after conventional physiotherapy and 22% after physiotherapy plus PEP (Campbell et al 1986). The PEP device used in this study is now commonly known as 'bubble' PEP as the end-expiratory pressure is maintained by the height of a column of water in a plastic bottle (Chapter

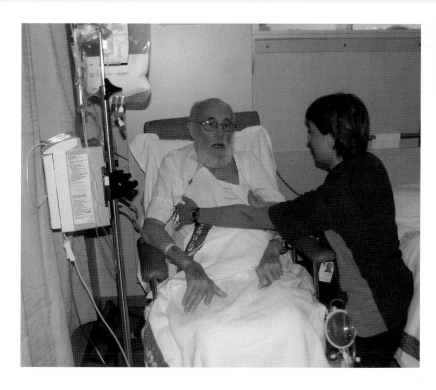

5). In this study no manometer was added to the circuit so that accurate PEP pressures could not be recorded. Comparison of PEP with continuous positive airway pressure (CPAP) and IS in a further study in UAS reported that both CPAP and PEP were more effective than IS in maintaining gas exchange and lung volumes postoperatively and lowering the incidence of atelectasis (Ricksten et al 1986). However, PEP and inspiratory resistance (IR) PEP have been used in previous research in patients having UAS with good effect, although comparison of techniques was not the main aim of the study (Olsen et al 1997). In patients undergoing oesophageal surgery a comparison of the use of IR-PEP and CPAP in the postoperative period showed that CPAP more effectively reduced the need for reintubation. The treatment with IR-PEP comprised 30 breaths every 2 hours and CPAP was applied for 30 minutes every 2 hours. Dosage and frequency of PEP application vary but commonly PEP is applied with physiotherapy treatments once or twice daily for 8–10 breaths in each of six cycles with a pressure of 10–20 cmH$_2$O.

Continuous positive airway pressure (CPAP). The use of CPAP by physiotherapists is generally in the form of intermittent or periodic application by mouthpiece or mask (Fig. 12.9). The decision of whether to implement CPAP treatment in postoperative patients is frequently made by the physiotherapist in conjunction with the medical team. In some centres, physiotherapists do not use CPAP on the wards as a treatment technique, giving a variable profile of use internationally.

The effects of CPAP application on lung volumes have been well documented. These include an increase in VC, a reduction in respiratory rate, reduced minute ventilation (MV) and increased FRC. The application of CPAP following UAS has been demonstrated to increase FRC when compared with other forms of respiratory prophylaxis (Lindner et al 1987). There is also support for the improvement of atelectasis with CPAP application after UAS (Andersen et al 1980).

The indications for the use of CPAP will to some extent depend on the unit and team structures of different centres and the role of the physiotherapist within them. Indications are derived from the physiological benefits of CPAP (Keilty & Bott 1992), but CPAP is generally considered a second-line treatment intervention for patients following major surgery. Indications include a significant fall in FRC and a significant deterioration in respiratory function and gas exchange as a result of atelectasis, most particularly acute hypoxaemia. The types of patient conditions seen therefore may include upper abdominal, thoracic, or cardiac surgery, especially for those high-risk patients not responding to voluntary lung expansion techniques such as mobilization and deep breathing exercises. Uncooperative or confused patients who develop significant respiratory

12

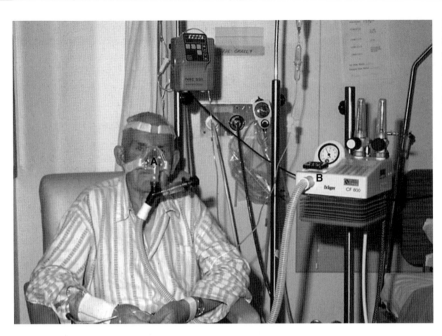

Figure 12.9 A patient receiving continuous positive airway pressure (CPAP) via (**A**) nasal mask with Ambu® positive expiratory pressure valve and Velcro® head straps, (**B**) Dräger CPAP unit.

12

problems after surgery may also benefit from application of CPAP as it requires no cooperation from the patient. In patients admitted to intensive care with acute hypoxaemia, the application of CPAP reduced the requirement for intubation and the incidence of severe complications (Squadrone et al 2005). The use of CPAP in intensive care units is generally considered to be a medical intervention and therefore physiotherapists may not be involved in the decision-making process or application of the technique.

To date, no specific treatment regimens have been compared to establish efficacy. Therefore the pressures used, length of treatment and frequency of application varies in different centres. In general, following surgery, CPAP should be applied as soon as a deterioration in the patient's condition is evident and used until clinical improvement is achieved. A suggested protocol is application of 7.5–10 cmH$_2$O CPAP for 30 minutes every 2–4 hours initially. Three continuous hours of application daily has also been associated with benefits (Denehy et al 2001).

Positive pressure devices in patients having thoracic or oesophageal surgery should be applied with caution. Flow rates and pressures used should be as low as possible to achieve effectiveness. Precautions with CPAP treatment may include an unstable cardiovascular system and recent oesophageal surgery. Swallowing air may overdistend the oesophagus at the site of the anastomosis, affecting its integrity. The presence of a nasogastric tube during CPAP administration to decompress the oesophagus is recommended. In a study of patients having oesophageal surgery, no adverse effects of CPAP application were reported (Olsen et al 2002).

Bilevel positive airway pressure. This can also be used in the management of surgical patients but generally is used in the treatment of hypercapnia rather than acute hypoxaemia. The evidence for its use in treating hypercapnia is strong (Chapter 11). In surgical patients bilevel devices may be used with the main aim of treatment being to improve lung volumes and gas exchange, particularly hypoxaemia.

Intermittent positive pressure breathing (IPPB). In postoperative patients the efficacy of IPPB has been compared with IS, breathing strategies and respiratory physiotherapy. The results from this extensive research were equivocal, with IPPB conferring no added benefit when compared with other methods of postoperative prophylaxis. Intermittent positive pressure breathing may be a useful tool in the management of postoperative patients who are unable or unwilling to inspire maximally (O'Donohue 1992). For patients with reduced lung volumes, improvement in vital capacity may provide the patient with a more effective cough, thereby improving secretion clearance. The aims of IPPB need to be directed toward improving volumes; the pressure and flow rate settings must therefore be set accordingly for individual patients and will depend on their body position and underlying lung pathology (O'Donohue 1992).

Positioning and mobilization

The cardiovascular and respiratory effects of immobility and bed rest have been well documented (Dean 1985, 1993). These include reduced lung volumes and capacities especially FRC, reduced PaO_2, decreased maximal oxygen consumption ($\dot{V}O_2max$), cardiac output (CO) and stroke volume, increased heart rate (HR) and orthostatic intolerance. The goal of mobilization of postoperative patients is to exercise at a sufficient level to increase minute ventilation and CO while still being within safe physiological limits.

Mobilization is a term used to describe a change from the supine or slumped posture in bed to sitting out of bed, standing or walking, although physiotherapists often use the terms positioning (sitting, standing) and ambulating (walking). A systematic review supports the benefits of upright positioning compared with the supine posture in improving FRC, oxygen saturation, PaO_2 and reducing $PaCO_2$ (Nielsen et al 2003). In surgical patients, sitting upright out of bed is an important component of postoperative management (Fig. 12.10). This technique is used by both nursing staff and physiotherapists. In a study of 15 subjects it was shown that ambulation on the third to fifth day after surgery increased tidal volume and respiratory rate, but that this increase was not significant once the effects of change in body position from bed to standing had been taken into account (Orfanos et al 1999).

Early mobilization is an important and widely practised component of postoperative patient care following surgery. In the early postoperative period, the ability of patients to mobilize is limited by the presence of intravenous lines and surgical drains, pain, decreased arousal, anxiety, surgical incisions and medication and a large proportion of patients become newly dependent on assistance to mobilize at this time (Denehy & Browning 2007). At two large Australian hospitals it was found that 52% of patients required at least standby assistance in order to mobilize safely on the fifth postoperative day (Mackay et al 2005). The same study reported that patients who received significantly higher numbers of physiotherapy treatments including more physiotherapy-assisted mobilization had better mobility outcomes, faster rates of resolution of PPC, and that a greater proportion of these patients were discharged earlier from hospital.

The benefits of mobilization in cardiac surgery patients have been established and research supports the benefits of mobilization without the additional need for deep breathing exercises or IS (Jenkins et al 1989). For patients having open UAS the addition of deep breathing exercises to a physiotherapist-directed program of early mobilization was found to have no effect on further reducing the incidence of PPC in 45 patients (Mackay et al 2005).

Despite the established important place of mobilization following surgery, little research has been aimed at identifying the intensity or frequency of mobilization that is most effective. Prescription of exercise such as walking a patient after surgery should be based on scientific principles. More research is needed to measure

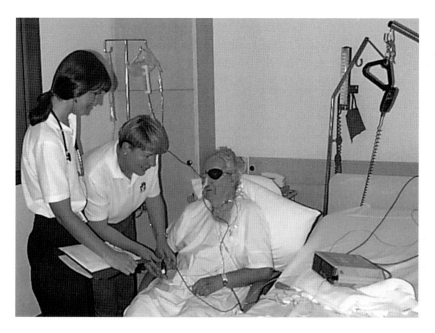

Figure 12.10 A postoperative patient who has just been sat out of bed in a chair to facilitate improvement in lung volumes and mobility.

12

the intensity at which physiotherapists can safely mobilize patients and how often this should be undertaken. Close monitoring is essential during and immediately following mobilization, especially at the first treatment session. Specific exercise guidelines must be based upon the individual patient's assessment findings and regular reassessment by the physiotherapist is important. Use of physiological outcomes could be included such as SpO_2, Borg rating of perceived exertion and heart and respiratory rate. It is possible that greater improvements in acute outcomes such as length of stay and incidence of PPC may be achieved with increased intensity and frequency of mobilization. In research conducted at a large tertiary hospital in Australia it was found that the average time that patients were standing or walking on the first day after open UAS was only 3 minutes (Browning et al 2005).

With advances in anaesthesia, surgical techniques and perioperative care, older people are having surgery that may not have been possible in the past. Not only are these patients at a higher risk of developing PPC but they are also at risk of a significant decline in physical function for some time following surgery. The functional recovery of patients aged over 60 years following abdominal surgery may be significantly reduced at 3–6 months. Prevention of PPC and improving functional status of older patients before surgery may enhance recovery (Lawrence et al 2004). In addition the use of 'fast-track' pathways, pioneered by Kehlet & Mogensen (1999), where attention is paid to nutrition and early mobilization, are being implemented more frequently around the world as they have been shown to reduce length of stay and hospital costs. Physiotherapy plays an important part in the early mobility of all major surgical patients (Fig. 12.11) and physiotherapists need to investigate the use of intensive rehabilitation both in the pre-, early and later postoperative periods to provide sound evidence upon which to direct treatment in the future.

Box 12.12 shows key points in physiotherapy treatment techniques.

Specialist surgery

In this section several other types of surgery encountered by physiotherapists will be briefly described; these are chest trauma, head and neck surgery, adult liver transplantation and vascular surgery.

Chest trauma

Sternal and rib fractures are commonly sustained after road traffic accidents. Sternal fractures are generally managed conservatively, but may require internal

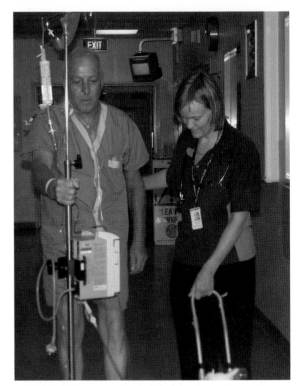

Figure 12.11   A physiotherapist ambulating a postoperative patient on a hospital ward.

fixation. Effective pain management is one of the most important aims of treatment for both sternal and rib fractures. When several ribs are fractured both anteriorly and posteriorly a 'flail' segment of chest wall may be evident. This creates paradoxical movement of the ribs such that the flail segment moves inward on inspiration, asynchronously with the chest wall. The underlying lung is therefore not ventilated adequately. Patients with a flail segment are at high risk for developing atelectasis and subsequent respiratory failure unless managed well. This means that pain control needs to be optimal and the physiotherapist should consider use of CPAP (after discussion with medical staff) to splint the flail segment and allow it to move in synchrony with the chest wall. The level of positive pressure is titrated so that synchrony is achieved. Underlying pneumothorax should be looked for on the chest radiograph before instituting positive pressure. Serial chest X-rays may be necessary in cases where a small untreated pneumothorax exists. Patients with chest trauma may also have underlying lung contusion and they can deteriorate quickly on the ward if not assessed and treated vigilantly.

Box 12.12   Key points in physiotherapy treatment techniques

- To date no specific treatment techniques have been found to be superior to any another.
- Preoperative treatment allows physiotherapists to assess patient risk factors and may be an effective treatment in its own right.
- The additional value of incentive spirometry over other forms of postoperative prophylaxis has not been supported in surgical patients.
- Continuous positive airway pressure is most commonly used as a second-line treatment intervention in the management of surgical patients.
- Mobilization of patients has been included in most of the research assessing effectiveness of physiotherapy treatment as a whole. The effectiveness of mobilization alone after abdominal, thoracic and oesophageal surgery needs further investigation.
- In cardiac surgery, pre- and postoperative assessment ± mobilization may be the only treatment required in the acute postoperative period.
- The place of physiotherapy in the postoperative rehabilitation and fast tracking of surgical patients needs further clarification.

Head and neck surgery

Most surgery performed in the head and neck region is for malignancy, predominately squamous cell carcinoma. Metastases to cervical lymph nodes are common and significantly impact prognosis. There has been a shift away from radical surgery such as total laryngectomy with the emphasis of treatment on organ preservation (particularly the larynx) where possible (Judson 2006). Multimodality treatments including chemotherapy and radiotherapy are used together with more selective surgery that spares sternomastoid, the internal jugular vein and the accessory nerve. Additionally, endoscopic laser techniques are now used for endolaryngeal and hypopharyngeal disease. Free tissue transfer techniques (flaps) allow tissue with a better blood supply to be used for reconstruction after more radical surgery. Where flaps have been used there may be precautions with specific movements and liaison with medical staff is essential. The use of these techniques leads to a better functional and cosmetic outcome for patients (Judson 2006). Following some surgical procedures, patients may have a temporary tracheostomy in situ to protect the airway from swelling and compression. For radical laryngectomy a permanent tracheostomy is necessary and speech therapists will be involved in the management of speech and swallowing problems. The physiotherapist will need to use suction to remove secretions from patients with tracheostomies and should understand how to care for patients with tracheostomies (Chapter 8).

Vascular surgery

Atherosclerosis accounts for most peripheral arterial disease and is usually coexistent with coronary and cerebrovascular disease. For physiotherapists, the most commonly encountered patients have undergone aortic aneurysm repair. An aneurysm is a permanent localized dilatation of an artery to one and a half times the normal diameter. When an artery dilates it may rupture or a thrombus may form. The incidence of aneurysms is higher in smokers, patients with hypertension and in Caucasians, and presentation can be asymptomatic until pending rupture. Abdominal aortic aneurysms are usually resected when they are larger than 5 cm in diameter as seen on ultrasound or computed tomography (CT) scan (as an incidental finding). Open repair involves an extensive midline laparotomy, clamping of the aorta and sewing in a prosthetic arterial graft to replace the area of aneurysm either using a straight or bifurcated method. Endoluminal repair involves insertion of a graft through the common femoral artery but not all patients are suitable to be treated using this method, as narrow and calcified arteries can pose technical problems. Further refinement of this technique in the future may overcome these problems (Harris 2006). Perioperative mortality is less with the endoluminal approach than open. Thoracic aortic aneurysms are less common than infrarenal aneurysms.

Liver transplantation

Liver transplantation is indicated in irreversible end-stage liver diseases caused by infections such as viral hepatitis A, B, C and E, immune or metabolic disorders, alcohol or drug abuse. Potential recipients are referred to a multidisciplinary transplant unit and are admitted to a waiting list for a suitable donor. While on the transplant list, clinical stability is maintained and nutritional deficiencies identified and treated in order to increase the probability of a successful outcome of the transplant. Patients who have liver failure may have a number of complications, including jaundice, portal hypertension, coagulopathy, varices, ascites, hepatopulmonary syndrome causing hypoxaemia, muscle wasting, deconditioning and fatigue. Sometimes the patients are

12

in the intensive care unit (ICU) before transplantation. It is important to remember that they have a coagulopathy and treatment should be performed carefully and only when indicated.

Transplant surgery is a difficult procedure due to the premorbid problems associated with liver failure. The operation usually lasts about 8–10 hours, but may be as long as 23 hours. Large amounts of blood replacement products are usually needed but cell saving is also used. The liver is accessed via a reverse 'L' incision; clamping of the inferior vena cava below the liver reduces cardiac output by 50% and is tolerated for 10–15 minutes. Venovenous bypass via the femoral vein, or inferior vena cava may be used if the patient is very sick or cardiovascularly unstable. Split liver transplants are performed where the left lobe of the liver of a donor may be used for a child and the right for an adult.

Postoperatively patients are admitted to the ICU for mechanical ventilation, haemodynamic monitoring and monitoring of liver function tests. If the patient's temperature increases to >37.5°C a full septic work-up is performed. The most common postoperative complications are rejection, infection (respiratory, wound, biliary tract, blood), renal failure and graft ischaemia. Antirejection and antiviral drugs are given postoperatively.

Physiotherapy management of the respiratory status of the patient is important because of prolonged anaesthesia, poor premorbid patient condition and since the liver is under the right hemidiaphragm, right lower lobe atelectasis and effusion are common. Musculoskeletal management is also important with the aims of increasing muscle bulk, strength and endurance. Back pain is common in this patient group and education about posture and lifting should be included in a comprehensive rehabilitation programme postoperatively (Stockton 2001). Research has shown that patients can improve their 6-minute walking distance and $\dot{V}O_2$ with exercise programmes. In the 1996 United States Transplant Games, 16 athletes with liver transplants competed. Their exercise capacity was 101% of age-matched controls, demonstrating that they are capable of achieving high levels of physical functioning (J Luke, Personal Communication, 2006).

Box 12.13 shows key physiotherapy points for specialist surgery.

> **Box 12.13 Physiotherapy key points for specialist surgery**
>
> - The same principles of physiotherapy management are indicated for special surgery: to prevent or minimize respiratory complications and rehabilitate the patient.
> - Ensure patients with rib and sternal fractures have effective pain management and are able to take deep breaths.
> - Be vigilant with patients who have a flail segment as their respiratory status can deteriorate rapidly.
> - Continuous positive airway pressure is an effective treatment for a patient with a flail segment.
> - Head and neck surgery can be difficult for patients to deal with when facial and neck muscles have been resected, causing disfigurement, and patients have a tracheostomy, preventing speech.
> - Heated humidification is required for patients with a tracheostomy.
> - Coagulopathy complicates preoperative management of patients awaiting liver transplant.
> - Arterial hypoxaemia is common in liver disease.
> - Immunosuppression increases risks of infection after liver transplant.
> - Long anaesthetic, high incision and poor preoperative health put liver transplant patients at high risk for developing postoperative complications.

Acknowledgement

I wish to acknowledge the help of several physiotherapists in the preparation of this chapter: Sarah Ridley for her diagrams carried through from the third edition; and current PhD students Laura Browning and Annemarie Lee for their suggestions on content. Additionally, I would like to acknowledge the clinicians of the University of Melbourne Clinical Schools who jointly contributed the information presented from the cardiorespiratory practical manuals of the School of Physiotherapy.

References

AIHW (Australian Institute of Health and Welfare) & AACR (Australasian Association of Cancer Registries) 2007. Cancer in Australia: an overview, 2006. Cancer series no. 37. Cat. no. CAN 32. (*www.aihw.gov.au/ publications/can/ca06/ca06.pdf*) (Accessed July 23 2007)

American Society of Anesthesiologists (ASA) 1963 New classification of physical status. Anesthesiology 24: 111

Andersen J, Olesen B, Eikhard B et al 1980 Periodic continuous positive airway pressure, CPAP, by mask in the treatment of atelectasis. European Journal of Respiratory Disease 61: 20–25

Bakow E 1977 Sustained maximal inspiration – a rationale for its use. Respiratory Care 22: 379–382

Barrat S 1997 Advances in acute pain management. International Anesthesiology Clinics 35: 27–33

12

Berrisford R, Brunelli A, Rocco G et al 2005 The European Thoracic Surgery Database project: modelling the risk of in-hospital death following lung resection. European Journal of Cardiothoracic Surgery 28: 306–311

Blaney F, Sawyer T 1997 Sonographic measurement of a diaphragmatic motion after upper abdominal surgery: a comparison of three breathing manoeuvres. Physiotherapy Theory and Practice 13: 207–215

Brasher P, McClelland K, Denehy L et al 2003 Does removal of deep breathing exercises from a physiotherapy program including pre-operative education and early mobilization after cardiac surgery alter patient outcomes? Australian Journal of Physiotherapy 49: 165–173

Brooks D, Crowe J, Kelsey C et al 2001 A clinical practice guideline on peri-operative physical therapy. Physiotherapy Canada 53: 9–25

Brooks-Brunn JA 1995 Postoperative atelectasis and pneumonia. Heart and Lung 24: 94–115

Browning L, Denehy L, Scholes R 2005 Quantitative measurement of mobility following upper abdominal surgery. Australian Journal of Physiotherapy 52: S8

Campbell T, Ferguson N, McKinlay R 1986 The use of a simple self-administered method of positive expiratory pressure (PEP) in chest physiotherapy after abdominal surgery. Physiotherapy 72: 498–500

Celli B, Rodriguez K, Snider G 1984 A controlled trial of intermittent positive pressure breathing incentive spirometry, and deep breathing exercises in preventing pulmonary complications after abdominal surgery. American Review of Respiratory Disease 130: 12–15

Chumillas S, Ponce J, Delgado F et al 1998 Prevention of postoperative pulmonary complications through respiratory rehabilitation: a controlled clinical study. Archives of Physical Medicine and Rehabilitation 79: 5–9

Condie E, Hack K, Ross A 1993 An investigation of the value of routine provision of post-operative chest physiotherapy in non-smoking patients undergoing elective abdominal surgery. Physiotherapy 79: 547–552

Craig DB 1981 Postoperative recovery of pulmonary function. Anesthesia and Analgesia 60: 46–52

Darbee J, Ohtake P, Grant B et al 2004 Physiologic evidence for the efficacy of positive expiratory pressure as an airway clearance technique in patients with cystic fibrosis. Physical Therapy 84: 524–536

Dean E 1985 Effect of body position on pulmonary function. Physical Therapy 65: 613–618

Dean E 1993 Bedrest and deconditioning. Neurology Report 17: 6–9

Dean E, Ross J 1992 Discordance between cardiopulmonary physiology and physical therapy: towards a rational basis for practice. Chest 101: 1694–1698

Denehy L, Browning L 2007 Abdominal surgery: the evidence for physiotherapy intervention. In: Partridge C (ed) Recent advances in physiotherapy. John Wiley and Sons, Chichester

Denehy L, Carroll S, Ntoumenopoulos G et al 2001 A randomized controlled trial comparing periodic mask CPAP with physiotherapy after abdominal surgery. Physiotherapy Research International 6: 236–250

Denehy L, van de Leur J 2004 Postoperative mucus clearance. In: Rubins B, van der Schans C (eds) Therapy for mucus-clearance disorders. Marcel Dekker, New York

Dodson M 1985 The management of postoperative pain. Edward Arnold Ltd, London

Duggan M, Kavanagh B 2005 Pulmonary atelectasis – a pathogenic perioperative entity. Anesthesiology 102: 838–854

El-Ansary D, Adams R, Ghandi A 2000 Musculoskeletal and neurological complications following coronary artery bypass graft surgery: a comparison between saphenous vein and internal mammary artery grafting. Australian Journal of Physiotherapy 46: 19–25

Euliano T, Gravenstein J 2004 Essential anaesthesia – from science to practice. Cambridge University Press, Cambridge

Fairshter R, Williams J 1987 Pulmonary physiology in the postoperative period. Critical Care Clinics 3: 286–306

Ferris B, Pollard D 1960 Effect of deep and quiet breathing on pulmonary compliance in man. Journal of Clinical Investigation 39: 143–149

Fisher B, Majumdar S, McAllister F 2002 Predicting pulmonary complications after non-thoracic surgery: a systematic review of blinded studies. American Journal of Medicine 112: 219–225

Ford GT, Rosenal TW, Clergue F et al 1993 Respiratory physiology in upper abdominal surgery. Clinics in Chest Medicine 14: 237–252

Gosselink R, Schrever K, Cops P et al 2000 Incentive spirometry does not enhance recovery after thoracic surgery. Critical Care Medicine 28: 679–683

Hassan I 2006 Lung cancer: staging. www.emedicine.com/radio/topic807.htm (Last updated 28 September 2006, accessed 16 July 2007)

Harris J 2006 Disorders of the arterial system. In: Tjandra J, Clunie G, Kaye A, Smith J (eds) Textbook of surgery. Blackwell Publishing, Massachusetts

Herbert R, Jamtvedt G, Mead J et al 2005 Practical evidence based physiotherapy. Elsevier Butterworth-Heinemann, London

Jenkins S, Moxham J 1991 The effects of mild obesity on lung function. Respiratory Medicine 85: 309–311

Jenkins S, Soutar S, Loukota J et al 1989 Physiotherapy after coronary artery surgery: are breathing exercises necessary? Thorax 44: 634–639

Jonasson B, Timmermans C 2001 The effect of incentive spirometry on postoperative pulmonary complications: a systematic review. Chest 120: 971–978

Judson R 2006 Tumours of the head and neck. In: Tjandra J, Clunie G, Kaye A, Smith J (eds) Textbook of surgery, 3rd edn. Blackwell Publishing, Massachusetts

Katz J 1993 Preoperative analgesia for postoperative pain. Lancet 342: 65–66

Kehlet H, Kennedy R 2006 Laparoscopic colonic surgery – mission accomplished or work in progress. Colorectal Disease 8: 514–517

Kehlet H, Mogensen T 1999 Hospital stay of 2 days after open sigmoidectomy with a multimodal rehabilitation programme. British Journal of Surgery 86: 227–230

Keilty S, Bott J 1992 Continuous positive airways pressure. Physiotherapy 78: 90–92

Kim WD 1997 Lung mucus: a clinician's view. European Respiratory Journal 10: 1914–1917

King D 1933 Postoperative pulmonary complications. Surgery, Gynecology and Obstetrics 56: 43–47

LaPier T, Schenk R 2002 Thoracic musculoskeletal considerations following open-heart surgery. Cardiopulmonary Physical Therapy Journal 13: 16–20

Law S, Wong J 2006 Tumours of the oesophagus In: Tjandra J, Clunie G, Kaye A, Smith J (eds) Textbook of surgery. Blackwell Publishing, Massachusetts

Law S, Wong K, Kwok K et al 2004 Predictive factors for postoperative pulmonary complications and mortality after esophagectomy for cancer. Annals of Surgery 240: 791–800

Lawrence V, Cornell J, Smetana G 2006 Strategies to reduce postoperative pulmonary complications after noncardiothoracic surgery: systematic

12

review for the American College of Physicians. Annals of Internal Medicine 144: 596–608

Lawrence V, Hazuda H, Cornell J et al 2004 Functional independence after major abdominal surgery in the elderly. Journal of the American College of Surgeons 199: 762–772

Levenson C 1982 Breathing exercises. Pulmonary management in physical therapy. Churchill Livingstone, New York

Lindner K, Lotz P, Ahnefeld F 1987 Continuous positive airway pressure effect on functional residual capacity, vital capacity and its subdivisions. Chest 92: 66–70

Mackay M, Ellis E, Johnston C 2005 Randomized clinical trial of physiotherapy after open abdominal surgery in high risk patients. Australian Journal of Physiotherapy 51: 151–159

Macnaughton PD 1994 Posture and lung function in health and disease. International Journal of Intensive Care Winter: 133–137

Marini JJ 1984 Postoperative atelectasis: pathophysiology, clinical importance and principles of management. Respiratory Care 29: 516–528

Menkes H, Traystman, R 1977 Collateral ventilation. American Review of Respiratory Disease 116: 287–309

Miller K, Sahn S 1987 Chest tubes. Chest 91: 258–264

Moore S 1997 Effects of interventions to promote recovery in coronary artery bypass surgical patients. Journal of Cardiovascular Nursing 12: 59–70

Morran C, Finlay I, Mathieson M et al 1983 Randomized controlled trial of physiotherapy for postoperative pulmonary complications. British Journal of Anaesthesia 55: 1113–1116

National Health and Medical Research Council 2005 Acute pain management: scientific evidence *www.nhmrc.gov.au/publications/synopses/cp104syn.htm* (accessed 16 July 2007)

Nielsen K, Holte K, Kehlet H 2003 Effects of posture on postoperative pulmonary function. Acta Anaesthesiologica Scandinavica 47: 1270–1275

Noble A, Johnson R, Thomas A et al 2005 The cardiovascular system. Basic science and clinical conditions. Elsevier Churchill Livingstone, London

Nunn J 1993 Nunn's applied respiratory physiology. Butterworth-Heinemann, Oxford

O'Donohue W 1992 Postoperative pulmonary complications. Postgraduate Medicine 91: 167–175

Olsen M 2000 Chest physiotherapy in open and laparoscopic abdominal surgery. Physical Therapy Reviews 5: 125–130

Olsen MF, Hahn I, Nordgren S et al 1997 Randomized controlled trial of prophylactic chest physiotherapy in major abdominal surgery. British Journal of Surgery 84: 1535–1538

Olsen MF, Wennberg E, Johnsson E et al 2002 Randomized clinical study of the prevention of pulmonary complications after thoracoabdominal resection by two different breathing techniques. British Journal of Surgery 89: 1228–1234

Orfanos P, Ellis E, Johnston C 1999 Effects of deep breathing exercises and ambulation on pattern of ventilation in postoperative patients. Australian Journal of Physiotherapy 45: 173–182

Overend T, Anderson C, Lucy S et al 2001 The effect of incentive spirometry on postoperative pulmonary complications: a systematic review. Chest 120: 971–978

Pasquina P, Tramer M, Walder B 2003 Prophylactic respiratory physiotherapy after cardiac surgery: systematic review. British Medical Journal 1379–1381

Pasquina P, Tramer M, Granier J et al 2006 Respiratory physiotherapy to prevent pulmonary complications after abdominal surgery: a systematic review. Chest 130: 1887–1899

Peeters-Asdourian C, Gupta S 1999 Choices in pain management following thoracotomy. Chest 115: 122S–124S

Platell C, Hall J 1997 Atelectasis after abdominal surgery. Journal of the American College of Surgeons 185: 584–592

Ready L 1985 Acute postoperative pain. Anesthesia 69: 2135–2143

Richardson J, Sabanathan S 1997 Prevention of respiratory complications after abdominal surgery. Thorax 52: S35–S40

Ricksten S, Bengtsson A, Soderberg C et al 1986 Effects of periodic positive airway pressure by mask on postoperative pulmonary function. Chest 89: 774–781

Roukema J, Carol E, Prins J 1988 The prevention of pulmonary complications after upper abdominal surgery in patients with non-compromised pulmonary status. Archives of Surgery 123: 30–34

Sabanathan S, Shah R, Tsiamis A et al 1999 Oesophagogastrectomy in the elderly high-risk patients: role of effective regional analgesia and early mobilization. Journal of Cardiovascular Surgery 40: 153–156

Sackett D, Strauss S, Richardson W et al 2000 Evidence-based medicine. Churchill Livingstone, Edinburgh

Scholes R, Denehy L, Sztendur E et al 2006 Development of a risk assessment model to predict pulmonary risk following upper abdominal surgery. Australian Journal of Physiotherapy 52: S26

School of Physiotherapy University of Melbourne 2006a Cardiorespiratory physiotherapy 1 student clinical Manual. Parkville

School of Physiotherapy University of Melbourne 2006b Cardiorespiratory physiotherapy 2 student clinical manual. Parkville

Sharma K, Brandstetter R, Brensilver J et al 1996 Cardiopulmonary physiology and pathophysiology as a consequence of laparoscopic surgery. Chest 110: 810–815

Smetana G, Lawrence V, Cornell J 2006 Preoperative pulmonary risk stratification for non-cardiothoracic surgery: systematic review for the American college of physicians. Annals of Internal Medicine 144: 581–595

Smith J 2006 Common topics in thoracic surgery. In: Tjandra J, Clunie G, Kaye A, Smith J (eds) Textbook of surgery, 3rd edn. Blackwell Publishing, Massachusetts

Smith MCL, Ellis E 2000 Is retained mucus a risk factor for the development of postoperative atelectasis and pneumonia? – Implications for the physiotherapist. Physiotherapy Theory and Practice 16: 69–80

Squadrone V, Coha M, Cerutti E et al 2005 Continuous positive airway pressure for treatment of postoperative hypoxaemia. Journal of the American Medical Association 293: 589–595

Stiller K, McInnes M, Huff N et al 1997 Do exercises prevent musculoskeletal complications after cardiac surgery? Physiotherapy Theory and Practice 13: 117–126

Stiller K, Montarello J, Wallace M et al 1994 Efficacy of breathing and coughing exercises in the prevention of pulmonary complications after coronary artery surgery. Chest 105: 741–747

Stockton K 2001 Exercise training in patients with chronic liver disease. Physiotherapy Theory and Practice 17: 29–38

Tatoulis J, Smith J 2006 Principles and practice of cardiac surgery. In: Tjandra J, Clunie G, Kaye A, Smith J (eds) Textbook of surgery, 3rd edn. Blackwell Publishing, Massachusetts

Thomas J, McIntosh J 1994 Are incentive spirometry, intermittent positive pressure breathing, and deep breathing exercises effective in the prevention of postoperative pulmonary complications after upper abdominal surgery? A systematic overview and meta-analysis. Physical Therapy 74: 3–16

Tjandra J 2006 Colorectal cancer and adenoma. In: Tjandra J, Clunie G, Kaye A, Smith J (eds) Textbook of surgery, 3rd edn. Blackwell Publishing, Massachusetts

Tjandra J, Chan M 2006 Systematic review of the short-term outcome of laparoscopic resection for colon and rectosigmoid cancer. Colorectal Disease 8: 375–388

Trauma.org 2004 Pulmonary contusion. *www.trauma.org/index.php?/main/article/398/* (Accessed 16 July 2007)

Tucker B, Jenkins S 1996 The effect of breathing exercises with body positioning on regional lung ventilation. Australian Journal of Physiotherapy, 42: 219–227

Wahba R 1991 Perioperative functional residual capacity. Canadian Journal of Anaesthesia 38: 384–400

Werawatganon T, Charuluxanun S 2005 Patient-controlled intravenous opioid analgesia versus continuous epidural analgesia for pain after intra-abdominal surgery. Cochrane Database of Systematic Reviews 2005, Issue 1. Art. No: CD004088. DOI: 10.1002/14651858.CD004088.pub2

Westerdahl E Lindmark B, Eriksson T et al 2005 Deep-breathing exercises reduce atelectasis and improve pulmonary function after coronary bypass surgery. Chest 128: 3482–3488

Wightman JAK 1968 A prospective survey of the incidence of postoperative pulmonary complications. British Journal of Surgery 55: 85–91

12

Chapter **13**

Pulmonary rehabilitation in chronic respiratory disease

Fabio Pitta, Vanessa Probst, Rachel Garrod

INTRODUCTION

Physical training for patients with respiratory disease is not a new concept and was recognized as beneficial in the early 19th century, although routine prescription of exercise has only recently become widely used. In fact, as Thomas Petty puts it:

'Over 40 years ago, oxygen was considered contraindicated, and exercise was prohibited for fear of straining the right heart'

(Petty 1993)

In the early 1980s there was scepticism regarding the value of physical training, due partly to one study that demonstrated negative results after an exercise training programme in patients with chronic obstructive pulmonary disease (COPD) (Belman & Kendregan 1981). These negative results may in part be explained by inadequate intensity of training. Fortunately, scientific advances have led to widespread recognition of the value of exercise in COPD. There is now a strong body of evidence showing that exercise training by itself or as part of a pulmonary rehabilitation programme results in improvements in disease-related problems of dyspnoea, reduced exercise intolerance, muscle weakness and poor health-related quality of life (Lacasse et al 2002). Despite the strong evidence supporting the benefits of physical training, survey data suggest that less than 2% of appropriate patients receive pulmonary rehabilitation (British Lung Foundation 2002). It is hoped that this chapter, publications, reviews and the impending National Service Framework for COPD will help to redress the balance and improve delivery of pulmonary rehabilitation to all patients with COPD.

Pulmonary rehabilitation is defined as:

'. . . a multidisciplinary continuum of services directed to persons with pulmonary disease and their families, usually by an interdisciplinary team of specialists, with the goal of achieving and maintaining the individual's maximum level of independence and functioning in the community'
(National Institutes of Health 1994)

Pulmonary rehabilitation programmes are delivered ideally by a multidisciplinary team whose structure varies according to patient population, programme budget, availability of team members and resources (Nici et al 2006). For many years, physiotherapists have been an important part of this multidisciplinary approach and have played an important role in the management of patients with respiratory disease. Effective positioning, mobilization, functional exercises, relaxed breathing and techniques to aid the removal of secretions are recognized physiotherapeutic treatment interventions for these patients. Physiotherapists have also traditionally been active in the education of patients with respiratory disease. The aim now must be to promote healthy attitudes and recognition of the benefits of exercise.

Pulmonary rehabilitation requires a holistic approach to the treatment of patients and their families with respiratory disease; it involves the participation of different health professionals. Physiotherapists may supervise and deliver the exercise programme while specialist input is provided from occupational therapists, nurses, dieticians, social workers and psychologists. All patients should be assessed by a physician before entry to an exercise training programme and then followed up regularly in order to optimize medical and drug therapy. Furthermore, the therapeutic focus of the disease has steadily changed from expiratory flow-related outcomes to other parameters, such as symptoms, exercise tolerance, nutritional status, quality of life and exacerbation frequency. This opens a broad window of therapeutic options other than pharmacological therapy alone. Since pulmonary rehabilitation aims to improve this whole range of parameters, it plays a fundamental role in the optimal management of patients with chronic obstructive disease.

RATIONALE FOR REHABILITATION IN CHRONIC OBSTRUCTIVE PULMONARY DISEASE

COPD is a major cause of morbidity and mortality worldwide, and individuals with COPD constitute the largest proportion of patients referred for pulmonary rehabilitation. One of the major limiting symptoms reported by patients with COPD is dyspnoea: the distressing and fearful sensation of breathlessness. Patients with COPD report significant limitations during daily life and reductions in exercise tolerance. One study has shown high levels of disability in patients with COPD, with 50% of patients studied requiring assistance with household chores (Garrod et al 2000a). Almost all the patients investigated reported some degree of breathlessness during washing and dressing. Other studies have shown that most patients with severe COPD are breathless even when performing simple activities of daily living (ADL) or walking around at home (Bestall et al 1999, Restrick et al 1993). Reduced tolerance to exercise is also a feature of COPD, and may be attributable to the illness itself (e.g. ventilatory limitation), cardiac dysfunction, gas exchange limitations, pre-existing levels of cardiovascular fitness and muscle dysfunction. In fact, while dyspnoea remains a striking and important symptom of COPD, weakness in the peripheral muscles (and possibly respiratory muscles) contributes strongly to exercise inefficiency (Gosselink et al 1996, Koppers et al 2006, Lotters et al 2002). It is increasingly apparent that muscle weakness and muscle fatigue play an important part in the disability evidenced in COPD patients. Fat-free mass in particular has been identified as an important predictor of muscle mass and associated with peak oxygen uptake during exercise (Gosker et al 2003). Peripheral muscle dysfunction in COPD is characterized by reduced muscle strength, reduced muscle endurance, impaired muscle oxidative capacity, and a shift toward a glycolytic fibre-type distribution; that is, a decrease in type I (slow oxidative) fibres and an increase in type IIb (fast glycolytic) fibres (Allaire et al 2004, Gosker et al 2002, Gosselink et al 2000, Janaudis-Ferreira et al 2006, Mador et al 2003, Maltais

13

et al 1999, Whittom et al 1998). Janaudis-Ferreira and co-workers compared quadriceps muscle strength and endurance in 42 patients with COPD with 53 age-matched healthy controls and showed significantly reduced muscle strength in the COPD group (Janaudis-Ferreira et al 2006). In addition, endurance was lower in the COPD group compared with their healthy age-matched controls. This supports earlier observations that leg fatigue is experienced at lower work intensities in COPD patients compared with healthy subjects (Killian et al 1992). The quadriceps muscle may therefore be significantly weaker and more prone to fatigue in patients with COPD compared with healthy subjects.

Patients with COPD are exposed to a number of factors that may contribute to peripheral muscle dysfunction. An extremely sedentary lifestyle is observed in this population (Pitta et al 2005a, Sandland et al 2005). Donaldson and co-workers showed that time spent outdoors declines markedly over time and deteriorates acutely during exacerbations (Donaldson et al 2005). Pitta and co-workers showed that patients with COPD are severely inactive not only during hospitalization for an acute exacerbation but also after discharge (Pitta et al 2006a). While it is clear that physical inactivity is an important factor, other factors such as the use of corticosteroids, malnutrition, disequilibrium in protein balance, chronic hypoxia and hypercapnia, oxidative stress, muscle apoptosis and genotype profile contribute to muscle impairment (American Thoracic Society/European Respiratory Society (ATS/ERS) 1999, Troosters et al 2005). There is now much interest in the place of inflammation in COPD and the part it plays in the development of muscle dysfunction. It has been shown that systemic inflammation is associated with loss of fat-free mass and muscle weakness both in stable patients and in patients during an acute exacerbation (Schols et al 1996, Spruit et al 2003). Importantly, data have shown relationships between inflammatory markers such as C-reactive protein (CRP), interleukin 6 (IL-6) and tumour necrosis factor alpha (TNFα) and health status, muscle weakness and exercise tolerance (Broekhuizen et al 2006, de Torres et al 2006, Garrod et al 2005a, Yende et al 2006). The mechanisms and contribution of inflammation to disability, reduced exercise tolerance and response to training are not yet clear (Spruit et al 2005), although it has been suggested that the intensity of systemic inflammation is linked to the severity of airflow obstruction (Gan et al 2004, Takabatake et al 2000). Furthermore, inactivity, oxidative stress, lactic acidosis and inflammatory cytokines may work congruently to disrupt the local anabolic/catabolic mechanisms (Debigare et al 2001). The current body of evidence demonstrates that peripheral muscle dysfunction in COPD is multifactorial, and factors mentioned above may act in combination. Owing to this multidimensional character, determining the severity of the disease based only on pulmonary function measurements has been questioned and a multidimensional index has been used to characterize COPD patients. Besides pulmonary function, this index includes also body composition, level of dyspnoea and functional exercise capacity (6 minute walking test – 6MWT) (Celli et al 2004). These developments in our understanding of the causes of myopathy in COPD reinforce the fact that strategies aimed at maximizing functional performance and peripheral muscle strength are of utmost importance in the pathophysiology of COPD.

The aims of pulmonary rehabilitation are to:

- reduce dyspnoea
- increase muscle endurance and strength (peripheral and respiratory)
- increase exercise capacity
- improve daily functioning and ensure long-term commitment to exercise
- help allay fear and anxiety and improve health-related quality of life
- increase knowledge of lung condition and promote self-management.

EXERCISE PRESCRIPTION

Exercise training is considered the cornerstone of a pulmonary rehabilitation programme (Lacasse et al 1997). Reconditioning of patients with respiratory disease reflects the same principles as those applied in healthy subjects, although programmes should be adapted to the individual limitations of the patient and take into consideration ventilatory, cardiovascular and muscular abnormalities (Troosters et al 2005). Based on solid evidence, it is now widely accepted that exercise training is beneficial to patients with chronic respiratory disease. It is also known that the training effects depend on different factors including duration and frequency of the training programme, training intensity and training modality. The extent of the benefits obtained will depend on the management of these factors.

Duration and frequency of the training programme

There is as yet no consensus as to the optimal duration of an exercise training programme for patients with COPD. Evidence suggests that longer programmes yield larger and more endurable training effects (Lacasse et al 2002). Twenty sessions of pulmonary rehabilitation have been shown to produce better results than 10 sessions in outcomes such as exercise tolerance and health-related quality of life (Rossi et al 2005). Furthermore, various studies have demonstrated that exercise pro-grammes lasting at least 7 weeks (7–12 weeks) result in greater benefits than programmes of shorter duration (Bendstrup et al 1997, Carrieri-Kohlman et al 2005, Green et al 2001, Lake et al 1990). It has therefore been suggested that programmes of at least 8 weeks are advisable to result in substantial positive effects (Fabbri & Hurd 2003, Troosters et al 2005). A meta-analysis has shown strong trends for improved results in functional exercise capacity from longer programmes with close supervision (Lacasse et al 2002). Programmes of 6 months or longer also seem to result in better long-term effects (Berry et al 2003, Guell et al 2000, Salman et al 2003, Troosters et al 2000).

Ideal training frequency is also a topic that has been much debated but there is as yet insufficient evidence to identify the optimal frequency. The scarce evidence available suggests that patients should exercise at least three times per week, and that regular supervision is fundamental (Puente-Maestu et al 2000, Ringbaek et al 2000, Wadell et al 2005). However, many programmes with twice-weekly supervision and encouragement of 'home exercise' have shown good results (Lacasse 2006). One intensive programme with 20 sessions condensed into 3–4 weeks showed positive results (Fuchs-Climent et al 1999), suggesting that frequency may be as impor-tant as duration of the programme.

Training intensity

Determining training intensity

A further element of exercise prescription concerns the intensity of exercise. A number of early studies of pul-monary rehabilitation had methodological flaws con-cerning the description of exercise intensity. Before considering appropriate levels of intensity, it is neces-sary to revisit relevant assessment tools. Two common methods of prescribing intensity are used: symptom-limited exercise prescription and physiological testing derived from maximal oxygen consumption (or related measures). In the first method patients are instructed to exercise to a prescribed symptom level, for example 'moderately or somewhat short of breath' (scores of 4–6) on the Borg breathlessness score (Borg 1982, Horo-witz et al 1996). Although this provides an effective training stimulus for most patients, problems may occur when patients demonstrate very high levels of dysp-noea, thus limiting the intensity of training. Dyspnoea is very much a subjective perception, meaning that fear and anxiety at the start of a programme may heighten scores. If this method is used, it may be necessary to reassess dyspnoea levels halfway through the pro-gramme and set a higher training target if appropriate.

Calculating the exercise intensity from maximum oxygen consumption ($\dot{V}O_2max$) is probably more reli-able and is easily performed using cycle ergometry or derived from an associated measure such as the shuttle walk test (Dyer et al 2002). However, for patients with COPD, a true $\dot{V}O_2max$ may be unattainable due to ventilatory limitations. An effective compromise is to determine the initial exercise prescription at 70–80% of the derived $\dot{V}O_2max$ and then to use breathlessness scores to monitor the training and adjust accordingly (Mahler et al 2003).

Power output has also been used as an option to determine training intensity, and an intensity of 60–80% of the maximal workload has been frequently used with positive results. However, the peak work rate obtained during the maximal incremental exercise test is deter-mined by the work rate increment used in the test and this must be taken into consideration (Debigare et al 2000). Another option to determine training intensity is using a percentage of the maximal heart rate. Caution is necessary because this may result in inadequate training stimulus (Brolin et al 2003, Pitta et al 2004, Zacarias et al 2000). This inadequacy may occur because maximal exercise capacity is often not affected by the cardiocirculatory system in COPD patients, and heart rate is also influenced by various medications com-monly prescribed to COPD patients.

Ideal training intensity

Casaburi and colleagues (1991) demonstrated greater physiological and cardiovascular benefits in patients who exercise at higher intensities when compared with patients exercising for a longer duration but at a lower intensity. The same research group, in another study, targeted patients with more severe COPD and obtained similar results (Casaburi et al 1997). Puente-Maestu and colleagues have also shown that supervised higher-intensity training programmes were more effective than lower-intensity self-monitored training (Puente-Maestu et al 2000). Others studies have also highlighted the positive effects of high-intensity exercise training (Gimenez et al 2000, Punzal et al 1991). These studies recommend training intensities of 60–80% of peak work rate or maximal oxygen consumption in order to achieve the greatest effects, although the rate of work increment during the maximal incremental test is an important factor in determining whether a patient is able to achieve a training target of 80% of peak work rate (Debigare et al 2000, Maltais et al 1997, Neder et al 2000). Low-intensity training has also been shown to result in significant improvements in symptoms and quality of life (Normandin et al 2002) and even in exercise tolerance (Clark et al 1996, Roomi et al 1996). Wedzicha and colleagues stratified a group of COPD

13

patients according to their degree of dyspnoea and instructed them to exercise until moderately to severely shortness of breath (Wedzicha et al 1998). They reported that the improvement in exercise performance and health status following an exercise programme depends on the initial degree of dyspnoea. Therefore, a cautionary note concerns the relative severity of the patients.

Findings from a systematic review highlight the fact that in very severe patients, there is a lack of evidence to indicate that high-intensity exercise is the ideal mode of training. (Puhan et al 2005). Applicability of high-intensity training in these most severe and symptomatic COPD patients requires further study in order to determine the ideal training intensity and to achieve better results. In summary, the most recent consensus statement by the American Thoracic Society and European Respiratory Society states that:

> '. . . although low-intensity training results in improvements in symptoms, health-related quality of life and some aspects of performance in ADL, greater physiological training effects occur at higher intensity. Training programs, in general, should attempt to achieve maximal physiologic training effects, but this approach may have to be modified because of disease severity, symptom limitation, co-morbidities and level of motivation. Furthermore, even though high intensity targets are advantageous for inducing physiologic changes in patients who can reach these levels, low intensity targets may be more important for long term adherence and health benefits for a wider population'
>
> (Nici et al 2006)

In cases where high-intensity exercise is advocated for the more symptomatic patients with severe COPD, interval training may prove to be more comfortable (Vogiatzis et al 2005).

From a clinical perspective there are probably a few practical issues to remember regarding exercise training. First, patients need to be very clear about the importance of exercising at home between supervised sessions and the importance of a long-term exercise routine. Secondly, training the peripheral muscles (in particular quadriceps) is likely to lead to greater effects on exercise tolerance and long-term benefits. Walking remains an important therapeutic exercise. Additionally, despite a lack of data it may be necessary to adopt different training strategies for patients with different baseline levels of airflow obstruction, dyspnoea, exercise capacity and even body composition. As implied by the consensus statement mentioned above, the influence of baseline severity on acceptability, tolerance and adherence of exercise regimens requires further investigation.

Training modality

A variety of training modalities has been employed in the management of patients with COPD, all with generally good results. The British Thoracic Guidelines recommend including functional exercises (Morgan et al 2001). Most programmes use continuous (or endurance) exercise training, incorporating an element of walking and/or cycling for 20–30 minutes per session. An alternative approach is interval training, where the 20- or 30-minute exercise session is divided into short bouts of high-intensity exercise for 30 seconds to 2–3 minutes, interspersed with equal periods of rest. One study compared interval training with continuous training in COPD patients and showed a different pattern of physiological response (Coppoolse et al 1999). Continuous training resulted in an improvement in maximal oxygen consumption, reduction in minute ventilation and a more pronounced decrease in lactic acid production, whereas interval training resulted in improvement in peak workload and a decrease in leg pain. This difference in training response may be a reflection of specific training effects in either oxidative or glycolytic muscle metabolic pathways. Vogiatzis and colleagues (2005) compared high-intensity interval training (bouts of 30 seconds at 125% maximal cycle ergometry and 30 seconds rest for 45 minutes) with equivalent constant load (at 75% of maximum for 30 minutes constantly) 3 times per week for 10 weeks. Both groups showed significant training effects; however, during the training sessions, symptoms of dyspnoea and leg discomfort were significantly lower for the high-intensity interval group. These data suggest that in order to minimize discomfort associated with exercise training (and hence aid long-term adherence) patients may be advised to exercise in short, high-intensity bursts of activity. Furthermore, interval training may allow more severe patients to achieve higher work rates and to exercise for longer with fewer symptoms, due to less dynamic hyperinflation and a higher stable ventilation (Sabapathy et al 2004, Vogiatzis et al 2004). When using interval training, it is important that the total exercise time is not reduced but kept to 20–30 minutes.

The relative benefits of generalized training programmes have been compared with individualized training programmes (Sewell et al 2005). General exercises consisted of three strength training activities for the lower limbs (step-ups, sit to standing and stationary cycling), thoracic exercises and upper limb activities (wall pushes, arm circling and shrugging). Individualized exercises were based on patient goals identified using the Canadian Occupational Performance Measure (2005). After the 7-week programme, there were no differences in any outcome measure between the 59

13

patients randomized to general training and the 64 randomized to individualized training. The sample size was large in this study with adequate power suggesting that targeting exercise specifically to patient-identified goals is unnecessary assuming that adequate attention is made to ensure that both upper and lower limb exercises are included at an appropriate intensity.

As data have become available from studies investigating the relative merits of different training regimens in pulmonary rehabilitation, it may be concluded that the most important aspect of exercise is that strengthening exercises are routinely incorporated into programmes. Strength training has the potential to increase muscle mass and muscle force, both of which are common therapeutic aims in COPD patients. Training is generally performed with 2 to 4 sets of 6 to 12 repetitions, at intensities ranging from 50% to 85% of the one repetition maximum (O'Shea et al 2004). A systematic review evaluating a number of comparative study designs concluded that strength training resulted in greater improvements in health-related quality of life than endurance training, although the benefits of strength over endurance are equivocal when considering the relative change in exercise tolerance (Puhan et al 2005). Interestingly, a randomized controlled trial reported no difference in change in muscle strength, distance walked or health-related quality of life between those who performed a strength training regimen compared with endurance training (Spruit et al 2002). In addition, Probst and colleagues showed that a major advantage of strength training is that the cardiopulmonary stress during this kind of exercise is lower than during whole-body endurance exercise and results in fewer symptoms (Probst et al 2006). As muscle weakness contributes to reductions in maximal walking test but not to endurance walking, there is probably a place for both types of training (Steiner et al 2005). Guidelines for pulmonary rehabilitation in COPD patients currently recommend a combination of endurance and strength training as it has multiple beneficial effects and is well tolerated (Nici et al 2006).

Although the focus of most studies of exercise training in COPD patients has been the lower limbs, it has been shown that upper limbs are also affected (Franssen et al 2005, Gosselink et al 2000) and that upper limb activity influences dynamic hyperinflation and pulmonary mechanics (Dourado et al 2006, Gigliotti et al 2005, McKeough et al 2003). Due to the fact that improvement is specific to the muscles trained, the inclusion of exercise for the upper limbs in a programme is justified, particularly exercises that reflect activities of daily living. Examples of such exercises include arm cycle ergometer, multigyms, free weights and elastic bands.

When training the upper limbs, it is important to consider the principles of positioning during exercise. Exercise endurance is less during unsupported upper limb compared with supported upper limb work (Astrand et al 1968), especially when the arms are elevated above the head such as in 'reaching' or 'arching the arms'. Stabilization of the accessory muscles occurs only during movements where the shoulder girdle is fixed. These principles can be utilized during training. Unsupported upper limb work may achieve greater desensitization of dyspnoea, while strength training will be performed best with the upper limbs supported in order to minimize dyspnoea and maximize the number of repetitions possible. Guidelines for exercise prescription in pulmonary rehabilitation for patients with COPD are outlined in Box 13.1.

> **Box 13.1 Practice guidelines for exercise prescription in pulmonary rehabilitation for patients with COPD**
>
> - A training programme consisting of between 14 and 24 sessions, supervised at least twice a week, should be offered: longer programmes generally result in better long-term effects.
> - Encourage patients to exercise independently in addition to supervised sessions.
> - 20–30 minutes of high-intensity endurance exercise training (walking, cycling) generally produces greater physiological benefit. Intensity of 60–80% of the peak work rate is a useful target. However, low-intensity training can also be effective for the more severe and symptomatic patients who cannot achieve this intensity level.
> - In more severe patients, interval training (i.e. short bouts of high-intensity exercise interspersed by rest) is a valid alternative to endurance training in order to allow patients to exercise at higher intensities, but total exercise time should be kept to 20–30 minutes.
> - Progression of the training load should be based on the patient's tolerance (symptom scores).
> - Strength training is indicated for most patients, especially for those with severe muscle weakness. Training can be performed with 2–4 sets of 6–12 repetitions at intensities ranging from 50 to 85% of one repetition maximum.
> - A combination of endurance and strength training is recommended.
> - Both upper and lower extremities should be trained.

13

PHYSIOLOGICAL TRAINING RESPONSES

Physiological training effects differ according to the training regimen. The first aspect of training that occurs is a learning effect or improved neuromuscular coordination. This is not associated with physiological training effects per se, but may result in improved gait efficiency and increased stride length after a programme involving repeated walks (McGavin et al 1977).

Significant improvements in lung function are not expected after a training programme in patients with COPD. However, training does result in fundamental benefits to the individual, that occur independently of improvements in lung function. The effects may be classified under three headings:

- improved mechanical efficiency
- cardiovascular adaptations
- muscle changes.

Improved mechanical efficiency

Mechanical efficiency is reduced in patients with chronic respiratory disease when compared with a healthy elderly population (Baarends et al 1997, Richardson et al 2004). The explanation for this seems to be linked to the elevated number of less efficient type II fibres (Richardson et al 2004) and the increased oxygen cost of breathing observed in COPD (Baarends et al 1997). Arm efficiency seems to be relatively preserved in comparison to the lower limbs (Franssen et al 2002).

Much of the improvement in exercise tolerance following pulmonary rehabilitation is likely to be a result of improvements in mechanical efficiency (O'Donnell 1994). Measures that may suggest an improvement in efficiency include stride length and gait coordination. McGavin and co-workers (1977) showed improvements in exercise tolerance after a 12-week home programme of low-intensity exercise. They reported a modest increase of approximately 8% in walking distance which was probably attributable to improvements in mechanical efficiency rather than cardiovascular changes per se. Similarly a group of patients housebound because of dyspnoea, showed some improvement in exercise tolerance after an 8-week home-based programme although this was not significant when compared with a control group (Wedzicha et al 1998). Another programme of home exercise, continued over a period of 1 year showed larger changes, suggesting that when exercise intensity is low a longer period of time may be needed to achieve true physiological training effects (Sinclair & Ingram 1980). Improvements in efficiency of the skeletal muscles after exercise training may lead to reduced alveolar ventilation during exercise, therefore reducing dynamic hyperinflation and reducing exertional dyspnoea (Nici et al 2006).

Cardiovascular adaptations

Cardiovascular adaptations that might be expected in a normal subject after training include a reduction in the heart rate after training for a given level of work, reductions in minute ventilation, a lowering of the onset of lactic acidosis and a lower maximum oxygen uptake ($\dot{V}O_2$max) for a given work rate. Numerous studies show evidence of these changes in patients with COPD, with both moderate and severe obstruction (Casaburi et al 1991, Griffiths et al 2000, Ries et al 1995).

Muscle changes

Studies have shown that the peripheral muscles in COPD respond to training in a similar manner to muscles in healthy individuals (Casaburi et al 1991). This suggests that the contractile mechanism of the peripheral muscles in patients with COPD remains intact and muscle strength can be improved with an appropriate training programme (Bernard et al 1999, Maltais et al 1997, Simpson et al 1992). Recently Vogiatzis and colleagues performed muscle biopsies of COPD patients before and after pulmonary rehabilitation (Vogiatzis et al 2005) and demonstrated that training, both interval and continuous, achieved physiological changes in muscle fibres of COPD patients. The improved oxidative capacity of muscles, evident by changes in cross-sectional area of both type I and type II fibres and by a shift from type II b fibres (glycolytic) to type IIa (oxidative) fibres, supports previous observations that showed delayed onset of lactic acidosis with training. The result of this is an improvement in oxygen uptake and the ability to maintain aerobic muscle metabolism for a prolonged period (Casaburi et al 1991).

In addition, there is evidence that type I fibres increase in size and number and that the concentration of mitochondrial enzymes is greater after training (Maltais et al 1996). Strength training is predominantly associated with an increase in size of muscle cells and number of myofibrils. Most importantly, muscle capillaries and myoglobin levels within a trained muscle are higher after training, thus improving the transport of oxygen to exercising muscles. In summary, adequate exercise training leads to improvements in the capacity to generate and to sustain contraction. However, it is important to remember that peripheral muscles of patients with COPD are responsive to training but factors other than deconditioning also contribute to dysfunction, namely nutritional status, hypoxia and hyper-

13

capnia, inflammatory mediators and circulating hormones.

PRACTICAL ASPECTS OF TRAINING

Location

There are arguments in favour of rehabilitation in a number of settings, from the hospital inpatient setting to the outpatient, home or community setting. Hospital inpatient programmes (Goldstein et al 1994) are better suited to patients with severe deconditioning and/or limited transportation resources. These programmes may offer a multidisciplinary approach and intensive training, but are costly and may lack insurance coverage in some countries. Outpatient programmes seem to be the most cost-effective in producing optimal effects especially in moderate to severe patients, as a multidisciplinary approach, adequate equipment and careful supervision are possible at more reasonable costs (Nici et al 2006). Most studies involving rehabilitation programmes that resulted in significantly positive effects were developed in hospital-based outpatient settings (Fig. 13.1) (Lacasse et al 2002, Nici et al 2006). The advantage of home-based programmes relates to improved adherence and prolonged benefits with an additional focus on functional and meaningful activities (Strijbos et al 1996). The disadvantages relate to the lack of peer group support (Wedzicha et al 1998), the potentially limited space for mobilization and the limited availability of a multidisciplinary team, exercise equipment and proper supervision. Individual supervision is required and patients may need input for a longer period of time when compared with outpatient programmes (Sinclair & Ingram 1980). The pros and cons of pulmonary rehabilitation at home are reviewed (Garrod 1998) and summarized in Table 13.1.

Other avenues are being explored, from community care settings (Cambach et al 1997) to primary care interventions in local surgeries and sports centres, but further trials will be needed to evaluate the role of rehabilitation in primary care. Recent advances in 'exercise on prescription' schemes run in conjunction with local sports facilities and general practitioner surgeries point towards greater community involvement and better use of private sector resources. In recognition of patient wishes and significant underresourcing of pulmonary rehabilitation, future developments will need to make greater use of community facilities (Garrod & Backley 2006). Physiotherapists are ideally placed to lead the way with referrals, support and training of local members.

The most appropriate location for pulmonary rehabilitation should be determined by the needs of the patient. Patients with moderate to severe COPD and exercise hypoxaemia may require assessment and training at a specialist centre with a view to oxygen requirements and adequate monitoring during exercise. However, patients with mild to moderate disease may perform all aspects of training at home or in the community, requiring only initial supervision from a physiotherapist.

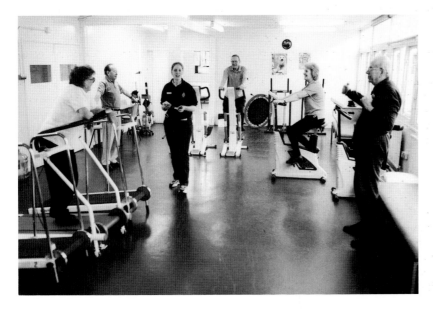

Figure 13.1   A pulmonary rehabilitation group provides peer support.

13

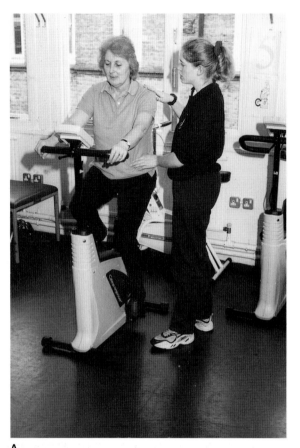
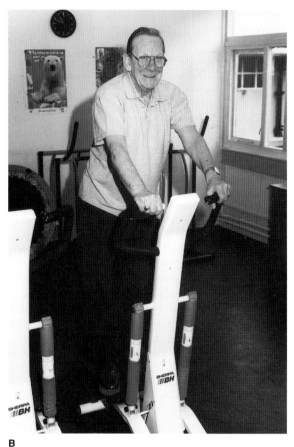

A **B**

Figure 13.2 (A) Cycle ergometry. (B) Stepping machine.

Table 13.1 The pros and cons of pulmonary rehabilitation at home

Pros	Cons
• Encourages lifestyle changes • Helps education on ADL • Greater accessibility for patients • Individual supervision enables cognitive and behavioural approach to exercise • Cost-effective in severe COPD	• Practical constraints, i.e. space • Makes multidisciplinary approach more difficult to manage • Requires supervision (at least weekly?) related to intensity • Requires a longer duration to achieve maximal changes • Less cost-effective than outpatient rehab for moderate COPD • Lack of group support

(Adapted from Garrod 1998)

Timing

Perhaps of more importance than where pulmonary rehabilitation should take place, is the issue of when rehabilitation is initiated. Pitta and co-workers showed that physical activity is markedly reduced not only during hospitalization for an acute COPD exacerbation, but also continued to be low after discharge (Pitta et al 2006a). In this study, the amount of time spent being active was related to the degree of muscle weakness. A study by Man et al (2004) has shown positive benefits of a training programme delivered within 10 days of discharge from hospital. In this randomized controlled trial a large clinical and statistically significant difference was seen in change in exercise tolerance after rehabilitation, compared with usual care only. No adverse events were reported and the drop out rate was similar in each group. Although the trial was small there were trends towards a reduction in hospital admissions and a significant difference in emergency room visits was observed. These are important findings, since they highlight two factors: firstly that rehabilitation early after discharge is safe and secondly that with usual care alone, exercise tolerance at 3 months following discharge does not improve (and in fact shows a small decline), suggesting that patients may deteriorate over time rather than improve without rehabilitation. A study involving pulmonary rehabilitation and neuromuscular electrostimulation initiated immediately after a hospital admission for acute exacerbation has also highlighted the benefits of early initiation of rehabilitation after exacerbation (Vivodtzev et al 2006). A higher level of physical activity has also been shown to be associated with a 46% reduction in readmission in COPD (Garcia-Aymerich et al 2003), further emphasizing the clinical importance of early rehabilitation. Preliminary data from Probst et al (2005) have shown that an exercise protocol based on strength training can be safely applied even during hospitalization, resulting in improvement in muscle force and counteracting the deleterious effects of immobilization.

Whether rehabilitation programmes should be repeated for individuals is an important clinical question. At the moment data suggest there is little value in repeating a programme 1 year after attendance (Foglio et al 2001), although there has been some suggestion that the number of hospitalizations may be reduced as a result of repeat rehabilitation. Another trial also showed that in severe and disabled COPD patients, a more frequently repeated inpatient programme resulted in only modest additional benefits over 1 year (Romagnoli et al 2006). These benefits were mostly linked to self-reported symptoms and health-related quality of life. The issue is made more complex when consideration is given to the fact that patients often request additional sessions, while many more known people with COPD do not have the opportunity to attend even one course of rehabilitation.

Equipment

As mentioned previously, functional exercise programmes are of the utmost importance to the success of pulmonary rehabilitation. Simple exercises aid clarity, and practical measures to include exercise in daily life may aid long-term adherence. Moreover, for older patients with COPD exercise must be seen as 'appropriate'; for patients with less severe disease, swimming, bike riding, golfing, bowling and walking are all appropriate forms of exercise. The type of equipment will depend primarily on the type of training to be performed and local financial resources. Equipment requirements may be as simple as a mat for floor exercises, dumbbells or hand weights and space to perform aerobic training. Where endurance training is the main objective, equipment such as cycle ergometry (Fig. 13.2A) and a treadmill may be helpful. However, walking practice, devices to simulate stair climbing (Fig. 13.2B), or actual stairs have high functional applicability. In order to achieve long-term benefits, patients must be able to continue exercising effectively after the programme has ended. For strength training a multigym may be ideal but simple hand and ankle weights will also be sufficient. It is important to note the necessity of training both the upper and lower limbs (Lake et al 1990, Sivori et al 1998) and the use of breathing control throughout exercise (see *Other adjuncts to rehabilitation* later in this chapter).

Changing attitudes towards exercise and dyspnoea

Fear and anxiety influence the breathing pattern. For many patients, the thought of exercise exacerbates dyspnoea. The underlying philosophy of pulmonary rehabilitation is that exercise is beneficial. During the programme the therapist attempts to help the patient to replace negative thought processes with positive ones. Teaching patients to perceive breathlessness as a positive effect of 'good' exercise rather than a negative effect of their health may enhance the training effect (Atkins et al 1984). This philosophy must, of course, extend to relatives and demands the education and involvement of the families of those with respiratory disease.

13

Supplemental oxygen during exercise training

The use of supplemental oxygen during training remains a complex question, one that in many cases is further complicated by the issue of available resources. It is widely accepted that oxygen supplementation leads to significant acute improvement in exercise tolerance in hypoxaemic patients (O'Donnell et al 2001), even in patients without appreciable exercise desaturation (Somfay et al 2001). Despite this, studies in which oxygen was provided during an exercise training programme have not been able to show additional benefits directly linked to oxygen supplementation. An early study by Zack & Palange (1985) showed an improvement in exercise tolerance after a 12-week outpatient training programme in which all patients trained with supplemental oxygen. However, there was no control group and it is not known whether additional benefits resulted from the use of supplemental oxygen. One randomized study investigated the role of oxygen in patients with severe COPD and exercise desaturation (Garrod et al 2000a). This showed an improvement in dyspnoea after rehabilitation that was greater in the patients who trained with oxygen compared with those who did not. However, as in an earlier study (Rooyackers et al 1997), there was no difference in the changes in exercise tolerance between the two groups. This suggests that although additional oxygen may augment desensitization to dyspnoea, it does little to enhance changes in exercise tolerance. Further data from 2001 showed similar results and concluded there were minimal benefits of oxygen as a training adjunct (Wadell et al 2001).

Hoo (2003) has undertaken a comprehensive review of this issue. Emtner and colleagues (2003) performed a randomized evaluation of the effects of oxygen on training in 29 non-hypoxaemic COPD patients. Breathing oxygen significantly increased endurance time compared with the air-trained group. Furthermore the rate of improvement was greater in the oxygen-trained patients. These data support previous observations that supplemental oxygen has a greater effect on submaximal exercise, improving endurance rather than intensity and reinforcing the likelihood that oxygen benefits are accrued largely through reductions in dynamic hyperinflation rather than correction of hypoxia per se (Somfay et al 2001). At the present time it is prudent to advise that patients who are on long-term oxygen therapy (LTOT) should exercise with supplemental oxygen. In addition, training with oxygen both for hypoxaemic and non-hypoxaemic patients may allow them to exercise at higher intensity and with less dyspnoea, although it is still unknown whether this translates into significant clinical benefits following a training programme.

The routine use of oxygen during pulmonary rehabilitation has implications. Instruction to exercise with supplemental oxygen during rehabilitation for patients not already prescribed LTOT or ambulatory oxygen could relay a confused message. This may adversely affect adherence both to the rehabilitation programme and the use of oxygen. Patients with exercise desaturation, even without resting daytime hypoxaemia, should ideally have saturation levels monitored throughout training. Where desaturation occurs and a clear benefit is shown, they should train with oxygen and be provided with ambulatory oxygen for home use.

Safety issues in rehabilitation

Many elderly people perceive exercise at 'their age' to be dangerous (O'Brien et al 1995). Issues of safety are obviously compounded in older people with respiratory disease and considerable reassurance may be required concerning safety. The issues of safety are somewhat unknown in the field of pulmonary rehabilitation. Although full exercise testing with ECG heart monitoring is recommended as routine for patients with COPD (American Thoracic Society 1999), a maximal incremental cycle ergometry test is unrealistic for many patients with severe disease. Even unloaded cycling can be exhausting for these patients, while adding incremental loads may cause distressing dyspnoea, ultimately preventing further exercise and disheartening the patient.

Most programmes exclude patients with unstable angina. For most patients, a field walking test with pulse oximetry (Fig. 13.3) and heart rate monitoring will identify oxygen needs and enable prescription of exercise intensity. In the hospital setting, resuscitation equipment and oxygen should be readily available and the personnel involved trained in the use of this equipment. However, a more pragmatic approach is required in the community setting where patients may be exercising at home or in local centres. There is evidence that patients with COPD demonstrate arterial desaturation during routine activities. The long-term effects of temporary falls in arterial saturation are unknown and warrant further investigation (Schenkel et al 1996). Patients with COPD often demonstrate ventilatory limitation or report fatigue before there is significant cardiovascular stress. However, this will not be the same for all groups of patients with respiratory disease and further research is required in this area. Anecdotally the only complications of exercise in these patients have been related to minor musculoskeletal injuries.

RESPIRATORY MUSCLE TRAINING

A considerable amount of research has focused on specific training for the respiratory muscles, hypothesizing that increased respiratory muscle strength will translate into increased exercise tolerance via a reduction in dyspnoea (Belman et al 1994). In theory, by improving the strength or endurance of the diaphragm, greater inspiratory loads may be tolerated, thereby prolonging exercise tolerance. Inspiratory muscle training can be performed by inspiratory resistive training, threshold loading and normocapnic hyperpnoea, and currently there is no sufficient evidence to support one method over another. Studies have found that inspiratory muscle training (IMT) significantly increases inspiratory muscle strength and endurance (Belman & Shadmehr 1988, Chen et al

13

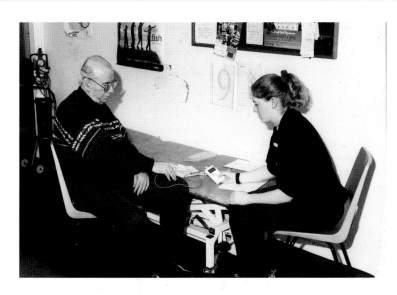

Figure 13.3 Assessment of oxygen saturation using a pulse oximeter.

1985, Harver et al 1989), whereas others did not (Belman et al 1986, Guyatt et al 1992). Positive results on muscle force and dyspnoea have been reported using high-intensity IMT, that is IMT performed at the highest tolerable inspiratory threshold load (Hill et al 2006). Other studies have evaluated the place of respiratory muscle training together with general body training and once again variable results have been reported. Wanke and co-workers (1994) showed an additional effect of IMT in COPD patients compared with cycle endurance alone. In contrast, studies by Berry et al (1996) and Larson et al (1999) showed no significant additive effects of IMT compared with general training alone. The differences in these results may be due to the different characteristics of the training, i.e. type, duration and intensity of programmes, since these characteristics will influence the response. In many studies training intensity is below that required to achieve physiological effects. In addition, changes in breathing pattern during training alter the resistance provided (Reid & Samrai 1995). Goldstein (1993) reported that in many studies no attempt to control breathing pattern was made and measurements of endurance were therefore often unreliable. Future work in respiratory muscle training must ensure standardization of breathing frequency and pattern with training regimens of sufficient intensity to achieve a training effect.

The most recent meta-analysis of inspiratory muscle training has shown that, overall, improvements in muscle strength, endurance and dyspnoea can be achieved (Lotters et al 2002). However, these benefits are not always translated into improvement in functional outcomes such as exercise tolerance. Furthermore, this meta-analysis identified that patients with inspiratory muscle weakness improve significantly more in

comparison to patients without inspiratory muscle weakness. This suggests that patients with low inspiratory pressures are the preferential target for inspiratory muscle training, since positive results are mostly linked to the presence of inspiratory muscle weakness.

Specific training of the expiratory muscles has been reported to increase exercise performance, symptoms and health-related quality of life (Mota et al 2006, Weiner et al 2003a). However, Weiner et al (2003b) showed no additional benefits in terms of functional exercise capacity and dyspnoea sensation when comparing expiratory and inspiratory muscle training in comparison with inspiratory muscle training alone.

EDUCATION AS PART OF REHABILITATION

The focus of educating the patient has evolved over the years from single lectures to a self-management approach that encourages and teaches skills involved in disease control: namely, health behaviour modification and improved self-efficacy. To educate the patient should be a shared responsibility between the family and all health professionals involved. Guidelines state that:

> '. . . patient education remains a core component of comprehensive pulmonary rehabilitation, despite the difficulties in measuring its direct contribution to overall outcomes'
>
> (Nici et al 2006)

There are few trials specifically evaluating the benefit of education programmes as part of pulmonary rehabilitation. Education alone (i.e. outside the context of a rehabilitation programme) appears to do little to reduce

13

the sensation of dyspnoea (Hunter & Hall 1989), improve quality of life (Gallefoss et al 1999, Ries et al 1995) or exercise tolerance (Sassi-Dambron et al 1995, Wedzicha et al 1998). Moreover, a review by Folgering and co-workers (1994) suggested that education programmes in COPD patients show ambiguous results and compare poorly with asthmatic patient education on the grounds of cost-effectiveness. Control groups for research studies often comprise groups of patients receiving education alone on the grounds that they have little effect on exercise tolerance (Ries et al 1995, Wedzicha et al 1998).

Appropriate assessment of health education requires evaluation of the benefits on patient knowledge, therapeutic compliance, cost-effectiveness and dyspnoea. Mackay (1996) reported that patients with COPD displayed improved knowledge and understanding after receiving dietary advice at home. However, no follow-up assessment was made of the change in eating habits. In a review of patient education Mazzuca (1982) stated that although general education may have little benefit:

> *'Behaviour (regimen orientated) instruction has therapeutic value'*

Regimen-orientated instruction includes interactive sessions such as medical management with instruction on inhaler technique, teaching relaxation techniques, practical demonstrations of energy conservation techniques and stress management. These approaches clearly have beneficial effects on rescue medication, use of steroids and antibiotics and yet the data do not always show any reduction in hospitalizations or exacerbation rate, nor any improvements in other outcomes such as health-related quality of life and lung function (Monninkhof et al 2003). While it seems strange that better use of medication does not impact on morbidity it is likely that the combined approach, which includes physical training, is more successful. This has been demonstrated by a multicentre randomized trial that showed evidence of effectiveness of a self-management programme including an exacerbation action plan and home exercise training (Bourbeau et al 2003). The programme significantly improved health-related quality of life, reduced hospital admissions due to an exacerbation of COPD (by 40%), reduced admissions for other health problems (by 57%), emergency department visits (by 41%) and unscheduled physician visits (by 58%). It is therefore not surprising that this form of self-management programme is considered cost-effective (Bourbeau et al 2006).

Psychosocial education

A meta-analysis of psychoeducational components of COPD management has shown a significant beneficial effect of behavioural education on inhaler use and a small non-significant effect on healthcare utilization (Devine & Pearcy 1996). Previous studies have shown reductions in dyspnoea after training in relaxation skills (Renfroe 1988) and coping strategies (Sassi-Dambron et al 1995). Eiser and colleagues (1997) reported improvements in exercise tolerance after group psychotherapy. In another study investigating psychosocial interventions, a combined behavioural and cognitive approach to exercise in COPD patients achieved greater improvements in walking distance than single interventions alone (Atkins et al 1984). Since the prevalence of depression and anxiety in COPD patients is very high (van Manen et al 2002), psychological counselling in addition to pulmonary rehabilitation renders additional benefits to patients with these characteristics (i.e. 20–40% of the patients) (Nguyen & Carrieri-Kohlman 2005, Withers et al 1999). Behaviour-orientated approaches to pulmonary rehabilitation such as goal setting may improve adherence and task performance (Locke et al 1981). Education programmes must be task-orientated, specific to the population and provided in a manner that is accessible to the patient. Analysis of the effects of education should focus on patient knowledge and its translation into improved self-management, prompt identification of problems and reductions in hospitalization. An educational programme, combined with physical training, optimizes functional ability as well as self-mastery. The main targets for self-management education programmes are patients with reduced health-related quality of life and frequent exacerbations.

OTHER ADJUNCTS TO REHABILITATION

Breathing techniques

Breathing control is defined as:

> *'. . . gentle breathing using the lower chest with relaxation of the upper chest and shoulders; it is performed at normal tidal volume, at a natural rate and expiration should not be forced'*
>
> (Partridge et al 1989)

Patients should be encouraged to breathe slowly and naturally. Appropriate terminology may help instruction, with words such as 'let the air flow in' rather than 'breathe in' which implies that a forced breath in is required. Effective positioning can reduce the work of breathing (O'Neill & McCarthy 1983) and should be utilized during exercise. Patients may use the 'lean forward position' in standing, against walls or equipment or in sitting (Bott 1997). Breathing control can be used during stair climbing (inhale while climbing up one step, exhale while climbing up the next two steps) to reinforce a rhythmical breathing pattern and minimize breath holding during activities. Although there is little empirical evidence for the value of these techniques, anecdotal and physiological evidence supports their use (Sharp et al 1980).

More recently investigators have studied the role of pursed lips breathing (PLB) as a component of rehabilitation. The subject performs a moderately active expiration through the half-opened lips, inducing expiratory mouth pressures of about 5 cmH$_2$O (van der Schans et al 1995). Data from Garrod and colleagues (2005b) show significant reductions in respiratory frequency and a speedier recovery after a maximal walk test when exercise is performed using PLB compared with tidal flow breathing. Other studies show evidence that during both rest and exercise PLB is associated with an increase in tidal volume and a reduction in minute ventilation (Jones et al 2003, Mueller et al 1970). Confirmation that PLB promotes a slower and deeper breathing pattern both at rest and during exercise, but has a variable effect on dyspnoea sensation when performed volitionally during exercise by patients with COPD, has been demonstrated by Spahija et al (2005).

Diaphragmatic breathing (DB) is a technique in which the patient is encouraged to allow forward movement of the abdominal wall during inspiration and to reduce upper rib cage motion. When performing DB, patients are able to voluntarily change their breathing pattern to a more abdominal movement, improve their blood gases, increase tidal volume, and decrease breathing frequency (Vitacca et al 1998). However, this happens at a high cost: DB can lead to increased asynchronous and paradoxical breathing movements, increased work of breathing, enhanced oxygen cost of breathing, reduced mechanical efficiency and ultimately to a worsening of dyspnoea sensation (Gosselink et al 1995, Sackner et al 1984, Vitacca et al 1998, Willeput et al 1983). In addition, no permanent changes of the breathing pattern are observed when DB training is stopped. Currently, there is no evidence from controlled studies to support the use of DB in COPD patients (Gosselink 2003).

In summary, there is evidence for the use of techniques such as pursed lips breathing and forward lean position, whereas the evidence for the benefits of diaphragmatic breathing is weak. Despite some evidence for the benefits of a few breathing techniques, the limited evidence for the transfer of their effects during resting conditions to exercise conditions remains unclear and questions have yet to be answered.

Specific training of activities of daily living

Specific training of activities of daily living (ADL) mainly concerns the optimization of the most common movements and activities performed in daily life, through energy conservation techniques. Physiotherapists and occupational therapists can teach patients how to perform their ADL in a way that induces less dyspnoea and fatigue, with the aim of maximal function and independence. Patients can also be taught to organize their home space and time schedule in order to facilitate ADL and functionality. Velloso and colleagues showed that the use of these energy conservation techniques lowers energy cost and dyspnoea perception (Velloso & Jardim 2006). In another study, addition of these techniques improved self-reported performance in ADL, although no additional benefits in exercise capacity (6MWD) were observed (Lorenzi et al 2004). Similar results were shown by Norweg and coworkers (Norweg et al 2005). They also found evidence for additional benefits in dyspnoea, fatigue and activity involvement after activity-specific training combined with exercise compared with exercise training alone, although the improvements were greater in the oldest patients. Conversely, Sewell and colleagues found no significant differences in exercise capacity, amount of physical activity performed in daily life and self-perceived domestic function when comparing a general exercise group with an individually targeted exercise group (Sewell et al 2005). The authors concluded that general exercise training is as effective as an ADL-targeted training in improving domestic function and physical activity in daily life. Evidence from the literature is contradictory and further research is required to determine the real benefits of adding specific ADL training to a pulmonary rehabilitation programme.

Walking aids

In order to improve walking ability, a rollator may be a useful option. A rollator is a walker with four wheels, equipped with swivel castors on the front wheels, brakes, a basket for carrying objects and a seat that allows sitting for rest (Fig. 13.4A). An alternative is a three-wheeled walker (Fig. 13.4B). Various studies have shown the acute benefits of using a rollator in more impaired individuals in terms of improved walking distance, ventilation, reduced dyspnoea and provision of a greater sense of safety (Probst et al 2004, Solway et al 2002). Despite these positive acute effects, the provision of a rollator for long-term use at home did not result in a significant effect on quality of life or exercise capacity (Gupta et al 2006). This was possibly because a large proportion of the patients did not use the rollator on a regular basis at home, that is less than three times per week. Regular users demonstrated better results than infrequent users. Therefore, the choice of which patient is most likely to use the rollator regularly is crucial in

13

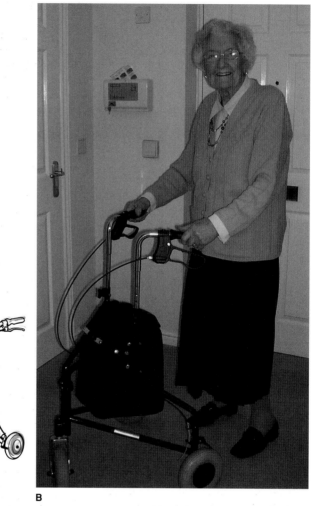

A   **B**

Figure 13.4 (A) Diagrammatic representation of a four-wheeled rollator (B) Using a three-wheeled walker.

13

order to obtain positive results. It is important to bear in mind that the most disabled patients are the ones who benefit most from the use of a rollator, and specific coaching should be provided in order to maximally increase walking efficiency when using the device (Probst et al 2004, Solway et al 2002).

Non-invasive positive pressure ventilation

The place of non-invasive positive pressure ventilation (NIPPV) as an adjunct to rehabilitation is based on the theory that unloading of the respiratory muscles during activity will enable higher work intensities to be reached, accruing greater benefit from exercise. For many patients with severe problems, dyspnoea may significantly limit the ability to exercise and NIPPV may be a valuable addition to rehabilitation. In a systematic review, rehabilitation experts from the Netherlands pooled data from seven critically appraised studies (van't Hul et al 2002) and found there was a significant benefit on exercise-induced dyspnoea and endurance time when NIPPV was applied during an acute exercise test.

However, there are practical difficulties to providing ventilation during a training session in terms of limiting the type of exercise and adherence to exercise. In a randomized controlled trial of overnight application of NIPPV plus daytime non-assisted rehabilitation, significant improvements in exercise tolerance and quality of life were found after rehabilitation in the home ventilated group compared with a non-ventilated group (Garrod et al 2000b). Improvement in exercise tolerance may have resulted from overnight relief of low-level fatigue of respiratory muscles caused during exhaustive exercise. Valid criticisms of this work concern the relatively short period of time spent using the ventilator (mean 2.5 hours) and the lack of placebo ventilation.

Although for most patients this additional aid will be unnecessary, for those severely disabled by dyspnoea this treatment may enable them to exercise at sufficient intensity to achieve an effective training response. Patients with cystic fibrosis or emphysema, awaiting lung transplantation, or those recently discharged from intensive care with significant ventilatory limitation may be suitable candidates for additional support.

Pharmacological agents

The effects of anabolic steroids and exercise training, especially in male patients with COPD, have been studied. The use of steroids was shown to increase muscle strength, enhancing the effects of strength training programmes (Casaburi et al 2004). A gain in bodyweight was also identified and this was said to be due mainly to an increase in fat-free mass rather than fat mass (Creutzberg et al 2003, Schols et al 1995). The main targets for this kind of intervention are male hypogonadal patients with COPD and patients receiving oral corticosteroids (Creutzberg et al 2003). The ideal dose of anabolic steroids, to balance the risks and benefits, deserves further investigation.

The effects of growth hormone administration have been investigated in patients with COPD as it had been hypothesized that hormone therapy may enhance muscle changes following rehabilitation. However, Burdet et al (1997) did not show a significant effect of added growth hormone on either exercise tolerance or muscle strength. Currently, the lack of evidence of functional benefit does not support the use of human growth hormone combined with a pulmonary rehabilitation programme.

Guidelines recommend the initiation of maintenance long-acting bronchodilator therapy in patients with moderate-to-severe disease (Fabbri & Hurd 2003). Evidence from a meta-analysis suggested that initiation of long-acting bronchodilator therapy with tiotropium, at earlier stages of the disease, may result in improvements in lung function and health-related quality of life (Barr et al 2006). In addition, there is evidence that the effects of exercise training may be amplified in patients with COPD receiving the long-acting anticholinergic agent tiotropium (Casaburi et al 2005). Cautious interpretation of this data is required since the placebo group were not previously optimized for pharmacological therapy. In addition, other classes of drugs show benefits on hyperinflation and exercise endurance such as combined corticosteroid and bronchodilator therapy

(O'Donnell et al 2006). This is a promising approach for respiratory rehabilitation.

There is still a need to identify those patients within the large heterogeneous group of patients with COPD who may benefit from corticosteroid administration. Complications from long-term corticosteroid use are important considerations (e.g. muscle weakness, osteoporosis) but they appear to be less of a problem when the corticosteroid is given via the inhaled route (Goldstein et al 1999, MacIntyre 2006). Guidelines recommend the use of inhaled corticosteroids in patients with severe disease and frequent exacerbations (Fabbri & Hurd 2003). There is strong clinical evidence to support the use of inhaled corticosteroids to prevent exacerbations and oral corticosteroids to reduce the duration and impact of exacerbations (MacIntyre 2006).

Nutrition

It has been demonstrated that there is a significant relationship between exercise tolerance and nutritional status in patients with COPD (Schols et al 1991). Low bodyweight and low body mass index (BMI) are each known to be poor prognostic factors of disease severity (Landbo et al 1999). Weight loss, muscle wasting and reduced fat-free mass often occur, and are linked to the lack of balance between ingestion and energy expenditure (decreased dietary intake, high energy requirements, and disturbances in metabolism caused by altered anabolic and catabolic mediators such as hormones, cytokines and growth factors).

A systematic review of randomized controlled trials showed no significant effects of nutritional supplementation on anthropometric measures, lung function or exercise capacity in patients with stable COPD (Ferreira et al 2005). Therefore, currently there is insufficient evidence of benefit of nutritional support for outpatients. However, patients who are non-responsive to nutritional support seem to have a profile of older age, relative anorexia and elevated systemic inflammatory response (Creutzberg et al 2000), and future research should therefore focus on the potential positive effects in subgroups of patients.

Neuromuscular electrical stimulation

Using transcutaneous low-intensity currents, muscle contraction can be induced by neuromuscular electrical stimulation (NMES) and specific muscle groups can be trained. In stable patients with muscle weakness, NMES applied to the lower limbs muscles improved muscle strength, exercise tolerance and peak oxygen uptake (Bourjeily-Habr et al 2002, Neder et al 2002). The use of NMES has also been reported to result in a fast functional recovery in severely disabled patients receiving

13

mechanical ventilation who were bedbound for more than 30 days (Zanotti et al 2003). In patients with well-preserved functional status, however, the results were very modest (Dal Corso et al 2007). The use of NMES as an adjunct to rehabilitation in severely disabled patients with low BMI has been shown to result in improvements in dyspnoea, exercise tolerance and muscle strength (Vivodtzev et al 2006). This suggests that NMES may provide an additional stimulus for changes in muscle physiology for malnourished patients or those with severe ventilatory limitation. The intervention was provided early following discharge from a hospital admission for acute exacerbation. It is possible that malnourished patients show greater hospital-induced sarcopenia than those with adequate BMI and that this may have contributed to the improved effects found in this study. One cautionary point is the fact that the rehabilitation programme lasted only 4 weeks rather than the recommended minimum of 8 weeks, and these early differences may not be evident in the longer term or after prolonged training.

Smoking cessation

There are different approaches for sustained smoking cessation, from counselling to pharmacological tools (nicotine replacement therapy and non-nicotine agents such as bupropion) (Marlow & Stoller 2003). Although smokers are more likely to decline invitations to rehabilitation programmes and may be less adherent (Young et al 1999), there is no evidence that continued smoking reduces the response to pulmonary rehabilitation. There has been much debate over whether patients who refuse to stop smoking should be eligible for pulmonary rehabilitation. However, in clinical practice, it is common to observe that for many smokers, the combined positive influence of pulmonary rehabilitation and the effect of peer pressure have helped a number of patients to stop smoking. Until trials show clearly that the benefit of training is reduced in current smokers, it is recommended that smokers be supported throughout pulmonary rehabilitation programmes and offered appropriate smoking cessation help (Kawane 1997).

Acupressure

One interesting study has evaluated the effect of acupressure practised daily in conjunction with a 6-week exercise programme (Maa et al 1997). The study was randomized with the control group receiving 'sham' acupressure. Significant benefits of acupressure on dyspnoea were reported although these were not reflected in differences in exercise tolerance. Unfortunately, the study was single blinded and the investigator, who met with the patients weekly to reinforce 'sham' or 'real'

acupressure, was aware of the randomization. A repeat of this study with a double-blind design would be of interest.

ASSESSMENT TOOLS IN PULMONARY REHABILITATION

Assessment tools are used to measure various outcomes and to characterize a population. Assessment tools enable reflection on practice, provide insight into the mechanisms of improvement and therefore aid development of programmes, allowing the health professional and the patient the opportunity to monitor progress in meaningful terms. The choice of assessment tool remains predominantly that of the investigator with consideration for the basic principles of validity, reliability and sensitivity.

Assessment of exercise tolerance and muscle function

Assessment of exercise tolerance is required in order to assess risks, characterize initial disability, set targets of training intensity, assess the benefit of rehabilitation programmes and motivate patients to continue with training regimens. All patients should perform a standardized test of exercise capacity before and after training. Evidence-based guidelines indicate that patients undergoing a period of rehabilitative training show improvements in exercise tolerance without evidence of adverse complications (American College of Chest Physicians (ACCP)/ American Association of Cardiovascular and Pulmonary Rehabilitation (AACVPR) 1997). These improvements are observed both in laboratory tests and field tests.

Laboratory incremental maximal tests versus field tests

Laboratory tests measuring maximal oxygen consumption ($\dot{V}O_2max$), heart rate, workload, arterial oxygenation and blood lactate levels remain the gold standard in exercise testing and are appropriate in patients with COPD for having the potential to provide a variety of vital information (e.g. the cause of exercise limitation) in this rather limited population (Palange et al 1994). However, where resources are limited, 'field tests' (tests of exercise tolerance applied in the clinical setting rather than the laboratory) may be performed, but these tests may be more susceptible to bias. Laboratory tests may have limited application, particularly in patients with severe disease where work capacity is very reduced, resulting in an inability to reach ventilatory threshold levels (Midorikawa et al 1997). The functional ability of patients will not necessarily reflect the true daily activi-

13

ties they can perform (Pitta et al 2005a). Field tests may have advantages over laboratory measurements due to simplicity and functional appropriateness, but disadvantages include the effects of motivation and the lack of physiological correlates. Overall, maximal incremental tests and field tests provide different and complementary information concerning exercise capacity in patients with COPD (Ong et al 2004, Turner et al 2004). Measurements of muscle strength and endurance have a central place in the assessment of patients with COPD (American Thoracic Society/European Respiratory Society 1999). These measurements are useful to identify muscle dysfunction, determine training load and assess improvements after interventions such as pulmonary rehabilitation.

The 6-minute walking test

In early rehabilitation trials, the 12-minute walking test (12MWT) was used to assess exercise tolerance (Cockcroft et al 1981, McGavin et al 1977, Sinclair & Ingram 1980). Over the years it has been replaced by a shorter version, the 6-minute walking test (6MWT). The 6MWT has been widely used in pulmonary rehabilitation (American Thoracic Society 2002). It is a simple test that measures the distance walked over 6 minutes. Subjects undergoing the test typically increase their oxygen consumption until the 3rd minute, when a plateau is observed (Troosters et al 2002). Pinto-Plata and coworkers (2004) showed that, in severe COPD, the 6MWT predicts mortality better than other traditional markers of disease severity such as spirometric variables. Furthermore, it also reflects the patient's functional capacity (Carter et al 2003) and is the best correlate of time spent actively in daily life, especially in those patients with reduced exercise capacity (Pitta et al 2005a). However, its limitations include dependence upon patient motivation, the susceptibility to practice effects and the lack of standardization of the test procedure throughout studies in the literature. To reduce these disadvantages, an American Thoracic Society guideline statement (2002) suggests a number of useful standardization measures in order to minimize the test's shortcomings. These measures include the length of the hallway (minimum of 30 metres), the need for standardized encouragement and the value of a practice test. Predicted normal values according to age, gender, height and weight are available (Troosters et al 1999).

Statistically significant changes in the 6MWT need to be interpreted in the light of clinically significant changes: 'how big is big?' (Guyatt et al 1991). The threshold for clinical differences is a measured value that equates to a level of change at which the patient perceives either an improvement in symptoms or deterioration. Redelmeier et al (1997) have identified the clinical threshold of the 6MWT as an increase or decrease of 54 metres following an intervention. Many results of rehabilitation trials in COPD patients fall short of this threshold (Cambach et al 1997, Wijkstra et al 1996), although many others have reached clinically important levels of improvement (de Torres et al 2002, Spruit et al 2002). Improvements in the 6MWD after pulmonary rehabilitation programmes vary considerably depending on the duration, frequency, intensity and location of the exercise training, as well as the modalities applied.

The shuttle walking tests

A 'field walking' test that is less susceptible to motivation is the shuttle walking test (SWT) (Singh et al 1992). This incremental test is externally paced, enhancing standardization, does not include patient stops and correlates to $\dot{V}O_2max$ (Singh et al 1994). The SWT demonstrates validity with other measures of exercise tolerance and is reliable on test–retest, requiring only one practice walk (Singh et al 1992). It has been shown to be a sensitive measure of change after rehabilitation in patients with severe COPD (Wedzicha et al 1998) and has been validated for use in elderly patients with COPD (Dyer et al 2002). A further test from this group of researchers measures endurance in a standardized manner, the endurance shuttle walk test (ESWT) (Revill et al 1999). Comparisons between the 6MWT and ESWT suggest that ESWT may be more responsive to change after pulmonary rehabilitation than the 6MWT (Eaton et al 2006) but much will depend upon individual programmes, resources and assessor preference.

In summary, field tests (Chapter 3) are an appropriate measure of exercise capacity in these patients and, although they may not provide full understanding with respect to the physiological mechanisms of improvement, when combined with other functional assessments they help to provide a practical evaluation of pulmonary rehabilitation. A comparison between the SWT and the 6MWT is summarized in Table 13.2.

Peripheral muscle strength and endurance

In previous years, this topic has been given considerably less attention than the assessment of maximal and submaximal exercise capacity. The reason for this may be due to the perception of the requirement for expensive complicated equipment. While it is true that many studies evaluating muscle function following rehabilitation have used equipment not always available in respiratory therapy departments, this has gradually changed as different methods to assess peripheral muscle strength and endurance have emerged.

13

Table 13.2 Comparison between the shuttle walking test (SWT) and the 6-minute walking test (6MWT)

SWT	6MWT
Standardized	Partially standardized
Facility to extrapolate $\dot{V}O_2$max from results	Evidence of validity and weak association with $\dot{V}O_2$max
Externally paced	Susceptible to patient motivation
Requires one practice walk	One practice test advised
Maximal test	Submaximal timed test
Requires tape and recorder	Requires no equipment
No clinical threshold	Clinical threshold identified

Muscle strength

Electromagnetic stimulation avoids the volitional effects of other motivation-dependent techniques by assuring maximal activation of the muscle (Man et al 2003), but is methodologically complex and not used in everyday practice. In clinical practice, muscle strength is commonly assessed by maximal voluntary contraction, and different types of dynamometers (handheld, motorized, electronic) are available. If adequate standardization and encouragement are used, the measurements should be appropriate for the clinical assessment of individuals before and after training. Grip strength, measured by simple handgrip devices, may be useful to assess upper limbs. In repetition maximum (RM) tests, subjects lift progressive loads until they are unable to complete the movement across a range of motion or use compensatory mechanisms to undertake the movement. This test can be performed with free weights or in multigyms.

Muscle endurance

The classical test for assessment of muscle endurance is that of the subject performing regular repetitions of movement against a determined weight, equivalent to a percentage of their maximal strength. The test is stopped when the subject is unable to sustain the repetitions, and the duration of the test (or the number of the repetitions) is the main outcome (Coronell et al 2004). Another endurance index is the total work (e.g. in Joules) executed during a certain time (Neder et al 2002). Exogenous electrical stimulation can also be used when assessing muscle endurance, in order to induce fatigue of limb muscles from which mechanical output can be measured.

As a key aim of rehabilitation is to improve muscle function (in particular quadriceps), assessment of muscle strength and endurance should be considered an essential part of a rehabilitation programme.

Assessment of activities of daily living, health-related quality of life and dyspnoea

Activities of daily living (ADL)

Increasing participation in daily activities is one of the main goals of pulmonary rehabilitation programmes (Global Initiative for Chronic Obstructive Lung Disease (GOLD) 2001). Currently the improvement in daily activities following rehabilitation programs remains poorly studied in patients with COPD, although there have been significant advances in the development of assessment tools both subjective and objective.

Subjective tools (questionnaires and scales)

Lareau and coworkers (1994) developed a 70-item activities of daily living (ADL) assessment tool, employed as a measure of outcome following pulmonary rehabilitation. The tool was modified to form a shorter questionnaire of 40 items and has been successful in identifying improvements in daily activities after pulmonary rehabilitation (Lareau et al 1998). Using this questionnaire, Trappenburg and colleagues (2005) showed significant improvements in functional status after 3 months of pulmonary rehabilitation. The short 15-item questionnaire, the London Chest Activity of Daily Living Scale has been validated in patients with COPD (Garrod et al 2000c) (Table 13.3). Significant improvements in dyspnoea during ADL were documented following pulmonary rehabilitation and the change in ADL was associated with change in exercise tolerance (Garrod et al 2002). Self-reported performance in ADL has also been shown to improve after pulmonary rehabilitation in other studies (Bendstrup et al 1997, Yohannes et al 2000).

Improvement in ADL, assessed by subjective methods, provides a useful and recognizable measure of the benefit of pulmonary rehabilitation to an individual's daily functioning. However, the above-mentioned ADL questionnaires and scales do not aim primarily at quantifying the amount and intensity of activity performed in daily life. In other words, these subjective tools assess whether the patient is less impaired by dyspnoea, more independent and able to perform better in daily activities, but this does not necessarily equate to the patient being more active in quantitative terms. Quantification of the amount and intensity of physical activity assessed by subjective methods has been shown to be inaccurate in patients with COPD (Pitta et al 2005b). The reasons for this are that questionnaires

13

Table 13.3   London Chest Activity of Daily Living Scale

THE LONDON CHEST ACTIVITY OF DAILY LIVING SCALE

NAME ....   DATE OF BIRTH ....

DO YOU LIVE ALONE?   YES ☐   NO ☐

Please tell us how breathless you have been during the last few days whilst doing the following activities.

SELF-CARE

Drying	0	1	2	3	4	5
Dressing upper body	0	1	2	3	4	5
Putting shoes / socks on	0	1	2	3	4	5
Washing hair	0	1	2	3	4	5

DOMESTIC

Make beds	0	1	2	3	4	5
Change sheet	0	1	2	3	4	5
Wash windows / curtains	0	1	2	3	4	5
Clean / dusting	0	1	2	3	4	5
Wash up	0	1	2	3	4	5
Vacuuming / sweeping	0	1	2	3	4	5

PHYSICAL

Walking up stairs	0	1	2	3	4	5
Bending	0	1	2	3	4	5

LEISURE

Walking in home	0	1	2	3	4	5
Going out socially	0	1	2	3	4	5
Talking	0	1	2	3	4	5

How much does your breathing affect you in your normal activities of daily living?

A lot ☐   A little ☐   Not at all ☐

The London Chest Activity of Daily Living Scale (score sheet)

Please read carefully and circle the relevant number next to each activity.
This questionnaire is designed to find out whether there are activities that you can no longer do because of your breathlessness and how breathless the things that you still do make you. All answers are confidential.

If you do not do an activity because it is not relevant, or you have never done it, please answer:
0 – Wouldn't do anyway

If an activity is easy for you, please answer:
1 – Do not get breathless

If the activity makes you a bit breathless, please answer:
2 – I get moderately breathless

If the activity makes you very breathless, please answer:
3 – I get very breathless

If you have stopped doing this **because of your breathlessness** and *have no one else to do it for you*, please answer:
4 – I can't do this anymore.

If someone else does this for you, or helps you, BECAUSE you are too breathless, e.g. the home help does your shopping, please answer:
5 – I need someone else to do this.

13

quantifying physical activity in daily life depend on factors such as cognitive capacity, age, cultural factors, accurate perception and memory, in addition to the questionnaire design (Pitta et al 2006b).

Objective tools (motion sensors)

Increasing attention has been given to the objective monitoring of daily physical activity in different populations, including patients with COPD. Motion sensors are devices used to detect body movement, which can be used to objectively quantify physical activity in daily life over a period of time. There are different types of motion sensors: pedometers (to count steps and estimate the distance walked and energy expenditure) and accelerometers (technologically more advanced devices that allow the quantity and intensity of movements to be determined). Some accelerometers are able to detect a variety of physical activities and outcomes, and are often described as activity monitors.

In contrast to ADL assessment by subjective tools, literature concerning objective quantification of improvement in physical activity in daily life after rehabilitation yields conflicting results. Two studies demonstrated very modest or no improvement in the motion sensors' output after programmes lasting 3 and 8 weeks (Coronado et al 2003, Steele et al 2003). It is not clear whether these disappointing results derived from actual lack of improvement by the patients due to characteristics of the rehabilitation programme (e.g. duration, intensity, frequency) or from methodological issues of the assessment method (e.g. the outcomes used). In contrast, two other studies found significant improvements after programmes of 7 and 8 weeks of duration (Mercken et al 2005, Sewell et al 2005). Differences in the populations involved and the types of programmes may explain the conflicting results among these studies. It is not yet possible to identify which patients are more physically active following pulmonary rehabilitation or the characteristics of the programmes that will induce changes in day-to-day physical activity behaviour. This is an area in which further research is required.

Health-related quality of life

A broad definition of quality of life includes factors that health care may not affect directly (although there may be indirect effects on health). Such factors include financial status, housing, employment and social support. Health-related quality of life (HRQoL) instruments can vary from disease-specific questionnaires, which measure a single item such as dyspnoea or numerous items, to generic measures intended for use in any disease. Generic questionnaires were originally designed to define the health of populations and not to measure therapeutic efficacy. They are considered useful

Table 13.4 Examples of disease-specific and generic health-related quality of life tools

Disease-specific	Generic
Chronic Respiratory Disease (CRQ)	Sickness Impact Profile Questionnaire (SIP)
St George's Respiratory Questionnaire (SGRQ)	MOS Short-Form 36 Disease (SF36)
Breathing Problems Questionnnaire (BPQ)	Quality of Well-Being Scale (QWB)
Oxygen Cost Diagram (OCD)	Nottingham Health Profile (NHP)

when comparing different populations of patients. Disease-specific questionnaires were designed to detect and quantify health gain following treatment (Table 13.4).

HRQoL instruments have been useful in assessing benefits of pulmonary rehabilitation programmes. There have been numerous reports of improvements in health status after such programmes (Garrod et al 2000a, 2000c, Goldstein et al 1994, Griffiths et al 2000, Lacasse et al 2002, Wedzicha et al 1998). In a study from the Netherlands (Wijkstra et al 1994), HRQoL was measured using the disease-specific Chronic Respiratory Questionnaire (CRQ) which measures four aspects of HRQoL: dyspnoea, mastery, emotion and fatigue (Guyatt et al 1987). Another commonly used questionnaire is the St George's Respiratory Questionnaire (SGRQ) (Jones et al 1991), which comprises symptoms, activities and impact domains and has provided strong evidence of a change in health status after rehabilitation (Griffiths et al 2000). The clinical threshold for the CRQ has been identified as requiring a change of at least 0.5 point per item (Jaeshchke et al 1989) while a change of 4 points or more, in the total score of the SGRQ, is required to achieve a clinical effect (Jones 2005). An empirical comparison between the SGRQ and CRQ showed strong similarities between the questionnaires in terms of validity and reliability, suggesting that either would be an appropriate measurement tool (Rutten-van Mölken et al 1999). Two studies have shown that these two disease-specific questionnaires are more responsive to changes than generic questionnaires, and suggest that the CRQ has superior responsiveness (Puhan et al 2007). It should also be acknowledged that informing patients about their pre-treatment scores does not significantly improve the responsiveness of the CRQ or the SGRQ after rehabilitation (Schunemann et al 2002).

Dyspnoea

Repeated trials of rehabilitation have shown improvement in dyspnoea using validated measures (Goldstein et al 1994, Reardon et al 1994, Ries et al 1995). A meta-analysis by Lacasse and colleagues (1997) concluded that training resulted in significant relief of dyspnoea. Dyspnoea can be measured in a variety of ways and graded scales such as the Baseline and Transition Dyspnoea Index (BDI) (Mahler et al 1984) and the Medical Research Council (MRC) Breathlessness Score (Fletcher 1960) are examples.

The MRC Breathlessness Score, which is self-administered, grades dyspnoea during walking according to five levels, with grade 5 representing patients who consider themselves to be housebound due to breathlessness. It is a valid and reliable questionnaire that has been found to be useful in stratification of patients before entry to a pulmonary rehabilitation programme (Bestall et al 1999). However, the problem with such scales concerns the wide variation of disability evident between the grades, which – although improving the reliability of the questionnaire – reduces its sensitivity (Jones 1992).

Other scales used to measure dyspnoea include the Borg Scale of Perceived Dyspnoea (Borg 1982), the dyspnoea component of the CRQ (Guyatt et al 1987), the University of California, San Diego (UCSD) Shortness of Breath Questionnaire (Eakin et al 1998) and the visual analogue scale (VAS) (Aitken 1969).

DO ALL PATIENTS BENEFIT FROM PULMONARY REHABILITATION?

This is a contentious question and to some extent remains unanswered. It is probably fair to say that all patients have the potential to gain benefit in specific outcomes, albeit modest in some cases, and the majority of patients benefit significantly in terms of improvement in exercise tolerance (Troosters et al 2001). As yet, it has not been possible to describe fully the specific predictive factors. ZuWallack and co-workers (1991), investigating 50 patients with COPD following rehabilitation, were unable to show a relationship between improvements and age, gender, pulmonary function or initial walking distance. However, they did show that patients with the greatest ventilatory reserve at baseline had the greatest improvement in walking distance following training. More recent robust evidence, concerning response to rehabilitation, comes from Troosters et al (2001) who showed that the patients most likely to respond well to rehabilitation were those with relatively weak peripheral muscles and preserved ventilatory reserve on starting the programme. This reinforces the importance of quadriceps assessment before rehabilitation. Moreover, this study also showed that about 30% of the patients may not show a significant improvement in exercise capacity, but may improve their health-related quality of life to a clinically significant extent. Garrod and colleagues (2006) recently performed a similar study aiming to identify predictors of response to rehabilitation. The authors purposefully included patients with mild disease (Grade 1 & 2 on MRC Scale) since there had been little evaluation of rehabilitation in this group, meaning that previous regression analysis may not have included all relevant stages of disease. It was not possible to identify clear predictors of response, but the authors did report two important findings. First, patients with mild disease do very well with rehabilitation and, secondly, patients with more severe disease (grade 5) demonstrate a smaller magnitude of change. This is in accordance with earlier data (Wedzicha et al 1998) but contrasts with findings from Berry and colleagues, who showed that patients with mild, moderate and severe disease all have similar improvements in physical function and HRQoL (Berry et al 1999). Garrod et al's (2006) work also highlighted an important finding concerning drop-out of pulmonary rehabilitation: patients who were depressed at baseline were eight times more likely to drop out compared with those who were not depressed. This further highlights the need for optimal medicalization of the condition before entry to pulmonary rehabilitation.

In summary, rehabilitation will benefit most patients, provided that the intensity and duration of exercise are sufficient. It is likely that patients with more severe disease will require longer training periods and/or specific adjuncts for meaningful benefits to result. At present there is no evidence to support denying access to rehabilitation programmes for older patients or those with severe/very severe lung function impairment or hypercapnia. Absence of improvements in exercise tolerance should not be regarded as an overall unsuccessful programme result, as patients may have gains in other important outcomes. Additionally, patients with mild COPD should be encouraged to receive early rehabilitation, as this is when lifestyle and behaviour modification is likely to have the greatest impact on progression of the disease.

LONG-TERM EFFECTS OF PULMONARY REHABILITATION – IS BENEFIT MAINTAINED?

Many studies have assessed the short-term benefits of pulmonary rehabilitation. These studies have shown that patients can gain significant benefits in exercise capacity, health status and dyspnoea immediately following a rehabilitation programme. However, full

13

assessment of pulmonary rehabilitation requires an evaluation of the long-term benefits of such programmes. As previously mentioned, one of the ways to obtain longer-lasting effects is to increase the programme's duration and another is to provide a follow-up programme. Vale et al (1993) assessed the maintenance of improvements in exercise tolerance and health status approximately 1 year after training. They compared two groups of patients; the first group had participated in a structured exercise maintenance follow-up programme, whereas the second group had no follow-up programme. Both groups showed a decline in outcome measures with no significant difference evident between the groups. The authors suggested that follow-up programmes were of little benefit and that other strategies are required to prolong the beneficial effects. However, interpretation of these findings should be made with caution as no control group (those who did not receive rehabilitation) was included.

Contrasting results were found in a study performed by Berry and coworkers (2003), in which patients had an initial programme of 3 months and were divided in two groups: a follow-up programme comprising sessions three times per week for 15 months and an exercise advice programme for the same period of time (Berry et al 2003). The exercise group showed superior results, demonstrating the value of long-term follow-up including regular exercise training. Another study has reported that participation in regular walking, after completing a pulmonary rehabilitation programme, is associated with slower declines in overall HRQoL and walking self-efficacy as well as less progression of dyspnoea during ADL (Heppner et al 2006). The conflicting results between these different studies may be due to the characteristics of the exercise follow-up programme. Repeated short-term programmes do not seem to achieve effective results, except for a reduction in exacerbation rates (Foglio et al 2001). Regular telephone support and monthly visits or meetings with health professionals have very modest effects (Brooks et al 2002, Ries et al 2003).

HRQoL improvements are still evident 12 months following rehabilitation (Griffiths et al 2000), and seem to be preserved for longer than improvements in exercise tolerance (Foglio et al 1999, Guell et al 2000, Troosters et al 2000). Wijkstra and colleagues (1995) demonstrated that positive results in HRQoL can be maintained for up to 18 months after a 2-month home-based programme followed by a programme comprising monthly home physiotherapy sessions. One of the most extensive follow-up studies has been carried out by Ries et al (1995), who reported on patients receiving an 8-week rehabilitation programme followed by monthly reinforcement sessions for 1 year and patients were followed for 6 years. They showed that improvements in exercise tolerance, dyspnoea and daily activity obtained following the initial 8-week programme were partially maintained for 1 year, but tended to diminish after that. Improvements in self-efficacy and perceived breathlessness were maintained for a few months longer. Overall the literature is conflicting and the available evidence does not allow definitive conclusions to be drawn on the ideal design of a follow-up programme, although periodic supervised exercise sessions seem advisable.

CONCLUSIONS

Pulmonary rehabilitation is an effective therapy. There is evidence to support that pulmonary rehabilitation programmes result in:

- improvement in exercise tolerance
- improvement in the sensation of dyspnoea
- improvement in the ability to perform routine activities of daily living
- improvement in health-related quality of life
- improvement in muscle strength, endurance and mass
- reductions in number of days spent in hospital.

With the majority of evidence in favour of pulmonary rehabilitation it should be considered an important therapeutic intervention. Cost and resources will remain obstacles to overcome, but pulmonary rehabilitation is a relatively low-budget intervention. The solid body of evidence currently available is, without any doubt, sufficient to support the provision of pulmonary rehabilitation for all patients for whom it is indicated. A multidisciplinary combined approach will spread the workload and ensure that we offer the most effective and evidence-based treatments to our patients.

References

Aitken RB 1969 A growing edge of measurement of feelings. Procedings of the Royal Society of Medicine, 62: 989–993

Allaire J, Maltais F, Doyon JF et al 2004 Peripheral muscle endurance and the oxidative profile of the quadriceps in patients with COPD. Thorax 59: 673–678

American College of Chest Physicians (ACCP)/American Association of Cardiovascular and Pulmonary Rehabilitation (AACVPR) 1997 Pulmonary rehabilitation guidelines panel. Pulmonary rehabilitation. Joint ACCP/AACVPR Evidence-based guidelines. Chest 112: 1363–1396

American Thoracic Society 1999 Pulmonary rehabilitation: an official statement. American Journal of Respiratory and Critical Care Medicine 159: 1666–1682

American Thoracic Society Committee on Proficiency Standards for Clinical Pulmonary Function Laboratories. 2002 ATS statement: guidelines for the six-minute walk test. American Journal of Respiratory and Critical Care Medicine 166(1): 111–117

American Thoracic Society and European Respiratory Society 1999 Skeletal muscle dysfunction in chronic obstructive pulmonary disease. American Journal of Respiratory and Critical Care Medicine 159(4): S1–S40

Astrand I, Guharay A, Wahren J 1968 Circulatory responses to arm exercise with different arm positions. Journal of Applied Physiology 25: 528–532

Atkins CJ, Kaplan RM Timms RM et al 1984 Behavioural exercise programmes in the management of chronic obstructive pulmonary disease. Journal of Consulting and Clinical Psychology 52(4): 591–603

Baarends EM, Schols AM, Akkermans MA et al 1997 Decreased mechanical efficiency in clinically stable patients with COPD. Thorax 52(11): 981–986

Barr RG, Bourbeau J, Camargo CA et al 2006 Tiotropium for stable chronic obstructive pulmonary disease: a metaanalysis. Thorax 61(10): 854–62

Belman MJ, Kendregan BA 1981 Exercise training fails to increase skeletal muscle enzymes in patients with chronic obstructive pulmonary disease. American Review of Respiratory Disease 123: 256–261

Belman MJ, Shadmehr R 1988 Targeted resistive muscle training in COPD. Journal of Applied Physiology 65: 2726–2735

Belman MJ, Thomas S, Lewis M 1986 Resistive breathing training in patients with chronic obstructive pulmonary disease. Chest 90: 662–669

Belman MJ, Botnick WC, Nathan SD et al 1994 Ventilatory load characteristics during ventilatory muscle training. American Journal of Respiratory and Critical Care Medicine 149(4): 925–929

Bendstrup KE, Ingemann JJ, Holm S et al 1997 Out-patient rehabilitation improves activities of daily living, quality of life and exercise tolerance in COPD. European Respiratory Journal 10: 2801–2806

Bernard S, Whittom F, Leblanc P et al 1999 Aerobic and strength training in patients with chronic obstructive pulmonary disease. American Journal of Respiratory and Critical Care Medicine 159: 896– 901

Berry M, Norman A, Sevensky S et al 1996 Inspiratory muscle training and whole body reconditioning in COPD. American Journal of Respiratory and Critical Care Medicine 153: 1812–1816

Berry MJ, Rejeski WJ, Adair NE et al 1999 Exercise rehabilitation and COPD stage. American Journal of Respiratory and Critical Care Medicine 160: 1248–1253

Berry MJ, Rejeski WJ, Adair NE et al 2003 A randomized controlled trial comparing long-term and short-term exercise in patients with COPD. Journal of Cardiopulmonary Rehabilitation 23: 60–68

Bestall JC, Paul EA, Garrod R et al 1999 Usefulness of the Medical Research Council (MRC) dyspnoea scale as a measure of disability in patients with COPD. Thorax 54: 581–586

Borg C 1982 Psychophysical basis of perceived exertion. Medicine and Science in Sports and Exercise 14: 377–381

Bott J 1997 Physiotherapy. In: Singh SJ, Morgan MDL (eds) Practical pulmonary rehabilitation. Chapman & Hall, London, pp 156–176

Bourbeau J, Collet JP, Schwartzman K et al 2006 Economic benefits of self-management education in COPD. Chest 130(6): 1704–1711

Bourbeau J, Julien M, Maltais F et al 2003 Reduction of hospital utilization in patients with chronic obstructive pulmonary disease: a disease-specific self-management intervention. Archives of Internal Medicine 10: 163(5): 585–591

Bourjeily-Habr G, Rochester C, Palermo F et al 2002 Randomized controlled trial of transcutaneous electrical muscle stimulation of the lower extremities in patients with chronic obstructive pulmonary disease. Thorax 57: 1045–1049

British Lung Foundation/British Thoracic Society Pulmonary Rehabilitation Survey 2002 *www.lunguk.org/downloads/BLF_pul_rehab_survey.pdf* (Accessed 16 July 2007)

Broekhuizen R, Wouters EF, Creutzberg EC, Schols AM 2006 Raised CRP levels mark metabolic and functional impairment in advanced COPD. Thorax 61(1): 17–22

Brolin SE, Cecins NM, Jenkins SC 2003 Questioning the use of heart rate and dyspnea in the prescription of exercise in subjects with chronic obstructive pulmonary disease. Journal of Cardiopulmonary Rehabilitation 23(3): 228–234

Brooks D, Krip B, Mangovski-Alzamora S et al 2002 The effect of post-rehabilitation programmes among individuals with chronic obstructive pulmonary disease. European Respiratory Journal 20(1): 20–29

Burdet L, Muralt B, Schutz Y et al 1997 Administration of growth hormone to underweight patients with chronic obstructive pulmonary disease. A prospective randomized, controlled study. American Journal of Respiratory and Critical Care Medicine 156: 1800–1806

Cambach W, Chadwick-Straver RVM, Wagenaar RC et al 1997 The effects of a community based pulmonary rehabilitation programme on exercise tolerance and quality of life: a randomized controlled trial. European Respiratory Journal 10: 104–113

Canadian Occupational Performance Measure 2005 *www.caot.ca/copm/index.htm* (Accessed 17 July 2007)

Carrieri-Kohlman V, Nguyen HQ, Doneski-Cuenco D et al 2005 Impact of brief or extended exercise training on the benefit of a dyspnea self-management program in COPD. Journal of Cardiopulmonary Rehabilitation 25(5): 275–284

Carter R, Holiday DB, Nwasuruba C et al 2003 6-minute walk work for assessment of functional capacity in patients with COPD. Chest 123(5): 1408–1415

Casaburi R, Bhasin S, Cosentino L et al 2004 Effects of testosterone replacement and strength training in men with COPD. American Journal of Respiratory and Critical Care Medicine 170: 870–878

Casaburi R, Kukafka D, Cooper CB et al 2005 Improvement in exercise tolerance with the combination of tiotropium and pulmonary rehabilitation in patients with COPD. Chest 127(3): 809–817

Casaburi R, Patessio A, Ioli F et al 1991 Reductions in exercise lactic acidosis and ventilation as a result of exercise training in patients with obstructive lung disease. American Review of Respiratory Disease 143: 9–18

Casaburi R, Porszasz J, Burns MR et al 1997 Physiologic benefits of exercise training in rehabilitation of patients with severe COPD. American Journal of Respiratory and Critical Care Medicine 155: 1541–1551

Celli BR, Cote CG, Marin JM et al 2004 The body-mass index, airflow obstruction, dyspnea, and exercise capacity index in chronic obstructive pulmonary disease. New England Journal of Medicine 350(10): 1005–1012

Chen H, Dukes R, Martin B 1985 Inspiratory resistance training in patients with COPD. American Review of Respiratory Disease 131: 251–255

Clark CJ, Cochrane L, Mackay E 1996 Low intensity peripheral muscle conditioning improves exercise tolerance and breathlessness in

13

COPD. European Respiratory Journal 9(12): 2590–2596

Cockcroft AE, Saunders MJ, Berry G 1981 Randomized controlled trial of rehabilitation in chronic respiratory disability. Thorax 36: 200–203

Coppoolse R, Schols A, Baarends E et al 1999 Interval versus continuous training in patients with severe COPD: a randomized controlled trial. European Respiratory Journal 14: 258–263

Coronado M, Janssens JP, de Muralt B et al 2003 Walking activity measured by accelerometry during respiratory rehabilitation. Journal of Cardiopulmonary Rehabilitation 23: 357–334

Coronell C, Orozco-Levi M, Mendez R et al 2004 Relevance of assessing quadriceps endurance in patients with COPD. European Respiratory Journal 24(1): 129–136

Creutzberg EC, Schols AM, Weling-Scheepers CA et al 2000 Characterization of nonresponse to high caloric oral nutritional therapy in depleted patients with COPD. American Journal of Respiratory and Critical Care Medicine 161(3 Pt 1): 745–752

Creutzberg EC, Wouters EF, Mostert R et al 2003 A role for anabolic steroids in the rehabilitation of patients with COPD? A double-blind, placebo-controlled, randomized trial. Chest 124(5): 1733–1742

Dal Corso S, Nápolis L, Malaguti C et al 2007 Skeletal muscle structure and function in response to electrical stimulation in moderately impaired COPD patients. Respiratory Medicine 101(6): 1236–43

de Torres JP, Cordoba-Lanus E, Lopez-Aguilar C et al 2006 C-reactive protein levels and clinically important predictive outcomes in stable COPD patients. European Respiratory Journal 27: 902–907

de Torres JP, Pinto-Plata V, Ingenito E et al 2002 Power of outcome measurements to detect clinically significant changes in pulmonary rehabilitation of patients with COPD. Chest 121(4): 1092–1098

Debigare R, Cote CH, Maltais F 2001 Peripheral muscle wasting in chronic obstructive pulmonary disease: clinical relevance and mechanisms. American Journal of Respiratory and Critical Care Medicine 164: 1712–1717

Debigare R, Maltais F, Mallet M et al 2000 Influence of work rate incremental rate on the exercise responses in patients with COPD. Medicine and Science in Sports and Exercise 32: 1365–1368

Devine E, Pearcy J 1996 Meta-analysis of the effect of psycho-educational care

in adults with COPD. Patient Education and Counselling 29(2): 167–178

Donaldson GC, Wilkinson TM, Hurst JR et al 2005 Exacerbations and time spent outdoors in chronic obstructive pulmonary disease. American Journal of Respiratory and Critical Care Medicine 171: 446–452

Dourado VZ, Antunes LC, Tanni SE et al 2006 Relationship of upper-limb and thoracic muscle strength to 6-min walk distance in COPD patients. Chest 129(3): 551–557

Dyer CA, Singh SJ, Stockley RA et al 2002 The incremental shuttle walking test in elderly people with chronic airflow limitation. Thorax 57: 34–38

Eakin E, Resnikoff P, Prewitt L et al 1998 Validation of a new dyspnoea measure: the UCSD shortness of breath questionnaire. Chest 113: 619–624

Eaton T, Young P, Nicol K et al 2006 The endurance shuttle walking test: a responsive measure in pulmonary rehabilitation for COPD patients Chronic Respiratory Disease 3: 3–9

Eiser N, West C, Evans S et al 1997 Effects of psychotherapy in moderately severe COPD: a pilot study. European Respiratory Journal 10(7): 1581–1584

Emtner M, Porszasz J, Burns M et al 2003 Benefits of supplemental oxygen in exercise training in nonhypoxemic chronic obstructive pulmonary disease patients. American Journal of Respiratory and Critical Care Medicine 168: 1034–1042

Fabbri LM, Hurd SS, GOLD Scientific Committee 2003 Global strategy for the diagnosis, management and prevention of COPD: 2003 update. European Respiratory Journal 22(1): 1–2

Ferreira IM, Brooks D, Lacasse Y et al 2005 Nutritional supplementation for stable chronic obstructive pulmonary disease. Cochrane Database of Systematic Reviews 2002; (1): CD000998

Fletcher CM 1960 Standardised questionnaire on respiratory symptoms: a statement prepared and approved by the MRC committee on the aetiology of chronic bronchitis (MRC Breathlessness Score). British Medical Journal 2: 1665

Foglio K, Bianchi L, Ambrosino N 2001 Is it really useful to repeat outpatient pulmonary rehabilitation programs in patients with chronic airway obstruction? A 2-year controlled study. Chest 119: 1696–1704

Foglio K, Bianchi L, Bruletti G et al 1999 Long-term effectiveness of pulmonary rehabilitation in patients with COPD. European Respiratory Journal 13: 125–132

Folgering H, Rooyakkers J, Herwaarden C 1994 Education and cost benefit ratios in pulmonary patients. Monaldi Archives of Chest Disease 49(2): 166–168

Franssen FM, Broekhuizen R, Janssen PP et al 2005 Limb muscle dysfunction in COPD: effects of muscle wasting and exercise training. Medicine and Science in Sports and Exercise 37(1): 2–9

Franssen FM, Wouters EF, Baarends EM et al 2002 Arm mechanical efficiency and arm exercise capacity are relatively preserved in chronic obstructive pulmonary disease. Medicine and Science in Sports and Exercise 34(10): 1570–1576

Fuchs-Climent D, Le Gallais D, Varray A et al 1999 Quality of life and exercise tolerance in COPD: effects of a short and intensive inpatient rehabilitation program. American Journal of Physical Medicine and Rehabilitation 78: 330–335

Gallefoss F, Bakke PS, Kjaersgaard P 1999 Quality of life assessment after patient education in a randomized controlled study on asthma and chronic obstructive pulmonary disease. American Journal of Respiratory and Critical Care Medicine 159: 812–817

Gan WQ, Man SF, Senthilselvan A et al 2004 The association between chronic obstructive pulmonary disease and systemic inflammation: a systematic review and a meta-analysis. Thorax 59: 574–580

Garcia-Aymerich J, Farrero E, Felez MA et al 2003 Risk factors of readmission to hospital for a COPD exacerbation: a prospective study. Thorax 58: 100–105

Garrod R 1998 Pulmonary rehabilitation: the pros and cons of rehabilitation at home. Physiotherapy 84(12): 603–607

Garrod R, Backley J 2006 Community-based pulmonary rehabilitation: meeting demand in chronic obstructive pulmonary disease. Physical Therapy Reviews 11: 57–61

Garrod R, Paul EA, Wedzicha JA 2000a Supplemental oxygen during pulmonary rehabilitation in patients with COPD and exercise hypoxaemia. Thorax 55: 539–543

Garrod R, Mikelsons C, Paul EA, Wedzicha JA 2000b Randomized controlled trial of domiciliary noninvasive positive pressure ventilation and physical training in severe chronic obstructive pulmonary disease. American Journal of Respiratory and Critical Care Medicine 162(41): 1335–1341

Garrod R, Bestall J, Wedzicha JA et al 2000c Development and validation of a standardised measure of activity of

13

daily living in patients with COPD: the London Chest Activity of Daily Living Scale (LCADL). Respiratory Medicine 94(6): 589–596

Garrod R, Paul EA, Wedzicha JA 2002 An evaluation of the reliability and sensitivity of the London Chest Activity of Daily Living Scale (LCADL). Respiratory Medicine 96: 725–730

Garrod R, Dallimore K, Cook J et al 2005b An evaluation of the acute impact of pursed lips breathing on walking distance in nonspontaneous pursed lips breathing chronic obstructive pulmonary disease patients. Chronic Respiratory Disease 2: 67–72

Garrod R, Marshall J, Barley E et al 2006 Predictors of success and failure in pulmonary rehabilitation. European Respiratory Journal 27: 788–794

Garrod R, Marshall J, Fredericks S et al 2005a CRP as a marker of impairment and disability in chronic obstructive pulmonary disease (COPD). Proceedings of The American Thoracic Society 2: A639

Gigliotti F, Colli C, Bianchi R et al 2005 Arm exercise and hyperinflation in patients with COPD: effect of arm training. Chest 128(3): 1225–1232

Gimenez M, Serverra E, Vergara P et al 2000 Endurance training in patients with COPD: a comparison of high versus moderate intensity. Archives of Physical Medicine and Rehabilitation 81: 102–109

Global Initiative for Chronic Obstructive Lung Disease (GOLD) 2001. Global Strategy for the diagnosis, management and prevention of COPD. NHLBI/WHO workshop report. Bethesda, National Heart, Lung and Blood Institute, 2001. *www. goldcopd.org/Guidelineitem. asp?l1=2&l2=1&intId=989.* Date last updated: November 2006, accessed 16 July 2007

Goldstein MF, Fallon JJ Jr., Harning R 1999 Chronic glucocorticoid therapy-induced osteoporosis in patients with obstructive lung disease. Chest 116(6): 1733–1749

Goldstein R 1993 Ventilatory muscle training. Thorax 48: 1025–1033

Goldstein RS, Gort EH, Stubbing D et al 1994 Randomized controlled trial of respiratory rehabilitation. Lancet 344: 1394–1397

Gosker HR, Lencer NH, Franssen FM et al 2003 Striking similarities in systemic factors contributing to decreased exercise capacity in patients with severe chronic heart failure or COPD. Chest 123(5): 1416–1424

Gosker HR, van Mameren H, van Dijk PJ et al 2002 Skeletal muscle fibre-type shifting and metabolic profile inpatients with COPD. European Respiratory Journal 19: 617–625

Gosselink R 2003 Controlled breathing and dyspnea in patients with chronic obstructive pulmonary disease (COPD). Journal of Rehabilitation Research and Development 40(5 Suppl 2): 25–33

Gosselink R, Troosters T, Decramer M 1996 Peripheral muscle weakness contributes to exercise limitation in COPD. American Journal of Respiratory and Critical Care Medicine 153(3): 976–980

Gosselink R, Troosters T, Decramer M 2000 Distribution of muscle weakness in stable patients with COPD. Journal of Cardiopulmonary Rehabilitation 20: 353–360

Gosselink RA, Wagenaar RC, Sargeant AJ et al 1995 Diaphragmatic breathing reduces efficiency of breathing in COPD. American Journal of Respiratory and Critical Care Medicine 151: 1136–1142

Green RH, Singh SJ, Williams J et al 2001 A randomized controlled trial of 4 weeks versus 7 weeks of pulmonary rehabilitation in COPD. Thorax 56: 143–145

Griffiths TL, Burr ML, Campbell IA et al 2000 Results at 1 year of out-patient multidisciplinary pulmonary rehabilitation: a randomized controlled trial. Lancet 355: 362–368

Guell R, Casan P, Belda J et al 2000 Long-term effects of outpatient rehabilitation of COPD: a randomized trial. Chest 117: 976–983

Gupta RB, Brooks D, Lacasse Y et al 2006 Effect of rollator use on health-related quality of life in individuals with COPD. Chest 130: 1089–1095

Guyatt GH, Feeny D, Patrick D 1991 Issues in quality of life measurement in clinical trials. Controlled Clinical Trials 81S–90S

Guyatt GH, Keller J, Singer J et al 1992 Controlled trial of respiratory muscle training in chronic airflow limitation. Thorax 47: 598–602

Guyatt GH, Townsend M, Berman L et al 1987 A measure of quality of life for clinical trials in chronic lung disease. Thorax 42: 773–778

Harver A, Mahler D, Daubenspeck J 1989 Targeted inspiratory muscle training improves respiratory muscle function and dyspnoea in patients with COPD. Annals of Internal Medicine 111(2): 117–124

Heppner PS, Morgan C, Kaplan RM et al 2006 Regular walking and long-term maintenance of outcomes after pulmonary rehabilitation. Journal of Cardiopulmonary Rehabilitation 26(1): 44–53

Hill K, Jenkins SC, Philippe DL et al 2006 High-intensity inspiratory muscle training in COPD. European Respiratory Journal 27(6): 1119–1128

Hoo GW 2003 Non-pharmacologic adjuncts to training during pulmonary rehabilitation: the role of supplemental oxygen and non-invasive ventilation. Journal of Rehabilitation Research and Development 40(5): S2 81–98

Horowitz MB, Littenberg B, Mahler DA 1996 Dyspnoea ratings for prescribing exercise intensity in patients with COPD. Chest 109(5): 1169–1175

Hunter S, Hall S 1989 The effect of an educational support programme on dyspnoea and the emotional status of COPD clients. Rehabilitation Nursing Journal 14 (4): 200–202

Jaeshchke R, Singer J, Guyatt GH 1989 Measurement of health status. Ascertaining the minimal clinically important difference. Controlled Clinical Trials 10(4): 407–415

Janaudis-Ferreira T, Wadell K, Sundelin G et al 2006 Thigh muscle strength and endurance in patients with COPD compared with healthy controls. Respiratory Medicine 100(8): 1451–1457

Jones AY, Dean E, Chow CC 2003 Comparison of the oxygen cost of breathing exercises and spontaneous breathing in patients with stable chronic obstructive pulmonary disease. Physical Therapy 83: 424–431

Jones PW 1992 Measurement of health in asthma and chronic obstructive airways disease. Pharmaceutical Medicine 6: 13–22

Jones PW 2005 St. George's Respiratory Questionnaire: MCID. COPD 2(1): 75–79

Jones PW, Quirk FH, Baveystock CM 1991 The St George's Respiratory Questionnaire (SGRQ). Respiratory Medicine 85(Suppl B): 25–31

Kawane H 1997 Smoking cessation in comprehensive pulmonary rehabilitation. Lancet 349: 285

Killian KJ, Leblanc P, Martin DH et al 1992 Exercise capacity and ventilatory, circulatory, and symptom limitation in patients with chronic airflow limitation. American Review of Respiratory Disease 146: 935–940

Koppers RJ, Vos PJ, Boot CR 2006 Exercise performance improves in patients with COPD due to respiratory muscle endurance training. Chest 129(4): 886–892

Lacasse Y, Brosseau L, Milne S et al 2002 Pulmonary rehabilitation for chronic obstructive pulmonary disease. Cochrane Database of Systematic Reviews No 3 CD003793

Lacasse Y, Goldstein R, Lasserson TJ et al 2006 Pulmonary rehabilitation for

13

chronic obstructive pulmonary disease. Cochrane Database of Systemic Reviews, Issue 4, Art. No.: CD0003793

Lacasse Y, Guyatt GH, Goldstein RS 1997 The components of a respiratory rehabilitation programme. Chest 111: 1077–1088

Lake F, Henderson K, Briffa T et al 1990 Upper limb and lower limb exercise training in patients with chronic airflow obstruction. Chest 97: 1077–1082

Landbo C, Prescott E, Lange P et al 1999 Prognostic value of nutritional status in COPD. American Journal of Respiratory and Critical Care Medicine 160(6): 1856–1861

Lareau SC, Carrieri-Kohlmon V, Janson-Bjerklie S et al 1994 Development of the Pulmonary Functional Status and Dyspnea Questionnaire (PFSDQ). Heart and Lung 23(3): 242–250

Lareau SC, Meek PM, Roos PJ 1998 Development and testing of the modified version of the Pulmonary Functional Status and Dyspnea Questionnaire (PFSDQ-M). Heart and Lung 27(3): 159–168

Larson J, Kim J, Sharp T et al 1999 Inspiratory muscle training with a pressure threshold breathing device in patients with COPD. American Review of Respiratory Disease 138: 689–96

Locke E, Shaw K, Sari L et al 1981 Goal setting and task performance 1969–1980. Psychological Bulletin 90(1): 125–152

Lorenzi CM, Cilione C, Rizzardi R et al 2004 Occupational therapy and pulmonary rehabilitation of disabled COPD patients. Respiration 71(3): 246–251

Lotters F, van Tol B, Kwakkel G et al 2002 Effects of controlled inspiratory muscle training in patients with COPD: a meta-analysis. European Respiratory Journal 20(3): 570–576

Maa SH, Gauthier D, Turner M 1997 Acupressure as an adjunct to a pulmonary rehabilitation programme. Journal of Cardiopulmonary Rehabilitation 17(4): 268–276

MacIntyre NR 2006 Corticosteroid therapy and chronic obstructive pulmonary disease. Respiratory Care 51(3): 289–296

Mackay L 1996 Health education and COPD rehabilitation: a study. Nursing Standard 10(40): 34–39

Mador MJ, Deniz O, Aggarwal A et al 2003 Quadriceps fatigability after single muscle exercise in patients with chronic obstructive pulmonary disease. American Journal of Respiratory and Critical Care Medicine 168(1): 102–108

Mahler DA, Ward J, Mejia-Alfaro R 2003 Stability of dyspnea ratings after exercise training in patients with COPD. Medicine and Science in Sports and Exercise 35(7): 1083–1087

Mahler DA, Weinberg DH, Wells CK et al 1984 The measurement of dyspnea; contents, inter-observer agreement and physiologic correlates of two new clinical indexes. Chest 85: 751–758

Maltais F, Leblanc P, Simard C et al 1996 Skeletal muscle adaptation to endurance training in patients with COPD. American Journal of Critical Care Medicine 154: 442–447

Maltais F, Leblanc P, Jobin J et al 1997 Intensity of training and physiologic adaptation with COPD. American Journal of Respiratory and Critical Care Medicine 155: 555–561

Maltais F, Sullivan MJ, LeBlanc P et al 1999 Altered expression of myosin heavy chain in the vastus lateralis muscle in patients with COPD. European Respiratory Journal 13: 850–854

Man WD, Polkey MI, Donaldson N et al 2004 Community pulmonary rehabilitation after hospitalisation for acute exacerbations of chronic obstructive pulmonary disease: randomized controlled study. British Medical Journal 329: 1209

Man WD, Soliman MG, Gearing J et al 2003 Symptoms and quadriceps fatigability after walking and cycling in chronic obstructive pulmonary disease. American Journal of Respiratory and Critical Care Medicine 168(5): 562–567

Marlow SP, Stoller JK 2003 Smoking cessation. Respiratory Care 48(12): 1238–1254

Mazzuca S 1982 Does patient education in chronic disease have therapeutic value? Journal of Chronic Diseases 35 (7): 521–529

McGavin CR, Gupta SP, Lloyd EL et al 1977 Physical rehabilitation for the chronic bronchitic: results of a controlled trial of exercises in the home. Thorax 32: 307–311

McKeough ZJ, Alison JA, Bye PT. 2003 Arm exercise capacity and dyspnea ratings in subjects with chronic obstructive pulmonary disease. Journal of Cardiopulmonary Rehabilitation 23(3): 218–225

Mercken EM, Hageman GJ, Schols AM et al 2005 Rehabilitation decreases exercise-induced oxidative stress in COPD. American Journal of Respiratory and Critical Care Medicine 172: 994–1001

Midorikawa J, Hida W, Taguchi O et al 1997 Lack of ventilatory threshold in patients with COPD. Respiration 64: 76–80

Monninkhof EM, van der Valk PDLPM, van der Palen J et al 2003 Self-management education for chronic obstructive pulmonary disease. Cochrane Database of Systematic Reviews No.1 CD002990

Morgan MD, Calverley PM, Clark C et al 2001 British Thoracic Society Statement on Pulmonary Rehabilitation. Thorax 56: 827–834

Mota S, Güell R, Barreiro E et al 2007 Clinical outcomes of expiratory muscle training in severe COPD patients. Respiratory Medicine 101(3): 516–524

Mueller RE, Petty TL, Filley GF 1970 Ventilation and arterial blood gas changes induced by pursed lips breathing. Journal of Applied Physiology 28(6): 784–789

National Institutes of Health 1994 Pulmonary rehabilitation research. National Institutes of Health workshop summary. American Review of Respiratory Disease 149: 825–893

Neder JA, Jones PW, Nery LE et al 2000 Determinants of the exercise endurance capacity in patients with COPD: the power-duration relationship. American Journal of Respiratory and Critical Care Medicine 162: 497–504

Neder JA, Sword D, Ward SA et al 2002 Home based neuromuscular electrical stimulation as a new rehabilitative strategy for severely disabled patients with chronic obstructive pulmonary disease (COPD). Thorax 57(4): 333–337

Nguyen HQ, Carrieri-Kohlman V 2005 Dyspnea self-management in patients with chronic obstructive pulmonary disease: moderating effects of depressed mood. Psychosomatics 46(5): 402–410

Nici L, Donner C, Wouters E et al 2006 American Thoracic Society/ European Respiratory Society Statement on Pulmonary Rehabilitation. American Journal of Respiratory and Critical Care Medicine 173: 1390–1413

Normandin EA, McCusker C, Connors M et al 2002 An evaluation of two approaches to exercise conditioning in pulmonary rehabilitation. Chest 121(4): 1085–1091

Norweg AM, Whiteson J, Malgady R et al 2005 The effectiveness of different combinations of pulmonary rehabilitation program components: a randomized controlled trial. Chest 128(2): 663–672

O'Brien Cousins S, Keating N 1995 Life cycle patterns of physical activity among sedentary and older women. Journal of Ageing and Physical Activity 3: 340–359

13

O'Donnell D 1994 Breathlessness in patients with chronic airflow limitation. Chest 106: 905–912

O'Donnell DE, D'Arsigny C, Webb KA 2001 Effects of hyperoxia on ventilatory limitation in advanced COPD. American Journal of Respiratory and Critical Care Medicine 163: 892–898

O'Donnell DE, Sciurba F, Celli B et al 2006 Effect of fluticasone propionate/salmeterol on lung hyperinflation and exercise endurance in COPD. Chest 130(3): 647–656

O'Neill S, McCarthy DS 1983 Postural relief of dyspnoea in severe chronic airflow limitation. Thorax 38: 595–600

Ong KC, Chong WF, Soh C et al 2004 Comparison of different exercise tests in assessing outcomes of pulmonary rehabilitation. Respiratory Care 49(12): 1498–1503

O'Shea SD, Taylor NF, Paratz J 2004 Peripheral muscle strength training in COPD: a systematic review. Chest 126: 903–914

Palange P, Carlone S, Forte S et al 1994 Cardiopulmonary exercise testing in the evaluation of patients with ventilatory vs circulatory causes of reduced exercise tolerance. Chest 105: 1122–1126

Partridge C, Pryor J, Webber B 1989 Characteristics of the forced expiration technique. Physiotherapy 73(3): 193–194

Petty TL 1993 Pulmonary rehabilitation in chronic respiratory insufficiency. 1. Pulmonary rehabilitation in perspective: historical roots, present status, and future projections. Thorax 48(8): 855–862

Pinto-Plata CM, Cote C, Cabral H et al 2004 The 6-min walk distance: change over time and value as a predictor of survival in severe COPD. European Respiratory Journal 23(1): 28–33

Pitta FO, Brunetto AF, Padovani CR et al 2004 Effects of isolated cycle ergometer training on patients with moderate-to-severe chronic obstructive pulmonary disease. Respiration 71(5): 477–483

Pitta F, Troosters T, Probst VS et al 2006a Physical activity and hospitalization for exacerbation of COPD. Chest 129: 536–544

Pitta F, Troosters T, Probst VS et al 2006b Quantifying physical activity in daily life with questionnaires and motion sensors in COPD. European Respiratory Journal 27: 1040–1055

Pitta F, Troosters T, Spruit MA et al 2005a Characteristics of physical activities in daily life in chronic obstructive pulmonary disease. American Journal of Respiratory and Critical Care Medicine 171: 972–977

Pitta F, Troosters T, Spruit MA et al 2005b Activity monitoring for assessment of physical activities in daily life in patients with chronic obstructive pulmonary disease. Archives of Physical Medicine and Rehabilitation 86(10): 1979–1985

Probst VS, Troosters T, Celis G et al 2005 Effects of resistance exercise training during hospitalization due to acute exacerbation of COPD – preliminary results [abstract]. European Respiratory Journal 26(Suppl 49): 432S

Probst VS, Troosters T, Coosemans I et al 2004 Mechanisms of improvement in exercise capacity using a rollator in patients with COPD. Chest 126: 1102–1107

Probst VS, Troosters T, Pitta F et al 2006 Cardiopulmonary stress during exercise training in patients with COPD. European Respiratory Journal 27(6): 1110–1118

Puente-Maestu L, Sanz M, Sanz P et al 2000 Comparison of effects of supervised versus self-monitored training programmes in patients with chronic obstructive pulmonary disease. European Respiratory Journal 15(3): 517–525

Puhan MA, Guyatt GH, Goldstein R et al 2007 Relative responsiveness of the Chronic Respiratory Questionnaire, St. Georges Respiratory Questionnaire and four other health-related quality of life instruments for patients with chronic lung disease. Respiratory Medicine 101(2): 308–316

Puhan MA, Schunemann HJ, Frey M et al 2005 How should COPD patients exercise during respiratory rehabilitation? Comparison of exercise modalities and intensities to treat skeletal muscle dysfunction. Thorax 60(5): 367–375

Punzal PA, Ries AL, Kaplan RM et al 1991 Maximum intensity training in patients with COPD. Chest 100: 618–623

Reardon J, Awad E, Normandin E et al 1994 The effect of comprehensive outpatient pulmonary rehabilitation on dyspnea. Chest 105: 1046–1052

Redelmeier D, Bayoumi A, Goldstein R et al 1997 Interpreting small differences in functional status: the Six Minute Walk test in chronic lung disease patients. American Journal of Respiratory and Critical Care Medicine 155(4): 1278–1282

Reid W, Samrai B 1995 Respiratory muscle training for patients with COPD. Physical Therapy 75(11): 70–79

Renfroe K 1988 Effect of progressive relaxation on dyspnoea and state anxiety in patients with COPD. Heart and Lung 17: 408–413

Restrick LJ, Paul EA, Braid GM et al 1993 Assessment and follow-up of patients prescribed long-term oxygen treatment. Thorax 48: 708–713

Revill SM, Morgan MDL, Singh SJ et al 1999 The endurance shuttle walk: a new field test for the assessment of endurance capacity in chronic obstructive pulmonary disease. Thorax 54: 213–220

Richardson RS, Leek BT, Gavin TP et al 2004 Reduced mechanical efficiency in chronic obstructive pulmonary disease but normal peak $\dot{V}O_2$ with small muscle mass exercise. American Journal of Respiratory and Critical Care Medicine 169(1): 89–96

Ries AL, Kaplan RM, Limberg TM et al 1995 Effects of pulmonary rehabilitation on physiologic and psychosocial outcomes in COPD. Annals of Internal Medicine 122(11): 823–831

Ries AL, Kaplan RM, Myers R et al 2003 Maintenance after pulmonary rehabilitation in chronic lung disease: a randomized trial. American Journal of Respiratory and Critical Care Medicine 167(6): 880–888

Ringbaek TJ, Broendum E, Hemmingsen L et al 2000 Rehabilitation of patients with chronic obstructive pulmonary disease: exercise twice a week is not sufficient! Respiratory Medicine 94: 150–154

Romagnoli M, Dell'Orso D, Lorenzi C et al 2006 Repeated pulmonary rehabilitation in severe and disabled COPD patients. Respiration 73(6): 769–776

Roomi J, Johnson MM, Waters K et al 1996 Respiratory rehabilitation, exercise capacity and quality of life in chronic airways disease in old age. Age and Ageing 25: 12–16

Rooyakers JM, Dekhuijzen PNR, Van Herwaarden CLA et al 1997 Training with supplemental oxygen in patients with COPD and hypoxaemia at peak exercise. European Respiratory Journal 10: 1278–1284

Rossi G, Florini F, Romagnoli M et al 2005 Length and clinical effectiveness of pulmonary rehabilitation in outpatients with chronic airway obstruction. Chest 127: 105–109

Rutten-van Mölken M, Roos B, Van Noord JA 1999 An empirical comparison of the St George's Respiratory Questionnaire (SGRQ) and the Chronic Respiratory Disease Questionnaire (CRQ) in a clinical trial setting. Thorax 54(11): 995–1003

Sabapathy S, Kingsley RA, Schneider DA et al 2004 Continuous and intermittent exercise responses in individuals with chronic obstructive pulmonary disease. Thorax 59(12): 1026–1031

Sackner MA, Gonzales HF, Jenouri G et al 1984 Effects of abdominal and

13

thoracic breathing on breathing pattern components in normal subjects and in patients with COPD. American Review of Respiratory Disease 130: 584–587

Salman GF, Mosier MC, Beasley BW et al 2003 Rehabilitation for patients with chronic obstructive pulmonary disease. Journal of General Internal Medicine 18: 213–221

Sandland CJ, Singh SJ, Curcio A et al 2005 A profile of daily activity in chronic obstructive pulmonary disease. Journal of Cardiopulmonary Rehabilitation 25(3): 181–183

Sassi-Dambron DE, Eakin EG, Ries AL et al 1995 Treatment of dyspnea in COPD. A controlled clinical trial of dyspnea management strategies. Chest 107: 724–729

Schenkel NS, Muralt BB, Fitting JW 1996 Oxygen saturation during daily activities in chronic obstructive pulmonary disease. European Respiratory Journal 9: 2584–2589

Schols AM, Buurman WA, Staal van den Brekel AJ et al 1996 Evidence for a relation between metabolic derangements and increased levels of inflammatory mediators in a subgroup of patients with COPD. Thorax 51: 819–824

Schols A, Mostert R, Soeters P et al 1991 Body composition and exercise performance in patients with chronic obstructive pulmonary disease. Thorax 46 (10): 695–699

Schols AM, Soeters PB, Mostert R et al 1995 Physiologic effects of nutritional support and anabolic steroids in patients with chronic obstructive pulmonary disease. A placebo-controlled randomized trial. American Journal of Respiratory and Critical Care Medicine 152(4 Pt 1): 1268–1274

Schunemann HJ, Guyatt GH, Griffith L et al 2002 A randomized controlled trial to evaluate the effect of informing patients about their pretreatment responses to two respiratory questionnaires. Chest 122(5): 1701–1708

Sewell L, Singh SJ, Williams JE et al 2005 Can individualized rehabilitation improve functional independence in elderly patients with COPD? Chest 128(3): 1194–1200

Sharp JT, Drutz WS, Moisan T et al 1980 Postural relief of dyspnoea in severe COPD. American Review of Respiratory Disease 122: 201–211

Simpson K, Killian K, McCartney N et al 1992 Randomized controlled trial of weightlifting exercise in patients with chronic airflow limitation. Thorax 47: 70–75

Sinclair DJM, Ingram CG 1980 Controlled trial of supervised exercise training in chronic

bronchitis. British Medical Journal 280: 519–521

Singh SJ, Morgan MDL, Hardman AE et al 1994 Comparison of oxygen uptake during a conventional treadmill test and the shuttle walk test in chronic airflow limitation. European Respiratory Journal 7: 2016–2020

Singh SJ, Morgan MDL, Scott S et al 1992 Development of a shuttle walking test of disability in patients with chronic airways obstruction. Thorax 47: 1019–1024

Singh SJ, Sodergren SC, Hyland ME et al 2001 A comparison of three disease-specific and two generic health-status measures to evaluate the outcome of pulmonary rehabilitation in COPD. Respiratory Medicine 95(1): 71–77

Sivori M, Rhodius E, Kaplan P et al 1998 Exercise training in chronic obstructive pulmonary disease. Comparative study of aerobic training of lower limbs vs combination with upper limbs. Medicina 58(6): 712–727

Solway S, Brooks D, Lau L et al 2002 The short-term effect of a rollator on functional exercise capacity among individuals with severe COPD. Chest 122: 56–65

Somfay A, Porszasz J, Lee SM et al 2001 Dose-response effect of oxygen on hyperinflation and exercise endurance in nonhypoxaemic COPD patients. European Respiratory Journal 18: 77–84

Spahija J, de Marchie M, Grassino A 2005 Effects of imposed pursed-lips breathing on respiratory mechanics and dyspnea at rest and during exercise in COPD. Chest 128(2): 640–650

Spruit MA, Gosselink R, Troosters T et al 2002 Resistance versus endurance training in patients with COPD and peripheral muscle weakness. European Respiratory Journal 19: 1072–1078

Spruit MA, Gosselink R, Troosters T et al 2003 Muscle force during an acute exacerbation in hospitalised COPD patients and its relationship with CXCL8 and IGF1. Thorax 58: 752–756

Spruit MA, Troosters T, Gosselink R et al 2005 Low-grade systemic inflammation and the response to exercise training in patients with advanced COPD. Chest 128(5): 3183–3190

Steele BG, Belza B, Hunziker J et al 2003 Monitoring daily activity during pulmonary rehabilitation using a triaxial accelerometer. Journal of Cardiopulmonary Rehabilitation 23: 139–142

Steiner MC, Singh SJ, Morgan MD 2005 The contribution of peripheral

muscle function to shuttle walking performance in patients with chronic obstructive pulmonary disease. Journal of Cardiopulmonary Rehabilitation 25(1): 43–49

Strijbos JH, Postma DS, Van Altena R et al 1996 A comparison between an outpatient hospital based pulmonary rehabilitation program and a home care pulmonary rehabilitation program in patients with COPD. Chest 109: 366–372

Takabatake N, Nakamura H, Abe S et al 2000 The relationship between chronic hypoxemia and activation of the tumor necrosis factor-alpha system in patients with chronic obstructive pulmonary disease. American Journal of Respiratory and Critical Care Medicine 161: 1179–1184

Trappenburg JC, Troosters T, Spruit MA et al 2005 Psychosocial conditions do not affect short-term outcome of multidisciplinary rehabilitation in chronic obstructive pulmonary disease. Archives of Physical Medicine and Rehabilitation 86(9): 1788–1792

Troosters T, Casaburi R, Gosselink R et al 2005 Pulmonary rehabilitation in chronic obstructive pulmonary disease (state of the art). American Journal of Respiratory and Critical Care Medicine 172: 19–38

Troosters T, Gosselink R, Decramer M 1999 Six minute walking distance in healthy elderly subjects. European Respiratory Journal 14(2): 270–274

Troosters T, Gosselink R, Decramer M 2000 Short and long-term effects of outpatient rehabilitation in patients with COPD: a randomized trial. American Journal of Medicine 109: 207–212

Troosters T, Gosselink R, Decramer M 2001 Exercise training in COPD: how to distinguish responders from non-responder. Journal of Cardiopulmonary Rehabilitation 21: 10–17

Troosters T, Vilaro J, Rabinovich R et al 2002 Physiological responses to the 6-min walk test in patients with chronic obstructive pulmonary disease. European Respiratory Journal 20(3): 564–569

Turner SE, Eastwood PR, Cecins NM et al 2004 Physiologic responses to incremental and self-paced exercise in COPD: a comparison of three tests. Chest 126(3): 766–773

Vale F, Reardon J, ZuWallack R 1993 The long-term benefits of outpatient pulmonary rehabilitation on exercise endurance and quality of life. Chest 103: 42–45

van der Schans CP, De Jong W, Kort E et al 1995 Mouth pressures during

13

pursed lip breathing. Physiotherapy Theory and Practice 11: 29–34

van Manen JG, Bindels PH, Dekker FW et al 2002 Risk of depression in patients with COPD and its determinants. Thorax 57: 412–416

van't Hul A, Kwakkel G, Gosselink R 2002 The acute effects of noninvasive ventilatory support during exercise on exercise endurance and dyspnea in patients with chronic obstructive pulmonary disease. Journal of Cardiopulmonary Rehabilitation 22: 290–297

Velloso M, Jardim JR 2006 Study of energy expenditure during activities of daily living using and not using body position recommended by energy conservation techniques in patients with COPD. Chest 130(1): 126–132

Vitacca M, Clini E, Bianchi L et al 1998 Acute effects of deep diaphragmatic breathing in COPD patients with chronic respiratory insufficiency. European Respiratory Journal 11: 408–415

Vivodtzev I, Pepin JL, Vottero G et al 2006 Improvement in quadriceps strength and dyspnea in daily tasks after 1 month of electrical stimulation in severely deconditioned and malnourished COPD. Chest 129(6): 1540–1548

Vogiatzis I, Nanas S, Kastanakis E et al 2004 Dynamic hyperinflation and tolerance to interval exercise in patients with advanced COPD. European Respiratory Journal 24: 385–390

Vogiatzis I, Terzis G, Nanas S et al 2005 Skeletal muscle adaptations to interval training in patients with advanced COPD. Chest 128: 3838–3845

Wadell K, Henriksson–Larsen K, Lundgren R 2001 Physical training with and without oxygen in patients with chronic obstructive pulmonary disease and exercise-induced hypoxaemia. Journal of Rehabilitation Medicine 33(5): 200–205

Wadell K, Henriksson-Larsen K, Lundgren R et al 2005 Group training in patients with COPD – long-term effects after decreased training frequency. Disability and Rehabilitation 27(10): 571–581

Wanke TH, Formanek D, Lahrmann H et al 1994 Effects of combined inspiratory muscle and cycle ergometer training on exercise performance in patient with COPD. European Respiratory Journal 7: 2205–2211

Wedzicha JA, Bestall JC, Garrod R et al 1998 Randomized controlled trial of pulmonary rehabilitation in severe chronic obstructive pulmonary disease patients, stratified with the MRC scale. European Respiratory Journal 12: 363–369

Weiner P, Magadle R, Beckerman M et al 2003a Specific expiratory muscle training in COPD. Chest 124(2): 468–473

Weiner P, Magadle R, Beckerman M et al 2003b Comparison of specific expiratory, inspiratory, and combined muscle training programs in COPD. Chest 124(4): 1357–1364

Whittom F, Jobin J, Simard PM et al 1998 Histochemical and morphological characteristics of the vastus lateralis muscle in patients with chronic obstructive pulmonary disease. Medicine and Science in Sports and Exercise 30(10): 1467–1474

Wijkstra PJ, Mark TW, Kraan J et al 1996 Long-term effects of home rehabilitation on physical performance in chronic obstructive pulmonary disease. American Journal of Respiratory and Critical Care Medicine 153: 1234–1241

Wijkstra PJ, Ten Vergert EM, Van Altena R et al 1995 Long-term effects of rehabilitation at home on quality of life and exercise tolerance in patients with chronic obstructive pulmonary disease. Thorax 50: 824–828

Wijkstra PJ, Van Altena R, Kraan J et al 1994 Quality of life in patients with COPD improves after rehabilitation at home. European Respiratory Journal 7: 269–273

Willeput R, Vachaudez JP, Lenders D et al 1983 Thoracoabdominal motion during chest physiotherapy in patients affected by chronic obstructive lung disease. Respiration 44: 204–214

Withers NJ, Rudkin ST, White RJ 1999 Anxiety and depression in severe COPD: the effects of pulmonary rehabilitation. Journal of Cardiopulmonary Rehabilitation 19: 362–365

Yende S, Waterer GW, Tolley EA et al 2006 Inflammatory markers are associated with ventilatory limitation and muscle dysfunction in obstructive lung disease in well functioning elderly subjects. Thorax 61(1): 10–16

Yohannes AM, Roomi J, Winn S et al 2000 The Manchester Respiratory Activities of Daily Living questionnaire: development, reliability, validity, and responsiveness to pulmonary rehabilitation. Journal of the American Geriatric Society 48(11): 1496–1500

Young P, Dewse M, Fergusson W et al 1999 Respiratory rehabilitation in COPD: predictors of non-adherence. European Respiratory Journal 13: 855–859

Zacarias EC, Neder JA, Cendom SP et al 2000 Heart rate at the estimated lactate threshold in patients with COPD: effects on the target intensity for dynamic exercise training. Journal of Cardiopulmonary Rehabilitation 20: 369–376

Zack MB, Palange AV 1985 Oxygen-supplemented exercise of ventilatory and non-ventilatory muscles in pulmonary rehabilitation. Chest 88(5): 669– 675

Zanotti E, Felicetti G, Maini M et al 2003 Peripheral muscle strength training in bedbound patients with COPD receiving mechanical ventilation: effect of electrical stimulation. Chest 124: 292–296

ZuWallack RL, Patel K, Reardon J et al 1991 Predictors of improvement in the 12-minute walking distance following a 6-week outpatient pulmonary rehabilitation programme. Chest 99(4): 805–808

Further reading

Garrod R 2004 Pulmonary rehabilitation: an interdisciplinary approach. Whurr Ltd, London

13

Chapter **14**

Cardiac rehabilitation and secondary prevention

Ann Taylor, Jenny Bell, Fiona Lough

INTRODUCTION

Cardiac rehabilitation is an accepted form of management for people with cardiac disease. Initially rehabilitation was offered mainly to people recovering from a myocardial infarction (MI), but now encompasses a wide range of cardiac problems. More than 275 000 people have a MI each year in England and, while more than 40% of these are fatal, the survival rate is improving (Department of Health 2006). With more people surviving the peri-infarct period, the incidence of people with chronic heart failure (CHF) is increasing. These changes in mortality and morbidity present challenges for health professionals involved in organizing and delivering rehabilitation programmes. The aim of cardiac rehabilitation is to enable people to regain full physical, psychological and social status and, in order to optimize long-term prognosis, to promote and implement coronary heart disease (CHD) secondary prevention measures. Cardiac rehabilitation should be an integral part of both acute care and long-term follow-up, but provision and uptake remains inconsistent (Beswick et al 2004, Bittner & Sanderson 2006, Brodie et al 2006). In the United Kingdom (UK), the National Service Framework for CHD (Department of Health 2000) was written to provide guidance on the management of people with coronary heart disease. One of the standards of recommended care is the provision of a multidisciplinary programme of cardiac rehabilitation and secondary prevention. There is large variation in the format and organization of rehabilitation programmes, both within and between countries, but traditionally most encompass a period of exercise training, education sessions, psychosocial support and advice/counselling for both the patient and their family. In addition to people with a MI or CHF, participants may include those with an implanted cardioverter defibrillator (ICD), pacemaker and following coronary artery bypass graft surgery (CABG) and transplantation. Demographic changes mean there is greater involvement of elderly people, which is both a reflection of an ageing population and expansion of health care, and there is also a gradual increase in the uptake of cardiac rehabilitation amongst women. The secondary prevention aspect of the programmes has an important place in the reduction of risk factors. Physically inactive people have approximately double the risk of CHD compared with active people and the implementation of regular exercise is considered to decrease their risk factor profile by the same magnitude as smoking cessation (Albu et al 2006, Department of Health 2004).

This chapter describes the exercise component of cardiac rehabilitation which is the aspect in which physiotherapists are mainly involved and is divided into five parts:

- evidence base for comprehensive rehabilitation
- provision of cardiac rehabilitation
- benefits of exercise training
- exercise prescription
- programme implementation.

EVIDENCE BASE FOR CARDIAC REHABILITATION

With the increased evidence base for the benefits of cardiac rehabilitation, and particularly exercise training, many clinical guidelines for the management of people with cardiac problems recommend participation in a rehabilitation programme (National Institute for Clinical Excellence 2001, 2003, Scottish Intercollegiate Guidelines Network 2002). While there is a plethora of research supporting the benefits of cardiac rehabilitation programmes, the era in which the information was obtained has to be taken into consideration. Early studies concentrated on the benefits of exercise for post-MI patients in whom traditional management had restricted early activity – which differs from the early resumption of activity practised today. Early studies did not include the benefits of revascularization, thrombolysis and protective drug therapy (Franklin 2004, Kovoor et al 2006, Zwisler et al 2005). The restriction of studies to exercise training also limits their applicability to comprehensive cardiac rehabilitation programmes, as the sum of a programme may be greater than its individual parts. Additionally, women and the elderly were often excluded from research (Witt et al 2004). Consequently, most of the research findings in the 1960s and 1970s are no longer directly applicable to the management of people following a MI. The meta-analyses of Oldridge et al

(1988) and O'Connor et al (1989) which have been used extensively to promote cardiac rehabilitation are now of limited usefulness and have been superseded by more recent studies (Jolliffe et al 2000, Rees et al 2004, Taylor et al 2004).

Current research continues to suggest that rehabilitation programmes confer benefit to participants in all domains of their lives, with a focus on patient selection and organization of the programme. Unfortunately the methodology of some research studies is of low quality (i.e. small sample number, restricted age/gender, lack of randomization), which limits extrapolation of their findings to clinical practice. Another problematic area for interpreting research findings is the choice of outcome measures (Sanderson et al 2004). The importance of improvement in health-related quality of life is recognized in many studies, but there is lack of consensus as to the most appropriate measuring tool (Shephard & Franklin 2001, Taylor et al 1998). The SF-36 and SF-12 Health Status Questionnaires have been widely used, but concern has been expressed as to their ability to detect change when used for serial measurements (Ni et al 2000, Smith et al 2000). Some studies suggest anxiety and depression improve after a period of rehabilitation and have been commonly measured by the Hospital and Depression Scale (Zigmond & Snaith 1983), but this is thought to be relatively insensitive to change in this group of patients (McGee et al 1999). With the difficulties in selecting robust and appropriate outcome measures for quality of life issues, studies frequently use physiological or exercise endurance indices to measure responses to exercise training. However, these also have methodological issues concerning the influence of motivation and relevance of results (Ingle et al 2005). It has been suggested that a suitable measure for people with ICDs is the confidence to exert themselves physically (Sears et al 2004). Measurements of general activity, using pedometers, are considered to demonstrate a close relationship with changes in functional status (Evangelista et al 2005) and may be a more appropriate outcome for determining the response to rehabilitation programmes.

The organization of cardiac rehabilitation programmes is varied, with some focusing primarily on education and psychosocial intervention (Mendes de Leon et al 2006) and others offering only exercise training. The World Health Organization (WHO) (Frye 1993) definition of cardiac rehabilitation encompasses the concept of comprehensive cardiac rehabilitation programmes. Research suggests the inclusion of exercise training is a key element in eliciting benefits both in facilitating return to function and secondary prevention (Leon et al 1991, National Institute for Clinical Excellence 2003, Taylor et al 2004). There is considerable

14

variation across and between patient groups in the type and setting of exercise training (Hansen et al 2005). Many studies have concentrated on aerobic exercise owing to concerns regarding the effects of resistance training on cardiac function, but there is growing evidence that a mix of endurance and strength exercises are both safe and optimize the benefits (Adams et al 2006, Delagardelle et al 2002, Jonsdottir et al 2005, Levinger et al 2005). Concern that some patients may develop myocardial remodelling, as a result of participating in early activity (Jugdutt et al 1988, Kloner & Kloner 1983), has been alleviated by other work indicating that exercise does not contribute to the onset of remodelling (Cannistra et al 1999, DuBach et al 1997, Giannuzzi et al 1993, Myers et al 2000). The benefits of low-intensity exercise in the early stages of a programme are thought be similar to those of higher intensity (Blumenthal et al 1988, Goble et al 1991, Worcester et al 1993) and adoption of low-intensity exercise would facilitate both adherence and safety. Women have previously been under-represented in cardiac rehabilitation and may require specific programmes, based in the community or at home, to improve their uptake and adherence (Sanderson & Bittner 2005, Todaro et al 2004, Witt et al 2004). Some studies recommend inspiratory muscle training in people with chronic heart failure (Dall'Ago et al 2006).

The duration of the period of exercise training is influenced by many factors, such as physiological and psychological state (Kovoor et al 2006), objectives and adherence. Secondary prevention requires a prolonged period of training (Brubaker et al 2000) and adherence and uptake to a programme may be influenced by social support (Husak et al 2004), age, gender (Todaro et al 2004) and location of training (Grace et al 2005). The lack of consensus on an optimal period of exercise training for different groups of patients and an absence of a robust prediction model to determine the magnitude of benefit each patient may receive from a rehabilitation programme (Pierson et al 2004, Shen et al 2006) places an emphasis on assessment, joint goal setting and regular re-evaluation of response. Few studies have included a prolonged follow-up period, but any benefits appear to be quickly lost on cessation of regular exercise training.

The diversity of programmes and client groups makes it difficult to determine the cost-effectiveness of cardiac rehabilitation and this is compounded by differences in health provision among countries where this has been investigated. A survey within the UK calculated the cost per patient to be of the order of £490 (Beswick et al 2004) while an American review had higher average costs of $2054 and determined that participation prolonged survival by an additional 1.82 years at a cost of $1773 per/life-year saved (Georgiou et al 2001). It has been suggested that cardiac rehabilitation is more cost-effective than thrombolytic therapy and coronary bypass surgery (Ades et al 1997).

There has not been any reported increase in adverse events during either supervised or unsupervised exercise training following the inclusion of people who were previously considered a high risk: i.e. CHF and ICDs (Davids et al 2005, Fitchet et al 2003, Pashkow et al 1997) However, there is a paucity of information on the occurrence of adverse events outside research studies, which usually include highly selected patients who undergo formal exercise tests.

PROVISION OF CARDIAC REHABILITATION

Goals

Cardiac rehabilitation should meet the emotional, educational and physical needs of cardiac patients and their families in the acute hospital phase, through outpatient care and long-term follow-up in the community. It should be an integral part of cardiological management, with common goals to:

- decrease cardiac morbidity and relieve symptoms
- promote risk modification and secondary prevention
- decrease anxiety and increase knowledge and self-confidence
- increase fitness and the ability to resume normal activities.

Cardiological management involves assessment, risk stratification (the 'risk' of further cardiac events), diagnostic testing, drug therapy and revascularization interventions, e.g. percutaneous coronary intervention (PCI) and CABG. There should be close collaboration between cardiology and rehabilitation professionals on risk stratification, levels of prescribed exercise and discussion of treatment plans for symptomatic patients.

Rehabilitation should combine exercise with patient education and counselling, which provide:

- reassurance, support and information
- risk factor modification and an appropriate behavioural change programme
- assessment and risk stratification
- exercise prescription and an activity programme.

Patients should be offered an individually tailored package from this menu of care, according to their needs and preferences (Scottish Intercollegiate Guidelines Network 2002). Individual packages are usually described as spanning four phases of care (Coats et al 1995):

Phase I   in-hospital period (average 3–5 days)

Phase II   immediate post-discharge/convalescence stage (2–6 weeks)

Phase III   supervised outpatient programme (6–12 weeks)

Phase IV   long-term maintenance programme in the community.

However, there is now less emphasis on a fixed time scale; patients are increasingly offered a more seamless transition of care between outpatient follow-up and long-term lifestyle maintenance in the community.

Considerable variation exists in the model, timing, content and delivery of outpatient cardiac rehabilitation. Rehabilitation may be offered in supervised groups, within a hospital or community setting, or as part of a home-based package. Some programmes include education, psychosocial and exercise components while others provide only exercise training; some programmes are confined to 4–6 weeks' duration while others last for up to a year. In order to maximize benefit and adherence, the rehabilitation professional must match the appropriate model of care to each patient's individual needs. Increasing use of national clinical guidelines and audit tools have led to increased standardization, quality and effectiveness of cardiac rehabilitation services (American Association of Cardiovascular and Pulmonary Rehabilitation 2004, American College of Sports Medicine 2006, Fletcher et al 2001, Leon et al 2005, Scottish Intercollegiate Guidelines Network 2002).

To whom should cardiac rehabilitation be made available?

Cardiac rehabilitation should be offered to all cardiac patients who would benefit. Traditionally programmes have been targeted at post-MI and CABG patients with limited and variable service provision for patients following PCI, with angina, CHF or those who have undergone cardiac transplantation. Uptake of service is often poor among women, multi-pathology patients, some ethnic groups and the elderly. As a consequence, issues relating to access, distance, timing and flexibility of cardiac rehabilitation programmes are crucial considerations when trying to optimize service provision for such under-represented groups.

By whom should cardiac rehabilitation be delivered?

A broad spectrum of care requires the combined skills and close collaboration of a multidisciplinary team of professionals. The team should be led by a cardiologist and include nursing, physiotherapy, dietetic, occupa-

tional therapy, pharmacy and psychology staff, who have specialist training in cardiology and rehabilitation. Additional input may be required from social services and vocational guidance staff. Continuation of care in the community includes the primary healthcare team (principally general practitioner and practice nurse), Phase IV exercise instructor and possibly attendance at a cardiac patient support group. Long-term risk factor monitoring and management, coupled with a regular activity programme, is promoted at Phase IV to reinforce the need for ongoing secondary prevention.

Exercise rehabilitation should be delivered by a team of clinical and exercise specialists who are skilled in cardiovascular assessment, risk stratification, patient monitoring, exercise prescription, goal setting and behavioural management. The team needs to be able to deal with concurrent medical and psychosocial issues and combine the art and science of exercise prescription and delivery, i.e. the art of integrating strategies for behaviour change in order to enhance exercise compliance and long-term adherence, with the science of exercise prescription (American College of Sports Medicine 2006). There should also be joint working and close liaison with British Association of Cardiac Rehabilitation (BACR) Phase IV instructors (or their equivalent) who accept patients for long-term exercise in the community. Physiotherapists are key members of the team as they have specialist skills in the assessment, exercise prescription and rehabilitation management of multi-pathology patients, as well as being health educators and exercise advisors (Association of Chartered Physiotherapists in Cardiac Rehabilitation 2006, Jolliffe et al 2000). The Association of Chartered Physiotherapists Interested in Cardiac Rehabilitation (ACPICR) in the UK has developed guidelines for practice (Association of Chartered Physiotherapists in Cardiac Rehabilitation 2006) and a competency document outlining the physiotherapist's role and required knowledge, skills and standard of performance in cardiac rehabilitation.

BENEFITS OF EXERCISE TRAINING

Improved exercise capacity

The development of cardiovascular endurance is the primary objective for CHD patients. Endurance training, defined as any activity which uses large muscle groups, can be sustained for a prolonged period and is rhythmic and aerobic in nature, results in an increase in maximal oxygen uptake ($\dot{V}O_2$max), i.e. the highest rate of oxygen consumption attainable during maximal exercise. Maximal oxygen uptake is limited:

14

- centrally by cardiac output (CO), which is a function of heart rate (HR) and stroke volume (SV)

- peripherally, in particular by the capacity of skeletal muscle to extract oxygen from the blood. This is represented as the difference between the oxygen content of arterial blood and mixed venous blood (arteriovenous oxygen difference $[(a-\bar{v})O_2 diff]$. Consequently an increase in $\dot{V}O_2 max$ depends on the potential for inducing central and/or peripheral adaptations.

Central changes

In healthy individuals, endurance training results in a significant increase in maximal cardiac output. Maximum heart rate does not alter with training and so the increase in CO must arise from a training-induced increase in maximal SV. This is achieved primarily through:

- increased left ventricular mass and chamber size
- increased total blood volume
- reduced total peripheral resistance at maximal exercise.

Peripheral changes

Training-induced changes within skeletal muscle, which contribute to increased extraction and utilization of oxygen, include:

- increased number and size of mitochondria
- increased oxidative enzyme activity
- increased capillarization
- increased myoglobin.

In cardiac patients, the increase in $\dot{V}O_2 max$ is attributed predominantly to peripheral adaptation. Central changes are associated with prolonged periods of high-intensity training and although in selected patients central changes have been provoked (Ehsani et al 1986, Schuler et al 1992), the high intensity of the training regimen would be inappropriate for the heterogeneous group of patients eligible for cardiac rehabilitation programmes.

Consequences of an increase in maximal oxygen uptake

The significance of an increase in $\dot{V}O_2 max$ for cardiac patients is not that it permits a higher level of maximal effort (as this is rarely demanded in everyday life) but that repeated submaximal activities of daily living constitute a smaller percentage of the increased maximal capacity and therefore impose relatively less physiological stress. This is reflected in a reduction in heart rate (attributed to both increased vagal tone and reduced sympathetic outflow), blood pressure and plasma catecholamine concentrations at rest and at submaximal

workloads. Since myocardial oxygen consumption ($M\dot{V}O_2$) is determined by heart rate and systolic blood pressure (referred to as rate pressure product (RPP) or double product), a reduction in either or both delays the onset of ischaemia and lessens the potential for arrhythmias. A further benefit of the training-induced bradycardia is that, at any reference submaximal workload, the period of diastole is extended and, since 80% of coronary blood flow occurs during the relaxation phase of the cardiac cycle, myocardial perfusion is significantly enhanced.

Risk factor modification

In cardiac patients exercise may have an important secondary prevention role. The rationale for aggressive risk factor modification, as part of optimal care of coronary heart disease patients, is based on the premise that the factors that contribute to initial development of disease will also influence the progression of established disease and the likelihood of future events. The 'acute' effects of each bout of exercise in healthy people include:

- a raised post-exercise metabolic rate

- changes in lipoprotein metabolism with consequent increased synthesis of high-density lipoprotein (HDL)

- improved insulin sensitivity

- decreased blood pressure.

These effects all relate to local changes in the previously exercised muscle and are evident even after light to moderate exercise, suggesting that a general increase in physical activity is likely to contribute to the patient's continued well-being and to the reduced mortality and morbidity associated with exercise rehabilitation.

In addition, exercise training is known to reduce known triggers for cardiac events including:

- preventing thrombus formation
- improving endothelial function
- reducing potential for serious arrhythmias.

EXERCISE PRESCRIPTION

Principles of exercise prescription

When individual bouts of exercise are repeated regularly, and in accordance with established principles of training, a series of longer-term cardiovascular and metabolic adaptations occur; for instance, as described earlier, an increase in $\dot{V}O_2 max$ results from aerobic endurance training.

14

The principles of exercise training are:

Individuality – heredity plays a major part in how quickly and to what extent an individual's body adapts to a training programme: i.e. no two individuals (other than identical twins) will exhibit the same adaptations in response to the same training programme.

Progressive overload – overload refers to placing greater demands on the body than it is accustomed to, thereby provoking adaptations. In order to continue to stimulate training adaptations, the overload must be progressively increased.

Regression or reversibility – this principle is often referred to as the principle of 'use it or lose it': i.e. if the stimulus to change (the overload) is withdrawn, the adaptations conferred will diminish until the level of functional capacity is once again sufficient to meet only the demands imposed by general activities of daily life.

Specificity – the adaptations conferred by training are highly specific to:

- the volume of training, which includes the **F**requency and duration (or **T**ime) of training
- the **I**ntensity of training
- the mode or **T**ype of training

The effectiveness and appropriateness of all exercise prescriptions will depend upon manipulation of the **FITT** principle: i.e. the frequency, intensity, time and type of training.

Intensity of exercise

The intensity of exercise is a critical issue because vigorous activity carries a greatly increased risk of precipitating adverse events such as myocardial infarction or arrhythmias (Willich et al 1993). Frequent, moderate-intensity exercise is recommended for CHD patients since it will optimize benefits without increasing the risk of adverse events (Dafoe & Huston 1997). For individuals with greatly diminished functional capacity, several short bouts (as little as 5–10 minutes) throughout the day may be advisable. There are a number of established methods for prescribing and monitoring intensity, which may be used separately or in combination with one another.

Use of heart rate

Ideally, training heart rate is based on information derived from a maximal or symptom-limited exercise electrocardiogram test (ETT) (Box 14.1). Where a maximal test has been achieved, training heart rate should be set at 60–75% of maximal heart rate (HRmax). If the test was symptom limited, training intensity should be set at 10–20 beats per minute (bpm) below the

---

Box 14.1   Exercise tolerance testing

In the cardiology setting, an exercise ECG using an incremental protocol is the most common method for determining cardiac perfusion and function. Its major applications are:

- diagnosis – to identify patients with CHD and the severity of their disease
- prognosis – to identify high-, moderate- and low-risk patients
- evaluation – to establish the effectiveness of a selected intervention
- measurement of functional capacity – on which advice about activities of daily living and a formal exercise prescription may be based
- measurement of acute exercise responses including blood pressure, heart rate, ventilatory responses and detection of exercise-induced arrhythmias.

Numerous exercise protocols have been developed which utilize a variety of different exercise modes, but in the United Kingdom an incremental treadmill protocol is the traditional test mode. Before acceptance into a Phase III programme, usually 2–6 weeks post MI, a symptom-limited test (i.e. the patient continues until signs or symptoms, which necessitate test termination, are evident) is customary; the Bruce protocol is the most common. Submaximal tests that use a predetermined endpoint such as an age-predicted maximum heart rate are usual before discharge. The modified Bruce protocol is the most commonly used since it introduces two preliminary, less strenuous stages (Table 14.1).

Criteria for terminating an exercise test include:

- horizontal or down-sloping ST segment depression greater than 2 mm, indicating ischaemia
- marked drop in systolic blood pressure (>20 mmHg) indicating poor left ventricular function or severe coronary disease
- serious arrhythmias, e.g. ventricular tachycardia
- patient fatigue and/or excessive breathlessness at low workloads, which may simply indicate poor functional capacity but may also be suggestive of serious problems such as heart failure.

In general an exercise ECG test is considered to be negative if haemodynamic responses to the increasing workload are normal and the patient satisfactorily completes a workload equivalent to the second stage of the full Bruce protocol (7 METs). The test is considered positive if the patient is symptomatic at low workloads, if there are significant ECG changes or there is an inappropriate heart rate/blood pressure response to the incremental workload.

14

Stage		Speed (mph)	Grade %	Duration (min)	METs
Modified Bruce	Full Bruce				
1	–	1.7	0	3	1.7
2	–	1.7	5	3	2.9
3	1	1.7	10	3	4.7
4	2	2.5	12	3	7.1
5	3	3.4	14	3	10.2
6	4	4.2	16	3	13.5
7	5	5.0	18	3	17.3
8	6	5.5	20	3	24.6
9	7	6.0	22	3	28.4

Table 14.1 Commonly used treadmill exercise protocols

(Adapted from Bruce 1973)

heart rate at which symptoms were apparent and the patient's heart rate should be monitored throughout each exercise session. ECG test information is, however, not always available to health professionals. In the absence of test data or if, for diagnostic purposes, a patient performs the exercise test 'off-medication', other methods for establishing appropriate training intensity have to be used.

Age-adjusted predicted maximal rates can be used (220 bpm minus age in years is one formula) and the training heart rate set at 60–75% of the predicted maximum; this is equivalent to 40–65% $\dot{V}O_2$max. However, the standard deviation (SD) for maximal heart rate during exercise is ± 10 bpm and some individuals will, therefore, have an actual maximum heart rate 20 bpm higher or lower (2 SD above or below the population mean) than predicted. An alternative approach is to prescribe training at 40–65% of heart rate reserve (HRR – the difference between resting and maximal heart rate). This HRR approach (also known as the Karvonen method) is convenient since it is known that 40–65% of heart rate reserve is equivalent to about 40–65% of $\dot{V}O_2$max (60–75% of maximal heart rate) although, across the entire range of fitness levels, it is more closely linked to the percentage of oxygen uptake reserve ($\dot{V}O_2$R): i.e. the difference between resting oxygen consumption and maximal oxygen consumption (American College of Sports Medicine 2006). An example of the HRR method for calculating training heart rate is shown

below for an individual with a resting heart rate of 60 bpm and maximal heart rate of 150 bpm.

150 – 60 = 90 (heart rate reserve, HRR)

Training heart rate = 40–65% of heart rate reserve + resting heart rate (RHR)

90 × 0.40 = 36 + 60 (RHR) = 96 bpm (40%)

90 × 0.65 = 59 + 60 (RHR) = 119 bpm (65%)

Note: The formula is intended for use with known maximal heart rates. In the absence of these data, the substitution of age-adjusted predicted maxima introduces the same potential for error as previously mentioned. Consequently, any prescription that is based on predicted maximal heart rates should be used in conjunction with a rating of perceived exertion scale (RPE).

Since the relationship between exercise intensity and the per cent of maximal heart rate is preserved in patients on beta-blockers, the above formula can be adopted for calculating a training heart rate for this group but the maximal or peak heart rate must be established from an exercise test performed on medication.

Use of rating of perceived exertion

Cardiorespiratory and metabolic variables are strongly related to perceived exertion, which is accepted as a valid and reproducible indicator of the intensity of steady-state exercise. Physiotherapists and exercise specialists working in a cardiac rehabilitation setting are recommended to familiarize themselves with the scales of perceived exertion developed by Borg (1998). The Borg 15-point scale and the Borg CR10 scale of perceived exertion, together with patient instructions, are published in the Appendix of Borg's Perceived Exertion and Pain Scales (Borg 1998). In order to preserve the validity and reproducibility of these scales, their format should not be altered and the patient instructions should be closely followed.

On the 15-point scale a rating of 12–13 (equivalent to 3–4 on the Borg CR10 scale) corresponds to approximately 40% of heart rate reserve or $\dot{V}O_2$max (60% HRmax). A rating of 15 on the 15-point scale (equivalent to 5–6 on the Borg CR10 scale) corresponds to approximately 65% of heart rate reserve or $\dot{V}O_2$max (75% HRmax).

Use of metabolic equivalent values (METs)

Exercise may also be regulated by choice of activities according to their known MET (metabolic equivalent) values (for which tables are available in most exercise physiology texts). If an individual assesses walking at 3 miles per hour (mph) as 12–13 on the Borg RPE scale (corresponding to 60% of $\dot{V}O_2$max), then activities of

14

comparable MET value can be prescribed in the knowledge that they will present an appropriate training stimulus. Knowledge of MET values is also important in terms of excluding those activities that might pose a risk to certain individuals. Skipping (8–12 METs) or freestyle swimming (9–10 METs), for example, would be entirely inappropriate for someone with a peak capacity of 7 METs.

Some activities have a wide range of MET values, while others are relatively constant between individuals, mainly because they permit little variation in individual execution, e.g. there is very little difference in the way individuals walk or cycle. In contrast, there can be great variation in the way 'free-moving' activities such as dancing, skipping or rebounding on a mini-trampoline are executed. Because precise control of the exercise prescription in a cardiac population is necessary (particularly in early recovery post-event and for stable angina patients) activities that can be maintained at prescribed workloads and which permit uniform modification, e.g. altering the speed of walking or jogging or the resistance on a cycle ergometer, are preferred to those that are not amenable to standardized prescription.

Regardless of the objective method used for monitoring intensity, it is important to observe individuals for signs of excessive breathlessness, loss of quality of movement, unusual pallor or excessive sweating, all of which are inappropriate responses to moderate levels of exertion. Indications for ceasing exercise and contraindications to initiating exercise are included in the section on programme implementation.

Type of training

The inclusion of a variety of training modes within the individual prescription or the class format will minimize the incidence of overuse injuries, maximize peripheral adaptation (as, for example, when activities which require a contribution from both upper and lower body musculature are included) and increase patient motivation and adherence.

It is well documented that CHD patients who expend about 250–300 kcal per session and 1000–1500 kcal per week in additional physical activity will improve their aerobic capacity by 15–30% over a 4–6-month period (Balady et al 1994). There appears to be a continuous gradient in the benefits conferred and there is evidence that a minimum of 1600 kcal per week may halt the progression of CHD, whereas atherosclerotic regression may be achieved with a weekly energy expenditure of about 2200 kcal (Hambrecht et al 1994). Within the recommended ranges of frequency, intensity and time (or duration) of training, similar conditioning effects can be expected from any programme that realizes comparable weekly energy expenditure. Consequently the FITT components may be adjusted to provide an optimal prescription for individuals of varying cardiovascular and general medical status.

Programme format

Warm-up

Preparation for activity in older adults and especially in the cardiac population must be more gradual than for apparently healthy individuals. Fifteen minutes devoted to the warm-up component is recommended (Association of Chartered Physiotherapists in Cardiac Rehabilitation 2006). Low-impact, dynamic movements which use large muscle groups and which take all major joint complexes through their normal range of motion should be incorporated. A gradual increase in the size and range of movements performed will delay the onset of ischaemia by allowing adequate time for coronary blood flow to increase in response to the greater myocardial demand. Gradual increments in myocardial workload will also lessen the risk of arrhythmias, which can be a consequence of abrupt increases in demand and concomitant elevated sympathetic activity. As a guideline, individuals should be within 20 bpm below the lower end of their prescribed training heart rate range at the end of the warm-up or, if RPE is used in place of heart rate monitoring, a rating no higher than 3 on the Borg CR10 scale or 10–11 on the original scale.

Although evidence of the benefit is equivocal, preparing for exercise has traditionally included static stretches, which are performed after the pulse raising and mobility phase. Because static stretches are used, the need to maintain pulse rate and body temperature during this time must be addressed.

Aerobic conditioning

The type of aerobic activity used for conditioning may adopt a continuous or interval approach. Continuous training, as the name implies, involves uninterrupted activity usually performed at a constant submaximal intensity. Its advantage is the ease with which intensity may be prescribed and monitored. Walking, jogging, cycling, rowing, bench stepping and swimming all lend themselves to a continuous approach. Interval training entails bouts of relatively intense work separated by periods of rest or less intense activity. Its main advantage is that, especially for debilitated patients, the total volume of work accomplished is generally greater than when exercise is continuous; consequently the stimulus to physiological change is greater. In an older cardiac population, the transition from one activity to another also provides a time for social interaction and support, which probably aids long-term compliance.

14

In group rehabilitation programmes, various approaches to circuit training have proved popular; an activity is undertaken for a fixed period of time after which participants all move onto a different activity. Depending on cardiac status and individual functional capacity, participants may be prescribed an interval approach in which relatively intense periods of activity are followed by a period of less intense exercise, or alternatively, they may undertake activities all of which are of similar intensity. Circuits can be performed using little or no equipment or, if sufficient equipment is available to accommodate the whole group, cycles, rowing machines, treadmills, etc., can be used throughout the exercise session. Two approaches to group training are provided; Figure 14.1 presents a circuit design that requires only minimal equipment and Box 14.2 provides an example of how a group circuit might operate when extensive equipment is available.

In the design shown in Figure 14.1, participants spend a fixed time (ranging from 30 seconds to 2 minutes) at 'aerobic/cardiovascular (CV) stations' and either rest or perform a lower intensity activity before moving on to the next aerobic station. The lower intensity or 'active recovery' stations are usually designed to increase the strength and endurance of specific muscle groups (MSE), e.g. triceps, pectorals, trapezius, used in activities of daily living. Individualization of the cardiovascular component of the programme is achieved through variation in:

- the duration at each CV station
- the intensity (by changing the resistance or the speed or range of movement)
- the period of rest between stations
- the overall duration of conditioning.

In general the duration of activity is extended before increasing the intensity.

Exercises involving a recumbent position are discouraged because:

- some older participants have difficulty in getting up and down
- following vigorous activity, the increase in venous return on lying down enhances preload and thereby myocardial workload, which increases the risk of arrhythmias and angina in some individuals
- on return to an upright position the potential for orthostatic hypotensive episodes is dramatically increased in cardiac patients, most of whom are on medication that lowers blood pressure, e.g. beta-blockers and angiotensin-converting enzyme (ACE) inhibitors. Consequently, it is recommended that any recumbent work (e.g. for the abdominals or erector spinae) should be performed after completion of the circuit and a cool-down period.

Resistance training

Traditionally, training to increase strength (as opposed to endurance) of specific muscle groups was considered to be inappropriate for individuals with established heart disease. This was because resistance training is associated with an increase in arterial blood pressure, which increases myocardial workload. Some early studies suggested that the isometric component caused reduced ejection fraction, left ventricle wall motion abnormalities and increased incidence of arrhythmias. Further studies (Squires et al 1991, Williams 1994) have generally reported that cardiovascular and haemodynamic responses to resistance training in CHD patients and in normal subjects are similar and, because of increased diastolic pressure, may even enhance myocardial perfusion. However, in the United Kingdom, it is rare to incorporate strength training into clinically supervised programmes unless it is indicated for vocational reasons.

The American College of Sports Medicine (2006) advocates a single set of 10–15 repetitions to 'moderate fatigue' using 8–10 exercises. This is based on evidence that strength gains derived from one set are very similar to those reported when several are performed and adherence to programmes that are less time consuming is increased.

Contraindications for resistance training are:

- abnormal haemodynamic responses with exercise
- ischaemic changes during graded exercise testing
- poor left ventricular function
- uncontrolled hypertension or arrhythmias
- exercise capacity less than 6 METs.

Cool-down

A period of 10 minutes is recommended for cool-down at the end of the cardiovascular component. This is because:

- there is an increased risk of hypotension in this group – for some this is a specific side effect of their medication. In addition, there is an age-related slowing of baroreceptor responsiveness which increases the risk of venous pooling following sustained exercise
- in older adults heart rates take longer to return to pre-exercise rates
- raised sympathetic activity during vigorous exercise increases the risk of arrhythmias during the immediate period following cessation of exercise.

The cool-down should incorporate movements of diminishing intensity and passive stretching of the

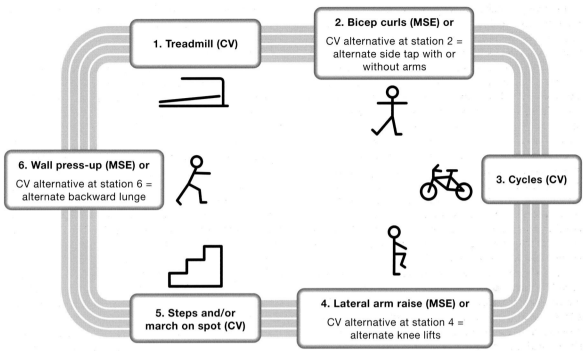

Figure 14.1   An example of interval-style circuit training suitable for a phase III cardiac rehabilitation programme. CV, cardiovascular work; MSE, muscle strength and endurance work.

Class management

Patients spend 2 minutes on stations 1, 3 and 5. At stations 2, 4 and 6, 1 minute is spent on the MSE work followed by 1 minute walking round the outside of the circuit. The patient's attention needs to be drawn to the start of each 2-minute activity period and (for the benefit of those at the even MSE stations) when the first minute has passed. One full circuit constitutes 12 minutes and 2 circuits, 24 minutes.

Individualization and progression

The emphasis should be on improving cardiovascular endurance. Greater duration of cardiovascular work may be achieved if individuals (as and when appropriate) are encouraged to adopt some of the CV alternatives at even station numbers. The intensity of the cardiovascular component may also be progressed at:

station 1   via speed and / or gradient of the treadmill
station 3   via resistance setting of the cycle
station 5   via progression from 2 minutes marching on spot to 1 minute of stepping and 1 minute marching and finally to 2 minutes stepping. To any of these arm work may be added. The height of the step may also be increased.

Progression on the *alternative* CV stations is achieved at:

station 2   via increased range of movement and/or lifting arms up to shoulder level as alternate legs go out to side
station 4   via increased range of movement and/or lifting arms up between each knee lift
station 6   via increased range of movement and/or lifting arms in front as alternate legs are extended back.

The *intensity* of *the MSE component* may be progressed by introducing dumbbells or resistance bands or, in the case of station 6, taking the feet further from the wall or introducing backward extension of the arm at the elbow (triceps 'kick-back') using a dumbbell.

Determining appropriate workloads using fixed equipment

Although individuals will vary considerably in the amount of cardiovascular work they can achieve, it is suggested that for:

- the treadmill – a walking speed of 2.5–3.0 miles per hour (mph) or 4.0–4.8 kilometres per hour (kph) is prescribed with the *gradient altered* to elicit a heart rate response within the target training heart rate range
- the cycle – 50–55 revolutions per minute (rpm) is prescribed with the *resistance altered* to elicit a heart rate response within the target training heart rate range
- the steps – a stepping speed of between 18 and 24 cycles per minute is prescribed (1 cycle – 4 footfalls; i.e. up, up, down, down) and the *step height altered* to elicit a heart rate response within the target training heart rate range.

The circuit when completed *twice* provides a minimum of 12 minutes CV work and a maximum of 24 minutes (if all CV alternatives at even numbered stations are used).

14

Box 14.2   An example of circuit training using gym equipment in which both interval and continuous training may be incorporated according to individual need

Treadmill for 6 minutes – speed (kph) and gradient (% grade) is individually prescribed

	Patient 1 (70 kg)	Patient 2 (70 kg)	Patient 3 (70 kg)
Minute 1,2	3.2 kph, 0%	4.8 kph, 0%	4.8 kph, 2.5%
Minute 3	2.5 kph, 0%	3.2 kph, 0%	4.8 kph, 2.5%
Minute 4,5	3.2 kph, 0%	4.8 kph, 0%	4.8 kph, 2.5%
Minute 6	2.5 kph, 0%	3.2 kph, 0%	4.8 kph, 2.5%

Cycle for 6 minutes @ 50–60 rpm – resistance (watts) individually prescribed

Minute 1,2	30 watts	50 watts	60 watts
Minute 3	no resistance	30 watts	60 watts
Minute 4,5	30 watts	50 watts	60 watts
Minute 6	no resistance	30 watts	60 watts

Stepping for 3 minutes – height of step (m) and rate of stepping (rpm) individually prescribed
Note: a cycle is 1st foot up, 2nd foot up, 1st foot down, 2nd foot down

Minute 1	0.10 m, 12 rpm	0.15 m, 16 rpm	0.15 m, 20 rpm
Minute 2	march on spot	0.15 m, 12 rpm	0.15 m, 20 rpm
Minute 3	0.10 m, 12 rpm	0.15 m, 16 rpm	0.15 m, 20 rpm

Repeat each activity to achieve a total conditioning period of 30 minutes or repeat selected activities in accordance with individual needs and abilities.

Note: On a treadmill and during stepping, relative $\dot{V}O_2$ (ml O_2/min) may be estimated on the basis of speed and gradient or speed and height of stepping, respectively, because the individual is carrying his own bodyweight and this contributes to the amount of work performed. On a cycle body weight has no influence on the cycle workload. It is important to start exercise at a relatively low level and to adjust the prescription in accordance with training heart rates and rating of perceived exertion.

kg, kilograms; kph, kilometres per hour; m, metres; rpm, rate per minute in cycles (1 cycle of stepping is 4 footfalls, i.e. up, up, down, down)

14

major muscle groups used during the conditioning phase. Patient observation for up to 30 minutes after the exercise session is recommended. Many programmes follow the exercise session with an education or relaxation component, which affords the opportunity for extended observation and supervision of participants.

Progression of training

The duration, frequency or intensity of training can be increased in order to maintain the training stimulus. Ideally serial exercise testing will form the basis on which the prescription is modified, in order to ensure that it provokes physiological adaptation. In the absence of exercise testing, heart rate monitoring and rating of perceived exertion, at reference workloads, may be used to establish the appropriateness of increasing any of the three variables, either singly or in combination with one another. The way in which exercise prescrip-tion is progressed and the rate at which it is progressed will be highly variable between individuals with CHD and will be a function of many factors including age, severity of disease, motivation, dual pathology and compliance.

PROGRAMME IMPLEMENTATION

Initial convalescence phase

In-hospital activity component

Graduated mobilization of cardiac patients following acute MI, coronary artery bypass graft or unstable heart failure is initiated by nursing or physiotherapy staff on acute units as part of overall patient care. Activities in the first 24–48 hours are usually restricted to breathing exercises, simple arm/leg range of movement exercises and limited self-care activities. Patients are encouraged to sit out of bed, take short walks, shower and dress over the next 2–3 days, depending on their cardiac status. Although the physiotherapist may be involved in the earlier stages with a multi-pathology patient, their customary role is to supervise the patient's mobilization plan, e.g. pre-discharge walk or stair assessments to determine individual exercise capacity, symptoms and/or limitations. By discharge, all patients should be conversant with the signs and symptoms of excessive exertion and be able to rate level of effort using, for example, the validated Borg scale (Borg 1998) or a locally developed scale. Both the patient and family should be advised on how to manage chest pain, symptoms of overexertion and encouraged to keep symptom diaries to discuss with staff at follow-up appointments.

A home exercise programme, which gives guidance on convalescence and household activities during the first 6 weeks and written advice on specific 'do and don't activities', should be provided. Walking is recommended as the main mode of exercise and means of increasing functional capacity. An individual schedule suggesting distance/speed ratios and progressions and a home activity diary should be incorporated. The British Heart Foundation provides a wide range of professionally produced written material if none is available locally.

Although the starting level and progression of activity is always dependent on individual clinical status, symptoms and medical history, the following exercise prescription may be used as a guideline at discharge:

Type/mode: an interval rather than a continuous approach may be required initially; encourage walking and performance of sitting/standing functional activities, including active, non-resisted general arm and leg exercises

Frequency and Timing: initially, short intermittent bouts of 5–10 minutes of activity interspersed with rest periods, 2–3 times per day. Overall duration of activity may be progressed from 5 to 20 minutes, 1–2 times per day

Intensity: RPE <11 (6–20 Borg scale) or to individual tolerance, i.e. symptom limited by breathlessness/angina/fatigue at or below these suggested targets:

- resting HR + 20–30 bpm post-MI and CABG (arbitrary target); *or*
- 40–50% of HRR if an exercise capacity test was completed before discharge.

Immediate post–discharge convalescence phase

This home-based period may typically last from 2 to 6 weeks, depending on local protocols and resources as well as the patient's fitness to attend the supervised outpatient programme. The immediate post-discharge phase is a time of high anxiety for patients and families

and unfortunately rehabilitation services vary considerably and range from either no or limited contact to regular phone follow-up and home visits in some areas. A home programme for MI and CABG patients in the form of a workbook or exercise videos, *The Heart Manual* (Lewin et al 1992) and *Road to Recovery* – a British Heart Foundation publication (www.bhf.org.uk) – may be used as either a complete rehabilitation package or as an interim measure or adjunct to a programme. Contact from rehabilitation staff at this stage provides the opportunity to answer questions, discuss symptoms, reinforce home exercises and daily walking as appropriate: e.g. uncomplicated post-MI and CABG patients should have increased the duration and frequency of activities and may be achieving up to 30 minutes of walking once or twice daily. Telephone contact also facilitates the review of risk factor modification goals and achievements.

Supervised outpatient exercise programme

The onset and duration of outpatient rehabilitation programmes vary considerably and are usually dependent on local resources. Programmes typically start any time from 3 to 6 weeks post-event and last for up to 6–12 weeks and include patients at different stages in their recovery. They may be hospital based, but there are increasing numbers of clinically supervised programmes in the community. For the purposes of this chapter, supervised exercise programmes are used as a model of exercise training.

The challenge for the exercise professional is to devise a safe and effective training programme that enables a patient to achieve a gradual transition from low-level convalescence activity through to an incremental exercise prescription. Although there is a perception that exercise training could be dangerous, the evidence is that rehabilitation programmes result in very few complications and the incidence of death is one per 1.3 million exercise hours (Franklin et al 1998, Van Camp & Peterson 1986, Vongvanich et al 1996). Indeed, if agreed guidelines and protocols for exercise training that relate to assessment, risk stratification, health and safety, patient induction, management and exercise prescription are implemented, then a safe, systematic approach, which minimizes risk and maximizes benefit, may be achieved (American Association of Cardiovascular and Pulmonary Rehabilitation 2004, American College of Sports Medicine 2006, Association of Chartered Physiotherapists in Cardiac Rehabilitation 2006).

Assessment and risk stratification

Local protocols referring patients for exercise training should include appropriate screening and consent from

14

a hospital physician or cardiologist. The following information should be available to the rehabilitation health professional as part of the assessment and risk stratification process:

- current clinical status, symptoms, progress since discharge and any complications

- current cardiac status, e.g. site and size of the infarct, revascularization details, results of investigations, e.g. exercise tolerance test (see Box 14.1), echocardiogram

- cardiac history and relevant previous medical history, e.g. musculoskeletal problems, respiratory or neurological conditions

- risk stratification, to enable appropriate patient management and exercise prescription

- current medication and CHD risk factor profile.

Clinical risk stratification, i.e. determining the prognosis and relative risk of future cardiac events and complications, as well as the risk of complications during exercise, should be carried out in accordance with AACVPR guidelines (American Association of Cardiovascular and Pulmonary Rehabilitation 2004; Fig. 5.1, page 63). The stratification of patients into low-, medium- or high-risk groups for the occurrence of events during exercise depends on their current cardiac status, including cardiac damage, complications and associated signs and symptoms. Patients who have a low ejection fraction consistent with impaired left ventricular function, serious arrhythmias or left ventricular failure are at greater risk of complications and future cardiac events and would be classified as high risk. Also the prognosis for these patients is much poorer than for the general cardiac patient; 50% of heart failure patients die within 4 years and in patients with severe heart failure 50% of those will die within 1 year (Swedberg et al 2005) compared with the mortality for patients in the first 4 weeks post-MI of 10–15% and 5% annually thereafter.

Patient safety during exercise is the main consideration for health professionals. The main risk to cardiac patients attending an exercise programme is ventricular fibrillation. When 'predicting' risk from clinical evidence and exercise ECG assessment, the patients who have suffered extensive cardiac damage, have residual ischaemia and demonstrate ventricular arrhythmias on exercise, for example, a patient with a significantly positive exercise ECG test (ETT) or poor functional capacity and low $\dot{V}O_2$ max, would be considered to be at higher risk of cardiac events and consequently prescribed a lower level, more cautious rehabilitation exercise programme. Limits for exercise prescription may be deter-

mined by onset of symptoms during the ETT, e.g. breathlessness or fatigue, and very importantly by evidence of ischaemia, with or without the presence of angina (silent ischaemia). Peak exercise prescription should always be set at least 10 bpm below the ischaemic threshold (American Association of Cardiovascular and Pulmonary Rehabilitation 2004, American College of Sports Medicine 2006). Distance achieved during a 6-minute walk test (6MWT) has also been used in risk assessment and exercise prescription, with a walking distance of less than 300m associated with poorer short-term survival.

Rehabilitation assessment and outcome measures

Assessment and outcome measures are essential, not only to determine risk stratification and functional capacity but also to set and evaluate the effectiveness of an exercise training programme, provide objective feedback to the patient and facilitate evidence-based practice. These measures can be used both as a baseline, entry assessment tool and as an exit outcome measure. They may include heart rate and blood pressure at rest, during exercise and at recovery, comparative ratings of perceived exertion (RPE) at given fixed workloads, bodyweight, body mass index, waist circumference measures, as well as measures of functional capacity. Direct measures of maximum functional capacity may be determined from $\dot{V}O_2$max derived from a cardiopulmonary exercise test (CPEX) and/or ETT. Indirect submaximal measures of functional capacity may be derived from the 6MWT (Steele 1994), shuttle walk test (Singh et al 1992) or Chester step test (Sykes & Roberts 2004). The measure of functional capacity used to set exercise prescription should then be successively monitored and adjusted to maintain the progressive, overload principle of exercise training. When using the walking distance achieved during a 6MWT to set an exercise prescription, the outcome may be used to calculate walk distance and speed for a home programme, the related METs level of daily activities and the general exercises which may be undertaken in a circuit training programme: e.g. 400 m walked in 6MWT is equivalent to 24 min per mile i.e. 2.5 mph pace equivalent to 2.9 METs.

Assessment

In addition to the initial screening and risk stratification on entry to the programme, there should be ongoing clinical assessment before each exercise session. Patients should be screened by the rehabilitation professional for changes and/or compliance with medication, symptoms and home activity levels. It is recommended that patients should not exercise if they are generally unwell, symptomatic or clinically unstable on arrival (Fletcher et al 2001), e.g. if they present with:

14

- fever and acute systemic illness
- unresolved/unstable angina
- resting blood pressure (BP) systolic >200 mmHg and diastolic >110 mmHg
- significant unexplained drop in blood pressure
- symptomatic hypotension
- resting or uncontrolled tachycardia (>100 bpm)
- uncontrolled atrial or ventricular arrhythmias
- new or recurrent symptoms of breathlessness, lethargy, palpitations, dizziness
- unstable heart failure, e.g. swelling of ankles and/or weight gain >2 kg over 2 days
- unstable/uncontrolled diabetes.

If any of these signs or symptoms is present, the patient should be seen by their general practitioner and/or cardiologist. Home activity and exercise goals should be adjusted appropriately and reviewed by rehabilitation staff before the patient restarts the exercise programme. For guidance on medication commonly used and prescribed for cardiac patients, and its associated relevance to exercise, see Table 14.2.

Programme delivery and management

Safe delivery of exercise also depends on patient supervision, appropriate education, induction and observance of health and safety protocols.

Patient supervision and staffing

- There should be an appropriate skill mix of staff with specialist training to lead and supervise exercise and deal with medical problems and emergencies.
- There should be a minimum of two trained staff present with staff:patient ratio dependent on the risk stratification of patients in the group. Current recommended ratio to ensure safe monitoring/management of patients is 1:5; inclusion of higher-risk patients may require a higher ratio (Association of Chartered Physiotherapists in Cardiac Rehabilitation 2006, Coats et al 1995, Scottish Intercollegiate Guidelines Network 2002).
- All staff should be skilled in monitoring the patient's HR, BP, symptoms and pacing of exercise.
- All staff should be competent and regularly updated in basic life support and be able to access and use an automated defibrillator (AED). Preferably one professional should have advanced life support training.

Patient induction

An induction and education session should be conducted with each patient and cover:

- the aims of the exercise programme
- use of equipment
- importance of safety, self-monitoring and pacing of exercise
- setting exercise goals and maintaining a home exercise and activity log book.

Patients and their families should also be advised on educational issues such as:

- signs and symptoms of exertion, e.g. 'listen to your body'
- warm-up and cool-down advice
- caution with isometric activities
- relative haemodynamic responses to arm-work versus leg-work
- environmental issues, e.g. excessive heat/cold, dehydration
- avoiding exercise after a heavy meal, during systemic illness and when fatigued
- the importance of remaining until surveillance of all patients in the immediate post-exercise period (for up to 30 minutes) is completed.

Health and safety protocols

Relevant considerations:

- There should be a local written policy, clearly displayed, for managing emergency situations, e.g. collapse of patient, and management of medical problems, e.g. chest pain, hypoglycaemic episode.
- There should be rapid access to an emergency team either in hospital or via ambulance, with access to a telephone for raising emergency help.
- Appropriate emergency equipment should be available. It should be regularly maintained in accordance with local protocols and staff should have regular practice in emergency drills and procedures.
- Exercise equipment should be regularly checked and maintained by staff.
- Drinking water and glucose drinks or supplements should be available for patients as required.
- Venue access, emergency exits, toilet and changing facilities, lighting, floor surface and room space should be checked by staff to be safe and appropriate. There should be adequate space for a free exercise area and patient traffic around exercise room, and safe placement of equipment meeting recommended requirements, e.g. floor space for aerobic exercise of 1.8–2.3 m^2 per patient and 0.6 m^2 of space

14

Table 14.2 A guide to medication

Drug group/name	When used	Possible side effects	Exercise considerations
ACE inhibitors Captopril Enalapril Fosinopril Lisinopril Perindopril Ramipril Trandolapril	**Standard drug therapy for post-MI patients, especially those who are at increased risk of deteriorating LV function and heart failure.** • Hypertension • Heart failure • Post MI to improve LV function and as secondary prevention	• Dry annoying cough • Hypotension • Skin rash • Metallic taste • Reduced kidney function • Allergic reaction involving swelling of the lips and tongue (angio-oedema)	• Possible increase in exercise capacity in individuals with heart failure • Rapid changes in posture or abrupt cessation of exercise will increase risk of hypotension
Alpha-blockers Doxazosin Indoramin Prazosin	• Hypertension (not controlled by other drugs)	• Postural hypotension • Headache • Palpitations	• Fatigue
Angiotensin II receptor blockers Candesartan Irbesartan Losartan Telmisartan Valsartan	• Hypertension (often used when the dry cough associated with ACE inhibitors cannot be tolerated) • Heart failure	• Fatigue • Hypotension • Taste disturbance • Skin rash	• Rapid changes in posture or abrupt cessation of exercise will increase risk of hypotension
Antiarrhythmics Amiodarone	Arrhythmias • Atrial fibrillation • Atrial flutter • Ventricular arrhythmias	• Photosensitivity – avoid direct sun on skin • Night glare • Metallic taste • Nightmares • Thyroid disorders	• Possible slower heart rate response to exercise • Reduced exercise capacity due to depressant effect on myocardium
Digoxin	• Atrial fibrillation • Limited use in heart failure	• Nausea, vomiting • Loss of appetite • Fatigue • Slow pulse • Ventricular arrhythmias • Vision disturbances	
Anticoagulants Warfarin	Reduce the risk of embolism forming in: • Atrial fibrillation • Valve disease • Valve surgery (taken for life if mechanical valve used and for about 3 months if tissue valve used) • Following large anterior MI if, as a consequence of poor ventricular contraction, there is a risk of thrombus formation within the left ventricle	• Haemorrhage as a result of external damage, e.g. cuts • Internal bleeding, e.g gastrointestinal	• Care with equipment to avoid accidents • Avoid contact sports or sports where there is a high risk of injury **Note:** unless under medical advice, patients should not take products containing aspirin when taking anticoagulants

table continues

Drug group/name	When used	Possible side effects	Exercise considerations
Antiplatelets Aspirin	**Standard drug therapy for all patients with cardiovascular disease and anyone at high risk of developing CHD or other vascular disease.** Also used in acute phase of MI	• Gastrointestinal upset/bleed • Bronchospasm in susceptible individuals • Other internal haemorrhage	
Clopidogrel	• Acute coronary syndrome • Standard therapy post PCI for limited period	• Lower incidence of gastrointestinal upset/bleed than with aspirin • Blood disorders	
Beta-blockers Atenolol Bisoprolol* Carvedilol* Metoprolol* Propanolol Sotalol *licensed for use in heart failure	**Standard drug therapy for post-MI patients who are at increased risk of further MI and sudden cardiac death.** **Also** • Hypertension • Angina • Arrhythmias • Tachycardia • Heart failure	• Reduced pulse rate • Reduced blood pressure • Dizziness • Tiredness / lethargy • Airway constriction • Cold fingers/toes • Male impotence • Sleep disturbance/ nightmares **Note:** beta-blockers should not be stopped suddenly without medical advice as this may lead to rebound angina and possibly MI	• Rapid changes in posture or abrupt cessation of exercise will increase risk of hypotension • Unless a training HR has been established from an ECG ETT done 'on medication', appropriate training intensity is best determined using a combination of RPE and HR responses • Estimated HRmax rate will be about 20–30 bpm lower than for those not on beta-blockers
Calcium-channel blockers			• Possible reduced HR response to exercise in verapamil and diltiazem
Type 1 Verapamil	• Angina • Hypertension • Arrhythmias	• Hypotension • Facial flushing • Palpitations • Pounding headaches • Constipation (mostly verapamil)	• Rapid changes in posture or abrupt cessation of exercise will increase risk of hypotension
Type 2 Amlodipine Felodipine Nicardipine Nifedipine	• Angina • Hypertension • Amlodopine is used when the radial artery is used in CABGS as it helps to maintain vasodilation of the grafted vessel	• Mild ankle swelling (mostly nifedipine)	Nifedipine may cause a reflex increase in HR in response to reduced BP
Type 3 Diltiazem	• Angina • Hypertension		

14

table continues

Drug group/name	When used	Possible side effects	Exercise considerations

Diuretics
Amiloride
Bendroflumethiazide
Bumetanide
Burinex A
  (bumetanide)
Frumil (co-amilofruse)
Furosemide
Hydrochlorothiazide
Metolazone
Moduretic
  (co-amilozide)
Spironolactone
Triamterene
	• Heart failure
	• Hypertension
	• Oedema
		• Loss of potassium (in some types)
		• Ventricular arrhyhmias
		• Tiredness
		• Muscle weakness and cramps
		• Elevated cholesterol and triglycerides
		• Loss of appetite
		• Gout
		• Diabetes
		• Impotence
			• Dehydration effects – keep encouraging fluids during exercise, especially in hot weather.
			• Dehydration increases potential for hypotension
			• Aching legs and /or tiredness may affect exercise capacity

Lipid–lowering drugs	Standard drug therapy for all CVD patients and anyone at high risk of developing CHD or other vascular disease. Hyperlipidaemia • Potent at lowering LDL-C • Moderate increase in HDL-C • Moderate reduction in elevated triglyceride levels	• Gastrointestinal upsets • Muscle pain • Headache	• Possible aching legs
Statins Atorvastatin Fluvastatin Pravastatin Rosuvastatin Simvastatin	In combination with statin therapy when further reduction of LDL-C is sought or on their own in patients who do not tolerate statin therapy		
Ezetimibe	• Mainly elevated triglyceride • Also to reduce LDL-C levels and raise HDL-C	• Gallstones • Rash • Acute pain in calf or thigh muscle if kidney function is impaired	• Possible aching legs
Fibrates Bezafibrate Clofibrate Fenofibrate Gemfibrozil	• To raise HDL-C levels alone or in combination with drugs listed above	• Flushing • Gastrointestinal upset	
Nicotinic acid	• Also has profound effect on triglyceride levels		
Nitrates Isosorbide dinitrate Isosorbide mononitrate	• Angina Longer-acting nitrates are given to prevent angina	• Hypotension • Facial flushing • Headache • Dizziness • Nausea	• Rapid changes in posture or abrupt cessation of exercise will increase risk of hypotension

table continues

Drug group/name	When used	Possible side effects	Exercise considerations
Glyceryl trinitrate (GTN tablets or spray)	• 'Breakthrough' angina When, despite the use of long-acting nitrates, angina occurs, GTN is used to alleviate the angina. GTN can also be used to prevent angina, e.g. prior to exercise	• Possible severe interaction with Viagra (sildenafil) and other medication used for erectile dysfunction	• Improved exercise tolerance as the ischaemic threshold is improved Clients must never exercise with or through an episode of angina as it may indicate the onset of MI
Potassium–channel activators Nicorandil	• Angina (especially when angina is resistant to other medication)	• Dizziness • Headaches • Hypotension • Tachycardia • Interaction with Viagra (sildenafil) as described above	• Rapid changes in posture or abrupt cessation of exercise will increase risk of hypotension • Possible tachycardia

(Adapted with permission from the British Association for Cardiac Rehabilitation (BACR) Training Module for Phase IV Exercise Instructors (2006), 4th edn. Human Kinetics, Leeds)

ACE, angiotensin-converting enzyme; LV, left ventricular; MI, myocardial infarction; CHD, coronary heart disease; PCI, percutaneous coronary intervention; ECG, electrocardiograph; ETT, exercise tolerance test; HR, heart rate; CABGS, coronary artery bypass grafting surgery; BP, blood pressure; CVD, cardiovascular disease; LDL-C, low-density lipoprotein cholesterol; HDL-C, high-density lipoprotein cholesterol

per individual using equipment (American Association of Cardiovascular and Pulmonary Rehabilitation 2004, Tharrett & Peterson 1997).

■ Temperature and ventilation of the room should be maintained at 18–23°C (65–72°F) and humidity at 65%.

Exercise class management

A skilled clinical exercise team will be able to create a safe, positive and non-intimidating environment in which a wide spectrum of patients are encouraged to participate and benefit from exercise. Supervised gym-based work or group exercise in a circuit training format are popular modes of delivering training. Each format requires rehabilitation professionals with excellent interpersonal and behaviour management skills to engage patients in exercise and develop their trust, confidence and participation. The exercise professional needs to establish an empathetic relationship with the patient and deal with emotional and psychological responses, which may vary from fearful, depressed, overdependent to aggressive, cavalier or in denial. Good interactive class management and group dynamics can create a positive atmosphere of social support and camaraderie which can result in a rewarding 'care of the group by the group' ethos and provide an opportunity to introduce exercise-related teaching points.

Exercise prescription and progression

The main objective of the exercise programme is to increase cardiorespiratory fitness through a cardiovascular and muscular endurance training programme. Patients report that the consequent improvement in functional capacity and strength enables them to perform activities with less effort, fewer symptoms, more confidence and an enhanced quality of life. The evidence and related pathophysiology, for endurance training in higher-risk patients with poor functional capacity, is that this is best achieved by increasing peripheral stimulus while minimizing cardiovascular stress (Swedberg et al 2005).

The principles of exercise training applied to a clinically supervised programme may be summarized as follows:

Type or mode

■ Aerobic and muscular strength and endurance training that involves large muscle groups in dynamic movement, e.g. walk, cycle, circuit training.

■ Initial adoption of an interval approach with eventual progression to low/moderate intensity continuous aerobic exercise.

■ Caution should be exercised over:
— The introduction of resistance training; exercises should be relatively low in resistance and high

14

in repetitions (American College of Sports Medicine 2006). Debilitated, higher-risk heart failure patients may require seated or very low intensity alternative exercises during the conditioning component.

— Abrupt posture shifts, e.g. upright work to recumbent position and recumbent to upright.

— Excessive use of arm/upper body exercise relative to leg work as arm work (at a given workload) results in a higher systolic and diastolic BP than when the same work is performed by a larger muscle mass such as the legs.

Timing and progression

■ Limit time initially to 5–10 min if patient is compromised (<3 METs).

■ Gradually increase time to 20–30 min conditioning, excluding warm-up (15–20 min) and cool-down (>10 min).

■ Consider progression in 3 stages; initial period <4 weeks, improvement phase >16 weeks and long-term maintenance >26 weeks.

Frequency

■ 1–2 times per week at a supervised rehabilitation class.

■ Additional, independent home-based exercise twice per week.

■ Walking and other leisure activities should be incorporated on remaining days.

Intensity

■ *Aerobic exercise:* 40–65% HRR or 60–75% maximal HR derived from an agreed age-estimated formula). A lower intensity prescription at 40–50% of functional capacity may be necessary for debilitated patients.

■ *Resistance training:* 1 set of between 3–20 repetitions (e.g. 10–15) of 8–10 major muscle groups 2–3 times per week @ RPE 15–16 (stop 2–3 repetitions before volitional fatigue, while maintaining good technique).

There should be close observation of all cardiac patients for up to 30 minutes post-exercise.

Exercise considerations for special cardiac groups

Considerations for prescribing and delivering exercise for various groups within the CHD population, e.g. patients with diabetes, hypertension and peripheral vascular disease, are summarized in Table 14.3. Exercise issues for specific cardiac patient groups, i.e. patients with heart failure and implantable cardioverter defibrillators, are described below.

Heart failure

Heart failure patients are among those deemed at highest risk of further cardiac events during exercise according to the AACVPR stratification criteria (American Association of Cardiovascular and Pulmonary Rehabilitation 2004), fulfilling one of the essential criteria for high-risk patients of an ejection fraction of less than 40%, but may additionally present with other criteria, e.g. significant symptoms at low levels of activity of less than 5 METs or the presence of abnormal haemodynamics with exercise testing. Quantifying functional capacity further stratifies relative risk; a peak $\dot{V}O_2$ of less than 10 millilitres of oxygen per kilogram of bodyweight per minute (<10 ml kg^{-1} min^{-1}) is associated with a relatively higher risk, a peak $\dot{V}O_2$ of >18 ml kg^{-1} min^{-1} categorizes a patient at lower risk, while a walking distance of <300 m in the 6MWT is associated with poorer short-term survival (Cahalin et al 1996, Likoff et al 1987, Lipkin et al 1986, Swedberg et al 2005). When undertaking exercise training with higher-risk patients, rigorous patient assessment, individual exercise prescription and monitoring, coupled with safe management and delivery of exercise, are paramount (Hunt et al 2005, Pina et al 2003).

In addition to the previously discussed exercise contraindications and cautions that apply to cardiac patients, heart failure patients should report:

■ significant weight gain of >2 kg over 2 days
■ deterioration in exercise tolerance or increased breathlessness on exertion
■ any recent implantable cardioverter defibrillator (ICD) event or change in pacemaker status.

Issues relating to the monitoring and safety of exercise include:

■ staff:patient supervision ratio should be reviewed dependent on higher risk stratification; consider 3:1

■ rigorous monitoring of individual patient's heart rate, blood pressure and use of RPE (i.e. Borg CR 0-10 scale) and dyspnoea scales

■ for those with ICDs, heart rate thresholds should be incorporated into the exercise prescription.

Additional training considerations include:

■ aim for low/ moderate intensity of training; may be as low as 40% of $\dot{V}O_2$R/HRR and/or 11–13 RPE

Table 14.3   Considerations for prescribing exercise for special groups within the coronary heart disease population

	Management	Precautions/other considerations
Diabetes	• Diabetes must be stable • Blood sugar levels should be checked twice before exercising: 30 minutes prior to exercise and again immediately before commencement of exercise. 20–30 g of additional carbohydrate should be ingested if pre-exercise blood glucose is <5.5 mmol/l • If new to exercise or increasing the intensity or duration of exercise, levels should be monitored every 30 minutes during exercise • Check blood glucose levels at least twice after exercise to ensure that hypoglycaemia is not developing • Those on insulin medication may experience 'exercise-induced hyperglycaemia'. Exercise should not be commenced if pre-exercise blood glucose levels are >13 mmol/l. If glucose levels pre-exercise are >10 mmol/l, check again 10 minutes after starting exercise and only continue to exercise if the level has fallen	• Carry medical information about condition in case of adverse incidents • 'Silent' ischaemia is more common in diabetics • Insulin may need to be reduced on exercise days • Insulin uptake may be increased if it is injected into exercising limbs, e.g. use the abdomen rather than the thigh • Have rapid-acting glucose source available • Late evening exercise is inadvisable • Autonomic neuropathy may lead to abnormal HR and BP responses • Peripheral neuropathy may cause sensory loss, impaired balance and coordination. • Peripheral neuropathy highlights the need for good foot care. Patients should check their feet before and after exercise • The effect of a single bout of exercise on blood glucose levels lasts less than 72 hours, so exercise needs to be frequent and regular • Specific benefits of aerobic exercise for diabetic patients include: 　— improved glycaemic clearance 　— increased insulin sensitivity 　— reduction in body fat while preserving lean muscle mass
Hypertension	• Do not exercise if SBP >180 mmHg or DBP >100 mmHg • Follow FITT principles but adopt lower end of training intensity with compensatory increase in the frequency and/or duration • Reduce resistance and increase number of repetitions for muscular strength and endurance exercises	• Medication is likely to lead to hypotension. Ensure that: 　— during upright exercise, feet are constantly moving to aid venous return 　— there is an extended post-exercise recovery period • Avoid Valsalva manoeuvre • Avoid high-intensity arm work and overgripping of equipment, e.g. cycle handlebars. • A specific benefit of exercise for hypertensive patients is that total peripheral resistance is reduced for several hours following a single bout of exercise. Consequently, an increase in frequency of exercise ensures that the overall time spent in a relative 'hypotensive' state is increased

table continues

14

	Management	Precautions/other considerations

Peripheral vascular disease	• Promote daily walking and other weightbearing exercise
	• Increase duration before intensity
	• Interval training may be better tolerated than continuous exercise
	• Use supplementary non-weightbearing exercise, e.g. cycling, if pain is severe and/or motivation is poor and an adequate CV dose is unlikely to be achieved through weightbearing exercises alone
	• Reassure and support patient to exercise despite discomfort and teach PVD scale of discomfort (ACSM 2006)
		• Cold weather, leading to vasoconstriction, may worsen symptoms; encourage extended warm-up period, e.g. slow walking gradually increasing to individually prescribed pace
		• Monitor for injuries to legs that could lead to leg ulcers or gangrene
		• Specific benefits of weightbearing exercise for patients with PVD may include:
		  – increase in peripheral blood flow and oxygen delivery
		  – improved oxygen extraction
		  – changed gait and, thereby, efficiency, i.e. less effort at same workload

Ageing population	• FITT principles apply for CV training but at lower intensity until ability is established. • Extended warm-up and cool-down is required. • Promote strength work for major muscle groups used in activities of daily living • Include flexibility and general mobility work within the programme	• Avoid exercises in extreme temperatures • Monitor hydration, especially if diuretics have been prescribed • Avoid using partners for support or in resistance work • Instructions must be especially clear/precise/unhurried and should be enhanced by good visual demonstration • Avoid exercises that might exacerbate urinary incontinence

g, gram; mmol/l, millimoles per litre; HR, heart rate; BP, blood pressure; SBP, systolic blood pressure; mmHg, millimetres of mercury; DBP, diastolic blood pressure; FITT, frequency, intensity, time and type of training; CV, cardiovascular; l, litre; PVD, peripheral vascular disease; ACSM, American College of Sports Medicine

■ adopt an interval training approach with initial work phases of 1–6 minutes of activity and rest phases of 1–2 minutes (American College of Sports Medicine 2006)

■ include respiratory and posture training; very deconditioned patients may suffer gross fatigue with arm and upper body exercise and accessory muscle use compromises breathing pattern.

Exercise issues following implantation of a cardioverter defibrillator

Exercise rehabilitation plays an important part in enabling patients to regain the confidence to resume activity following implantation of an ICD device (Lampman & Knight 2000). Significant benefits in cardiorespiratory fitness, confidence and psychological well-being have been demonstrated in patients participating in rehabilitation following implantation of an ICD device (Fitchet et al 2003). The following specific points should be considered when prescribing and delivering exercise for ICD patients:

■ knowledge of ICD heart rate settings

■ knowledge of ICD therapy settings

■ knowledge of medication used to control heart rate, e.g. beta-blockade

■ avoidance of excesssive shoulder range of movement and/or highly repetitive vigorous shoulder movement.

Transition of patients to long-term community-based exercise provision

When medically and psychologically stable, CHD patients should progress from the clinically supervised rehabilitation environment to a community-based, long-term Phase IV exercise programme. They should demonstrate:

■ significant improvement in functional capacity (achieving approximately 5 METs is recommended)

■ psychological adaptation to chronic disease

- the foundation of behavioural and lifestyle changes required for continued risk factor modification.

Rehabilitation staff discharging the patient to their general practitioner and Phase IV instructor should be satisfied that the patient is able to:

- exercise safely and effectively, according to an individual exercise prescription

- monitor own heart rate or use scale of perceived exertion effectively

- recognize warning signs and symptoms and take appropriate action (e.g. stop/reduce exercise level, take glyceryl trinitrate)

- identify specific goals for long-term maintenance of lifestyle change and risk factor reduction, relating to own personal history

- take responsibility to monitor risk factors (i.e. smoking, blood pressure, cholesterol and diabetes) with their general practitioner and the practice nurse

- report results of any ongoing investigations and possible implications for exercise prescription to the Phase IV instructor.

A discharge communication should be provided to the patient's general practitioner, summarizing rehabilitation outcomes, CHD risk factor status and future plans regarding exercise follow-up before the patient moves on to Phase IV. Either a similar version of this discharge summary or the recommended British Association of Cardiac Rehabilitation Information Sheet (www. bacrphaseiv.co.uk), for transition between Phases III and IV, should be completed and given to the patient so that he may take this information to the proposed Phase IV instructor.

CONCLUSION

Cardiac rehabilitation, and specifically exercise training, is an effective form of management for people with cardiac disease and is endorsed by numerous clinical guidelines. It has a large and increasing evidence base to support its implementation in a variety of settings and for a variety of cardiac conditions. Challenges remain to increase the uptake of all people who would benefit from participation in programmes and to ensure programmes and research evidence reflect changes in the medical management of this group of people.

References

Adams J, Cline MJ, Hibbard M, McCullough T, Hartman J 2006 A new paradigm for post-cardiac event resistance exercise guidelines. American Journal of Cardiology 97: 281–286

Ades PA, Pashkow FJ, Nestor JR 1997 Cost-effectiveness of cardiac rehabilitation after myocardial infarction. Journal of Cardiopulmonary Rehabilitation 17: 222–231

Albu J, Gottlieb SH, August P et al 2006 Modifications of coronary risk factors. American Journal of Cardiology 97(12): 41–52

American Association of Cardiovascular and Pulmonary Rehabilitation 2004 Guidelines for cardiac rehabilitation and secondary prevention programmes, 4th edn. Human Kinetics, Champaign, IL

American College of Sports Medicine 2006 ACSMs guidelines for exercise testing and prescription, 7th edn. Williams and Wilkins, Baltimore

Association of Chartered Physiotherapists in Cardiac Rehabilitation 2006 Standards for the exercise component of the phase III cardiac rehabilitation. CSP, London

Balady GJ, Fletcher BJ, Froelicher ES et al 1994 Cardiac rehabilitation programs. A statement for healthcare professionals from the American Heart Association. Circulation 90: 1602–1610

Beswick AD, Rees K, Griebsch I et al 2004 Provision, uptake and cost of cardiac rehabilitation programmes: improving services to under-represented groups. Health Technology Assessment 8: 1–152

Bittner V, Sanderson B 2006 Cardiac rehabilitation as a secondary prevention centre. Coronary Artery Disease 17: 211–218

Blumenthal JA, Rejeski WJ, Walsh-Riddle M et al 1988 Comparison of high- and low-intensity exercise training early after acute myocardial infarction. American Journal of Cardiology 61: 26–30

Borg G 1998 Borg's perceived exertion and pain scales. Human Kinetics, Champaign, IL

Brodie D, Bethell H, Bren S 2006 Cardiac rehabilitation in England: a detailed national survey. European Journal of Cardiovascular Prevention and Rehabilitation 13: 122–128

Brubaker PH, Rejeski WJ, Smith MJ et al 2000 A home-based maintenance exercise program after centre-based cardiac rehabilitation: effects on blood lipids, body composition and functional capacity. Journal of Cardiopulmonary Rehabilitation 20: 50–56

Bruce RA 1973 Principles in exercise testing. In: Naughton JP, Heuerstein HK (eds) Exercise testing and exercise training in coronary heart disease. Academic Press, New York

Cahalin LP, Mathier MA, Semigran MJ et al 1996 The six minute walk test predicts peak oxygen uptake and survival in patients with advanced heart failure. Chest 110: 325–332

Cannistra LB, Davidoff R, Picard MH, Balady GJ 1999 Moderate-high intensity exercise training after myocardial infarction: effect on left ventricular remodeling. Journal of Cardiopulmonary Rehabilitation 19: 373–380

Coats A, McGee H, Stokes H, Thompson D 1995 BACR Guidelines for cardiac rehabilitation. Blackwell Science, Oxford

Dafoe W, Huston P 1997 Current trends in cardiac rehabilitation. Canadian

14

Medical Association Journal 156: 527–532

Dall'Ago P, Chiappa GRS, Guths H et al 2006 Inspiratory muscle training on patients with heart failure and inspiratory muscle weakness. Journal of American College of Cardiology 47: 757–763

Davids JS, McPherson CA, Early C et al 2005 Benefits of cardiac rehabilitation in patients with implantable cardioverter-defibrillators: a patient survey. Archives of Physical Medicine Rehabilitation 86: 1924–1928

Delagardelle C, Feiereisen P, Autier P et al 2002 Strength/endurance training versus endurance training in congestive heart failure. Medicine and Science in Sports and Exercise 34: 1868–1872

Department of Health 2000 National Service Framework: Coronary Heart Disease. Modern standards and service models. *www.dh.gov.uk/en/ Policyandguidance/ Healthandsocialcaretopics/ Coronaryheartdisease/DH_4108602* (last updated 14 April 2005, accessed 17 July 2007)

Department of Health 2004 At least five a week: evidence on the impact of physical activity and its relationship to health

Department of Health 2006 Coronary Heart Disease. *www.dh.gov.uk/ PolicyAndGuidance/ HealthAndSocialCareTopics/ CoronaryHeartDisease/fs/en* (Accessed 17 July 2007)

DuBach P, Myers J, Dziekan G et al 1997 Effect of exercise training on myocardial remodeling in patients with reduced left ventricular function after myocardial infarction. Circulation 95: 2060–2067

Ehsani AA, Biello DR, Schultz J et al 1986 Improvement of left ventricular contractile function in patients with coronary artery disease. Circulation 74: 350–388

Evangelista LS, Dracup K, Erickson V et al 2005 Validity of pedometers for measuring exercise adherence in heart failure patients. Journal of Cardiac Failure 11: 366–371

Fitchet A, Doherty PJ, Bundy C et al 2003 Comprehensive cardiac rehabilitation programme for ICD patients – a randomized controlled trial. Heart 89: 155–160

Fletcher GF, Balady GJ, Amsterdam EA et al 2001 Exercise standards for testing and training: a statement for healthcare professionals from the American Heart Association. Circulation 104: 1694–1781

Franklin B 2004 An alternative approach to the delivery of cardiac rehabilitation services: a 'Hybrid' model for patient care. Journal of Cardiopulmonary Rehabilitation 2: 383–386

Franklin BA, Bonzheim K, Gordon S, Timmis GC 1998 Safety of medically supervised outpatient cardiac rehabilitation exercise therapy: a 16 year follow-up. Chest 114: 902–906

Frye BA 1993 Review of the World Health Organization's report on disability prevention and rehabilitation. Rehabilitation Nursing 18: 43–44

Georgiou D, Chen Y, Appadoo S et al 2001 Cost-effectiveness analysis of long-term moderate exercise training in chronic heart failure. American Journal of Cardiology 87: 984–988

Giannuzzi I, Tavazzi L, Temporelli PL et al for EAMI 1993 Long-term physical training and left ventricular remodeling after anterior myocardial infarction: results of the Exercise in Anterior MI (EAMI) trial. Journal of the American College of Cardiology 22: 1821–1829

Goble AJ, Hare DL, MacDonald PS et al 1991 Effect of early programmes of high and low intensity exercise on physical performance after transmural acute myocardial infarction. British Heart Journal 65: 126–131

Grace SL, McDonald J, Fishman D, Caruso V 2005 Patient preferences for home-based versus hospital-based cardiac rehabilitation. Journal of Cardiopulmonary Rehabilitation 25: 24–29

Hambrecht R, Niebauer J, Marburger C et al 1994 Various intensities of leisure time physical activity in patients with coronary atherosclerotic lesions. Journal of Cardiopulmonary Rehabilitation 14: 167–168

Hansen D, Dendale P, Berger J, Meeusen R 2005 Rehabilitation in cardiac patients: what do we know about training modalities. Sports Medicine 35: 1063–1084

Hunt SA, Abraham WT, Chin MH et al 2005 A report of the American College of Cardiology and American Heart Association (ACC/AHA) Task Force on Practice Guidelines 'Guideline Update for the Diagnosis and Management of Chronic Heart Failure in the Adult – Summary Article'. Journal of American College of Cardiology 46: 1116–1143

Husak L, Krumholz HM, Qiutin Z et al 2004 Social support as a predictor of participation in cardiac rehabilitation after coronary artery bypass surgery.

Journal of Cardiopulmonary Rehabilitation 24: 19–25

Ingle L, Shelton RJ, Rigby AS et al 2005 The reproducibility and sensitivity of the 6 minute walk test in elderly patients with chronic heart failure. European Heart Journal 26: 742–751

Jolliffe JA, Rees K, Taylor RS et al 2000 Exercise-based rehabilitation for coronary heart disease. Cochrane Database of Systematic Reviews, Issue 1. Art. No.: CD001800. DOI: 10.1002/14651858.CD001800

Jonsdottir S, Anderson KK, Sigurosson AF, Sigurosson SB 2005 The effect of physical training in chronic heart failure. European Journal of Heart Failure 8: 97–101

Jugdutt BI, Michorowski BL, Kappagoda CT 1988 Exercise training after anterior Q wave myocardial infarction: importance of regional left ventricular function and topography. Journal of the American College of Cardiology 12: 362–372

Kloner RA, Kloner JA 1983 The effect of early exercise on myocardial infarct scar formation. American Heart Journal 106 (5, part 1): 1009–1013

Kovoor P, Lee AK, Carrozzi F et al 2006 Return to full normal activities including work after acute myocardial infarction. American Journal of Cardiology 97: 952–958

Lampman, RM, Knight BP 2000 Prescribing exercise training for patients with defibrillators. American Journal of Physical Medicine and Rehabilitation 79(3): 292–297

Leon AS, Certo C, Comoss P et al 1991 Scientific evidence of the value of cardiac rehabilitation services with emphasis on patients following myocardial infarction. Journal of Cardiopulmonary Rehabilitation 10: 79–87

Leon AS, Franklin BA, Costa F et al 2005 Cardiac Rehabilitation and Secondary Prevention of CHD: American Heart Association Scientific Statement. Circulation 111: 369–376

Levinger I, Bronks R, Cody DV et al 2005 Resistance training for chronic heart failure patients on beta-blocker medications. International Journal of Cardiology 102: 493–499

Lewin B, Robertson IH, Cay EL et al 1992 Effects of self-help post-myocardial infarction rehabilitation on psychological adjustment and use of health services. Lancet 339: 1036–1040

Likoff MJ, Chandler SL, Kay HR 1987 Clinical determinants of mortality in chronic congestive heart failure secondary to idiopathic dilated or ischaemic cardiomyopathy. American

Journal of Cardiology 59: 634–638

Lipkin DP, Scriven AJ, Crake T, Poole-Wilson PA 1986 Six minute walking test for assessing exercise capacity in chronic heart failure patients. British Medical Journal 292: 653–655

McGee HM, Hevey D, Horgan JH 1999 Psychological outcome assessments for use in cardiac rehabilitation service evaluation: a 10 year systematic review. Social Science and Medicine 48: 1373–1393

Mendes de Leon CF, Czajkowski SM, Freeland KE, Bang H for ENRICHD Investigators 2006 The effect of a psychosocial intervention and quality of life after an acute myocardial infarction. Journal of Cardiopulmonary Rehabilitation 26: 9–13

Myers J, Goebbels U, Dzeikan G 2000 Exercise training and myocardial remodelling in patients with reduced ventricular function: one-year follow-up with magnetic resonance imaging. American Heart Journal 139: 252–261

National Institute for Clinical Excellence (NICE) 2001 Prophylaxis for patients who have experienced a myocardial infarction: drug treatment, cardiac rehabilitation and dietary manipulation. London

National Institute for Clinical Excellence (NICE) 2003 Chronic Heart Failure, Guideline No 5, Royal College of Physicians, London

Ni H, Toy W, Burgess D et al 2000 Comparative responsiveness of Short Form 12 and Minnesota Living With Heart Failure Questionnaire in patients With heart failure. Journal of Cardiac Failure 6: 83–91

O'Connor GT, Buring JE, Yusuf S et al 1989 An overview of randomized trials of rehabilitation with exercise after myocardial infarction. Circulation 80: 234–244

Oldridge NB, Guyatt GH, Fischer ME, Rimm AA 1988 Cardiac rehabilitation after myocardial infarction. Combined experience of randomized clinical trials. Journal of the American Medical Association 260: 945–950

Pashkow FJ, Schweikert RA, Wilkoff BL 1997 Exercise testing and training in patients with malignant arrhythmias. Exercise and Sport Sciences Reviews 25: 235–269

Pierson LM, Miller LE, Herbert WG 2004 Predicting exercise training outcome from cardiac rehabilitation. Journal of Cardiopulmonary Rehabilitation 24: 113–118

Pina IL, Apstein CS, Balady GJ et al 2003 Exercise and heart failure – a statement from the American Heart Association Committee on Exercise, Rehabilitation and Prevention. Circulation 107(8): 1210–1229

Rees K, Taylor RS, Singh S et al 2004 Exercise based rehabilitation for heart failure. Cochrane Database of Systematic Reviews, Issue 3: CDOO3331

Sanderson KB, Bittner V 2005 Women in cardiac rehabilitation: outcomes and identifying risk for dropout. American Heart Journal 150: 1052–1058

Sanderson KB, Southard D, Oldridge N 2004 Outcomes evaluation in cardiac rehabilitation/secondary prevention programmes: improving patient care and programme effectiveness. Journal of Cardiopulmonary Rehabilitation 24: 68–79

Schuler G, Hambrecht R, Schlierf G et al 1992 Regular physical exercise and low-fat diet. Effects on progression of coronary artery disease. Circulation 86: 1–11

Scottish Intercollegiate Guidelines Network (SIGN) 2002 Cardiac rehabilitation: Guideline 57 *www.sign.ac.uk/guidelines/fulltext/57/index.html* (Accessed 17 July 2007)

Sears SF, Kovacs AH, Conti JB, Handberg E 2004 Expanding the scope of practice for cardiac rehabilitation: managing patients with implantable cardioverter defibrillators. Journal of Cardiopulmonary Rehabilitation 24: 209–215

Shen BJ, Myers HF, McCreary CP 2006 Psychological predictors of cardiac rehabilitation quality-of-life outcomes. Journal of Psychosomatic Research 60: 3–11

Shephard RJ, Franklin B 2001 Changes in the quality of life: a major goal of cardiac rehabilitation. Journal of Cardiopulmonary Rehabilitation 21: 189–200

Singh SJ et al 1992 Developments of a shuttle walking test of disability in patients with chronic airways obstruction. Thorax 47: 1019–1024

Smith HJ, Taylor R, Mitchell A 2000 A comparison of four quality of life instruments in cardiac patients: SF-36, QLI, QLMI and SEIQoL. Heart 84: 390–394

Squires RW, Muri AJ, Anderson LJ et al 1991 Weight training during phase II (early outpatient) cardiac rehabilitation: heart rate and blood pressure responses. Journal of Cardiac Rehabilitation 11: 360–364

Steele B 1994 The six minute walk. In AACVPR Proceedings 9th Annual Meeting Portland, OR. AACVPR, Chicago, 383–388

Swedberg K, Cleland J, Dargie H 2005 Task Force for the Diagnosis and Treatment of Chronic Heart Failure of the European Society of Cardiology Guidelines for the diagnosis and treatment of chronic heart failure: full text (update 2005). European Heart Journal 26: 1115–1140

Sykes K, Roberts A 2004 The Chester step test – a simple yet effective tool for the prediction of aerobic capacity. Physiotherapy 90: 183–188

Taylor R, Kirby B, Burdon D, Caves R 1998 The assessment of recovery in patients after myocardial infarction using three generic quality-of-life measures. Journal of Cardiopulmonary Rehabilitation 18: 139–144

Taylor RS, Brown A, Ebrahim S et al 2004 Exercise-based rehabilitation for patients with coronary heart disease: a systematic review and meta-analysis of randomized controlled trials. American Journal of Medicine 11: 682–692

Tharrett SJ, Peterson JA 1997 ACSM's health/fitness facility standards and guidelines. Human Kinetics, Champaign, IL

Todaro JF, Shen BJ, Niaura R et al 2004 Do men and women achieve similar benefits from cardiac rehabilitation. Journal of Cardiopulmonary Rehabilitation 24: 45–50

Van Camp SP, Peterson RA 1986 Cardiovascular complications of outpatient cardiac rehabilitation programmes. Journal of American Medical Association 256: 1160–1163

Vongvanich P, Paul-Labrador MJ, Merz C 1996 Safety of medically supervised exercise in a cardiac rehabilitation centre. American Journal of Cardiology 77: 1383–1385

Williams MA 1994 Exercise testing and training in the elderly cardiac patient. Current issues in cardiac rehabilitation series. Human Kinetics, Champaign, IL

Willich SN, Lewis M, Lowel H et al 1993 Physical exertion as a trigger of acute myocardial infarction. New England Journal of Medicine 329: 1684–1690

Witt BJ, Jacobsen SJ, Weston SA et al 2004 Cardiac rehabilitation after myocardial infarction in the community. Journal of American College of Cardiology 44: 988–996

Worcester MC, Hare DL, Oliver RG et al 1993 Early programmes of high and low intensity exercise and quality of life after acute myocardial infarction.

14

British Medical Journal 307: 1244–1247

Zigmond AS, Snaith RP 1983 The hospital anxiety and depression scale. Acta Psychiatrica Scandinavica 67: 361–370

Zwisler A-DO, Schoul L, Soja AMB et al 2005 A randomized clinical trial of hospital-based, comprehensive cardiac rehabilitation versus usual care for patients with congestive heart failure, ischaemic heart disease or high risk ischaemic heart disease. American Heart Journal 150: 899e7–899e16

Chapter 15

Thoracic organ transplantation

Prue E Munro, Kate J Hayes, Paul Aurora

INTRODUCTION

Thoracic organ transplantation is a well-established treatment for patients with end-stage heart and lung disease. It aims to improve the quality of life and survival of those patients who are already managed optimally, often with maximal medical therapy. Physiotherapists are key members of the transplant team, providing expertise in the physical and functional assessment, respiratory management and rehabilitation of patients both before and after surgery.

This chapter discusses the physiotherapy management before and after heart, heart-lung and lung transplantation. The historical context, assessment and selection of appropriate candidates, surgical procedures, key concepts of immunosuppression, rejection, infection and denervation are also considered. Issues specific to paediatric patients are identified.

HISTORY

The first human thoracic organ transplants were performed in the 1960s. In 1963 Dr James Hardy (Jackson, USA) performed a single lung transplant in a lung cancer sufferer. Controversially, the following year he transplanted a chimpanzee heart into a human recipient. In 1967 Dr Christiaan Barnard (Cape Town, South Africa) performed the first human heart transplant. More than a hundred heart transplants were performed in 1968–69, but almost all patients died within 60 days.

The 1980s heralded a new era in thoracic organ transplantation with the first long-term survivors of heart-lung (Reitz et al 1982), single lung (Cooper et al 1987) and double lung (Patterson et al 1988) transplantation. The advent of cyclosporin (Borel 1980) as the principal immunosuppressant, with a greater ability to prevent acute rejection, was considered pivotal to improved survival outcomes.

From the late 1980s to the mid 1990s there was steady growth in both the overall numbers of transplants performed and the number of centres performing them. These numbers have now stabilized and reflect the ongoing shortage of donor organs. Internationally, over 4000 heart transplants, 60 heart-lung transplants and 1600 lung transplants are performed in adults each year (Taylor et al 2005, Trulock et al 2005). The number of paediatric transplants is much smaller, with approximately 350 heart transplants, 10 heart-lung transplants, and 80 lung transplants performed (Boucek et al 2005).

Over the last 30 years, significant advances have been made in all aspects of the care of thoracic organ transplant recipients. There have been improvements in operative techniques, organ preservation and cross matching. New, less toxic immunosuppressants have been developed. There is a greater understanding of immunology and a greater ability to bridge to transplant with mechanical support devices. Current survival outcomes for patients receiving heart transplantation are more favourable than for lung transplantation with 81%, 67% and 48% survival at 1, 5 and 10 years compared with 76%, 49% and 24%, respectively (Taylor et al 2005, Trulock et al 2005). Outcomes in children are similar to those in adults.

SELECTION OF CANDIDATES

A variety of criteria have been developed to identify patients who will live longer and function better with transplantation than with medical therapy. Through a rigorous evaluation process, the transplant team assesses the patient's severity of organ failure, screen for comorbidities that may negatively affect survival, and assess psychosocial variables necessary for successful outcomes following transplantation.

INDICATIONS FOR TRANSPLANTATION

Thoracic organ transplantation is indicated in patients with various end-stage diseases where survival is limited and quality of life poor (Table 15.1).

Heart transplant

The distribution of indications for cardiac transplantation has not changed significantly over the last 10 years (Taylor et al 2005). The most common indications in adults continue to be ischaemic and non-ischaemic heart failure (45% each). Valvular disease (3–4%), adult congenital heart disease (2%) and allograft failure requiring retransplantation (2%) make up the remaining indica-

tions. What has changed is the increasing number of patients bridged to transplant using intravenous inotropic support (48%) and some type of mechanical circulatory support (21%) with a left ventricular assist device (LVAD).

Lung transplant

The main indications of adult lung transplant are chronic obstructive pulmonary disease (38%), idiopathic pulmonary fibrosis (17%), cystic fibrosis (17%) and α_1-antitrypsin deficiency emphysema (9%). The most common indications in childhood differ by age group. In infants, congenital heart disease is the most common indication (47%). In older children, cystic fibrosis (72%), primary pulmonary hypertension (10%) and retransplantation (6%) are the main indications. Interstitial lung disease, pulmonary vascular disease and bronchiolitis obliterans less commonly lead to transplantation in children (Boucek et al 2005). Lung transplant is rarely appropriate in critically ill patients in desperate clinical situations (i.e. intubated in the intensive care unit).

Heart-lung transplant

Primary pulmonary hypertension and pulmonary hypertension associated with Eisenmenger's syndrome/congenital heart disease have been the main indications for heart-lung transplantation in adults and children (see Table 15.1).

Table 15.1 Indications for thoracic organ transplantation	

Heart	Ischaemic cardiomyopathy
	Non-ischaemic cardiomyopathy:
	  idiopathic, drug toxicity, postpartum,
	  hypertrophic, restrictive
	Other: valvular disease, congenital heart
	  disease, allograft failure requiring
	  retransplantation

Heart-lung	Congenital heart diseases (Eisenmenger's
	  syndrome)
	Primary pulmonary hypertension
	Pulmonary parenchymal disease with
	  non-reversible cardiac dysfunction

Single lung	Chronic obstructive pulmonary disease Interstitial lung disease
Bilateral lung	Cystic fibrosis Bronchiectasis Chronic obstructive pulmonary disease Pulmonary vascular disease

15

Contraindications to transplantation

Patients with comorbidities that may seriously compromise the outcome of transplantation are excluded. There are few absolute contraindications to thoracic organ transplantation, and consideration of relative contraindications is usually made on an individual basis (Box 15.1).

Box 15.1   Potential contraindications for thoracic organ transplantation

- Irreversible dysfunction of other organ systems (e.g. hepatic, renal)
- Malignancy with a high risk of recurrence
- Older than 65 years
- Complicated diabetes mellitus
- Active systemic infection
- Active systemic illness that would significantly limit survival or rehabilitation
- Peripheral or cerebrovascular disorders
- Active substance abuse including cigarette smoking, alcohol and illicit drugs
- Severe psychiatric disorders
- Non-compliance with medical regimen
- Body mass index outside the healthy weight range
- Inadequate social supports
- Immobility with poor potential for rehabilitation

ASSESSMENT

Potential recipients are assessed by an experienced multidisciplinary team at a transplant centre (Box 15.2). This process involves extensive physiological, functional and psychological assessment in order to:

- evaluate the severity of cardiac and/or pulmonary dysfunction (e.g. pulmonary function testing, perfusion scan, echocardiography, gated blood pool scan)

Box 15.2   Multidisciplinary transplant team

- Physician
- Surgeon
- Transplant coordinator
- Physiotherapist
- Nurse
- Social worker
- Psychiatrist
- Dietician
- Occupational therapist

- identify contraindications to transplantation (Box 15.1)
- assess immunological status (ABO group, human leucocyte antigens, tissue typing)
- identify previous exposure to potentially complicating infection: cytomegalovirus (CMV), toxoplasmosis, hepatitis B, hepatitis C, methicillin-resistant *Staphylococcus aureus* (MRSA), Epstein–Barr virus (EBV) and human immunodeficiency virus (HIV)
- evaluate nutritional status
- evaluate psychological status
- assess functional and exercise capacity.

The assessment is usually performed as an inpatient over a 2–3 day period. Once the evaluation has been compiled, all members of the transplant team meet to discuss the findings and come to a consensus regarding the patient's appropriateness for listing.

Physiotherapy assessment

Physiotherapy assessment of the potential transplant candidate is similar to that of any cardiorespiratory medical or surgical patient. It focuses on the impact of cardiac, respiratory and musculoskeletal limitations on exercise, functional capacity and social performance. The medical history and results of relevant investigations (e.g. imaging, arterial blood gases, lung function, angiography) should be reviewed before seeing the patient so that the patient's unique pathophysiology and clinical status is understood.

Subjective assessment

The subjective assessment should elucidate detail of:

- clinical course (e.g. duration of illness, rate of decline, hospital admissions)
- symptoms experienced
- main limitations to activities
- ability to perform activities of daily living
- current/previous exercise and rehabilitation
- recreational pursuits, employment
- social supports
- patient goals and expectations of transplant.

Musculoskeletal assessment

The screening assessment should include:

- posture
- joint range of movement
- muscle length
- muscle strength
- muscle bulk.

15

A more in-depth assessment is required if musculoskeletal abnormalities are found. Structural and postural thoracic kyphosis, shoulder pathologies (rotator cuff impingement syndromes), shortened calf, hamstrings and iliopsoas muscles and reduced muscle bulk are commonly seen in thoracic transplant candidates.

Exercise capacity

- six-minute walk test (6MWT)
  - distance walked, response to exercise (i.e. SpO_2, HR, BP, symptoms), limitation to exercise
  - may be used as a predictor of survival in cardiac disease and also in some diagnostic groups (e.g. cystic fibrosis, idiopathic pulmonary fibrosis, pulmonary arterial hypertension)
  - general guidelines: In adults a 6MWT distance <300–400 m is suggested as appropriate for listing for both heart and lung transplantation (Kadikar et al 1997, Raul et al 1998), whereas in children desaturation on 6MWT is a better predictor of survival (Aurora et al 2000).
- maximal exercise testing
  - $\dot{V}O_2$ peak ≤ 14 ml kg^{-1} min^{-1} is an indication for listing for cardiac transplant (Mancini et al 1991). There is little evidence that this test predicts prognosis in pulmonary disease.

Respiratory assessment

- breathing pattern
  - extent and use of accessory muscles
  - work of breathing
- auscultation
- effectiveness of cough and huff
- ventilatory support
  - oxygen therapy
  - non-invasive ventilation
- airway clearance
  - sputum quantity and quality
  - evaluation of effectiveness of current techniques
  - preferences of techniques
  - adherence.

The physiotherapist should:

- determine whether an exercise programme is indicated
- give advice regarding exercise and the importance of maintaining physical fitness preoperatively
- provide education regarding the commitment required for rehabilitation post transplant with emphasis on incorporating exercise into lifestyle with long-term maintenance the goal

- refer on to local physiotherapist, or other members of multidisciplinary team
- provide advice on energy conservation strategies
- inform the team as to patient adherence with previous/current exercise and airway clearance regimens.

SURGICAL PROCEDURES

Heart transplantation

Orthotopic heart transplantation

Preparation of the heart (and heart-lung) transplant recipient is similar to that for any patient undergoing cardiac surgery (anaesthesia, median sternotomy and cardiopulmonary bypass). When the donor heart is present in the recipient theatre and has passed a final inspection, the recipient heart is removed, by incising the atria, pulmonary artery and aorta. The posterior walls of both atria, including the sinoatrial node, are left intact. The donor heart is sutured in place. The anastomoses join the recipient and donor atria, the pulmonary arteries and the aortas (Keogh et al 1986) (Fig. 15.1).

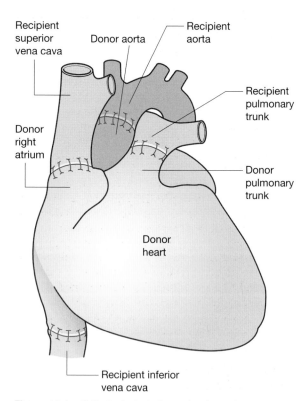

Figure 15.1 Orthotopic technique: the donor heart following implantation.

More recently, the bicaval anastomosis technique has been carried out at some centres. Potential advantages of this technique, which maintains the anatomic integrity of the donor right atrium, include a reduction in the incidence and severity of tricuspid regurgitation, preservation of right atrial function and facilitation of restoration of sinus rhythm (Morgan & Edwards 2005).

Heterotopic heart transplantation

Heterotopic transplantation is rarely performed, but is occasionally indicated in patients with cardiac dysfunction resulting in severe pulmonary hypertension. In this 'piggyback' procedure the recipient heart is left in place and the donor heart is positioned in the right chest. The donor heart is connected to the recipient's in parallel by anastomoses made between the two hearts at the atria, pulmonary arteries and aortas (Newcomb et al 2004). Both hearts contribute to the cardiac output and share the work required to overcome the increased pulmonary pressures (Newcomb et al 2004, Novitzky et al 1983). Inherent problems with this procedure include pulmonary compression of the recipient's right lung, difficulty obtaining endomyocardial biopsy and need for anticoagulation.

Lung transplantation

Single lung transplantation

In single lung transplantation, the native lung with the poorest pulmonary function according to the preoperative quantitative perfusion scan is excised. If both the lungs have similar function, then the right side is preferred as surgical exposure and the institution of cardiopulmonary bypass is easier.

The operation is performed via a posterolateral thoracotomy through the fourth or fifth intercostal space. The recipient's lung is removed and the donor lung positioned in the chest. The bronchial anastomosis is performed first, followed by the pulmonary artery anastomosis. After completion of these anastomoses, the lung is reinflated and perfusion is re-established. Following resumption of ventilation to the donor lung, haemostasis is obtained, two intercostal catheters are placed (apical and basal) and the chest is closed. Following reintubation with a single lumen tube, flexible bronchoscopy is performed to inspect the bronchial anastomosis and clear the airway of blood or residual secretions. Cardiopulmonary bypass is rarely needed during this operation.

Double lung/bilateral sequential lung transplantation

The most commonly performed double lung transplantation (DLT) procedure is bilateral sequential lung transplantation. The early experiences of double lung transplantation involved the implantation 'en bloc' of both lungs via a median sternotomy, utilizing an omental wrap to secure the tracheal anastomosis (Patterson et al 1988). In an effort to avoid the high incidence of airway complications associated with the original procedure, the technique of bilateral sequential lung transplantation via bilateral anterolateral thoracotomies through the fourth or fifth intercostal space connected with a transverse sternotomy or 'clamshell incision' is now preferred. Mobilization and pneumonectomy of the native lung and the implantation of the lung graft are conducted in the same manner as described for single lung transplantation.

Heart–lung transplantation

This operation can be performed via a median sternotomy or a clamshell incision. Following the institution of cardiopulmonary bypass, the heart and lungs are excised separately, allowing identification and protection of the phrenic, recurrent laryngeal and vagus nerves. The heart is removed, leaving the posterior wall of the right atrium. The left and then right lungs are removed (following stapling of the bronchi, to minimize the risk of contaminating the area) and the trachea is divided. The donor heart-lung block is implanted, starting with the tracheal, then the atrial and aortic anastomoses (Fig. 15.2). Ventilation is established (ensuring the patency of the airway anastomosis) and the heart resuscitated (Jamieson et al 1984). To improve donor availability, recipients with primary lung disease who receive heart-lung blocks (e.g. patients with cystic fibrosis) may be asked to donate their hearts to a cardiac patient. This is termed the 'domino' procedure.

Other lung techniques

The scarcity of donor lungs, especially for small and paediatric recipients, has led to the development of operations that allow larger lungs to be downsized. These techniques are not considered standard practice.

The *split-lung technique* (Couetil et al 1997) utilizes individual lobes from the donor. It may be indicated if there is localized pathology in one lobe of the donor lung or if the donor organ is larger than expected.

Living donor lobar lung transplantation (Date et al 2003, Starnes et al 1999) involves two donors (usually relatives) each donating a single lobe (usually lower lobe) for bilateral lung transplantation. The recipient is usually critically ill and cannot wait for cadaveric transplantation. It is most often performed in adolescents or young adults with cystic fibrosis.

15

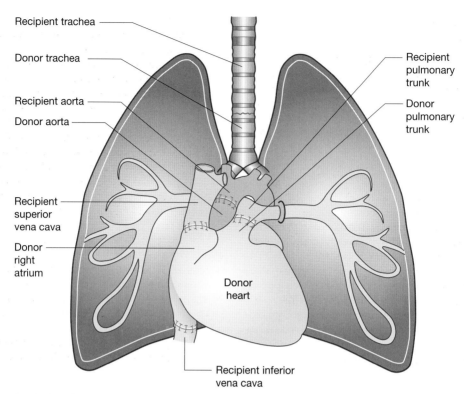

Figure 15.2 The donor heart–lung block following implantation.

KEY CONCEPTS

Organ donation

Organ donation for transplantation is performed in the setting of brain death. Brain death is defined as a complete and irreversible cessation of brain activity. The main causes are severe head injury from physical trauma, often from road traffic accidents and from subarachnoid haemorrhage. In most countries, consent from family members or next-of-kin is required. It is normal practice for consent to be sought even if the brain-dead individual had expressed the wish to donate. In some countries (e.g. Spain, Belgium, Poland, France) potential donors are presumed to have given consent, although some jurisdictions allow opting out from the system. Once consent is obtained, the non-living donor is kept on ventilatory support until the organs have been surgically removed. The donor is given expert medical and nursing care to optimize organ performance. Physiotherapists sometimes assist in the removal of retained lung secretions and help to optimize ventilation (Gabbay et al 1999).

A very small number of living and non-heart beating donors are used for lung transplantation internationally. Living donor lobar transplantation remains a second-line treatment due to the inevitable risk of lobectomy to the donors. Non-heart-beating donors are individuals who do not meet brain death criteria but for whom further medical intervention is futile. Organs can be rapidly retrieved after certification of death following withdrawal of support and asystole.

Timing of organ retrieval and implantation is important and necessitates a high level of coordination between the donor and recipient transplant teams. Organ procurement occurs at the hospital where the donor is managed. The organ is kept in preservation solution while it is transported to the transplant centre for implantation into the selected recipient. Most cardiac teams aim for an ischaemic time of less than 4 hours, from the time of cross-clamping the aorta in the donor to reperfusing the organ in the recipient. Lung teams aim for less than 8 hours. Longer ischaemic times are associated with poorer early graft function (Del Rizzo et al 1999, Thabut et al 2005).

The recipient team selects the appropriate recipient based upon:

- blood group
- size (weight and height)
- cytomegalovirus (CMV) serological status (lungs)

- prospective cross matching
- clinical status.

Organ allocation systems vary worldwide. In Australia and the UK, severity of illness and medical urgency are taken into account. In the United States of America, the system for allocation of heart and lungs has recently been changed, in an attempt to direct scarce organs to individuals who will derive the most benefit from them.

Immunosuppression and rejection

Rejection is a specific immune response to the donor tissue (allograft) and is part of the normal host defence system against foreign antigens. The response can occur by humoral (B lymphocyte) or cell-mediated (T lymphocyte) immune mechanisms. Immunosuppression is required to manage rejection.

The majority of thoracic organ transplant recipients remain on two or three lifelong maintenance immunosuppressive agents. Typically, one of these will be a calcineurin inhibitor (e.g. cyclosporin, tacrolimus), one will be a cell-cycle inhibitor (e.g. mycophenolate mofetil,

azathioprine), and the third will be a glucocorticoid (e.g. prednisone). Immunosuppression protocols vary widely from centre to centre.

Immunosuppressants have a number of specific side effects, which are listed in Table 15.2. It is important that physiotherapists working with thoracic organ transplant recipients are familiar with these side effects. Many agents impact on the musculoskeletal system and may cause bone morbidities such as avascular necrosis, osteoporosis and reduced tissue healing. Side effects of some agents affect the patient's ability to participate in exercise training (e.g. hypertension, nausea) or have practical implications (e.g. fine hand tremor affecting writing ability and difficulty fitting into footwear due to fluid retention).

Immunosuppressive therapy must be carefully balanced to prevent rejection without the development of serious adverse effects of the immunotherapy itself. Excessive immunosuppression increases the risk of infection, kidney and liver dysfunction and malignancies. Inadequate immunosuppression may result in rejection.

Graft rejection can be divided into three subcategories: hyperacute, acute and chronic rejection.

Table 15.2 Immunosuppression and side effects

Immunosuppressant	Side effects
Calcineurin inhibitors	
Cyclosporin	Nephrotoxicity, hepatic dysfunction, hirsutism, tremor, hypertension, susceptibility to malignant neoplasms
Tacrolimus	Hypertension, diabetes, nephrotoxicity, increased risk of malignancy, neurotoxicity, tremor, headache, diarrhoea, nausea
Cell cycle inhibitors	
Azathioprine	Bone marrow suppression, hepatic dysfunction, nausea, anorexia
Mycophenolate mofetil (MMF)	Diarrhoea, bone marrow suppression, opportunistic infection (especially invasive CMV)
Sirolimus	Diarrhoea, haematological disturbances, hyperlipidaemia, arthralgia, opportunistic infection (PCP, CMV), epistaxis, rash, abnormal healing, hepatic dysfunction, renal impairment, increases malignancy especially skin, bone necrosis
Everolimus	Increased malignancy especially skin, haematological disturbances, opportunistic infection (PCP, CMV), gastrointestinal upset, hepatic dysfunction, hyperlipidaemia, myalgia, hypertension
Corticosteroids	
Prednisolone	Sodium and fluid retention, hypokalaemia, hyperglycaemia, gastrointestinal ulceration, osteoporosis, skin fragility, increased appetite, mood changes
Methylprednisolone	As above

PCP, *Pneumocystis carinii* pneumonia; CMV, cytomegalovirus

15

Hyperacute rejection

Hyperacute, or primary graft failure, generally occurs within the first 72 hours postoperatively. Primary graft failure generally results from ischemia–reperfusion injury. The presenting features of the heart transplant recipient may be similar to a patient in cardiogenic shock, while the features of the lung transplant recipient may be similar to a patient with acute respiratory distress syndrome. Both may require total mechanical support in the form of extracorporeal membrane oxygenation (ECMO).

Acute rejection

Acute rejection (Fig. 15.3) is characterized by a host T-cell response toward the transplanted organ and is a common complication in the first weeks to months following transplant. The diagnosis is based on both clinical and histological criteria. Often, mild to moderate rejection is not associated with any reliable signs or symptoms.

In lung transplant recipients, rejection often mimics an upper respiratory tract infection or bronchitis. The spectrum of clinical features is non-specific and includes dyspnoea, fever, non-productive cough, hypoxaemia, or malaise. The chest radiograph may show new opacifications or pleural effusions. There may be a drop in lung function. As it is difficult to differentiate rejection and infection on the basis of clinical, radiological or physiological criteria, bronchoscopy with bronchoalveolar lavage (BAL) and transbronchial biopsy (TBB) are often required. Acute lung rejection is graded from A0 (none) to A4 (severe) based on a standardized grading system (Yousem et al 1996). In addition, the presence of airway inflammation is graded from B0 (no airway inflammation) to B4 (severe airway inflammation). Grade A2 and above is generally treated with augmented immunosuppression, usually intravenous pulsed methylprednisolone. A1 rejection is usually not treated.

Heart transplant recipients with moderate to severe rejection may present with arrhythmias, hypotension, fever, increased weight/fluid retention, malaise or dyspnoea. Routine endomyocardial biopsies via right heart catheter are the mainstay for monitoring rejection in these patients. Criteria for grading these biopsies have recently been modified, but the principles of grading and treatment are similar to those for lung transplantation.

Chronic graft impairment

Chronic graft impairment, sometimes called chronic rejection, manifests as airway disease in lung transplant recipients, and cardiac allograft vasculopathy in cardiac recipients. In both cases the causes are not completely understood, but are likely to be a result of scarring following acute rejection, infection, and other triggers, combined with chronic low-grade inflammation.

In the lung, chronic graft dysfunction is characterized histologically by bronchiolitis obliterans and physiologically by airflow limitation (Cooper et al 1993). High-resolution computed tomography typically shows traction bronchiectasis, decreased peripheral vascular markings and gas trapping (Moorish et al 1991). Transbronchial biopsy rarely produces enough tissue to confirm the diagnosis, so the surrogate diagnosis of bronchiolitis obliterans syndrome (BOS) is used instead. BOS is defined by an irreversible fall in lung function when other causes have been excluded, and is graded from BOS 0 to BOS 3.

Until recently, BOS was described as untreatable and irreversible. However, it is now believed that some patients who were previously diagnosed with BOS had some degree of reversible airway dysfunction caused by non-immune insults such as gastro-oesophageal reflux or airway infection. Specifically, a number of centres have now reported a very high prevalence of gastro-oesophageal reflux in transplant recipients, with a gratifying improvement in outcomes following surgical

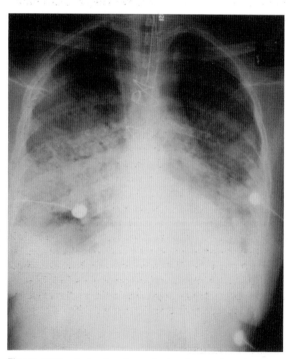

Figure 15.3 A chest radiograph showing acute pulmonary rejection in a heart-lung recipient.

15

treatment of this reflux (Button et al 2005, Cantu et al 2004, Davis et al 2003). In addition, reports from more than one centre have described how low-dose macrolide therapy can improve graft function in some patients with BOS. The mechanism is not fully understood, but the observation that patients who respond are usually those who have evidence of neutrophilic airway inflammation suggests that the anti-inflammatory properties of macrolides are responsible for the improvement (Crowley & Egan 2005).

Patients who have established BOS, which does not respond to such measures, are of considerable concern, as by definition there is no effective treatment. Some of these patients stabilize, and can continue for many years with limited lung function. Others develop steadily worsening graft dysfunction and progress to respiratory failure. BOS is the most common cause of late death following lung transplantation and is the main reason why improvements in long-term outcome have been slow.

Cardiac allograft vasculopathy is the main cause of late graft failure and death in heart transplant recipients (Taylor et al 2005). The coronary arteries develop a progressive concentric hyperplasia leading to vessel lumen obliteration. This can develop as early as 3 months after transplantation and is detected by angiography or increasingly, by intravascular ultrasound. The cause of the process is unclear, though long graft ischaemic time and recurrent rejection episodes have been identified as contributing factors. A recent study from a paediatric centre suggests that chronic low-grade CMV infection or reactivation may be a major cause (Hussain et al 2006). Treatment options are limited, although statin therapy may be of some benefit (Grigioni et al 2006) and is therefore now prescribed to all heart transplant recipients, including those with no evidence of vasculopathy. Angioplasty may be undertaken for diseased vessels if there is a discrete lesion, but is considered palliative and has not been shown to alter the natural history of cardiac allograft vasculopathy (Jonas et al 2006). The only definitive therapy is retransplantation.

Infection

Chronic immunosuppression renders transplant recipients more susceptible to infections (Box 15.3). The frequency of bacterial infections tends to peak within the first 3 months, while immunosuppressive therapy is often at a maximum level. The most frequent sites of infection are the lungs and blood. Infection is the major cause of morbidity and mortality in both the early and late post-transplant periods.

Box 15.3   Infectious organisms in thoracic organ transplant recipients

- Bacterial
  - Gram negative
  - Gram positive
  - Atypical
- Viral
  - Cytomegalovirus (CMV)
  - Herpes simplex virus (HSV)
- Fungal
  - *Aspergillus*
  - *Candida albicans*
  - *Pneumocystis carinii*
- Mycobacteria
  - Tuberculosis
  - Atypical

Denervation

Cardiac denervation

The pathophysiology of the transplanted heart is unique. The denervation of the organ makes it dependent on its intrinsic rate. It will therefore have a higher than normal resting heart rate secondary to the lack of inhibitory vagal influence. An alteration in the physiological response to exercise is also seen. In the normally innervated heart it is predominantly changes in heart rate that account for the increase in cardiac output in response to dynamic exercise. In contrast, the denervated heart increases cardiac output by increasing stroke volume (based on the Frank–Starling mechanism). The heart rate rises more gradually following the start of exercise, does not reach a similar peak and slows more gradually once exercise is stopped. This pattern of heart rate response is primarily the result of changing levels of circulating catecholamines (i.e. adrenaline and noradrenaline). In addition, transmission of ischaemic pain is prevented in the denervated heart (Weber 1990). Although partial reinnervation occurs in some recipients, the majority of patients will not experience anginal symptoms and should be advised against unsupervised exercise at high intensities for long periods. This is especially important if angiography indicates the presence of coronary artery disease (Hosenpud 1999, Kavanagh 1996).

Lung denervation

Similarly, lung and heart-lung transplantation involves denervation of the lungs below the airway anastomosis,

15

with associated loss of all pulmonary innervation except post-ganglionic efferent nerves. Although the laryngeal expiration reflex is preserved, the cough response is severely impaired (Higenbottam et al 1989). In addition, ciliary function in the graft is abnormal, possibly because of the loss of the normal blood supply. Taken together, these two defects predispose the recipient to retained airway secretions and lower respiratory tract infection, particularly in the early postoperative period. Some clinicians believe that loss of afferent feedback results in loss of the Hering–Breuer reflex. This may lead to an erratic breathing pattern soon after extubation in some patients (Mattila et al 1987).

PREOPERATIVE REHABILITATION

Pre-transplant rehabilitation for heart and lung transplant candidates closely follows cardiac and pulmonary rehabilitation models of care, respectively. It involves the active collaboration between the patient, his family/supports and the multidisciplinary team. Exercise training, education, nutritional intervention and psychosocial support are key components. As cardiac and pulmonary rehabilitation programmes are now widely recognized as part of the routine management of patients with chronic cardiac and respiratory disease, most patients assessed for transplant will have participated in a rehabilitation programme before transplant assessment (Lloyd-Williams et al 2002).

Pre-transplant rehabilitation aims to optimize physical and functional performance and quality of life. Addressing the deconditioning that results from the preoperative disease state is considered essential for survival to transplant and recovery afterwards.

Exercise training

The heterogeneous nature of transplant candidates means that the individual patient's unique pathophysiology, time in clinical course, symptoms, needs, goals and response to exercise must be taken into consideration when undertaking exercise training. All patients waiting for heart, heart-lung and lung transplants are encouraged to remain as active as possible. A careful assessment is required to ensure that each patient is safe to exercise. Physiotherapists working in this area may be exposed to conditions rarely seen. Caution must be taken with all patients. Patients who demonstrate profound desaturation despite oxygen therapy, hypotension or any other markedly abnormal response may not be able to exercise, or will be restricted to gentle stretches or activities of daily living only. Overall, the vast majority of patients are safe to participate in an exercise training programme.

General guidelines for exercise training in cardiac rehabilitation and pulmonary rehabilitation have been discussed (Chapters 13 & 14). It is important to note that currently there are no formal evidence-based guidelines regarding exercise training in lung disease populations other than COPD. Expert opinion based on knowledge of the underlying pathophysiology and clinical experience underpins clinical practice in this area.

Some disease groups have unique features that must be taken into consideration when planning and conducting exercise training programmes. Patients who experience dynamic hyperinflation may benefit from using a four-wheeled frame to support their upper limbs during lower limb training (Solway et al 2002). The prevention of cross-infection and ensuring an adequate salt intake is essential for patients with cystic fibrosis (Lands & Coates 1999, Saiman & Siegel 2004). Patients with interstitial lung disease often experience dyspnoea but may be able to perform interval training regimens with high-flow oxygen. High-intensity exercise is generally not recommended for patients with pulmonary arterial hypertension (Nici et al 2006).

Cardiac transplant candidates are generally able to exercise within the limits of standard haemodynamic guidelines. Close monitoring of symptoms, in particular dyspnoea, dizziness, light-headedness and chest pain, in addition to heart rate and blood pressure, is required. If they have an inappropriate response to exercise (e.g. a decrease in systolic blood pressure >20 mmHg), exercise should be ceased (Fletcher et al 2001).

Exercise tolerance in heart failure patients is poorly correlated with the degree of cardiac dysfunction (Myers et al 1998). The major limitation to exercise capacity stems from secondary, peripheral adaptations. These include impaired muscle structure and function, vascular and metabolic abnormalities (Clark et al 1996). Recent studies suggest that $\dot{V}O_2$ peak, a measure of cardiopulmonary exercise capacity, strongly predicts prognosis in heart failure, exhibiting a higher correlation with mortality than measures of left ventricular function (Myers et al 1998). The positive effect of endurance training on $\dot{V}O_2$ peak in patients with heart failure is well recognized (Lloyd-Williams et al 2002); however, it is known that endurance training alone does not enhance skeletal muscle strength (Delagardelle et al 2002). Resistance training has been shown to be safe and is recommended for patients with stable heart failure, as it directly targets the peripheral impairments demonstrated by this patient population (King et al 2000, Werber-Zion et al 2004). Studies have shown that 1-repetition maximum (RM) testing should be performed to ensure effective and safe dosage of resistance training (Werber-Zion et al 2004). A combined model of training would appear to be superior to either isolated endurance or resistance training, with improvements in $\dot{V}O_2$ peak, muscle strength, endurance, vascular function and quality of life (Maiorana et al 2000).

In lung transplant candidates, many factors contribute to exercise limitation, including ventilatory limitations, gas exchange abnormalities, skeletal muscle dysfunction and respiratory muscle dysfunction. It has been shown that patients with severe chronic respiratory disease can sustain the necessary training intensity and duration for skeletal muscle adaptation (Maltais et al 1996, Whittom et al 1998).

Close monitoring of symptoms, particularly shortness of breath, in addition to oxygen saturation and heart rate is required. An appropriate target for oxygen saturation during exercise for each individual should be determined before starting exercise. Supplemental oxygen is often required. It is clinical practice to maintain oxygen saturation at greater than 90% during exercise where possible. Non-invasive ventilation may help achieve a greater training intensity by unloading the respiratory muscles in some patients (Hoo 2003, van 't Hul et al 2006).

Most adult transplant centres offer dedicated preoperative exercise training classes for transplant candidates. Patients living close to the transplant centre attend the gymnasium 2–3 times a week and continue elements of the programme in a home routine. Patients who regularly attend other centres for ongoing outpatient treatment should be supervised by their local physiotherapist. Patient progress should be reported back to the transplant team. Patients who live beyond the reach of regular hospital attendance often benefit from regular telephone contact. The use of a diary to maintain motivation and for adequate monitoring is often beneficial.

Experience suggests that an ongoing, supervised exercise programme performed with other transplant candidates is ideal. Supervision by an experienced physiotherapist allows for alterations in exercise prescription as physical performance and symptoms change. Patient behavioural patterns, particularly adherence to therapies and the ability to cope with stressors, can be observed and strategies to facilitate modification put in place where needed. In a supportive, encouraging environment, patient motivation and self-management can be fostered and maintained during the often long waiting period (Craven et al 1990). Exercise training classes are often a key referral point for care from other members of the multidisciplinary team.

Pre-transplant exercise guidelines

- Exercise 3–5 times per week
- Supervision of exercise where possible

- Combination of endurance and strength training
- Training intensity:
  - lung patients: aim for Borg 4 for dyspnoea or fatigue
  - cardiac patients: aim for Borg rate of perceived exertion (RPE) 9–12 (Chapter 14)
- 30 minutes total time endurance training (treadmill, stationary cycle ergometer)
- Interval training may be useful in more symptomatic patients
- Stretch/ maintain muscle length, particularly of lower limb muscles
- Maintain range of movement of shoulders and chest wall
- Include functional exercises (e.g. step ups, squats).

Education

Pre-transplant education is facilitated by various members of the multidisciplinary team. Some units have a structured, group education programme while others provide one-to-one (individual patients and carer) education.

Topics may include:

- keeping active
- nutrition
- practical aspects of being on the waiting lists (notification, what to bring to hospital, how to get to hospital)
- understanding the patient's role in transplantation
- appliances to assist with activities of daily living (ADLs) and energy conservation strategies
- constructive use of time to improve quality of life while awaiting transplant
- stress management.

Timing to transplantation is variable, with more hearts being available than lungs. Time on the waiting list can vary from weeks to years. Once on the waiting list, patients are monitored closely by the transplant team to ensure that candidates continue to meet selection criteria. Periodic review also allows for fine-tuning of patient management.

Bridge to transplant

In an effort to optimize therapy and improve survival while on the waiting list, a number of management strategies including pharmacological therapies, device therapies and surgical intervention are considered.

15

Device therapies have been shown to decrease mortality and improve cardiac function in patients with end-stage heart failure. Device therapies used in cardiac transplant candidates include implantable cardioverter-defibrillators (ICDs), cardiac resynchronization therapy (CRT) and ventricular assist devices (VADs).

The left ventricular assist device (LVAD) has been increasingly utilized as a bridge to cardiac transplantation and is now being used as destination therapy (Peterzen et al 2002). The first bridge to transplant with a LVAD was performed more than 20 years ago. Since that time, devices have continued to evolve. Increased knowledge about patient selection, the timing of implantation and improved patient management has resulted in improved outcomes with decreasing adverse events.

LVAD implantation has been shown to have a significant impact on exercise capacity, with improvements in haemodynamic, ventilatory and neurohormonal measures (Mancini et al 1998, Peterzen et al 2002). Both submaximal and peak exercise capacity have been shown to improve. It seems logical therefore, that if the general health and fitness of these patients can be improved before transplantation, this may improve outcome following surgery.

Exercise prescription for LVAD patients is a particular challenge given the nature and position of the equipment and the often very poor functional capacity of these patients prior to implantation. Several studies (Morrone et al 1996, Reedy et al 1992) have demonstrated that early submaximal exercise is not only safe in this population but improves morbidity and mortality. A structured training programme has been shown to improve exercise capacity (Mettauer et al 2001); however, more work is needed in this area to determine the optimum type and intensity of exercise.

In lung transplant candidates, surgery, pharmaceutical agents and mechanical support are also used. Lung volume reduction surgery may be used to delay the need for transplant in highly selected patients with emphysema (Cordova & Criner 2002). Inhaled nitric oxide may be used in the setting of severe pulmonary hypertension (Olsson et al 2005, Yung et al 2001) and non-invasive ventilation for those with hypercapnic respiratory failure (British Thoracic Society 2002) and cystic fibrosis (Madden et al 2002).

POSTOPERATIVE MANAGEMENT

The aim of medical management in the early transplant period is to initiate effective immunosuppression, to minimize the risk of infection and to protect other organ systems, such as the renal system.

Post-transplant physiotherapy management is similar to that of other thoracic surgery patients. All physiotherapy interventions must be based on thorough assessment and treatment individualized for each patient. Subjective and objective assessment findings must be reviewed along with the latest microbiology results, arterial blood gases, chest radiograph, cardiovascular measures and oxygen saturation. Treatment choice, frequency and duration will depend on the individual patient presentation. Patients vary according to a number of factors, including:

- graft function
- pain control
- preoperative physical condition
- presence of comorbidities (diabetes – unstable blood sugar levels)
- emotional adjustment
- postoperative complications (Box 15.4).

Physiotherapy treatment in the postoperative period aims to:

- optimize ventilation
- clear retained lung secretions
- promote independent function (i.e. bed mobility, transfers, ambulation)
- improve fitness/activity tolerance
- facilitate self-management.

Management in the intensive care unit

The physiotherapy programme is initiated in the intensive care unit (ICU) as early as the first postoperative day. Acutely, the goals are to prevent perioperative complications of bedrest. Airway clearance techniques, joint range of motion and positioning are implemented as indicated. Once the cardiovascular and respiratory

---

Box 15.4 Postoperative complications impacting on rehabilitation

- Pain control
- Acute rejection
- Chest infection
- Renal insufficiency
- Steroid myopathy
- Psychiatric disturbance secondary to steroid therapy
- Persistent air leak*
- Phrenic nerve injury*
- Poor healing of airway anastomosis*

*Lung transplant

---

systems are stabilized, the patient is rapidly weaned from the ventilator and extubated. Delay in extubation can occur for a number of reasons. Primary graft failure is one of the most common reasons. As the intubation period increases, so too does the risk of nosocomial pneumonia. Non-invasive ventilatory support may be useful in assisting patients who have experienced difficulties in weaning and extubation.

It is important for patients to have sufficient analgesia to allow effective huffing, coughing and for early mobilization. Patients are commonly taught thoracic expansion exercises, huffing and coughing routines to detect and clear secretions. It is common for lung and heart-lung transplant recipients to expectorate old blood and slough from the bronchial/tracheal anastomosis during the first few days to a week. Secretions may also originate from the donor (donor-acquired infection) or recipient's native airways (common in cystic fibrosis).

Lung transplant patients often have a poor ability to perceive the presence of secretions and this may persist in the long term. The loss of neural innervation and abnormal mucociliary function are amongst a number of factors that predispose the lung transplant recipient to lung infections (Chaparro & Kesten 1997). If sputum retention becomes a problem for a recipient, inhalation therapy and an appropriate airway clearance technique should be instituted. Positioning, combined with an airway clearance technique (e.g. active cycle of breathing techniques), are the primary forms of initial treatment. If other airway clearance techniques are deemed necessary (i.e. treatments involving positive pressure), this is usually undertaken following consultation with the medical team. The place of regular airway clearance in the absence of excessive secretions has not yet been established but is currently under investigation.

Once extubated and stable, the emphasis is on early mobilization, with patients assisted to sit out of bed often within 24 hours of surgery (Fig. 15.4). Ambulation is initiated in the ICU when the patient shows adequate muscle strength, testing a minimum of grade 3 out of 5 in selective lower limb muscles (Clarkson & Gilewich 1989). The length of stay in ICU can be as short as 1 day or extend to prolonged periods depending on complications.

Ward management

On the ward, physiotherapy treatment focuses on achieving independence with activities of daily living, increasing endurance (walking, stationary cycling, stair climbing), and exercises addressing any specific musculoskeletal deficits. Stationary cycling in the patient's room is particularly useful in the early stages following lung and heart-lung transplant when

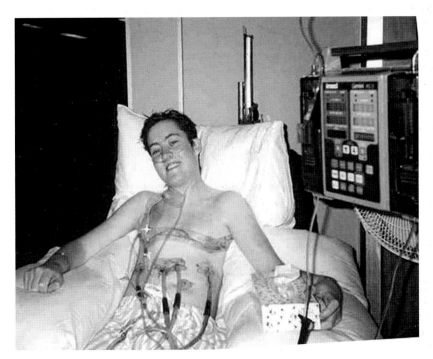

Figure 15.4 Sitting out of bed soon after bilateral sequential lung transplantation.

15

intercostals drains are on suction. Full range of upper limb elevation should be encouraged once drain tubes are removed. Postural re-education is also often required. Motivation and self-management may be enhanced by using charts to provide a measure of improvement in function.

Regular airway clearance may be necessary only in the presence of infection and retained secretions. Routine bronchoscopy is used to assess airway anastomotic healing and patency, the presence of infection (from bronchoalveolar lavage) and rejection (from transbronchial biopsy). Bronchoscopic findings are very useful to the physiotherapist and assist in clinical decision making and in determining appropriate treatments.

The average length of hospital stay following heart or lung transplantation is 2–3 weeks. Some patients are discharged as early as 1 week postoperatively, while others may spend weeks to months in hospital secondary to complications.

Before discharge from hospital, patients must have a good understanding of the signs and symptoms of rejection and infection, their medications and chest wall/sternal precautions. Patients are advised not to lift greater than 5 kg for 10–12 weeks. Rehabilitation usually continues on an outpatient basis at the transplant centre.

OUTPATIENT REHABILITATION

Many patients attend a formal outpatient rehabilitation programme comprising exercise training and education at the transplant centre. The primary goals in the rehabilitation phase after transplantation are to:

- improve the patient's physical condition (strength, endurance, posture)

- promote independence in maintaining and monitoring their physical condition

- improve the patient's confidence in becoming involved in a full range of activities of daily living and appropriate exercise activities

- nurture realistic expectations for employment, sport and leisure activities

- facilitate the integration back into social and vocational roles.

Ideally patients would attend the gymnasium three times per week for supervised exercise training, commonly in a group setting with other transplant recipients (Fig. 15.5). By approximately 12 weeks, most patients have achieved a good level of fitness and func-

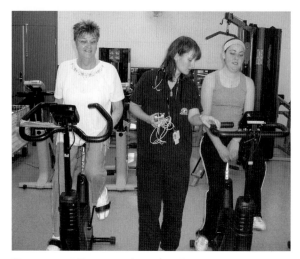

Figure 15.5   Post-transplant gym class.

tion and are able to be discharged from physiotherapy with a maintenance home exercise programme to be undertaken independently. Patients are encouraged to maintain an active lifestyle (Fig. 15.6) and those who require further rehabilitation are referred closer to their local area where access to services is more convenient.

Exercise training programmes post-transplant are similar to those previously described pre-transplant. Special considerations for exercise training are outlined in Box 15.5.

Education continues for the patient and carer in the outpatient setting facilitated by the multidisciplinary team. Common topics include:

- medication
- recognizing rejection and infection
- getting fit and staying fit
- food hygiene
- returning to work
- organ donation.

Regular medical follow-up continues until most patients can be reviewed on a 6–12 monthly basis. Improvements in functional exercise capacity and quality of life reflect the multimodal nature of the management of the transplant recipient (e.g. surgery, rehabilitation, lifestyle changes). Specific outcome measures for physiotherapy interventions should relate to each physiotherapy goal. Current clinical practice is variable and there is no consensus as to which key outcomes should be used (Maher & Williams 2005). It has been suggested that functional exercise capacity and level of activity should be measured before and after postoperative rehabilitation and then yearly as a minimum.

15

Box 15.5   Special considerations for exercise training post-transplant

Closely monitor signs and symptoms
- Heart transplant: HR, BP, Borg SOB, RPE
- Lung transplant: HR, SpO$_2$, Borg SOB, RPE
- Transplant complications (e.g. rejection, infection) often manifest as a reduction in exercise tolerance or abnormal exercise response. Concerns should be reported immediately to the transplant unit

Heart transplant recipients have an abnormal response to exercise due to denervation
- Do not use HR as the primary indicator of response to exercise
- Ensure adequate warm up and cool down to allow adequate time for the effects of catecholamine levels on cardiac output (Niset et al 1991)

Consider the musculoskeletal side effects of immunosuppressant drugs
(see Table 15.2)

Observe chest wall/sternal precautions

Bone morbidity – osteoporosis, pathological fracture and avascular necrosis are common
- Progressive resistance training should be included in post-transplant exercise programmes to optimize bone mineral density (Braith et al 1996, Mitchell et al 2003)
- Pathological fracture (particularly vertebral compression) and avascular necrosis (commonly head of femur) should be considered as potential causes of pain. Imaging techniques such as bone scan may be required so that appropriate management is undertaken (Henderson et al 1997)

Care must be taken when progressing activity
- Most patients are unaccustomed to exercise and are at risk of overuse injuries if activity is progressed too rapidly (e.g. achilles tendinitis, shin splints)

Modify exercise during episodes of acute rejection
- Mild rejection – continue with close monitoring of patient's signs and symptoms
- Moderate rejection – patients should not exercise during the short period in which they are receiving high-dose steroids. Exercise should be gradually increased and symptom-limited when recommenced
- Severe rejection – no exercise; activity limited to self-care only

HR, heart rate; BP, blood pressure; SOB, shortness of breath; RPE, rate of perceived exertion

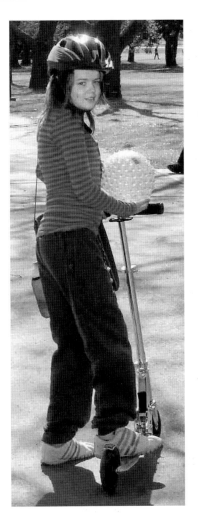

Figure 15.6   An active lifestyle is strongly encouraged.

FUNCTIONAL OUTCOMES POST-TRANSPLANT

Exercise capacity improves significantly after heart, heart-lung and lung transplantation; however, it remains below normal predicted values.

Heart transplant recipients demonstrate an improvement in $\dot{V}O_2$ peak for up to 2 years post-transplant; however, this value is only approximately 50% of normal values. The main determinant of this lower exercise capacity appears to be chronotropic incompetence of the denervated heart (Mandak et al 1995, Quigg et al 1988).

Substantial exercise limitation is seen almost universally in lung transplant recipients with a $\dot{V}O_2$ peak of 40–60% predicted normal (Howard et al 1994, Levy

15

et al 1993, Theodore et al 1987, Williams et al 1992). Patients demonstrate an adequate heart rate reserve, no significant gas exchange abnormalities and a normal breathing reserve. Peripheral muscle limitation, with leg tiredness the predominant symptom at exercise termination, is thought to be due to a number of factors including skeletal muscle deconditioning, dysfunction and atrophy (Wang et al 1999) and myotoxic effects of immunosuppressants (Mercier et al 1995).

Perceived functional status also improves following thoracic organ transplantation (Grady & Lanuza 2005, Lanuza et al 2000). Eighty to ninety per cent of paediatric transplant recipients report no limitation to activity levels for at least 5 years following transplant (Boucek et al 2005). Adult recipients demonstrate variable return to work rates (12–74%), which appear to increase over time. Patients report high global quality of life and these perceptions improve over pre-transplant levels (Cupples et al 2006).

LONG-TERM MANAGEMENT

Improved survival outcomes have led to significant growth in the demand for physiotherapy management of long-term morbidity. Long-term survivors experience a range of problems requiring hospital admission or outpatient follow-up. These include:

- acute rejection
- chronic graft dysfunction
- steroid myopathy
- renal dysfunction
- acute or chronic infection
- hypertension
- hyperlipidaemia
- malignancy.

Many transplant recipients maintain near-normal function for many years post-transplant. Others develop complications that require long-term medical or physiotherapy input. Physiotherapists commonly address problems such as:

- respiratory tract infection
- musculoskeletal morbidities
- reduced functional mobility
- declining exercise capacity
- changes in social and vocational roles.

In such cases there is a need to set realistic goals and to assist the patient and family to accept the decline in functional performance. Optimizing quality of life remains the primary goal. Inevitably, the care of these patients shifts away from acute medical management towards chronic disease management and palliative care. This transition is often difficult for both the patient and the health care team.

SPECIFIC CONSIDERATIONS FOR PAEDIATRIC PATIENTS

Most of the information presented above applies to both paediatric and adult heart and lung transplant recipients. However, there are a few additional issues that are specific to children. These are listed in Table 15.3.

CONCLUSION

Over the past two decades, thoracic organ transplantation has changed from a highly experimental surgical procedure to a widely accepted therapeutic option for end-stage cardiac and pulmonary failure. Continuing advances in all aspects of pre- and post-transplant management (e.g. immunosuppressive therapy, medical management, operative techniques) have led to significant improvements in morbidity and mortality. As long-term survival improves, there is greater recognition of the importance of optimizing the physical condition of potential candidates pre-transplant and the need to actively manage long-term comorbidities. Physiotherapists have a key and enduring role in the management of these patients that extends from pre-transplant assessment through to the palliative care of long-term survivors. Patients undergoing thoracic organ transplantation present with a broad range of complex medical issues, which necessitate management by a highly specialized team. Physiotherapists are an integral part of that team, and as such require a high level of knowledge and a range of specialist skills in the management of cardiorespiratory, orthopaedic and neurological pathologies.

Acknowledgement

The authors would like to thank Catherine E Bray for the sections taken from 'Cardiopulmonary transplantation' in the third edition of *Physiotherapy for respiratory and cardiac problems*.

15

Table 15.3 Specific considerations for children undergoing heart or lung transplantation

Lung function testing	All lung transplant recipients use spirometry to monitor lung function. This is possible in all children aged 4 years or more, though techniques may need to be modified. Different lung function techniques are needed for children less than 4 years
Biopsy	Endocardial and transbronchial biopsies are essential for detecting graft rejection. In all children these procedures are usually performed under general anaesthetic, rather than sedation. They are technically more difficult in younger children
Infections	Many children will not have had previous exposure to common viruses, and the incidence of primary infection is much higher than for adults. It is therefore essential that immunization status is optimized prior to listing for transplantation
Malignancy	Post-transplant lymphoproliferative disease (PTLD) is far more common in children than in adults. Other tumours, especially skin and lung, are rarer in children
Psychosocial issues	Many children coming to transplant are physically and emotionally immature because of their chronic illness. A successful transplant allows a child to transform their life and to catch up on many of the activities that were previously denied to them. Some children find this change in lifestyle difficult, particularly if it coincides with puberty. Non-adherence to therapy is an important cause of poor outcome, especially in teenage patients, and appears worst in those who have a chronic illness like cystic fibrosis. Most centres stress that adolescents should steadily take more responsibility for their own care and are given practical assistance to boost adherence to therapy

References

Aurora P, Wade A, Whitmore P, Whitehead B 2000 A model for predicting life expectancy of children with cystic fibrosis. European Respiratory Journal 16(6): 1056–1060

Borel JF 1980 Immunosuppressive properties of ciclosporin A (CY-A). Transplantation Proceedings 12(2): 233

Boucek MM, Edwards LB, Keck BM et al 2005 Registry of the International Society for Heart and Lung Transplantation: Eighth Official Pediatric Report – 2005. Journal of Heart and Lung Transplantation 24(8): 968–982

Braith RW, Mills RM, Welsch MA, Keller JW, Pollock ML 1996 Resistance exercise training restores bone mineral density in heart transplant recipients. Journal of the American College of Cardiology 28(6): 1471–1477

British Thoracic Society Standards of Care Committee 2002 Non-invasive ventilation in acute respiratory failure. Thorax 57(3): 192–211

Button BM, Roberts S, Kotsimbos TC et al 2005. Gastroesophageal reflux (symptomatic and silent): a potentially significant problem in patients with cystic fibrosis before

and after lung transplantation. Journal of Heart and Lung Transplantation 24(10): 1522–1529

Cantu E 3rd, Appel JZ 3rd, Hartwig MG et al 2004 J. Maxwell Chamberlain Memorial Paper. Early fundoplication prevents chronic allograft dysfunction in patients with gastroesophageal reflux disease. Annals of Thoracic Surgery 78(4): 1142–1151

Chaparro C, Kesten S 1997 Infections in lung transplant recipients. Clinics in Chest Medicine 18(2): 339–351

Clark A, Poole-Wilson P, Coats A 1996 Exercise limitation in chronic heart failure: central role of the periphery. Journal of the American College of Cardiology 28: 1092–1102

Clarkson H, Gilewich G 1989 Musculoskeletal assessment. Joint range of motion and manual muscle strength. Williams & Wilkins, Baltimore

Cooper JD, Billingham M, Egan T et al 1993 A working formulation for the standardization of nomenclature and for clinical staging of chronic dysfunction in lung allografts. International Society for Heart and

Lung Transplantation. Journal of Heart and Lung Transplantation 12(5): 713–716

Cooper JD, Pearson FG, Patterson GA et al 1987 Technique of successful lung transplantation in humans. Journal of Thoracic and Cardiovascular Surgery 93(2): 173–181

Cordova FC, Criner GJ 2002 Lung volume reduction surgery as a bridge to lung transplantation. American Journal of Respiratory Medicine 1(5): 313–324

Couetil JP, Tolan MJ, Loulmet DF et al 1997 Pulmonary bipartitioning and lobar transplantation: a new approach to donor organ shortage. Journal of Thoracic and Cardiovascular Surgery 113(3): 529–537

Craven JL, Bright J, Dear CL 1990 Psychiatric, psychosocial, and rehabilitative aspects of lung transplantation. Clinics in Chest Medicine 11(2): 247–257

Crowley S, Egan JJ 2005 Macrolide antibiotics and bronchiolitis obliterans following lung transplantation. Expert Review of Anti-infective Therapy 3(6): 923–930

15

Cupples S, Dew MA, Grady KL et al 2006 Report of the Psychosocial Outcomes Workgroup of the Nursing and Social Sciences Council of the International Society for Heart and Lung Transplantation: present status of research on psychosocial outcomes in cardiothoracic transplantation: review and recommendations for the field. Journal of Heart and Lung Transplantation 25(6): 716–725

Date H, Aoe M, Nagahiro I et al 2003 Living-donor lobar lung transplantation for various lung diseases. Journal of Thoracic and Cardiovascular Surgery 126(2): 476–481

Davis RDJ, Lau CL, Eubanks S et al 2003 Improved lung allograft function after fundoplication in patients with gastroesophageal reflux disease undergoing lung transplantation. Journal of Thoracic and Cardiovascular Surgery 125(3): 533–542

Del Rizzo DF, Menkis A H, Pflugfelder PW et al 1999 The role of donor age and ischemic time on survival following orthotopic heart transplantation. Journal of Heart and Lung Transplantation 18(4): 310–319

Delagardelle C, Feiereisen P, Autier P et al 2002 Strength/endurance training versus endurance training in congestive heart failure. Medicine and Science in Sports and Exercise 34(12): 1868–1872

Fletcher G, Balady G, Amsterdam E et al 2001 Exercise standards for testing and training: a statement for healthcare professionals from the American Heart Association. Circulation 104: 1694–1740

Gabbay E, Williams TJ, Griffiths AP et al 1999 Maximizing the utilization of donor organs offered for lung transplantation American Journal of Respiratory and Critical Care Medicine 160(1): 265–271

Grady KL, Lanuza DM 2005 Physical functional outcomes after cardiothoracic transplantation. Journal of Cardiovascular Nursing 20(5 Suppl): S43–50

Grigioni F, Carigi S, Potena L et al 2006 Long-term safety and effectiveness of statins for heart transplant recipients in routine clinical practice. Transplant Proceedings 38(5): 1507–1510

Henderson K, Marshall G, Sambrook P, Keogh A, Eisman J 1997 Two cases of hip pain in patients with heart transplantation. Australian Journal of Physiotherapy 43(2): 131–133

Higenbottam T, Jackson M, Woolman P, Lowry R, Wallwork J 1989 The cough response to ultrasonically nebulized distilled water in heart-lung transplantation patients. American Review of Respiratory Disease 140(1): 58–61

Hoo GWS 2003 Nonpharmacologic adjuncts to training during pulmonary rehabilitation: the role of supplemental oxygen and noninvasive ventilation. Journal of Rehabilitation Research and Development 40(5 Suppl 2): 81–97

Hosenpud J 1999 Coronary artery disease after heart transplantation. American Heart Journal 138(5 part 2): 469–472

Howard DK, Iademarco EJ, Trulock EP 1994 The role of cardiopulmonary exercise testing in lung and heart-lung transplantation. Clinics in Chest Medicine 15(2): 405–420

Hussain T, Fenton MJ, Burch M et al 2006 Pre-transplant cytomegalovirus serology is a risk factor for cardiac allograft vasculopathy in children. Journal of Heart and Lung Transplantation 25(2)(Suppl): 85

Jamieson S, Stinson D, Oyer PE, Baldwin JC, Shumway NE 1984 Operative technique for heart-lung transplantation. Journal of Thoracic and Cardiovascular Surgery 87: 930–935

Jonas M, Fang JC, Wang JC et al 2006 In-stent restenosis and remote coronary lesion progression are coupled in cardiac transplant vasculopathy but not in native coronary artery disease. Journal of the American College of Cardiology 48(3): 453–461

Kadikar A, Maurer J, Kesten S 1997 The six-minute walk test: a guide to assessment for lung transplantation. Journal of Heart and Lung Transplantation 16(3): 313–319

Kavanagh T 1996 Physical training in heart transplant recipients. Journal of Cardiovascular Risk 3: 154–159

Keogh A, Baron D, Spratt P, Esmore DS, Chang V 1986 Cardiac transplantation in Australia. Australian Family Physician 15(11): 1474–1481

King M, Dracup, K, Fonarow G, Woo MA 2000 The hemodynamic effects of isotonic exercise using hand-held weights in patients with heart failure. Journal of Heart and Lung Transplantation 19: 1209–1218

Lands L, Coates A 1999 Cardiopulmonary and skeletal muscle function and their effects on exercise limitation. In: Yankaskas J, Knowles M (eds) Cystic fibrosis in adults. Lippincott-Raven, New York, pp 365–379

Lanuza DM, Lefaiver CA, Farcas GA 2000 Research on the quality of life of lung transplant candidates and recipients: an integrative review. Heart and Lung 29(3): 180–195

Levy RD, Ernst P, Levine SM et al 1993 Exercise performance after lung transplantation. Journal of Heart and Lung Transplantation 12(1, Pt 1): 27–33

Lloyd-Williams F, Mair FS, Leitner M 2002 Exercise training and heart failure: a systematic review of current evidence. British Journal of General Practice 52(474): 47–55

Madden BP, Kariyawasam H, Siddiqi AJ et al 2002 Noninvasive ventilation in cystic fibrosis patients with acute or chronic respiratory failure. European Respiratory Journal 19(2): 310–313

Maher C, Williams M 2005 Factors influencing the use of outcome measures in physiotherapy management of lung transplant patients in Australia and New Zealand. Physiotherapy Theory and Practice 21(4): 201–217

Maiorana A, O'Driscoll G, Cheetham C et al 2000 Combined aerobic and resistance exercise training improves functional capacity and strength in chronic heart failure. Journal of Applied Physiology 88: 1565–1570

Maltais F, LeBlanc P, Simard C et al 1996 Skeletal muscle adaptation to endurance training in patients with chronic obstructive pulmonary disease. American Journal of Respiratory and Critical Care Medicine 154(2 Pt 1): 442–447

Mancini D, Goldsmith R, Levin H et al 1998 Comparison of exercise performance in patients with chronic severe heart failure versus left ventricular assist devices. Circulation 98(12): 1178–1183

Mancini DM, Eisen H, Kussmaul W et al 1991 Value of peak exercise oxygen consumption for optimal timing of cardiac transplantation in ambulatory patients with heart failure. Circulation 83(3): 778–786

Mandak J, Aaransen K, Mancini D 1995 Serial assessment of exercise capacity after heart transplantation. Journal of Heart and Lung Transplantation 14(3): 468–478

15

Mattila S, Mattila I, Viljanen B, Viljanen A 1987 Reappearance of Hering–Breuer reflex after bilateral autotransplantation of the lungs. Scandinavian Journal of Thoracic and Cardiovascular Surgery 21(1): 15–20

Mercier JG, Hokanson JF, Brooks GA 1995 Effects of ciclosporine A on skeletal muscle mitochondrial respiration and endurance time in rats. American Journal of Respiratory and Critical Care Medicine 151(5): 1532–1536

Mettauer B, Geny B, Lonsdorfer-Wolf E et al 2001 Exercise training with a heart device: a hemodynamic, metabolic, and hormonal study. Medicine and Science in Sports and Exercise 33(1): 2–8

Mitchell MJ, Baz MA, Fulton MN, Lisor CF, Braith RW 2003 Resistance training prevents vertebral osteoporosis in lung transplant recipients. Transplantation 76(3): 557–562

Moorish W, Herman S, Weisbrod G, Chamberlain D 1991 Bronchiolitis obliterans after lung transplantation: findings at chest radiography and high-resolution CT. Radiology 179: 487–490

Morgan JA, Edwards NM 2005 Orthotopic cardiac transplantation: comparison of outcome using biatrial, bicaval and total techniques Journal of Cardiac Surgery 20: 102–106

Morrone T, Buck L, Catanese K et al 1996 Early progressive mobilization of patients with left ventricular assist devices is safe and optimizes recovery before heart transplantation. Journal of Heart and Lung Transplantation 15: 423–429

Myers J, Gullestad L, Vagelos R et al 1998 Clinical, hemodynamic, and cardiopulmonary exercise test determinants of survival in patients referred for evaluation of heart failure. Annals of Internal Medicine 129: 286–293

Newcomb AE, Esmore DS, Rosenfeldt FL, Richardson M, Marasco S F 2004 Heterotopic heart transplantation: an expanding role in the twenty-first century? Annals of Thoracic Surgery 78(4): 1345–1350

Nici L, Donner C, Wouters E et al 2006 American Thoracic Society/European Respiratory Society statement on pulmonary rehabilitation. American Journal of Respiratory and Critical Care Medicine 173(12): 1390–1413

Niset G, Hermans L, Depelchin P 1991 Exercise and heart transplantation. A

review. Sports Medicine 12(6): 359–379

Novitzky D, Cooper DK, Barnard CN 1983 The surgical technique of heterotopic heart transplantation. Annals of Thoracic Surgery 36(4): 476–482

Olsson JK, Zamanian RT, Feinstein JA, Doyle RL 2005 Surgical and interventional therapies for pulmonary arterial hypertension. Seminars in Respiratory and Critical Care Medicine 26(4): 417–428

Patterson GA, Cooper JD, Goldman B et al 1988 Technique of successful clinical double-lung transplantation. Annals of Thoracic Surgery 45(6): 626–633

Peterzen B, Lonn U, Jansson K et al 2002 Long-term follow-up of patients treated with an implantable left ventricular assist device as an extended bridge to heart transplantation. Journal of Heart Transplantation 21: 604–607

Quigg R, Salyer J, Mohanty P, Simpsen P 1988 Impaired exercise capacity late after cardiac transplantation: influence of chronotropic incompetence, hypertension, and calcium channel blockers. American Heart Journal 136(3): 465–473

Raul G, Germain P, Bareiss P 1998 Does the 6-minute walk test predict prognosis in patients with NYHA class II or III chronic heart failure? American Heart Journal 136(3): 449–457

Reedy JE, Swartz MT, Lohmann DP et al 1992 The importance of patient mobility with ventricular assist device support. American Society for Artificial Internal Organs Journal 38(3): M151–153

Reitz BA, Wallwork JL, Hunt SA et al 1982 Heart-lung transplantation: successful therapy for patients with pulmonary vascular disease. New England Journal of Medicine 306(10): 557–564

Saiman L, Siegel J 2004 Infection control in cystic fibrosis. Clinical Microbiology Review 17(1): 57–71

Solway S, Brooks D, Lau L, Goldstein R 2002 The short-term effect of a rollator on functional exercise capacity among individuals with severe COPD. Chest 122(1): 56–65

Starnes VA, Woo MS, MacLaughlin EF et al 1999 Comparison of outcomes between living donor and cadaveric lung transplantation in children. Annals of Thoracic Surgery 68(6): 2279–2283; discussion 2283–2274

Taylor DO, Edwards LB, Boucek MM et al 2005 Registry of the International Society for Heart and Lung Transplantation: Twenty-second Official Adult Heart Transplant Report – 2005. Journal of Heart and Lung Transplantation 24(8): 945–955

Thabut G, Mal H, Cerrina J et al 2005 Graft ischemic time and outcome of lung transplantation: a multicenter analysis. American Journal of Respiratory and Critical Care Medicine 171(7): 786–791

Theodore J, Morris AJ, Burke CM et al 1987 Cardiopulmonary function at maximum tolerable constant work rate exercise following human heart-lung transplantation. Chest 92(3): 433–439

Trulock EP, Edwards LB, Taylor DO et al 2005 Registry of the International Society for Heart and Lung Transplantation: Twenty-second Official Adult Lung and Heart-lung Transplant Report – 2005. Journal of Heart and Lung Transplantation 24(8): 956–967

van't Hul A, Gosselink R, Hollander P, Postmus P, Kwakkel G 2006 Training with inspiratory pressure support in patients with severe COPD. European Respiratory Journal 27(1): 65–72

Wang XN, Williams TJ, McKenna MJ et al 1999 Skeletal muscle oxidative capacity, fiber type, and metabolites after lung transplantation. American Journal of Respiratory and Critical Care Medicine 160(1): 57–63

Weber, B 1990 Cardiac surgery and heart transplantation. In: Hudak C, Gallo B, Benz J (eds) Critical care nursing: a holistic approach, 5th edn. JB Lippincott, Philadelphia, PA

Werber-Zion G, Goldhammer E, Shaar A, Pollock M 2004 Left ventricular function during strength testing and resistance exercise in patients with left ventricular dysfunction. Journal of Cardiopulmonary Rehabilitation 24 100–109

Whittom F, Jobin J, Simard PM et al 1998 Histochemical and morphological characteristics of the vastus lateralis muscle in patients with chronic obstructive pulmonary disease. Medicine and Science in Sports and Exercise 30(10): 1467–1474

Williams TJ, Patterson GA, McClean PA, Zamel N, Maurer JR 1992 Maximal exercise testing in single and double lung transplant recipients. American Review of Respiratory Disease 145(1): 101–105

15

Yousem SA, Berry GJ, Cagle PT et al 1996 Revision of the 1990 working formulation for the classification of pulmonary allograft rejection: Lung Rejection Study Group. Journal of Heart and Lung Transplantation 15(1 Pt 1): 1–15

Yung GL, Kriett JM, Jamieson SW et al 2001 Outpatient inhaled nitric oxide in a patient with idiopathic pulmonary fibrosis: a bridge to lung transplantation. Journal of Heart and Lung Transplantation 20(11): 1224–1227

Chapter 16

Spinal cord injury

Kathryn Harris, Trudy Ward

INTRODUCTION

The prognosis for the patient sustaining spinal cord injury was poor until the latter part of the 20th century. An unknown Egyptian physician of 2500 BC describing spinal cord injury in the Edwin Smith Papyrus wrote:

> 'An ailment not to be treated'
>
> (Grundy & Swain 1996)

This view continued until the work of Guttmann and others encouraged development of special centres throughout the world and saw the problems associated with spinal cord injury at last being addressed, although mortality from tetraplegia until the 1960s remained at 35% (Grundy & Swain 1996). Improvements in administering care at the time of the accident, technological advances in diagnosis and management have contributed to a continuing fall in mortality and morbidity rates over recent years. Kemp & Krause (1999) state that there has been a 2000% increase in life expectancy following spinal cord injury in the past 50 years compared with a 30% increase for the non-disabled population. Mortality is significantly higher during the first year after injury, especially for those with higher-level injuries. Life expectancy tables and other facts and figures are available online from the National Spinal Cord Injury Statistical Center at the University of Alabama, USA (see *Further reading*).

In a 50-year study in the United Kingdom, Frankel et al (1998) found that 92.3% of spinal cord injuries survived, the primary cause of death being attributed to respiratory complications. Another study has shown a projected mean life expectancy of 84% of normal for paraplegia and 70% for tetraplegia (Yeo et al 1998).

The respiratory care of patients with spinal cord injury is discussed in this chapter. It should, however, be remembered that effective management of patients requires a holistic, multidisciplinary approach, preferably in a spinal cord injuries unit, to ensure optimal rehabilitation.

MECHANICS OF RESPIRATION AND THE EFFECT OF SPINAL CORD INJURY

Normal respiration

An understanding of normal respiratory mechanics is needed to appreciate the effect of a spinal cord injury. Figure 16.1 lists the muscles of respiration and their level of innervation.

The contraction and downward movement of the diaphragm and contraction of the intercostal muscles cause normal inspiration by generation of negative intrapleural and subsequent negative intrathoracic pressure (Lucke 1998). The intercostal muscles also work to stabilize the rib cage against the tendency for paradoxical inward movement caused by the negative intrathoracic pressure during inspiration.

Expiration is normally a passive process except during a forceful manoeuvre such as coughing or sneezing. This force is generated mainly by the abdominal muscles, assisted by the intercostals at large lung volumes (De Troyer & Heilporn 1980).

Respiratory complications are a major cause of death in the early stages of spinal injury (Lanig & Peterson 2000, Van Buren et al 1994), and those at the highest risk are:

- tetraplegic patients
- patients with associated injuries such as rib fractures or chest trauma
- patients who have pre-existing lung disease.

Effects of spinal cord injury

Following a spinal cord injury the muscles below and, not uncommonly, at the level of the injury are paralysed. The higher the level of injury, the greater the effect on respiration (Linn et al 2000). To gain a more precise picture of the muscles affected, the physiotherapist should refer to the level of innervation of the respiratory muscles and relate this to the neurological level of injury.

Tetraplegic patients (i.e. those with an injury affecting T1 or above) will have lost the use of their intercostal muscles, which has a profound effect on respiratory function. Depending on the level of their injury, only part of the diaphragm may be spared, yet it has to provide them with all of their respiratory effort (Cohn 1993).

Paradoxical breathing

Tetraplegic patients injured at or below C4 will have partial or total innervation of the diaphragm and some

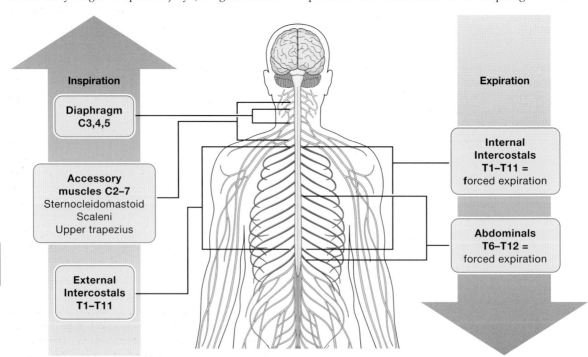

Figure 16.1　Spinal innervation of the respiratory muscles.

Inspiration

Diaphragm
C3,4,5

Accessory
muscles C2–7
Sternocleidomastoid
Scaleni
Upper trapezius

External
Intercostals
T1–T11

Expiration

Internal
Intercostals
T1–T11 =
forced expiration

Abdominals
T6–T12 =
forced expiration

accessory muscles of respiration and can be totally independent of mechanical ventilation. However, in the initial spinal shock stage, tetraplegic patients will have paralysis of their intercostal muscles, which, when flaccid, causes disruption to the mechanics of respiration. The usual splinting function of the intercostal muscles is lost and the negative intrathoracic pressure during inspiration causes paradoxical inward depression of the ribs (Lucke 1998, Menter et al 1997) (Fig. 16.2). This may lead to microatelectasis and an increase in the work of breathing (Fishburn et al 1990). With time the tendons, ligaments and joints of the rib cage stiffen owing to decreased active movement. This, together with spasticity of the intercostals, will provide some compensation for the loss of active control of these muscles and stabilize the rib cage, so that paradoxical breathing lessens (Axen et al 1985, Mansel & Norman 1990).

Cough

The ability to produce an effective cough is severely impaired in patients with cervical or high thoracic spinal cord injury (Roth et al 1997, Wang et al 1997). This is most marked when the intercostals are flaccid and the rib cage is at its most mobile. Patients who have loss of innervation to the abdominal muscles and the internal intercostals lose the ability to produce a forced expiration (Gouden 1997). De Troyer & Estenne (1991) have shown that patients with injuries at C5-8 can utilize the clavicular portion of pectoralis major to generate an expulsive force, although the extent to which this is functional is not clear. Linn et al (2000) found that in a group of patients with high tetraplegia (above C5) loss of peak expiratory flow rate was greater than 50% predicted. An effective cough for these patients requires external compression to produce the necessary large intrathoracic pressures; assisted coughing is discussed later.

The effect of position

In the normal subject, mechanisms exist to ensure that adequate ventilation is maintained in all positions. In the supine position, contraction of the diaphragm displaces the abdominal contents without significantly expanding the rib cage, as the abdomen is more compliant than the rib cage. In standing, abdominal tone increases to support the abdominal contents, thereby decreasing abdominal wall compliance. Contraction of the diaphragm, intercostal and accessory muscles causes greater rib cage expansion, resulting in an increase in vital capacity in standing of about 5% (Chen et al 1990).

Positional changes will, however, affect the respiratory function of the tetraplegic patient. In supine, the weight of the abdominal contents forces the diaphragm to a higher resting level so that contraction produces greater excursion of the diaphragm. In sitting or standing, the weight of the unsupported abdominal contents increases the demand on the diaphragm, which now rests in a lower and flatter position (Chen et al 1990, Lucke 1998), decreasing effectiveness and restricting available excursion for creating negative intrapleural pressure (Fig. 16.3). Chen et al (1990) recorded a 14% drop in predicted vital capacity in the tetraplegic patient on changing position from supine to sitting or standing. Conversely, vital capacity of a tetraplegic patient rises by 6% when the bed is tipped 15° head down from supine (Bromley 1998). Linn et al (2000) showed a statistically significant decrease in forced vital capacity (FVC) in the erect position as compared with supine. It is therefore important with these patients not to assume that their respiratory ability will be sufficient in all positions.

Abdominal binders

Elasticated abdominal binders have been used on patients with high spinal cord injury for many years, both to minimize the effect of postural hypotension and aid respiration (Goldman et al 1986, McCool et al 1986,

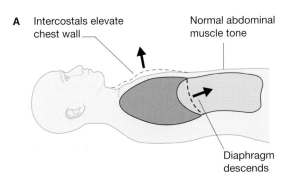

A Intercostals elevate chest wall

Normal abdominal muscle tone

Diaphragm descends

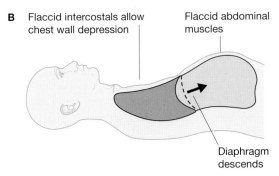

B Flaccid intercostals allow chest wall depression

Flaccid abdominal muscles

Diaphragm descends

Figure 16.2   Paradoxical breathing in tetraplegia.

16

A

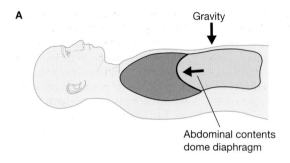

B

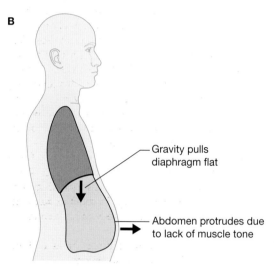

Figure 16.3 The effect of position on diaphragm function in tetraplegia: **(A)** Lying; **(B)** Sitting or standing.

Scott et al 1993). Their effect is achieved by providing support to the abdominal contents, decreasing the compliance of the abdominal wall and thereby allowing the diaphragm to assume a more normal resting position in the upright posture (Alvarez et al 1981). Goldman et al (1986) investigated the effect of abdominal binders on breathing in tetraplegic patients and concluded that in the supine position there was no change, but when sitting there was a trend for improvement in lung volumes. This may help the patient considerably during the early stages of mobilization.

Incomplete injuries and position

If a spinal cord lesion is incomplete, i.e. there is sensation and/or movement below the level of injury, there are specific circumstances where the effect of position as described above can be reversed. A high-level C3–C5 incomplete lesion of the spinal cord can result in diaphragm paralysis but sparing of the intercostal muscles. Paradoxical breathing will not be observed. The patient

will experience respiratory compromise in supine, which may be relieved by the sitting position, enabling the intercostal muscles to work more effectively. This scenario further emphasizes the need for accurate assessment of vital capacity in all positions where possible (see *Respiratory assessment*, below).

Sleep–disordered breathing and sleep apnoea syndrome after spinal cord injury

Sleep apnoea has been widely reported in patients with spinal cord injury and is known to be twice as prevalent as compared with the general population (Cahan et al 1993, McEvoy et al 1995, Young et al 1993). Stockhammer and colleagues (2002) defined two factors of sleep-disordered breathing and sleep apnoea. If a patient had more than 5 apnoeas per hour of sleep – the apnoea index (AI) and a respiratory disturbance index (RDI) of 15 or more, they were defined as having sleep apnoea syndrome (SAS). If their RDI was 15 or more but AI was less than 5 then they were defined as having sleep-disordered breathing (SDB). In this study of tetraplegic patients 62% had SDB. Forty-eight per cent (55% of the men studied and 20% the women) had SAS. This is comparable with other studies that have found the prevalence of SAS to be 40% (Burns 2000) and 45% (Short et al 1992). Stockhammer et al (2002) found no correlation of level of lesion or spirometry values with the presence of RDI. They did, however, find a significant correlation of age, time since injury, body mass index (BMI) and neck circumference with RDI. They concluded that SAS incidence is high in tetraplegia, especially in older men with long-standing spinal cord injury. They also noted that patients with a high RDI did not complain of daytime drowsiness and were not obese, and therefore these individuals may not be investigated for SAS. Graham et al (2004) reported on two paraplegic men who had sleep apnoea who were aged 54 and 55 and were 37 and 25 years, respectively, post injury.

Berlowitz et al (2005) studied patients during the first year after cervical spinal cord injury. They found a high prevalence of SDB, which was first apparent 2 weeks following injury (60%) and peaked at 13 weeks or 3 months (83%). This then improved but remained significantly elevated (62%) at 1-year post injury. It should be noted that these outcomes cannot be compared directly with the studies quoted above, because this study reported on SDB whereas the others reported on SAS. Treatment for SAS with non-invasive ventilation is discussed later.

RESPIRATORY ASSESSMENT

Accurate assessment and regular review of respiratory status are vital. Initial assessment must be carried out

16

as soon as possible to establish a baseline against which future deterioration or improvement can be monitored. Assessment is discussed in Chapter 1; however, in patients with spinal cord injury, the following details should also be considered:

1. Motor and sensory neurological examination, relating this to the respiratory muscle innervation and hence likely function (Roth et al 1997).
2. Associated injuries – rib fractures and flail segments are commonly seen in the patient with thoracic spinal injury and these may require modification of treatment techniques. Patients involved in diving accidents may present with the additional respiratory complications of water aspiration. The presence of intra-abdominal trauma or complications such as paralytic ileus, acute gastric dilatation or gastrointestinal bleeding will also require modification of the techniques used by the physiotherapist, especially assisted coughing.
3. Associated lung trauma – common injuries include pneumothorax, haemothorax and pulmonary contusion.
4. Pre-existing lung disease – problems such as asthma or chronic airflow limitation may exist and should be treated as indicated.
5. Presence of an endotracheal tube, tracheostomy tube, nasal or facemask and/or ventilatory support.
6. Psychological state – major psychological adjustment is required by the patient with spinal cord injury, not only to the injury itself but also to the necessary treatment procedures. Sensory deprivation may cause loss of orientation, made worse by enforced immobilization and restricted visual input. Anxiety and interrupted sleep patterns caused by frequent turns and other procedures can result in confusion and fatigue. These factors will all affect respiratory function and must be considered by the physiotherapist to enable the most effective and appropriate planning of respiratory treatment.
7. Results of the chest radiograph and arterial blood gases, if available.
8. Altered levels of consciousness.
9. Respiratory rate at rest – with normal diaphragm activity the rate remains regular at 12–16 breaths/min. In the presence of a weak or fatiguing diaphragm the rate will increase (Alvarez et al 1981).
10. Assessment of breathing pattern to establish the degree of paradoxical movement or presence of unequal movement of the chest wall.
11. Assessment of diaphragm function, by inspection or palpation of the upper abdomen.
12. Assessment of cough to ascertain effectiveness.
13. Measurement of vital capacity – repeated measurements of vital capacity provide an indication of trends developing in respiratory function and should be recorded in all the positions in which the patient may be nursed, to detect postural variations (Lucke 1998). This will be especially pronounced in the presence of unilateral phrenic nerve damage, and incomplete high cervical injuries where the intercostal muscles are functioning but the diaphragm is not (see *Incomplete injuries and position*). Values will vary depending on the level of injury. Lucke (1998) reports observed initial vital capacities of 24% of predicted normal values in mid-cervical injuries and 31% in lower cervical injuries. This can rise to 50% after spinal shock has resolved. Vital capacity may fall over the first few days following injury owing to factors such as muscle or patient fatigue, respiratory complications or oedema within the spinal cord which results in a rise in neurological level (Alderson 1999). Improvement is usually seen as this oedema resolves and respiratory function stabilizes (Axen et al 1985, Ledsome & Sharp 1981). Vital capacity values of less than 15 ml per kilogram of bodyweight may, in con-junction with clinical assessment, indicate the need for ventilation (Thomas & Paulson 1994).
14. Auscultation of the chest to detect areas of lung collapse, pleural effusion or secretions.

PHYSIOTHERAPY TREATMENT

Respiratory management of the patient with spinal cord injury requires the application of the same principles as other respiratory problems; the skills used are discussed in Chapters 4 and 5. The goals of treatment include:

- clearance of secretions from the lungs
- improvement in breath sounds
- increase in lung volumes
- strengthening of the available muscles of respiration
- improvement of pulmonary and rib cage compliance
- education of the patient and their carer.

Treatment may be prophylactic or aimed at specific problems.

16

PROPHYLACTIC TREATMENT

This should include breathing exercises, modified postural drainage by regular turning and assisted coughing.

Breathing exercises

Breathing exercises to encourage maximal inspiration must be established at an early stage, but the therapist should be aware of the implications of lack of sensation of the chest wall. Exercises are directed to improve lateral basal and apical chest wall expansion and diaphragmatic excursion, but care must be taken to avoid tiring the diaphragm. Patients with intercostal paralysis are usually unable to perform localized breathing exercises.

Respiratory muscle training

Many authors have reported the use of respiratory muscle training for tetraplegia but there is a lack of randomized controlled trials, which makes the findings of the (often small) studies difficult to apply to the general patient group. Neither Stiller & Huff (1999) nor Brooks & O'Brien (2005) could recommend routine use of respiratory muscle training for tetraplegic patients (Chapter 5).

There have been some favourable findings. Liaw et al (2000) found that resistive inspiratory muscle training in tetraplegic patients, who were between 30 days and 6 months of injury, improved ventilatory function but noted that the patients needed to be highly motivated to gain benefit. Uijl et al (1999) reported on nine tetraplegic patients who underwent target flow endurance training and showed enhanced endurance capacity and an increase in aerobic exercise performance. Wang et al 2002 conducted a home programme of resistive inspiratory muscle training (RIMT) with a group of 14 tetraplegic patients who had sleep-disordered breathing and found that it had a positive effect on respiratory muscle strength and endurance. They suggested that this may reduce the patients' sleep-disordered breathing. As with any training, the effect is soon lost when training ceases so this must be a lifelong commitment for long-term benefit to be maintained.

Incentive spirometry

Incentive spirometry enables respiratory training with immediate visual feedback to reinforce success. However, caution is needed in providing acutely injured tetraplegic patients with such a device, as a balance is needed between maintaining and improving lung volumes and respiratory muscle fatigue in the early days and weeks following injury.

Glossopharyngeal breathing

Glossopharyngeal breathing is another technique that can be used to increase lung volumes and assist secretion clearance (Chapter 5) in the high tetraplegic. Vital capacity may be increased by as much as 1000 ml (Alvarez et al 1981). Bach refers to the technique for augmenting inspired volume for patients with neuromuscular disorders to the extent where they can achieve a vital capacity of up to 1.7 litres (Bach 1993, Bach & McDermott 1990, Bach et al 1993). Pryor (1999) suggests that glossopharyngeal breathing (GPB) is a useful technique for increasing cough effectiveness in tetraplegia. In the high tetraplegic patient dependent on mechanical ventilation, other important benefits of GPB are to provide security in case of ventilator failure and independence from the ventilator for periods of time (Chapter 5).

TREATMENT OF THE PATIENT WITH RESPIRATORY PROBLEMS

In the presence of respiratory problems such as retained secretions or lung collapse, sputum clearance is of paramount importance and vigorous, aggressive treatment is often needed. Physiotherapy treatment plans will be determined by ongoing monitoring and assessment. Unless contraindicated by other complications, postural drainage either with an electric turning bed or manual turn into supported side lying, should be used as appropriate. Great care must be taken to maintain spinal alignment and cervical traction throughout treatment. The effect of positioning on lung ventilation and perfusion must be considered (Chapter 4). Patients should never be left unsupervised during postural drainage in case of sudden sputum mobilization, which could cause the patient to choke unless secretions are cleared by assisted coughing.

Treatment may consist of the active cycle of breathing techniques (Pryor 1999), vibration, shaking and chest clapping as necessary, followed by assisted coughing. 'Little and often' is the general rule as acutely injured patients will tire quickly, but treatment must be effective, using two physiotherapists if necessary. Where possible, treatment should link in with planned turn times to allow some rest between various procedures. Some authors recommend the use of the mechanical in-exsufflator (or CoughAssist™ machine), which has been used to great effect for many years (Bach 1993, Bach et al 1993, Tzeng & Bach 2000) (see *Mechanical aids for assisted coughing*, below).

Assisted coughing

Assisted coughing is a vital inclusion in any respiratory programme. Patients may be able to clear sputum from small to large airways, but will need assistance to produce an effective cough for expectoration. Assistance is provided by the application of a compressive force directed inwards and upwards against the thorax to create a push against the diaphragm, thus replacing the work of the abdominal and internal intercostal muscles. The sound of the resultant cough is the best indicator of the force required, but care must be taken to avoid movement of any fracture. Pressure directed down through the abdomen must be avoided, especially in the acute patient, owing to the possibility of associated abdominal injury or paralytic ileus. Care should also be taken in the presence of rib fractures or other chest injuries and therapists should position their hands away from the problem area to perform an assisted cough.

Bromley (1998) describes various methods of achieving assisted cough. Assisted coughing remains one of the most important techniques for airway clearance in the patient with an acute spinal cord injury. The technique needs to be relatively forceful and for this reason it is advisable for the therapist to lower the bed to gain the most advantageous position from which to perform the technique. However, great care must be taken not to allow any weights used for cervical traction to touch the floor.

The spinal stability of the patient must be carefully considered and for the patient with an unstable cervical spine, a shoulder hold should be used to counter any movement of the fracture site. Figure 16.4 shows the methods that may be used in the supine patient requiring a shoulder hold.

If one person is assisting with the cough, hands should be placed so that one rests on the near side of the thorax and the other on the opposite side of the thorax, with the forearm resting across the lower ribs (Fig. 16.4A). As the patient attempts to cough the physiotherapist pushes inwards and upwards with the forearm and stabilizes the thorax with the hands. Alternatively, the hands are positioned bilaterally over the lower thorax (Fig. 16.4B) and, with elbows extended, the physiotherapist pushes inwards and upwards evenly through both arms. In the case of the patient with a large thorax or having particularly tenacious sputum, two people may be required to produce an effective cough (Fig. 16.4C & D).

Care must be taken to synchronize the applied compressive force with the expiratory effort of the patient. Once the cough is completed, pressure must be lifted momentarily from the lower ribs, thus enabling the patient to use their diaphragm to initiate the next breath. In the presence of paralytic ileus or internal injury, extreme care must be taken during assisted coughing to avoid the application of pressure over the abdomen. Patients should be encouraged to cough 3–4 times per day, with nursing staff involved in this process. If possible, patients should be taught self-assisted coughing

when in a wheelchair and relatives should learn how to assist the patient to cough in both lying and sitting.

Mechanical aids for assisted coughing

The use of a mechanical in-exsufflation device to assist coughing has been documented in the literature as being effective with patients with neuromuscular disorders and respiratory muscle weakness (Chatwin et al 2003, Sancho et al 2004, Vianello et al 2005, Whitney et al 2002). Many of these studies used a device called the CoughAssist™ (JH Emerson Co, Cambridge, MA, USA). Whitney et al suggest using pressures in the range of 25 cmH$_2$O positive pressure and −30 cmH$_2$O negative pressure, while Chatwin & Simonds (2002) have reported effective coughs at pressures of +10 to +30 cmH$_2$O and −10 to −30 cmH$_2$O negative pressures.

There is an increasing body of literature which describes using electrical stimulation of the abdominal muscles to assist coughing (Langbein et al 2001, Lin et al 1998, Linder 1993, Stanic et al 2000, Taylor et al 2002, Zupan et al 1997). This technique, although often effective, is not widely available owing to the lack of standardized equipment available.

Airway suction

Nasopharyngeal suction may be used as a last resort if clearance by assisted cough alone is insufficient, but great care must be taken as pharyngeal suction can cause stimulation of the parasympathetic nervous system via the vagus nerve, resulting in bradycardia and even cardiac arrest. Hyperoxygenation of the patient with 100% oxygen before treatment will help to minimize this possibility (Wicks & Menter 1986). Atropine or an equivalent drug should be available for intravenous administration should profound bradycardia occur, defined as a heart rate of less than 50 with a continuing downward trend. Occasionally fibre-optic bronchoscopy may be necessary to treat unresolving lung or lobar collapse.

Intermittent positive pressure breathing and non-invasive ventilation

Intermittent positive pressure breathing (IPPB) and non-invasive ventilation (NIV) may be used in conjunction with other methods of treatment, particularly assisted coughing. Work by Rose et al (1987) concluded that increasing lung volumes had no major effect on lung function in stable tetraplegics. IPPB may be useful to aid the clearance of secretions by increasing inspiratory volume in patients with sputum retention and lung collapse (Chapter 5). The introduction of many new ventilators for NIV has overcome some of the

16

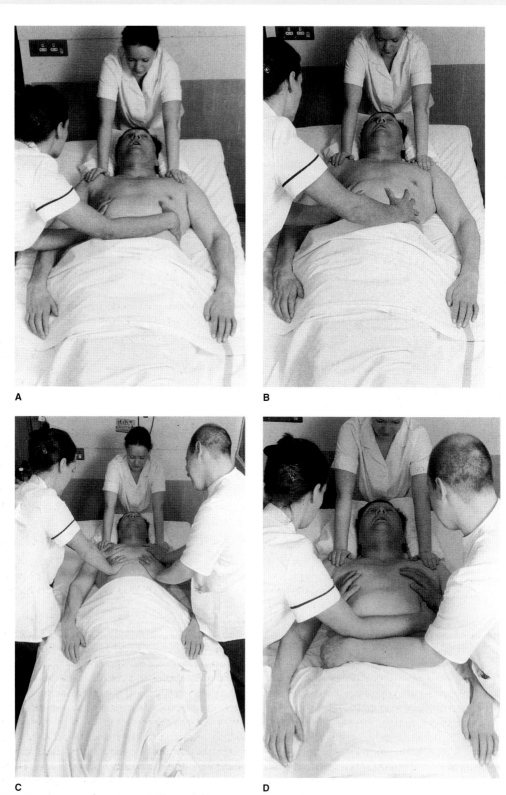

A

B

C

D

Figure 16.4   (A, B, C, D) Assisted coughing.

16

limitations of IPPB machines such as lack of choice of interface and requirement for pressurized gas (Bott et al 1992).

It is useful to initiate NIV at an early stage, before the onset of fatigue, to enable the patient to become familiar with the machine (Tromans et al 1998) and if the patient does tire it can be used to provide assistance for up to 24 hours if required. This has been shown to be an effective way of preventing intubation and ventilation in acute spinal cord injury (Tromans et al 1998).

Unfortunately, in the case of acute spinal cord injury the psychological impact is devastating. Acceptance of a face or nose mask by the patient is often poor when they are also dealing with profound sensory deprivation from immobility and sensory loss. Kannan (1999) acknowledges that patient comfort and mental status can be reasons for failure of NIV and this is supported by clinical experience.

Non-invasive ventilation treatment for sleep apnoea syndrome

NIV can also be used to treat sleep apnoea syndrome (SAS) in spinal cord injury. Stockhammer et al 2002 reported that out of 31 patients recommended for BiPAP treatment only 16 opted to receive it and of those five subsequently discontinued treatment. They did comment that there was a strong correlation between symptoms of daytime drowsiness and acceptance of treatment. The group who experienced improvement of their drowsiness symptoms using the BiPAP demonstrated good adherence with treatment. Patients with SAS, who did not complain of drowsiness during the day, were the least likely to both accept treatment in the first instance and to continue with it. Burns et al (2000) also reported acceptance problems, with only 25% of patients with SAS undertaking treatment.

Readmissions to hospital with a chest infection

As survival following spinal cord injury increases, the cohort rises. This has led to an increase in hospital readmission for chest infection (Burns et al 2004, Capoor and Stein 2005). Physiotherapists in general hospitals are increasingly seeing patients with chronic spinal cord injury. This is partly due to the pressure on beds in the spinal units for treatment of acutely injured patients.

Patients with a vital capacity of less than 2 litres are at greatest risk of developing late-onset respiratory failure (Peterson & Kirshblum 2002). Some patients with long-standing spinal cord injury develop an altered response to carbon dioxide levels in the blood, in a similar way to patients with chronic obstructive pulmonary disease. Characteristically these patients are those who chronically hypoventilate and develop a raised partial pressure of carbon dioxide in the blood which leads to decreased chemoreceptor sensitivity to the presence of carbon dioxide (Stockhammer et al 2002). Consequently these patients have only a hypoxic element to their respiratory drive and administration of high inspiratory concentrations of oxygen may result in apnoea and respiratory arrest. If a readmitted patient requires ventilation, the weaning should be similar to that described later in *Ventilation and weaning considerations* as weaning should generally be slow in order to be successful.

Care of the ventilated patient

Around 20% of acute cervical spinal cord injuries will require some form of respiratory support (DiMarco 2005). Mechanical ventilation may be necessary in the following circumstances:

- Injury to the upper cervical spine C1-3, resulting in paralysis of the diaphragm

- Deterioration in respiratory function as a result of oedema or bleeding within the spinal canal causing the neurological level to rise, so affecting the diaphragm. Patients are most at risk during the first 72 hours

- Respiratory muscle fatigue. The use of non-invasive ventilation, e.g. a bilevel positive pressure device, may be helpful in providing ventilatory assistance without the need for full ventilation (Tromans et al 1998) (see *Intermittent positive pressure breathing and non-invasive ventilation* above, and Chapter 10). Tracheostomy may be beneficial in reducing dead space by up to 50% (Bromley 1998)

- Associated chest or head injuries, which require management by elective ventilation.

Insertion of a minitracheostomy may be considered for patients with problems of retained secretions (Gupta et al 1989).

Physiotherapy goals for treatment of the ventilated patient are the same as those for the non-ventilated patient. Treatment will include modified postural drainage, vibration and shaking with manual hyperinflation, followed by suction to remove secretions. As previously stated, hyperoxygenation may be needed to prevent overstimulation of the vagus nerve resulting in bradycardia. Other methods for minimizing this are to use a suction catheter that is no more than half the diameter of the tracheostomy or endotracheal tube and to be as gentle and brief as possible (Carroll 1994, Dean 1997, Glass & Grap 1995). Frequency of treatment will be determined by assessment of the respiratory condition but should not exceed 15–20 minutes (Bromley 1998).

16

Patients requiring ventilation due to complications from spinal cord injury are often not sedated and a system of communication must be established before physiotherapy is started.

Ventilation and weaning considerations

Early intervention with a non-invasive ventilatory technique may avoid progression of respiratory failure and the need for sedation, intubation and full mechanical ventilation (Tromans et al 1998). Where intubation and ventilation are necessary, weaning will typically progress from IPPV to pressure support and then, in the neurologically intact patient, continuous positive airway pressure (CPAP) is often used. However, in patients with hypercapnic respiratory failure, as seen in spinal cord injury, CPAP is not indicated as it cannot influence tidal volume or respiratory rate and therefore will not lower arterial carbon dioxide (Keilty & Bott 1992). Bilevel positive pressure may be of use during the weaning period, as it assists both expiration and inspiration (Ashworth 1990). Many machines now have a very sensitive flow trigger, which decreases the work of breathing.

Weaning from the ventilator should start as soon as the patient's condition permits and is best performed with the patient supine, allowing the most effective diaphragm function (Chen et al 1990, Mansel & Norman 1990). Weaning must take into account the possibility that the patient's respiratory muscles will have atrophied if ventilation has been prolonged. Cohn (1993) suggests that weaning should be thought of as a conditioning process for the diaphragm and also warns that fatigue of the muscle should be avoided. The goal must therefore be to achieve spontaneous breathing for short periods, several times a day, to avoid fatigue. A vital capacity of at least 15 ml per kilogram of bodyweight is generally used as a goal for the weaning patient and conversely as a threshold for ventilation for a self-ventilating patient (Chevrolet & Deleamont 1991, Mahanes & Lewis 2004).

A study by Peterson et al (1994) compared weaning onto a T-piece for progressive periods of time with the synchronized intermittent mandatory ventilation (SIMV) mode of ventilation, the latter being used frequently in the neurologically intact patient (Cull & Inwood 1999). Compared with SIMV, the T-piece group was almost twice as likely to wean successfully from the ventilator. Tromans et al (1998) reported on the use of BiPAP for weaning 15 patients from ventilation, with success in 13 out of 15 patients who weaned in an average of 32 days using a gradual decrease in pressure. Menter et al (1997) quote average weaning times for 74 spinal cord injured patients to be 36 days using progres-

sive T-piece weaning. Peterson et al (1999) reported on the use of high tidal volumes to ventilate tetraplegic patients in association with T-piece weaning and concluded that tidal volumes of more than 20 ml per kilogram of bodyweight were most successful. McKinley (1996) reported one case of an initially ventilator-dependent tetraplegic patient with a C3-4 lesion who was successfully weaned from a ventilator after 5 years. Other authors support the view that weaning can be prolonged and can take months, if not years (Fromm et al 1999, Oo et al 1999). Gutierrez et al (2003) used resistance and endurance respiratory muscle training to wean tetraplegic patients from ventilation. Although the numbers were small they reported success in fully weaning five patients with C4-C7 who had been ventilated for between 4 months and 2 years. They also achieved improvement in 'off ventilator' breathing time for two C2 tetraplegic patients using their weaning protocol.

Irrespective of technique used, regular recording of vital capacity, oxygen saturation and respiratory rate are minimal requirements to effectively monitor the patient's progress (Menter et al 1997). If end-tidal carbon dioxide can be monitored, it is very useful and less traumatic than arterial blood gas sampling in the absence of arterial access (Cull & Inwood 1999). However, arterial blood gases are the gold standard and if the patient is unable to sustain his vital capacity, arterial carbon dioxide is likely to be rising and weaning should not be progressed until it has stabilized. The presence of other associated injuries and/or complications may have an effect on the success of the weaning process.

Long-term ventilation

For the patient on long-term ventilation, a battery-driven ventilator is attached to the wheelchair to enable mobility (Fig. 16.5). With increasing numbers surviving the initial injury owing to greater public awareness of resuscitation skills, home ventilation is now becoming more common, enabling these patients to undergo rehabilitation and to go home (Alderson 1999, Carter 1993). Planning must start at the earliest opportunity in conjunction with the patient's local and community services in order to achieve timely discharge to an appropriate location. Comprehensive training is needed for the family and care team, for each patient, in order to minimize the risks of being fully ventilator dependent within the community.

The ethical dilemmas surrounding the ventilation of the high tetraplegic patient have challenged and continue to challenge medical practice (Gupta et al 1989, Maynard & Muth 1987). Only the ventilated tetraplegic knows what it is like to be a ventilated tetraplegic and

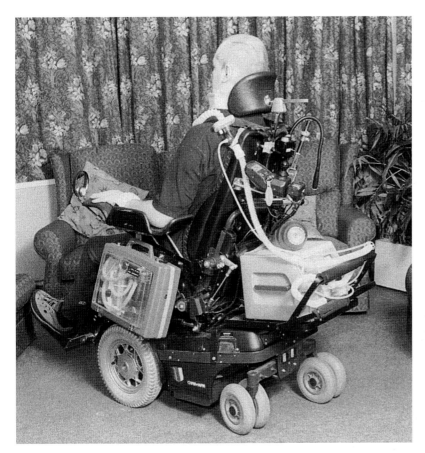

Figure 16.5   Ventilated patient in a wheelchair.

only his carer knows what it is like to care for him. In a review of 21 patients who had required artificial ventilation (Gupta et al 1989), 18 stated that they would prefer a further period of continuous ventilation to being allowed to die. Sixteen of the 21 nearest caring relatives indicated that they were glad that their relative had been kept alive by ventilation. The study concluded that patients with spinal cord injury should be ventilated, provided that total emotional, educational and physical support could be given and maintained to all involved. This would seem to be most important.

In a case study, Maynard & Muth (1987) reveal how one individual's request to cease life-supporting ventilation was met. They suggest that:

'If rehabilitation is defined as achieving optimal quality of life for people with severe disability then quality must be defined by the disabled individual'

An individual's perception of what constitutes acceptable quality of life will change over time (Purtilo 1986) and this poses the question of the feasibility of involvement of the newly injured patient and relatives in the decision regarding ventilation, as they are unable to appreciate the global implications of tetraplegia in the acute stage. However, 'Right to Die' issues have been in the media repeatedly in recent years, as individuals have challenged the established medical models of care (see *Further reading*). Physiotherapists must take great care to obtain consent and not to treat patients against their will.

Electrical and magnetic stimulation of breathing

A paralysed diaphragm can be electronically or magnetically stimulated if the phrenic nerve is intact and the cell bodies of C3, C4, C5 at the spinal cord are viable. The technique was first developed by Dr Glenn in the 1960s (Carter 1993). It should be noted, however, that many ventilator-dependent patients have sustained damage to the lower motor neurons and therefore are not suitable for this technique. Full preoperative assessment is required to ascertain a patient's suitability for stimulation (DiMarco 2005). Electrodes may be placed to stimulate the phrenic nerve in either the neck, thorax or intramuscularly directly into the diaphragm (DiMarco 2005). Stimulation is achieved by means of a radio transmitter placed over the receiver. Extensive postoperative training is necessary to increase diaphragmatic endurance and to teach the patient, his family and carers the necessary skills and understanding of the device. For some patients phrenic nerve pacing will provide a fulltime alternative to the ventilator and the tracheostomy will no longer be required, but for others the ventilator and tracheostomy will remain an emergency back-up.

Benefits include greater wheelchair mobility, elimination of the fear of accidental disconnection from the ventilator, loss of embarrassment and social stigma associated with being attached to a ventilator, improved speech, no noise from the ventilator, reduced need for carer input and improved well-being and overall health

– particularly when decannulation of the tracheostomy has occurred (DiMarco 1999, 2005). Disadvantages include the need for major surgery involving thoracotomy, a prolonged hospital stay for the postoperative training, risk of surgical damage to the phrenic nerve and failure of the implanted device (DiMarco 2005).

CONCLUSION

Greater understanding of the problems of the spinal cord-injured patient has led to continuing improvements in morbidity and mortality rates. Respiratory complications can be managed more effectively with increased understanding of the problems facing these patients. Physiotherapists have, and will continue to have, much to offer in the respiratory care of the patient with spinal cord injury.

References

Alderson JD 1999 Spinal cord injuries. Care of the Critically Ill 15(2): 48–52

Alvarez S, Peterson M, Lunsford B 1981 Respiratory treatment of the adult patient with spinal cord injury. Physical Therapy 61(12): 1737–1745

Ashworth LJ 1990 Pressure support ventilation. Critical Care Nurse 10(7): 20–25

Axen K, Pineda H, Shunfenthal I, Haas F 1985 Diaphragmatic function following cervical cord injury: neurally mediated improvement. Archives of Physical Medicine and Rehabilitation 66: 219–222

Bach JR 1993 Mechanical insufflation-exsufflation: comparison of peak expiratory flows with manually assisted and unassisted coughing techniques. Chest 104: 1553–1562

Bach JR, McDermott IG 1990 Strapless oral-nasal interface for positive-pressure ventilation. Archives of Physical Medicine and Rehabilitation 71(11): 910–913

Bach JR, Smith WH, Michaels J et al 1993 Airway secretion clearance by mechanical exsufflation for poliomyelitis ventilator-assisted individuals. Archives of Physical Medicine and Rehabilitation 74(2): 170–177

Berlowitz DJ, Brown DJ, Campbell DA, Pierce RJ 2005 A longitudinal evaluation of sleep in the first year after cervical spinal cord injury. Archives of Physical Medicine and Rehabilitation 86(6): 1193–1199

Bott J, Keilty SJ, Noone L 1992 Intermittent positive pressure breathing – a dying art? Physiotherapy 78(9): 656–660

Bromley I 1998 Tetraplegia and paraplegia: a guide for

physiotherapists, 5th edn. Churchill Livingstone, Edinburgh

Brooks D, O'Brien K 2005 Is inspiratory muscle training effective for individuals with cervical spinal cord injury? A qualitative systematic review. Clinical Rehabilitation 19: 237–246

Burns SP, Little JW, Hussey JD et al 2000 Sleep apnea syndrome in chronic spinal cord injury: associated factors and treatment. Archives of Physical Medicine and Rehabilitation 81: 1334–1339

Burns SP, Weaver FM, Parada JP et al 2004 Management of community-acquired pneumonia in persons with spinal cord injury. Spinal Cord 42: 450–458

Cahan C, Gothe B, Decker MJ et al 1993 Arterial oxygen saturation over time and sleep studies in quadriplegic patients. Paraplegia 31: 172–179

Capoor J, Stein AB 2005 Aging with spinal cord injury. Physical Medicine and Rehabilitation Clinics of North America 16: 109–128

Carroll P 1994 Safe suctioning. Registered Nurse 57(5): 32–36

Carter RE 1993 Experience with ventilator dependent patients. Paraplegia 31: 150–153

Chatwin M, Ross E, Hart N et al 2003 Cough augmentation with mechanical insufflation-exsufflation in patients with neuromuscular weakness. European Respiratory Journal 21: 502–508

Chatwin M, Simonds A 2002 Mechanical technique for assisted cough (Correspondence). Physiotherapy 88(6): 381–382

Chen C, Lien I, Wu M 1990 Respiratory function in patients with spinal cord

injuries: effects of posture. Paraplegia 28: 81–86

Chevrolet J, Deleamont P 1991 Repeated vital capacity measurements as predictive parameters for mechanical ventilation need and weaning success in Guillain–Barré syndrome. American Review of Respiratory Disease 144: 814–818

Cohn JR 1993 Pulmonary management of the patient with spinal cord injury. Trauma Quarterly 9(2): 65–71

Cull C, Inwood H 1999 Weaning patients from mechanical ventilation. Professional Nurse 14(8): 535–538

De Troyer A, Estenne M 1991 Review article: the expiratory muscles in tetraplegia. Paraplegia 29: 359–363

De Troyer A, Heilporn A 1980 Respiratory mechanics in quadriplegia. The respiratory function of the intercostal muscles. American Review of Respiratory Disease 122: 591–600

Dean B 1997 Evidence-based suction management in accident and emergency: a vital component of airway care. Accident and Emergency Nursing 5: 92–97

DiMarco AF 1999 Diaphragm pacing in patients with spinal cord injury. Topics in Spinal Cord Injury Rehabilitation 5(1): 6–20

DiMarco AF 2005 Restoration of respiratory muscle function following spinal cord injury: review of electrical and magnetic stimulation techniques. Respiratory Physiology and Neurobiology 147: 273–287

Fishburn MJ, Marino RJ, Ditunno JF 1990 Atelectasis and pneumonia in acute spinal cord injury. Archives of Physical Medicine and Rehabilitation 71: 197–200

16

Frankel HL, Coll JR, Charlifue SW et al 1998 Long-term survival in spinal cord injury: a fifty year investigation. Spinal Cord 36(12): 868–869

Fromm B, Hundt G, Gerner HJ et al 1999 Management of respiratory problems unique to high tetraplegia. Spinal Cord 37: 239–244

Glass CA, Grap MJ 1995 Ten tips for safer suctioning. American Journal of Nursing 5: 51–53

Goldman J, Rose L, Williams S et al 1986 Effect of abdominal binders on breathing in tetraplegic patients. Thorax 41: 940–945

Gouden P 1997 Static respiratory pressures in patients with post-traumatic tetraplegia. Spinal Cord 35: 43–47

Graham LE, Maguire SM, Gledhill IC 2004 Two case reports of sleep apnoea in patients with paraplegia. Spinal Cord 42: 603–605

Grundy D, Swain A 1996 ABC of spinal cord injury, 3rd edn. BMJ Books, London

Gupta A, McClelland M, Evans A, El Masri W 1989 Minitracheostomy in the early respiratory management of patients with spinal cord injury. Paraplegia 27: 269–277

Gutierrez CJ, Harrow J, Haines F 2003 Using an evidence-based protocol to guide rehabilitation and weaning of ventilator-dependent cervical spinal cord injury patients. Journal of Rehabilitation Research and Development 40(5 Suppl 2): 99–110

Kannan S 1999 Practical issues in non-invasive positive pressure ventilation. Care of the Critically Ill 15(3): 76–79

Keilty SEJ, Bott J 1992 Continuous positive airways pressure. Physiotherapy 78(2): 90–92

Kemp BJ, Krause JS 1999 Depression and life satisfaction among people aging with post-polio and spinal cord injury. Disability Rehabilitation 21: 241–249

Langbein WE, Maloney C, Kandare F et al 2001 Pulmonary function testing in spinal cord injury: effects of abdominal muscle stimulation. Journal of Rehabilitation Research and Development 38(5): 591–598

Lanig IS, Peterson WP 2000 The respiratory system in spinal cord injury. Physical Medicine and Rehabilitation Clinics of North America 11(1): 29–43

Ledsome J, Sharp J 1981 Pulmonary function in acute cervical cord injury. American Review of Respiratory Disease 124: 41–44

Liaw MY, Lin MC, Cheng PT, Wong MKA, Tang FT 2000 Resistive inspiratory muscle training: its effectiveness in patients with acute complete cervical cord injury. Archives of Physical Medicine and Rehabilitation 81: 752–756

Lin VWH, Singh H, Chitkara RK, Perkash I 1998 Functional magnetic stimulation for restoring cough in patients with tetraplegia. Archives of Physical Medicine and Rehabilitation 79: 517–522

Linder SH 1993 Functional electrical stimulation to enhance cough in quadriplegia. Chest 103: 166–169

Linn WM, Adkins RH, Gong H, Waters RL 2000 Pulmonary function in chronic spinal cord injury: a cross-sectional survey of 222 Southern California adult outpatients. Archives of Physical Medicine and Rehabilitation 81: 757–763

Lucke KT 1998 Pulmonary management following acute SCI. Journal of Neuroscience Nursing 30(2): 91–103

Mahanes D, Lewis R 2004 Weaning of the neurologically impaired patient. Critical Care Nursing Clinics of North America 16: 387–393

Mansel J, Norman J 1990 Respiratory complications and management of spinal cord injuries. Chest 97(6): 1446–1452

Maynard F, Muth A 1987 The choice to end life as a ventilator-dependent quadriplegic. Archives of Physical and Medical Rehabilitation 68: 862–864

McCool FD, Pichurko BM, Slutsky AS et al 1986 Changes in lung volume and rib configuration with abdominal binding in quadriplegia. Journal of Applied Physiology 60(4): 1198–1202

McEvoy DR, Mykytyn I, Sajkov D et al 1995 Sleep apnoea in patients with quadriplegia. Thorax 50: 613–619

McKinley WO 1996 Late return of diaphragm function in a ventilator-dependent patient with a high tetraplegia: case report, and interactive review. Spinal Cord 34: 626–629

Menter RR, Bach JR, Brown DJ et al 1997 A review of the respiratory management of a patient with high level tetraplegia. Spinal Cord 35: 805–808

Oo T, Watt J, Soni BM, Sett PK 1999 Delayed diaphragm recovery in 12 patients after high cervical spinal cord injury. A retrospective review of the diaphragm status of 107 patients ventilated after acute spinal cord injury. Spinal Cord 37: 117–122

Peterson P, Kirshblum S 2002 Pulmonary management of spinal cord injury. In: Kirshblum S, Campagnolo D, DeLisa J (eds) Spinal cord medicine. Lippincott, Williams & Wilkins Philadelphia, PA, 136–155

Peterson W, Barbalata L, Brooks CA et al 1999 The effect of tidal volumes on the time to wean persons with high tetraplegia from ventilators. Spinal Cord 37: 284–288

Peterson W, Charlifue MA, Gerhart A, Whiteneck G 1994 Two methods of weaning persons with quadriplegia from mechanical ventilators. Paraplegia 32: 98–103

Pryor JA 1999 Physiotherapy for airway clearance in adults. European Respiratory Journal 14(6): 1418–1424

Purtilo R 1986 Ethical issues in the treatment of chronic ventilator dependent patients. Archives of Physical and Medical Rehabilitation 67: 718–721

Rose L, Geary M, Jackson J, Morgan M 1987 The effect of lung volume expansion in tetraplegia. Physiotherapy Practice 3: 163–167

Roth EJ, Lu A, Primack S et al 1997 Ventilatory function in cervical and high thoracic spinal cord injury. American Journal of Physical Medicine and Rehabilitation 76(4): 262–267

Sancho J, Servera E, Diaz J et al 2004 Efficacy of mechanical insufflation-exsufflation in medically stable patients with amytrophic lateral sclerosis. Chest 125: 1400–1405

Scott MD, Frost F, Supinski G 1993 The effect of body position and abdominal binders in chronic tetraplegic subjects more than 15 years post-injury. Journal of the American Paraplegia Society 16(2): 117

Short DJ, Stradling JR, Williams SJ 1992 Prevalence of sleep apnoea in patients over 40 years of age with spinal cord lesions. Journal of Neurology, Neurosurgery, and Psychiatry 55: 1032–1036

Stanic U, Kandare F, Jaeger R, Sorli J 2000 Functional electrical stimulation of abdominal muscles to augment tidal volume in spinal cord injury. IEEE Transactions on Rehabilitation Engineering 8(1): 30–34

Stockhammer E, Tobon A, Michel F et al 2002 Characteristics of sleep apnea syndrome in tetraplegic patients. Spinal Cord 40: 286–294

Stiller K, Huff N 1999 Respiratory muscle training for tetraplegic patients: a literature review. Australian Journal of Physiotherapy 45: 291–299

Taylor PN, Tromans AM, Harris KR, Swain ID 2002 Electrical stimulation of abdominal muscles for control of blood pressure and augmentation of cough in a C3/4 level tetraplegic. Spinal Cord 40: 34–36

Thomas E, Paulson SS 1994 Protocol for weaning the SCI patient. SCI Nursing 11(2): 42–45

Tromans AM, Mecci M, Barrett FH et al 1998 The use of the BiPAP biphasic positive airway pressure system in acute spinal cord injury. Spinal Cord 36: 481–484

Tzeng AC, Bach JR 2000 Prevention of pulmonary morbidity for patients with neuromuscular disease. Chest 118(5): 1390–1396

Uijl SG, Houtman S, Folgering HTM, Hopman MTE 1999 Training of the respiratory muscles in individuals with tetraplegia. Spinal Cord 37: 575–579

Van Buren R, Lemons MD, Franklin C, Wagner MD Jr 1994 Respiratory complications after cervical spinal cord injury. Spine 19(20): 2315–2320

Vianello A, Corrado A, Arcaro G et al 2005 Mechanical insufflation-exsufflation improves outcomes for neuromuscular disease patients with respiratory tract infections. American Journal of Physical Medicine and Rehabilitation 84(2): 83–88

Wang AY, Jaeger RJ, Yarkony GM, Turba RM 1997 Cough in spinal cord injured patients: the relationship between motor level and peak expiratory flow. Spinal Cord 35: 299–302

Wang TG, Wang YH, Tang FT et al 2002 Resistive inspiratory muscle training in sleep-disordered breathing of traumatic tetraplegia. Archives of Physical Medicine and Rehabilitation 83(4): 491–496

Whitney J, Harden B, Keilty S 2002 Assisted cough: a new technique. Physiotherapy 88(4): 201–207

Wicks A, Menter R 1986 Long-term outlook in quadriplegic patients with initial ventilator dependency. Chest 3: 406–410

Yeo JD, Walsh J, Rutkowski S et al 1998 Mortality following spinal cord injury. Spinal Cord 36: 329–336

Young T, Palta M, Dempsey J et al 1993 The occurrence of sleep-disordered breathing among middle-aged adults. New England Journal of Medicine 328: 1230–1235

Zupan A, Savrin R, Erjavec T et al 1997 Effects of respiratory muscle training and electrical stimulation of abdominal muscles on respiratory capabilities in tetraplegic patients. Spinal Cord 35: 540–545

Further reading

Facts and figures at a glance. University of Alabama, Spinal Cord Injury Information Network. Online. (*www.spinalcord.uab.edu/show. asp?durki=21446*)(updated June 2006, accessed 18 July 2007)

Woman welcomes 'right to die' ruling. *news.bbc.co.uk/1/hi/health/1887281.stm* (accessed 18 July 2007)

Chapter 17

Dysfunctional breathing

Diana M Innocenti, Fiona Troup

INTRODUCTION

To breathe is the bedrock of our mortal life. It is the activity on which our physiological and our psychological being depends. Most of the time we are unaware of breathing, yet as soon as something physical or psychological causes it to change, it immediately impinges on our conscious sense of well-being and causes a range of sensations from discomfort, through dyspnoea, to fear of death. This chapter looks in detail at some aspects of overbreathing, or hyperventilation and the reordering of this disordered pattern. It will also consider more briefly the re-education of disordered breathing patterns in asthma and emphysema and in relation to musculoskeletal dysfunction.

The term 'dysfunctional breathing' is, in itself, confusing. One would expect it to mean that a particular breathing pattern does not fulfil its function, yet it appears to be used as a synonym for hyperventilation. In a review Morgan (2002) remarks on 'this new term', that:

> 'Dysfunctional breathing is therefore just the latest imprecise description of a behaviour and symptom-complex which remains unexplained . . . definition of dysfunctional breathing and methods for identifying it require careful validation'

Since the previous edition of this book, the term dysfunctional breathing has become more popular. Papers relating to dysfunctional breathing in asthma and chronic obstructive pulmonary disease (COPD) have been published and the work relating to hyperventilation has become more varied. A deeper understanding of how musculoskeletal dysfunction can restrict the normal free pattern of breathing is resulting in new approaches to treatment.

However, there is still no clear understanding of the relationships between the psychological, anatomical, physiological, pathological and behavioural variables as they appear to affect the central breathing pattern generator and/or disrupt the physical movements of breathing in differing ways.

CONTROL OF BREATHING

The respiratory system is the only autonomic function that can be controlled voluntarily. This complex system (Fig. 17.1) is self-sustaining and is centred on the respiratory-pacemaker-generator in the brain stem. It is moderated by oxygen and carbon dioxide chemoreceptors, lung tissue reflexes, mechanoreceptors in the ventilatory and the peripheral muscles and joints, emotion, temperature and vestibular influences. This sensory feedback may be filtered through, and integrated by, the reticular formation and limbic autonomic system or be transmitted directly to the breathing centre. Voluntary and behavioural stimuli from the cerebral cortex also feed back to the breathing centre and can influence the respiratory muscles directly by bypassing or overriding the reflex pathways. The cerebral cortex is also responsible for perceiving dyspnoea. Adaptation of any of the components of these motor or sensory pathways or

centres of respiration could influence or concentrate disordered responses, breathing patterns and carbon dioxide levels. This results, in time, in what appears to be a resetting of the respiratory centre's triggering mechanisms and the formation of new conditioned patterns of breathing.

Why are some people more prone to respond to physiological, psychological or environmental stimuli with grossly altered breathing patterns? Clark & Cochrane (1970), considering patients with chronic bronchitis and emphysema, concluded that the sensitivity of the respiratory centres is personality linked and related to mood-state and disposition. Papp et al (1993) discuss the theory of an inherently unstable autonomic nervous system and a hypersensitive respiratory control system. Cowley & Roy-Byrne (1987) suggest that this underlying biological and often inherited vulnerability, leading to a hypersensitive central nervous 'alarm system', may be triggered inappropriately, causing a premature 'fight or flight' response.

HYPERVENTILATION

Hyperventilation may be acute, it may coexist with organic disease or may occur in a chronic idiopathic form. In the past few years, together with ongoing

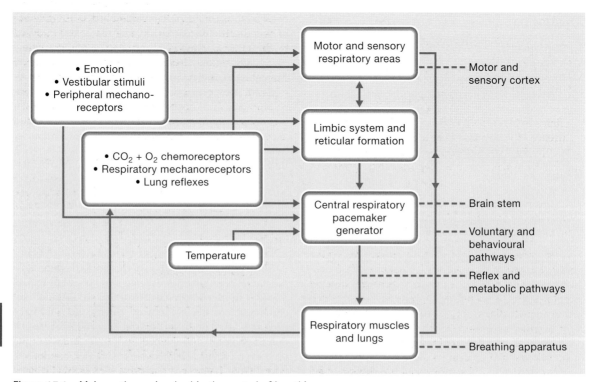

Figure 17.1 Major pathways involved in the control of breathing.

research into the relationships between hyperventilation and panic disorders, researchers and practitioners have noted strong relationships between hyperventilation and vestibular and musculoskeletal disorders. These findings have now influenced some treatment programmes and investigative procedures.

Acute hyperventilation

Acute hyperventilation or breathing in excess of metabolic requirements results in a lowering of alveolar partial pressure of carbon dioxide ($PACO_2$), arterial partial pressure of carbon dioxide ($PaCO_2$) and a respiratory alkalosis. It is a normal response to pain or psychological or emotional states such as stress, anxiety, anger or fright. It may result in self-regulatory paraesthesia, dizziness, palpitation and, in extreme circumstances, tetany.

Chronic hyperventilation

The chronic fluctuating disorder of chronic hyperventilation or idiopathic hyperventilation is difficult to define. It has been characterized as:

'. . . sustained arterial and alveolar hypocapnia [commonly to levels below 30 mmHg] with no discernable aetiology'

(Jack et al 2003)

and as:

'. . . a physiological response to abnormally increased respiratory "drive" which can be caused by a wide range of organic, psychiatric and physiological disorders or a combination of these'

(Gardner & Bass 1989)

Clinically it can be recognized by the spontaneous occurrence of multiple and alarming symptoms.

In 1937 Kerr et al described a group of patients who, in addition to their anxious tensional state, presented with:

'. . . a variety of symptoms referable to many structures in the body; and in whom hyperventilation precipitates and maintains a state of hyperirritability'

In the table of their laboratory work they coined the term 'hyperventilation syndrome' (Kerr et al 1937). A syndrome is, by definition, identified by its combination of symptoms and is therefore not able to be contained within a single diagnostic measurement. The difficulty regarding the understanding of the various mechanisms producing the symptoms, of finding a definitive form of diagnostic test and agreeing a more appropriate name for this disorder, is still creating some discussion in the literature, as views change regarding the possible causes

and effects (Gardner 2000, Hornsveld et al 1996, Howell 1997, Malmberg et al 2000, Troosters et al 1999). Howell (1997) and Tweeddale et al (1994) considered that 'behavioural breathlessness' may be a more appropriate term, but as many patients do not experience breathlessness as their main symptom (if at all) Howell considered at the time, that there was nothing to be gained by changing the name.

Although anxiety was a component in Kerr's original description of hyperventilation syndrome, anxiety is not always present. Also, there may not always be a hyperventilation component in anxiety. With no universally agreed term for this subtle form of chronically disturbed breathing, the terms hyperventilation syndrome (HVS), idiopathic symptomatic hyperventilation (IH) and behavioural breathlessness continue to be used.

HYPERVENTILATION SYNDROME

The diagnosis was not uncommon in the past (Baker 1934, Wood 1941) but in the present technological era, hyperventilation in its various chronic recurrent forms often tends to go unrecognized and the diverse symptoms are labelled as functional. Even though it has been shown that severe chronic hyperventilation with profound hypocapnia can be present in the absence of psychiatric, respiratory or other organic abnormalities (Bass & Gardner 1985), patients may attend a succession of clinics, presenting with increasingly disturbing symptoms and yet receive little help. The new anxiety aroused by the situation increases the hyperventilation–anxiety spiral, which may already be in operation. The spiral may be perpetuated by physiological and/or psychological causes, setting up conditioned reflexes of new and incorrect habitual patterns of breathing and a resetting, or loss of fine tuning, of the respiratory centre's trigger mechanisms (Fig. 17.2).

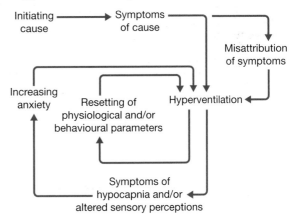

Figure 17.2 Factors contributing to the hyperventilation–anxiety spiral.

17

Hyperventilation is today likely to be recognized more often in association with panic disorders or phobic states because of its causal, consequential or perpetuating relationships (Cowley & Roy-Byrne 1987). Patients presenting with panic disorder or anxiety (van den Hout et al 1992) or anxiety and evidence of depression (Jack et al 2003) have been shown to have lower resting levels of carbon dioxide than normal. Some may demonstrate a greater than normal sensitivity of the basilar artery's response to hypocarbia (Ball & Shekhar 1997).

Hyperventilation has been shown to be prevalent in patients with vestibular dysfunction. This could be caused by the anxiety of the condition, but for some patients neither the hyperventilation nor the vestibular dysfunction provokes anxiety (Humphriss et al 2004). Ongoing work demonstrates a relationship between the vestibular and respiratory pathways in the brain stem, the contribution of the vestibular system to respiratory muscle activity and cardiovascular control during changes of posture and movement, and posture instability following hyperventilation (Yates & Bronstein 2005, Yates & Miller 1998, Yates et al 2002). Stress, acute pain and chronic pain may often result in hyperventilation producing hypocapnia (Terekhin & Forster 2006).

SIGNS AND SYMPTOMS

The vast array of commonly reported signs and symptoms can be loosely grouped as they affect different systems (Table 17.1). Timmons (1994) suggests that it would be useful to have a comprehensive validated list of symptoms, in order to hasten history taking and to facilitate comparisons of therapeutic trials. Few, if any, studies have looked at the association of symptoms with age, sex, personality traits and causal factors.

Some patients present with a constant resting level of hypocapnia and others present with resting levels of carbon dioxide within the normal range. Both groups feel generally unwell and experience 'attacks' featuring a galaxy of symptoms, which appear to occur sometimes with no apparent reason. Further hypocapnia may or may not be recorded at these times. In some patients the symptoms seem to precede the event of hypocapnia rather than be a consequence (Hornsveld et al 1996). If symptoms in some patients are not generated by hypocapnia, we must ask what other mechanisms could be the cause. Could the symptoms be a direct consequence of the disordered movements of overbreathing and their abnormal feedback? And if so, which sensory, motor or behavioural mechanisms could be involved?

Hypocapnia induces vascular constriction, resulting in decreased blood flow, and as a response to the Bohr effect there is also inhibition of transfer of oxygen from

Table 17.1 Commonly reported signs and symptoms

System	Signs and symptoms
Cardiovascular	Palpitation Chest pain (pseudoangina) Vasoconstriction
Gastrointestinal	Dysphagia Dyspepsia Epigastric pain Diarrhoea
General	Exhaustion Lethargy Weakness Headache Sleep disturbance Excessive sweating Disturbance of concentration and memory
Musculoskeletal	Altered muscle tone Muscle pains Tremors Involuntary contractions Cramps Tetany (rarely)
Neurological	Paraesthesia Lack of coordination Dizziness Disturbance of vision and hearing Syncope (rarely)
Respiratory	Breathlessness Bronchospasm Difficulty in taking a satisfying breath Excessive sighing/yawning Chest pain Irregular breathing pattern
Psychological/psychiatric	Anxiety Panic attacks Feelings of unreality Phobic states Depersonalization

haemoglobin in the circulating blood to the tissue cells. Hypocapnic vasoconstriction is probably the cause of the characteristic range of cerebral, peripheral and cardiac symptoms. As the cerebral symptoms of hypoglycaemia are similar to those of hypocapnia, the cerebral effects of hyperventilation are highlighted at times of low blood sugar and it has been suggested that hyperventilation increases circulating histamine, which may be the cause of the high incidence of allergies reported (Lum 1994). Fluctuations in $PaCO_2$ can have a destabilizing effect on the autonomic system resulting in a sympathetic dominance (Freeman & Nixon 1985). The patients are often in a state of arousal. It has been shown that the mean urinary excretion of adrenaline in a group of persons who hyperventilate was three times as high as in a group of normals (Folgering et al 1983). Mogyoros et al (1997) suggest that hyperventilation has a selective action on nerve conduction, which is greater on sensory than motor fibres. This may explain why hyperventilation induces paraesthesia before fasciculation.

Altered patterns of breathing can cause musculoskeletal dysfunction. The combination of habitual overuse, ischaemia and increased sympathetic drive increases myofascial tone via smooth muscle cell contraction and leads to the evolution of active myofascial trigger points (Chaitow 2002). Pain thresholds are also reduced. Patients with dysfunctional breathing may describe a history of neck and/or thoracic pain and stiffness, headaches, low back pain and temporomandibular joint dysfunction. Orofacial pain is also associated with this patient group (Hruska 1997).

The diaphragm has a place in postural control and spinal stability, such that control of intra-abdominal pressure occurs through coordinated activity of the diaphragm, pelvic floor and transversus abdominis muscles (Hodges & Gandevia 2000, Hodges et al 1997). Dysfunction in this stabilizing mechanism has been implicated in recurrent low back pain. Postural activity in the diaphragm (and transversus abdominis) was shown to be reduced or absent after only 60 seconds of experimentally induced hypercapnia, suggesting that stability of the spine may be compromised in some respiratory disease or dysfunction (Hodges et al 2001). It is hypothesized that such a compromise may lead to increased potential for injury to spinal structures and reduced postural control (Hodges et al 2001); however, further research is indicated. Disorders of breathing (and continence) have been shown to have a higher association with low back pain than obesity and physical activity (Smith et al 2006).

Alternatively, acute or chronic musculoskeletal disorders may precipitate breathing dysfunction due to pain, postural compensations, and structural and functional changes in the fascial, neural, muscular and skeletal systems. The typical flexed posture of a person in pain impedes normal respiratory function. Musculoskeletal dysfunction such as thoracic spine hypomobility, rib immobility, and short overactive accessory respiratory muscles can directly cause dysfunctional breathing patterns to develop (Chaitow 2002).

The relationship between chronic fatigue syndrome (CFS) and hypocapnia is questioned and Naschitz et al (2006) suggest that unrecognized hypocapnia is common in CFS. Interestingly, patients with CFS also frequently experience chronic musculoskeletal pain (Nijs et al 2006). Patients with hypermobility syndrome commonly present with dysfunctional breathing patterns and chronic pain. Hypermobility syndrome may have an effect on ventilation because of abnormally compliant lungs, disordered lung receptors, hypermobility of the thoracovertebral joints and/or pain. Hypermobility syndrome has been shown to be associated with fibromyalgia (Ofluoglu et al 2006) and CFS (Nijs et al 2006). Could dysfunctional breathing be the common link between these three conditions?

CAUSES OF HYPERVENTILATION

The many circumstances that may stimulate a hyperventilatory response (Box 17.1) may or may not become a chronic disorder. Other than HVS being the primary cause of the patient's symptoms, we have seen that it is not uncommon for chronic hyperventilation to coexist with other conditions and to be a sustaining factor within the complex interaction of a number of physiological, organic and psychological disorders (Gardner 1994). Before embarking on a treatment programme, it is necessary to ensure that the patient has been suitably investigated in order to diagnose any underlying treatable disease or disorder and to recognize any other possible coexisting factors. Where pain is believed to be a causative or contributing factor, appropriate management strategies should be investigated.

DIAGNOSTIC TESTS

There are no generally accepted measurable diagnostic criteria and it is probably not possible to devise a satisfactory or conclusive diagnostic test for HVS because of the multifactorial effects and complex systemic interactions. Various tests have been described but time has shown that *none should be used alone*. Each test can be useful when used with other information.

The voluntary hyperventilation provocation test (HVPT)

The hyperventilation provocation test (HVPT) (Hardonk & Beumer 1979) records end-tidal $PACO_2$ and all symptoms provoked during and after the test. Using end-tidal $PACO_2$ recordings, the patient is requested to hyperventilate for 3 minutes. If the $PACO_2$ falls by at least 1.33 kPa (10 mmHg) and the level of recovery is less than two-thirds of the former resting level after

17

Box 17.1   Some causes of hyperventilation

Drugs	Drug ingestion (causing acidosis or respiratory dyskinesia)
	Alcohol
	Caffeine
	Nicotine
Organic disorder	Anaemia
	Asthma
	Chronic severe pain
	Central nervous system disorders
	Cerebral tumour
	Diabetes mellitus
	Head trauma
	Musculoskeletal disorders
	Nasal congestion
	Pneumonia
	Pulmonary embolus
	Pulmonary oedema (LVF)
	Recurrent laryngeal nerve paralysis
	Vestibular disorder
Physiological	Altitude
	Pyrexia
	Pregnancy
	Luteal phase of the menstrual cycle
Psychiatric	Anxiety
	Depression
Psychological	Anger
	Anxiety
	Effects of torture
	Panic disorders
	Phobic states

3 minutes, the result is recorded as a positive diagnosis of a hyperventilation syndrome. Nevertheless, as about a quarter of 'normals' also show this phenomenon, a lowering of $PACO_2$ and slow recovery is not in itself diagnostic. Immediately after the completion of the recordings the patient is asked to compare any symptoms provoked during the test with recognized complaints. When two or more major symptoms are reproduced, the HVPT is considered positive. Generally, tingling of fingers and dizziness are not included because these symptoms occur in 'normal' subjects. However, some patients report that some provoked symptoms are only 'similar' but not the 'same'. Sometimes provoked symptoms are new experiences and not related to the patient's complaints. Others may be helped by recognizing that altered breathing can precipitate their symptoms. Caution should be exercised on using this test if the patient complains of cardiac symp-

toms or pseudoangina. As yet this test has not been standardized.

The Nijmegen questionnaire

This was first drawn up as a list of 16 complaints chosen by a team of specialists from different disciplines, from 45 clinically relevant symptoms related to hyperventilation syndromes (van Doorn et al 1982). The complaints fall into three categories or dimensions, corresponding with the classic triad of breathing disruption, paraesthesiae and central nervous system effects. The list does not include fatigue or behavioural disturbances. Patients score on a five-point scale from 0–4 (0 = never, 1 = rare, 2 = sometimes, 3 = often, 4 = very often) against each of the 16 listed symptoms and a score over 23 is recognized as positive (Box 17.2). The efficacy of the questionnaire was investigated by comparing patients who hyperventilate with persons who do not. It showed a high ability to differentiate between the two groups (van Dixhoorn & Duivenvoorden 1985) and, although not conclusive, it was recognized that the questionnaire was suitable to be used as a screening instrument in diagnosing HVS when used with additional information. A correlation has been shown between positively rated Nijmegen questionnaire results (score of 24 or more) and positive HVPT results (recognition of at least two major symptoms) (Vansteenkiste et al 1991).

Humphriss et al (2004) found that, despite some limitations, the Nijmegen questionnaire is a quick and easy to administer assessment tool to detect HVS in patients seen for vestibular assessment. It is important to diagnose the condition in vestibular disease as it has been suggested that hyperventilation disrupts vestibular compensation and increases postural sway. Conventional vestibular rehabilitation may be only suboptimally successful until a normal breathing pattern has been re-established. The questionnaire has been used to diagnose HVS in some patients complaining of nasal congestion and subsequent breathing re-education has been successful in correcting the nasal congestion without further surgery (Bartley 2005).

The questionnaire can be useful for physiotherapists to record symptoms and, if used at regular intervals, to record the changing status in relation to treatment. A final score at discharge could be used as a semi-objective outcome measure.

The 'think test'

The 'think test' (Nixon & Freeman 1988) provides a patient-specific stimulation, which can have an advantage over unspecific challenges in testing for episodic hypocapnia or a change in the breathing pattern. The patient is invited to close the eyes and then to recall the

17

Box 17.2   Nijmegen questionnaire

	NEVER 0	RARE 1	SOMETIMES 2	OFTEN 3	VERY OFTEN 4
Chest pain					
Feeling tense					
Blurred vision					
Dizzy spells					
Feeling confused					
Faster or deeper breathing					
Short of breath					
Tight feelings in chest					
Bloated feelings in stomach					
Tingling fingers					
Unable to breathe deeply					
Stiff fingers or arms					
Tight feelings around mouth					
Cold hands or feet					
Palpitations					
Feelings of anxiety					

emotions and sensations surrounding certain situations that have caused distress or provoked symptoms. A change in the breathing pattern and/or a fall in $PaCO_2$ greater than 1.33 kPa (10 mmHg) is considered to be significant.

Ambulatory monitoring of transcutaneous carbon dioxide

The transcutaneous sensor is attached to the patient who is instructed how to press the 'event button' and in the use of a diary. The 'event button' marks the recording tape and the diary entry records:

- type of symptom
- severity of symptoms (on a visual analogue scale 0–8)

- type of activity or non-activity
- the extent of the physical exertion (visual analogue scale 0–8) (Pilsbury & Hibbert 1987).

Prolonged monitoring may produce helpful data (Hibbert & Pilsbury 1988).

Patients with recurrent laryngeal nerve palsy can become fatigued during prolonged phonation, due to excessive breath loss while trying to maintain sufficient subglottal pressure for speech. Transcutaneous carbon dioxide ($P_{Tc}CO_2$) recordings have shown significant decreases in $PaCO_2$ in these patients. Education of the disrupted pattern and control of the expiratory phase during vocalization has produced improvement in $PaCO_2$ levels on $P_{Tc}CO_2$ and a decrease in symptoms (Miyazaki et al 1999).

17

Breath-holding time

This is a semi-objective measure that generally shows a direct relationship between the maximum breath-holding time (BHT) and the resting $PaCO_2$ (short breath-holding time is usually associated with a low or unstable resting $PaCO_2$). Breath-holding time tends to increase as the breathing pattern becomes more regular and stable. The patient is given a description of the method and then asked to take a normal breath in, followed by a normal breath out and to hold the breath in the resting phase until it becomes too uncomfortable to hold any longer. This breath-holding time is recorded. Some ask for the breath-hold after a full inspiration and a full expiration. Whichever method is used, it is essential to use a similar process and a similar posture each time. Standardization of the procedure would be helpful. The average BHT is suggested to be approximately 30 seconds (Bradley 2002). The patient will hope to increase the BHT if it is low but it is not helpful to know the norm at this time, as it may cause a forced hold time, which could be damaging to the process. If breath-holding time is recorded at regular intervals it could be used as a semi-objective outcome measure.

PATTERNS OF BREATHING

Quiet normal breathing patterns at approximately 8–14 breaths per minute at rest involve three phases:

- an active inspiratory phase
- a passive expiratory phase
- a slight pause at the end of expiration.

During inspiration, the active descent of the diaphragm is reflected as a gentle forward swelling of the abdomen and there may be minimal movement outwards of the lower ribs. On natural passive expiration the abdomen and lower chest return to the resting position. During exercise, the minimal lower thoracic movement increases and as exercise increases so does the thoracic involvement. Rate, volume and place of movement change with posture, motion, exercise, varying stimuli, disease or dysfunction. The act of inspiration naturally draws air in through the nose where it is warmed, filtered, moistened and the flow controlled before entering the airways. Air that is drawn in through the mouth bypasses this conditioning.

Breathing patterns, related to the chronic hyperventilation syndromes or idiopathic symptomatic hyperventilation, vary widely from gross upper thoracic movement with sternocleidomastoid and accessory muscle involvement at a rate as high as 50 breaths/min to a near-normal rate and volume and minimal upper thoracic movement. The degree of lower thoracic movement and abdominal movement also varies from almost nil to normal.

The respiratory rate and volume may be extremely irregular (Fig. 17.3) and the pattern interspersed with sighs, sniffs and yawns. At the other extreme, once habitual hypocapnia has been established, it may require only an occasional deep sigh to maintain the new low levels of carbon dioxide and the general breathing pattern may appear normal.

The breathing patterns vary with each patient and within the daily experience of each patient. The only constant feature in HVS is that the patient's breathing appears to respond inappropriately to the changing metabolic and emotional requirements of daily living and that symptoms generally vary throughout the day for no apparent reason. Often there are 'good days' and 'bad days'. There does not seem to be a strict correlation between the abnormality of the breathing pattern, the depression of $PaCO_2$ and the severity and type of symptoms.

REFERRAL FOR PHYSIOTHERAPY

There appear to be various groups of patients with symptoms related to overbreathing. Patients presenting for physiotherapy tend to fall into four main groups:

1. Hyperventilation syndrome (HVS) in the absence of psychiatric, respiratory or other organic abnormalities – generally there is low or fluctuating $PaCO_2$.
2. Chronic hyperventilation with associated physical symptoms, presenting with panic or phobic states, anxiety or other psychological disturbance. There may or may not be a low resting $PaCO_2$.
3. Chronic hyperventilation presenting as a conditioned physiological or behavioural pattern related to other organic conditions. Generally when the underlying condition is resolved, the hyperventilating component is also resolved. However, in some instances when the disordered breathing pattern has been conditioned, it needs to be addressed and treated in order to gain optimal resolution of any long-standing underlying problems as in chronic fatigue, vestibular, laryngeal, musculoskeletal and nasal congestive

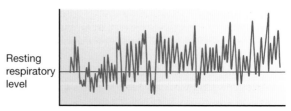

Resting respiratory level

Figure 17.3 Diagrammatic representation of an irregular pattern taken from a spirometry trace.

17

dysfunction. In order to prevent this perpetuating factor from obstructing resolution of the organic disorder an interdisciplinary approach should be followed. Whether the hyperventilation is the primary or secondary factor, an improvement of subjective symptoms, exercise tolerance, general fitness and quality of life can be gained by re-educating the breathing pattern, with the subsequent reordering of the patient's responses to the internal and external environment.

4. Dysfunctional breathing with a concurrent musculoskeletal complaint, or a musculoskeletal complaint with associated dysfunctional breathing. The direct relationship between pain and hyperventilation has long been documented (Glyn et al 1981) and is seen frequently in the clinical setting. The patient may initially present to outpatient physiotherapy with an acute injury that has affected the pattern of breathing such as a rib injury, whiplash, cervical, thoracic or lumbar pain, or following surgery. The physiotherapist should ensure that correction of the breathing pattern forms an early part of management. Alternatively the patient may complain of a complex chronic musculoskeletal problem whereby the dysfunctional breathing may be a causative factor, secondary to the pain or an integral factor in perpetuating the cycle. In this patient group, clinical findings suggest that both the breathing and musculoskeletal systems should be addressed for optimal outcome.

OVERVIEW

Re-education of the breathing pattern for all groups will follow similar lines, involving a conscious control of nose breathing, place of movement, rate, volume and regularity of the breathing cycle. If the $PaCO_2$ is low or labile, the programme will be devised to help to raise and stabilize the resting level. If low $PaCO_2$ is not an issue, attention will remain with making the pattern slow and regular and in correcting the place of movement. A predominantly relaxed, passive abdominal movement (reflecting the movement of the diaphragm) is preferred and movement directed away from the upper thorax and shoulder girdle. This abdominal pattern of movement may in turn help to induce physical and mental relaxation. Relaxation is often aided by a regular, slow pattern of breathing. It may be necessary with some patients to teach and practise a suitable relaxation technique before, during or after the breathing control. The long-term goal is to re-establish a more normal, slower and personally acceptable pattern of movement that decreases ventilation sufficiently to raise the resting $PaCO_2$ by a small measure.

In the short term, until the new pattern of breathing becomes the natural, constant, unconscious, spontaneous method of breathing, the patient is likely to continue to experience episodes of symptoms. Some symptoms may be provoked if the patient 'tries too hard' and, by overcompensating in one component of the new pattern, increases ventilation rather than decreases it. Early warning of these phenomena must be built into the sessions. Other symptoms may be related to certain recognizable situations, stresses or exercise, precipitating disordered breathing before the patient has mastered control of the new pattern. The patient needs to know of these frustrating possibilities and pitfalls and be taught to take 'first aid' measures of controlled breath-holding or rebreathing expired carbon dioxide from a bag or cupped hands. In time, with reassurance and perseverance, it should be possible to control the new way of breathing and ward off any episodes of falling carbon dioxide levels, or inappropriate breathing by identifying the provoking situations and practising precautionary measures.

Initially treatment sessions usually take approximately 1 hour. Outpatients should attend weekly at first. As the patient progresses the sessions become less frequent. Some patients who have been diagnosed early and who have no underlying pathology may need only 2 or 3 sessions; others, with organic disorders, will need more time and those with background psychological history may need 12 or 14 sessions spaced out over 12 or 18 months. At the time of discharge it is important for the patient to know that it is possible to keep in touch and to have a telephone number to call in an emergency for advice or review if necessary. Inpatients will probably be treated daily at first. Sessions will be given less frequently as soon as possible, to allow the patient to take more responsibility and to practise alone.

TREATMENT

Assessment

The assessment should include:

- history
- signs and symptoms
- personality
- physical examination.

History

The patient may have been referred for treatment with a breathing problem related to an organic cause. If not, it is helpful to ask open-ended questions to elicit when the patient first became aware of problems and the response to them. The giving of the history and the

17

description of the symptoms may trigger unpredictable responses from the patient which could slow up the process, yet help to bond an understanding relationship between patient and physiotherapist when handled sensitively (it is always helpful to have a box of tissues to hand). The first awareness of a problem may have been an acute 'attack', for instance driving home on the motorway on a Friday night after a stressful week and experiencing dizziness, tingling in the limbs and central chest pain. The response to this could be that of believing it to be a heart attack. This would be very understandable, especially if a member of the family had recently died of coronary disease. The anxiety would stimulate the respiratory rate further and the symptoms would increase, possibly to the point of admission to the nearest accident and emergency department. Misrepresentation of the symptoms of an acute short-term episode of stress may cause a single natural response to be transformed into a pattern of inappropriate responses thereafter.

Signs and symptoms may not present so dramatically. Commonly symptoms may be traced back to a history of glandular fever, a long viral illness or low-grade fever, bereavement, failed expectations, change of lifestyle or job or house, family breakdown, frightening experience, fear of inability to perform to targets and fear of failure or prolonged emotional pressures, conflicts or abuse. A definitive trigger point may not be found and the first experience of the disorder may be related to an array of stimuli or events that happened together or in close succession. History of musculoskeletal pain, previous injuries or accidents, past surgical history and generalized feelings of muscular tenderness, tension and stiffness should be recorded as any of these may be the underlying cause.

Family history. Any similar symptoms, allergy, anxiety, hypermobility syndrome, cardiac or respiratory disease experienced by other members of the family should be elicited. Not uncommonly, the habit of overbreathing can be traced back to family illness patterns or relationships.

Childhood history. History of premature birth; oxygen therapy or artificial ventilation immediately after birth are incidents which are increasingly reported. It is also helpful to record childhood general health, including any tonsil or adenoid problems, physical ability, exercise tolerance, allergy and some idea of the quality of the relationships at school and at home.

Signs and symptoms

There may be difficulty in describing the symptoms, as many of them are not usually within one's everyday experience. The symptoms generally occur when the brain is trying to function in a hypoxic condition or the patient is trying to respond to an abnormal situation, thus causing difficulty in perception, retention and recall of phenomena. A full list of symptoms, including any allergies, should be recorded, listed and numbered in relation to severity, occurrence and concern. The degree to which a symptom is incapacitating could rate 0–10 on a *disability scale* and the degree to which a symptom is fear provoking could rate 0–10 on a *distress scale*, while the frequency of occurrence of the symptom could also be rated 0–10. These records will give a guide to progress and ultimately could give a semi-objective outcome measure.

Assessment of personality

A detailed analysis of the personality is neither possible nor necessary in this setting. However, a simple assessment may be made by noticing the posture, facial expression, demeanour of the hands, manner in which the history is given and the patient's emotional responses and reactions to the situations related in the history. One patient may be overtly obsessive and perfectionist and obviously reacting against the uncertainties of life, while another may be superficially tranquil, masking the underlying burden of troubles and emotions that are being carried. These may come spilling out at any time during the treatment sessions when the patient begins to feel safe.

Physical examination

It is wise to complete a physical examination; however, it may not always be necessary if pertinent information is given in the referral. When examination is deemed necessary and with the patient's chest unclothed, note should be made of:

- general postural alignment including spinal alignment and head position

- the shape and posture of the chest and shoulder girdle, and abdominal and accessory muscle tone. Observe for pectus excavatum, asymmetries and any physical deformity

- relative breathing movements of the chest and abdomen

- the findings from auscultation.

Generally the pattern of breathing can be assessed with the patient dressed. The place of movement, size, regularity and rate of breathing should be recorded and whether the patient breathes through the nose or mouth. The physiotherapist should have a watch with a second hand available to record the breathing rate per minute. It will be helpful to make a record of the number of breaths per minute at each visit and ultimately this

17

record can be used as an outcome measure. The patient should not be informed at this stage that the rate is being recorded nor of the rate per minute, as the re-education of the pattern will take place at the level of the individual breath or phase of breath. A knowledge of the greater timescale, in the early stages, can be damaging as the patient may try to take fewer breaths per minute without regard to the size of the breath.

Treatment plan

The overall plan should be discussed with the patient. The transfer of oxygen and carbon dioxide should be described in lay terms and related to the patient's manner of moving air. Once patients are able to connect their symptoms to the manner of breathing and not to some life-threatening disease, they are usually only too delighted to make a firm commitment to learn more about the manner of breathing and its control and to take responsibility for the home treatment programme. They happily recognize that it is possible to help themselves and to gain a degree of mastery over symptoms and the environment.

Treatment is not a matter of learning 'breathing exercises', but of learning how to feel, alter and control the manner of breathing. The treatment plan in the short term (to control symptoms) and in the long term (spontaneously to maintain a corrected pattern of breathing) should be described and agreed. Agreement should also be sought to look constructively at the activities of the day and to try to identify possible factors influencing the onset of symptoms. A fitness programme may be discussed at this stage, but it should not be introduced until later in the plan when there is some semblance of breathing control.

Breathing awareness education

Probably the most comfortable position for learning about breathing is lying with suitable support. Most people with chronic hyperventilation do not have respiratory disease and therefore can lie flat without distress. The suggested position is supported with one or two pillows under the head and under the knees. The knee pillow(s) help to prevent tension in the abdominal muscles and thus enables a natural passive abdominal movement during the respiratory cycle. In lying, the abdominal contents move up somewhat into the thorax and during inspiration act as a stimulating natural resistance to the descent of the diaphragm. For patients who find that this position is uncomfortable or if it precipitates breathlessness or a feeling of vulnerability, another position should be found. Relaxed sitting with adequate support is usually acceptable to most people.

The first step of breathing awareness is to help to bring the breathing pattern into the consciousness by beginning to concentrate on the feeling of the body movements in relation to the flow of air while breathing. Sensory input and body awareness are increased if the patient rests both hands on the abdomen. Some prefer to place the dominant hand on the abdomen and the other on the upper chest, better to distinguish the place of movement. This position may be helpful at certain times during re-education to confirm the movement pattern. These possible positions are personal preference, but proprioceptive input may be more positive for retraining if both hands are rested on the abdomen. The physiotherapist lightly covers them with her hands. This light contact helps to bond the physiotherapist–patient relationship and allows the physiotherapist to feel, as well as observe, the movements related to the breathing cycle.

Again, a simple description of respiration should be given to help the patient observe sensations and movements relating to the flow of air in and out and to the chest, diaphragmatic and abdominal movements. The patient is helped to 'internalize' these descriptions of airflow and body movement by using the imagination. If the patient is a mouth breather, time should be spent describing the purpose of breathing through the nose and practising nose breathing. Tuition and discussion should continue in this position until the physiotherapist is satisfied that the patient has grasped a basic and simple anatomical and physiological understanding. Generally the patient will become more relaxed as the interaction distracts from excess self-awareness.

Having had the breathing described, the patient is asked to close the eyes and try to feel and sense what is happening to the body with regard to the breathing. It may be necessary for the physiotherapist to relate what is happening.

Care must be taken not to direct the pattern but merely to describe. For example:

> 'You are now breathing in . . . and now you are breathing out'

> 'You are breathing in and your abdomen is swelling . . . and now your abdomen is falling back to rest'

> 'Can you feel your upper chest moving?'

> 'Can you feel your abdomen moving as you breathe in?'

At this early stage, the patient is learning to establish the relationships between air movement and the associated body movement and to recognize that as the air moves 'in' the body moves 'out' to accommodate the air

17

and vice versa. By this stage a feeling of discomfort may be experienced and an explanation must be given relating to the subconscious, reflex and automatic nature of breathing. When the act of breathing is brought into the consciousness – as it has to be for re-education – there will be some discomfort, which has to be recognized, accepted and yet, at the same time, disregarded. It is within this forum that changes can voluntarily take place. The patient is then asked to focus on the 'in breath' and notice when and how it starts and finishes. This 'quiet attentiveness' is then transferred to the 'out breath' and note taken of the beginning and end of this phase. Particular attention should be given to the end of the phase to recognize when the breath gently stops. The spontaneous rest point is identified as the natural rest point in the breathing cycle and the patient is helped to feel it as a place of relaxation, a place of balance, not a place of tension. It may be helpful to practise general relaxation into this place of 'no movement'. Most patients can accept this experience and begin to recognize it as a welcome rest.

In order to recognize the full breathing capacity it is helpful to ask the patient to hold the breath at the upper point of the tidal volume and then to request a continuation of inspiration until full inflation is achieved. In this way it is possible to experience the inspiratory capacity. Similarly, the expiratory reserve can be experienced by breath-holding at the bottom of the tidal volume and then exhaling entirely by using all the expiratory muscles. Having practised these two manoeuvres, the patient will also realize that the relaxed tidal volume is relatively easy compared with the muscle work needed above and below the tidal flows. Patients may be able to use this information to perceive a change in their breathing pattern before symptoms occur. The learned corrective steps could then be made before full-blown symptoms take hold.

Breathing pattern re-education

The initial education and breathing awareness training is followed by re-education of any components that have been identified as being disordered. Any change, especially in volume or rate, must be balanced to attain a decrease in minute volume. The components are:

- tidal volume
- flow rate
- regularity
- place of movement.

The new breathing cycle may be of two or three phases, depending on the patient's body preference at the time. The two-phase cycle consists of a gentle inspiration followed by a slower expiration and hopefully, in time, progress to a more normal three-phase cycle. In a three-phase cycle the natural rest point at the end of expiration is inserted and/or extended. A gentle inspiration is followed by an easy (passive) expiration, which naturally changes into the rest period, which is comfortably extended until the next inspiration is gently initiated. Practice will help to lengthen this rest, but care has to be taken not to extend it to the point where a gasping inspiration is stimulated.

Method

By this stage the patient and physiotherapist should be aware of the volume and flow rate of each breath and the rhythm of the breathing pattern. The physiotherapist will describe these components and clarify with the patient what changes need to be made to decrease the minute volume and to regularize the pattern. Breathing is a very personal activity, and the new pattern should not be imposed by another from the outside. The changes should be made by the patient from within, guided carefully by the physiotherapist. They work together experimenting with changing certain aspects until a pattern evolves which fulfils the physiological requirements and which harmonizes with the patient's inner knowledge of well-being. The new pattern will be remade with the least possible interference.

As many patients who hyperventilate have a predominantly thoracic movement, this needs to be changed to a gentle passive movement of the abdominal wall. In general, most patients manage to recognize what is needed to change from a thoracic 'in and up' pattern to an abdominal 'in and down' pattern. However, some patients find it extremely difficult to obtain any abdominal movement and it may be necessary to spend several treatment sessions using different word combinations and images until a more relaxed abdominal movement is achieved. Should this not be the case then incorporation of manual therapy techniques, such as myofascial release techniques and mobilization, may be indicated. Large or forced breaths must be discouraged. Any increase in ventilation will increase or precipitate symptoms.

Some therapists like to place a heavy book or sandbag on the abdomen to give resistance and direction to the inspiratory movement. The weight is inanimate and therefore will need to be controlled during expiration; thus expiration cannot be a relaxed, passive, natural movement but rather the abdominal muscles will be called into an unnatural state of extrinsic work in order to control the expiratory phase, thus compromising the work of re-education. It is not physiological to pursue this practice. If resistance to inspiration is required to help centre the new movement of the abdomen, manual resistance given by the physiotherapist can be graded

17

and be flexible according to need. It is not wise for the patient to give manual resistance as this would recruit shoulder girdle muscles. The weight of both hands is usually sufficient but the use of a pillow over the abdomen on which the forearms are rested is often useful and comfortable.

Special care also needs to be taken in order not to increase the volume if the flow is slowed, nor to increase the flow rate if the volume is decreased. A new pattern is introduced by gradual and patient work. It will be very individual. Guidance should be given breath-by-breath and phase-by-phase, relating which movement is good and which incorrect, and thus reinforcing correct patterns of volume, movement and rest, which will of course be smaller and slower and more regular.

This decrease in body movement and ventilation may cause the patient an uncomfortable sensation akin to suffocation. This sensation is probably due to altered responses from the stretch reflexes in muscles, joints and lung tissue and from any rise in $PaCO_2$. The patient is helped to understand and accept this sensation of unease or discomfort, which will in time subside.

It is necessary to experience this sensation at a minimal level while practising the corrected pattern. It should be perceptible but acceptable. Changes should not be so great that they create an unacceptably strong sensation, as the new pattern would not be physiologically and psychologically sustainable and would stimulate a sense of anxiety. By maintaining the controlled pattern for as long as possible, the respiratory centres will be reprogrammed to trigger inspiration at a higher level of carbon dioxide and the reflexes involved in the new movement pattern will be reinforced. (The reprogramming is similar to that which occurs in patients with ventilatory insufficiency in COPD. An imperceptible increase in $PaCO_2$ over a period of time appears to condition the respiratory centre to accept higher levels before triggering inspiration and any altered patterns of movement become habitual.)

If the desire to breathe becomes too great to contain, simple swallowing may ease the discomfort. If this is not sufficient, a slow, controlled deep breath may be taken. To compensate for moving this large volume of air, a longer period of time must be used. It is helpful to hold the breath after expiration, if it is possible, for a count of five or six (3–4 seconds) or as long as is acceptable without stimulating an inspiratory gasp. In normal subjects the $PaCO_2$ drops as the result of a deep breath and takes 3–4 minutes to return to normal if no compensatory measures are taken. Patients need to learn of this phenomenon and to use the knowledge positively by compensating for deep breathing or sighing by breath-holding (preferably at the point of expiration) for a count of five or six. It is helpful to practise this slow deep breath, with a breath-hold on expiration, during treatment sessions.

Once a pattern has been found that fulfils the change criteria and suits the patient, it needs to be reinforced in the patient's mind. Some are able to recognize the pattern without external help; others find it difficult to recognize the timescale required. The correction in time may be helped by the physiotherapist guiding, by counting monotonously, the time span of the phases of each breath. The possibilities are many and individual. They may vary from *in out and in out and . . .* to a slower more natural pattern of *in and out two three and rest and in and out two three . . .* (Fig. 17.4). The use of a recording machine, to capture the timing of the pattern during a treatment session, may help the patient to practise more effectively at home. The chosen new pattern may be the ideal to control the symptoms and enable the patient to feel better. However, it is sometimes necessary to move forward more slowly and, having achieved a very small step, to make further corrective changes until a curative pattern can be accepted.

The patient will need to learn control of the breathing pattern in sitting, standing, walking and during and after exercise. Evidence to support this practice is offered by Malmberg et al (2000), who reported that when changing body posture from supine to standing, patients with HVS increase their pulmonary ventilation in excess of metabolic needs greater than healthy controls. The work of Yates (1998) and his colleagues has shown an important relationship between vestibular stimulation and respiratory control. It may be necessary to practise changing positions and exercising during treatment sessions. Natural breathlessness will occur on exercise and should be recognized and accepted as normal. Some patients may feel better on exercise, as the body's metabolic needs rise to equilibrate with the respiratory physiology. Others may overbreathe on exercise; this will be recognized by an increase in, or occurrence of, symptoms. Appropriate control measures will need to be introduced and practised. If the natural breathlessness does not subside within an acceptable time span after exercise (by the time the pulse rate is back to normal), control may be gained by changing one component of the breathing cycle at a time. First slow the rate, then decrease the volume, then slow the rate, etc., until control is achieved.

Compensatory procedures

The patient must become aware that the old habits of irregular large breaths, frequent sighs, yawns and sniffs, and also coughing and laughing, are likely to precipitate symptoms and will need to be compensated. An easy first aid measure is to respond immediately with a compensatory breath-hold followed by a normal

17

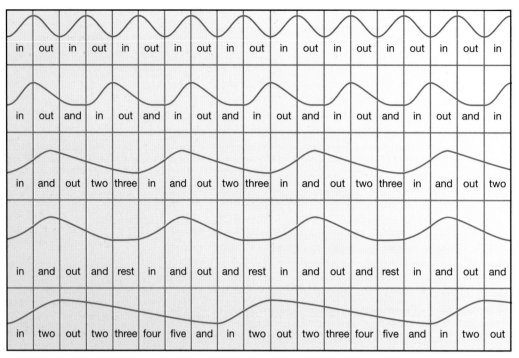

Figure 17.4 Some suggested breathing patterns demonstrating a regular small tidal volume with various flow rates and rest periods.

size breath. It is useful to form a habit of intermittent breath-holding during the day. The hold should not be anticipated by a deep breath; rather, the breathing cycle should be stopped anywhere in the cycle for a count of 2 or 3 or a longer time such as does not provoke a large following inspiration. It can also be practised and linked to simple everyday activities (like walking through a doorway) until it becomes a conditioned reflex. The hypothesis of this manoeuvre is to help lessen the risk of carbon dioxide falling to symptomatic levels.

Planned rebreathing

It has been recorded that paper bag rebreathing may carry the hazard of hypoxia (Callaham 1989). However, poorly programmed rebreathing in acute hyperventilators who may have undiagnosed cardiac or respiratory conditions should not rule out the careful, controlled use of rebreathing therapy for chronic hyperventilators. There is a small group of people who cannot control the breathing pattern when it is most needed. There may be many reasons for this. One possibility is that the low $PaCO_2$ and associated cerebral vasoconstriction have an effect on memory programming and recall. If the $PaCO_2$ can be raised by rebreathing, the patient becomes clearer-headed and can then remember the breathing control programme.

At times of acute distress or inability to control the disordered breathing, a bag (25 cm × 30 cm minimum) may be used as a rebreathing apparatus. The bag must be shaken out so that it is full of room air. The open end of the bag is placed loosely over the nose and mouth, allowing some free passage of air between face and bag. The patient should breathe freely within the bag. Rebreathing of the expired gases takes place, thus raising the $PaCO_2$. After approximately 6–8 breaths, the bag should be removed from the face and shaken out to refill it with fresh room air. The procedure should continue with regular shaking of the bag until the acute presenting symptoms subside or until the patient is capable of controlling the breathing pattern effectively. For safety reasons the rebreathing bag must only be used in the sitting or standing position and never in lying. Should the patient lose consciousness, the bag would fall away from the face and not remain in situ, with the risk of asphyxia. Cupped hands held over the nose and mouth form another suitable and less obvious rebreathing procedure.

Rebreathing only raises the $PaCO_2$ during the procedure and, if the breathing pattern is not changed, the $PaCO_2$ would fall back when rebreathing ceased. The purpose of the procedure is to raise the carbon dioxide sufficiently to calm the patient and to enable conscious correction of the breathing pattern to take place.

17

An ordinary oxygen mask with large holes, as used for inhalation therapy, may be used for patients who are unable to control the breathing sufficiently at certain times or who, as a result of hyperventilation, are housebound and unable to do household and personal routines. The facemask may be worn for the duration of the task. The $PaCO_2$ is artificially raised by the rebreathing function of the mask. The vent holes are left open so that room air can be drawn in to maintain sufficient oxygen concentration.

A facemask may be the short-term therapy of choice for patients who are terminally ill and hyperventilate with anxiety.

It is unwise to use bags or masks too freely, as some patients can become dependent on the aid and never learn to reorder the breathing cycle. They should only be used when the patient's personality and situation are understood and when all other avenues have been investigated.

Speech

Many patients report that speaking and singing provoke symptoms. Normal conversational speech occurs at the upper end of expiratory tidal flows and there is a delicate interplay between breathing and speaking. Complex coordination of the respiratory muscles is required to produce the necessary subglottal pressures and the intricate manipulations needed to produce and maintain sound.

Speech requires longer controlled expirations and shorter, faster inspirations than resting breathing. These inspirations need to be taken at suitable points in the sentence in order to maintain fluency and intelligibility. Often the old pattern of speech is very fast, as the patient tries to say as much as possible on one breath, before snatching at the next. The aim to amend this habit is to articulate each word more slowly, to say fewer words on each breath and to try not to move down into the expiratory reserve volume. The new pattern of breathing required to incorporate these needs has to be found and carried out. It is usually helpful if the physiotherapist works with the patient, while the patient practises reading aloud and listening carefully to the new pattern of speech. This process helps to re-educate the breathing control and the sensory feedback loop.

Home programme

Therapy is directed towards re-educating the breathing pattern, not to breathing exercises. Practice sessions should be as many and for as long as possible. By using a practical approach, an acceptable programme must be worked out by the physiotherapist and the patient. At first it may only be possible to practise for 5 minutes a day, but three or four sessions of 20–30 minutes each

is obviously more beneficial. Many patients find that as they change their lifestyle, more time can be made available for breathing control and relaxation sessions.

It is good to start the day with a period of conscious control of breathing. It is suggested that 10–15 minutes is spent in practice before rising in the morning. When travelling by bus or train, conscious breathing control and relaxation is time well spent, even if one is standing in a crowd. Car drivers can use their time constructively while waiting at traffic lights. Coffee, lunch and tea breaks could afford a few minutes of practice. Some people prefer to remember to practise breathing control for a few minutes each hour, on the hour, during the day. Fifteen or 20 minutes should be put aside when returning home from work or shopping, to relax and practise breathing control. It is worth spending this time after a working day to allow the body to equilibrate. The evening can be more enjoyable when not fighting symptoms. The last period of practice can be done having retired to bed using the favourite sleeping position.

Compensatory breath-holding, intermittent breath-holding and general physical and mental relaxation should become part of the normal day. People who have experienced HVS are probably always at risk, even after the presenting episode has been resolved. It would be judicious always to remember to practise breathing control before aggravating situations such as flying, travelling to a high altitude, heat, hot baths and periods of prolonged excitement, stress or risk.

Exercise and fitness programmes

As a result of the disordered breathing pattern, many patients have been unable to exercise and have become unfit, thus compounding the problem. Guidance in a slowly graded exercise scheme forms an important part of management. It may need to start with very simple movements in lying, such as arm raises, heel slides or knee fallouts at low repetitions. The progression must be carefully graded into more functional positions such as sitting and standing and activities such as walking. Swimming is another excellent form of exercise, which encompasses general movement synchronized with breathing. Most importantly, the physiotherapist should guide the patient to find an activity that is enjoyable and may be fitted easily into the daily routine. It should start with very short sessions of only a few minutes, interspersed with rest breaks as needed. Sessions can be gradually built up toward 20–30 minutes with close monitoring of symptoms. Realistic short-term goals should be set, such as walking an extra bus stop, or swimming one length of the pool at a time. The exercise programme should be clearly prescribed, monitored and gradually progressed by a physiotherapist. To err on the slow side is preferable to advancing too quickly

17

as impatience for progress may cause decline rather than improvement. Rehabilitative styles of Pilates or stability training, both performed with a physiotherapist on an individualized basis, can offer a safe and gentle approach to exercise. Breathing control, stability, balance, spinal mobility, postural alignment and body awareness can all be improved with this method. There is variation in the way Pilates is taught and the physiotherapist should review the teacher's qualifications and experience before referring patients. It is not appropriate to refer these patients to Pilates sessions or group classes until they have worked individually with a physiotherapist and can independently control their breathing with movement. Work within a group should never be competitive. Each person should be following an individual programme. These group sessions must be monitored carefully to ensure that they are not used for 'swapping symptoms'. With careful guidance they can help to give confidence and enhance the patient's ability to return to a more active life.

Discharge

At discharge the outcome could be measured by:

- Nijmegen questionnaire
- breath-hold time
- breathing rate
- tidal volume
- disability/distress records
- breathing pattern measured by spirography or Respi-Vest if these services are available
- thoracic mobility.

Those who habitually hyperventilate are often gifted and interesting people and are generally highly motivated and compliant with treatment. A high proportion of people with dysfunctional breathing are helped by a systematic, individual treatment programme and by an intelligent and sympathetic approach to the syndrome. The condition is a challenging one for the physiotherapist and the improvement is pleasing.

Breathing is a very complex system that is affected by many stimuli and appears to have effects other than the exchange of gases (van Dixhoorn 1996). Some patients' symptoms may be attributed to various dysfunctional aspects within the inherent mechanisms of the afferent and efferent responses of the breathing system, other than the variable or low levels of $PaCO_2$. Many phenomena are not yet understood and there are many areas inviting research. Work is currently in progress in a few centres, which should offer a greater understanding of the physiological sensitivities and complexities and the interplay of feedback loops in the breathing system in relation to individual responses to life events.

DYSFUNCTIONAL BREATHING IN ASTHMA AND COPD

Breathing pattern modulation

Based on the understanding that the pattern of breathing and the central control mechanisms can be changed (Grossman et al 1985), a programme of breathing pattern re-education should be a positive part of the total care management plan. The knowledge of the underlying causes of the breathing problem, the capacity to recognize the onset of acute problems and the ability to alter the method of breathing appropriately would not only decrease the anxiety that the patient experiences but also make a positive input to the actual process of ventilation.

HYPERVENTILATION AND ASTHMA

The relationship between hyperventilation and asthma is ambiguous. Papers regarding 'dysfunctional breathing and asthma' relate to overbreathing or a hyperventilatory component and not to the typical disrupted pattern of 'gasping in' and 'squeezing out' of acute asthma. Hyperventilation does appear to be one factor in acute asthma, either in cause or effect. Panic or anxiety could exacerbate the symptoms of asthma by their propensity to stimulate hyperventilation. Hammo & Weinberger (1999) have shown that chest discomfort and dyspnoea, in some children, precipitated by exercise are associated with hypocapnia from hyperventilation rather than a true exercise-induced asthma. They suggest that an atypical history in the form of late onset, the absence of other symptoms of asthma, the absence of response to inhaled β_2-agonist and a competitive personality should alert physicians to this alternative diagnosis of 'exercise-induced hyperventilation' rather than misdiagnose asthma.

Osborne et al (2000) have demonstrated that decreased airflow in a group of patients diagnosed with asthma was related to a low $PaCO_2$ and end-tidal PCO_2 in association with hyper-responsive airways, rather than to airway obstruction or mucosal inflammation. In some people with 'mild asthma', hypocapnia may be responsible for the increase in smooth muscle contractility rather than true asthma. These patients would benefit by learning breathing control, which includes the rest periods and breath-holds as described above.

Regulation of the breathing pattern with regard to true asthma should be taught ideally when the patient is in good health and would incorporate the techniques already described, when deemed appropriate. Finding a basic pattern together would give confidence and reduce the risk of panic. Control of air through the nose helps to regulate the pace, keeps the flow as laminar as possible and prevents any unnecessary irritation of the airways as when cold, fast moving air is drawn in through the mouth. Encouragement is given to move the air as smoothly as possible and to raise the respiratory level of each breath by not breathing out to the end and by starting inspiration a little sooner in the cycle. This should help to prevent excessive compression of the airways and allow a freer flow of air. Learning to cope with an acute attack would include changing the pattern of inspiration from the upper chest and shoulder girdle to the diaphragm. This would be encouraged by appropriate resistance, given by the physiotherapist's hands, to encourage a gentle swelling of the abdominal wall. A relaxed passive expiration is the norm, but during a period of extreme airways obstruction a degree of abdominal contraction will probably be necessary and it should be taught to be controlled rather than forced, and not extended too far towards full expiration. Greater control of this new pattern and some confidence to ward off attacks can be gained by practising changing back and forth between thoracic 'in and up' breathing and diaphragmatic 'in and down' breathing (Innocenti 1974). Free exercise and posture awareness will help to prevent the possibility of deformity in children.

Clinically relevant improvements in quality of life scores have been seen in patients who have received breathing retraining (Thomas et al 2003).

Kellet & Mullan (2002) comment that techniques regarding control of flow rate, tidal volume, cadence, place of movement and the three-phase cycle described here have similarities with those described by Buteyko. They suggest that physiotherapists are ideally placed to develop and research these techniques and if they are shown to be of value it may herald the dawn of a new era in the management of asthma.

The *Buteyko breathing technique* is spreading in Australia, New Zealand and United Kingdom. The technique is based on the theory that hyperventilation is a major cause of asthma and the technique of 'reducing the depth and frequency of respiration' and of breath-holding is taught, together with other input. It seems to be based on a similar understanding of the need to upregulate the $PaCO_2$ levels. The regimen appears to be a fixed formula, which is imposed on everyone in the group. The training occurs over 7 days; each session lasts 60–90 minutes and consists

'... of exercises in which subjects reduced the depth and frequency of respiration. Breath-holding exercises measured the impact of this training and gauged progress. Participants were encouraged to practise these exercises several times a day.'

'People experiencing difficulty with the technique were given extra breathing classes'

(Bowler et al 1998)

DYSFUNCTIONAL BREATHING IN EMPHYSEMA

Correspondence (Connolly 2003) on 'dysfunctional breathing in COPD' appears to relate to a general feeling of breathlessness. This may be so, but no comment is made regarding the different forms of breathing patterns that evolve due to the specific pathological changes effected in emphysema and chronic bronchitis. The typical pattern in emphysema is one of a prolonged 'push-out' expiration, frequently with pursed lips and a further tightening of the abdominal muscles, followed by a quick gasping inspiration.

There is little change in the volume of the emphysematous areas during the ventilatory cycle. They appear to act as space-occupying lesions. Prolonged expiration, therefore, does not produce significant emptying of the emphysematous spaces; rather, it compresses the normal lung tissue and the unsupported airways. Pursed lip breathing tries to keep the airways open longer by increasing the intraluminal pressure; this it does, but the work of breathing is increased and not much more air is moved.

Therefore more space and less expiratory pressure is required to prevent the early closure of the unsupported airways and to allow the unaffected lung tissue to participate more effectively in the ventilation. Airflow is freer and less expensive of energy, when the expiratory pattern with muscle contraction (with or without pursed lips) is reversed to an inspiratory pattern with a slightly raised resting respiratory level.

Re-education can take place in the sitting position and after attention has been drawn towards the upper chest expiratory pattern, it is then directed towards an abdominal inspiratory pattern. Appropriate manual resistance is given by the physiotherapist's hands on the abdomen throughout inspiration, to stimulate diaphragmatic descent. The resistance is gradually released as expiration takes over. This should not be prolonged; rather, the next inspiration is begun a little sooner than previously, thus raising the resting respiratory level a few cubic centimetres (Fig. 17.5) (Innocenti 1966). Care must be taken to ensure that the breathing rate is not slowed, such that the patient becomes more breathless. A comfortable pace and level of flow should be found to improve ventilation and comfort. Although these procedures have been reported as beneficial and practised for many years, there has been no formal research to replicate the original laboratory findings of improved air flows and reduced intrathoracic pressures (Innocenti 1966), and to test objectively the subjective reports of

17

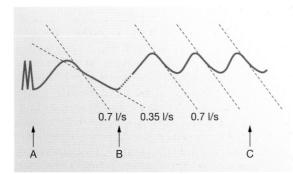

Figure 17.5 Tracing showing the effect of raising the resting respiratory level by approximately 300 cc. Note the velocity of airflow remains higher for a greater part of expiration (taken from the tracing of a severely disabled patient). **(A–B)**, old pattern level; **(B–C)**, new pattern level (from Innocenti 1966).

improved exercise tolerance, well-being and activities of daily living.

MUSCULOSKELETAL INTERVENTION

Dysfunctional breathing inevitably induces both structural and functional changes in the musculoskeletal system (Chaitow 2002). These changes, in turn, affect breathing function, thus perpetuating a chronic cycle. Where there is evidence of musculoskeletal compromise in this patient group and treatment includes breathing techniques only, it may be difficult for a patient to revert to, and maintain, a normal breathing pattern. Despite effective respiratory intervention, the patient may be unable to master the diaphragmatic pattern of breathing. This may be due to over-riding dominance in the accessory muscles of respiration, thoracic hypomobility, excessive activity in the rectus and oblique abdominals which restricts free descent of the diaphragm, costovertebral dysfunction or increased myofascial tone. Alternatively, the patient may be able to master the breathing pattern in a relaxed supported position, but it may not become functionally integrated and their symptoms persist. In clinical practice, when the musculoskeletal and postural dysfunction is addressed, which may include manual release techniques for the diaphragm in order to enhance its contraction and relaxation functions, the patient is often seen to revert more easily to the lower chest, diaphragmatic pattern of breathing. However, there is as yet little evidence to support this clinical finding.

The effects of dysfunctional breathing on the musculoskeletal system, and the importance of breathing retraining in musculoskeletal physiotherapy, are becoming more widely recognized. Re-education of the diaphragmatic pattern of breathing in a supported neutral spine position is the first stage in stability training for low back pain (Richardson et al 2004). Clinically, physiotherapists specializing in musculoskeletal work see a high incidence of postural-based musculoskeletal dysfunction in patients who spend prolonged periods driving, sitting at a desk or working on computers, particularly if the seating arrangements are not ergonomically sound. Invariably exacerbation of their symptoms is associated with an increase in work or family demands, poor sleep, stress and insufficient 'time-out'. A stressful meeting, phone call or commute can be enough to aggravate their symptoms. The patient may present to physiotherapy complaining of widespread (or localized) aches, pains and stiffness with or without a mechanical pattern. Often the symptoms are worse at the end of the day, and may fluctuate depending on factors such as stress, emotion and fatigue. In this group of patients there is very commonly an associated breathing dysfunction which, when addressed, can significantly contribute to their recovery and management of symptoms. When the breathing dysfunction is not addressed, the physiological consequences of hyperventilation (ischaemia, fatigue and pain, increased sympathetic arousal, spasm and reduced pain thresholds) will continue to drive the musculoskeletal complaint. As such, the patient may only derive temporary benefit from treatment or the problem may recur. A joint management approach may be required in this patient group for optimal outcome.

Posture

Normal breathing function relies upon correct postural alignment. The classic postural set described by Janda (1983) as the 'upper-crossed syndrome' with a forward head posture, thoracic kyphosis and anterior shift of the pelvis with reduced abdominal and gluteal tone can, over time, lead to breathing dysfunction, chronic musculoskeletal complaints and a cyclic link between the two. Poor postural habits are known to contribute to myofascial dysfunction (Edwards 2005). Assessment of posture and early education regarding the importance of correct alignment for the optimal functioning of the respiratory and musculoskeletal systems are integral parts of the rehabilitation process in this patient group. The patient should be in a relaxed state for postural re-education. Diaphragmatic breathing in a supported supine position, and appropriate manual therapy techniques should be applied before postural retraining in order to bring the body into an optimal state to accept the aligned posture. Re-education should occur in both sitting and standing. The patient should be encouraged to become aware of their individual postural habits and how these affect their respiratory function and musculoskeletal system. The patient should be taught to correct their alignment independently and this may take several sessions. Often in an enthusiastic attempt to achieve 'good posture' patients may overcorrect and extend excessively through the thoracolumbar junction. This is not favourable, can reinforce an upper chest-breathing pattern, and will ultimately lead to further musculoskeletal problems. We are aiming to normalize posture and movement, not overcorrect it. Any habit takes conscious retraining to change, and posture is no exception. At first the aligned posture will feel unnatural to the patient; however, over time, this will become their new norm. The patient should be encouraged to accept this change.

Assessment

It is useful to evaluate the musculoskeletal system as to whether it is the primary cause of, or consequential to, the breathing dysfunction. Referral to a musculoskeletal physiotherapist may be appropriate. A suggested guideline is as follows:

1. A detailed postural assessment should be undertaken. In particular spinal posture, scapular position, head/neck position, tone in the accessory muscles, abdominal tone should be noted and the breathing pattern observed.
2. In standing, evaluate the upper limb kinetic chain by observing scapulohumeral rhythm through active flexion and abduction, unilaterally and bilaterally. Note any overactivity in upper trapezius, levator scapulae, scalenes, and deficiencies in the stabilizing muscles. Note if there is a tendency to hinge through the thoracolumbar junction with upper limb movements, as this may indicate a lumbo-pelvic stability dysfunction.
3. Specific balance testing may be appropriate in standing.
4. In sitting, evaluate thoracic and cervical spine range and quality of movement.
5. In supine, complete specific length tests and palpate for myofascial tightness or trigger points in upper trapezius, sternocleidomastoid, scalene, pectorals, rectus and oblique abdominals, diaphragm and latissimus dorsi. Psoas palpation may be indicated. It may also be appropriate to assess first rib and anterior cervical spine mobility, and to assess function of the deep neck flexors, particularly if the patient reports associated neck pain.
6. In prone or side lying, palpate for myofascial restriction and evaluate intervertebral and costovertebral mobility. Palpate quadratus lumborum for trigger points.

Management

Treatment clearly depends on assessment findings. Manual techniques such as mobilization, muscle energy techniques (MET), proprioceptive neuromuscular facilitation (PNF), trigger point release and myofascial release can help to normalize joint, fascial and muscular restrictions. There are several books which describe these techniques in detail, including Cantu & Grodin (2000), Chaitow (2001), Chaitow et al (2002) and Maitland et al (2005), listed in 'Further reading'. A great number of techniques may be applied to each individual and their effectiveness needs to be assessed within and between treatment sessions. Outcome measures may include measurement of rib expansion, range of movement, observation of breath pattern and ease of postural alignment.

In conjunction, specific movement retraining may be necessary to improve stability with smooth execution and efficiency of movement. For example, a common habit is to fix or grip unnecessarily through the upper trapezius in activities of daily living (ADLs). This type of movement habit will encourage overactivity in the accessory respiratory muscles and reinforce the dysfunctional breathing pattern. This is just one example of a myriad of movement impairments with which the patient may present. A functional motor control approach whereby normal patterns of movement are facilitated from a well-aligned stable base is suggested. Specific stabilization training may be indicated in this group and the reader is referred to Richardson et al (2004).

CONCLUSION

It is clear that a close relationship exists between the respiratory and musculoskeletal systems. Dysfunction in one can lead directly to dysfunction in the other. In order to restore efficient functioning of each system, a holistic and coordinated approach is required. Patience and perseverance of physiotherapist and patient are necessary for the long-term re-education of the breathing pattern. Each patient's respiratory system is unique and each physiotherapist will learn new nuances of breathing patterns and new ways of helping to re-educate the system from each patient. The treatment programmes can never be exactly the same, nor should they be imposed rigidly. Each patient needs to be guided to find a personal corrected breathing arrangement, which suits and fulfils the basic physiological principles. The chosen pattern should eventually become the new, unconscious, habitual method of breathing. When pathological conditions are involved an important aspect of training is to control acute exacerbations as best as possible. Likewise, efficient move-

17

ment and postural alignment will become recognized as the norm and be integrated into everyday activities, thus helping to break the negative cycle between musculoskeletal and respiratory dysfunction. It is in the experience of many physiotherapists that patients can, and do, change the way they use their bodies and learn how to change their pattern of breathing and how to control it in moments of crisis. Reports of improvements are common. With increasing numbers of people reporting breathing difficulties, it is essential that research is undertaken to ascertain the merits of these procedures.

Patients are currently prescribed drugs, even though the breathing disorder may not have any associated pathology and the risk is that they may become established as the treatment of choice. Those who hyperventilate could be maintained indefinitely on addictive tranquillizers or inappropriate antidepressants (Timmons 1994) and long-term pain medications. In cases where symptoms can be minimized by controlling the breathing pattern and by addressing any related musculoskeletal dysfunction, drug therapy should be decreased to enable patients to attain their full recovery potential.

The effects of re-education of the breathing pattern and the place of musculoskeletal interventions in this group of patients merit further study and the field is wide open for physiotherapists to research.

References

Baker DM 1934 Sighing respiration as a symptom. Lancet 1: 174–177

Ball S, Shekhar A 1997 Basilar artery response to hyperventilation in panic disorder. American Journal of Psychiatry 154(11): 1603–1604

Bartley J 2005 Nasal congestion and hyperventilation syndrome. American Journal of Rhinology 19(6): 607–611

Bass C, Gardner WN 1985 Respiratory and psychiatric abnormalities in chronic symptomatic hyperventilation. British Medical Journal 290: 1387–1390

Bowler SD, Green A, Mitchell CA 1998 Buteyko breathing techniques in asthma: a blinded randomized controlled trial. Alternative Medicine 169: 575–578

Bradley D 2002 Patterns of breathing dysfunction in hyperventilation syndrome and breathing pattern disorders. In: Chaitow L, Bradley D, Gilbert C (eds) Multidisciplinary approaches to breathing pattern disorders. Churchill Livingstone, Edinburgh, p 51

Callaham M 1989 Hypoxic hazards of traditional paper bag rebreathing in hyperventilating patients. American Emergency Medicine 18(b): 622–628

Chaitow L 2002 Biomechanical influences on breathing. In: Chaitow L, Bradley D, Gilbert C (eds) Multidisciplinary approaches to breathing pattern disorders. Churchill Livingstone, Edinburgh, p 83

Clark TJH, Cochrane GN 1970 Effect of personality on alveolar ventilation in patients with chronic airways obstruction. British Medical Journal 1: 273–275

Connolly CK 2003 Dysfunctional breathing in COPD. Thorax 58: 460–461

Cowley DS, Roy-Byrne PP 1987 Hyperventilation and panic disorder. American Journal of Medicine 83: 929–937

Edwards J 2005 The importance of postural habits in perpetuating myofascial trigger point pain. Acupuncture Medical Journal 23(2): 77–82

Folgering H, Ruttern H, Rouman Y 1983 Beta-blockade in the hyperventilation syndrome. A retrospective assessment of symptoms and complaints. Respiration 44(1): 19–25

Freeman LJ, Nixon PGF 1985 Chest pain and the hyperventilation syndrome: some etiological considerations. Postgraduate Medical Journal 61: 957–961

Gardner WN 1994 Diagnosis and organic causes of symptomatic hyperventilation. In: Timmons BH, Ley R (eds) Behavioural and psychological approaches to breathing disorders. Plenum Press, New York, pp 99–112

Gardner W 2000 Orthostatic increase of respiratory gas exchange in hyperventilation syndrome. Thorax 55: 257–259

Gardner WN, Bass C 1989 Hyperventilation in clinical practice. British Journal of Hospital Medicine 41(1): 73–81

Glyn C, Lloyd JW, Folkard S 1981 Ventilatory responses to intractable pain. Pain 11(2): 201–211

Grossman P, De Swart JCG, Defares PB 1985 A controlled study of a breathing therapy for treatment of hyperventilation syndrome. Journal of Psychosomatic Research 29(1): 49–58

Hammo AH, Weinberger MM 1999 Exercise-induced hyperventilation: a pseudoasthma syndrome. Annals of Allergy, Asthma and Immunology 82(6): 574–578

Hardonk HJ, Beumer HM 1979 Hyperventilation syndrome. In: Vinken PJ, Bruyn GW (eds) The handbook of clinical neurology. North Holland, Amsterdam, pp 309–360

Hibbert G, Pilsbury D 1988 Hyperventilation in panic attacks. Ambulant monitoring of transcutaneous carbon dioxide. British Journal of Psychiatry 153: 76–80

Hodges PW, Butler JE, McKenzie DK, Gandevia SC 1997 Contraction of the human diaphragm during rapid postural adjustments. Journal of Physiology 505(Pt 2): 539–548

Hodges PW, Gandevia SC 2000 Activation of the human diaphragm in a repetitive postural task. Journal of Physiology 522(Pt 1): 165–175

Hodges PW, Heijnen I, Gandevia SC 2001 Postural activity in the diaphragm is reduced in humans when respiratory demand increases. Journal of Physiology 537(Pt 3): 999–1008

Hornsveld HK, Garssen B, Fiedeldij Dop MJC, Van Spiegel PI, De Haes JCJM 1996 Double blind placebo-controlled study of the hyperventilation provocation test and the validity of the hyperventilation syndrome. Lancet 348: 154–158

Howell JBL 1997 The hyperventilation syndrome: a syndrome under threat? Thorax 52(3): S30–S34

Hruska RJ Jr 1997 Influences of dysfunctional respiratory mechanics on oro-facial pain. Dental Clinics of North America 41(2): 211–227

Humphriss RL, Baguley DM, Anderson G, Wagstaff S 2004 Hyperventilation in the vestibular clinic: use of the Nijmegen questionnaire. Clinical Otolaryngology and Allied Sciences 29(3): 232–237

Innocenti DM 1966 Breathing exercises in the treatment of emphysema. Physiotherapy 52(12): 437–441

Innocenti DM 1974 Physiotherapy in the management of acute asthma. Nursing Mirror July 12: 77–79

Jack S, Rossiter HB, Warburton CJ, Whipp BJ 2003 Behavioural influences and psychological indices of ventilatory control in subjects with idiopathic hyperventilation. Behaviour Modification 27(5): 637–652

Janda V 1983 Muscle function testing. Butterworths, London

Kellet C, Mullan J 2002 Breathing control techniques in the management of asthma. Physiotherapy 88(12): 751–758

Kerr WJ, Dalton JW, Gliebe PA 1937 Some physical phenomena associated with the anxiety states and their relation to hyperventilation. Annals of Internal Medicine 11: 961–992

Lum LC 1994 Hyperventilation syndromes: physiological considerations in clinical management. In: Timmons BH, Ley R (eds) Behavioural and psychological approaches to breathing disorders. Plenum Press New York, pp 113–123

Malmberg LP, Tamminen K, Sovijarvi ARA 2000 Orthostatic increase of respiratory gas exchange in hyperventilation syndrome. Thorax 55: 295–301

Miyazaki H, Yamashita H, Masuda T, Yamamoto T, Komiyama S 1999 Transcutaneous PCO_2 monitoring in the evaluation of hyperventilation of patients with recurrent nerve paralysis. European Archives of Otorhinolaryngology 256(1): S47–S50

Mogyoros I, Kiernan MC, Burke D, Bostock H 1997 Excitability changes in human sensory and motor axons during hyperventilation and ischaemia. Brain 120(Pt 2): 317–325

Morgan MDL 2002 Dysfunctional breathing in asthma: is it common, identifiable and correctable? Thorax 57(Suppl 11): ii31–ii35

Naschitz JE, Mussafia-Preselac R, Koalev Y et al 2006 Patterns of hypocapnia on tilt in patients with fibromyalgia, chronic fatigue syndrome, non-specific dizziness and neurally mediated syncope. American Journal of Medical Science 331(6): 295–303

Nijs J, Meeus M, De Meirleir K 2006 Chronic musculoskeletal pain in chronic fatigue syndrome: recent developments and therapeutic implications. Manual Therapy 11(3): 187–191

Nixon PGF, Freeman LJ 1988 The 'think test': a further technique to elicit hyperventilation. Journal of the Royal Society of Medicine 81: 277–279

Ofluoglu D, Gunduz OH, Kul-Panza E, Guven Z 2006 Hypermobility in women with fibromyalgia syndrome. Clinical Rheumatology 25(3): 291–293

Osborne CA, O'Connor BJ, Lewis A, Kanabar V, Gardner WN 2000 Hyperventilation and asymptomatic chronic asthma. Thorax 55: 1016–1022

Papp LA, Klein DF, Gorman JM 1993 Carbon dioxide hypersensitivity, and panic disorder. American Journal of Psychiatry 150(8): 1149–1157

Pilsbury D, Hibbert GA 1987 An ambulatory system for long term continuous monitoring of transcutaneous PCO_2. Clinical Respiratory Physiology 23: 9–13

Richardson C, Hodges P, Hides J 2004 Therapeutic exercise for lumbopelvic stabilisation. Churchill Livingstone, Edinburgh, pp 185–219

Smith MD, Russell A, Hodges PW 2006 Disorders of breathing and continence have a stronger association with low back pain than obesity and physical activity. Australian Journal of Physiotherapy 52(1): 11–16

Terekhin P, Forster C 2006 Hypocapnia-related changes in pain-induced brain activation as measured by functional MRI. Neuroscience Letters 400(1–2): 110–114

Thomas M, McKinley RK, Freeman E et al 2003 Breathing retraining for dysfunctional breathing in asthma: a randomised controlled trial. Thorax 58: 110–115

Timmons BH 1994 Breathing-related issues in therapy. In: Timmons BH, Ley R (eds) Behavioral and psychological approaches to breathing disorders. Plenum Press, New York, pp 261–292

Tweedale PM, Rowbottom I, McHardy GJR 1994 Breathing retraining: effect on anxiety and depression scores in behavioural breathlessness. Journal of Psychosomatic Research 38(1): 11–21

Troosters T, Verstraete A, Ramon K et al 1999 Physical performance of patients with numerous psychosomatic complaints suggestive of hyperventilation. European Respiratory Journal 14: 1314–1319

van den Hout MA, Hoekstra R, Arntz A et al 1992 Hyperventilation is not diagnostically specific to panic patients. Psychosomatic Medicine 54(2): 182–191

van Dixhoorn J 1996 Hyperventilation and dysfunctional breathing. A presentation at the Third Annual Meeting of the International Society

for the Advancement of Respiratory Psychophysiology (ISARP), University of Nijmegen

van Dixhoorn J, Duivenvoorden HJ 1985 Efficacy of Nijmegen questionnaire in recognition of the hyperventilation syndrome. Journal of Psychosomatic Research 29(2): 199–206

van Doorn P, Colla P, Folgering H 1982 Control of end-tidal PCO_2 in the hyperventilation syndrome: effects of biofeedback and breathing instructions compared. Bulletin Europeen de Physiopathologie Respiratoire 18: 829–836

Vansteenkiste J, Rochette M, Demedts M 1991 Diagnostic tests of hyperventilation syndrome. European Respiratory Journal 4: 393–399

Wood P 1941 Da Costa's syndrome (or effort syndrome). British Medical Journal 1: 767–772, 805–811, 845–851

Yates BJ, Bronstein AM 2005 The effects of vestibular system lesions on autonomic regulation: observations, mechanisms and clinical implications. Journal of Vestibular Research. 15(3): 119–129

Yates BJ, Miller AD 1998 Physiological evidence that the vestibular system participates in autonomic and respiratory control. Journal of Vestibular Research 8(1): 17–25

Yates BJ, Billig I, Cotter LA, Mori RL, Card JP 2002 Role of the vestibular system in regulating respiratory muscle activity during movement. Clinical and Experimental Pharmacology and Physiology 29(5): 112–117

Further reading

Cantu RI, Grodin AJ 2000 Myofascial manipulation. Aspen Publishers Inc., USA

Chaitow L 2001 Muscle energy techniques, 2nd edn. Churchill Livingstone, Edinburgh

Chaitow L, Bradley D, Gilbert C 2002 Multidisciplinary approaches to breathing pattern disorders. Churchill Livingstone, Edinburgh

Lum LC 1976 The syndrome of chronic hyperventilation. In: Hill O (ed) Modern trends in psychosomatic medicine. Butterworths, London, pp 196–230

Maitland G, Hengelfeld E, Banks K, English K 2005 Maitland's vertebral manipulation, 7th edn. Butterworth-Heinemann Ltd, Edinburgh

Timmons BH, Ley R 1994 (eds) Behavioral and psychological approaches to breathing disorders. Plenum Press, New York

17

Chapter 18

Bronchiectasis, primary ciliary dyskinesia and cystic fibrosis

Mary E Dodd, A Kevin Webb

BRONCHIECTASIS

For many years, non-cystic fibrosis (CF) bronchiectasis has been a poorly evaluated condition for which management has been somewhat empirical and the patients have been included in a general respiratory clinic. The British Thoracic Society Bronchiectasis Guidelines (2007) have been developed with three aims:

- to identify all relevant studies in non-CF bronchiectasis
- to provide medical management consensus guidelines based on these studies
- to identify knowledge gaps and therefore the direction of future studies.

With over a thousand references, these guidelines are an excellent resource for managing non-CF bronchiectasis. The recently published guidelines by the American College of Physicians have emphasized the paucity of evidence-based clinical information for the management of non-CF bronchiectasis (Rosen 2006).

'Bronchiectasis' is the term used for permanent dilatation of one or more bronchi, whereby the elastic and muscular tissue of the bronchial walls is destroyed by acute or chronic infection (Cole 1995). This damage leads to impaired drainage of bronchial secretions. These secretions often become chronically infected, producing a persistent host inflammatory response. The combination of infection and a chronic inflammatory host response results in a progressive destructive lung disease. Depending upon the aetiology, bronchiectasis can affect specific lobes or both lungs.

The incidence and prevalence of bronchiectasis are unknown. Chest radiography – although usually the first investigation – is an insensitive method for evaluating bronchiectasis. Computed tomography (CT) is the gold standard in the detection of bronchiectasis (Smith & Flower 1996), but population screening using CT is not justified. With the decline in childhood tuberculosis, measles and whooping cough there is an impression that bronchiectasis is less prevalent. However, treatment of bronchiectasis has improved and it is important to try and establish the exact cause. Diagnosing the cause may define a specific approach to treatment and provide a prognosis as in the case of cystic fibrosis. A survey of the causative factors of bronchiectasis identified that 29% of cases were post infectious, 8% due to an immune defect and 7% due to allergic bronchopulmonary aspergillosis (ABPA), but for 53% of patients no cause was found (Pasteur et al 2000). A list of the common causes of bronchiectasis is set out in Table 18.1.

Delivery of care for complex diseases requires experience, expertise and teamwork. This maxim applies to lung cancer, transplantation and interstitial lung disease and it may improve the outcome for patients with bronchiectasis if they are cared for by a specialist multidisciplinary team, in a similar way to patients with cystic fibrosis.

Clinical features

The range of disease expression may vary from patients who are totally asymptomatic to those who have severe disease with a cough productive of large amounts of purulent sputum, which is sometimes bloodstained. The latter require treatment of high intensity with frequent hospital attendance. Severe exacerbations may be accompanied by chest pain, breathlessness and fevers.

Table 18.1 Common causes of bronchiectasis	
Post-infective	Tuberculosis
	Measles
	Whooping cough
Mucociliary clearance defects	Cystic fibrosis
	Primary ciliary dyskinesia
	Young's syndrome
Immune defects	Immunoglobulin deficiency
	Cellular defects
Allergic bronchopulmonary aspergillosis	
Localized bronchial obstruction	Foreign body
	Benign tumour
	External compression
Gastric aspiration	

Patients with inherited diseases such as cystic fibrosis and primary ciliary dyskinesia will often have accompanying sinus disease with nasal blockage, a purulent discharge and facial pain.

Clinical signs are non-specific. On auscultation there may be localized or widespread inspiratory and expiratory crackles with occasional wheezing. Clubbing is infrequent except with severe disease and cystic fibrosis.

Diagnosis and investigations

- *Assessment* using subjective and objective findings, as discussed in Chapter 1.

- *The chest radiograph* may be normal or there may be signs of thickened bronchial walls (tramlining), crowding of vessels with loss of volume and cyst-like shadows with fluid levels. The chest radiograph on its own is an insensitive test, detecting less than 50% of patients with bronchiectasis (Currie et al 1987).

- *High-resolution CT* is the imaging method of choice as a diagnostic tool in bronchiectasis. It has a high specificity, greater than 90% (Smith & Flower 1996).

- *Sputum specimens* for examination and culture to identify the micro-organisms and their sensitivity to antibiotics. The most common bacteria found in bronchiectatic sputum are *Haemophilus influenzae* (70%), *Streptococcus pneumoniae* and *Pseudomonas (Ps) aeruginosa*. The latter is found in patients with diffuse bronchiectasis and associated with accelerated lung disease (Evans et al 1996). Patients infected with *Ps. aeruginosa* require a higher intensity of treatment.

- *Bronchoscopy* should be considered if a foreign body or tumour is suspected.

- *Lung function tests* are used to assess severity of airflow obstruction and airway reversibility.

- *Serum immunoglobulins* will detect patients with hypogammaglobulinaemia.

- The diagnosis of allergic bronchopulmonary aspergillosis (ABPA) is difficult. The routine investigations should include: skin prick tests, eosinophil count, *Aspergillus* precipitins, total IgE levels with specific IgG and IgE levels to *Aspergillus*. Plain radiography may show fleeting shadows responsive to steroids. CT scanning may show the typical proximal bronchiectasis.

- *Gene mutation analysis.* This should be performed on all cases of idiopathic bronchiectasis to exclude some of the more benign mutations of cystic fibrosis (Pasteur et al 2000).

18

- *Electron microscopy* of the cilia (if the diagnosis of primary ciliary dyskinesia (PCD) is being considered) and evaluation of the patient in a specialist centre (Ferkol et al 2006).

Medical management

Progression of bronchiectasis is related to poor clearance of infected secretions. Physiotherapy (see below) is probably the most important component of long-term treatment. Antibiotics are fundamental to treating infective exacerbations and controlling the severity of bronchiectasis. The choice of antibiotic will be determined by the frequency and sensitivity of micro-organisms grown in sputum culture. The route and frequency of delivery will be decided by the severity of the disease. Antibiotics can be given orally, nebulized and intravenously. The best results will depend on the skill and experience of the team looking after the patient.

Indications for antibiotics

Oral antibiotics can be given as prophylaxis, for occasional infective exacerbations or continuously for repeated severe infections. Viral infections can produce a bacterial infective exacerbation, which will often require a course of prophylactic oral antibiotics. Patients with severe disease and persistent purulent sputum, who repeatedly relapse following a short course of antibiotics, can be maintained on long-term oral antibiotics. Those commonly used are the penicillins and more recently the macrolides.

Nebulized antibiotics may be used for patients with severe bronchiectasis whose disease is progressive and difficult to control (Currie 1997). Nebulized antibiotics can delay persistent infection with *Ps. aeruginosa* in patients with cystic fibrosis if instituted at the time of first colonization (Valerius et al 1991). Although there are no randomized clinical trials, this practice may be used in bronchiectasis as acquisition of *Ps. aeruginosa* is associated with greater morbidity (Evans et al 1996). Randomized controlled trials, using nebulized antibiotics for bronchiectatic patients chronically infected with *Ps. aeruginosa*, have shown a reduction in sputum density of *Ps. aeruginosa* (Barker et al 2000) and a lessening of disease severity (Oriols et al 1999). Tobramycin solution for inhalation (TOBI) has been used in a pilot study in patients with severe bronchiectasis (Scheinberg & Shore 2005). Although there was an improvement in respiratory symptoms, there was a significant intolerance of the medication, with 10 withdrawals from the study (n = 41). Intravenous antibiotics are used for severe disease, patients who fail to respond to oral antibiotics and those chronically infected with *Ps. aeruginosa*.

Other treatment measures

Influenza vaccination should be given annually to all patients with bronchiectasis unless there is a medical contraindication.

Topical medication may be indicated for chronic mucopurulent rhinosinusitis and the recommended technique for inhaled topical deposition of drugs is the head-down and forward position to encourage entry of the drops to the ethmoid and maxillary sinuses (Wilson et al 1987).

Where there is an immunoglobulin deficiency, replacement therapy should be given in an attempt to prevent further lung damage.

Surgical resection should be considered only if the bronchiectasis is localized, but there are no randomized controlled trials to compare surgical versus conservative treatment in the decision-making process (Corless & Warburton 2000). In very severe widespread bronchiectasis with respiratory failure, lung transplantation may be considered.

The inhalation of recombinant human deoxyribonuclease (rhDNase) does not appear to improve ciliary transportability, spirometry, dyspnoea or quality of life in patients with non-CF bronchiectasis (Wills et al 1996).

Inhaled steroids have been evaluated, with a trend to improving some respiratory parameters, but larger studies are needed (Kolbe & Wells 2000). A subset of bronchiectatic patients respond to bronchodilators and all patients should be tested for a response (Hassan et al 1999).

Physiotherapy management

Physiotherapy may help in the treatment of patients' problems of excess bronchial secretions, breathlessness, reduced exercise tolerance and chest wall pain of musculoskeletal origin.

Excess bronchial secretions

It is important that the patient understands the pathology of the condition and the reasons for treatment. Clinically, effective physiotherapy should reduce the episodes of superimposed infection and may help to minimize further lung damage.

An airway clearance technique (ACT), for example the active cycle of breathing techniques (ACBT) or autogenic drainage (AD) (Chapter 5), should be introduced and self-treatment encouraged (Rosen 2006). Each patient should be assessed to determine the positions that may increase the efficiency of secretion clearance and a CT scan, if available, may facilitate this. The sitting position may be adequate for patients with minimal secretions. The horizontal position may be a more

18

acceptable and comfortable alternative to the head-down tipped position and has been shown to be equally effective in patients who expectorate >20 g of sputum per day (Cecins et al 1999).

In patients who present with gastro-oesophageal reflux (GOR) there may be concern that the head-down tipped position will exacerbate the problem. The head-down tipped position is now rarely indicated. Chen et al (1998) reported no difference in the duration or frequency of symptoms in the various drainage positions. Other techniques that may be used to facilitate airway clearance have proven efficacy when used in gravity-assisted positions, e.g. Flutter and the active cycle of breathing techniques (Eaton et al 2007, Thompson et al 2002) and Acapella (Patterson et al 2004, 2005, 2007). These are discussed in Chapter 5. It has been suggested that a test of incremental respiratory endurance (TIRE) may be a useful method of airway clearance. In a single treatment session comparing the TIRE with ACBT, significantly more sputum was expectorated with ACBT (Patterson et al 2004). In contrast, Chatham et al (2004) demonstrated that TIRE was more effective than the ACBT. Further research is needed in this field.

Regular daily treatment is often necessary, but the frequency will vary among individuals. For many patients, treatment once a day is sufficient but the frequency should be increased during episodes of superimposed infection. Some patients find their chest is 'dry' at the beginning of the day. The timing of treatment should take into consideration both the time of day that the chest is most productive and the patient's lifestyle. Adherence may be increased by agreeing a suitable home programme with the patient. Elderly or frail patients may require assistance from a relative or carer who should be carefully instructed by a physiotherapist.

It is important that physiotherapy techniques and positions for treatment are reassessed at regular intervals (Currie et al 1986). Most patients should be reassessed within 3 months of initial instruction and then at least annually. A diagnosis of bronchiectasis may be confirmed in the absence of a daily productive cough. For these patients it would seem advisable to teach an ACT to be used during acute exacerbations of pulmonary infection (British Thoracic Society Guidelines 2007). In some patients with bronchiectasis it may be the increase in ventilation to the bronchiectatic area (use of the dependent position) rather than any 'drainage' from the area in an uppermost position that will increase airway clearance. Individual assessment is imperative for effective management and the endpoint of a treatment session must be recognized by self-assessment.

Hypertonic saline

Hypertonic saline has been shown to increase the ciliary transportability of bronchiectatic sputum, probably through its action of altering sputum rheology (Wills & Greenstone 2006). Kellet et al (2005) compared ACBT with three other treatment arms: ACBT preceded by nebulized terbutaline alone or in combination with either isotonic or 7% saline, in stable bronchiectatic patients producing less than 10 mg sputum per day. Hypertonic saline was shown to improve sputum weight, ease of expectoration, and lung function and reduce viscosity compared with the other treatment arms. Longer-term studies are required to determine the place of hypertonic saline on infection rates, quality of life and lung function.

Acute exacerbation of infection

Patients may be admitted to hospital with an acute exacerbation of pulmonary infection. The patient will probably be expectorating an increased amount of more purulent sputum, may be febrile, dehydrated and breathless. Haemoptysis is not uncommon and pleuritic chest pain may be present. The most severely affected may present with respiratory failure.

Mechanical adjuncts will be required in addition to an airway clearance technique to assist the clearance of excess bronchial secretions. A nebulized bronchodilator and/or humidification (Conway et al 1992) before treatment may help in the mobilization of tenacious secretions. Intermittent positive pressure breathing (IPPB) may help both in the clearance of secretions and in reducing the work of breathing. Patients who, many years ago, received the more radical treatment of resection of more than one lobe will probably have very poor respiratory reserve by the time they reach middle age. A superimposed infection in these patients may precipitate respiratory failure. Modified positioning, for example side lying or high side lying, combined with IPPB may be an effective form of treatment in minimizing the effort of clearing secretions. Non-invasive ventilation (Chapter 11) may be indicated in acute respiratory failure, although the outcome may be less successful in the presence of excess bronchial secretions.

Following resection of lung tissue, the anatomy of the bronchial tree may alter and the traditional positions for drainage of segments of the remaining lobes may be unsuitable or inappropriate. The physiotherapist should try various positions until the optimal ones are found.

The presence of blood streaking in the sputum is not a contraindication to physiotherapy and treatment should be continued. If there is frank haemoptysis, physiotherapy should be temporarily discontinued but resumed as soon as the sputum is only mildly blood-

18

stained to avoid retention of old blood and mucus. Before discharge from hospital, it is important that the patient is able to take the responsibility for their treatment and is confident with the positions and techniques required to continue regularly at home. If a bronchodilator has been prescribed, this should be taken before treatment and a few patients with bronchiectasis may also be prescribed nebulized antibiotic drugs, which should be inhaled after airway clearance. A breath-enhanced nebulizer or adaptive aerosol delivery (AAD) device is recommended for delivery of antibiotics (Chapter 5). If a patient is on the waiting list for lung transplantation, a preoperative rehabilitation programme should be established and postoperative treatment would be as outlined in Chapter 15.

Breathlessness

Some patients with bronchiectasis also demonstrate a degree of bronchospasm and may benefit from the inhalation of a bronchodilator before physiotherapy to clear secretions. Instruction in the use of an appropriate device for drug delivery is important.

A minority of patients with bronchiectasis complain of breathlessness. For these patients rest positions to relieve breathlessness and breathing control while walking and stair climbing should be included in the treatment programme (Chapter 5).

Reduced exercise tolerance

Exercise should be encouraged to improve general physical fitness. It will also assist the mobilization of bronchial secretions. Patients with severe bronchiectasis may benefit from a group pulmonary rehabilitation programme (Chapter 13). There is little research evaluating the place of exercise in bronchiectasis although there is a suggestion that inspiratory muscle training (IMT) may improve endurance exercise and quality of life (Bradley et al 2002). Newall et al (2005) evaluated an 8-week high-intensity pulmonary rehabilitation programme in combination with IMT or IMT sham or a control group. Both exercise groups showed significant improvements in exercise performance and inspiratory muscle strength. This was maintained at 3 months only in the IMT group. In the short term there would appear to be no advantage of including IMT in an exercise programme although it may prove beneficial in the longer term.

Chest wall pain of musculoskeletal origin

The management of this problem is discussed in Chapter 5.

Evaluation of physiotherapy

Effective treatment can be recognized by a decrease in the quantity and purulence of sputum, absence of fever, improvements in spirometry, a reduction in breathlessness, an increase in exercise tolerance, increased energy levels and a reduction or absence of chest wall pain. Improvements in oxygen saturation and blood gas tensions may also be identified.

PRIMARY CILIARY DYSKINESIA

Primary ciliary dyskinesia (PCD) is an autosomal recessive disorder with an incidence of between 1 in 15 000 and 1 in 30 000 (Cole 1995) and an expected prevalence of 3000 cases in the United Kingdom. Many cases are underdiagnosed. However, there is an increasing understanding of the complex genetics of PCD (Bush & Ferkol 2006) and therefore an improvement in the diagnosis and understanding of the phenotypic features (Noone et al 2004).

PCD is characterized by abnormal structure of the cilia; normal structure of the cilia but with abnormal function; absence of the cilia. These abnormalities result in recurrent infections in the nose, ears, sinuses and lungs. Fertility may be affected, both in the female because the fallopian tubes are lined with cilia and in the male due to reduced sperm motility. In 50% of cases, PCD is associated with dextrocardia or situs inversus. Kartagener described a syndrome of bronchiectasis, sinusitis and situs inversus in 1933. Later it was recognized that there was also a ciliary abnormality and this could occur without situs inversus. Cilia defects were described first in spermatozoa and later in nasal and bronchial cilia and the term 'immotile cilia syndrome' was applied to this group of conditions. With the discovery of a range of cilial defects, with variation in beat frequency and ultrastructure and the recognition that not all abnormal cilia are immotile, the term primary ciliary dyskinesia was adopted (Greenstone et al 1988).

The age of presentation can vary from newborn to 51 years (Turner et al 1981). Chronic sputum production and nasal symptoms are the main presenting symptoms. Other presentations include pneumonia and rhinitis in the newborn, 'asthma' with a productive cough, chronic and severe secretory otitis media (with associated hearing problems), severe oesophageal reflux in the older child and problems of infertility and ectopic pregnancy in the adult. Specific investigations which may clarify the diagnosis of PCD include a nasal mucociliary clearance test such as the saccharin test (Stanley et al 1984), photometric determination of ciliary beat frequency (Rutland & Cole 1980) and electron micrographic analysis. Genetic testing should be undertaken to exclude the diagnosis of cystic fibrosis. Exhaled and nasal nitric oxide is very low in PCD (Karadag et al 1997) but increased in bronchiectasis and asthma. Although the measurement is not recommended as a diagnostic test, if levels are low in a patient with bronchiectasis then the diagnosis of PCD should be excluded.

Medical management

Early diagnosis is essential and medical treatment centres around the prevention of lung damage and bronchiectasis with aggressive use of antibiotics and daily chest physiotherapy. Intravenous treatment may be necessary for unresponsive infections and long-term nebulized antibiotics should be considered for patients colonized with *Ps. aeruginosa*. In childhood, careful regular assessment and monitoring of hearing should indicate the requirement for hearing aids or grommet insertion due to the build-up of fluid in the middle ear. Hearing aids are considered preferable because grommets may cause additional discharge. Hearing loss is temporary and resolves spontaneously later in childhood.

Recent studies have focused on the influence of drugs on cough clearance (Houtmeyers et al 1999, Noone et al 1999). In PCD airway clearance is dependent on cough, but an increased amount of secretion is necessary to ensure effective clearance with coughing. Aerolized uridine-5'-triphosphate has been shown to improve whole lung clearance during cough after a single dose when compared to 0.12% saline (Noone et al 1999). Further trials of this drug are required to determine the clinical significance of long-term administration. Two case reports have suggested benefit from inhalation of rhDNase in the acute situation (Desai et al 1995, ten Berge et al 1999). However, its use has not been validated in PCD in a controlled trial. Inhaled β_2-agonists are frequently prescribed in PCD for their effect on bronchodilation, mucociliary transport and thinning of secretions (Rubin 1988). Regular use in asthma may be associated with increased bronchial responsiveness and decreased airway calibre. Koh et al (2000) have shown that no such adverse effects or decrease in lung function were seen in PCD over a 6-week period. Severe gastro-oesophageal reflux, which can compromise airway clearance, is a problem for some patients and requires appropriate management with a proton pump inhibitor.

Referral for assisted conception may be necessary for both males and females who are infertile or subfertile. Psychosocial support will include help with benefits, liaison with schools about infections and possible deafness and counselling may be appropriate to cope with the problem of infertility. Care centres around daily airway clearance and the control of infection by the general practitioner. Periodic review in a specialist centre by a multidisciplinary team, with expertise in respiratory disorders, is recommended.

Physiotherapy management

Daily physiotherapy is usually necessary in the child with PCD. It is important that parents are taught to recognize signs of infection early: for example, the child may be lethargic, 'off colour' and feel abnormally hot (pyrexia). In a study to examine cough frequency in children who were clinically stable, parental scoring equated to ambulatory monitoring. The cough frequency was shown to correlate with inflammatory markers but not with FEV_1 (Zihlif et al 2005). Physiotherapy should be increased during infective episodes and parents must understand that effective treatment is not achieved by antibiotics alone.

Due to the cilial defect, secretions are most likely to collect in the dependent areas: the lower lobes and often the middle lobe and lingula. The middle lobe, which may be situated on the left side owing to situs inversus, is more commonly affected than the lingula. The goal of treatment should be to assist clearance of secretions from the dependent parts of the lungs using an effective airway clearance technique. Both children and adults should be encouraged to blow their noses regularly.

Huffing games and airway clearance devices can usually be introduced at an early age and by 8 or 9 years the child can begin to do most of the treatment themselves, gradually becoming independent. It has been suggested that the PEP mask may be a useful technique, based on the theoretical benefits of peripheral mobilization of secretions, and can be used at any age including babies (Gremmo & Guenza 1999). Some patients may require nebulized antibiotics and inhaled β_2-agonists for their beneficial effect on mucociliary clearance. Beta-2 agonists should be inhaled before and antibiotics after airway clearance. Exercise, which increases bronchodilation to a greater extent than β_2-agonists (Phillips et al 1996), should be encouraged from the time of diagnosis and its importance emphasized to parents and patients (Fig. 18.1). Even with grommets in place children can enjoy swimming (Pringle 1992).

Very occasionally, nasopharyngeal suction may be indicated in the infant when it is impossible to clear nasal and bronchial secretions by any other means.

Regular assessment of techniques, remotivation of the patient and support for the parents are important aspects of physiotherapy. It is probable that chronic lung damage will be minimized if physiotherapy is continued on a regular basis.

Evaluation of physiotherapy

In the young patient with PCD, effective treatment in the stable condition may be recognized by the presence

18

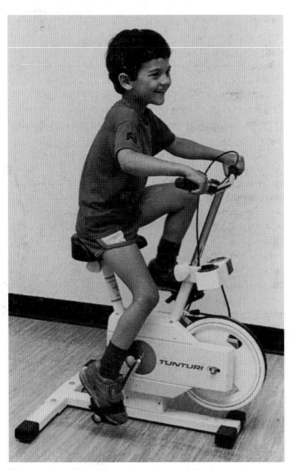

Figure 18.1 Exercise on a stationary bicycle.

of only minimal coughing on exertion. During an infective episode signs and symptoms of effective treatment include a reduction in shortness of breath, coughing, wheeze and fever if either or both have been present.

In the older patient, a constant volume of sputum is usually expectorated while stable. During an infective episode, the increased volume of expectorated sputum should lessen with effective treatment.

CYSTIC FIBROSIS

Cystic fibrosis (CF) is the most frequent cause of suppurative lung disease in Caucasian children and young adults and is characterized by chronic pulmonary disease, pancreatic insufficiency and increased concentrations of electrolytes in the sweat (Høiby & Koch 1990).

Cystic fibrosis is an autosomal recessive condition most commonly found in Caucasian populations with a carrier rate of 1 in 25 and the disease occurring in approximately 1 in 2500 live births (Dodge et al 1993). Carriers of the genetic defect show no signs of cystic fibrosis, but if both parents carry the abnormal gene each child born has a 1 in 4 chance of inheriting the condition. When the condition was first described by Anderson (1938), life expectancy was less than 2 years. Increased recognition of the disease, especially in its milder forms, and improved treatment has resulted in a median age of survival of approximately 31 years (Shale 1997a). Current survival figures from the Cystic Fibrosis Foundation (2006) report a median survival in the USA of over 35 years of age. Over the last 20 years in the Manchester Centre (United Kingdom), the number of patients living into the fourth and fifth decade of life has increased from 5% to 35%. Cohort survival graphs indicate an improvement in survival, with time, in the UK in all age groups (Dodge et al 1993). If the trend for improved survival continues, many of the patients born in 2000 now have a predicted median survival exceeding 50 years (Dodge et al 2007).

Before identification of the gene in 1989, a diagnosis of cystic fibrosis was made using the sweat test, which measures the amount of sodium in the sweat (Di Sant'Agnese & Davis 1979). The basic defect for CF lies on chromosome 7 and was identified in 1989 (Rommens et al 1989). The faulty gene in CF codes for the transmembrane conductance regulator (CFTR). The abnormality in this protein leads to changes in ion transport (McBride 1990), which produce changes in the nature of the mucus and serous secretions produced by the exocrine glands, cells of the respiratory system and digestive tract.

Ion transport in human airways is dominated by the absorption of sodium ions from the mucosal surface (Alton et al 1992), and this is associated with the movement of water into the epithelial cells. The balance between the movement of sodium and chloride probably determines the volume and composition of the airway surface liquid and may affect mucociliary clearance (Alton et al 1992).

It has proved extremely difficult to provide an accepted unifying hypothesis as to how defective CFTR function translates into the lethal pathophysiology of the lung. In particular, how it results in the aggressive suppurative lung disease so characteristic of CF and different from the indolent non-CF bronchiectasis. Two conflicting theories currently prevail. One is the airway surface liquid (ASL) *tonicity* hypothesis (Zabner et al 1998), which relates the pathophysiology to altered tonicity (high salt content) of the ASL layer. However, the weight of evidence now favours the ASL *volume* hypothesis, which suggests that a depletion of the volume of the ASL is a significant factor in the pathogenesis of CF pulmonary disease (Coakley & Boucher 2007).

18

The lungs are structurally normal at birth (Reid & De Haller 1967), but studies have demonstrated evidence of inflammation and infection in infants and children with CF (Birrer et al 1994, Khan et al 1995) and in asymptomatic adults with normal lung function (Konstan et al 1994). Infection stimulates further mucus secretion and a generalized obstructive, suppurative cycle becomes established. Repeated infections result in a neutrophil bronchiolitis. The neutrophils are ineffective at eliminating the micro-organisms which chronically infect the small airways. They break down, releasing numerous peptides, and in particular neutrophil elastase, which destroy lung tissue. The consequences are a destructive progressive suppurative bronchiectasis. The cycle of infection and inflammation impairs ciliary function and reduces mucus clearance.

As the suppurative bronchiectasis progresses, chronic hypoxia may lead to pulmonary hypertension. The majority of patients die from respiratory failure when they no longer respond to medical treatment or they do not receive a transplant.

Diagnosis and presentation

Newborn screening for CF is now possible and, where available, it most often uses measurement of immunoreactive trypsin (IRT) (which is abnormally high in CF) followed by DNA testing for a limited number of CFTR mutations. National newborn screening programmes for CF currently exist in New Zealand, France and Denmark, and will be available nationally in the United Kingdom by 2008. Regional or local programmes exist in parts of the United States of America, Australia and other areas of Europe. The results of a large randomized controlled trial of newborn screening for CF reported improved height, weight and head circumference in a screened group compared with a non-screened group (Farrell et al 2001) as well as higher cognitive function (Koscik et al 2004).

In the absence of newborn screening, the majority of patients continue to be diagnosed early in life with symptoms related to either the respiratory or gastrointestinal systems. Gastrointestinal abnormalities are often the earliest and most common presenting feature. The finding of echogenic bowel, during routine antenatal ultrasound, is associated with CF (although only in a minority of cases). Karyotyping and CF screening should be considered in this situation. In the neonate failure to pass meconium (meconium ileus) is the most common presenting feature, occurring in about 10–15% of cases (Park & Grand 1981). Signs of intestinal obstruction usually occur within 48 hours of birth. The infant fails to pass meconium after birth because the bowel is obstructed by sticky inspissated intestinal contents. In milder cases there may only be a delay in the passage of meconium. Blood should be taken for genotyping in infants with meconium ileus, as this condition can also occur in infants who do not have CF.

Another presenting sign in infants and young children is a voracious appetite and failure to thrive due to pancreatic insufficiency and malabsorption. Abnormalities in ion transport in the pancreas lead to inflammation and later to fibrosis of the acinar portion of the gland and to hyposecretion of the major digestive enzymes secreted by the pancreas. The presenting symptom is steatorrhoea with the passage of characteristically fatty and offensive stools. The majority of patients (85%) with CF are pancreatic insufficient (Davidson 2000). The remaining 15% usually have better nutrition and pulmonary function and a better survival prognosis. Occasionally older children present, having been managed for other respiratory conditions, for example asthma. In adulthood a late diagnosis may be made when the patient presents with infertility.

Classically the diagnosis is based on clinical findings, a high concentration of sweat chloride (>60 mmol/l) and/or identification of two disease-associated CFTR mutations. Early diagnosis is important to facilitate early access to specialist services in order to initiate appropriate treatment and to access prognostic and genetic services.

Signs and symptoms

Respiratory

The respiratory signs and symptoms of cystic fibrosis vary. The majority of older children and adults have a cough productive of sputum with varying degrees of purulence. The respiratory pathogens most commonly isolated in sputum are *Pseudomonas aeruginosa* (61%), *Staphylococcus aureus* (28.3%), *Haemophilus influenzae* (8.9%) and *Burkholderia cepacia* (3.2%) (FitzSimmons 1993). Infection with *B. cepacia* is often associated with accelerated pulmonary disease and a worse prognosis (Muhdi et al 1996).

Chest pain is common as the disease progresses and may be musculoskeletal or pleuritic. Breathlessness may be associated with infective exacerbations and increasing disease severity. Pneumothorax should be considered if there is an acute onset of breathlessness and pain. As breathlessness increases, appetite may fall and weight loss is common. Haemoptysis is common in adults but is usually mild, although episodes of frank haemoptysis may occur. Most patients develop finger clubbing which is associated with more severe disease.

Auscultation is often unrewarding when compared with the severity of radiological disease. Coarse inspira-

18

tory crackles are often heard. A pleural rub may be heard in association with infective exacerbations. The chest radiograph is often normal at birth but early changes include bronchial wall thickening, initially in the upper zones. As the disease progresses, hyperinflation may be noticeable with ill-defined nodular shadows, numerous ring and parallel line shadows indicating bronchial wall thickening and bronchiectasis (Chapter 2). High-resolution computed tomography (HRCT) imaging provides detailed evaluation of the lungs in CF (Chapter 2). Studies using HRCT in infants with CF have demonstrated early structural changes, even in those who have minimal symptoms (Long et al 2004).

Pulmonary function tests initially show signs of airways obstruction, but with advanced disease a restrictive pattern may be superimposed on the obstructive defect and a diffusion abnormality will also become apparent. Pulmonary function tests in infants with CF have shown early changes with diminished airway function soon after diagnosis, even in infants with no clinical history of clinical infection. These changes seem to persist during early childhood (Ranganathan et al 2001, 2004). More recently the use of multiple breath washout techniques to measure lung clearance index (LCI) (Chapter 3) have been shown to be effective and sensitive in terms of detecting early lung disease in cystic fibrosis (Aurora et al 2005a, Lum et al 2007). Pulmonary function measurements (FEV_1, PaO_2, $PaCO_2$) have been shown to be predictors of mortality (Kerem et al 1992). As the disease progresses ventilation/perfusion imbalance occurs, leading to hypoxaemia and pulmonary hypertension. Carbon dioxide retention occurs in patients with severe disease.

Asthma is as common in patients with CF as it is among the general population. Many patients with CF have a positive skin test to *Aspergillus fumigatus*. This is often seen in the sputum of patients and can be isolated in 40–60% of patients (Chen et al 2001). Colonization of the lower airway with *Aspergillus fumigatus* and the complication of allergic bronchopulmonary aspergillosis (ABPA) is well recognized in patients with cystic fibrosis (Skov et al 2005) and occurs in up to 10% of patients (Mastella et al 2000). ABPA is recognized by recurrent wheezing, deteriorating chest symptoms, fleeting fluffy shadows on the chest radiograph and elevated IgE levels which are specifically raised to *Aspergillus*.

Some patients develop nasal polyps. These may grow rapidly, are frequently recurrent and may require surgical removal. They may be related to chronic sinus infection.

Gastrointestinal

Distal intestinal obstruction syndrome (DIOS) is obstruction of the small bowel occurring in children and adults and is similar to that seen in neonates presenting with meconium ileus. This may be related to poor adherence with pancreatic supplements. It presents as small bowel obstruction with abdominal distension and discomfort, vomiting and reduced or absent bowel signs. Diagnosis is confirmed by the classic radiographic appearances of small bowel obstruction.

Cystic fibrosis-related diabetes (CFRD) has become a significant complication as a consequence of improved survival and is a result of progressive fibrosis damaging the endocrine cells that produce insulin (Bridges & Spowart 2006). The onset of diabetes, if not detected and treated promptly, can result in a decline in the patient's clinical condition (Lanng et al 1992). The basic defect also affects the hepatobiliary system, which can result in a biliary cirrhosis. Patients with severe disease can develop portal hypertension. The main complication is bleeding from gastric or oesophageal varices. Liver transplantation may be required.

Other

Puberty may be delayed for both male and female patients. Most women with cystic fibrosis have normal or near-normal fertility. Improving survival has resulted in an increasing number of the female population having children. Outcome of pregnancy is improved if pulmonary function is greater than 60% predicted (Edenborough et al 1995). Pregnancy has been reported to have a slight adverse effect on the health of women with CF (Gillet et al 2002). Women with CF require a greater intensity of treatment during pregnancy (McMullen et al 2006).

Most males are infertile because of developmental defects of the vas deferens, which is either absent or blocked, but they can produce sperm. Improved technology, whereby sperm can be aspirated from either the testis or epididymal sac in conjunction with intracytoplasmic sperm injection (ICSI), has resulted in CF biological fathers (Phillipson et al 2000).

Approximately one-third of adult patients with CF develop rheumatic symptoms (Bourke et al 1987). The two most common forms are an episodic and recurrent arthralgia /arthritis and hypertrophic pulmonary osteoarthropathy. They are characterized by joint pain, tenderness, swelling and limitation of movement, usually symmetrical and affecting particularly the knees, ankles and wrists (Johnson & Knox 1994). More important has been the recent recognition of the high prevalence of low bone mineral density in children and adults (Bachrach et al 1994, Bhudmkanok et al 1996, Haworth et al 1999), which leads to a high incidence of fractures. Rib fractures can result in considerable pain, sputum retention and morbidity.

18

Medical management

Paediatric and adult patients with CF should receive care from a specialist CF centre. Pulmonary function and nutrition, the two main prognostic indicators for survival, are better when care is delivered from paediatric and adult CF centres (Mahadeva et al 1998). Models for shared care, between the CF centre and the district hospital, at the paediatric level have worked extremely well for many years but this process is not commonly practised at the adult level. Most specialist units have a system of annual review when comprehensive assessment and testing is undertaken.

Cystic fibrosis is an extremely complex disease. Care is best delivered by a multidisciplinary team comprising doctors, physiotherapists, dietitians, nurses, social workers, psychologists and other disciplines who will complement each other in their individual areas of expertise. The patient should also be closely involved in choice of care and self-care at home.

Morbidity and mortality are primarily related to chronic progressive respiratory infection. Therefore the mainstay of treatment is oral, nebulized and intravenous antibiotics.

Long-term oral anti-staphylococcal antibiotics are given in the early years to treat *Staphylococcus aureus*, which is often the main micro-organism causing chronic infection. A considerable advance over the last few years has been the introduction of the macrolides as a long-term treatment for cystic fibrosis. Although an antibiotic, it is probable that the modulatory anti-inflammatory properties of the drug are responsible for the improvement in clinical status and preserved pulmonary function demonstrated in well-conducted clinical trials (Equi et al 2002, Saiman et al 2003, Wolter et al 2002).

Subsequently patients become chronically infected with *Ps. aeruginosa*, which increases treatment requirements and morbidity. The practice of starting nebulized and oral antibiotics at time of first culture of *Ps. aeruginosa* has been shown to be effective in eradicating and delaying persistent infection (Valerius et al 1991).

Nebulized antibiotics (Webb & Dodd 1997) have been shown to be effective in the treatment of chronic *Ps. aeruginosa* infection (Mukhopadhyay et al 1996, Touw et al 1995). Antibiotics are usually inhaled twice daily and should follow airway clearance. For many years, colistin has been the standard drug used for nebulization but there have been no large randomized controlled trials to unequivocally demonstrate benefit. High-dose preservative-free tobramycin (TOBI) has been used for inhalation with demonstrated benefit in CF patients (Ramsey et al 1999). However, the high cost and occasional intoler-ance may preclude its use in all CF patients infected with *Ps. aeruginosa*.

Intravenous antibiotics are frequently used for acute infective exacerbations but opinions differ as to the regular or symptomatic use of intravenous antibiotics (Elborn et al 2000). Treatment usually needs to continue for at least 14 days and can be evaluated by monitoring respiratory function, sputum quantity, bodyweight, blood gases and blood inflammatory markers such as C-reactive protein (Hodson 1996).

Patients needing frequent or prolonged antipseudomonal treatment, and who have poor venous access, may require implantable intravenous access devices. These devices can maintain continuity of antibiotic infusions and quality of life for the patient undertaking treatment at home (Shale 1997b, Stead et al 1987).

Segregation of patients colonized with *Burkholderia cepacia*, from other patients with cystic fibrosis, limits the spread of the organism by social contact (Govan et al 1993, LiPuma et al 1990, Muhdi et al 1996). It is now recognized that organisms classified as *B. cepacia* comprise a number of distinct genomic species each known as a genomovar of the *B. cepacia* complex (BCC). Currently there are 10 different described genomovars in the BCC. Disease progression and survival may be influenced by the genomovar status of the CF patient (Jones et al 2004). In some units adults are segregated in outpatient clinics according to their genomovar status on the basis that some genomars are transmissible and can superinfect patients with non-transmissible genomovars (Ledson et al 1998).

Many CF units adopt a general segregation policy for outpatient clinics. This is based either according to microbiological status or on a total segregation approach (where all patients are segregated regardless of microbiological culture). Health professionals must pay particular attention to hygiene and thorough hand washing between examining patients (Cystic Fibrosis Trust 2004a).

There has been concern regarding the emergence of transmissible strains of *Ps. aeruginosa* in large CF centres despite the use of the correct infection control measures (Jones et al 2001, McCallum et al 2001). As a consequence, many CF clinics practice inpatient and outpatient segregation by microbiological status (Cystic Fibrosis Trust 2004b). At the Manchester Centre (United Kingdom), a 4-year prospective surveillance demonstrated ongoing transmissible *Ps. aeruginosa* cross-infection between inpatients despite established conventional infection control measures. As a consequence, communal areas such as the day room and kitchen were closed and the patients are now required to stay in their rooms and not mix irrespective of their individual microbiological status (Jones et al 2005).

18

Contamination of nebulizers is common and patients must be given instruction in the cleaning and care of nebulizer equipment. To minimize contamination, cleaning and drying of this equipment after use are essential (Hutchinson et al 1996).

Some patients benefit from the inhalation of bronchodilator drugs. Steroids may be indicated if asthma or ABPA complicates cystic fibrosis. The use and value of inhaled steroids, to treat the inflammatory component of airflow obstruction in the long-term management of cystic fibrosis, are still under review with prospective controlled trials.

As a consequence of lung infection, there are large quantities of DNA from the breakdown of inflammatory cells, e.g. neutrophils. The inhalation of rhDNase acts on the DNA in the purulent lung secretions (Range & Knox 1995). It has been shown to improve lung function (Shah et al 1996), reduce viscoelasticity of the mucus (Shah et al 1996) and decrease exacerbations of bronchopulmonary infection (Fuchs et al 1994). Occasionally alteration in voice and episodes of pharyngitis may be experienced, but these are usually minor and transient (Hodson & Shah 1995). Alternate day therapy may be as effective as daily treatment in some patients (Suri 2005).

Hypertonic saline, inhaled before physiotherapy, may also assist in clearance of secretions (Eng et al 1996, Robinson et al 1996). There is a potential logic in the use of hypertonic saline for inhalation, whereby it will restore to normal the disrupted airway surface liquid of the CF airways. Two randomized trials have shown, in a small number of CF patients, preservation of lung function and in one of the trials a reduction in infective exacerbations (Donaldson et al 2006, Elkins et al 2006a). Hypertonic saline is inexpensive, safe and there is a reasonably high level of evidence to support its use. However, it does have an unpleasant taste and adds another treatment burden to the already overloaded self-care plan of all CF patients.

There is little evidence to support the use of other mucolytic agents such as acetylcysteine (Parvolex®). Some mucolytic agents may induce bronchoconstriction and a bronchial challenge should be undertaken at the time of the first inhalation.

In CF a high energy intake is needed as a result of malabsorption and the increased metabolic requirements during infection. The dietary energy intake should exceed the normal daily recommendation to sustain and maintain adequate weight, muscle bulk and function (Poole 1995). Supplements of fat-soluble vitamins and vitamin K are usually necessary in addition to pancreatic enzymes, which should be taken with all meals and snacks (Wolfe & Collins 2007). When nasal obstruction by polyps is incomplete, a corticosteroid nasal spray may be tried. Complete obstruction is unusual and polypectomy may be indicated.

Haemoptysis will usually stop spontaneously, but if bleeding is severe and prolonged, bronchial artery embolization by an experienced operator in a specialist centre can be a life-saving procedure (Ashleigh & Webb 2007) The current use of short courses of oral or intravenous tranexamic acid for moderate haemoptysis is effective.

Pneumothorax can occur spontaneously in the older patient. Small pneumothoraces may resolve without treatment, but most pneumothoraces require the insertion of an intercostal drain. Surgical intervention is required for large non-resolving leaks. Video-assisted thorascopic surgery (VATS) may be used to avoid a thoracotomy.

Heart-lung and double lung transplantation (Chapter 15) have been successfully carried out in patients with end-stage lung disease but there is a critical shortage of donor organs. Non-invasive ventilation may be life-saving and indicated for patients developing severe respiratory failure to bridge the waiting time to transplantation (Hodson et al 1991, Madden et al 2002).

If medical treatment has failed and the patient is distressed, palliative care must be expertly employed to allow the patient to die comfortably and with dignity. It is important not to withhold such care even if the patient is listed for transplantation.

Home treatment

In many countries the emphasis on treatment is moving from hospital to home. The benefits for patients of treatment at home include less disruption to school, work and family life while avoiding the isolation from friends and family that hospitalization incurs. Increasing numbers of CF patients are receiving their intravenous antibiotics at home usually because quality of life is better, but clinical outcome is better for the patient treated in hospital and patients treated at home require close supervision (Nazer et al 2006, Thornton et al 2004).

For the newly diagnosed or newly referred patient, home visits by members of the specialist team (usually the clinical nurse specialist) provide an opportunity for advice, education and support for the patient and family, as necessary. Domiciliary physiotherapy services are sometimes available and can provide the opportunity for discussion and demonstration of physiotherapy techniques in the home, an opportunity for a more effective assessment of the necessity and appropriateness of equipment and the possibility of specialist physiotherapy during terminal care. There is also evidence of improved adherence with treatment and a reduction in the stress of coping with the disease (Rogers & Goodchild 1996).

Many patients awaiting heart-lung transplantation can be cared for at home, with a clinical nurse specialist visiting to provide assessment and to identify the need for changes in treatment to maintain optimal health status. It may be appropriate for a patient to receive either a course of intravenous antibiotics at home or to continue a course started in hospital.

The future

Cystic fibrosis is a complex disease. An enormous amount of effort is being expended to improve standards of care (de Boeck 2000), provide guidelines for antibiotic treatment (Cystic Fibrosis Trust 2002a, Doring et al 2000) and evidence, based upon controlled trials, for different aspects of treatment (Cheng et al 2000). More patients (but not enough) are being transplanted and survival figures are improving with greater experience (Vizza et al 2000). The physicians and scientists are continuously evaluating current care (Davis et al 1996) and searching for new therapies to improve quality of life and long-term survival (Rubin 1998).

Gene therapy aims to correct the basic defect by inserting the appropriate DNA or RNA to compensate for the defective gene. The gene is transferred via a 'carrier' or vector. To date both viral and non-viral vectors have been extensively investigated but difficulties have been experienced with both. Viral vectors such as the adenovirus can stimulate an inflammatory response and non-viral vectors such as liposomes are not as efficient (Du Bois 1995). Theoretically the transfer of sufficient normal copies of the CFTR gene, to sufficient numbers of affected cells, should result in the production of enough normal protein to reduce the clinical manifestations of cystic fibrosis (Stern & Geddes 1994). Despite several in-vitro and in-vivo studies it has been difficult to convert this theory into practice. Significant advances have, however, been made and there is considerable research in progress which may lead to effective gene therapy in the future (Boyd 2006).

Stem cell therapy aims to permanently correct the genetic defect by developing a cell line that continually produces cells to re-establish a normal epithelium. To date research in stem cell therapy for CF is in its infancy and little is known about the stem cell biology of the lung. Stem cell research is attracting interest and is a hope for future treatment (Boyd 2006).

Physiotherapy management

Advances in the medical management of cystic fibrosis have increased the expectation of survival into the fifth decade of life (Dodge et al 2007). As the science of the basic defect is translated into a greater understanding of the pathophysiology of the disease and novel complications of an ageing population emerge, the physiotherapist's role is continually challenged. The management encompasses the treatment from birth through childhood and adolescence into adulthood and parenting. It is adapted through changing lifestyles, disease severity and the changes of the acute exacerbation and stable state of the disease. Physiotherapy requires detailed accurate assessment and treatment, tailored to the individual as lifestyle and disease severity change. In parallel with the advances in the medical management, the role of the physiotherapist has expanded from the clearance of bronchial secretions to include the assessment of exercise capacity and the prescription of safe and effective exercise programmes, assessment and education of inhalation therapy and in the later stages of the disease the use of oxygen therapy and non-invasive ventilation (NIV).

More recently the problems of musculoskeletal pain, low bone mineral density and urinary incontinence have emerged. The physiotherapist's treatment is confounded by the many complications of this multisystem disease, e.g. diabetes, distal intestinal obstruction syndrome and arthropathy. Improved survival is also attributed to the enormous burden of self-care imposed on patients. To enhance adherence to this treatment regimen it is crucial that the physiotherapist works with the patient and their family/carers to encourage an effective but realistic treatment plan, balanced with their wishes to lead a normal life.

Infants and small children

Historically a diagnosis of CF was confirmed in babies at some time during the first year of life, often following a symptomatic presentation of respiratory infection and failure to thrive. Traditionally 'chest physiotherapy' was instigated twice daily as soon as the diagnosis had been confirmed and treatment comprised the use of gravity-assisted positions and chest clapping. In the absence of specific radiological signs, most physiotherapists adopted a general drainage regimen (alternate side lying and prone in a head-down tipped position and supine flat) with the addition of the sitting position for the apical segments of the upper lobes in infants, as they spend much of their time lying down. Once the child began to sit and stand, the apical segments were omitted from treatment.

In the past few years, the approach to airway clearance in babies with CF has changed considerably. Many other airway clearance techniques have been developed (Chapter 5) and some of these, such as positive expiratory pressure (PEP) applied via a facemask, assisted autogenic drainage (AD) and physical activity are now

18

used in the infant/paediatric population. Many centres throughout the world have modified the traditional approach by omitting the use of gravity-assisted positioning in the drainage regimen. This has been to a large extent due to growing clinical concerns regarding gastro-oesophageal reflux. Gravitational effects in the tipped position theoretically lead to a lowering of intra-abdominal pressure and an increase in intrathoracic pressure. This, together with the increase in diaphragmatic activity, may enhance the competence of the oesophageal sphincter (Sindel et al 1989). Despite this theoretical assumption, infants with CF are known to have a higher incidence of gastro-oesophageal reflux (GOR) and studies have suggested that this is exacerbated by use of the head-down tipped position during airway clearance (Button et al 1997). Other groups have not reproduced these findings, albeit in slightly differing cohorts (Phillips 1996, Taylor & Threlfall 1997). Longer-term follow-up data from the subjects included in the study by Button et al (1997) suggest that GOR may result in both short- and long-term sequelae in terms of respiratory status (Button et al 2003, 2004). These results have led many centres to discontinue using the head-down tipped position. This remains a slightly contentious issue, and there are centres that continue to use gravity-assisted positioning judiciously. When GOR is suspected, it should be investigated rigorously and if confirmed the airway clearance regimen may need to be modified and anti-reflux medication should be started.

Whichever airway clearance treatment is chosen, it is usually advised that it be undertaken before feeds and for approximately 10–15 minutes. If an infant or child has specific radiological signs, or in the presence of a lower respiratory tract infection, treatment may need to be intensified in terms of frequency and duration.

Early diagnosis of CF, particularly since the introduction of neonatal screening in many parts of the world, along with early and aggressive multidisciplinary care, has led to a novel cohort of infants who are apparently free of any respiratory symptoms and are nutritionally healthy. The appropriateness of implementing a routine daily airway clearance regimen in this cohort of infants has raised much debate. Unfortunately there are no studies that have evaluated whether the routine instigation of airway clearance regardless of clinical status is beneficial. The debate continues widely on the international stage and opinion remains divided (Prasad & Main 2006).

Arguments for routine treatment are threefold. First, many feel it is essential to establish a daily routine in order to ensure adherence to therapy in the long term. Secondly, the anatomical and physiological differences in the infant respiratory system (Chapter 10) may make them more vulnerable to chest complications. Finally, there is conclusive evidence that pathophysiological changes in the lungs occur very early, before the onset of clinical signs, with evidence of early inflammation and infection (Armstrong et al 1995), altered respiratory function (Ranganathan et al 2001) and structural changes radiologically (Martinez et al 2005).

However, while the evidence that pathophysiological changes occur early in the disease process is compelling, the early picture is usually not one associated with copious secretions. The value of a daily airway clearance regimen is therefore unclear (Bush & Gotz 2006). In addition there is no doubt that a significant burden of care is imposed on families by routine treatment regimens.

There is little robust evidence with respect to best physiotherapy practice in this group of infants (Button 1999, Constantini et al 2001). The few existing studies that attempt to evaluate the efficacy of airway clearance or to compare the various airway clearance modalities have been undertaken in older populations with established disease (Desmond et al 1983), as have the majority of studies comparing the efficacy of the various techniques (Elkins et al 2006b, Main et al 2005). It is unlikely to be appropriate to extrapolate findings from these studies to a healthy infant who shows no overt signs of respiratory involvement. In the United Kingdom the proposal of a national neonatal screening programme provided a unique opportunity to undertake a randomized controlled trial of the efficacy of routine daily chest physiotherapy in screened infants with CF. Unfortunately this trial did not come to fruition but in attempting to address this important issue, the Association of Chartered Physiotherapists in Cystic Fibrosis (United Kingdom) undertook a consensus exercise based on the Delphi process (Jones & Hunter 1995) in order to provide expert opinion and guidance for the future care of these infants (Prasad et al 2008). The results of the Delphi process have resulted in guidelines which state that physiotherapists are not required to initiate routine airway clearance if, following careful assessment, the child is well and felt not to have symptoms which would respond to respiratory physiotherapy. It is important to stress that all parents and carers should be taught an appropriate airway clearance regimen, and this is practised and revised to maintain competency. Airway clearance is instigated whenever there are respiratory symptoms and an assessment tool is being developed to assist parents with assessment (Fergusson, personal communication 2007). The Delphi process has also recognized that the more recently developed airway clearance modalities may be more appropriate for these

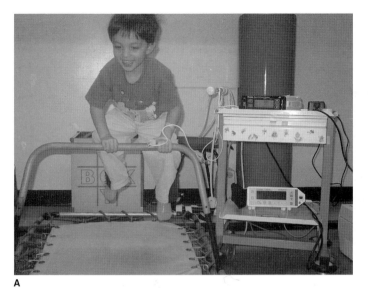
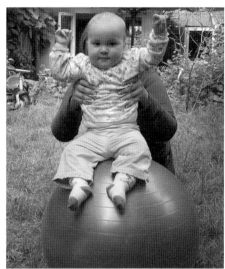

A   B

Figure 18.2   (A) Jumping on a mini-trampoline. (B) Exercise on a gym ball.

infants, rather than traditional postural drainage or modified postural drainage and percussion, and that physical activity should be greatly emphasized from the outset. The suggestion is *not* that treatment should be withdrawn, but that a different emphasis be placed on the management to include physical activity and a more flexible and holistic approach supported by an easily accessible specialist physiotherapy service.

Even at a young age treatment should be fun. The young child can be bounced up and down on the parent's knees, exercises such as 'wheelbarrows', jumping on a mini-trampoline (Fig. 18.2A) or the use of a gym ball (Fig 18.2B). Laughing often also stimulates coughing. From the age of 2 years the child can be encouraged to actively participate in breathing techniques in the form of play and other airway clearance modalities (Chapter 5) can be introduced as the child grows. PEP can be made more enjoyable if administered in the form of bubble PEP (Chapter 5). From as early an age as possible children should be encouraged to play a more active role in their treatment. With increased cooperation, the child can be introduced to various airway clearance techniques and become independent with treatment (Box 18.1).

Infants and small children swallow their bronchial secretions, but as soon as possible expectoration should be encouraged. Nasopharyngeal suction should only be used in babies if it is essential to obtain a sputum specimen or if the infant is distressed by secretions. Learning to blow the nose is also important, to keep the upper airways clear.

Airway clearance

The removal of bronchial secretions remains the mainstay of physiotherapy management as bronchial infection and respiratory failure continue to be the major causes of morbidity and mortality.

Infected bronchial secretions are responsible for many complications in the airways and lung tissue (Fig. 18.3). Obstruction occurs initially in the small airways, with repeated infections and hypersecretion resulting in damage to the airway wall, central airway instability and hyperreactivity. Infected secretions in cystic fibrosis are dehydrated, hyperadhesive and hyperviscoelastic. Studies of airway clearance techniques have attempted to identify characteristics to address some of the problems of the airway and secretions. The presenting pathological problem should be considered when choosing an airway clearance technique (Lapin 2000).

The physiological principles of airway clearance are discussed in Chapter 5. In order to achieve effective treatment, secretions should be mobilized and removed without causing an increase in airway obstruction or fatigue. The evidence-based airway clearance techniques (see Box 18.1) all aim to enhance airflow, increase lung volume and may alter the rheological properties of mucus. In people with CF who have bron-

18

Box 18.1 Airway clearance techniques

Active cycle of breathing techniques (ACBT)

Autogenic drainage (AD)

Modified autogenic drainage (M AD)

Exercise

High-frequency chest wall oscillation (HFCWO)

Intrapulmonary percussive ventilation (IPV)

Oscillating positive expiratory pressure:
- Acapella®
- Flutter®
- R-C Cornet®

Positive expiratory pressure (PEP):
- PEP
- High PEP

Postural drainage and percussion

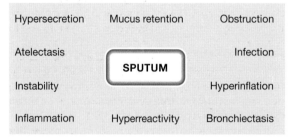

Figure 18.3 The pathophysiological consequences of sputum.

chial wall instability, expiratory airflow is likely to be reduced when intrathoracic pressures are high (Zach et al 1985). Huffing generates lower intrathoracic pressure than coughing (Langlands 1967) and it has been suggested that it is as effective as coughing for mucociliary clearance (Hasani et al 1994). By altering the intrathoracic pressure and the lung volume at which the expiratory manoeuvre is performed, the physiotherapist can tailor the point of compression to the area of obstruction without causing airway collapse. Autogenic drainage prevents airway collapse by maximizing airflow at different lung volumes and avoiding high-pressure peaks (Schöni 1989).

The changing clinical picture of people with CF, with improved clinical status and a generally more active lifestyle, together with an increased understanding of the pathophysiological concepts of airway clearance techniques, have obviated the emphasis on gravity-assisted positioning for airway clearance. Research has shown that ventilation to the dependent area of the lung may be more effective than gravity-assisted 'drainage' from the uppermost lung (Lannefors & Wollmer 1992). Elkins et al (2005a) have shown that huffing and coughing are compromised in the 'head-down tilt' and side-lying positions.

Currently there is a lack of robust evidence to support the long-term benefit of airway clearance. Trials are confounded by small numbers, inconsistency of techniques and no control population (Prasad & Main 1998). To date the majority of trials have been short term and undertaken mainly in adults. A meta-analysis of chest physiotherapy suggested that airway clearance produced significantly greater sputum expectoration than no treatment and the addition of exercise further improved lung function (Thomas et al 1995). However, a systematic review was not able to demonstrate a benefit for treatment compared with no treatment, although short-term studies indicate that there may be deterioration in lung function during periods without treatment in those with established disease (van der Schans et al 2000).

Systematic reviews have not identified any single airway clearance technique as being superior (Elkins et al 2006b, Main et al 2005) and longer-term RCTs support these findings (Accurso et al 2004, Pryor et al 2006a). However, patient preference is likely to be an important factor in terms of adherence. Constant review of techniques is essential to determine the most effective regimen to meet changing lifestyles and disease progression during the clinically stable and acute state.

Exercise offers an important contribution to sputum expectoration (Baldwin et al 1994, Sahl et al 1989), but in the majority of patients it should be complementary and not exclusive (Bilton et al 1992). Patients perceive exercise differently to other forms of treatment (Abbott et al 1996) and some prefer this method of airway clearance. It is important for the physiotherapist to be sensitive to the patient's beliefs (Carr et al 1996), but encourage formal airway clearance during an acute exacerbation when the patient is unable to exercise at his normal level.

The frequency and duration of treatment will vary. When secretions are minimal, treatment once a day may be sufficient but additionally some form of exercise should be encouraged. Many patients will require treatment two or three times a day, but the programme should be realistic and allow for other normal activities. Some techniques may be more time consuming to perform, difficult to learn and may be position depen-

18

dent. Others involve equipment that requires meticulous cleaning. The choice of technique should be individualized to suit the patient's age, lifestyle, preference and disease severity.

Maintenance / increase in exercise tolerance

The value of exercise in the management of CF is now well established. Short-term studies of exercise training programmes in cystic fibrosis have been shown to have considerable therapeutic benefit and the majority of patients wish to include exercise in their routine self-care (Webb & Dodd 2000). Studies have shown improved exercise tolerance (Andreasson et al 1987, Edlund et al 1986, Freeman et al 1993), ventilatory muscle endurance (Keens et al 1977), cardiorespiratory fitness (Orenstein et al 1981), muscle bulk and body image (Strauss et al 1987), decreased breathlessness (O'Neill et al 1987) and improved quality of life (de Jong et al 1997). Two randomized controlled trials of home exercise programmes have demonstrated the long-term value of exercise (Moorcroft et al 2004, Schneiderman-Walker et al 2000). Early studies demonstrated that patients with mild to moderate disease ($FEV_1 = 55\%$ predicted) could exercise to the same level as their peers, but those with more severe disease ($FEV_1 < 55\%$ predicted) would require individualized recommendations and supervised exercise programmes (Cropp et al 1982). Everyone can exercise and no patient should be excluded because of disease severity (Webb & Dodd 2000). The benefits of exercise should be introduced and emphasized from a very early age.

Assessment of exercise capacity

The patient's baseline exercise capacity should be assessed, when the patient is clinically stable, to determine their level of fitness and limitations. The results will give guidance for effective and safe exercise recommendations. The test will provide a baseline measure for further testing to monitor improvement or change in any values and evaluate an intervention. Assessment should consider the choice of protocol, the type of test and the measurements required. The choice of protocol (Table 18.2) depends on the information required, the facilities available and the patient's clinical condition. It may be desirable to determine a functional level of exercise in preference to peak performance (Jones 1988).

Space may be limited and a cycle ergometer may therefore be more appropriate than the modified shuttle test (Bradley et al 1999). The patient may be too breathless to perform a maximal test and some tests may be too difficult for children to perform. The step test may be a validated alternative to measure functional exercise capacity (Balfour-Lynn et al 1998). The measurements and equipment required are outlined in

Table 18.2 Types of exercise test	
Endurance exercise	Progressive maximal • Treadmill • Cycle ergometer • Modified shuttle walk Sub maximal • Treadmill • Cycle ergometer • Step test
Peak power output	Wingate protocol
Strength	Isokinetic dynamometer Isometric dynamometer Maximal weight that can be lifted comfortably (1RM)

Table 18.3. The standard measures of work capacity (distance walked, wattage), pulse, oxygen saturation and a subjective measure of breathlessness and muscle fatigue are sufficient for routine assessment (Fig. 18.4). More sophisticated measures give additional information but are not necessary for routine use. Safety precautions during testing should include personnel trained in resuscitation; oxygen and appropriate drugs for resuscitation should be immediately available in the exercise area. From the results of the test, the physiotherapist can recommend a level of exercise to provide an appropriate training effect that is safe. It is also useful to establish the pattern of habitual activity. Some patients are unwilling to participate in formal exercise programmes, but are happy to increase everyday activity.

Exercise programmes

Exercise is limited by the symptoms of breathlessness or muscle fatigue. The aim of an exercise programme is to improve exercise performance, make a given level of exercise more comfortable and increase the activities of daily living. It is important to establish the goals of an exercise programme for the individual patient, which may be different for carer and patient (Table 18.4). Exercise programmes must be tailored to the individual, based on disease severity, level of fitness and patient preference.

Types of exercise

An exercise progamme should combine endurance and strength-training exercises for upper and lower body. Attention has also been paid to the value of anaerobic exercise and strength training, especially in children whose natural activity patterns are characterized by

18

Table 18.3 Measurements and equipment required for assessing exercise capacity

Measurements	Equipment
Peak work capacity	• Bicycle – resistance • Treadmill – speed and incline • Walking – speed and distance
Peak heart rate	• Cardiac monitor • Pulse meter • Fingers
Oxygen saturation	• Pulse oximeter
Spirometry (pre- and post-exercise)	• Spirometer
Perceived breathlessness	• Borg or VAS scores • 15-count breathlessness score
Perceived muscular fatigue	• Borg or VAS scores
Respiratory rate	• Count or 'on-line'
Ventilation ($\dot{V}_E$, V_T, TiTOT, RR) Oxygen uptake CO_2 output End-tidal CO_2	• On-line system
Blood lactate	• Lactate analyser or blood to laboratory
PaO_2 and $PaCO_2$	• Arterial line

VAS, visual analogue scale; $\dot{V}_E$, minute ventilation; V_T, tidal volume; TiTOT, ratio of time spent in inspiration to total respiratory time; RR, respiratory rate; CO_2, carbon dioxide; PaO_2, partial pressure of oxygen in arterial blood; $PaCO_2$, partial pressure of carbon dioxide in arterial blood

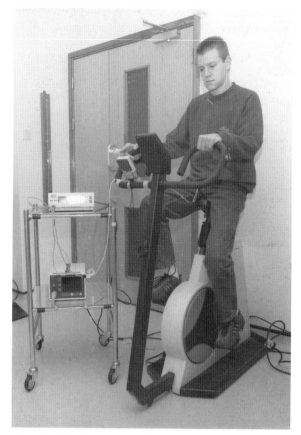

Figure 18.4 Assessing exercise capacity with cycle ergometry and pulse oximetry monitoring.

Table 18.4 The differing aims of exercise programmes for the patient and carer

Aims of carer	Aims of patient
• ↑ Maximal exercise performance, endurance and strength • ↓ Breathlessness • ↑ Nutritional status • ↑ Quality of life • ↓ Respiratory tract infections • Preserve lung function • ?↓ Mortality	• Healthy lifestyle • Enjoyment and social interaction • Improved body image • Improved stamina for socializing • Improved fitness for a sporting activity • A replacement for chest clearance

short bursts of vigorous physical activity (Klijn et al 2004, Orenstein et al 2004).

■ *Endurance exercise* aims to improve the capacity to endure more exercise without discomfort, e.g. swimming, running, cycling, skipping, aerobic classes, step aerobics, trampolines (Edlund et al 1986, Orenstein et al 1981, Sahl et al 1989) (Fig. 18.5).

■ *Strength training* aims to increase muscle mass and strength, e.g. weights and sprint training (Strauss et al 1987) (Fig. 18.6).

■ *Interval training* may be useful for those patients unable to sustain long periods of exercise. Short bursts of exercise at higher rates will enhance a train-

ing response. It may be of benefit for those patients with prolonged periods of desaturation.

■ The evidence for inspiratory muscle training (IMT) has previously been conflicting (Asher et al 1982, Sawyer & Clayton 1993) and to date has shown no

18

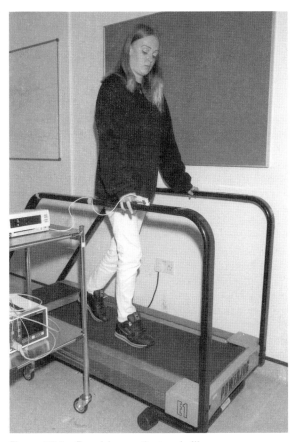

Figure 18.5   Exercising on the treadmill.

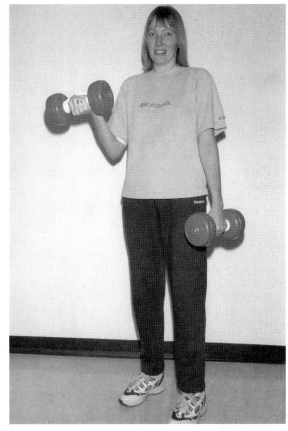

Figure 18.6   Exercising with dumbbells.

advantage over general upper body muscle training (Keens et al 1977). Two randomized controlled trials of IMT in adults and children have shown a positive outcome on exercise performance and quality of life (Albini et al 2004, Enright et al 2004)

- There are no studies to date evaluating the benefits of a lifestyle change. Parents of children and adolescents with CF have been reported to be less positive about the benefits of exercise than the parents of healthy children (Boas et al 1999). It is essential to establish from the time of diagnosis the importance of the contribution that exercise makes to a healthy lifestyle and to encourage participation of the whole family. There is a decline in physical activity in late adolescence (Britto et al 2000). Careful consideration and encouragement should be given to this age group at this time. Contact by the physiotherapist with local gym and sports facilities may offer reduced fees for exercise sessions.

Intensity, duration and frequency

Endurance exercise.   An effective exercise programme should make reasonable demands on the patient's physical capacity and be progressive. The intensity can be derived from the results of the exercise test. Various recommendations have been suggested:

- 50% of peak work capacity is below the anaerobic threshold for most patients and represents a functional level of activity (Marcotte et al 1986)

- 50–60% peak oxygen consumption ($\dot{V}O$peak) is necessary to improve physical fitness (Astrand & Rodahl 1977) and the patient's capability is related to the percentage of their individual $\dot{V}O_2$peak

- 70–85% of the measured maximum heart rate is sufficient to achieve a training effect (Orenstein et al 1981)

18

- 70% of the maximum speed attained on a maximal field test (Pryor et al 2006b)

- 'breathlessness without distress' for those patients with severe disease who are limited by ventilatory mechanics (Godfrey & Mearns 1971).

Exercise should begin at the chosen intensity for a period of time sufficient to cause breathlessness or muscle fatigue without undue stress and progress to 20–30 minutes 3–4 days a week. Progression for the patient who is limited by breathlessness will be at a slower rate than the unfit patient who is limited by muscular fatigue.

Strength training. This should begin with a weight that can be lifted comfortably 10–15 times and progressed by increasing the repetitions to 20–30 and then by increasing the weight. The intensity should be sufficient to leave the patient 'pleasantly tired without soreness'. The duration and frequency can progress to 15–30 minutes on alternate days. It is important to ensure correct positioning, correct technique and coordination of breathing for each exercise. A warm-up, stretching exercises and cool-down should be incorporated into each session to avoid injury. A more aerobic programme would include low weights and high repetitions whereas high weights and low repetitions constitute an anaerobic programme.

Strength training in children should be approached with care. Growing bones are sensitive to repetitive loading and the epiphysial plate is susceptible to injury before full growth is complete. Overstrenuous resistance training is as dangerous for children as it is for adults and joints should not be subjected to repetitive stress. Heavy weights and high resistance eccentric exercises should be avoided and machines are generally safer than free weights. To minimize the risk, a resistance should be selected which can be lifted 10–15 times without fatigue (or 8–12 repetitions in children). As with adults, exercises should be carefully planned and well performed in a correct position.

Precautions

There are no absolute contraindications but exercise should cease temporarily for the following medical problems: abdominal obstruction, an acute bronchopulmonary exacerbation associated with fever, transient arthralgia and arthritis, pneumothorax, persistent haemoptysis and surgery including a Caesarean section. Exercise-induced bronchoconstriction is rare in CF, but can usually be controlled with pre-exercise bronchodilators. Patients undertaking exercise in hot climates should be well hydrated and advised to supplement their salt intake (Bar-Or et al 1992). Exercise for the diabetic patient should be encouraged (see section on CF related diabetes). Certain sporting activities carry a medical risk (Webb & Dodd 1999). Contact sports, bungee jumping and parachute jumping are not advised for those patients with diagnosed low bone mineral density, portal hypertension and significant enlargement of the spleen and liver. Scuba diving could be hazardous for patients with air trapping and sinus disease. In the hypoxic patient, exercise at altitude poses a potential risk (Speechly-Dick et al 1992). Careful advice should be given to patients contemplating skiing and any strenuous/high-intensity aerobic and anaerobic exercise at altitude.

Exercising the patient with advancing disease

There is no evidence that carefully tailored and supervised exercise is harmful in these patients and they should not be excluded from a training programme. For patients with severe disease and those awaiting transplantation, deconditioning occurs rapidly. Maintaining mobility is crucial and strength and endurance exercises should be encouraged (Webb et al 1996). A maximal exercise test will define the limits of breathlessness and muscle fatigue. Exercise programmes should then be planned with these in mind. Positions for breathing control (Chapter 5) should be introduced to alleviate exertion breathlessness and increase mobility.

Studies have reported the benefits of oxygen supplementation for patients with severe disease (Heijerman et al 1992, Marcus et al 1992). Oxygen may be required to ease the symptom of breathlessness and increase exercise performance. Many patients are reluctant to use oxygen for activity, especially outdoors. Considerable benefits are achieved using oxygen before and after exercise for recovery. Patients can use small oxygen cylinders discreetly to enable them to travel and socialize in the community. During exercise and periods of recovery, inspiratory flow rates increase, so the oxygen prescription and delivery device should be adjusted to relieve exercise-induced breathlessness. Patients mouth breathe during exercise and periods of breathlessness and a fixed concentration mask at low concentration and high flows may provide greater relief than nasal cannulae (Dodd et al 1998). The oxygen flow should be titrated to a level of comfort which provides an arterial oxygen saturation >90% (Heijerman et al 1992). For patients who are dependent on non-invasive ventilation, exercise should also be performed using the equipment (Webb et al 1996). This can take the form of weight training in sitting and step-ups in standing or walking on a treadmill (Fig. 18.7). Careful assessment with attention to respiratory rate, perceived breathlessness and

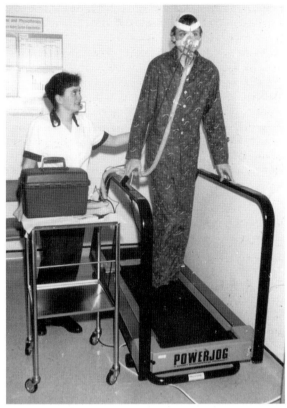

Figure 18.7 Exercising with non-invasive ventilation. (Reproduced with permission from Webb et al 1996.)

exertion can provide a comfortable level of exercise without undue breathlessness, with or without oxygen to maintain mobility and quality of life.

Inhalation therapy

Patients are prescribed an ever-increasing number of medications delivered by inhalation. Delivery is potentially maximized by matching the patient's inspiratory flow rate and drug characteristics to the delivery device. Inhalers are more convenient and less time consuming than nebulizers, but some drugs can be delivered only by the nebulized route.

Bronchodilators

Bronchodilators are prescribed to relieve airway obstruction. Careful evaluation by reversibility testing and subjective benefit will determine the response and the merits of the inhaled or nebulized route for the individual patient. Beta-adrenergic drugs increase cilial

action, improve mucociliary clearance (Wood et al 1975) and may be of benefit before chest clearance (Kuhn & Nahata 1985). During an acute exacerbation, when secretions are excessive and obstruction is increased, the nebulized route may be more effective (Conway & Watson 1997). Inhalers are available in a range of doses. It is preferable and less time consuming for the patient to be prescribed a device that will deliver a higher dose of medication than to increase the number of puffs of a lower dose.

The value of long-acting β_2-agonists has been described (Bargon et al 1997) but the place of inhaled corticosteroids is questionable (Balfour-Lynn et al 1997, 2000, Bisgaard et al 1997). Withdrawing steroids in selective patients would however appear to be safe and not affect respiratory exacerbation rates (Balfour-Lynn et al 2006). CF patients often show a dip in PEFR and report symptoms of tightness in the early evening. One can speculate that this is because drugs are metabolized faster in patients with CF so that the benefits of long-acting drugs are shortened. It is important to select a device that is both acceptable to the individual patient and matches their inspiratory flow rate. Generally CF patients have high inspiratory flow rates. There are various teaching devices to assess patient technique and suitability for the required flow rate of the device, but careful consideration must be given to the risk of cross-infection in this patient group. Some commercially prescribed devices require specific inspiratory flow rates for effective deposition. The Accuhaler®(GlaxoSmith-Kline) is a dry powder inhaler, which is less dependent on inspiratory flow (Hill & Slater 1998). It is less confusing for the patient if the same device is prescribed for all medications. It is sometimes possible to combine two types of drug in one preparation, e.g. Seretide® (Glaxo-SmithKline) combining a corticosteroid and long-acting bronchodilator. The physiotherapist should always be mindful of the treatment burden on CF patients.

Mucolytic agents

Inhalation of hypertonic saline by an ultrasonic nebulizer has been shown to improve lung function and perceived effectiveness of chest physiotherapy over a 2-week period (Eng et al 1996) and to improve mucociliary clearance after one inhalation (Robinson et al 1996). In both of these studies the positive effects were significantly increased when compared with 0.9% saline. Hypertonic saline may induce bronchoconstriction (Rodwell & Anderson 1996). A test dose should be given, with recordings of PEFR or FEV_1 before and 5 minutes after inhalation, to identify any increase in airflow obstruction. In a large controlled long-term study of twice daily 7% saline, respiratory exacerbations

18

were reduced and the treatment was considered to be safe if preceded by a bronchodilator (Elkins et al 2006a).

The optimal drug effect of rhDNase is different for each individual and can vary from 30 minutes to several hours. It is recommended initially that inhalation should be performed before early evening to avoid coughing during sleeping hours and 30 minutes to 2 hours before chest clearance (Conway & Watson 1997). Some patients who have difficulty clearing sputum in the morning gain considerable benefit from inhalation of rhDNase at night, without coughing during sleeping hours. Treatment regimens should therefore be individualized and frequently assessed as the disease changes. When the optimum time has been determined, inhalation in relation to chest clearance can be recommended. The effect on lung function has been shown to be equally as effective with alternate day dosing as daily (Suri et al 2002). This may decrease the treatment burden and cost, but the effect on sputum viscosity should be carefully monitored. rhDNase should not be mixed with other drugs as it requires isotonic conditions and a neutral pH for maximal activity. If nebulized antibiotics or inhaled steroids are part of the treatment regimen, the pH of these solutions is acidic and may denature the protein (Ramsey & Dorkin 1994). At least 30 minutes should separate antibiotic and rhDNase inhalation (Conway & Watson 1997). A sidestream nebulizer (Respironics) has been recommended for inhalation (Shah et al 1997). The nebulizer chamber used for rhDNase should not be used for any other drug. rhDNase should be stored at 0–4°C and should be removed from the refrigerator and brought to room temperature (approximately 15 minutes) before inhalation to avoid bronchoconstriction. Other mucolytic agents, for example acetylcysteine (Parvolex®), are also said to reduce mucus viscosity, but have been less frequently used since the introduction of rhDNase and hypertonic saline.

Antibiotics

Aerosolized antibiotics should be inhaled following airway clearance. Studies have shown that bronchoconstriction may be induced by some preparations of inhaled antibiotics. (Chua et al 1990, Cunningham et al 2001, Maddison et al 1994, Nikolaizik et al 1996). A test dose should be performed when the patient is clinically stable, to detect any increase in airflow obstruction. Spirometry should be performed before, immediately and up to 30 minutes following inhalation (Webb & Dodd 1997). Bronchoconstriction may be prevented by altering the tonicity of the solution to iso- or hypotonic (Dodd et al 1997). The long-term effects of repeated bronchoconstriction are unknown and it is now recommended that the inhalation of antibiotics should be preceded by an inhaled bronchodilator (Chua et al 1990, Webb & Dodd 1997).

The details of inhaling several drugs can be complex. It is crucial that the patient is given verbal and written instructions of how to use (including the cleaning and maintenance of any equipment), when to use and the order of use in relation to airway clearance and other drugs. This complexity may be simplified by the admixture of inhaled solutions /suspensions (Wolfgang et al 2006). While the physico-chemical compatibility is known, the aerodynamic characteristics of a mixture require further study.

Intelligent nebulizers

The development of a new generation of nebulizer delivery devices utilizing vibrating mesh technology e.g. eFlow® rapid (PARI), I-neb™ AAD® System (Respironics UK), has revolutionized the efficiency and efficacy of drug delivery, deposition and patient acceptability of this burdensome treatment. Treatment times are shorter with audible feedback on completion of inhalation. The devices are small, silent and battery driven. Incorporated within this technology in some devices (e.g. I-neb™ AAD®) is an adaptive aerosol delivery (AAD) and 'controlled inhalations'. These devices adapt to the individual's breathing pattern and deliver a preset dose during a proportion of the inhalation phase only. A precise dose is always delivered irrespective of the breathing pattern and environmental contamination is minimized. A controlled inhalation by the device restricts the patient to a slow deep inhalation to maximize peripheral airway deposition (Mullinger et al 2004).

Acute bronchopulmonary infection

Increased cough and sputum production with a fall in spirometry, decreased exercise tolerance, weight loss, lack of energy and increased breathlessness are common signs and symptoms of an acute exacerbation. Fever and chest pain may also be present. It is likely that during an acute infection, the duration and frequency of airway clearance will need to be increased and, if necessary, assistance given with manual techniques. Periods of breathing control may need to be lengthened to avoid fatigue and the treatment should be discontinued before the patient feels exhausted. Positions for treatment may need to be modified to reduce breathlessness. During periods of rest the positions of high side lying and forward lean sitting may facilitate contraction of the diaphragm, by altering the length–tension status (Sharp et al 1980), and ease the work of breathing. There are

18

such wide variations in pathology, signs and symptoms that for the inexperienced physiotherapist it is very difficult to know when to discontinue a treatment session. As a guide, a treatment session may range from about 15 to 45 minutes. This may include the use of devices: for example, non-invasive ventilation and intermittent positive pressure breathing.

Airway obstruction should be minimized before instigating airway clearance. Regular nebulized bronchodilators may be recommended (Conway & Watson 1997) and benefits have been reported following the use of intravenous terbutaline (Finnegan et al 1992) or aminophylline (Hodson 2000).

Mucolytic agents such as hypertonic saline and rhDNase have been shown to be effective mucolytic agents (Fuchs et al 1994) as discussed above. Although rhDNase is recognized to be the treatment of choice (Suri et al 2002), there is individual variability and both drugs are worthy of consideration. There is little evidence that inhaling bland aerosols, e.g. normal saline as a mucolytic is effective in improving the rheological properties of mucus, increasing ciliary clearance or increasing mucus transport in CF (Wanner & Rao 1980).

Intermittent positive pressure breathing (IPPB) or non-invasive ventilation (NIV) may be indicated for the tiring breathless patient who is having difficulty clearing secretions because of compromised ventilatory mechanics. Short-term trials of NIV in adults and children have shown improved oxygen saturation and muscle pressure during airway clearance, compared with the active cycle of breathing techniques (ACBT) and the forced expiration technique (FET) alone. There was no difference in lung function or sputum expectoration, but NIV was preferred by the patients (Fauroux et al 1999, Holland et al 2003). It is important to note, however, that in both studies supplemental oxygen was not used during airway clearance. Careful consideration must be given in patients who have had a previous pneumothorax.

Supplemental oxygen, during airway clearance, is advised if the PaO_2 is below 8.0 kPa (60 mmHg) or SpO_2 is below 92%. Theoretically, improving hypoxia should decrease respiratory rate and improve tidal volume, thus promoting a more effective treatment. Airway clearance techniques may be better tolerated and breathlessness reduced with the use of supplemental oxygen. The high total gas flows of low-concentration Venturi masks may be more acceptable, and provide greater relief than nasal cannulae for recovery from coughing (Dodd et al 1998).

Oxygen therapy for respiratory failure

CF patients have a supra-normal drive to breathe, with an increased ventilatory response to increasing hypoxia resulting in a lower than usual $PaCO_2$. Inspiratory time is increased, which further increases the work of breathing. Patients are therefore unlikely to chronically retain carbon dioxide, but at a PaO_2 below 50 mmHg, ventilation decreases and respiratory failure easily ensues (Bureau et al 1981) (presumably due to muscle fatigue in the presence of an increasing respiratory drive). Patients with CF have high inspiratory flow rates and the normal recommended flow rates of fixed-concentration masks may be insufficient to meet that demand. It is important to increase the normal recommended flow rate to meet the peak inspiratory flow rate, i.e. a 24% mask may require settings of 2–4 litres or more and a 28% mask 4–6 litres or more. Failure to increase the flow rate will result in a decreased oxygen concentration and increased work of breathing. For the severely breathless patient requiring >28% concentration, oxygen delivery by a high-flow generator at low concentrations of oxygen (e.g. 32%) may be necessary (Dodd et al 1998).

CF patients with severe disease may hypoventilate at night, leading to a significant rise in $PaCO_2$ (Spier et al 1984). The ventilatory response to hypercapnia is blunted in CF and although the long-term consequences of increasing hypercapnia are unclear, it is possible that ventilatory drive and CO_2 sensitivity may be blunted (Gozal 1997). A fixed-concentration mask should be considered for the safe delivery of oxygen at night-time, but NIV may be required for those patients with increasing levels of $PaCO_2$ in response to oxygen. CF patients may not be hypercapnic during the day, but may retain carbon dioxide at night and may therefore respond differently to supplemental oxygen administered at night than during the day. An accurate prescription will be necessary for night-time, exercise and rest with details of delivery device, concentration and flow rate.

Non-invasive ventilation

Non-invasive ventilation (NIV) has reported benefits for patients who are listed for transplantation (Hill et al 1998, Hodson et al 1991) and for the stable hypercapnic patient at home (Piper et al 1992). The physiotherapist may be involved with introducing the patient to the ventilator and adjusting the settings to meet the patient's comfort and give adequate oxygenation. For some patients NIV may be continued during airway clearance with appropriate adjustment to the settings, but for others airway clearance alone or in conjunction with IPPB is just as effective. There is evidence, from short-term studies, for the use of NIV in airway clearance but

18

the long-term effect is unknown (Bradley et al 2006). The development of a pneumothorax in patients who are dependent on NIV causes a medical management dilemma. If a patent intercostal tube is in situ, NIV can be delivered safely with a pressure preset ventilator. Each patient will require supervised and individualized management with the risks of mechanical ventilation being balanced against the potential benefits (Haworth et al 2000).

Humidification of oxygen

It is recommended that oxygen should be humidified in CF, due to the basic defect in the airway. It is suggested that water vapour humidity is preferable to nebulized humidity for maintenance of PaO_2 (Kuo et al 1991). Oxygen delivered by nasal cannulae can be humidified with a bubble through water vapour humidifier to a maximum flow of 6 litres. A heated humidifier (e.g. Aerodyne, Kendall, Basingstoke, Hampshire; Fisher & Paykel, Maidenhead, Berkshire) is necessary to humidify the large volumes of gas delivered by 24% and 28% concentration masks and a high-flow generator because the time interval for moisture transfer decreases as flow rate increases above 20 l/min.

The large volumes of air delivered by NIV may cause drying of secretions and require humidification by a heated water vapour source. This may increase the problem of breakdown of the skin on the bridge of the nose, and in those patients humidification may have to be reserved for an acute exacerbation. In the terminal stage of the disease, when secretions are very tenacious, it may be necessary to humidify the oxygen delivered to the nasal mask with a bubble-through humidifier.

Domiciliary oxygen

Transferring oxygen into the community can be a challenge (Dodd et al 1998). Oxygen concentrators are usually prescribed for night-time use. The driving pressure is much lower than that of a cylinder and although adequate for use with nasal cannulae and NIV, there may be difficulties with the use of Venturi masks. Cylinders and 24% or 28% Venturi masks are recommended for relief of breathlessness. Liquid oxygen is the ideal system for CF patients and allows mobility outside the home. Careful assessment is required for overnight, ambulatory and short-burst oxygen to determine the required flow rate, concentration and hours of use. In the United Kingdom, explicit details are given to the contractors for domiciliary oxygen to enable them to work with the patient to decide which technology would best suit their therapeutic need (Department of Health 2004).

Complications of cystic fibrosis

Advanced cystic fibrosis

The late stages of the disease are characterized by repeated exacerbations, often with continuous intravenous antibiotics and increased hospitalization, respiratory failure and reduced mobility. It is essential to maximize the reversal of airway obstruction with airway clearance techniques, nebulized and intravenous bronchodilators and steroids. Sputum viscosity is reduced with rhDNase and intravenous fluids, and expectoration facilitated with hypertonic saline.

Shortness of breath may be reduced with the use of humidified oxygen, careful positioning and relaxation techniques. Type I respiratory failure requires meticulous evaluation at rest and during mobility for the requirements of oxygen. Hypercapnic respiratory failure may be reversed with NIV. Mobility is crucial for patients who are listed for transplantation and to maintain quality of life. Some patients have difficulty coming to terms with their loss of independence and input from a clinical psychologist experienced in the treatment of cystic fibrosis may prove beneficial.

Despite optimal medical and physiotherapeutic care, the terminal stage of the disease will ensue. It is inappropriate to withdraw support in the terminal stages even though physiotherapy may no longer be effective. Assistance can be given with positioning breathless patients in high side lying or sitting leaning forward, to make them as comfortable as possible. Occasionally IPPB can be used to assist the clearance of secretions from the upper airways, but care must be taken to use it only as a part of physiotherapy treatment and not as a form of pseudoventilation. Nasotracheal suction is not indicated as it would serve no useful purpose at this stage. Morphine or one of its derivatives will help to relieve anxiety and breathlessness.

Allergic bronchopulmonary aspergillosis

Allergic bronchopulmonary aspergillosis (ABPA) leads to airway narrowing, gas trapping and small airways disease. Tenacious mucus plugs, often brown in colour, and wheezing are common presenting symptoms of ABPA. Airway obstruction is increased and there is often a marked reduction in lung function (Kraemer et al 2006). Medical management includes oral steroids and antifungal agents (e.g. itraconazole or voriconazole). Mucus plugging can lead to lobar or segmental collapse. Bronchodilators may be helpful and airway clearance techniques should be adapted to minimize airway obstruction. IPPB may be indicated. Exercise tolerance may be reduced (Simmonds et al 1990) and programmes may need to be modified.

Arthropathy and joint pain

CF-related arthropathy can present as hypertrophic pulmonary osteoarthropathy (HPOA) or periodic arthritis (Koch & Lanng 2000). HPOA is related to pulmonary disease and presents most frequently in adults. Episodes of transient arthritis appear to be unrelated to pulmonary disease. HPOA is characterized by pain, swelling and warmth of the involved area and occasionally small joint effusions. Arthritis can be associated with fever and vasculitis. Active physiotherapy is not generally indicated. Joints should be rested and gentle mobilization encouraged, within the limits of the symptoms. The medical management for a pulmonary exacerbation may lead to a resolution of symptoms (Rush et al 1986) and CF arthritis usually resolves spontaneously (Turner et al 1997).

Cystic fibrosis-related diabetes

The specific changes in glucose metabolism in CF are well described (Bridges & Spowart 2006, Koch & Lanng 2000). The incidence increases with age and it is suggested that survival is reduced in this group. Hyperglycaemia causes polyuria, which leads to dehydration and a possible increase in sputum viscosity. Expectoration is difficult and lung function declines. The physiotherapist should be alert to the results of blood glucose monitoring (BM) in the analysis of chest symptoms and formulation of a treatment plan. It is essential that the medical management includes control of blood sugar and rehydration with intravenous fluids. When diabetes is difficult to control, attention should be directed to the application of airway clearance techniques which reduce viscosity and the consideration of rhDNase.

Insulin requirements will change with exercise. Exercise can sometimes improve overall blood glucose control by reducing insulin requirements. When diabetes is well controlled, exercise may induce hypoglycaemia either during exercise or up to 24–36 hours after exercise (Cystic Fibrosis Trust 2004c). The balance of insulin requirement and carbohydrate intake should be discussed with the CF dietitian and physician and individualized for both normal activity and exercise programmes. It is important to maintain exercise during admission to hospital because reduced activity will result in an increase in BM values. If the diabetes is labile during an acute exacerbation, a pre-exercise BM is advisable in addition to close liaison with the dietitian.

Distal intestinal obstruction syndrome

This complication describes intestinal obstruction occurring after the neonatal period (Davidson 2000). It is characterized by abdominal pain, distension, vomiting, palpable fecal masses and partial or complete intestinal obstruction. Urgent medical management includes intravenous rehydration, Gastrografin® and possibly a balanced electrolyte solution. The symptoms of immobility, pain, decreased functional residual capacity and dehydration compromise the clearance of secretions. It is important for airway clearance to continue, but techniques should be modified until the problem resolves. Mobilization is encouraged and may help bowel movement. For patients with a persistent problem, a lower body exercise programme may be useful.

Gastro-oesophageal reflux

This is well recognized in CF with a higher incidence in infants. The cause and effect of physiotherapy positioning for this group is unclear and has been discussed earlier. Treatment is directed at medical management with the use of prokinetic agents and/or gastric suppressants, thickening of feeds and appropriate positioning. The adult is often unaware that gastro-oesophageal reflux (GOR) is a complication of CF and the symptoms may be under-reported. The physiotherapist may be alerted to the possibility of GOR if the patient reports symptoms during airway clearance (for example upper gastrointestinal discomfort). In adults with more severe disease GOR, both silent and symptomatic, can be a significant problem (Button et al 2005a). Oxygenation and reflux scores have been shown to deteriorate in the head-down tilt position. This may be of significance when undertaking airway clearance treatments, particularly in the acutely unwell individual with CF (Elkins et al 2005a).

Haemoptysis

Blood streaking of sputum frequently occurs, especially at the time of an acute pulmonary exacerbation. It is appropriate to continue with the normal airway clearance regimen and to reassure the patient. Frank haemoptysis can be considered moderate at <250 ml or severe at >250 ml (Hodson 1994) and it is important to establish the volume expectorated over 24 hours to determine the treatment plan (Table 18.5). It is important to continue with chest clearance to remove the blood and infected secretions (Hodson 1994). Management is aimed at clearing secretions without increasing the bleeding. Noting the activity and position at the time of haemoptysis will provide a clue to the cause and influence management. The weakened artery may rupture due to increasing heart rate or increasing the flow of blood when the area of lung supplied by the artery is dependent (the bronchial arteries lie posteriorly). If the patient can establish the location of the bleed, it is advisable to avoid chest clearance with the affected lobe dependent (Bilton et al 1990).

18

Table 18.5	The treatment of haemoptysis
Mild Streaking	• Normal airway clearance regimen
Moderate <250 ml	• Careful positioning • Thoracic expansion exercises • Gentle huffing to low lung volume • Minimize coughing. Airway clearance techniques should minimize increases in intrathoracic pressure • Exercise advice (avoid sudden increases in heart rate)
Severe >250 ml	• Oxygen/humidification • When the bleeding has subsided resume treatment as for moderate
Embolization	• Chest clearance can resume after the procedure in consultation with the radiologist

When haemoptysis is severe, the location of the bleeding should be dependent to avoid asphyxiation (Jones & Davis 1990). When the bleeding has subsided, chest clearance can be resumed. Bronchoscopy will locate the bleeding for those patients with persistent haemoptysis and the management usually requires embolization (King et al 1989, Vidal et al 2006). Chest clearance can resume following the procedure in consultation with the radiologist. Implantable venous access devices, which require flushing with an anticoagulant to maintain patency, may increase the risk of haemoptysis during intravenous therapy. If this occurs, the use of normal saline for flushing may lead to cessation of bleeding.

Liver disease

Liver disease usually presents as biliary cirrhosis, but fatty infiltration is a recognized feature. Hepatosplenomegaly and portal hypertension ensue with the development of oesophageal varices and potentially life-threatening haematemesis (Westaby 2000). Liver transplantation is an increasing feature of adult CF care. An enlarged liver and spleen will compromise respiratory mechanics and cause breathlessness. Careful consideration should be given to positioning during airway clearance. Airway clearance should be discontinued during acute haemorrhage. Careful exercise advice is recommended (see exercise section).

Low bone mineral density

Low bone mineral density (BMD) is a recognized complication of CF in both children and adults (Bachrach

et al 1994, Bhudmkanok et al 1996). The correlates of low BMD include poor absorption of vitamins, minerals and protein from the gut, oral steroids, inactivity, increased cytokines from infection and hypogonadism (Haworth et al 1999). The problem is one of reduced bone accretion in childhood and early and increased rate of bone resorption in adult life. Bone mineral density appears to be normal until the age of about 10 years and seems to decrease during the adolescent years (Cystic Fibrosis Trust 2007). Lack of physical activity is a known correlate, but there is no direct evidence that lack of physical activity leads to low BMD and it is currently unknown if weight-bearing activities can increase peak bone mass, preserve BMD or increase BMD in those with low BMD. However, it would seem prudent to encourage weight-bearing exercises based on studies in the healthy population (Cystic Fibrosis Trust 2007) There is an increased risk of rib fractures (Bachrach et al 1994) and there is some concern that manual techniques during airway clearance could cause a rib fracture. While there are no reports to date of manual techniques causing rib fractures in CF, there are other methods of airway clearance with proven efficacy which should be considered as alternatives (Cystic Fibrosis Trust 2002b). Coughing has been reported to cause a rib fracture in CF (Elkin et al 2001). A regular review of airway clearance techniques is essential in this vulnerable group of patients.

Rib and vertebral fractures are extremely painful and inhibit airway clearance and mobility. A chest X-ray should always be performed to exclude a pneumothorax. Mucus plugging and an infective exacerbation may quickly ensue. Effective analgesia is a priority before airway clearance and mobilization. Effective coughing should be facilitated by support to the chest wall and the use of antibiotics and rhDNase should reduce sputum volume and ease the mobilization of secretions.

Musculoskeletal dysfunction

Patients with CF develop alterations in chest wall mechanics and spinal deformities due to progressive lung disease, malnutrition and poor bone mineralization (Tattersall et al 2000). This leads to abnormal posture, pain and poor quality of life (Dodd & Prasad 2005). Postural screening and specific testing will direct the design of targeted interventions to improve musculoskeletal and neuromuscular impairments (Massery 2005). Musculoskeletal abnormalities are secondary to respiratory impairment. An understanding of the relationship between the respiratory and postural muscles of the trunk is critical to planning an effective strategy to address the musculoskeletal problems in CF. Current clinical evidence would suggest that an optimum time to screen and intervene, to minimize or prevent musculoskeletal problems, would be during the prepubescent years. Postural adjustments may correct kyphosis and lordosis, but the value of postural therapy needs further evaluation in CF. The flexible ruler technique has been validated in adults with CF to assess spinal deformity and may provide a simple non-invasive tool for routine use in the clinical setting (Boyle et al 2003). Other outcome measures to be considered would include optimal postural development, improved breathing mechanics, prevention of joint conditions, development of fewer pulmonary complications and functional and quality of life issues (Massery 2005). Manual therapy techniques may increase thoracic mobility and may improve lung function (Vibekk 1991). Musculoskeletal abnormalities are a consequence of improved survival and the physiotherapist should be proactive in addressing postural concerns and symptoms and treat appropriately. Flexibility and postural exercises should be introduced in childhood as part of an exercise regimen to prevent the problems that are reported with increasing age and disease severity.

Pneumothorax

In people with CF a pneumothorax usually occurs with advanced disease and chronic *Pseudomonas* infection (Penketh et al 1982). It is associated with increased mortality and may be an independent indicator of prognosis. A pneumothorax may occur due to rupture of a subpleural bleb through the visceral pleura or, rarely, as a result of misplacement of a central line. The physiotherapist may be alerted to the problem by a sudden increase in breathlessness and shoulder tip pain.

The aim of physiotherapy management is to clear secretions, aid re-expansion of the collapsed lung and prevent infection in the re-expanding lung (Table 18.6). It is usual for prophylactic intravenous antibiotics to be given at this time because airway clearance and mobility are compromised. When the pneumothorax is small (<20% of lung volume) treatment is conservative and airway clearance should continue with the aim of clearing secretions without increasing the size of the pneumothorax. Techniques that increase intrathoracic pressure and paroxysmal coughing should be avoided and positive pressure devices should be used with caution. Mobility is encouraged but exercise programmes should temporarily cease. An increase in symptoms may be an indication that the pneumothorax has increased in size. This should be immediately reported and an urgent chest X-ray requested.

Larger pneumothoraces will require an intercostal drain and, if persistent, video-assisted thoracoscopic surgery (VATS) is the preferred treatment. In the light of lung transplantation, pleurodesis should be avoided. While the drain is in situ, airway clearance techniques

Table 18.6	The treatment of a pneumothorax
Small (up to 20% of lung volume)	Chest clearance techniques are aimed at clearing secretions without increasing the size of the pneumothorax. ↑ Intrathoracic pressure should be minimized. • Position the patient with affected side uppermost • Thoracic expansion exercises and 'hold' • Gentle huffing • Minimize coughing • Exercise advice
Large (with intercostal drain)	Treatment is aimed at clearing secretions of all lung areas with adequate pain relief. • Thoracic expansion exercises and 'hold' • Huffing • Coughing • Exercise advice • Care with moving and handling. Drainage bottle should always be lower than the patient
Removal of intercostal drain	• Treatment as for small pneumothorax • Care is taken in the short-term to prevent any reoccurrence of the resolving pneumothorax
Unresolved	• VATS or thoracotomy

VATS, video-assisted thoracoscopic surgery

are reintroduced as indicated at assessment and with appropriate analgesia. Mobilization and gentle exercise are encouraged. When the intercostal tube is removed, care should be taken with airway clearance, in the short term, to prevent any reoccurrence of the resolving pneumothorax. Normal activities are advised, but strenuous exercise and lifting are not recommended. Patients should be cautioned about driving and air travel is contraindicated for 6 weeks (British Thoracic Society 2004). Following surgery, airway clearance should be restarted as soon as possible with adequate analgesia.

Pregnancy

Improved survival has resulted in more females reaching reproductive age. Pregnancy is well tolerated by patients with an FEV_1 >60% predicted, but associated with increased maternal and fetal complications in those

18

with an FEV_1 <60% predicted (Edenborough et al 1995). As pregnancy can stress the pulmonary, nutritional and cardiovascular reserves of the patient with CF, knowledge of the normal changes (Elkus & Popovich 1992, Weinberger et al 1980) and their implications in CF (Kotloff et al 1992) is useful (Table 18.7). Airway clearance techniques should continue throughout pregnancy and be modified as pregnancy progresses with consideration of the degree of breathlessness and discomfort. Breathlessness commonly occurs in the first and second trimesters and may be normal. Careful monitoring of the vital capacity is essential to identify the onset of an acute exacerbation. Elevation of the diaphragm reduces functional residual capacity and causes early airway closure. Attention should be paid to clearance of the lung bases to prevent the possibility of trapped secretions.

Gentle exercise during pregnancy should be encouraged and established aerobic programmes may be continued. Non-weight-bearing exercises, e.g. swimming and cycling, have a lower energy cost than weight-bearing exercises (Kotloff et al 1992). Weight training should not be introduced during pregnancy, but an established programme should be modified and discussed with the medical team. The importance of pelvic floor exercises should be stressed at the beginning of pregnancy and reinforced at each clinic visit. Leakage of urine is a problem for many women (Orr et al 2001) and pregnancy will further stress the pelvic floor. Abdominal supports are available for patients who suffer lower back pain or sacroiliac strain, in combination with postural advice and gentle exercise. Gastro-oesophageal reflux may present for the first time. Medication should relieve symptoms and prevent potential aspiration.

Following the birth, airway clearance begins immediately and physiotherapy may be required while the patient is in the delivery room. It is important to liaise

Table 18.7 The normal changes of pregnancy and the implications for patients with cystic fibrosis

Normal changes	Implications in cystic fibrosis
Thoracic cage • 4 cm elevation of diaphragm with ↓ abdominal tone • ↑ AP and transverse diameter due to laxity of ligaments • Normal pressures of respiratory muscles	• Normal excursion of the diaphragm
Cardiovascular • ↑ Cardiac output by 30–40% • ↑ Blood volume by 50%	• In the presence of cor pulmonale and pulmonary hypertension the risk of cardiovascular collapse is greater, due to the inability to cope with the increased circulating blood volume, particularly during and immediately following delivery
Hormones (peak in the 3rd trimester) • ↑ Oestrogen results in hypersecretion and mucosal oedema of airways • ↑ Progesterone = ↑ respiratory drive, ↑ minute ventilation, resulting in chronic hyperventilation by ↑ TV • ↑ PaO_2 ↓ $PaCO_2$ • ↓ Bronchomotor tone • Threefold ↑ in cortisol level and prostaglandins	• Potential ↑ airway obstruction • Breathlessness most commonly occurs in the 1st and 2nd trimesters and may be normal • Careful monitoring of vital capacity determines the cause, i.e. normal mechanism of pregnancy or ↑ disease severity • Instability of airways may be increased • This may improve airway obstruction
Lung volumes • ↓ ERV ↓ RV ↓ FRC (due to diaphragmatic displacement) • Normal VC ↓ TLC	• ↓ FRC results in early airway closure at lung bases and possible retention of secretions • Hypoxaemia may result from ventilation–perfusion mismatch

AP, anteroposterior; TV, tidal volume; PaO_2, partial pressure of oxygen in arterial blood; $PaCO_2$, partial pressure of carbon dioxide in arterial blood; ERV, expiratory reserve volume; RV, residual volume; FRC, functional residual capacity; VC, vital capacity; TLC, total lung capacity

18

with the midwife and medical team to ensure that pain relief is adequate. Sputum production may increase as the diaphragm descends and ventilation to the lower lobes improves. Gravity-assisted positioning, if indicated, can resume as soon as the mother feels comfortable. Pelvic floor exercises should continue and foot and leg exercises are introduced while the mother is immobile. Mobility begins as soon as the mother feels comfortable. The return to physical activity depends on prenatal fitness, maternal health during pregnancy and progress during the postnatal period. It is usual to begin with gentle forms of exercise such as walking and to build up to low-impact aerobics. Returning to an established programme will depend on the discomfort of the women's abdomen and perineum; every mother will require individualized advice. In the postnatal period pelvic floor exercises should continue for at least 12 weeks, but many mothers give up after the postnatal check up at 6 weeks.

Surgery

Routine surgical procedures, for example insertion of totally implantable venous access ports and gastrostomy, have become increasingly common. In addition the improved longevity of people with CF has led to an increased frequency of surgical interventions either directly or indirectly associated with the disease. Careful pre- and postoperative assessment of this patient group is essential to minimize postoperative pulmonary complications. A preoperative admission for intravenous antibiotics and intensive physiotherapy is often undertaken before elective surgery. Physiotherapists in some centres use these elective surgical procedures as an opportunity to perform perioperative airway clearance during intubation and anaesthesia. Effective airway clearance during anaesthesia may in theory compensate for any postoperative respiratory deterioration related to the anaesthetic and surgery or compromised airway clearance techniques because of postoperative discomfort. In addition, bronchial lavage and suction during anaesthesia can provide valuable sputum samples for microbiological culture.

Relatively little is known about the immediate or postoperative effects of physiotherapy treatments under anaesthesia. A small paediatric study reported a significant reduction in lung function parameters (compliance and peak inspiratory pressure) associated with physiotherapy during anaesthesia compared with a group receiving airway care as deemed appropriate by the attending anaesthetist (Tannenbaum et al 2007). Both groups showed a non-significant decline in FEV_1 the day after surgery, compared with preoperative values, although there were no longer-term effects on FEV_1. Perioperative chest physiotherapy should not be per-

formed routinely in patients undergoing elective surgical procedures; however, it should be considered if the benefits of removing secretions are deemed to outweigh the short-term risk. In these circumstances it may be prudent for the anaesthetist to consider modifying ventilatory support to counteract any short-term negative effects of treatment (Tannenbaum et al 2007).

Transplantation

The physiotherapist should be involved both before and after heart-lung or lung transplantation as outlined in Chapter 15.

Urinary incontinence

Leakage of urine is recognized internationally as a problem for women and girls with CF (Cornaccia et al 2001, Orr et al 2001, Prasad et al 2006), with higher prevalence rates (30–68%) than the normal population (12.8% in women aged 16–20 years and 35% in women over 35 years of age) (Chiarelli et al 1999, Thomas et al 1980). The studies report no relationship between prevalence and age, with onset occurring as early as 10 years (Dodd & Langman 2005). Leakage in men is described in CF, with higher than normal prevalence rates of 16% (Gumery et al 2005) compared with 1.7% in the general population aged 15–64 years (Maral et al 2001). Coughing is the major cause of leakage for the majority of women with increased frequency and severity during acute pulmonary exacerbations.

Studies have addressed the assessment and treatment of the pelvic floor muscles (Button et al 2005b, 2005c, McVean et al 2003). Button and colleagues measured pelvic floor muscle activity using electromyographic (EMG) activity, and ultrasound imaging during coughing and huffing. The authors concluded that the problem of leakage was likely to be related to reduced endurance during prolonged coughing rather than the strength or the timing of the contraction. Following a 3-month intervention of pelvic floor muscle training (exercise, electrical stimulation, biofeedback and bladder training), EMG and ultrasound imaging measures all improved and patients reported significantly fewer incontinent episodes. The improvement was sustained over the following 3 months. Over the same time period, McVean et al (2003) reported an improvement in pelvic floor muscle endurance (Oxford grade), with no change in strength, in a self-selected group of patients.

Despite the physical and social implications of urinary incontinence (UI), women report the major impact of the problem to be their ability to perform airway clearance and spirometry. The physiotherapist should pay particular attention to teaching controlled

18

and effective coughing during ACTs (Langman et al 2006). Cornaccia et al reported no association between airway clearance and leakage, but all subjects were taught to practise 'the knack' (Miller et al 1998) before performing a cough. Continence during a cough depends on the complex interaction of the muscles of the abdomino-pelvic capsule, which work to their greatest advantage with the lumbar spine in a neutral lordotic position (Sapsford et al 2001). Careful positioning advice, to optimize cough and continence, will avoid the flexed spinal posture encouraged by the intense prolonged coughing in women with CF (Figs 18.8 and 18.9).

Studies have revealed that women and girls are rarely forthcoming about the problem, are tolerant of their symptoms and face assessment and treatment with apprehension and embarrassment. A sensitive and open approach with early recognition of symptoms needs to be developed to evaluate this distressing problem.

As a result of our emerging knowledge it would seem prudent to adopt both preventative and active strategies to the management of UI (Button et al 2005b, Dodd & Langman 2005). This requires the collaborative expertise of specialist respiratory, incontinence and musculoskeletal physiotherapists.

Infection control

The physiotherapist should have knowledge of the respiratory pathogen harboured by the patient, the risk of transmission and the potential for cross-infection. Infection control policies, specific to cystic fibrosis, should be in place and attention paid to the risk of cross-infection between patients and from physiotherapy equipment. All physiotherapy treatment sessions should be with individual patients (Cystic Fibrosis Trust 2004a, 2004b).

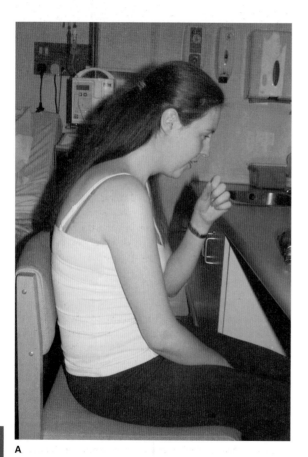

A

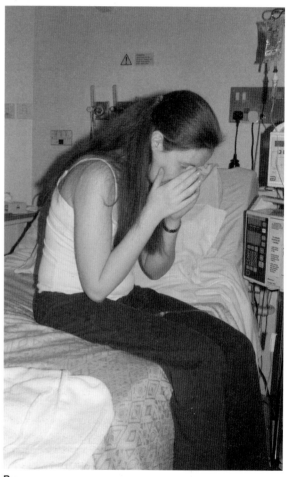

B

18

Figure 18.8 The flexed posture associated with coughing showing bulging of the abdominal wall.

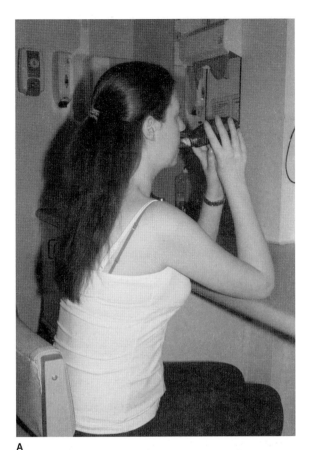
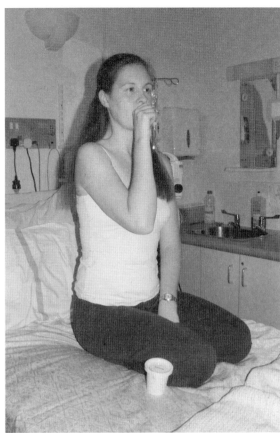

A   **B**

Figure 18.9   Corrected positioning during **A** ACT and **B** coughing. Support is given to the pelvic floor.

Evaluation of physiotherapy

Sputum weight

In clinical practice sputum weight or volume is a useful outcome measure of airway clearance in an individual in a stable state. It provides a baseline measure of the normal sputum production for the individual. Any increase in sputum, either during treatment or out of treatment, is a possible indication of an acute exacerbation of pulmonary infection. Total daily sputum weight during an acute exacerbation is less informative, but, together with lung function, will determine if the problem is one of increased infection or sputum retention (Table 18.8). During an admission for an acute exacerbation, the goal is to maximize sputum expectoration during periods of airway clearance and minimize expectoration at other times. Measures of treatment and out-of-treatment sputum weight will provide this information and indicate, to the less adherent patient, the

value of airway clearance techniques. Radiolabelled aerosols have been used to measure rate of mucus clearance in efficacy studies of airway clearance techniques (Elkins et al 2005b, Lannefors & Wollmer 1992), but remain a research tool rather than a practical clinical measurement.

Lung function

FEV_1 is considered a gold standard measure of lung function. However, as an outcome measure in airway clearance studies it is not ideal as it may not be sufficiently sensitive to detect changes caused by sputum clearance. In addition, there are a number of other confounding factors that may influence this outcome in patients with chronic respiratory disease such as CF (Gibson 2005, Prasad & Main 1998, van der Schans et al 1999). However, measurements of FEV_1 in an individual, as a clinical outcome tool, are useful, in terms of assessing the response to an intervention (for example

18

Table 18.8 The value of spirometry and sputum weight during an acute exacerbation

Outcome		Analysis	Action
↑ FEV$_1$	↓ Sputum weight	Treatment goal	Continue present treatment
↑ FEV$_1$	↑ Sputum weight	↑ Ventilation	↑ Airway clearance
↓ FEV$_1$	↑ Sputum weight	↑ Infection	↑ Airway clearance Review antibiotics
↓ FEV$_1$	↓ Sputum weight	Sputum retention	Review airway clearance techniques

initiation of rhDNase therapy), and longitudinal measurements are helpful in monitoring disease progression (rate of decline). In children particularly, measurement of FEV$_1$ depends on effort and cooperation and is not always a reliable or sensitive measure of early lung disease (Aurora et al 2004). It cannot therefore be considered a robust tool for paediatric physiotherapy intervention studies. Lung clearance index (LCI) calculated from multiple breath inert gas washout has recently been proposed as a more sensitive alternative measure of peripheral lung disease (Aurora et al 2005b). Measurement of lung function is now possible in infants and preschool children (Ranganathan 2006), although it is not widely available.

Other spirometric measurements are also used. The expiratory flow volume curve identifies the location of any flow limitation throughout expiration from total lung capacity (TLC) to residual volume (RV). This will vary from the early detection of small airway limitation to large airway collapse and gives the physiotherapist an invaluable insight into the problems of airway clearance. The manoeuvre is performed with an open glottis and therefore mimics a huff from TLC to RV. In the long term, measurements of small airway function (FEF$_{25}$ and FEF$_{75}$) are not comparable due to changes in TLC and RV and should therefore be interpreted with caution.

Arterial / capillary blood gases

Serial measurements of PaO_2 and $PaCO_2$ monitor decreases in oxygen tension and ensuing hypercapnia. $PaCO_2$ levels inform the physiotherapist of ventilatory drive and the work of breathing. Pulse oximetry gives a quick measure of oxygen saturation, but should not be used to prescribe oxygen as the corresponding $PaCO_2$ is unknown.

Subjective measures

Visual analogue scales (VAS) and Borg scores (Chapters 3 and 14) provide important subjective measures of breathlessness, chest tightness, muscle fatigue and pain. The 15-count breathlessness score and ease of breathing scores have been validated in children (Orenstein 2002, Prasad et al 2000).

Other useful measures include health status/quality of life questionnaires (Congleton et al 1997, Gee et al 2000, Orenstein et al 1989, Shepherd et al 1992) and activities of daily living. More recently emphasis has been placed on the importance of patient-reported outcomes that are disease-specific and one such measure has been validated in the CF population (Quittner et al 2000).

Adherence

The daily timetable of self-care can be an enormous burden for the patient and carer who are trying to balance treatment with family, work and social commitments. This can be particularly difficult for the adolescent and young adult, and studies show a decline in adherence with increasing age (Gudas et al 1991). Adherence has been shown to be treatment-specific in people with CF (Abbott et al 1994) and adherence with one treatment does not guarantee adherence with all self-care. Treatments that are complex, requiring time and effort with no immediate benefit, e.g. airway clearance and nebulized antibiotics, have lower adherence rates than other treatments that are quick and give immediate relief of symptoms (Dodd & Webb 2000). Over the years, studies have reported only 50% of patients to have 'good' adherence with airway clearance (Abbott et al 1994, Conway et al 1996, Passero et al 1981). Large sputum production, feeling better following treatment and help with treatment were significant factors influencing adherence with chest clearance (Abbott et al 1994).

Exercise is perceived differently; adherence is higher and should be encouraged for all its therapeutic benefits. Self-management and self-efficacy should be encouraged to improve adherence, but support and praise are essential to avoid the feeling of loneliness and isolation (McIlwaine & Davidson 1996).

Knowledge is considered an important precursor to adherence and it is important to appraise knowledge of treatments and correct any misunderstandings (Conway et al 1996). Assessing patients' understanding of specific treatments and providing individualized specific teaching has been shown to improve knowledge and reported adherence in the short term (Unsworth et al 1998).

The reasons for non-adherence are complex and the World Health Organization has identified interacting factors that may affect adherence (WHO 2003). Psychological influences, patients' perceptions and health beliefs (Abbott et al 1996) and coping styles (Abbott et al 2001) influence adherence (Prasad & Cerny 2002). It is important to recognize that non-adherence is normal and to encourage openness with self-reporting by adopting a non-judgmental approach. The multidisciplinary team should examine all levels of care from their centre policies, social and economic factors, treatment complexities and individual patient-related factors to seek opportunities to encourage adherence (Downs 2006). Treatment goals and plans tailored to daily lifestyle should be agreed and compromise accepted by the medical team.

Continuity of care

Continuous assessment and reassessment of patients with cystic fibrosis is essential for effective management. Patients' needs will change as they progress from infancy through school, higher education, work and parenting. The emphasis is on leading as normal a life as possible while making time to include the many aspects of treatment. Visits to schools to support individual patients and to increase the awareness and knowledge of the teachers are beneficial (Dyer & Morais 1996). Children should be encouraged to attend normal schools.

Although the majority of parents and patients can take the responsibility for physiotherapy treatments, it is essential that there is a regular review of the techniques by a physiotherapist. This also provides an opportunity to update the techniques and to discuss any problems. It is important for the physiotherapist to work with carers and patients to encourage autonomy with treatments from an early age and to ensure a successful transfer to adult care. There are times when the parents or patient are unable to cope effectively on their own and the need for assistance during these periods should be recognized and help should be arranged.

If the patient is treated at both a local hospital and a specialist cystic fibrosis unit, communication among physiotherapists is essential to avoid confusion about treatment.

The physiotherapist is part of a multidisciplinary team and must be aware of the roles of the other members. Good communication within the team is essential. Members of the team may experience considerable stress from long-term involvement with patients with a chronic progressive illness. Coping with this stress can be helped by the team members recognizing each other's needs and providing the necessary support.

In caring for the patient with cystic fibrosis, the physical care is important but the psychological effects on both the family and the patient must also be considered. Many countries have cystic fibrosis associations, which offer encouragement and support for patients and their families. In spite of the frequently high demands of treatment, most patients with cystic fibrosis are leading fulfilling lives and many adults are in full-time employment, homeowners and parents (Walters et al 1993).

References

Abbott J, Bilton D, Dodd M, Webb AK 1994 Treatment compliance in adults with cystic fibrosis. Thorax 59: 115–120

Abbott J, Dodd M, Webb AK 1996 Health perceptions and treatment adherence in adults with cystic fibrosis. Thorax 51: 1233–1238

Abbott J, Dodd M, Gee L, Webb AK 2001 Ways of coping with cystic fibrosis: implications for treatment adherence. Disability and Rehabilitation 23: 315–324

Accurso FJ, Sontag MK, Koenig JM et al 2004 Multi-centre airway secretion clearance study in cystic fibrosis. Pediatric Pulmonolology suppl 27: 314

Albini S, Rath R, Renner S et al 2004 Additional inspiratory muscle training intensifies the beneficial effects of cycle ergometer training in patients with cystic fibrosis. Journal of Cystic Fibrosis 3(Suppl 1): 63

Alton E, Caplen N, Geddes D, Williamson R 1992 New treatments for cystic fibrosis. British Medical Bulletin 48: 785–804

Anderson DH 1938 Cystic fibrosis of the pancreas and its relation to celiac disease: clinical and pathological study. American Journal of Disease in Childhood 56: 344–399

Andreasson B, Jonson B, Kornfalt R et al 1987 Long-term effects of physical exercise on working capacity and pulmonary function in cystic fibrosis. Acta Paediatrica Scandinavica 76: 70–75

Armstrong DS, Grimwood K, Carzino R et al 1995 Lower respiratory tract infection and inflammation in infants with newly diagnosed cystic fibrosis. British Medical Journal 310: 1571–1572

18

Asher MI, Pardy RL, Coates AL 1982 The effects of inspiratory muscle training in patients with cystic fibrosis. American Review of Respiratory Disease 126: 855–859

Ashleigh RJ, Webb AK 2007 Radiological intervention for haemoptysis in cystic fibrosis. Journal Royal Society of Medicine 100(Suppl 47): 38–45

Astrand PO, Rodahl K 1977 Text book of work physiology. McGraw-Hill, London

Aurora P, Bush A, Gustafsson P et al 2005a Multiple-breath washout as a marker of lung disease in preschool children with cystic fibrosis. American Journal of Respiratory and Critical Care Medicine 171(3): 249–256

Aurora P, Gustafsson P, Bush A et al 2004 Multiple breath inert gas washout as a measure of ventilation distribution in children with cystic fibrosis. Thorax 59(12): 1068–1073

Aurora P, Kozlowska W, Stocks J 2005b Gas mixing efficiency from birth to adulthood measured by multiple breath washout. Respiratory Physiology and Neurobiology 148: 125–134

Bachrach LK, Loutit CW, Moss RB 1994 Osteopenia in adults with cystic fibrosis. American Journal of Medicine 96: 27–34

Baldwin DR, Hill AL, Peckham KG et al 1994 Effect of addition of exercise to chest physiotherapy on sputum expectoration and lung function in adults with cystic fibrosis. Respiratory Medicine 88: 49–53

Balfour-Lynn IM, Klein NH, Dinwiddie R 1997 Randomized controlled trial of inhaled corticosteroids (fluticasone propionate) in cystic fibrosis. Archives of Disease in Childhood 77: 124–130

Balfour–Lynn IM, Lees B, Hall B et al 2006 Multicentre randomized controlled trial of withdrawal of inhaled corticosteroids in cystic fibrosis. American Journal of Respiratory Critical Care Medicine 173: 1356–1362

Balfour–Lynn IM, Prasad SA, Laverty A 1998 A step in the right direction: assessing exercise tolerance in cystic fibrosis. Pediatric Pulmonology 25: 78–84

Balfour-Lynn IM, Walters S, Dezateux C 2000 Inhaled corticosteroids for cystic fibrosis. Cochrane Database of Systemic Reviews. Issue 1. Art. No.: CD001915

Bargon J, Viel K, Dauletbaev N et al 1997 Short-term effects of regular salmeterol treatment on adult cystic fibrosis patients. European Respiratory Journal 10: 2307–2311

Barker AF, Couch L, Fiel SB et al 2000 Tobramycin solution for inhalation reduces sputum Pseudomonas aeruginosa density in bronchiectasis. American Journal of Respiratory and Critical Care Medicine 162: 481–485

Bar-Or O, Blimkie CJ, Hay JA et al 1992 Voluntary dehydration and heat intolerance in cystic fibrosis. Lancet 339: 696–699

Bhudmkanok GS, Lim J, Marcus R et al 1996 Correlates of osteopenia in patients with cystic fibrosis. Journal of Pediatrics 97: 103–111

Bilton D, Dodd ME, Abbot J et al 1992 The benefits of exercise combined with physiotherapy in the treatment of adults with cystic fibrosis. Respiratory Medicine 86: 507–511

Bilton D, Webb AK, Foster H et al 1990 Life threatening haemoptysis in cystic fibrosis: an alternative therapeutic approach. Thorax 45: 523–524

Birrer P, McElvaney N G, Rüdeberg A et al 1994 Protease-antiprotease imbalance in the lungs of children with cystic fibrosis. American Journal of Respiratory and Critical Care Medicine 150: 207–213

Bisgaard H, Pederson SS, Nielsen KG et al 1997 Controlled trial of inhaled budesonide in patients with cystic fibrosis and chronic Pseudomonas aeruginosa infection. American Journal of Respiratory and Critical Care Medicine 156: 1190–1196

Boas SR, Danduran MJ, McColley SA 1999 Parental attitudes about exercise regarding their children with cystic fibrosis. International Journal of Sports Medicine 20: 334–338

Bourke S, Rooney M, Fitzgerald M et al 1987 Episodic arthropathy in adult cystic fibrosis. Quarterly Journal of Medicine 64: 651–659

Boyd AC 2006 Gene and stem cell therapy In: Bush A, Alton EWFW, Davies J, Griesenbach J, Jaffe A (eds) Cystic fibrosis in the 21st century. Progress in Respiratory Research. Karger, Basel, Vol 34, pp 221–229

Boyle L, Bradley JM, McGregor K 2003 Thoracic kyphosis in cystic fibrosis. The flexible ruler technique. Pediatric Pulmonology 36: 331

Bradley J, Howard J, Wallace E et al 1999 The validity of a modified shuttle test in adult cystic fibrosis. Thorax 54: 437–439

Bradley JM, Moran FM, Greenstone M 2002 Physical training for bronchiectasis. Cochrane Database of Systematic Reviews 3: CD002166

Bradley JM, Moran FM, Elborn JS 2006 Evidence for physical therapies (airway clearance and physical training) in cystic fibrosis: an overview of five Cochrane Systematic

Reviews. Respiratory Medicine 100: 191–201

Bridges N, Spowart K 2006 Diabetes in cystic fibrosis In: Bush A, Alton EWFW, Davies J, Griesenbach J, Jaffe A (eds) Cystic fibrosis in the 21st century. Progress in Respiratory Research. Karger, Basel, Vol 34, pp 278–283

British Thoracic Society 2004 Recommendations: Managing patients with lung disease planning air travel. British Thoracic Society, London

British Thoracic Society 2007 Guidelines: Bronchiectasis. British Thoracic Society, London

Britto MT, Garrett JM, Konrad TR et al 2000 Comparison of physical activity in adolescents with cystic fibrosis versus age-matched controls. Pediatric Pulmonology 30: 86–91

Bureau MA, Lupien L, Begin R 1981 Neural drive and ventilatory strategy of breathing in normal children and in patients with cystic fibrosis and asthma. Pediatrics 68: 187–194

Bush A, Ferkol T 2006 The emerging genetics of primary ciliary dyskinesia. American Journal of Respiratory and Critical Care Medicine 174: 109–111

Bush A, Gotz M 2006 Cystic fibrosis. Respiratory Monograph 11(37): 234–291

Button BM 1999 Postural drainage techniques and gastro-oesophageal reflux in infants with cystic fibrosis. European Respiratory Journal 14: 456–1457.

Button BM, Heine RG, Catto-Smith AG et al 1997 Postural drainage and gastro-oesophageal reflux in infants with cystic fibrosis. Archives of Disease in Childhood 76: 148–150

Button BM, Heine RG, Catto-Smith AG et al 2003 Chest physiotherapy in infants with cystic fibrosis: to tip or not? A five-year study. Pediatric Pulmonology 35: 208–213

Button BM, Heine RG, Catto-Smith AG et al 2004 Chest physiotherapy, gastro-oesophageal reflux, and arousal in infants with cystic fibrosis. Archives of Disease in Childhood 89(5): 435–439

Button BM, Roberts S, Kotsimbos TC et al 2005a Gastroesophageal reflux (symptomatic and silent): a potentially significant problem in patients with cystic fibrosis before and after lung transplantation. Journal of Heart and Lung Transplantation 24: 1522–1529

Button BM, Sherburn M, Chase J et al 2005b Pelvic floor muscle function in women with chronic lung disease (cystic fibrosis and COPD) versus controls: relationship to urinary

18

incontinence. Pediatric Pulmonology 113 (Suppl 28): a368

Button BM, Sherburn M, Chase J et al 2005c Effect of a three-month physiotherapeutic intervention on incontinence in women with chronic cough related to cystic fibrosis and COPD. Pediatric Pulmonology 113 (Suppl 28): a369

Carr L, Smith RE, Pryor JA et al 1996 Cystic fibrosis patients' views and beliefs about chest clearance and exercise – a pilot study. Physiotherapy 82: 621–627

Cecins NM, Jenkins SC, Pengelly J et al 1999 The active cycle of breathing techniques – to tip or not to tip? Respiratory Medicine 93: 660–665

Chatham K, Ionescu AA, Nixon LS, Shale DJ 2004 A short-term comparison of two methods of sputum expectoration in cystic fibrosis. European Respiratory Journal 23(3): 435–439

Chen HC, Liu CY, Cheng HF et al 1998 Chest physiotherapy does not exacerbate gastroesophageal reflux in patients with chronic bronchitis and bronchiectasis. Respiratory Medicine 21: 409–414

Chen KY, Ko SC, Hsueh PR et al 2001 Pulmonary fungal infection: emphasis on microbiological spectra, patient outcome and prognostic factors. Chest 120: 177–184

Cheng K, Smyth RL, Motley J et al 2000 Randomized controlled trials in cystic fibrosis (1966–1997) categorised by time, design and intervention. Pediatric Pulmonology 29: 1–7

Chiarelli P, Brown W, McElduff P 1999 Leaking urine: prevalence and associated factors in Australian women Neurourology and Urodynamics 18: 567–577

Chua HL, Collis GG, Le-Souef PN 1990 Bronchial response to nebulized antibiotics in children with cystic fibrosis. European Respiratory Journal 3: 1114–1116

Coakley RD, Boucher RC 2007 Pathophysiology: epithelial cell biology, ASL channel functions including sweat gland and pancreas. In: Hodson M, Geddes D, Bush A (eds) Cystic fibrosis, 3rd edn. Hodder Arnold, London, pp 59–68

Cole P 1995 Bronchiectasis. In: Brewis RAL, Corrin B, Geddes DM, Gibson GJ (eds) Respiratory medicine, 2nd edn. WB Saunders, London, ch 39

Congleton J, Hodson M, Duncan-Skingle F 1997 Quality of life in adults with cystic fibrosis. Thorax 52: 397–400

Constantini D, Brivio A, Brusa D, et al 2001 PEP-mask versus postural drainage in CF infants: a long-term comparative trial. Pediatric Pulmonology Suppl 22: A400

Conway JH, Fleming JS, Perring S et al 1992 Humidification as an adjunct to chest physiotherapy in aiding tracheo-bronchial clearance in patients with bronchiectasis. Respiratory Medicine 86: 109–111

Conway SP, Pond MN, Watson A et al 1996 Knowledge of adult patients with cystic fibrosis about their illness. Thorax 51: 34–38

Conway SP, Watson A 1997 Nebulized bronchodilators, corticosteroids and rhDNase in adult patients with cystic fibrosis. Thorax 52(Suppl 2): S64–68

Corless JA, Warburton CJ 2000 Surgery vs non-surgical treatment for bronchiectasis. Cochrane Database Systematic Review 4: CD002180

Cornaccia M, Zenorini A, Braagion C et al 2001 Prevalence of urinary incontinence in women with cystic fibrosis. British Journal of Urology International 88: 44–48

Cropp GJA, Pullano TP, Cerny FJ et al 1982 Exercise tolerance and cardiorespiratory adjustments at peak work capacity in cystic fibrosis. American Review of Respiratory Disease 126: 211–216

Cunningham S, Prasad SA, Collyer L et al 2001 Bronchoconstriction following nebulized colistin in cystic fibrosis. Archives of Disease in Childhood 84: 432–433

Currie DC 1997 Nebulizers for bronchiectasis. Thorax 52(Suppl 2): S72–74

Currie DC, Cooke JC, Morgan AD et al 1987 Interpretation of bronchograms and chest radiographs in patients with chronic sputum production. Thorax 42: 278–284

Currie DC, Munro C, Gaskell D et al 1986 Practice, problems and compliance with postural drainage: a survey of chronic sputum producers. British Journal of Diseases of the Chest 80: 249–253

Cystic Fibrosis Foundation 2006 www.cff.org

Cystic Fibrosis Trust 2002a Antibiotic treatment for cystic fibrosis. Cystic Fibrosis Trust, Bromley

Cystic Fibrosis Trust 2002b Clinical guidelines for the physiotherapy management of cystic fibrosis. Cystic Fibrosis Trust, Bromley

Cystic Fibrosis Trust 2004a The Burkholderia cepacia complex Cystic Fibrosis Trust, Bromley

Cystic Fibrosis Trust 2004b Pseudomonas aeruginosa infection in people with cystic fibrosis. Cystic Fibrosis Trust, Bromley

Cystic Fibrosis Trust 2004c Management of cystic fibrosis related diabetes mellitus. Cystic Fibrosis Trust, Bromley

Cystic Fibrosis Trust 2007 Bone mineralisation in cystic fibrosis. Cystic Fibrosis Trust, Bromley

Davidson AGF 2000 Gastrointestinal and pancreatic disease in cystic fibrosis. In: Hodson ME, Geddes DM (eds) Cystic fibrosis. Arnold, London, pp 261–289

Davis PB, Drumm M, Konstan MW 1996 Cystic fibrosis: state of the art. American Journal of Respiratory and Critical Care Medicine 154: 1229–1256

de Boeck K 2000 Improving standards of clinical care in cystic fibrosis. European Respiratory Journal 16: 585–587

de Jong W, Kaptein AA, Van Der Schans CP et al 1997 Quality of life in patients with cystic fibrosis. Pediatric Pulmonology 23: 95–100

Department of Health 2004 Home oxygen therapy service: Service specifications. www.dh.gov.uk/en/Publicationsandstatistics/Publications/PublicationsPolicyAndGuidance/DH_4126268 (Accessed 19 July 2007)

Desai M, Weller PH, Spencer DA 1995 Clinical benefit from nebulized human recombinant DNase in Kartagener's syndrome. Pediatric Pulmonology 20: 307–308

Desmond KJ, Schwenk WF, Thomas E et al 1983 Immediate and long-term effects of chest physiotherapy in patients with cystic fibrosis. Journal of Pediatrics 103: 538–542

Di Sant'Agnese PA, Davis PB 1979 Cystic fibrosis in adults. American Journal of Medicine 66: 121–132

Dodd ME, Langman H 2005 Urinary incontinence in cystic fibrosis. Journal of Royal Society of Medicine 98(Suppl 45): 28–36

Dodd ME, Prasad SA 2005 Physiotherapy management of cystic fibrosis. Chronic Respiratory Disease 2: 139–149

Dodd ME, Webb AK 2000 Understanding non-compliance with treatment in adults with cystic fibrosis. Journal of the Royal Society of Medicine 93(Suppl 38): 2–8

Dodd ME, Abbott J, Maddison J et al 1997 The effect of the tonicity of nebulized colistin on chest tightness and lung function in adults with cystic fibrosis. Thorax 52: 656–658

Dodd ME, Haworth CS, Webb AK 1998 Practical application of oxygen therapy in cystic fibrosis. Journal of the Royal Society of Medicine 91(Suppl 34): 30–39

Dodge JA, Lewis PA, Stanton M, Wilsher J 2007 Cystic fibrosis mortality and survival in the UK: 1947–2003. European Respiratory Journal 29: 522–526

18

Dodge JA, Morison S, Lewis PA et al 1993 Cystic fibrosis in the United Kingdom, 1968–1988: incidence, population and survival. Paediatric and Perinatal Epidemiology 7: 157–166

Donaldson SH, Bennett WD, Zeman KL et al 2006 Mucus clearance and lung function in cystic fibrosis with hypertonic saline. New England Journal of Medicine 354: 241–250

Doring G, Conway SP, Heijerman HGM et al 2000 Antibiotic therapy against *Pseudomonas aeruginosa* in cystic fibrosis. European Respiratory Journal 16: 749–767

Downs AM 2006 ACT and the non-participating patient/family. Pediatric Pulmonology Suppl 29: S21.2

Du Bois RM 1995 Respiratory medicine – recent advances. British Medical Journal 310: 1594–1597

Dyer J, Morais JA 1996 Supporting children with cystic fibrosis in school. Professional Nurse 11: 518–520

Eaton T, Young P, Zeng, I, Kolbe J 2007 A randomized evaluation of the acute efficacy, acceptability and tolerability of Flutter and active cycle of breathing with and without postural drainage in non-cystic fibrosis bronchiectasis Chronic Respiratory Disease 4: 23–30

Edenborough FP, Stableforth DE, Webb AK et al 1995 Outcome of pregnancy in women with cystic fibrosis. Thorax 50: 170–174

Edlund LD, French RW, Herbst JJ et al 1986 Effects of a swimming program on children with cystic fibrosis. American Journal of Diseases of Childhood 140: 80–83

Elborn JS, Prescott RJ, Stack BH et al 2000 Elective versus symptomatic antibiotic treatment in cystic fibrosis patients with chronic *Pseudomonas* infection of the lungs. Thorax 55: 355–358

Elkin SL, Fairney A, Burnett S et al 2001 Vertebral deformities and low bone mineral density in adults with cystic fibrosis: a cross sectional study. Osteoporosis International 12: 366–372

Elkins MR, Alison JA, Bye PT 2005a Effect of body position on maximal expiratory pressure and flow in adults with cystic fibrosis. Pediatric Pulmonology 40: 385–391

Elkins MR, Eberl S, Constable C et al 2005b The effect of manual chest physiotherapy, positive expiratory pressure (PEP) and oscillating PEP on mucociliary clearance in subjects with cystic fibrosis. Pediatric Pulmonology 40(Suppl 28): A377

Elkins MR, Robinson M, Rose BR et al 2006a A controlled trial of long-term inhaled hypertonic saline in patients with cystic fibrosis. New England Journal of Medicine 354: 229–240

Elkins MR, Jones A, Schans C 2006b Positive expiratory pressure physiotherapy for airway clearance in people with cystic fibrosis. Cochrane Database of Systematic Reviews. Issue 2. Art. No.: CD003147

Elkus R, Popovich J 1992 Respiratory physiology in pregnancy. Clinics in Chest Medicine 13: 555–565

Eng PA, Morton J, Douglass JA et al 1996 Short-term efficacy of ultrasonically nebulized hypertonic saline in cystic fibrosis. Pediatric Pulmonology 21: 77–83

Enright S, Chatham K, Ionescu AA et al 2004 Inspiratory muscle training improves lung function and exercise capacity in adults with cystic fibrosis. Chest 126: 405–411

Equi A, Balfour-Lynn IM, Bush A, Rosenthal M 2002 Long-term azithromycin in children with cystic fibrosis: a randomized, placebo-controlled crossover trial. Lancet 360(9338): 978–984

Evans SA, Turner SM, Bosch BJ, Hardy MA, Woodhead MA 1996 Lung function in bronchiectasis: the influence of *Pseudomonas aeruginosa*. European Respiratory Journal 9: 1601–1604

Farrell PM, Kosorok MR, Rock MJ et al 2001 Early diagnosis of cystic fibrosis through neonatal screening prevents severe malnutrition and improves long-term growth. Paediatrics 107: 1–13

Fauroux B, Boule M, Lofaso F et al 1999 Chest physiotherapy in cystic fibrosis: improved tolerance with nasal pressure support ventilation. Pediatrics 103: 1–9

Ferkol T, Mitchison HM, O'Callaghan C et al 2006 Current issues in the basic mechanisms, pathophysiology, diagnosis and management of primary ciliary dyskinesia. European Respiratory Journal, Monograph 37: 291–313

Finnegan MJ, Hughes DV, Hodson ME 1992 Comparison of nebulized and intravenous terbutaline during acute exacerbations of pulmonary infection in patients with cystic fibrosis. European Respiratory Journal 5: 1089–1091

FitzSimmons SC 1993 The changing epidemiology of cystic fibrosis. Journal of Pediatrics 122: 1–9

Freeman W, Stableforth DE, Cayton R et al 1993 Endurance exercise capacity in adults with cystic fibrosis. Respiratory Medicine 87: 252–257

Fuchs HJ, Borowitz DS, Christiansen DH et al 1994 Effect of aerolized recombinant human DNase on exacerbations of respiratory symptoms and on pulmonary function in patients with cystic fibrosis. New England Journal of Medicine 331: 637–642

Gee L, Abbott J, Conway SP et al 2000 Development of a disease specific health related quality of life measure for adults and adolescents with cystic fibrosis. Thorax 55: 946–954

Gibson GJ Spirometry: then and now. Breathe 2005; 1: 206–216

Gillet D, de Braekeleer M, Bellis G, Durieu I 2002 French cystic fibrosis registry: cystic fibrosis and pregnancy. Report from French data (1980–1999). British Journal of Obstetrics and Gynaecology 109: 912–918

Godfrey S, Mearns M 1971 Pulmonary function and response to exercise in cystic fibrosis. Archives of Disease in Childhood 46: 144–151

Govan J, Brown PH, Maddison J et al 1993 Evidence for transmission of *Pseudomonas cepacia* by social contact in cystic fibrosis. Lancet 342: 15–18

Gozal D 1997 Nocturnal ventilatory support in patients with cystic fibrosis: comparison with supplemental oxygen. European Respiratory Journal 10: 1999–2003

Greenstone M, Rutman A, Dewar I et al 1988 Primary ciliary dyskinesia: cytological and clinical features. Quarterly Journal of Medicine 67(253): 405–430

Gremmo ML, Guenza MC 1999 Positive expiratory pressure in the physiotherapeutic management of primary ciliary dyskinesia in paediatric age. Monaldi Archives of Chest Disease 54: 255–257

Gudas LJ, Koocher GP, Wypij D 1991 Perceptions of medical compliance in children and adolescents with cystic fibrosis. Journal of Behaviour in Pediatrics 12: 236–242

Gumery L, Lee J, Whitehouse J et al 2005 The prevalence of urinary incontinence in adult cystic fibrosis males. Journal of Cystic Fibrosis 4: S97

Hasani A, Pavia D, Agnew JE, Clarke SW 1994 Regional lung clearance during cough and forced expiration technique (FET): effects of flow and viscoelasticity. Thorax 49: 557–561

Hassan JA, Saadiah S, Roslan H et al 1999 Bronchodilator response to inhaled beta 2-agonist and anticholinergic drugs in patients with bronchiectasis. Respirology 4: 423–426

Haworth CS, Dodd ME, Atkins M et al 2000 Pneumothorax in adults with cystic fibrosis dependent on nasal intermittent positive pressure ventilation (NIPPV): a management dilemma. Thorax 55: 620–662

18

Haworth CS, Selby PL, Webb AK et al 1999. Low bone mineral density in adults with cystic fibrosis. Thorax 54: 961–967

Heijerman HG, Bakker W, Sterk PJ et al 1992 Long-term effects of exercise training and hyperalimentation in adult cystic fibrosis patients with severe pulmonary dysfunction. International Journal of Rehabilitation and Respiration 15: 252–257

Hill AT, Edenborough FP, Cayton RM et al 1998 Long-term nasal intermittent positive pressure ventilation in patients with cystic fibrosis and hypercapnic respiratory failure (1991–1996). Respiratory Medicine 92: 523–526

Hill LS, Slater AL 1998 A comparison of the performance of two modern multidose dry powder asthma inhalers. Respiratory Medicine 92: 105–110

Hodson ME 1994 Adults. In: Hodson ME, Geddes DM (eds) Cystic fibrosis. Chapman & Hall, London, pp 237–253

Hodson ME 1996 Principles of antibiotic management. In: Issues in cystic fibrosis: antibiotic therapy. Report of a meeting held at Royal College of Pathologists, November (Zeneca), pp 6–14

Hodson ME 2000 The respiratory system: adults. In: Hodson ME, Geddes DM (eds) Cystic fibrosis. Arnold, London, pp 218–242

Hodson ME, Shah PL 1995 DNase trials in cystic fibrosis. European Respiratory Journal 8: 1786–1791

Hodson ME, Madden BP, Steven MH et al 1991 Non-invasive mechanical ventilation for cystic fibrosis patients – a potential bridge to transplantation. European Respiratory Journal 4: 524–527

Høiby N, Koch C 1990 Pseudomonas aeruginosa infection in cystic fibrosis and its management. Thorax 45: 881–884

Holland AE, Denehy L, Ntoumenopoulos G et al 2003 Non-invasive ventilation assists chest physiotherapy in adults with acute exacerbations of cystic fibrosis. Thorax 58: 880–884

Houtmeyers E, Gosselink R, Gayan-Ramirez G et al 1999 Effects of drugs on mucus clearance. European Respiratory Journal 14: 452–467

Hutchinson GR, Parker S, Pryor JA et al 1996 Home-nebulizers: a potential primary source of Burkholderia cepacia and other colistin-resistant, gram-negative bacteria in patients with cystic fibrosis. Journal of Clinical Microbiology 34: 584–587

Johnson S, Knox AJ 1994 Arthropathy in cystic fibrosis. Respiratory Medicine 88: 567–570

Jones AM, Dodd ME, Govan JRW et al 2004. Burkholderia cenocepacia and Burkholderia multivorans: influence on survival in cystic fibrosis. Thorax 59: 948–951

Jones AM, Dodd ME, Govan JRW et al 2005 Prospective surveillance for Pseudomonas aeruginosa cross-infection at a cystic fibrosis centre. American Journal of Respiratory and Critical Care Medicine 171: 257–260

Jones AM, Govan JR, Doherty C et al 2001 Spread of a multiresistant strain of Pseudomonas aeruginosa in an adult cystic fibrosis clinic. Lancet 358: 557–558

Jones DK, Davis RJ 1990 Massive haemoptysis. British Medical Journal 300: 889–890

Jones J, Hunter D 1995 Consensus methods for medical and health services research. British Medical Journal 311: 376–80

Jones NL 1988 Clinical exercise testing, 3rd edn. WB Saunders, Philadelphia, pp 306–307

Karadag B, Gultekin E, Wilson N et al 1997 Exhaled nitric oxide (NO) in children with primary ciliary dyskinesia (abstrct). European Respiratory Journal 10(Suppl 25): 339s

Kartagener M 1933 Zur Pathogenese der Bronchiektasien. Beitrage zur Klinik der Tuberkulose 83: 489–501 B

Keens TG, Krastins IRB, Wannamaker EM et al 1977 Ventilatory muscle endurance training in normal subjects and patients with cystic fibrosis. American Review of Respiratory Disease 116: 853–860

Kellett F, Redfern J, Niven RM 2005 Evaluation of nebulized hypertonic saline (7%) as an adjunct to physiotherapy in patients with stable bronchiectasis. Respiratory Medicine 99: 27–31

Kerem E, Reisman J, Corey M et al 1992 Prediction of mortality in patients with cystic fibrosis. New England Journal of Medicine 326: 1187–1191

Khan TZ, Wagener JS, Bost T et al 1995 Early pulmonary inflammation in infants with cystic fibrosis. American Journal of Respiratory and Critical Care Medicine 151: 1075–1082

King AD, Cumberland DC, Brennan SR 1989 Management of severe haemoptysis by bronchial artery embolisation in a patient with cystic fibrosis. Thorax 44: 523–524

Klijn PH, Oudshoorn A, van der Ent CK et al 2004 Effects of anaerobic training in children with cystic fibrosis: a randomized controlled study. Chest 125: 1299–1305

Koch C, Lanng S 2000 Other organ systems In: Hodson ME, Geddes DM (eds) Cystic fibrosis. Arnold, London, pp 314–328

Koh YY, Park Y, Jeong JH et al 2000 The effect of regular salbutamol on lung function and bronchial responsiveness in patients with primary ciliary dyskinesia. Chest 117: 427–433

Kolbe J, Wells A 2000 Inhaled steroids for bronchiectasis. Cochrane Database of Systematic Reviews 2: CD000996

Konstan MW, Hilliard KA, Norvell TM et al 1994 Bronchoalveolar lavage findings in cystic fibrosis patients with stable, clinically mild lung disease suggest ongoing infection and inflammation. American Journal of Respiratory and Critical Care Medicine 150: 448–454

Koscik RL, Farrell PM, Kosorok MR et al 2004 Cognitive function of children with cystic fibrosis: deleterious effect of early malnutrition. Pediatrics 113: 1549–1558

Kotloff RM, Fitzsimmons SC, Fiel SB 1992 Fertility and pregnancy in patients with cystic fibrosis. Clinics in Chest Medicine 13: 623–635

Kraemer R, Delosea N, Baliinari P et al 2006 Effects of allergic bronchopulmonary aspergillosis on lung function in children with cystic fibrosis. American Journal of Respiratory and Critical Care Medicine 74: 1211–1220

Kuhn RJ, Nahata MC 1985 Therapeutic management of cystic fibrosis. Clinical Pharmacology 4: 555–565

Kuo C, Lin S, Wang J 1991 Aerosol, humidity and oxygenation. Chest 99: 1352–1356

Langlands J 1967 The dynamics of cough in health and in chronic bronchitis. Thorax 22: 88–96

Langman HB, Webb AK, Jones AM et al 2006 Airway clearance therapy and urinary incontinence. Pediatric Pulmonology (Suppl 29): S21.3

Lannefors L, Wollmer P 1992 Mucus clearance with three chest physiotherapy regimes in cystic fibrosis: a comparison between postural drainage, PEP and physical exercise. European Respiratory Journal 5: 748–753

Lanng S, Thorsteinsson B, Nerup J et al 1992 Influence of the development of diabetes mellitus on clinical status in patients with cystic fibrosis. European Journal of Paediatrics 151: 684–687

Lapin CD 2000 Mixing and matching airway clearance techniques to patients. Pediatric Pulmonology Supplement 20: S12.3

Ledson MJ, Gallagher MJ, Corkhill JE et al 1998 Cross infection between cystic

18

fibrosis patients colonized with *Burkholderia cepacia*. Thorax 53: 432–436

LiPuma JJ, Dasen SE, Nielson DW et al 1990 Person-to-person transmission of *Pseudomonas cepacia* between patients with cystic fibrosis. Lancet 336: 1094–1096

Long FR, Williams RS, Castille RG 2004 Structural airway abnormalities in infants and young children with cystic fibrosis. Journal of Pediatrics 144(2): 154–161

Lum S, Gustafsson P, Ljungberg H et al 2007 Early detection of cystic fibrosis lung disease: multiple breath washout versus raised volume tests. Thorax 62(4): 341–347

Madden BP, Kariyawasam H, Siddiqi AJ et al 2002 Non-invasive ventilation in cystic fibrosis patients with acute or chronic respiratory failure. European Respiratory Journal 19: 310–313

Maddison J, Dodd M, Webb AK 1994 Nebulized colistin causes chest tightness in adults with cystic fibrosis. Respiratory Medicine 88: 145–147

Mahadeva R, Webb AK, Westerbeek RC et al 1998 Clinical outcome in relation to care in centres specialising in cystic fibrosis: cross-sectional study. British Medical Journal 316: 1771–1775

Main E, Prasad A, Schans C 2005 Conventional chest physiotherapy compared to other airway clearance techniques for cystic fibrosis. Cochrane Database of Systematic Reviews 25(1): CD002011

Maral I, Ozkardes H, Peskircioglu L, Bumin MA 2001 Prevalence of stress urinary incontinence in both sexes at or after age 15 years: a cross-sectional study. Journal of Urology 165(2): 408–412

Marcotte JE, Grisdale RK, Levison H et al 1986 Multiple factors limit exercise in cystic fibrosis. Pediatric Pulmonology 2: 274–281

Marcus CL, Bader D, Stabile M et al 1992 Supplemental oxygen and exercise performance in patients with cystic fibrosis with severe pulmonary disease. Chest 105: 52–57

Martinez TM, Llapur CJ, Williams TH et al 2005 High-resolution computed tomography imaging of airway disease in infants with cystic fibrosis. American Journal of Respiratory and Critical Care Medicine 172: 1133–1138

Massery M 2005 Musculoskeletal and neuromuscular interventions: a physical approach to cystic fibrosis. Journal of the Royal Society of Medicine 98(Suppl 45): 55–66

Mastella G, Rainisio M, Harms HK et al 2000 Allergic bronchopulmonary aspergillosis in cystic fibrosis: a European epidemiological study. European Respiratory Journal 16: 464–471

McBride G 1990 More progress in cystic fibrosis. British Medical Journal 301: 627

McCallum SJ, Corkhill J, Gallagher M et al 2001 Superinfection with a transmissible strain of a *Pseudomonas aeruginosa* in adults with cystic fibrosis chronically colonized by *P aeruginosa*. Lancet 358: 558–560

McIlwaine MP, Davidson GF 1996 Airway clearance techniques in the treatment of cystic fibrosis. Current Opinion in Pulmonary Medicine 2: 447–451

McMullen AH, Pasta DJ, Frederick PD et al 2006 Impact of pregnancy on women with cystic fibrosis. Chest 129: 706–711

McVean R, Orr A, Webb AK et al 2003 Treatment of urinary incontinence in cystic fibrosis. Journal of Cystic Fibrosis 2: 171–176

Miller JM, Ashton-Miller JA, DeLancey JO 1998 A pelvic muscle contraction can reduce cough-related urine loss in selected women with mild SUI. Journal of the American Geriatric Society 46(7): 870–874

Moorcroft AJ, Dodd ME, Webb AK 2004 Individualised unsupervised exercise training in adults with cystic fibrosis: a one-year randomized controlled trial. Thorax 59: 1074–1080

Muhdi K, Edenborough FP, Gumery L et al 1996 Outcome for patients colonised with *Burkholderia cepacia* in a Birmingham adult cystic fibrosis clinic and the end of an epidemic. Thorax 51: 374–377

Mukhopadhyay S, Singh M, Cater JI et al 1996 Nebulized antipseudomonal antibiotic therapy in cystic fibrosis: a meta-analysis of benefits and risks. Thorax 51: 364–368

Mullinger B, Sommerer K, Herpich C et al 2004 Inhalation therapy can be improved in CF patients by controlling the breathing pattern during inspiration. Journal of Cystic Fibrosis 3: S65

Nazer D, Abdulhamid I, Thomas R, Pendleton S 2006 Home versus hospital intravenous antibiotic therapy for acute pulmonary exacerbations in children with cystic fibrosis. Pediatric Pulmonology 41(8): 744–749

Newall C, Stockley RA, Hill SL 2005 Exercise training and inspiratory muscle training in patients with bronchiectasis. Thorax 60: 943–948

Nikolaizik WH, Jenni-Galovie V, Schoni MH 1996 Bronchial constriction after nebulized tobramycin preparations and saline in patients with cystic fibrosis. European Journal of Pediatrics 155: 608–611

Noone PG, Bennett WD, Regnis JA et al 1999 Effect of aerolised uridine-5′-triphosphate on airway clearance with cough in patients with primary ciliary dyskinesia. American Journal of Respiratory and Critical Care Medicine 160: 144–149

Noone PG, Leigh MW, Sannuti A et al 2004 Primary ciliary dyskinesia; diagnostic and phenotypic features. American Journal of Respiratory and Critical Care Medicine 169: 459–467

O'Neill PA, Dodd M, Phillips B et al 1987 Regular exercise and reduction of breathlessness in cystic fibrosis. British Journal of Diseases of the Chest 81: 62–66

Orenstein DM, Franklin BA, Doershuk CF et al 1981 Exercise conditioning and cardiopulmonary fitness in cystic fibrosis. Chest 80: 392–398

Orenstein DM, Holt LS, Rebovich P et al 2002 Measuring ease of breathing in young patients with cystic fibrosis. Pediatric Pulmonology 34(6): 473–477

Orenstein DM, Hovell MF, Mulvihill M et al 2004 Strength vs aerobic training in children with cystic fibrosis. Chest 126: 1204–1214

Orenstein DM, Nixon PA, Ross EA et al 1989 The quality of well-being in cystic fibrosis. Chest 95: 344–347

Oriols R, Roig J, Ferrer J et al 1999 Inhaled antibiotic therapy in non-cystic fibrosis patients with bronchiectasis and chronic bronchial infection by *Pseudomonas aeruginosa*. Respiratory Medicine 93: 476–480

Orr A, McVean R, Webb AK et al 2001 A questionnaire survey of the prevalence of urinary incontinence in females with cystic fibrosis: a marginalised and undertreated problem. British Medical Journal 322: 1521

Park RW, Grand RJ 1981 Gastrointestinal manifestations of cystic fibrosis: a review. Gastroenterology 81: 1143–116

Passero MA, Remor B, Salomon J 1981 Patient-reported compliance with cystic fibrosis therapy. Clinical Pediatrics 20: 264–268

Pasteur MC, Heliwell SM, Houghton SJ et al 2000 An investigation into the causative factors in patients with bronchiectasis. American Journal of Respiratory and Critical Care Medicine 162: 1277–1284

Patterson JE, Bradley JM, Elborn JS 2004 Airway clearance in bronchiectasis: a randomized crossover trial of active cycle of breathing techniques (incorporating postural drainage and vibration) versus test of incremental respiratory endurance. Chronic Respiratory Disease 1: 127–130

Patterson JE, Bradley JM, Hewitt O et al 2005 Airway clearance in bronchiectasis: a randomized crossover trial of active cycle of breathing techniques versus Acapella® Respiration 72: 239–242

Patterson JE, Bradley JM, Hewitt O, Kent L et al 2007 Acapella vs 'usual airway clearance' during acute exacerbation in bronchiectasis: a randomized crossover trial. Chronic Respiratory Disease 4: 67–74

Penketh ARL, Knight RK, Hodson M et al 1982 Management of pneumothorax in adults with cystic fibrosis. Thorax 37: 850–853

Phillips G 1996 To tip or not to tip? Physiotherapy Research International 1: 1–6

Phillips GE, Thomas S, Heather S, Bush A 1996 Airway responsiveness in primary ciliary dyskinesia: intrasubject variability and the effects of exercise and bronchodilator therapy (abstract). European Respiratory Journal 9(Suppl 23): 36s

Phillipson GTM, Petrucco OM, Mathews CD 2000 Congenital absence of the vas deferens, cystic fibrosis mutational analysis and intracytoplasmic sperm injection. Human Reproduction 15: 431–435

Piper AJ, Parker S, Torzillo PJ et al 1992 Nocturnal nasal IPPV stabilizes patients with cystic fibrosis and hypercapnic respiratory failure. Chest 102: 846–850

Poole S 1995 Dietary treatment of cystic fibrosis. In: Hodson ME, Geddes DM (eds) Cystic fibrosis. Chapman & Hall, London, pp 383–395

Prasad SA, Cerny FJ 2002 Factors that influence adherence to exercise and their effectiveness: application to cystic fibrosis. Pediatric Pulmonology 34(1): 66–72

Prasad SA, Main E 1998 Finding evidence to support airway clearance techniques in cystic fibrosis. Disability and Rehabilitation 20: 235–246

Prasad SA, Main E 2006 Routine airway clearance in asymptomatic infants and babies with cystic fibrosis in the UK: obligatory or obsolete? Physical Therapy Reviews 11(1): 11–20

Prasad SA, Balfour-Lynn IM, Carr S et al 2006 A comparison of the prevalence of urinary incontinence in girls with cystic fibrosis, asthma and healthy controls. Pediatric Pulmonology 41: 1065–1068

Prasad SA, Dodd M, Main E 2008 Finding consensus on the physiotherapy management of asymptomatic infants with cystic fibrosis. Pediatric Pulmonology In Press

Prasad SA, Randall SD, Balfour-Lynn I 2000 Fifteen-count breathlessness score: an objective measure for children. Pediatric Pulmonology 30: 56–62

Pringle MB 1992 Swimming and grommets. British Medical Journal 304: 198

Pryor JA, Tannenbaum E, Cramer D et al 2006a A comparison of five airway clearance techniques in the treatment of people with cystic fibrosis. Journal of Cystic Fibrosis 5: S 76

Pryor JA, Main E, Agent P et al 2006b Physiotherapy. In: Bush A, Alton EWFW, Davies JC, Griesenbach U, Jaffe A (eds) Cystic fibrosis in the 21st century. Progress in Respiratory Research. Karger, Basel, pp 303–305

Quittner AL, Sweeny S, Watrous M et al 2000 Translation of a linguistic validation of a disease specific quality of life measure for cystic fibrosis. Journal of Pediatric Psychology 25: 403–414

Ramsey BW, Dorkin HL 1994 Consensus conference: practical applications of Pulmozyme. Pediatric Pulmonology 17: 404–408

Ramsey BW, Pepe MS, Quan JM et al 1999 Intermittent administration of inhaled tobramycin in patients with cystic fibrosis. New England Journal of Medicine 340: 23030

Ranganathan S 2006 Recent advances in infant and pre-school lung function. In: Bush A, Alton EWFW, Davies JC, Griesenbach U, Jaffe A (eds) Cystic fibrosis in the 21st century. Progress in Respiratory Research. Karger, Basel

Ranganathan SC, Dezateux C, Bush A et al 2001 London Collaborative Cystic Fibrosis Group: airway function in infants newly diagnosed with cystic fibrosis. Lancet 358: 1964–1965

Ranganathan SC, Stocks J, Dezateux C et al 2004 The evolution of airway function in early childhood following clinical diagnosis of cystic fibrosis. American Journal of Respiratory and Critical Care Medicine 169: 928–933

Range SP, Knox AJ 1995 rhDNase in cystic fibrosis. Thorax 50: 321–322

Reid L, De Haller R 1967 The bronchial mucous glands – their hypertrophy and changes in intracellular mucus. Bibliotheca Pediatrica 86: 195–200

Robinson M, Regnis JA, Bailey DL et al 1996 Effect of hypertonic saline, amiloride, and cough on mucociliary clearance in patients with cystic fibrosis. American Journal of Respiratory and Critical Care Medicine 153: 1503–1509

Rodwell LT, Anderson SD 1996 Airway responsiveness to hyperosmolar saline challenge in cystic fibrosis: a pilot study. Pediatric Pulmonology 21: 282–289

Rogers D, Goodchild MC 1996 Role of a domiciliary physiotherapist in the treatment of children with cystic fibrosis. Physiotherapy 82: 396–402

Rommens JM, Iannuzzi MC, Kerem B et al 1989 Identification of the cystic fibrosis gene: chromosome walking and jumping. Science 245: 1059–1065

Rosen MJ 2006 Chronic cough due to bronchiectasis. ACCP evidence-based clinical practice guidelines. Chest 129: 122S–131S

Rubin BK 1988 Immotile cilia syndrome (primary ciliary dyskinesia) and inflammatory lung disease. Clinics of Chest Medicine 9: 657–668

Rubin K 1998 Emerging therapies for cystic fibrosis lung disease. Chest 115: 1120–1126

Rush PJ, Shore A, Coblentz C et al 1986 The musculoskeletal manifestations of C.F. Seminars in Arthritis and Rheumatism 15(3): 213–225

Rutland J, Cole PJ 1980 Non-invasive sampling of nasal cilia for measurement of beat frequency and study of ultrastructure. Lancet ii: 564–565

Sahl W, Bilton D, Dodd M, Webb AK 1989 Effect of exercise and physiotherapy in aiding sputum expectoration in adults with cystic fibrosis. Thorax 44: 1006–1008

Saiman L, Marshall BC, Mayer-Hamblett N et al 2003 Azithromycin patients with cystic fibrosis chronically infected with *Pseudomonas aeruginosa*. A randomized clinical controlled trial. Journal of the American Medical Association 290: 1749–1756

Sapsford RR, Hodges PW, Richardson CA et al 2001 Co-activation of the abdominal and pelvic floor muscles during voluntary exercises. Neurourology and Urodynamics 20: 31–42

Sawyer E, Clayton TL 1993 Improved pulmonary function and exercise tolerance with inspiratory muscle conditioning in children with cystic fibrosis. Chest 104: 1490–1497

Scheinberg P, Shore E 2005 A pilot study of the safety and the efficacy of tobramycin solution for inhalation in patients with severe bronchiectasis. Chest 127: 1420–1426

Schneiderman-Walker J, Pollack SL, Corey M et al 2000 A randomized controlled trial of a 3-year home exercise program in cystic fibrosis. Journal of Pediatrics 136: 304–310

Schöni MH 1989 Autogenic drainage – a modern approach to chest physiotherapy in cystic fibrosis. Journal of the Royal Society of Medicine 82(Suppl 16): 32–37

Shah PL, Scott SF, Knight RA et al 1996 In vivo effects of recombinant human DNase I on sputum in patients with cystic fibrosis. Thorax 51: 119–125

18

Shah PL, Scott SF, Geddes DM et al 1997 An evaluation of two aerosol delivery systems for rhDNase. European Respiratory Journal 10: 1261–1267

Shale DJ 1997a Predicting survival in cystic fibrosis. Thorax 52: 309

Shale DJ 1997b Commentary. Thorax 52: 95–96

Sharp JT, Drutz WS, Moisan T, Forster J, Machnach W 1980 Postural relief of dyspnea in severe chronic obstructive pulmonary disease. American Review of Respiratory Disease 122: 201–211

Shepherd SL, Hovell MF, Slymen DJ et al 1992 Functional status as an overall measure of health in adults with cystic fibrosis: a further validation of a generic health measure. Journal of Clinical Epidemiology 45: 117–125

Simmonds EJ, Littlewood JM, Evans EGV 1990 Cystic fibrosis and allergic bronchopulmonary aspergillosis. Archives of Disease in Childhood 65: 507–511

Sindel BD, Maisels MJ, Ballantine TVN 1989 Gastroesophageal reflux to the proximal esophagus in infants with bronchopulmonary dysplasia. American Journal of Disease in Childhood 143: 1103–1106

Skov M, McKay K, Koch C, Cooper PJ 2005 Prevalence of allergic bronchopulmonary aspergillosis in cystic fibrosis in an area with a high frequency of atopy. Respiratory Medicine 99: 887–893

Smith IE, Flower CDR 1996 Review article: imaging in bronchiectasis. British Journal of Radiology 69: 589–593

Speechly-Dick ME, Rimmer SJ, Hodson ME 1992 Exacerbation of cystic fibrosis after holidays at high altitude: a cautionary tale. Respiratory Medicine 86: 55–56

Spier S, Rivlin J, Hughes D et al 1984 The effect of oxygen on sleep, blood gases and ventilation in cystic fibrosis. American Review of Respiratory Disease 129: 712–718

Stanley P, MacWilliam L, Greenstone M et al 1984 Efficacy of a saccharin test for screening to detect abnormal mucociliary clearance. British Journal of Diseases of the Chest 78: 62–65

Stead RJ, Davidson TI, Duncan FR et al 1987 Use of a totally implantable system for venous access in cystic fibrosis. Thorax 42: 149–150

Stern M, Geddes D 1994 Gene therapy for cystic fibrosis. Respiratory Disease in Practice Winter: 18–23

Strauss GD, Osher A, Wang C et al 1987 Variable weight training in cystic fibrosis. Chest 92: 273–276

Suri R 2005 The use of human deoxyribonuclease (rhDNase) in the management of cystic fibrosis. BioDrugs 19(3): 135–144

Suri R, Grieve R, Normand C et al 2002 Effects of hypertonic saline, alternate day and daily rhDNase on healthcare use, costs and outcomes in children with cystic fibrosis. Thorax 57: 841–846

Tannenbaum E, Prasad SA, Dinwiddie R, Main E 2007 Chest physiotherapy during anaesthesia for children with cystic fibrosis: effects on respiratory function. Pediatric Pulmonology 42(12): 1152–1158

Tattersall R, Callaghan H, Groves D, Walshaw MJ 2000 Assessment of posture by Quantec scanning in adult cystic fibrosis (CF) patients. Proceedings of the XIIIth International Cystic Fibrosis Congress, Stockholm S237, p 148

Taylor CJ, Threlfall D 1997 Postural drainage techniques and gastro-oesophageal reflux in cystic fibrosis. Lancet 349: 1567–1568

ten Berge M, Brinkhorst G, Kroon AA et al 1999 DNase treatment in primary ciliary dyskinesia – assessment by nocturnal pulse oximetry. Pediatric Pulmonology 27: 59–61

Thomas J, Cook DJ, Brooks D 1995 Chest physical therapy management of patients with cystic fibrosis: a meta-analysis. American Journal of Respiratory and Critical Care Medicine 151: 846–885

Thomas TM, Plymat KR, Blannin J, Meade TW 1980 Prevalence of urinary incontinence. British Medical Journal 281: 1243–1124

Thompson CS, Harrison S, Ashley J et al 2002 Randomized crossover study of the Flutter device and the active cycle of breathing technique in non-cystic fibrosis bronchiectasis. Thorax 57: 446–448

Thornton J, Elliot R, Tully MP, Dodd M, Webb AK 2004 Long-term clinical outcome of home and hospital intravenous antibiotic treatment in adults with cystic fibrosis Thorax 59: 242–246

Touw DJ, Brimicombe RW, Hodson ME et al 1995 Inhalation of antibiotics in cystic fibrosis. European Respiratory Journal 8: 1594–1604

Turner JA, Corkey CW, Lee JY et al 1981 Clinical expression of immotile cilia syndrome. Pediatrics 67: 805–810

Turner M, Baildam E, Patel L et al 1997 Joint disorders in CF. Journal of the Royal Society of Medicine 90(Suppl 31): 13–20

Unsworth R, Davis A, Dodd ME et al 1998 Does education improve patient understanding and adherence with airway clearance techniques? Proceedings of 22nd European Cystic Fibrosis Conference

Valerius NH, Koch C, Høiby N 1991 Prevention of chronic *Pseudomonas aeruginosa* colonisation in cystic fibrosis by early treatment. Lancet 338: 725–772

van der Schans CP, Postma KS, Koeter GH, Rubin BK 1999 Physiotherapy and bronchial mucus transport. European Respiratory Journal 13: 1477–1486

van der Schans C, Prasad A, Main E 2000 Chest physiotherapy compared to no chest physiotherapy for cystic fibrosis. Cochrane Database of Systematic Reviews 2000, Issue 2. Art. No.: CD001401. DOI: 10.1002/14651858.CD001401

Vibekk P 1991 Chest mobilization and respiratory function. In: Pryor JA (ed) Respiratory care. Churchill Livingstone, Edinburgh, pp 103–119

Vidal V, Therasse E, Berthiaume Y et al 2006 Bronchial artery embolization in adults with cystic fibrosis: impact on the clinical course and survival. Journal of Vascular and Interventional Radiology 17(6): 953–958

Vizza CD, Yusen RD, Jynch JP et al 2000 Outcome of patients with cystic fibrosis awaiting lung transplantation. American Journal of Respiratory and Critical Care Medicine 162: 819–825

Walters S, Britton J, Hodson ME 1993 Demographic and social characteristics of adults with cystic fibrosis in the United Kingdom. British Medical Journal 306: 549–552

Wanner A, Rao A 1980 Clinical implications for and effects of bland, mucolytic and antibiotic aerosols. American Review of Respiratory Diseases 122: 79–87

Webb AK, Dodd ME 1997 Nebulized antibiotics for adults with cystic fibrosis. Thorax 52(Suppl 2): S69–71

Webb AK, Dodd ME 1999 Exercise and sport in cystic fibrosis: benefits and risks. British Journal of Sports Medicine 33: 77–78

Webb AK, Dodd ME 2000 Exercise and training for adults with cystic fibrosis. In: Hodson ME, Geddes DM (eds) Cystic fibrosis. Arnold, London, pp 433–444

Webb AK, Egan J, Dodd ME 1996 Clinical management of cystic fibrosis patients awaiting and immediately following lung transplantation. In: Dodge A, Brock DJH, Widdecombe JH (eds) Cystic fibrosis: current topics, vol 3. John Wiley, Chichester, pp 311–337

Weinberger JBL, Weiss ST, Cohen WR et al 1980 Pregnancy and the lung. American Review of Respiratory Disease 121: 559–581

Westaby D 2000 Liver and biliary disease. In: Hodson ME, Geddes DM (eds) Cystic fibrosis. Arnold, London, pp 289–300

Wills P, Greenstone M 2006 Inhaled hyperosmolar agents for bronchiectasis. Cochrane Database of Systematic Reviews 2006, Issue 2. Art. No.: CD002996. DOI: 10.1002/14651858.CD002996.pub2

Wills PJ, Wodehouse T, Corkery K et al 1996 Short-term recombinant human DNase in bronchiectasis. American Journal of Respiratory and Critical Care Medicine 154: 413–417

Wilson R, Sykes DA, Chan KL et al 1987 Effect of head position on the efficacy of topical treatment of chronic mucopurulent rhinosinusitis. Thorax 42: 631–663

Wolfe S, Collins S 2007 Nutritional aspects. In: Hodson M, Geddes D, Bush A (eds) Cystic fibrosis, 3rd edn. Hodder Arnold, London

Wolfgang K, Schwabe A, Kramer I 2006 Inhalation solutions – which ones are allowed to be mixed? Physico-chemical compatibility of drug solutions in nebulizers. Journal of Cystic Fibrosis 5: 205–213

Wolter J, Seeney S, Bell S et al 2002 Effect of long-term treatment with azithromycin on disease parameters in cystic fibrosis: a randomized trial Thorax 57: 212–216

Wood RE, Wanner A, Hirsch J et al 1975 Tracheal muco-ciliary transport in cystic fibrosis and its stimulation by terbutaline. American Review of Respiratory Disease 111: 733–738

World Health Organization Report 2003 Adherence to long-term therapies. O3.01

Zabner JJJ, Smith PH, Karp J, Widdicombe JH, Welsh MJ 1998 Loss of CFTR chloride channels alters salt absorption by cystic fibrosis airway epithelia in vitro. Molecular Cell 2(3): 397–403

Zach MS, Oberwaldner B, Forche G et al 1985 Bronchodilators increase airway instability in cystic fibrosis. American Review of Respiratory Disease 131: 537–543

Zihlif N, Paraskakis E, Lex C, Van de Pohl LA, Bush A 2005 Correlation between cough frequency and airway inflammation in children with primary ciliary dyskinesia. Pediatric Pulmonology 39(6): 551–557

Further reading

Bush A, Alton EWFW, Davies JC, Griesenbach U, Jaffe A (eds) 2006 Cystic fibrosis in the 21st century. Karger, Basel

Bluebond-Langner M, Lask B, Angst D 2001 Psychosocial aspects of cystic fibrosis. Arnold, London

Hodson M, Geddes D, Bush A (eds) 2007 Cystic fibrosis, 3rd edn. Hodder Arnold, London

18

Appendix
Normal values, conversion table and abbreviations

NORMAL VALUES

Age group	Heart rate mean (range) (beats/min)	Respiratory rate range (breaths/min)	Blood pressure systolic/diastolic (mmHg)
Preterm	150 (100–200)	40–60	39–59 / 16–36
Newborn	140 (80–200)	30–50	50–70 / 25–45
<2 years	130 (100–190)	20–40	87–105 / 53–66
>2 years	80 (60–140)	20–40	95–105 / 53–66
>6 years	75 (60–90)	15–30	97–112 / 57–71
Adults	70 (50–100)	12–16	95–140 / 60–90

Arterial blood

pH	7.35–7.45 [H^+] 45–35 nmol/l
PaO_2	10.7–13.3 kPa (80–100 mmHg)
$PaCO_2$	4.7–6.0 kPa (35–45 mmHg)
HCO_3^-	22–26 mmol/l
Base excess	−2 to +2

Venous blood

pH	7.31–7.41 [H^+] 46–38 nmol/l
PO_2	5.0–5.6 kPa (37–42 mmHg)
PCO_2	5.6–6.7 kPa (42–50 mmHg)

Ventilation/perfusion

Alveolar–arterial oxygen gradient A–aPO_2:

Breathing air	0.7–2.7 kPa (5–20 mmHg)
Breathing 100% oxygen	3.3–8.6 kPa (25–65 mmHg)

Pressures

		mmHg	kPa
Right atrial (RA) pressure	Mean	−1 to +7	−0.13 to 0.93
Right ventricular (RV) pressure	Systolic	15–25	2.0–3.3
	Diastolic	0–8	0–1.0
Pulmonary artery (PA) pressure	Systolic	15–25	2.0–3.3
	Diastolic	8–15	1.0–2.0
	Mean	10–20	1.3–2.7
Pulmonary capillary wedge pressure (PCWP)	Mean	6–15	0.8–2.0
Central venous pressure (CVP)		3–15 cmH$_2$O	
Intracranial pressure (ICP)		<10	<1.3
Peak inspiratory mouth pressure (PiMax)	Male	103–124 cmH$_2$O (age dependent)	
	Female	65–87 cmH$_2$O (age dependent)	
Peak expiratory mouth pressure (PeMax)	Male	185–233 cmH$_2$O (age dependent)	
	Female	128–152 cmH$_2$O (age dependent)	

Blood chemistry

Albumin	37–53 g/l
Calcium (Ca^{2+})	2.25–2.65 mmol/l
Creatinine	60–120 µmol/l
Glucose	4–6 mmol/l
Potassium (K$^+$)	3.4–5.0 mmol/l
Sodium (Na$^+$)	134–140 mmol/l
Urea	2.5–6.5 mmol/l
Haemoglobin (Hb)	14.0–18.0 g/100 ml (men)
	11.5–15.5 g/100 ml (women)
Platelets	150–400 × 10^9/l
White blood cell count (WBC)	4–11 × 10^9/l
Urine output	1 ml/kg/h

CONVERSION TABLE

0.133 kPa = 1.0 mmHg		pH = 9 − log [H$^+$] where [H$^+$] is in nmol/l	
kPa	mmHg	pH	[H$^+$]
1	7.5	7.52	30
2	15.0	7.45	35
4	30.0	7.40	40
6	45.0	7.35	45
8	60.0	7.30	50
10	75.0	7.26	55
12	90.0	7.22	60
14	105.0	7.19	65

ABBREVIATIONS

6MWD	6-minute walk distance		BiPAP	bilevel positive airway pressure
6MWT	6-minute walk test		BIVAD	biventricular device
			BM	blood glucose monitoring
AAA	abdominal aortic aneurysm		BMD	bone mineral density
AACVPR	American Association of Cardiovascular and Pulmonary Rehabilitation		BMI	body mass index
			BOS	bronchiolitis obliterans syndrome
AAD	adaptive aerosol delivery		BP	blood pressure
A–aO₂	alveolar–arterial oxygen gradient		BPD	bronchopulmonary dysplasia
ABG	arterial blood gases		BPF	bronchopleural fistula
ABPA	allergic bronchopulmonary aspergillosis		bpm	beats per minute
A–C	assist–control mode		BSA	body surface area
ACBT	active cycle of breathing techniques		BTPS	body temperature and pressure saturated
ACE	angiotensin-converting enzyme			
ACPICR	Association of Chartered Physiotherapists in Cardiac Rehabilitation		Ca²⁺	calcium ion
			CABG	coronary artery bypass graft
ACSM	American College of Sports Medicine		CAD	coronary artery disease
ACT	airway clearance technique		CAL	chronic airflow limitation
AD	autogenic drainage		CAVG	coronary artery vein graft
ADH	antidiuretic hormone		CBCL	Child Behaviour Check List
ADL	activities of daily living		CBF	cerebral blood flow
AF	atrial fibrillation		CC	closing capacity
AHRF	acute hypoxaemic respiratory failure		CCAM	congenital cystic adenomatoid malformation
AI	apnoea index			
AIDS	acquired immune deficiency syndrome		CF	cystic fibrosis
ALI	acute lung injury		CFA	cryptogenic fibrosing alveolitis
AMBER	advanced multiple beam equalization radiography		CFRD	cystic fibrosis-related diabetes
			CFS	chronic fatigue syndrome
AP	anteroposterior		CFTR	cystic fibrosis transmembrane conductance regulator
APACHE	acute physiology and chronic health evaluation			
			CHD	coronary heart disease
APRV	airway pressure release ventilation		CHF	chronic heart failure
AQLQ	Asthma Quality of Life Questionnaire		CK	creatine kinase
ARDS	acute respiratory distress syndrome		C_L	lung compliance
ARF	acute renal failure		CLD	chronic lung disease
ASA	American Society of Anestheologists		CLDP	chronic lung disease of prematurity
ASD	atrial septal defect		CLE	congenital lobar emphysema
ASL	airway surface liquid		cm	centimetre
AT	anaerobic threshold		CMV	controlled mandatory ventilation
ATN	acute tubular necrosis		CMV	cytomegalovirus
ATPS	ambient temperature and pressure saturated		CO	cardiac output
			CO₂	carbon dioxide
ATS	American Thoracic Society		COAD	chronic obstructive airways disease
AVAS	absolute visual analogue scale		COPD	chronic obstructive pulmonary disease
AVSD	atrioventricular septal defect		CPAP	continuous positive airway pressure
			CPB	cardiopulmonary bypass
BACR	British Association of Cardiac Rehabilitation		CPEX	cardiopulmonary exercise test
			CPP	cerebral perfusion pressure
BAL	bronchoalveolar lavage		CRF	chronic renal failure
BDI	baseline and transition dyspnoea index		CRP	C-reactive protein
BHR	bronchial hyper-reactivity		CRP	conditioning rehabilitation programme
BHT	breath-holding time			

CRQ	chronic respiratory disease questionnaire
CRT	cardiac resynchronization therapy
CSF	cerebrospinal fluid
CT	computed tomography
CTR	cardiothoracic ratio
CV	cardiovascular
CV	closing volume
CVP	central venous pressure
CWC	chest wall compliance
DBE	deep breathing exercises
DH	drug history
DIC	disseminated intravascular coagulopathy
DIOS	distal intestinal obstruction syndrome
dl	decilitre
DLCO	diffusing capacity for carbon monoxide
DL_{CO}	diffusing capacity for carbon monoxide
DLT	double lung transplant
DMD	Duchenne muscular dystrophy
DNA	deoxyribonucleic acid
$\dot{D}O_2$	oxygen delivery
DVT	deep vein thrombosis
EBV	Epstein–Barr virus
$ECCO_2R$	extracorporeal carbon dioxide removal
ECG	electrocardiograph
ECMO	extracorporeal membrane oxygenation
EECP	enhanced external counter pulsation
EEG	electroencephalogram
EIA	exercise-induced asthma
EIB	exercise-induced bronchospasm
EMG	electromyogram
EOG	electro-oculogram
EPAP	expiratory positive airway pressure
EPP	equal pressure point
ERCP	endoscopic retrograde choliangiopancreatography
ERS	European Respiratory Society
ERV	expiratory reserve volume
ESWT	endurance shuttle walking test
ET	endotracheal
$ETCO_2$	end-tidal carbon dioxide
ETT	endotracheal tube
ETT	exercise tolerance test
EVLWI	extravascular lung water index
FDG	fluorodeoxyglucose
FDP	fibrin degradation product
FEF_{50}	forced expiratory flow at 50% of forced vital capacity
FEF_{75}	forced expiratory flow at 75% of forced vital capacity
FET	forced expiration technique

FEV_1	forced expiratory volume in 1 second
FG	French gauge
FGF	fibroblast growth factor
FH	family history
FHF	fulminant hepatic failure
FiO_2	fractional inspired oxygen concentration
FITT	frequency, intensity, time and type of training
FRC	functional residual capacity
ft	feet
FVC	forced vital capacity
g	gram
g/dl	gram per decilitre
GA	general anaesthetic
GCS	Glasgow Coma Scale
GEDVI	global end-diastolic volume index
GOR	gastro-oesophageal reflux
GORD	gastro-oesophageal reflux disorder
GPB	glossopharyngeal breathing
GTN	glyceryl trinitrate
h	hour
H^+	hydrogen ion
$[H^+]$	hydrogen ion concentration
H_2O	water
Hb	haemoglobin
HCO_3^-	bicarbonate
Hct	haematocrit
HD	haemodialysis
HDL	high-density lipoprotein
HDU	high dependency unit
HFCC	high-frequency chest compression
HFCWO	high-frequency chest wall oscillation
HFJV	high-frequency jet ventilation
HFO	high-frequency oscillation
HFOV	high-frequency oscillatory ventilation
HFPPV	high-frequency positive pressure ventilation
HFV	high-frequency ventilation
Hg	mercury
HIV	human immunodeficiency virus
HLA	human leucocyte antigen
HLT	heart-lung transplantation
HME	heat and moisture exchanger
HPC	history of presenting condition
HPOA	hypertrophic pulmonary osteoarthropathy
HPV	hypoxic pulmonary vasoconstriction
HR	heart rate
HRCT	high-resolution computed tomography
HRQoL	health-related quality of life
HRR	heart rate reserve
HVPT	hyperventilation provocation test

HVS	hyperventilation syndrome
Hz	hertz
I:E	inspiratory:expiratory
IABP	intra-aortic balloon pump
ICC	intercostal catheter
ICD	implantable cardioverter defibrillator
ICG	impedance cardiography
ICP	intracranial pressure
ICU	intensive care unit
Ig	immunoglobulin
IgE	immunoglobulin E
IgG	immunoglobulin G
IH	idiopathic symptomatic hyperventilation
IHD	ischaemic heart disease
ILD	interstitial lung disease
IMA	internal mammary artery
IMT	inspiratory muscle training
IMV	intermittent mandatory ventilation
in	inches
INOS	inducible nitric oxide synthetase
INR	international normalized ratio
IPAP	inspiratory positive airway pressure
IPPB	intermittent positive pressure breathing
IPPV	intermittent positive pressure ventilation
IPS	inspiratory pressure support
IPV	interpulmonary percussive ventilation
IR–PEP	inspiratory resistance–positive expiratory pressure
IRT	immunoreactive trypsin
IRV	inspiratory reserve volume
IS	incentive spirometry
ISWT	incremental shuttle walking test
ITBVI	intrathoracic blood volume index
IV	intravenous
IVH	intraventricular haemorrhage
IVOX	intravenacaval oxygenation
IVUS	intravascular ultrasound
JVP	jugular venous pressure
K^+	potassium ion
Kcal	kilocalories
KCO	coefficient of gas transfer
K_{CO}	coefficient of gas transfer
kg	kilogram
kJ	kilojoule
kPa	kilopascal
kV	kilovoltage
kVp	kilovoltage
l	litre
LAP	left atrial pressure
LCI	lung clearance index

LED	light-emitting diode
LRTD	lower respiratory tract disease
LTOT	long-term oxygen therapy
LVAD	left ventricular assist device
LVEF	left ventricular ejection fraction
LVF	left ventricular failure
LVRS	lung volume reduction surgery
m	metre
μm	micrometre (10^{-6} m)
μs	microsecond
MAP	mean airway pressure
MAP	mean arterial pressure
MAPCA	major aortopulmonary collateral artery
MAS	minimal access surgery
MBTS	modified Blalock–Taussig shunt
MBW	multiple-breath inert gas washout
MCC	mucociliary clearance
mcg	microgram
MCH	mean corpuscular haemoglobin
MCID	minimal clinically important difference
MCV	mean corpuscular volume
MDCT	multidetector computed tomography
MDI	metered dose inhaler
MEF_{50}	maximal expiratory flow at 50% of forced vital capacity
MEF_{75}	maximal expiratory flow at 75% of forced vital capacity
MET	muscle energy technique
METs	metabolic equivalents
MHI	manual hyperinflation
mg	milligram
MHz	megahertz
MI	myocardial infarction
MIE	meconium ileus equivalent
min	minute
MIP	maximum inspiratory pressure
ml	millilitre
mm	millimetre
MMAD	mass median aerodynamic diameter
mmHg	millimetres of mercury
mmol/l	millimoles per litre
mph	miles per hour
MRA	magnetic resonance angiography
MRC	Medical Research Council
MRI	magnetic resonance imaging
MRSA	methicillin-resistant *Staphylococcus aureus*
ms	millisecond
MUGA	multi-gated acquisition (scans)
$M\dot{V}O_2$	myocardial oxygen consumption
MVV	maximum voluntary ventilation
n	number
Na^+	sodium ion

NAEPP	National Asthma Education and Prevention Programme		PCV	packed cell volume
			PCV	pressure controlled ventilation
NEPV	negative extrathoracic pressure ventilation		PCWP	pulmonary capillary wedge pressure
NIBP	non-invasive blood pressure		PD	peritoneal dialysis
NICO	non-invasive cardiac output		PD	postural drainage
NICU	neonatal intensive care unit		PDA	patent ductus arteriosus
NIV	non-invasive ventilation		Pdi	transdiaphragmatic pressure
nm	nanometre		PDP	postural drainage and percussion
NMES	neuromuscular electrical stimulation		PE	pulmonary embolus
nmol	nanomole		PEEP	positive end-expiratory pressure
NNU	neonatal unit		PEF	peak expiratory flow
NO	nitric oxide		PEFR	peak expiratory flow rate
NO_2	nitrogen dioxide		PeMax	peak expiratory mouth pressure
NPPV	non-invasive positive pressure ventilation		PEP	positive expiratory pressure
NPV	negative pressure ventilation		PERL	pupils equal and reactive to light
NREM	non-rapid eye movement		PET	positron emission tomography
NSAID	non-steroidal anti-inflammatory drug		pH	hydrogen ion concentration
NYHA	New York Heart Association		P_{high}	high pressure
			PI	pulsatility index
O_2	oxygen		PICU	paediatric intensive care unit
OB	obliterative bronchiolitis		PIE	pulmonary interstitial emphysema
OHFO	oral high-frequency oscillation		PIF	peak inspiratory flow
OHS	obesity hypoventilation syndrome		PIFR	peak inspiratory flow rate
OHS	open heart surgery		PiMax	peak inspiratory mouth pressure
OI	oxygen index		PIP	peak inspiratory pressure
OLT	orthotopic liver transplantation		PLB	pursed-lip breathing
OSA	obstructive sleep apnoea		P_{low}	low pressure
			PMDI	pressurized metered dose inhaler
PA	posteroanterior		PMH	previous medical history
PA	pulmonary artery		PMR	percutaneous myocardial revascularization
PaCO$_2$	partial pressure of carbon dioxide in alveolar gas		PN	percussion note
PaCO$_2$	partial pressure of carbon dioxide in arterial blood		PND	paroxysmal nocturnal dyspnoea
			PNF	proprioceptive neuromuscular facilitation
PACS	Picture Archiving and Communications Systems		POMR	problem oriented medical record
			PPC	postoperative pulmonary complication
PALISI	Pediatric Acute Lung Injury and Sepsis Investigators		PPHN	persistent pulmonary hypertension of the newborn
PaO$_2$	partial pressure of oxygen in arterial blood		PRVC	pressure regulated volume controlled
			PSI	Parenting Stress Index
PAO$_2$	partial pressure of oxygen in alveolar gas		PTB	pulmonary tuberculosis
PAOP	pulmonary artery occlusion pressure		PTCA	percutaneous transluminal coronary angioplasty
PAP	pulmonary artery pressure			
PAPVC	partial anomalous pulmonary venous connection		P_{Tc}CO$_2$	transcutaneous carbon dioxide tension
			PTFE	polytetrafluoroethylene
PAWP	pulmonary artery wedge pressure		PTLD	post-transplant lymphoproliferative disease
PCA	patient-controlled analgesia			
PCD	primary ciliary dyskinesia		PTT	partial thromboplastin time
PCI	percutaneous coronary intervention		PVC	polyvinyl chloride
PCIRV	pressure-controlled inverse ratio ventilation		PVH	periventricular haemorrhage
			PVL	periventricular leukomalacia
PCP	*Pneumocystis carinii* pneumonia		PvO$_2$	partial pressure of oxygen in venous blood
PCPAP	periodic continuous positive airway pressure		PVR	pulmonary vascular resistance
			PWC	peak work capacity

$\dot{Q}$	blood flow/perfusion
QoL	quality of life
RAP	right atrial pressure
R_{aw}	airway resistance
RBC	red blood cell
RCT	randomized controlled trial
RDI	respiratory disturbance index
RDS	respiratory distress syndrome
REM	rapid eye movement
RER	respiratory exchange ratio
rhDNase	recombinant human deoxyribonuclease
RIM	resistive inspiratory muscle training
R_{int}	resistance measured by the interruptor technique
RM	repetition maximum
RMS	respiratory mass spectrometer
RMT	respiratory muscle training
RNA	ribonucleic acid
ROP	retinopathy of prematurity
RPE	rating of perceived exertion
RPP	rate pressure product
RSV	respiratory syncytial virus
RTA	road traffic accident
RV	residual volume
RVF	right ventricular failure
s	second
SA	sinoatrial
SaO_2	arterial oxygen saturation
SAS	sleep apnoea syndrome
SDB	sleep-disordered breathing
SER	scanning equalization radiography
SG_{AW}	specific airway conductance
SGRQ	St George's Respiratory Questionnaire
SH	social history
SIGN	Scottish Intercollegiate Guidelines Network
SIMV	synchronized intermittent mandatory ventilation
SIRS	systemic inflammatory response syndrome
SMART	specific, measurable, achievable, realistic, timed
SOAP	subjective, objective, analysis, plan
SOB	shortness of breath
SpO_2	pulse oximetry arterial oxygen saturation
SV	saphenous vein
SVC	superior vena cava
SVO_2	mixed venous oxygen saturation
SVR	systemic vascular resistance
SVV	stroke volume variation
SWT	shuttle walk test

TAA	thoracic aortic aneurysm
TAPVC	total anomalous pulmonary venous connection
TBB	transbronchial biopsy
$TcCO_2$	transcutaneous carbon dioxide
TCD	transcranial Doppler
TcO_2	transcutaneous oxygen
TEB	thoracic electrical bioimpedance
TED	thromboembolic deterrent
TEE	thoracic expansion exercises
TENS	transcutaneous electrical nerve stimulation
TGA	transposition of the great arteries
TIRE	test of incremental respiratory endurance
TLC	total lung capacity
TLCO	transfer factor in lung of carbon monoxide
TMR	transmyocardial revascularization
TNF	tumour necrosis factor
TNM	tumour–nodes–metastases
TOBI	tobramycin solution for inhalation
TV	tidal volume
UAS	upper abdominal surgery
UWSD	underwater sealed drainage
$\dot{V}$	ventilation
$\dot{V}/\dot{Q}$	ventilation/perfusion ratio
$\dot{V}_A$	alveolar ventilation/alveolar volume
$\dot{V}_E$	minute ventilation
$\dot{V}O_2$	oxygen consumption
$\dot{V}O_2max$	maximum oxygen uptake/consumption
$\dot{V}O_2R$	oxygen uptake reserve
VAD	ventricular assist device
VAP	ventilatory acquired/associated pneumonia
VAS	visual analogue scale
VATS	video-assisted thoracoscopy surgery
VC	vital capacity
VCV	volume controlled ventilation
V_D	dead-space ventilation
VDS	verbal descriptor scales
VEGF	vascular endothelial growth factor
VF	ventricular fibrillation
VF	vocal fremitus
VHI	ventilator hyperinflation
VILI	ventilator induced lung injury
VR	vocal resonance
VRE	vancomycin-resistant enterococcus
VSD	ventricular septal defect
V_T	tidal volume
W	watt
WAnT	Wingate anaerobic test
WBC	white blood count
WCC	white cell count
WOB	work of breathing

Subject index